At the end of the session:

- When you have finished the touch therapy session, verbally let the client know that it is time to return gradually to the here-and-now, to begin to move around slowly, and to awaken fully.
- Anticipate that the client will take a few minutes to reorient to time and place after being in a deep state of relaxation.
- Allow a period of silence for the client to appreciate fully the experience and benefits of his or her relaxed body–mind.
- Stay in the room while the client rouses and sits up. Give necessary assistance to ensure a safe transfer to an ambulatory position.
- Allow time to receive the client's verbal feedback about the meaning of the session if the client feels the need to talk. If this does not occur spontaneously, ask for feedback. The insight gained provides guidelines for further sessions or specific ideas that the client can follow up in daily life.
- When the touch therapy is used for relaxation or sleep induction for hospitalized patients, close the session by softly pulling the bedcovers up over the patient's back and quietly turning off the light as the patient moves into sleep. Let the client know in advance that you will leave quietly at the end.

- Use the client outcomes that were established before the session (see Exhibit 19-1) and the client's subjective experience (**Exhibit 19-2**) to evaluate the session.

Case Study (Implementation)

CASE STUDY 1

Setting: Medical/surgical unit of a general hospital

Patient: E. S., a 68 year-old single man with COPD

Patterns/Challenges/Needs:

1. Anxiety
2. Altered comfort
3. Social isolation (related to chronic obstructive pulmonary disease [COPD] and pneumonia)

E. S. was oxygen dependent and [am]bulatory. After a history of hea[rt?] 40 years, his lungs continued spite of quitting smoking at a[ch?] ach frequently felt upset, and it him to eat much. He could n[ot?] nutritional supplements, he w[anted?] to breathe, and his weight ha[d?] 160 to 100 pounds over a 2-yea[r?] become very weak. Because E[. S.?] sedentary and very bony, he wa[s?] most of the time, with stiffness and body aches.

> ### CASE STUDIES
>
> Read and analyze real-life situations dealing with holistic nursing. Then use your critical thinking skills and knowledge from the text to answer questions. Case studies can also be found on the companion website at **http://go.jblearning.com/dossey.**

EXHIBIT 19-2   Evaluation of the Client's Subjective Experience of Touch Therapies

1. Was this a new kind of experience for you? Can you describe it?
2. Did this feel like a comforting or stimulating tactile sensation or both?
3. Was it pleasurable on all planes—physical, mental, emotional, and spiritual—or more focused in one area than another?
4. Were you aware of your surroundings during the experience, or did you sink into a sense of timelessness?
5. Did emotions surface during the experience? If so, what were they? Can you focus on them now?
6. Did you experience any imagery during the touch session?
7. Did you feel comfortable with the therapist? Is there anything that you want to do to increase your comfort level with the touch therapist?
8. Did you feel relaxed and refreshed after the experience?
9. Would you like to try this again?
10. What would be helpful to make this a better experience for you?
11. Can you develop a plan or strategy to integrate more of the touch therapies into your life on a regular basis?

weeks later. Her experience and testimony demonstrate how comfort can be brought into the lives of others through the use of energetic touch therapies and the practitioner's healing presence.

Evaluation

With the client, the nurse determines whether the client outcomes for touch therapies were successfully achieved (see Exhibit 19-1). To evaluate the session further, the nurse may again explore the subjective effects of the experience with the client using the evaluation questions in Exhibit 19-2.

Directions for
FUTURE RESEARCH

1. Develop valid and reliable tools to measure the effects of touch and hand-mediated therapies.
2. Investigate hand-mediated techniques practiced in conjunction with other modalities to mirror real-world usage of these modalities.
3. Continue to strengthen the evidence base for practicing touch and hand-mediated

ies are best suited for ns and populations.

f touch and hand-
in ambulatory and

cost-effectiveness of ated techniques.

riodic hand-mediated increase work perfor-

y, complications, and to the use of touch techniques.

9. Examine the responses to touch and hand-mediated therapies related to developmental stage.
10. Investigate how touch can be taught effectively in nursing schools and what methods are best suited to accomplish this.
11. Explore ways in which nursing students' cultural learning pertaining to touch affects performance of clinical care.
12. Measure parental and caregiver satisfaction when taught to offer touch and hand-mediated therapies to loved ones.

DIRECTIONS FOR
FUTURE RESEARCH

Think critically about the material in each chapter with these activities that conclude each chapter. Work in a group or individually to engage the material in new ways with these thought-provoking questions.

Nurse Healer
REFLECTIONS

After reading this chapter, the nurse healer will be able to answer or to begin the process of answering the following questions:

- How do I feel about using touch and hand-mediated therapies as healing interventions?
- What does th feel like?
- How does the experience of
- How astute a response to t
- How can I in use of touch a
- Who might b increase my re
- What other include to touch?

NURSE HEALER
REFLECTIONS

Develop your critical thinking skills with these questions at the end of each chapter. The "www" icon directs you to the companion website at **http://go .jblearning.com/dossey** to delve deeper into concepts by completing these exercises online.

 For a full suite of assignments and additional learning activities, use the access code located in the front of your book to visit this exclusive website: http://go.jblearning.com /dossey. If you do not have an access code, you can obtain one at the site.

NOTES

1. K. Fontaine, *Complementary and Alternative Therapies for Nursing Practice*, 3rd ed. (Upper Saddle River, NJ: Prentice Hall, 2010).
2. H. Harlow, "Love in Infant Monkeys," *Scientific American* 200 (1958): 68–74.
3. R. Spitz, *The First Year of Life* (New York: International Universities Press, 1965).
4. B. Grad, "Some Biological Effects of the Laying on of Hands: A Review of Experiments with Animals and Plants," *Journal of the American Society for Psychical Research* 59 (1965): 95–127.
5. M. J. Smith, "Enzymes Are Activated by the Laying on of Hands," *Human Dimensions* (1973): 46–48.
6. D. Leder and M.W. Krucoff, "The Touch That Heals: The Uses and Meanings of Touch in the Clinical Encounter," *Journal of Alternative and Complementary Medicine* 14, no. 3 (2008): 321–327.

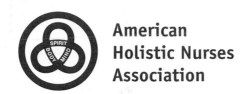

American
Holistic Nurses
Association

SIXTH EDITION

HOLISTIC NURSING

A Handbook for Practice

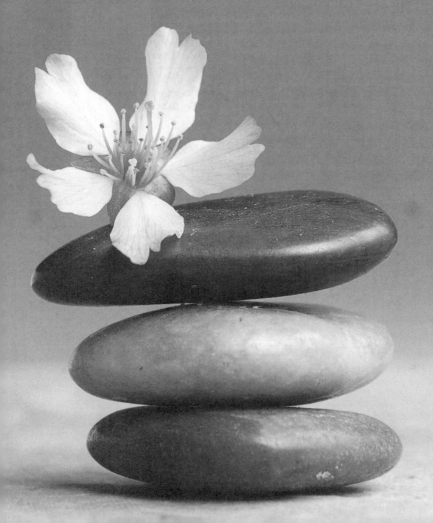

The Pedagogy

Holistic Nursing: A Handbook for Practice, Sixth Edition drives comprehension through various strategies that meet the learning needs of students, while also generating enthusiasm about the topic. This interactive approach addresses different learning styles, making this the ideal text to ensure mastery of key concepts. The pedagogical aids that appear in most chapters include the following:

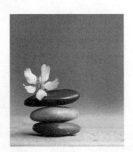

Chapter 19

Touch and Hand-Mediated Therapies

Christina Jackson and Corinne Latini

Nurse Healer
OBJECTIVES

Theoretical

- Describe various types of touch therapies.
- Compare and contrast the various touch therapies.
- [gic] changes that can [...] rapies.
- [...] tional changes that [...] therapies.

[www]

- [...]s to become calm and [...]se touch therapies in
- [...]thing music, guided [...] herapy as adjuncts to
- [...] nd objective changes [...]cing a touch therapy

Personal

- Examine the significance of touch in your personal and professional relationships.
- Notice whether there are any changes in your emotions and sense of well-being during or after you use touch therapy.
- Create opportunities to practice touch therapies in your clinical practice.

NURSE HEALER OBJECTIVES

Nurse Healer Objectives are divided into three sections: Theoretical, Clinical, and Personal. These objectives provide you with a snapshot of the key information you will encounter in each chapter, and serve as a checklist to focus your study. Nurse Healer Objectives can also be found on the companion website at **http://go.jblearning.com/dossey.**

DEFINITIONS

Acupressure (Shiatsu): The application of finger and/or thumb pressure to specific sites along the body's energy meridians for the purpose of relieving tension, reestablishing the flow of energy along the meridian lines, and restoring balance to the human energy system.

Body therapy and/or touch therapy: The broad range of [...] tioner uses in [...] near the body to [...] optimal functio[...]

Centering: A calm [...] relatedness tha[...] place of inner [...] within oneself [...] and focused.

Chakra or energy [...] consciousness i[...] that allows for [...] energy from ou[...] from the indiv[...] are seven major energy centers in relation to the spine and many minor centers at bone articulations in the palms of the hands and the soles of the feet.

Energy meridian: An energy circuit or line of force. Eastern theories describe meridian lines flowing vertically through the body, culminating at points on the feet, hands, and ears.

DEFINITIONS

Key words and terms are outlined and defined at the start of every chapter. These terms are also included in Animated Flashcards and Crossword Puzzles on the companion website to help you study and nail the definitions. Learn more at **http://go.jblearning.com/dossey.**

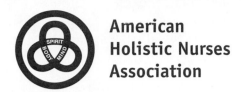

American Holistic Nurses Association

SIXTH EDITION

HOLISTIC NURSING
A Handbook for Practice

Barbara Montgomery Dossey, PhD, RN, AHN-BC, FAAN

Codirector, International Nurse Coach Association (INCA)
Codirector, Integrative Nurse Coach Certificate Program (INCCP)
Huntington, New York
International Codirector, Nightingale Initiative for Global Health
Washington, DC and Ottawa, Ontario, Canada
Director, Holistic Nursing Consultants
Santa Fe, New Mexico

Lynn Keegan, PhD, RN, AHN-BC, FAAN

Director, Holistic Nursing Consultants
Port Angeles, Washington
Partner, Absolutely: Business and Personal Strategic Consulting, LLC
Indianapolis, Indiana
Past President, American Holistic Nurses Association

ASSOCIATE EDITORS:

Cynthia C. Barrere, PhD, RN, CNS, AHN-BC

Professor of Nursing
Quinnipiac University School of Nursing
Hamden, Connecticut

Mary Blaszko Helming, PhD, APRN, FNP-BC, AHN-BC

Professor of Nursing
FNP Track Coordinator for MSN and DNP programs
Quinnipiac University School of Nursing
Hamden, Connecticut

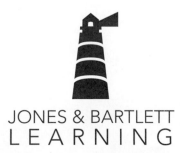

JONES & BARTLETT
LEARNING

World Headquarters
Jones & Bartlett Learning
5 Wall Street
Burlington, MA 01803
978-443-5000
info@jblearning.com
www.jblearning.com

Jones & Bartlett Learning books and products are available through most bookstores and online booksellers. To contact Jones & Bartlett Learning directly, call 800-832-0034, fax 978-443-8000, or visit our website, www.jblearning.com.

Production Credits

Publisher: Kevin Sullivan
Acquisitions Editor: Amanda Harvey
Editorial Assistant: Sara Bempkins
Associate Production Editor: Sara Fowles
Marketing Manager: Elena McAnespie
V.P., Manufacturing and Inventory Control: Therese Connell

Composition: Arlene Apone
Cover Design: Kristin E. Parker
Cover Image: © zimmytws/ShutterStock, Inc.
Printing and Binding: Edwards Brothers Malloy
Cover Printing: Edwards Brothers Malloy

To order this product, use ISBN: 978-1-4496-5175-6

Library of Congress Cataloging-in-Publication Data
Holistic nursing : a handbook for practice / [edited by] Barbara Montgomery Dossey,
Lynn Keegan. -- 6th ed.
    p. ; cm.
Includes bibliographical references and index.
ISBN 978-1-4496-4563-2 (pbk.)
I. Dossey, Barbara Montgomery. II. Keegan, Lynn.
[DNLM: 1. Holistic Nursing. WY 86.5]
610.73--dc23

                                  2011043985

6048

Printed in the United States of America
16 15 14 13 12   10 9 8 7 6 5 4 3 2

The Flame of Florence Nightingale's Legacy

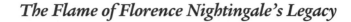

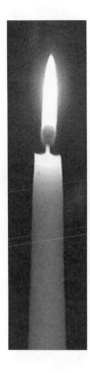

Today, our world needs healing and to be rekindled with Love.
Once, Florence Nightingale lit her beacon of lamplight
    to comfort the wounded
And her Light has blazed a path of service across a Century to us,
Through her example and through the countless Nurses and Healers
    who have followed in her footsteps.

Today, we celebrate the flame of Florence Nightingale's Legacy.
Let that same Light be rekindled to burn brightly in our hearts.
Let us take up our own Lanterns of Caring, each in our own ways.
To more brightly walk our own paths of service to the World.
To more clearly share our own Noble Purpose with each other.

May Human Caring become the Lantern for the 21st Century.
May we better learn to care for ourselves,
    for each other and for all Creation.
Through our Caring, may we be the Keepers of that Flame.
That Our Spirits may burn brightly
To kindle the hearts of our children and great-grandchildren
As they too follow in these footsteps.

Deva-Marie Beck, PhD, RN
International Codirector, Nightingale Initiative for Global Health
Washington, D.C., and Ottawa, Ontario, Canada
www.NightingaleDeclaration.net

To Our Colleagues in Nursing

When a nurse
Encounters another
Something happens
What occurs
Is never a neutral event

A pulse taken
Words exchanged
A touch
A healing moment
Two persons
Are never
The same

Contents

10   *Facilitating Change: Motivational Interviewing and Appreciative Inquiry*   205

Mary Elaine Southard, Darlene R. Hess, and Linda Bark

11   *Cognitive Behavioral Therapy*   221

Eileen M. Stuart-Shor, Carol L. Wells-Federman, and Esther Seibold

12   *Self-Reflection*   247

Jackie D. Levin and Jennifer L. Reich

25   *Aromatherapy*   **563**

Jane Buckle

26   *Relationship-Centered Care and Healing Initiative in a Community Hospital*   **583**

Pamela Steinke and Nancy Moore

27   *Exploring Integrative Medicine: The Story of a Large, Urban, Tertiary Care Hospital*   **609**

Lori L. Knutson

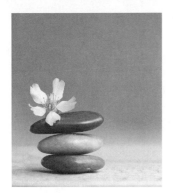

The sixth edition of *Holistic Nursing: A Handbook for Practice* continues the previous editions' tradition of providing holistic nursing students, practitioners, and scholars of holism the latest scientific and practical thinking in the field. This latest edition provides the most contemporary integral models for holistic caring healing practices. This evolving work has become the primary information source for holistic nursing in the world. It continues to be significant in that holistic nursing has attained and sustained recognition by the American Nurses Association (ANA) as a formal ANA nursing specialty with a defined scope of practice and standards, meriting certification.

The fact that this work is now in its sixth edition is a testimony to its use and importance. It continues to expand and deepen previous editions, moving from theory, knowledge, and values to skills and applications that integrate personal and professional competencies of being into authentic caring healing work.

This edition relates holistic nursing within the context of Wilber's model of integrality and the very contemporary philosophical scientific paradigm; thus, this paradigm is congruent for locating holistic thinking within a larger unitary field. It also represents the evolving consciousness of the public seeking more authentic caring healing. Likewise, this work represents the evolving consciousness of nurses practicing and studying holistic nursing. Further, what is important is that this sixth edition brings holistic nursing and the integral model to life through specific examples from the field.

In this expanded work, new visions of healing bring forth a deep authenticity, locating healing within circles of knowledge, experiences, and diverse ways of knowing. Thus, one can understand how Holistic Nursing Is Caring Science as Sacred Science. Holistic nursing offers expanded views of nursing generally, bringing forth the beauty, art, artistry, and ethics of the deeply human and humane dimensions of practice. The evolution of the work reflects the evolution of the nursing profession, calling forth not only the intellectual foundation but the ethical, values-guided aspect of deeper levels of commitment, compassion, love, and caring that underpin this kind of advanced practice: a holistic practice that is oriented toward the betterment of human health, healing, and humankind.

These latest developments of holistic nursing guide students, faculty, and practicing nurses with emancipatory breakthroughs, continuing the contribution for the more mature emergence of formal holistic standards and scopes of practice. At the same time, holistic nursing grounds these breakthroughs in the blueprint of timeless goals, values, and moral ideals consistent with the finest heritage and wisdom of Nightingale.

The authors are committed to the highest actualization of nursing, as an ancient, pioneering, yet futuristic profession. They practice what they teach by translating and integrating this latest thinking into scientific, theoretical, pragmatic, and concrete nursing actions, process, and artistic acts of caring and healing. They help us all to comprehend the critical nature of these practices and how they inform any "caring moment."

A consequence of this continuous work is that the self of the nurse is invited—and even reminded of the calling—to nursing, to self-care and self-healing, as essential for authentic living of this knowledge in their personal and professional lives. As such, then, the holistic nurse has the potential not only to transform self and system, but transform nursing itself.

In summary, this sixth edition provides a world-class philosophical and intellectual blueprint for all of nursing's holistic caring healing practices; it offers a guide and vision for personal and professional care within the holistic integral paradigm. The result: a major work of excellence that exceeds even previous editions as it responds to current demands for reform from within and without. At another level, this work transcends nursing, per se; it has relevance for transdisciplinary health education and practices, leading to greater authenticity and advancement of all health professionals and caring healing relationships with the public.

Jean Watson, PhD, RN, AHN-BC, FAAN
Distinguished Professor of Nursing
Murchinson-Scoville Endowed Chair
in Caring Science
College of Nursing and Anschutz
Medical Center
University of Colorado, Denver
Denver, Colorado
www.nursing.ucdenver.edu/caring

Founder and Executive Director
Watson Caring Science Institute
Boulder, Colorado
www.watsoncaringscience.org

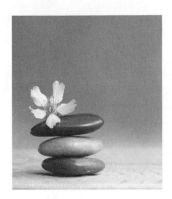

Preface

The American Holistic Nurses Association (AHNA) has joined with the authors, Barbara Montgomery Dossey and Lynn Keegan, associate editors Cynthia C. Barrere and Mary Blaszko Helming, and contributors of *Holistic Nursing: A Handbook for Practice, Sixth Edition* to develop further the knowledge base for holistic nursing and delineate the essence of contemporary nursing. The purposes of this book are threefold: (1) to expand an understanding of an integral worldview, healing, and the nurse as an instrument of healing; (2) to explore the unity and relatedness of nurses, clients, and others; and (3) to develop caring healing interventions to strengthen the whole person—local to global.

Health care in the 21st century requires a radically different type of nurse who understands an integral and holistic perspective, relationship-centered care, behavioral change strategies, health promotion, health maintenance, and disease prevention. In the United States, actual solutions to the thicket of the nation's health problems are guiding holistic nurses and healthcare professionals. In 2009, the Samueli Institute released its visionary report titled *Wellness Initiative for the Nation (WIN)*.[1] This report advocates new approaches to disease prevention and health promotion. Referring to a "broken disease treatment system," the authors state that a new vision of health is needed that is based on human flourishing.[1p4] It is clear that the current healthcare delivery practices, whether conventional or holistic, are seeking models of care that provide a wide range of choices for individuals that are efficient, effective, and reduce costs. This is fundamental to transforming health care from a disease model of care to one that focuses on health and wellness.

In March 2010, the Patient Protection and Affordable Care Act (PPACA) became law (HR3590).[2] In Section 4001, the language references partnerships with a diverse group of licensed health professionals including practitioners of integrative health, preventive medicine, health coaching, public education, and more. Holistic nurses as nurse coaches can address the health of the nation by assisting clients to take the steps that lead to improved health and well-being.

In October 2010, the Institute of Medicine (IOM), in collaboration with the Robert Wood Johnson Foundation, published a landmark document titled *The Future of Nursing* that presents four key messages:[3]

- Nurses should practice to the full extent of their education and training.
- Nurses should achieve higher levels of education and training through an improved education system that promotes seamless academic progression.
- Nurses should be full partners, with physicians and other healthcare professionals, in redesigning health care in the United States.
- Effective workforce planning and policy making require better data collection and information infrastructure.

In June 2011, the National Prevention, Health Promotion, and Public Health Council announced the release of the National Prevention and Health Promotion Strategy, a comprehensive plan that will help increase the number of Americans who are healthy at every stage of life.[4] These efforts are designed to stop disease before it starts and to create strategies for a healthy and fit nation, recognizing that prevention must become part of daily life. The National Prevention and Health Promotion Strategy report recognizes that good health comes not just from receiving high-quality medical care, but also from disease prevention, healthy behaviors, and stress management. The document addresses the importance of healthy foods, clean air and water, and safe worksites. Similarly, the *Healthy People 2020* initiative continues the work started in 2000 with the *Healthy People 2010* initiative for improving the nation's health.[5]

The world is calling for 21st-century nurses who can work autonomously and collaboratively to engage in interprofessional dialogues and projects—local to global—to create a healthy nation and a healthy world.

The American Nurses Association (ANA) recognizes holistic nursing as a specialty. The joint AHNA and ANA *Holistic Nursing: Scope and Standards of Practice* documents holistic practice to inform holistic nurses, the nursing profession, other healthcare providers and disciplines, employers, third-party payers, legislators, and the public about the unique scope of knowledge and standards of practice and professional performance of a holistic nurse.[6]

Today, nursing and health care are fragmented. The pace of life is faster than ever at both the professional and personal levels. Self-care is a low priority; time is not given or valued within practice settings to address basic self-care such as breaks for personal needs and meals. Professional burnout is extremely high and many nurses are very discouraged. Nurse retention in all settings is at a crisis level. Many nurses undervalue their power and their voice and often do not articulate their work and role in society. Often, there is a lack of respect for each other. We also do not consistently listen to the pain and suffering that nurses experience within the profession nor do we truly listen to the pain and suffering of the patient and family members or our colleagues.

Severe health needs exist in almost every community and nation throughout the world. We are presented with new common health concerns for humankind and global health imperatives; these are not isolated problems in far-off countries. With global warming and the globalization of the world, no natural or political boundaries can stop the spread of disease. Nurses are key in mobilizing new approaches in prevention education and healthcare delivery. The role of an integral and holistic perspective has never been so important.

The first priority of nursing is devotion to human health—of individuals, of communities, and of the world. Nurses are educated and prepared—physically, emotionally, mentally, and spiritually—to effectively accomplish the activities required—on the ground—with the care team for the health of people. An increasingly severe global nursing shortage is threatening nursing's ranks in almost every nation. Securing the health and happiness of people everywhere in the global community is the common ground for a creating a sustainable, prosperous future. Yet, a healthy world still requires nurses' knowledge, expertise, wisdom, and dedication. If today's nurses, midwives, and allied health professionals are nurtured and sustained in innovative ways, they can become, like Florence Nightingale, effective voices calling for and demonstrating the healing, leadership, and global action required to achieve a healthy world.[7-9] This can strengthen nursing's ranks and help the world to value and nurture nursing's essential contributions. The authors and contributors to this sixth edition believe that their combined effort provides guidelines to solve some of these challenges.

This book guides nurses in the art and science of holistic nursing and healing and in becoming more aware of an integral approach that is developed in the Theory of Integral Nursing in Chapter 1. This provides a comprehensive way to organize multiple phenomena of human experience and reality: the individual interior (intentional), individual exterior (behavioral), collective interior (cultural), and collective exterior (social). It offers ways of thinking, practicing, and responding both personally and professionally.

The National Center for Complementary and Alternative Medicine (NCCAM) has focused on consistent and cumulative research on holistic and integrative nursing and medicine.[10] Research findings reveal that holistic and integrative approaches and complementary and alternative therapies not only work and are extremely safe, but are also cost effective. At the present time, they should be considered complements to orthodox medical treatments and not a replacement for them. We advocate a "both/and" instead of an "either/or" approach in interfacing these healing modalities with contemporary medical and surgical therapies.

We challenge nurses to explore the following three questions:

1. What do you know about the meaning of healing?
2. What can you do each day to facilitate healing in yourself?
3. How can you be an instrument of healing and a nurse healer?

Healing is a lifelong journey into understanding the wholeness of human existence. Along this journey, our lives mesh with those of clients, families, and colleagues, where moments of new meaning and insight emerge in the midst of crisis. Healing occurs when we help clients, families, others, and ourselves embrace what is feared most. It occurs when we seek harmony and balance. Healing is learning how to open what has been closed so that we can expand our inner potentials. It is the fullest expression of oneself that is demonstrated by the light and shadow and the male and female principles that reside within each of us. It is accessing what we have forgotten about connections, unity, and interdependence. With a new awareness of these interrelationships, healing becomes possible, and the experience of the nurse as an instrument of healing and as a nurse healer becomes actualized. A nurse healer is one who facilitates another person's growth toward wholeness (body-mind-spirit) or who assists another with recovery from illness or transition to peaceful death. Healing is not just curing symptoms. Rather, it is the exquisite blending of technology with caring, love, compassion, and creativity.

Incorporating ideas of perennial philosophy, natural systems theory, and the holistic caring process expands this holistic approach. The information presented within this sixth edition of *Holistic Nursing: A Handbook for Practice* may be of additional interest to the nurse because it incorporates the following:

- Theory of Integral Nursing, an integral worldview and integral approaches
- American Holistic Nurses Association and American Nurses Association *Holistic Nursing: Scope and Standards of Practice* (2007)
- Two new chapters: "Nurse Coaching" and "Motivational Interviewing and Appreciative Inquiry"
- New integrative health and wellness assessments in eight categories: life balance and satisfaction, relationships, spiritual, mental, emotional, physical (nutrition, exercise, weight), environmental, health responsibility
- Exploration of ways to incorporate nursing diagnoses, the Nursing Interventions Classification, and the Nursing Outcomes Classification within a holistic nursing practice
- Guidelines for integrating holistic interventions in four areas: before, at the beginning, during, and at the close of the session
- Both basic and advanced strategies for integrating complementary and alternative interventions
- Client case studies in the acute care and outpatient settings
- Research and directions for future research

As we have explored new meanings of healing in our work and lives, we have interwoven the many diverse threads of knowledge from nursing as well as from other disciplines in this book. This integration has engendered a more vivid, dynamic, and diverse understanding of the nature of holism, healing, and its implications for nursing. Each chapter then begins with Nurse Healer Objectives to direct your learning within the theoretical, clinical, and personal domains. Each chapter has a glossary of definitions for easy reference. The term *patient* is used for acute care settings, and the term *client* is used in the outpatient settings. With both the patient and the client, we view persons as coparticipants in all phases of care. The challenge is to integrate all concepts in this text in clinical practice and daily life. As clinicians, authors, educators, and researchers, we have successfully used these holistic concepts and interventions in various settings, from the critical care unit and home health to the classroom.

Each chapter ends with Directions for Future Research specific to each topic. This section presents suggested research questions that are timely and in need of scientific exploration in nursing. In concluding each chapter, Nurse Healer Reflections are offered to nurture and spark a special self-reflective experience of body-mind-spirit and the inward journey toward self-discovery and healing.

This book is organized according to the five core values of holistic nursing contained within the AHNA and ANA *Holistic Nursing: Scope and Standards of Practice* (2007) as follows:

Core Value 1:   Holistic Philosophy, Theories, and Ethics

Core Value 2:   Holistic Caring Process

Core Value 3:   Holistic Communication, Therapeutic Environment, and Cultural Diversity

Core Value 4:   Holistic Education and Research

Core Value 5:   Holistic Nurse Self-Care

Core Value 1 presents the philosophic concepts that explore what occurs when the nurse honors, acknowledges, and deepens the understanding of inner knowledge and wisdom. It explores relationship-centered care. The *Holistic Nursing: Scope and Standards for Practice* are explored in depth. Trends and issues in holistic nursing are identified. The foundation for transpersonal human caring and the art of holistic nursing provides insight into how people create change and sustain these new health behavior changes related to wellness, values clarification, and motivation theory. Holistic nursing theorists and theories are developed to guide holistic nursing practice. Holistic ethics is also addressed in both personal and professional arenas.

Core Value 2 expands the nursing process to the holistic caring process and includes a detailed discussion of ways to explore the possible strategies to incorporate nursing diagnoses, the Nursing Interventions Classification, and the Nursing Outcomes Classification within a holistic nursing practice. The nursing process is a six-part circular process: assessment, patterns/challenges/ needs, outcomes, therapeutic care plan, implementation, and evaluation. Self-assessments and complementary and alternative strategies are developed to expand concepts relevant to healing and reaching human potential. Specific areas covered are nurse coaching, motivational interviewing and appreciative inquiry, cognitive therapy, self-reflection, nutrition, exercise and movement, humor, laughter, and play, relaxation, imagery, music, touch, relationships, and dying in peace and exploring grief, weight management, smoking cessation, addictions and recovering, aromatherapy, relationship-centered care and healing initiatives in a community hospital, and exploring integrative medicine and the healing environment in a large urban acute care hospital.

Core Value 3 explores therapeutic communication and the art and skills of helping. The necessary steps in creating an external as well as an internal healing environment are expanded to help nurses recognize that each person's environment includes everything surrounding the individual, both the external and the internal, as well as patterns not yet understood.

Concepts related to cultural diversity are presented so that the nurse can recognize each person as a whole body-mind-spirit being. Such recognition facilitates the development of a mutually cocreated plan of care that addresses the cultural background, health beliefs, sexual orientation, values, and preferences of each unique individual.

Core Value 4 addresses the psychophysiology of body-mind-spirit healing, spirituality, and health. Energetic healing is also developed to expand further one's understanding and practice of holism. Guidelines for holistic research are also explored to provide a framework for establishing evidence-based practice. Evidence-based holistic nursing practice guidelines are developed and are examined as the conscientious use of the best available evidence combined with the clinician's expertise and judgment, and the patient's preferences and values to arrive at the best decision that leads to quality outcomes. Steps for integrating holistic content into the undergraduate program to teach future nurses are provided.

Core Value 5 develops and explores the nurse as an instrument of healing. Concepts of therapeutic presence and the qualities and characteristics of becoming an instrument of healing are developed. It also explores the importance of self-care. It addresses our own self-healing so that we can offer new ways to others and practice in new ways in a time of great vulnerability. It presents expanded strategies for enhancing our psychophysiology using self-assessments, relaxation, imagery, nutrition, exercise, and aromatherapy. It also assists nurses in their challenging roles of bringing healing to the forefront of health care and helping to shape healthcare reform.

Our book is intended for students, clinicians, educators, and researchers who desire to expand their knowledge of holism, healing, and spirituality. The philosophical and conceptual frameworks are beginner, intermediate, and advanced. Therefore, the reader can approach this book as a guide for learning basic content or for exploring advanced concepts. The specific "how to" for implementing holistic interventions into clinical practice is divided into both basic and advanced levels. Some advanced interventions may require additional training that can be obtained in practicums under mentors or in elective or continuing education courses. Most chapters also present case studies that illustrate how to use and integrate the interventions into clinical practice.

The sixth edition of *Holistic Nursing: A Handbook for Practice* challenges nurses to explore the inward journey toward self-transformation and to identify the growing capacity for change and healing. This exploration creates the synergy and the rebirth of a compassionate power to heal ourselves and to facilitate healing within others. This inner healing allows us to return to our roots of nursing where healer and healing have always been understood and to carry Florence Nightingale's vision for healing, leading, and global action forward into the twenty-first century. As she said, "My work is my must." By her shining example, she invites each of us to find and know our "must" and to explore our own meaning, purpose, and spirituality.[7]

The radical changes necessary in healthcare reform are occurring rapidly. Change has always been the rule in health care. These changes provide us with a greater opportunity to integrate caring and healing into our work, research, and lives. It is up to us to help determine what these new changes will be. We challenge you to capture your essence and emerge as true healers as we navigate the rough waters in this dynamic period in health care. Best wishes to you in your healing work and life.

Barbara Montgomery Dossey
Lynn Keegan

NOTES

1. Samueli Institute. *Wellness Initiative for the Nation* (2009). http://www.siib.org/siib/509-SIIB.html.
2. J. Weeks, Reference Guide: Language and Sections on CAM and Integrative Practice in HR 3590/Healthcare Overhaul. *The Integrator Blog* (May 2010). http://theintegratorblog.com/site/index.php?option=com_content&task=view&id=658&Itemid=93.
3. Institute of Medicine, *The Future of Nursing: Leading Change, Advancing Health* (2010). http://www.iom.edu/Reports/2010/The-Future-of-Nursing-Leading-Change-Advancing-Health.aspx.
4. U.S. Department of Health and Human Services, "Obama Administration Releases National Prevention Strategy" (June 16, 2011). http://www.hhs.gov/news/press/2011pres/06/20110616a.html.
5. HealthyPeople.gov, "About Healthy People." http://www.healthypeople.gov/2020/about/default.aspx.
6. American Holistic Nurses Association and American Nurses Association, *Holistic Nursing: Scope and Standards of Practice* (Silver Spring, MD: NurseBooks.org, 2012).
7. B. Dossey, *Florence Nightingale: Mystic, Visionary, Healer* (Philadelphia, PA: F. A. Davis, 2010).
8. B. M. Dossey, L. C. Selanders, D. M. Beck, and A. Attewell, *Florence Nightingale Today: Healing, Leadership, Global Action* (Silver Spring, MD: NurseBooks.org, 2005).
9. NightingaleDeclaration.net, Nightingale Initiative for Global Health. http://www.nightingaledeclaration.net.
10. National Center for Complementary and Alternative Medicine. http://nccam.nih.gov.

■ RESOURCES

For more information about the American Holistic Nurses Association and the AHNA continuing education programs and home study courses, contact the association at the following address:

American Holistic Nurses Association (AHNA)
323 N. San Francisco Street, Suite 201
Flagstaff, AZ 86001
Telephone: 1-800-278-2462
Fax: 1-928-526-2752
Email: info@ahna.org
Website: http://www.ahna.org

For information on the holistic nursing certification examination and professional nurse coaching certification, use the following contact information:

**American Holistic Nurses'
Certification Corporation**
1350 Broadway, 17th Floor
New York, NY 10018
212-356-0672
Email: ahncc@flash.net
Website: http://www.ahncc.org

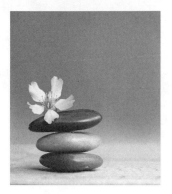

Contributors

Jeanne Anselmo, BSN, RN, BCIAC-SF, HN-BC
Holistic Nurse Educator/Consultant
Sea Cliff, New York
Cofounder, Faculty
Contemplative Urban Law Program
City University of New York School of Law
Queens, New York
Faculty
Iona Spirituality Institute
Iona College
New Rochelle, New York
Dharma Teacher
Order of InterBeing
Ordained by VietNamese Zen Master
    Venerable Thich Nhat Hanh
Green Island Sangha: Community of
    Mindful Living
Long Island, New York

**Carol M. Baldwin, PhD, RN, CHTP, CT,
AHN-BC, FAAN**
Associate Professor and Southwest
    Borderlands Scholar
Director, Center for World Health Promotion
    and Disease Prevention
Affiliate Faculty, Southwest Interdisciplinary
    Research Center of Excellence (SIRC)
Affiliate Faculty, North American Center for
    Transborder Studies (NACTS)
Arizona State University College of Nursing
    and Health Innovation
Phoenix, Arizona

Linda Bark, PhD, RN, MCC
Founder and President, Bark Coaching Institute
Alameda, California
Adjunct Faculty, John F. Kennedy University
Pleasant Hill, California
Adjunct Faculty, National Institute of
    Whole Health
Boston, Massachusetts

Cynthia C. Barrere, PhD, RN, CNS, AHN-BC
Professor of Nursing
Quinnipiac University School of Nursing
Hamden, Connecticut

Genevieve M. Bartol, EdD, RN, AHN-BC
Professor Emeritus
University of North Carolina, Greensboro
Greensboro, North Carolina

Deva-Marie Beck, PhD, RN
International Codirector, Nightingale Initiative
    for Global Health
Washington, DC, and Ottawa, Ontario, Canada

Jane Buckle, PhD, RN, Cert Ed, CCAP
Director, RJ Buckle Associates, LLC
Author, Clinical Aromatherapy in Nursing
    and Clinical Aromatherapy: Essential Oils
    in Practice
London, England and Hazlet, New Jersey

Margaret A. Burkhardt, PhD, FNP, AHN-BC
Associate Professor Emerita, Robert C. Byrd
    Health Sciences Center
West Virginia University, Charleston Division
Charleston, West Virginia

**Megan McInnis Burt, MS, RN, CARN,
PMH-BC, CARN**
Faculty, Huntington Meditation and
    Imagery Center
Huntington, New York

**Nancy F. Courts, PhD, RN,
NCC, LPCA**
Associate Professor Emeritus
School of Nursing
University of North Carolina, Greensboro
Greensboro, North Carolina

**Barbara Montgomery Dossey, PhD, RN,
AHN-BC, FAAN**
Codirector, International Nurse Coach
    Association (INCA)
Codirector, Integrative Nurse Coach
    Certificate Program (INCCP)
Huntington, New York
International Codirector, Nightingale
    Initiative for Global Health
Washington, DC and Ottawa, Ontario, Canada
Director, Holistic Nursing Consultants
Santa Fe, New Mexico

Joan C. Engebretson, DrPH, RN, AHN-BC
Judy Fred Professor in Nursing
University of Texas Health Science Center,
    Houston
Houston, Texas

**Noreen Cavan Frisch, PhD, RN, APHN,
AHN-BC, FAAN**
Professor and Director, School of Nursing
University of Victoria
Victoria, British Columbia, Canada
Past President, American Holistic
    Nurses Association

Francie Halderman, RN, BSN, HN-BC
Director, The Art of Universal Medicine
Integrative Health Management
Philadelphia, Pennsylvania

**Mary Blaszko Helming, PhD, APRN,
FNP-BC, AHN-BC**
Professor of Nursing
FNP Track Coordinator for MSN and
    DNP Programs
Quinnipiac University School of Nursing
Hamden, Connecticut

**Darlene R. Hess, PhD, RN, AHN-BC,
PMHNP-BC, ACC**
Psychiatric/Mental Health Nurse Practitioner,
    Consultant, Nurse Educator
Brown Mountain Visions
Los Ranchos, New Mexico
Practitioner Faculty
University of Phoenix
Albuquerque, New Mexico
Phoenix, Arizona

Shannon S. Spies Ingersoll, DNP, CRNA
Doctor of Nursing Practice
Staff Registered Nurse Anesthetist
Olmsted Medical Center
Rochester, Minnesota

Christina Jackson, PhD, APRN, AHN-BC
Professor of Nursing
Eastern University
St. Davids, Pennsylvania

Lynn Keegan, PhD, RN, AHN-BC, FAAN
Director, Holistic Nursing Consultants
Port Angeles, Washington
Partner, Absolutely: Business and Personal
    Strategic Consulting, LLC
Indianapolis, Indiana
Past President, American Holistic Nurses
    Association

Lori L. Knutson, BSN, RN, HN-BC
President, The Marsh
Minnetonka, Minnesota
Former Executive Director, Integrative Medicine
Penny George Institute for Health and Healing
Allina Hospitals and Clinics
Former Executive Director, Sister Kenny
    Rehabilitation Institute
Allina Hospitals and Clinics
Minneapolis, Minnesota

Corinne Latini, MEd, BSN, RN-BC, CSN
Reiki Master and Healing Touch
    Level 1 Student
Nursing Clinical Resource Laboratory
    Coordinator and Adjunct Faculty
Eastern University Department of Nursing
St. Davids, Pennsylvania

Jackie D. Levin, RN, MS, CHTP, AHN-BC
Holistic Nurse Consultant
Private Practice
Clinical Coordinator/Educator
Jefferson Healthcare Home Health and Hospice
Port Townsend, Washington

Susan Luck, RN, MA, HNC, CCN
Codirector, International Nurse Coach Association
    (INCA)
Codirector, Integrative Nurse Coach Certificate
    Program (INCCP)
Huntington, New York
Adjunct Faculty, School of Nursing
University of Miami
Miami, Florida
Director, Earthrose Institute
Miami, Florida

Carla Mariano, EdD, RN, AHN-BC, FAAIM
Adjunct Associate Professor
College of Nursing, New York University
New York City, New York
Consultant, Holistic Nursing Education
Past President, American Holistic Nurses
    Association

**Deborah McElligott, DNP, AHN-BC,
ANP-BC**
Nurse Practitioner
Southside Hospital
North Shore LIJ Health System
Bayshore, New York

**Bernadette Mazurek Melnyk, PhD, RN,
CPNP/PMHNP, FNAP, FAAN**
Associate Vice President for Health Promotion
University Chief Wellness Officer
Dean, College of Nursing
The Ohio State University
Columbus, Ohio

Nancy Moore, PhD, RN
Nancy Moore Consulting
Redmond, Oregon
Formerly, Chief Nursing Officer
St. Charles Medical Center
Bend, Oregon

Mary Gail Nagai-Jacobson, MSN, RN
Community Health Consultant
Director, Healing Matters
San Marcos, Texas

Melodie Olson, PhD, RN
Professor Emerita, College of Nursing
Medical University of South Carolina
Charleston, South Carolina

Sue Popkess-Vawter, PhD, RN
Professor of Nursing
University of Kansas School of Nursing
Kansas City, Kansas

Pamela J. Potter, DNSc, RN, CNS
Assistant Professor, School of Nursing
University of Portland
Portland, Oregon

Janet F. Quinn, PhD, RN, FAAN
Spiritual Director, Integrative Health and
    Healing Consultant/Educator
Director, HaelanWorks
Lyons, Colorado

Jennifer L. Reich, PhD, MA, MS, RN, ANP-BC
Part-time Faculty
College of Nursing
Department of Health Sciences
Northern Arizona University
Flagstaff, Arizona

**Jo Rycroft-Malone, PhD, MSc,
BSc(Hons), RN**
Professor of Health Services and
    Implementation Research
University Director of Research
Editor, *Worldviews on Evidence-Based Nursing*
Bangor University
Wales, United Kingdom

Ana Schaper, PhD, RN
Nurse Scientist
Gundersen Lutheran Health System
La Crosse, Wisconsin

Bonney Gulino Schaub, RN, MS, PMHCNS-BC
Codirector, International Nurse
    Coach Association (INCA)
Codirector, Integrative Nurse Coach
    Certificate Program (INCCP)
Codirector, Huntington Meditation
    and Imagery Center
Private Practice and Consultation
Huntington, New York

Alyce A. Schultz, RN, PhD, FAAN
Owner/Consultant, EBP Concepts
Alyce A. Schultz & Associates, LLC
Appraiser, Magnet Recognition Program,
    American Nursing Credentialing Center
Fulbright Senior Specialist
Boromarajonani College of Nursing
Nakhon Lampang (BCNLP), Thailand

Esther Seibold, DNSc, RN
Clinical Assistant Professor
University of Massachusetts, Boston
Boston, Massachusetts

Victoria E. Slater, PhD, RN, AHN-BC, CHTP/I
Holistic Nurse, Private Practice
Clarksville, Tennessee

Mary Elaine Southard, RN, MSN, APHN-BC
CEO, Integrative Health Consulting
    and Coaching
Scranton, Pennsylvania
Health Manager, Geisinger Health Plan
Danville, Pennsylvania

Pamela Steinke, RN, MSN-HCA
Chief Nurse Executive
St. Charles Health System
Bend, Oregon

Eileen M. Stuart-Shor, PhD, ANP, FAHA, FAAN
Assistant Professor
University of Massachusetts, Boston
Boston, Massachusetts
Nurse Practitioner
Cardiology/Anesthesia/Critical Care
Beth Israel Deaconess Medical Center
Boston, Massachusetts

Lucia Thornton, MSN, RN, AHN-BC
Faculty, Energy Medicine University
Associate Editor, *BRIDGES Magazine*
President, Innovations in Healthcare
Past President, American Holistic
    Nurses Association

Carol L. Wells-Federman, MEd, MSN, NP-BC
Northwest Regional Coordinator
Reach Out and Read, Colorado
Carbondale, Colorado

Patty Wooten, BSN, RN, PHN
Nurse Humorist and Speaker
Director, Jest for Health
Santa Cruz, California

Rothlyn P. Zahourek, PhD, PMHCNS-BC, AHN-BC
Holistic Nurse Researcher and Consultant
Adjunct Faculty, University of
    Massachusetts School of Nursing
Amherst, Massachusetts

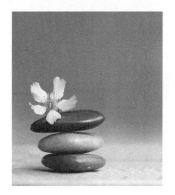

Acknowledgments

Our book flows out of the larger questions that have been raised for us in the health or illness of clients/patients, the professional community with which we have worked, the global community and our families and friends with whom we live and play.

We celebrate with our colleagues in nursing as we explore new meanings of healing in our work and life, as we acknowledge what we have done well, and as we anticipate what we must do better. We honor the collaboration with our Associate Editors, Cynthia C. Barrere and Mary Blaszko Helming, on *Holistic Nursing: A Handbook fro Practice, Sixth Edition*. Special thanks are due to Clayton E. Jones, Chief Executive Officer, Don Jones, Jr., Chief Operating Office, and Robert W. Holland, Jr., Executive Vice President and Publisher, at Jones & Bartlett Learning, who have provided a wonderful partnership for *Holistic Nursing: A Handbook for Practice, Sixth Edition*. We thank Kevin Sullivan, Publisher, and Amanda Harvey, Acquisitions Editor, who helped us keep our goals in sight and believed in the project; to Amanda Harvey for attention to editorial details; to Sara Bempkins, Editorial Assistant and Sara Fowles, Associate Production Editor; Katie Hennessy, Associate Marketing Manager; Arlene Apone, Composition; and Kristin E. Parker, for cover design.

Most of all, for their understanding, encouragement, and love in seeing us through one more book, we thank our families—Larry Dossey; and Gerald, Catherine Keegan Michael and Genevieve Keegan Bedano, who share our interconnectedness.

Holistic Philosophy, Theories, and Ethics

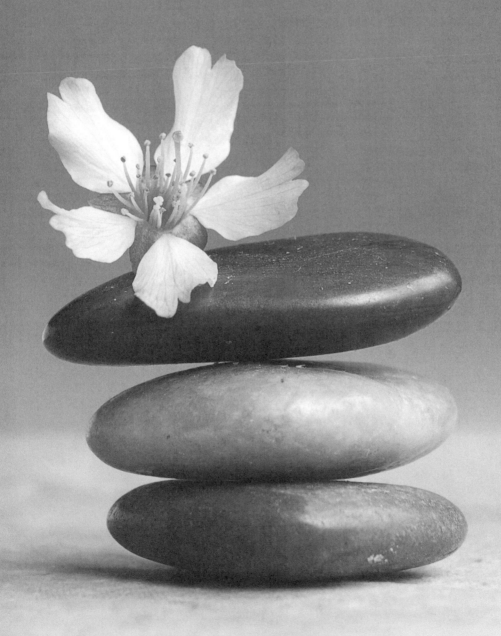

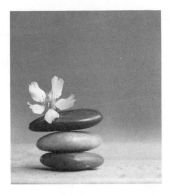

Chapter 1

Nursing: Integral, Integrative, and Holistic—Local to Global

Barbara Montgomery Dossey

Nurse Healer
OBJECTIVES

Theoretical

- Explore the Theory of Integral Nursing and its application to holistic nursing.
- Examine the United Nations Millennium Goals.
- Link Florence Nightingale's legacy of healing, leadership, global action, and her work as a nurse and citizen activist to 21st-century integral and holistic nursing.
- Analyze relationship-centered care and its three components.
- Examine optimal healing environments and their four domains.

Clinical

- Apply relationship-centered care principles and components in your practice.
- Compare and contrast the three eras of medicine.
- Examine the Theory of Integral Nursing, and begin the process of integrating the theory into your clinical practice.
- Determine whether you have an integral worldview and approach in your clinical practice and other education, research, hospital policies, and community endeavors.

Personal

- Create an integral self-care plan.
- Examine ways to enhance integral understanding in your personal endeavors.
- Develop short- and long-term goals related to increasing your commitment to an integral developmental process.

DEFINITIONS

Global health: Exploration of the emerging value base and new relationships and innovations that occur when health becomes an essential component and expression of global citizenship; an increased awareness that health is a basic human right and a global good that needs to be promoted and protected by the global community.

Holistic nursing: See Chapter 2 definitions.

Integral: Comprehensive way to organize multiple phenomena of human experience related to four perspectives of reality: (1) the individual interior (personal/intentional); (2) individual exterior (physiology/behavioral); (3) collective interior (shared/cultural); and (4) collective exterior (systems/structures).

Integral dialogue: Transformative and visionary exploration of ideas and possibilities across disciplines where the individual interior (personal/intentional), individual exterior (physiology/behavioral), collective interior (shared/cultural), and collective exterior (structures/systems) are considered as equally important to exchanges and outcomes.

Integral healing process: Contains both nurse processes and patient/family and healthcare worker processes (individual interior and individual exterior), and collective healing processes of individuals and of systems/structures (collective interior and exterior); an understanding of the unitary whole person interacting in mutual process with the environment.

Integral health: Process through which we reshape basic assumptions and worldviews about well-being and see death as a natural process of living; may be symbolically viewed as a jewel with many facets that is reflected as a "bright gem" or a "rough stone" depending on one's situation and personal growth that influence states of health, health beliefs, and values.

Integral health care: A patient-centered and relationship-centered caring process that includes the patient, family, and community and conventional, integrative, and integral healthcare practitioners and services and interventions; a process where the individual interior (personal/intentional), the individual exterior (physiology/behavioral), the collective interior (shared/cultural), and the collective exterior (structures/systems) are considered in all endeavors.

Integral nurse: A 21st-century Nightingale who is engaged as a "health diplomat" and an integral health coach who is coaching for integral health.

Integral nursing: A comprehensive integral worldview and process that includes holistic theories and other paradigms; holistic nursing is included (embraced) and transcended (goes beyond); this integral process and integral worldview enlarges our holistic understanding of body-mind-spirit connections and our knowing, doing, and being to more comprehensive and deeper levels.

Integral worldview: Process where values, beliefs, assumptions, meaning, purpose, and judgments are identified and related to how individuals perceive reality and relationships that includes the individual interior (personal/intentional), individual exterior (physiology/behavioral), collective interior (shared/cultural), and collective exterior (systems/structures).

Relationship-centered care: A process model of caregiving that is based in a vision of community where the patient–practitioner, community–practitioner, and practitioner–practitioner relationships, and the unique set of responsibilities of each are honored and valued.

■ NURSING: INTEGRAL, INTEGRATIVE, AND HOLISTIC

In the future, which I shall not see, for I am old, may a better way be opened! May the methods by which every infant, every human being will have the best chance at health—the methods by which every sick person will have the best chance at recovery, be learned and practiced. Hospitals are only an intermediate stage of civilization, never intended, at all events, to take in the whole sick population. . . .

May we hope that, when we are all dead and gone, leaders will arise who have been personally experienced in the hard, practical work, the difficulties, and the joys of organizing nursing reforms, and who will lead far beyond anything we have done! May we hope that every nurse will be an atom in the hierarchy of ministers of the Highest! But she [or he] must be in her [or his] place in the hierarchy, not alone, not an atom in the indistinguishable mass of thousands of nurses. High hopes, which shall not be deceived!"[1]

Florence Nightingale's (1893) words above empower us in our mission of service. In 2010, the Institute of Medicine *Future of Nursing* report published a landmark document that presented four key messages:[2]

- Nurses should practice to the full extent of their education and training.
- Nurses should achieve higher levels of education and training through an improved

education system that promotes seamless academic progression.

- Nurses should be full partners, with physicians and other healthcare professionals, in redesigning health care in the United States.
- Effective workforce planning and policy making require better data collection and information infrastructure.

To fulfill the challenges addressed in the IOM report an integral perspective has never been more important. At the forefront, nurses are now engaged as change agents to improve the health of the nation, to focus on increasing the "health span" of individuals rather than focusing on life span. Integral nursing can be described as a comprehensive integral worldview and process that includes holistic theories and other paradigms; holistic nursing practice is included (embraced) and transcended (goes beyond).[3-6] This integral process and the integral worldview enlarge our holistic understanding of body-mind-spirit connections and our knowing, doing, and being to more comprehensive and deeper levels (Note: See the section titled "Theory of Integral Nursing" later in this chapter for full discussion.)

Holistic nursing is defined as "all nursing practice that has healing the whole person as its goal."[7] As described and developed later in this text (Chapter 2), holistic nursing has attained new levels of acceptance and is now officially recognized by the American Nurses Association (ANA) as a nursing specialty with a defined scope and standards of practice.[7] Our holistic nursing challenges as described throughout this text include ways to learn and integrate new theories, models, and information, and how to articulate the science and art of holistic nursing, complementary and alternative modalities (CAM), integrative modalities, and healing in all areas and specialties of nursing. Our challenges and opportunities to interface in interprofessional conversations related to integral, integrative, and holistic nursing and integrative medicine with traditional and nontraditional healthcare professionals, healers, disciplines, and organizations can transform health care.[8-10] Integrative medicine (IM) is the practice of medicine that reaffirms the importance of the relationship between practitioner and patient, focuses on the whole person, is informed by evidence, and makes use of all appropriate therapeutic approaches, healthcare professionals, and disciplines to achieve optimal health and healing.[8] The next section provides an overview of how we can globally integrate and translate integral and holistic nursing concepts.

■ GLOBAL NURSING, NIGHTINGALE DECLARATION, AND UNITED NATIONS MILLENNIUM DEVELOPMENT GOALS

Severe health needs exist in almost every community and country. These are no longer isolated problems in far-off places. Across humankind, we all face common health concerns and global health imperatives. With globalization and global warming, no natural or political boundaries stop the spread of disease.[11-13] Yet, the health and well-being of people everywhere can be seen as common ground to secure a sustainable, prosperous future for everyone. In interdisciplinary and interprofessional collaboration with professional and allied health colleagues, as well as concerned citizens, nurses can play a major role in mobilizing new approaches to education, healthcare delivery, and disease prevention. Global health requires new leadership models in communication, negotiations, resource, management, work-life balance, and mentor-mentee models and relationships.[13-14]

Global health is the exploration of the emerging value base and new relationships and agendas that occur when health becomes an essential component and expression of global citizenship.[13] It is an increased awareness that health is a basic human right that is "decent care"[15] that addresses the body, mind, and spirit and is a global good that needs to be promoted and protected by the global community. Severe health needs exist in almost every community and nation throughout the world. Thus, all nurses are involved in some aspect of global health because their caring and healing endeavors assist individuals to become healthier, which leads to healthy people living in a healthy world by 2020.[16,17]

Currently, there are 17.6 million nurses and midwives engaged in nursing and providing health care around the world.[18] Together, we are collectively addressing human health—the health of individuals, of communities, of environments (interior and exterior), and the world as our first priority. We are educated and prepared—physically, emotionally, socially, mentally, and spiritually—to accomplish effectively the activities required to create a healthy world. Nurses are key in mobilizing new approaches in health education and healthcare delivery in all areas of nursing. Solutions and evidence-based practice protocols can be shared and implemented around the world through dialogues, the Internet, and publications, which are essential as we address the global nursing shortage.[19]

We are challenged to act locally and think globally and to address ways to create healthy environments. For example, we can address global warming in our own personal habits at home as well as in our workplace (using green products, using energy-efficient fluorescent bulbs, turning off lights when not in the room) and simultaneously address our own personal health and the health of the communities where we live. As we expand our awareness of individual and collective states of healing consciousness and integral dialogues, we can explore integral ways of knowing, doing, and being.

We can unite 17.6 million nurses (**Figure 1-1**) and midwives, along with concerned citizens through the Internet to create a healthy world through many endeavors such as signing the Nightingale Declaration (at www.nightingale declaration.net), as shown in **Figure 1-2**.[16] (See the section titled "Theory of Integral Nursing" later in this chapter.)

During the year 2000, world leaders convened a United Nations Millennium Summit to establish eight Millennium Development Goals (MDGs), as shown in **Figure 1-3**, that must be achieved for the 21st century to progress toward a sustainable quality of life for all of humanity.[20] These goals are an ambitious agenda for improving lives worldwide. Of these eight MDGs, three—MDG 4, Reduce Child Mortality, MDG 5, Improve Maternal Health, and MDG 6, Combat HIV/AIDS—are directly related to health and nursing. The other five goals, MDG 1, Eradicate Extreme Poverty and Hunger, MDG 2, Achieve Universal Primary Education, MDG 3, Promote Gender Equality and Empower Women, MDG 7, Ensure Environmental Sustainability, and MDG 8, Develop a Global Partnership for Development are factors

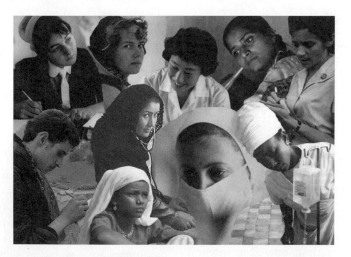

FIGURE 1-1   Global nurses collage.
Source: Global Nurses collage from the World Health Organization (WHO)
Source: Photo Credits: Site, Source, Photographer; clockwise from upper left: Switzerland, WHO, John Mohr; Finland, WHO, John Mohr; Japan, WHO, T. Takahara; India, WHO, T.S. Satyan; Brazil, WHO, L. Nadel; Niger, WHO, M. Jacot; Sweden, WHO, John Mohr; Afghanistan, Wikimedia, Ben Barber of USAID; India, Wikimedia, Oreteki; Morocco, WHO, P. Boucas. All World Health Organization (WHO) photos used with attribution as required. Wikimedia Commons: Afghanistan, in the public domain; India, used under the terms of the GNU Free Documentation License.

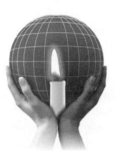

Nightingale Declaration for A Healthy World

"We, the nurses and concerned citizens of the global community, hereby dedicate ourselves to achieve a healthy world by 2020.

We declare our willingness to unite in a program of action, to share information and solutions and to improve health conditions for all humanity—locally, nationally and globally.

We further resolve to adopt personal practices and to implement public policies in our communities and nations—making this goal achievable and inevitable by the year 2020, beginning today in our own lives, in the life of our nations and in the world at large."

www.NightingaleDeclaration.net

FIGURE 1-2   Nightingale declaration for a healthy world by 2020.
Source: Used with permission, Nightingale Initiative for Global Health (NIGH), http://www.nightingaledeclaration.net

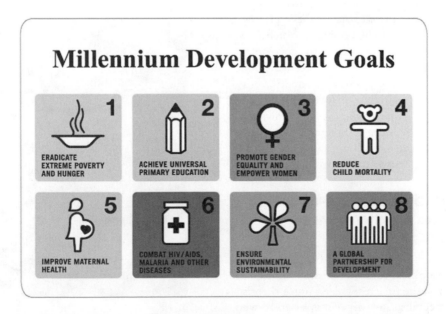

FIGURE 1-3   United Nations millennium development goals and targets.
Source: World Health Organization, WHO Assembly Report: Millennium Development Goals and Targets (Geneva, WHO: 2000), http://www.who.int/mdg/en.

that determine the health or lack of health of people. For each goal, one or more targets, which used the 1990 data as benchmarks, are set to be achieved by 2015. *Health* is the common thread running through all eight UN MDGs. The goals are directly related to nurses, as they work today to achieve them at grassroots levels everywhere and many are engaged in sharing local solutions at the global level.

An integral approach can help nurses conceptualize and map what is missing from caregiving and care delivery. With an integral worldview, collectively we can move closer to achieving global health. Ensuring basic survival needs has been identified as the single most important factor in building responsive and effective health systems in all countries. The health and happiness of people everywhere in the global community are the only common ground for a secure and sustainable prosperous future.[3] Yet a healthy world still requires nurses' knowledge, expertise, wisdom, and dedication. If today's nurses, midwives, and allied health professionals are nurtured and sustained in innovative ways, they can become like Nightingale—effective voices calling for and demonstrating the healing, leadership, and global action required to achieve a healthy world. This can strengthen nursing's ranks and help the world to value and nurture nursing's essential contributions.[3] As Nightingale said, "We must create a public opinion, which must drive the government instead of the government having to drive us . . . an enlightened public opinion, wise in principle, wise in detail."[21]

Nurses aim to initiate new approaches and connect the dots by empowering both individuals and groups to *see through* integral nursing *lenses* and to revisit the integral approach to Nightingale's legacy in 21st-century terms.

■ PHILOSOPHICAL FOUNDATION: FLORENCE NIGHTINGALE'S LEGACY

Florence Nightingale (1820–1910) (**Figure 1-4**), the philosophical founder of modern secular nursing and the first recognized nurse theorist, was an integralist. An *integralist* is a person who focuses on the individual and the collective, the inner and outer, human and nonhuman con-

cerns. Nightingale was concerned with the most basic needs of human beings and all aspects of the environment (clean air, water, food, houses, etc.)—local to global.[22-26] She also experienced and recorded her personal understanding of the connection with the Divine as an awareness that something greater than her, the Divine, was a major connecting link woven into her work and life.[22] The entirety of her life, work, and insights clearly articulates and demonstrates the science and art of an integral worldview for nursing, health care, and humankind, as developed further in the section titled "Theory of Integral Nursing" and in Figure 1-9, later in this chapter.

Nightingale was a nurse, educator, administrator, communicator, statistician, and environmental activist.[22,26] Her specific accomplishments include establishing the model for nursing schools throughout the world and creating a prototype model of care for the sick and wounded soldiers during the Crimean War (1854–1856). She was an innovator for British Army medical reform that included reorganizing the British Army Medical Department, creating an Army Statistical Department, and collaborating on the first British Army medical school, including developing the curriculum and choosing the

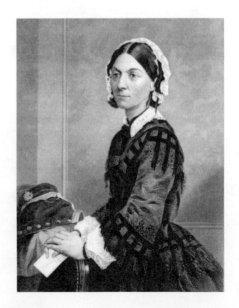

FIGURE 1-4   Florence Nightingale (1820–1910).

professors. She revolutionized hospital data collection and invented a statistical wedge diagram equivalent to today's circular histograms or circular statistical representation. In 1858, she became the first woman admitted to the Royal Statistical Society. She developed and wrote protocols and papers on workhouses and midwifery that led to successful legislation reform. She was a recognized expert on the health of the British Army and soldiers in India for more than 40 years; she never went to India but collected data directly from Army stations, analyzed the data, and wrote and published documents, articles, and books on the topic.

In 1902, besides her numerous other recognitions, she was the first woman to receive the Order of Merit. She wrote more than 100 combined books and official Army reports. Her 10,000 letters now make up the largest private collection of letters at the British Library with 4,000 family letters at the Wellcome Trust in London.[22,26] Today we recognize Nightingale's work as global nursing: She envisioned what a healthy world might be with her integral philosophy and expanded visionary capacities. Her work included aspects of the nursing process (see Chapter 7) as well; it has indeed had an impact on nurses today and will continue to affect us far into the future. Nightingale's work was social action that demonstrated and clearly articulated the science and art of an integral worldview for nursing, health care, and humankind. Her social action was also sacred activism,[27] the fusion of the deepest spiritual knowledge with radical action in the world.

In the 1880s, Nightingale began to write that it would take 100–150 years before educated and experienced nurses would arrive to change the healthcare system. We are that generation of 21st-century Nightingales who have arrived to transform health care and carry forth her vision of social action and sacred activism to create a healthy world. Using terms coined by Patricia Hinton-Walker, 21st-century Nightingales are "health diplomats" and "integral health coaches" who are "coaching for integral health."[28]

Nightingale was ahead of her time. Her dedicated and focused 40 years of work and service still inform and influence our nursing work and our global mission of health and healing for humanity today. **Table 1-1** lists the themes in her *Notes on Hospitals* (1859),[29] *Notes on Nursing* (1860),[30] her formal letters to her nurses (1872–1900),[31] and her article "Sick-Nursing and Health-Nursing" (1893).[32] **Table 1-2** shows Nightingale's themes recognized today as total healing environments. The next section presents an overview of the eras of medicine and application of this information to integral and holistic nursing.

■ ERAS OF MEDICINE

Three eras of medicine currently are operational in Western biomedicine (see **Table 1-3**).[33] Era I medicine began to take shape in the 1860s, when medicine was striving to become scientific. The underlying assumption of this approach is that health and illness are completely physical in nature. The focus is on combining drugs, medical treatments, and technology for curing. A person's consciousness is considered a byproduct of the chemical, anatomic, and physiologic aspects of the brain and is not considered a major factor in the origins of health or disease.

In the 1950s, Era II therapies began to emerge. These therapies reflected the growing awareness that the actions of a person's mind or consciousness—thoughts, emotions, beliefs, meaning, and attitudes—exerted important effects on the behavior of the person's physical body.[33] In both Era I and Era II, a person's consciousness is said to be "local" in nature; that is, confined to a specific location in space (the body itself) and in time (the present moment and a single lifetime).

Era III, the newest and most advanced era, originated in science. Consciousness is said to be nonlocal in that it is not bound to individual bodies. The minds of individuals are spread throughout space and time; they are infinite, immortal, omnipresent, and, ultimately, one. Era III therapies involve any therapy in which the effects of consciousness create bridges between different persons, as with distant healing, intercessory prayer, shamanic healing, so-called miracles, and certain emotions (e.g., love, empathy, compassion). Era III approaches involve transpersonal experiences of being. They raise a person above control at a day-to-day material level to an experience outside his or her local self.

TABLE 1-1   Florence Nightingale's Legacy and Themes for Today

Themes Developed in Notes on Hospitals (1859, 1863)

The hospital will do the patient no harm. Four elements essential for the health of hospitals:

- Fresh air
- Ample space
- Light
- Subdivision of sick into separate buildings or pavilions

Hospital construction defects that prevented health:

- Defective means of natural ventilation and warming
- Defective height of wards
- Excessive width of wards between the opposite windows
- Arrangement of the bed along the dead wall
- More than two rows of beds between the opposite windows
- Windows only on one side, or a closed corridor connecting the wards
- Use of absorbent materials for walls and ceilings, and poor washing of hospital floors

- Defective condition of water closets
- Defective ward furniture
- Defective accommodation for nursing and discipline
- Defective hospital kitchens
- Defective laundries
- Selection of bad sites and bad local climates for hospitals
- Erecting of hospitals in towns
- Defects of sewerage
- Construction of hospitals without free circulation of external air

Themes Developed in Notes on Nursing (1860)

Understand God's laws in nature
- Understanding that, in disease and in illness, nursing and the nurses can assist in the reparative process of a disease and in maintaining health

Nursing and nurses
- Describing the many roles and responsibilities of the nurse

Patient
- Observing and managing the patient's problems, needs, and challenges, and evaluating responses to care

Health
- Recognizing factors that increase or decrease positive or negative states of health, well-being, disease, and illness

Environment
- Both the internal (within one's self) and the external (physical space). (See the specifics listed in the next 12 categories.)

Bed and bedding
- Promote proper cleanliness.
- Use correct type of bed, with proper height, mattress, springs, types of blankets, sheets, and other bedding.

Cleanliness (rooms and walls)
- Maintain clean room, walls, carpets, furniture, and dust-free rooms using correct dusting techniques.
- Release odors from painted and papered rooms; discusses other remedies for cleanliness.

Cleanliness (personal)
- Provide proper bathing, rubbing, and scrubbing of the skin of the patient as well as of the nurse.
- Use proper handwashing techniques that include cleaning the nails.

Food
- Provide proper portions and types of food at the right time, and a proper presentation of food types: eggs, meat, vegetables, beef teas, coffee, jellies, sweets, and homemade bread.

Health of houses
- Provide pure air, pure water, efficient drainage, cleanliness, and light.

Light
- Provide a room with light, windows, and a view that is essential to health and recovery.

Noise
- Avoid noise and useless activity such as clanking or loud conversations with or among caregivers.
- Speak clearly for patients to hear without having to strain.
- Avoid surprising the patient.
- Only read to a patient if it is requested.

Petty management
- Ensure patient privacy, rest, a quiet room, and instructions for the person managing care of patient.

TABLE 1-1   Florence Nightingale's Legacy and Themes for Today *(continued)*

Themes Developed in Notes on Nursing (1860) *(continued)*

Variety

- Provide flowers and plants and avoid those with fragrances.
- Be aware of effects of mind (thoughts) on body.
- Help patients vary their painful thoughts.
- Use soothing colors.
- Be aware of positive effect of certain music on the sick.

Ventilation and warming

- Provide pure air within and without; open windows and regulate room temperature.
- Avoid odiferous disinfectants and sprays.

Chattering hopes and advice

- Avoid unnecessary advice, false hope, promises, and chatter of recovery.

- Avoid absurd statistical comparisons of patient to recovery of other patients, and avoid mockery of advice given by family and friends.
- Share positive events; encourage visits from a well-behaved child or baby.
- Be aware of how small pet animals can provide comfort and companionship for the patient.

Observation of the sick

- Observe each patient; determine the problems, challenges, and needs.
- Assess how the patient responds to food, treatment, and rest.
- Help patient with comfort, safety, and health strategies.
- Intervene if danger to patient is suspected.

Themes Developed in Letters to Her Nurses (1872–1900)

All themes above in Notes on Hospitals and Notes on Nursing plus:

Art of nursing

- Explore authentic presence, caring, meaning, and purpose.
- Increase communication with colleagues, patients, and families.
- Build respect, support, and trusting relationships.

Environment

- Includes the internal self as well as the external physical space

Ethics of nursing

- Engage in moral behaviors and values and model them in personal and professional life.

Health

- Integrate self-care and health-promoting and sustaining behaviors.
- Be a role model and model healthy behaviors.

Personal aspects of nursing

- Explore body-mind-spirit wholeness, healing philosophy, self-care, relaxation, music, prayers, and work of service to self and others.
- Develop therapeutic and healing relationships.

Science of nursing

- Learn nursing knowledge and skills, observing, implementing, and evaluating physicians' orders combined with nursing knowledge and skills.

Spirituality

- Develop intention, self-awareness, mindfulness, presence, compassion, love, and service to God and humankind.

Themes Developed in "Sick-Nursing and Health-Nursing" (1893 Essay)

All themes above in Notes on Nursing and Letters to Her Nurses (1872–1893) plus:

Collaboration with others

- Meet with nurses and women at the local, national, and global level to explore health education and how to support each other in creating health and healthy environments.

Health education curriculum and health missioners education

- Include all components discussed in Notes on Nursing.
- Teach health as proactive leadership for health.

Source: Used with permission. B. M. Dossey, "Florence Nightingale's Tenets: Healing, Leadership, Global Action," in *Florence Nightingale Today: Healing, Leadership, Global Action*, eds. B. M. Dossey et al. (Silver Spring, MD: Nurses books.org, 2005).

TABLE 1-2   Total Healing Environments Today: Integral and Holistic

The Internal Healing Environment

- Includes presence, caring, compassion, creativity, deep listening, grace, honesty, imagination, intention, love, mindfulness, self-awareness, trust, and work of service to self and others.
- Grounded in ethics, philosophies, and values that encourage and nurture such qualities as are listed above and in a way that:
  - Engages body-mind-spirit wholeness
  - Fosters healing relationships and partnerships
  - Promotes self-care and health-promoting and sustaining behaviors
  - Engages with and is affected by the elements of the external healing environment (below).

The External Healing Environment

Color and texture

- Use color that creates healing atmosphere, sacred space, moods, and that lifts spirits.
- Coordinate room color with bed coverings, bedspreads, blankets, drapes, chairs, food trays, and personal hygiene kits.
- Use textural variety on furniture, fabrics, artwork, wall surfaces, floors, ceilings, and ceiling light covers.

Communication

- Provide availability of caring staff for patient and family.
- Provide a public space for families to use television, radio, and telephones.

Family areas

- Create facilities for family members to stay with patients.
- Provide a comfortable family lounge area where families can keep or prepare special foods.

Light

- Provide natural light from low windows where patient can see outside.
- Use full-spectrum light throughout hospital, clinics, schools, public buildings, and homes.
- Provide control of light intensity with good reading light to avoid eye strain.

Noise control

- Eliminate loudspeaker paging systems in halls and elevators.
- Decrease noise of clanking latches, food carts and trays, pharmacy carts, slamming of doors, and noisy hallways.
- Provide 24-hour continuous music and imagery channels such as Healing Healthcare Systems Continuous Ambient Relaxation Environment (C.A.R.E., www.healinghealth.com) and Aesthetic Audio Systems (www.aestheticas.net), and other educational channels related to health and well-being.
- Decrease continuous use of loud commercial television.
- Eliminate loud staff conversations in unit stations, lounges, and calling of staff members in hallways.

Privacy

- Provide a Do Not Disturb sign for patient and family to place on door to control privacy and social interaction.
- Position bed for view of outdoors, with shades to screen light and glare.
- Use full divider panel or heavy curtain for privacy if in a double-patient room.
- Secure place for personal belongings.
- Provide shelves to place personal mementos such as family pictures, flowers, and totems.

Thermal comfort

- Provide patient control of air circulation, room temperature, fresh air, and humidity.

TABLE 1-2   Total Healing Environments Today: Integral and Holistic *(continued)*

The External Healing Environment *(continued)*

Ventilation and air quality

- Provide fresh air, adequate air exchange, rooftop gardens, and solariums.

- Avoid use of toxic materials such as paints, synthetic materials, waxes, and foul-smelling air purifiers.

Views of nature

- Use indoor landscaping, which may include plants and miniature trees.

- Provide pictures of landscapes that include trees, flowers, mountains, ocean, and the like for patient and staff areas.

Integral and integrative practice

Throughout hospitals, clinics, schools, and all parts of a community:

- Combine conventional medical treatments, procedures, and surgery with complementary and alternative therapies and folk medicine.

- Engage in integral and interdisciplinary dialogues and collaboration that foster deep personal support, trust, and therapeutic alliances.

- Offer educational programs for professionals that teach the specifics about the interactions of the healer and healee, holistic philosophy, patient-centered care, relationship-centered care, and complementary and alternative therapies.

- Develop and build community and partnerships based on mutual support, trust, values, and exchange of ideas.

- Use strategies that enhance the interconnectedness of persons, nature, inner and outer, spiritual and physical, and private and public.

- Use self-care and health-promoting education that includes prevention and public health.

- Provide support groups, counseling, and psychotherapy, specifically for cancer and cardiac support groups, lifestyle change groups, 12-step programs and support groups, for leisure, exercise, and nutrition and weight management.

- Use health coaches for staff, patients, families, and community.

- Provide information technology and virtual classroom capabilities.

Source: Used with permission. B. M. Dossey, "Florence Nightingale's Tenets: Healing, Leadership, Global Action," in *Florence Nightingale Today: Healing, Leadership, Global Action*, eds. B. M. Dossey et al. (Silver Spring, MD: Nurse-Books.org, 2005).

"Doing" and "Being" Therapies

Holistic nurses use both "doing" and "being" therapies, as shown in **Figure 1-5**. These are also referred to as holistic nursing therapies, complementary and alternative therapies, or integrative and integral therapies throughout this textbook. Doing therapies include almost all forms of modern medicine, such as medications, procedures, dietary manipulations, radiation, and acupuncture. In contrast, being therapies do not employ things, but instead use states of consciousness.[33,34] These include imagery, prayer, meditation, and quiet contemplation, as well as the presence and intention of the nurse. These techniques are therapeutic because of the power of the psyche to affect the body. They may be either directed or nondirected.[32,34] A person who uses a directed mental strategy attaches a specific outcome to the imagery, such as the regression of disease or the normalization of the blood pressure. In a nondirected approach, the person images the best outcome for the situation but does not try to direct the situation or assign a specific outcome to the strategy. This reliance on the inherent intelligence within oneself to come forth is a way of acknowledging the intrinsic wisdom and self-correcting capacity within.

It is obvious that Era I medicine uses doing therapies that are highly directed in their approach. It employs things, such as medications, for a specific goal. Era II medicine is a classic body–mind approach that usually does not require the use of things, except for biofeedback instrumentation, music therapy, and CDs and videos to enhance learning and experience an increase in awareness of body–mind connections. It employs being therapies that can be directed or nondirected, depending on the mental strategies selected (e.g., relaxation or meditation). Era III medicine is similar in this regard. It requires

TABLE 1-3 Eras of Medicine			
	Era I	**Era II**	**Era III**
Space-Time Characteristic	Local	Local	Nonlocal
Synonym	Mechanical, material, or physical medicine	Mind-body medicine	Nonlocal or transpersonal medicine
Description	Causal, deterministic, describable by classical concepts of space-time and matter-energy. Mind not a factor; "mind" a result of brain mechanisms.	Mind a major factor in healing within the single person. Mind has causal power; is thus not fully explainable by classical concepts in physics. Includes but goes beyond Era I.	Mind a factor in healing both within and between persons. Mind not completely localized to points in space (brains or bodies) or time (present moment or single lifetimes). Mind is unbounded and infinite in space and time—thus omnipresent, eternal, and ultimately unitary or one. Healing at a distance is possible. Not describable by classical concepts of space-time or matter-energy.
Examples	Any form of therapy focusing solely on the effects of things on the body is an Era I approach—including techniques such as acupuncture and homeopathy, the use of herbs, etc. Almost all forms of "modern" medicine—drugs, surgery, irradiation, CPR, etc.—are included.	Any therapy emphasizing the effects of consciousness solely within the individual body is an Era II approach. Psychoneuroimmunology, counseling, hypnosis, biofeedback, relaxation therapies, and most types of imagery-based "alternative" therapies are included.	Any therapy in which effects of consciousness bridge between different persons is an Era III approach. All forms of distant healing, intercessory prayer, some types of shamanic healing, diagnosis at a distance, telesomatic events, and probably noncontact therapeutic touch are included.

Source: Reprinted with permission from L. Dossey, *Reinventing Medicine: Beyond Mind-Body to a New Era of Healing.* San Francisco: HarperSanFrancisco, 1999. Copyright Larry Dossey.

a willingness to become aware, moment by moment, of what is true for our inner and outer experience. It is actually a "not doing" so that we can become conscious of releasing, emptying, trusting, and acknowledging that we have done our best, regardless of the outcome. As the therapeutic potential of the mind becomes increasingly clear, all therapies and all people are viewed as having a transcendent quality. The minds of all people, including families, friends, and the healthcare team (both those in close proximity and those at a distance), flow together in a collective as they work to create healing and health.[35]

Rational Versus Paradoxical Healing

All healing experiences or activities can be arranged along a continuum from the rational domain to the paradoxical domain. The degree of doing and being involved determines these domains, as shown in **Figure 1-6**. Rational healing experiences include those therapies or events that make sense to our linear, intellectual thought processes, whereas paradoxical healing experiences include healing events that may seem absurd or contradictory but are, in fact, true.[34]

Doing therapies fall into the rational healing category. Based on science, these strategies conform to our worldview of commonsense notions. Often, the professional can follow an algorithm that dictates a step-by-step approach. Examples of rational healing include surgery, irradiation, medications, exercise, and diet. On the other hand, being therapies fall into the paradoxical healing category because they frequently happen without a scientific explanation. In psychological counseling, for example, a breakthrough is a paradox. When a patient has a psychological breakthrough, it is clear that there is a new meaning for the person. However, no clearly delineated steps led to the breakthrough. Such an event is called a breakthrough for the very reason that it is unpredictable—thus, the paradox.

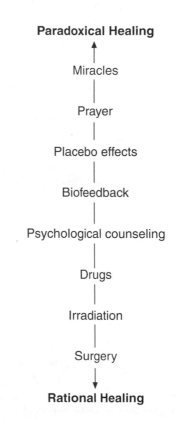

Paradoxical Healing

↑

Miracles

|

Prayer

|

Placebo effects

|

Biofeedback

|

Psychological counseling

|

Drugs

|

Irradiation

|

Surgery

↓

Rational Healing

FIGURE 1-5 "Being" and "Doing" Therapies
Source: Reprinted with permission from L. Dossey, *Meaning and Medicine: A Doctor's Tales of Breakthrough and Healing*, p. 204, New York, Bantam Books, 1991. Copyright Larry Dossey.

FIGURE 1-6 Continuum of Rational and Paradoxical Healing
Source: Reprinted with permission from L. Dossey, *Meaning and Medicine: A Doctor's Tales of Breakthrough and Healing*, p. 205, New York, Bantam Books, 1991. Copyright Larry Dossey.

Biofeedback also involves a paradox. For example, the best way to reduce blood pressure or muscle tension, or to increase peripheral blood flow, is to give up trying and just learn how to be. Individuals can enter into a state of being, or passive volition, in which they let these physiologic states change in the desired direction. Similarly, the phenomenon of placebo is a paradox. If an individual has just a little discomfort, a placebo does not work very well. The more pain a person has, however, the more dramatic the response to a placebo medication can be. In addition, a person who does not know that the medication is a placebo responds best. This is referred to as the "paradox of success through ignorance." Prayer and faith fall into the domain of paradox because there is no rational scientific explanation for their effectiveness. Many scientific studies have been conducted, however.[32,34]

Miracle cures also are paradoxical because there is no scientific mechanism to explain them.[32,34,35] Every nurse has known, heard of, or read about a patient who had a severe illness that had been confirmed by laboratory evidence but that disappeared after the patient adopted a being approach. Some say that it was the natural course of the illness; some die and some live. At shrines such as Lourdes in France and Medjugorje in Yugoslavia, however, people who experience a miracle cure are said to be totally immersed in a being state. They do not try to make anything happen. When interviewed, these people report experiencing a different sense of space and time; the flow of time as past, present, and future becomes an eternal now. Birth and death take on new meaning and are not seen as a beginning and an end. *Premonition* literally means "forewarning."[36] Premonitions are a heads-up about something just around the corner, something that is usually unpleasant. It may be a health crisis, a death in the family, or a national disaster. But premonitions come in all flavors. Sometimes they provide information about positive, pleasant happenings that lie ahead—a job promotion, the location of the last remaining parking space, or, in some instances, the winning lottery numbers.

These people go into the self and explore the "not I" to become empty so that they can understand the meaning of illness or present situations. To further integrate these concepts, relationship-centered care is discussed next.

■ RELATIONSHIP-CENTERED CARE

In 1994, the Pew Health Professions Commission published its landmark report on relationship-centered care.[37] This report serves as a guideline for addressing the bio-psycho-social-spiritual dimensions of individuals in integrating caring, healing, and holism into health care. The guidelines are based on the tenet that relationships and interactions among people constitute the foundation for all therapeutic activities.

In integral and holistic nursing, relationship-centered care serves as a model of caregiving that is based in a vision of community where three types of relationships are identified: (1) patient–practitioner relationships, (2) community–practitioner relationships, and (3) practitioner–practitioner relationships.[37] The three components of relationship-centered care are shown in **Table 1-4**, **Table 1-5**, and **Table 1-6**. Each of these interrelated relationships is essential within a reformed system of health care, and each involves a unique set of tasks and responsibilities that address self-awareness, knowledge, values, and skills.

Patient–Practitioner Relationship

In integral health care, the patient–practitioner relationship is crucial on many levels. The practitioner incorporates comprehensive biotechnologic care with psycho-social-spiritual care. To work effectively within the patient–practitioner relationship, the practitioner must develop specific knowledge, skills, and values, as shown in Table 1-4.[37] This includes an expanding self-awareness, understanding the patient's experience of health and illness, developing and maintaining caring relationships with patients, and communicating clearly and effectively.

Active collaboration with the patient and family in the decision-making process, promotion of health, and prevention of stress and illness within the family are also part of the relationship. A successful relationship involves active listening and effective communication; integration of the elements of caring, healing, values, and ethics to enhance and preserve the dignity and

TABLE 1-4	Patient–Practitioner Relationship: Areas of Knowledge, Skills, and Values		
Area	**Knowledge**	**Skills**	**Values**
Self-awareness	Knowledge of self Understanding self as a resource to others	Reflect on self and work	Importance of self-awareness, self-care, self-growth
Patient experience of health and illness	Role of family, culture, community in development Multiple components of health Multiple threats and contributors to health as dimensions of one reality	Recognize patient's life story and its meaning View health and illness as part of human development	Appreciation of the patient as a whole person Appreciation of the patient's life story and the meaning of the health-illness condition
Developing and maintaining caring relationships	Understanding of threats to the integrity of the relationship (e.g., power inequalities) Understanding of potential for conflict and abuse	Attend fully to the patient Accept and respond to distress in patient and self Respond to moral and ethical challenges Facilitate hope, trust, and faith	Respect for patient's dignity, uniqueness, and integrity (mind-body-spirit unity) Respect for self-determination Respect for person's own power and self-healing processes
Effective communication	Elements of effective communication	Listen Impart information Learn Facilitate the learning of others Promote and accept patient's emotions	Importance of being open and nonjudgmental

Source: Pew Health Professions Commission at the Center for the Health Professions, University of California, San Francisco, 1388 Sutter Street, Suite 805, San Francisco, California 94109, (415) 476-8181. http://futurehealth.ucsf.edu/Content/2/1994-12_Health_Professions_Education_and_Relationship-centered_Care.pdf

integrity of the patient and family; and a reduction of the power inequalities in the relationship with regard to race, sex, education, occupation, and socioeconomic status.

Community–Practitioner Relationship

In integral health care, the patient and his or her family simultaneously belong to many types of communities, such as the immediate family, relatives, friends, coworkers, neighborhoods, religious and community organizations, and the hospital community. The knowledge, skills, and values needed by practitioners to participate effectively in and work with various communities are shown in Table 1-5. This includes understanding the meaning of the community, recognizing the multiple contributors to health and illness within the community, developing

TABLE 1-5   Community–Practitioner Relationship: Areas of Knowledge, Skills, and Values

Area	Knowledge	Skills	Values
Meaning of community	Various models of community Myths and misperceptions about community Perspectives from the social sciences, humanities, and systems theory Dynamic change—demographic, political, industrial	Learn continuously Participate actively in community development and dialogue	Respect for the integrity of the community Respect for cultural diversity
Multiple contributors to health within the community	History of community, land use, migration, occupations, and their effect on health Physical, social, and occupational environments and their effects on health External and internal forces influencing community health	Critically assess the relationship of healthcare providers to community health Assess community and environmental health Assess implications of community policy affecting health	Affirmation of relevance of all determinants of health Affirmation of the value of health policy in community services Recognition of the presence of values that are destructive to health
Developing and maintaining community relationships	History of practitioner–community relationships Isolation of the healthcare community from the community at large	Communicate ideas Listen openly Empower others Learn Facilitate the learning of others Participate appropriately in community development and activism	Importance of being open minded Honesty regarding the limits of health science Responsibility to contribute health expertise
Effective community-based care	Various types of care, both formal and informal Effects of institutional scale on care Positive effects of continuity of care	Collaborate with other individuals and organizations Work as member of a team or healing community Implement change strategies	Respect for community leadership Commitment to work for change

Source: Pew Health Professions Commission at the Center for the Health Professions, University of California, San Francisco, 1388 Sutter Street, Suite 805, San Francisco, California 94109, (415) 476-8181.

TABLE 1-6	Practitioner–Practitioner Relationship: Areas of Knowledge, Skills, and Values		
Area	**Knowledge**	**Skills**	**Values**
Self-awareness	Knowledge of self	Reflect on self and needs Learn continuously	Importance of self-awareness
Traditions of knowledge in health professions	Healing approaches of various professions Healing approaches across cultures Historical power inequities across professions	Derive meaning from others' work Learn from experience within healing community	Affirmation and value of diversity
Building teams and communities	Perspectives on team-building from the social sciences	Communicate effectively Listen openly Learn cooperatively	Affirmation of mission Affirmation of diversity
Working dynamics of teams, groups, and organizations	Perspectives on team dynamics from the social sciences	Share responsibility responsibly Collaborate with others Work cooperatively Resolve conflicts	Openness to others' ideas Humility Mutual trust, empathy, support Capacity for grace

Source: Pew Health Professions Commission at the Center for the Health Professions, University of California, San Francisco, 1388 Sutter Street, Suite 805, San Francisco, California 94109, (415) 476-8181.

and maintaining relationships with the community, and working collaboratively with other individuals and organizations to establish effective community-based care.[37]

Practitioners must be sensitive to the impact of these various communities on patients and foster the collaborative activities of these communities as they interact with the patient and family. The restraints or barriers within each community that block the patient's healing must be identified and improved to promote the patient's health and well-being.

Practitioner–Practitioner Relationship

Providing integral care to patients and families can never take place in isolation; it involves many diverse practitioner–practitioner relationships. To form a practitioner–practitioner relationship requires the knowledge, skills, and values shown in Table 1-6, including developing self-awareness; understanding the diverse knowledge base and skills of different practitioners; developing teams and communities; and understanding the working dynamics of groups, teams, and organizations that can provide resource services for the patient and family.[37]

Collaborative relationships entail shared planning and action toward common goals with joint responsibility for outcomes. There is a difference, though, between multidisciplinary care and interdisciplinary care. Multidisciplinary care consists of the sequential provision of discipline-specific health care by various individuals. Interdisciplinary care, however, also includes coordination, joint decision making, communication, shared responsibility, and shared authority.

Because the cornerstone of all therapeutic and healing endeavors is the quality of the relationships formed among the practitioners caring for the patient, all practitioners must understand and respect one another's roles. Conventional and alternative practitioners need to learn about the diversity of therapeutic and healing modalities that they each use. In addition, conventional practitioners must be willing to integrate complementary and alternative practitioners and their therapies in practice (i.e., acupuncture, herbs, aromatherapy, touch therapies, music therapy, folk healers). Such integration requires learning about the experiences of different healers, being open to the potential benefits of different modalities, and valuing cultural diversity. Ultimately, the effectiveness of collaboration among practitioners depends on their ability to share problem solving, goal setting, and decision making within a trusting, collegial, and caring environment. Practitioners must work interdependently rather than autonomously, with each assuming responsibility and accountability for patient care. In the next section, the role of the Pew report on relationship-centered care is discussed.

■ CORE COMPETENCIES FOR INTERPROFESSIONAL COLLABORATIVE PRACTICE

In 1998, following a decade of leadership and advocacy for health professions education, the Pew Health Professions Commission published its fourth and final report on relationship-centered care. The report assesses the challenges facing professionals in the 21st century and recommends general and professional-specific actions.[38]

In 2011, the Interprofessional Education Collaborative Expert Panel[9] came together with an inspired vision for identifying the necessary core competencies for interprofessional collaborative practice that would be safe, high quality, accessible, and inclusive of patient-centered care. The six organizations that comprise the expert panel were the American Association of Colleges of Nursing, American Association of Colleges of Osteopathic Medicine, American Association of Colleges of Pharmacy, American Dental Education Association, Association of American Medical Colleges, and Association of Schools of Public Health. To achieve its vision

the expert panel showed that health professions students need continuous development of interprofessional competencies as an essential part of their learning process. When this type of education occurs, they are more likely to enter the workforce ready to practice effective teamwork and team-based care.

Each expert panel group contributed its competencies, which resulted in interprofessional collaborative practice competencies identified in the following four domains: (1) values/ethics for interprofessional practice, (2) roles/responsibilities, (3) interprofessional communication, and (4) teams and teamwork.[9]

Teaching of these interprofessional collaborative competencies must extend beyond profession-specific education so that students are more likely to work effectively as members of clinical teams. In teaching interprofessional competencies and collaboration with the goal of practicing relationship-centered care, new theories must be applied such as complexity theories and positive psychology to transform organizations.[39,40] To cross the patient-centered divide and apply relationship-centered care, faculty development must include mindfulness practice, formation, and training in communication skills. The next section explores several examples of how these concepts are being translated.

■ CREATING OPTIMAL HEALING ENVIRONMENTS

The Samueli Institute for Information Biology (www.siib.org) studies relationship-centered care and ways to transform organizational culture through research and innovative projects that articulate and demonstrate a complete optimal healing environment (OHE) framework of actionable practices and evaluation methods.[41] The institute defines an optimal healing environment as one in which "the social, psychological, spiritual, physical and behavioral components of health care are oriented toward support and stimulation of healing and the achievement of wholeness." From this perspective, facilitating healing is thought to be a crucial aspect of managing chronic illness and the basis for sustainable health care.

Key concepts in optimal healing environments are awareness and intention. Awareness is a state of being conscious and "in touch" with one's interior and exterior self that is cultivated through reflective practices (meditation, prayer, mindfulness, spiritual practices, journaling, dialogue, art, etc.). **Table 1-7** shows that an OHE contains four environmental domains—internal, interpersonal, behavioral, external. Under these four domains are eight constructs that each have several elements. The shading shows how these components, elements, and specific areas are integrated with all others. **Figure 1-7** depicts this information, showing how all aspects are connected from the internal environment to the outer environments of the individual and the collective. Optimal healing environments always starts with the individual, whether it is the practitioner, healer, healee (client/patient), a significant other, and/or the community as an entity. When these steps are implemented it can lead to more cost-effective, efficient organizations in which the environment truly facilitates healing and where practitioners are fully supported to connect to the "soul of healing" and the mission of caring.

Another innovative organization is Planetree International, which is recognized as an international leader in healing environments and innovative patient-centered care models.[42] In healthcare settings throughout the United States, Canada, and Europe, Planetree demonstrates that patient-centered care is not only an empowering philosophy; it is a viable, vital, and cost-effective model. The Planetree model is implemented in acute and critical care departments, emergency departments, long-term care facilities, outpatient services, as well as in ambulatory care and community health centers. The Planetree model of care is a patient-centered, holistic approach to health care that promotes mental, emotional, spiritual, social, and physical healing. It empowers patients and families through the exchange of information and encourages healing partnerships with caregivers. It seeks to maximize positive healthcare outcomes by integrating optimal medical therapies and incorporating art and nature into the healing environment.

As interprofessional collaboration steadily increases and blends traditional health care with integrative health care and complementary and alternative therapies, the relationship-centered care model can assist traditional and integrative practitioners to achieve the highest level of care. This level of care requires new educational endeavors. An example is the Penny George Institute for Health and Healing, the

TABLE 1-7   Optimal Healing Environments (OHE).

OPTIMAL HEALING ENVIRONMENTS
MAKING HEALING AS IMPORTANT AS CURING

An Optimal Healing Environment is one that supports and stimulates patient healing by addressing the social, psychological, physical, spiritual and behavioral components of health care and enabling the body's capacity to heal itself.

INTERNAL		INTERPERSONAL		BEHAVIORAL		EXTERNAL	
DEVELOPING HEALING INTENTION	EXPERIENCING PERSONAL WHOLENESS	CULTIVATING HEALING RELATIONSHIPS	CREATING HEALING ORGANIZATIONS	PRACTICING HEALTHY LIFESTYLES	APPLYING COLLABORATIVE MEDICINE	BUILDING HEALING SPACES	FOSTERING ECOLOGICAL SUSTAINABILITY
Expectation Hope Understanding Belief	Mind Body Spirit Energy	Communication Compassion Social Support Empathy	Leadership Mission Teamwork Technology	Diet Exercise Relaxation Addiction Management	Integrative Person Centered Family Centered Culturally Sensitive	Color and Light Art and Architecture Aroma and Air Music and Sound	Eco-Friendly Green Energy Efficient Nature

INNER ENVIRONMENTS	TO	OUTER ENVIRONMENTS

Source: ©2011 Used with permission. Samueli Institute for Information Biology, 1737 King Street, Suite 600, Alexandria, VA (www.siib.org).

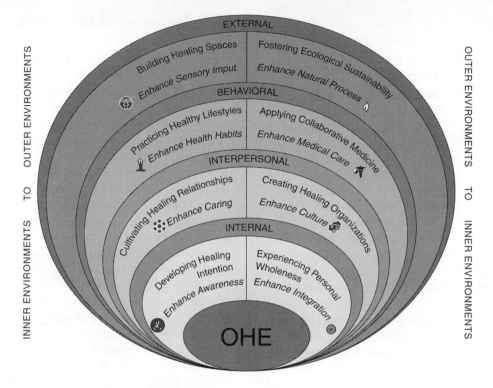

FIGURE 1-7 Optimal healing environments.
Source: ©2011 Used with permission. Samueli Institute for Information Biology, 1737 King Street, Suite 600, Alexandria, VA (www.siib.org).

largest hospital-based program of its kind in the country. It is setting national standards for enhancing health care through a holistic and integrative health approach as follows:[43]

- Blending complementary therapies, integrative medicine, and conventional Western medicine
- Providing services to inpatients and outpatients
- Educating healthcare professionals
- Teaching community members about health promotion and self-healing practices
- Conducting research to identify best practices of integrative health and the impact of these services on healthcare costs

The key to changing nursing practice is to embrace approaches that allow institutions to flourish and where healing emerges resulting in creative delivery models. The Transformative Nurse Training (TNT) Program (see Chapter 27) is one example of the Penny George Institute for Health and Healing Abbott Northwestern commitment to excellence in nursing.[43] The program brings nurses back to the essence of nurs-

ing practice and teaches the foundations and principles of holistic nursing.

Nurses are challenged to move into more expanded roles such as nurse coaching (see Chapter 9) to achieve the highest levels of care and service to patients and families. They understand optimal healing environments, relationship-centered care, healing awareness, and intention.[44-46] The time has never been greater for nurses and all healthcare practitioners to come together in interprofessional collaboration to fully implement their knowledge, skills, and expertise to achieve all parts of the Patient Protection Act[47] and the National Prevention Strategy.[48]

In the next section, the Theory of Integral Nursing is discussed. As you read about the Theory of Integral Nursing remember that the words *integral* and *integrally informed* are used often because this is a shift to a deeper level of understanding about being human as related to the four dimensions of reality. It is incorrect to substitute the word *holistic* because it does not mean the same thing. Consider where you are now in your life—as a novice, intermediate, or expert nurse, you bring a wealth of experiences that inform you at the professional and personal levels. Begin to explore the integral process in your thinking, projects, and endeavors. Examine whether your approaches are reductionistic, narrow, or limited, or whether you have an integral awareness and integral understanding that includes the four perspectives of reality.

■ THEORY OF INTEGRAL NURSING

Overview

The Theory of Integral Nursing is a grand theory that presents the science and art of nursing. It includes an integral process, integral worldview, and integral dialogues that are praxis—theory in action.[5] Concepts specific to the Theory of Integral Nursing are set in italics throughout this chapter. Please consider these words as a frame of reference and a way to explain what you have observed or experienced with yourself and others. An integral process is defined as a comprehensive way to organize multiple phenomena of human experience and reality from four perspectives: (1) the individual interior (personal/intentional); (2) individual exterior (physiology/behavioral); (3) collective interior (shared/cultural); and (4) collective exterior (systems/structures). Holistic nursing practice is included (embraced) and transcends (goes beyond).[5] An integral worldview examines values, beliefs, assumptions, meaning, purpose, and judgments related to how individuals perceive reality and relationships from the four perspectives. Integral dialogues are transformative and visionary explorations of ideas and possibilities across disciplines where these four perspectives are considered as equally important to all exchanges, endeavors, and outcomes. With an increased integral awareness and an integral worldview, nurses have new possibilities and ways to strengthen their capacities for integral dialogues with each other and other disciplines. We are more likely to raise our collective nursing voice and power to engage in social action in our professional roles and service work for society—locally to globally.

To decrease further fragmentation in the nursing profession the Theory of Integral Nursing incorporates existing theoretical work in nursing that builds on our solid holistic and multidimensional theoretical nursing foundation. This theory may be used with other holistic nursing and nonnursing caring concepts, theories, and research; it does not exclude or invalidate other nurse theorists who have informed this theory (see Chapter 5). This is not a freestanding theory because it incorporates concepts and philosophies from various paradigms including holism, multidimensionality, integral, chaos, spiral dynamics, complexity, systems, and many others.

An integral understanding allows us to more fully comprehend the complexity of human nature and healing; it assists nurses in bringing to health care and society their knowledge, skills, and compassion. The integral process and an integral worldview present a comprehensive map and perspective related to the complexity of wholeness and how to simultaneously address the health and well-being of nurses, the healthcare team, the patients, families and significant others, the healthcare system/structure, and the world.

The nursing profession asks nurses to wrap around "all of life" on so many levels with self and others that we often can feel overwhelmed. So, how do we get a handle on "all of life"? The question always arises "How can overworked nurses and student nurses use an integral approach or apply the Theory of Integral Nursing?" The answer is to start right now. By the time you finish reading this chapter you will find the answers to these questions. Be aware of healing, the core concept in this theory; it is the innate natural phenomenon that comes from within a person and describes the indivisible wholeness, the interconnectedness of all people and all things.

Reflect on this clinical situation. Imagine that you are caring for a very ill patient who needs to be transported to a radiology procedure. The current protocol for transportation between the medical unit and the radiology department lacks continuity. In this moment, shift your feelings and your interior awareness (and believe it!) to: "I am doing the best that I can in this moment," and "I have all the time needed to take a deep breath and relax my tight chest and shoulder muscles." This helps you connect these four perspectives as follows: (1) the interior self (caring for yourself in this moment); (2) the exterior self (using a research-based relaxation and imagery integral practice to change your physiology); (3) the self in relationship to others (shifting your awareness creates another way of being with your patient and the radiology team member); and (4) the relationship to the exterior collective of systems/structures (considering ways to work with the radiology team member and department to improve a transportation procedure in the hospital). An integral world-view and approach can help each nurse and student nurse increase her or his self-awareness, as well as the awareness of how one's self affects others—the patient, family, colleagues, and the workplace and community. As the nurse discovers her or his own innate healing from within, the nurse can model self-care and how to release stress, anxiety, and fear that manifest each day in this human journey.

All nursing curricula can be mapped to the integral quadrants (see the section on application of the theory later in this chapter). This teaches students to think integrally and to become aware of an integral perspective and how these four perspectives create the whole. Students can also learn the importance of self-care at all times as faculty also remember that they are role models and must model self-care and these integral ideas.

Developing the Theory of Integral Nursing: Personal Journey

As a young nurse attending my first nursing theory conference in the late 1960s, I was captivated by nursing theory and the eloquent visionary words of these theorists as they spoke about the science and art of nursing. This opened my heart and mind to the exploration and necessity to understand and to use nursing theory. Thus, I began my professional commitment to address theory in all endeavors as well as to increase my understanding of other disciplines that could inform me at a deeper level about the human experience. I realized that nursing was neither a science nor an art, but both/and. From the beginning of my critical care and cardiovascular nursing focus, I learned how to combine science and technology with the art of nursing. For example, I gave a patient with severe pain following an acute myocardial infarction pain medication while simultaneously guiding him in a relaxation practice to enhance relaxation and release anxiety. I also experienced a difference in myself when I used this approach combining the science and art of nursing.

In the late 1960s, I also began to study and attend workshops on holistic and mind–body related ideas as well as read in other disciplines such as systems theory; quantum physics; integral, Eastern, and Western philosophy and mysticism; and more. I also read nurse theorists and other discipline theorists that informed my knowing, doing, and being in caring, healing, and holism. My husband, an internist, who was also caring for critically ill patients and their families, was with me on this journey of discovery. As we cared for critically ill patients and their families, some of our greatest teachers, we were able to reflect on how to blend the art of caring, healing modalities with the science of technology and traditional modalities. I joined with a critical care and cardiovascular nursing colleague and soul mate, Cathie Guzzetta, with whom I could also discuss these ideas. We began to write teaching protocols and lecture in critical care courses as well as write textbooks and articles with other contributors.

My husband and I both had health challenges—mine was postcorneal transplant rejection and my husband's was blinding migraine headaches. We both began to take courses related to body-mind-spirit therapies (biofeedback, relaxation, imagery, music, meditation, and other reflective practices) and began to incorporate them into our daily lives. As we strengthened our capacities with self-care and self-regulation modalities, our personal and professional philosophies and clinical practices changed. We took seriously teaching and integrating these modalities into the traditional healthcare setting that today is called integrative and integral health care. From then till now, we have found many professional and interdisciplinary healthcare colleagues with whom to discuss concepts, protocols, and approaches for practice, education, and research.

In 1981, I was a founding member of the American Holistic Nurses Association (AHNA). In November 2006, with Lynn Keegan, Cathie Guzzetta, and many other colleagues, we obtained recognition by the American Nurses Association (ANA) of our collective holistic nursing endeavors as the specialty of holistic nursing. The AHNA and ANA *Holistic Nursing: Scope and Standards of Practice* were published in June 2007 and will be revised in 2012.[7] I now believe that the important specialty of holistic nursing can be expanded by using an integral lens.

Beginning in 1992 in London during my Florence Nightingale primary historical research studying and synthesizing her original letters, army and public health documents, manuscripts, and books, I deepened my understanding of Nightingale's relevance to holistic nursing. Nightingale was indeed an integralist. This revelation led to my Nightingale authorship[11, 22-25] and my collaborative Nightingale Initiative for Global Health and the Nightingale Declaration,[16] the first global nursing Internet signature campaign. My current professional mission is to articulate and use the integral process and integral worldview in my nursing, in integrative nurse coaching (see Chapter 9), and healthcare endeavors and to explore rituals of healing with many. My sustained nursing career focus with nursing colleagues on wholeness, unity, and healing and my Florence Nightingale scholarship have resulted in numerous protocols and standards for practice, education, research, and healthcare policy. My integral focus since 2000 and my many conversations with Ken Wilber[49-51] and the integral team and other interdisciplinary integral colleagues have led to my development of the Theory of Integral Nursing. It is exciting to see other nurses expanding the holistic process and incorporating the integral model as well.

Theory of Integral Nursing Intentions and Developmental Process

The intention (purpose) in a nursing theory is the aim of the theory. The Theory of Integral Nursing has three intentions: (1) to embrace the unitary whole person and the complexity of the nursing profession and health care; (2) to explore the direct application of an integral process and integral worldview that includes four perspectives of realities—the individual interior and exterior and the collective interior and exterior; and (3) to expand nurses' capacities as twenty-first-century Nightingales, health diplomats, and integral health coaches who coach for integral health—locally to globally. The Theory of Integral Nursing develops the evolutionary growth processes, stages, and levels of humans' development and consciousness to move toward a comprehensive integral philosophy and understanding. This can assist nurses to more deeply map human

capacities that begin with healing to evolve to the transpersonal self and connection with the Divine, however defined or identified, and their collective endeavors to create a healthy world.

The Theory of Integral Nursing development process at this time is to strengthen our 21st-century nursing endeavors so that we can expand personal awareness of our holistic and caring, healing knowledge and approaches with traditional nursing and health care. Nursing and health care are fragmented. Collaborative practice has not been realized because only portions of reality are seen as being valid within health care and society. Often there is a lack of respect for each other. We also do not consistently listen to the pain and suffering that nurses experience within the profession, and neither do we consistently listen to the pain and suffering of the patient and family members or our colleagues. Self-care is a low priority. Time is not given or valued within practice settings for nurses to address basic self-care such as short breaks for personal needs and meals; this is made worse by short staffing and overtime. Professional burnout is extremely high, and many nurses are very discouraged. Nurse retention is at a crisis level throughout the world. As nurses integrate an integral process and integral worldview and use daily integral life practices, they will be healthy and model health more consistently and understand the complexities of healing. This will then enhance nurses' capacities for empowerment, leadership, and being change agents for a healthy world.

Integral Foundation and the Integral Model

The Theory of Integral Nursing adapts work of Ken Wilber (1949–), one of the most significant American new-paradigm philosophers, to strengthen the core concept of healing. Wilber's integral model is an elegant, four-quadrant model that has been developed over 35 years. In his eight-volume *Collected Works of Ken Wilber*,[50-51] Wilber synthesizes the ideas and theories of the best-known and most influential researchers and theorists to show that no individual or discipline can determine reality or have all the answers.

Many concepts within this integral nursing theory have been researched or are in very formative stages and exploration within integral medicine, integral healthcare administration, integral business, integral healthcare education, integral psychotherapy, integral coaching, and more.[49,52-54] Within the nursing profession, other nurses are also exploring integral and related theories and ideas.[55-61] But as of yet, no theory of nursing combines Nightingale's philosophical foundation as an integralist with the integral process and integral worldview. When nurses consider the use of an integral lens they are more likely to expand nurses' roles in interdisciplinary dialogues, to explore commonalities, and to examine differences and how to address these across disciplines. Our challenge in nursing is to increase our integral awareness as we increase our nursing capacities, strengths, and voices in all areas of practice, education, research, and healthcare policy.

Content, Context, and Process

To present the Theory of Integral Nursing, Barbara Barnum's framework to critique a nursing theory provides an organizing structure that is most useful.[62] Her approach, which examines content, context, and process, highlights what is most critical to understand a theory, and it avoids duplication of explanations within the theory. In the next section, the Theory of Integral Nursing philosophical assumptions are provided. The reader is encouraged to integrate the integral process concepts and to experience how the word *integral* expands one's thinking and worldview. To delete the word *integral* or to substitute the world *holistic* diminishes the impact of the expansiveness of the integral process and integral worldview and its implications, as previously stated. The philosophical assumptions of the Theory of Integral Nursing are listed in **Table 1-8**.[5]

Content Components

Content of a nursing theory includes the subject matter and building blocks that give a theory form. It comprises the stable elements that are acted on or that do the acting. In the Theory of Integral Nursing, the subject matter and building blocks are as follows: (1) healing, (2) the meta-paradigm of nursing theory, (3) patterns of knowing, (4) the four quadrants that are adapted from Wilber's integral theory (individual interior [subjective, personal/intentional], individual exterior [objective, behavioral], collective interior

---

TABLE 1-8   Theory of Integral Nursing: Philosophical Assumptions

1. An integral understanding recognizes the wholeness of humanity and the world that is open, dynamic, interdependent, fluid, and continuously interacting with changing variables that can lead to greater complexity and order.

2. An integral worldview is a comprehensive way to organize multiple phenomena of human experience and reality and identifies these phenomena as the individual interior (subjective, personal), individual exterior (objective, behavioral), collective interior (intersubjective, cultural), and collective exterior (interobjective, systems/structures).

3. Healing is a process inherent in all living things; it may occur with curing of symptoms, but it is not synonymous with curing.

4. Integral health is experienced by individuals, and also groups, communities, nations, cultures, and ecosystems as wholeness with development towards personal growth and expanding states of consciousness to deeper levels of personal and collective understanding of one's physical, mental, emotional, social, spiritual, relational, sexual, and psychodynamic dimensions.

5. Integral nursing is founded on an integral worldview, using integral language and integral knowledge that are enacted in these integral life practices and skills.

6. Integral nursing has the capacity to include all ways of knowing and knowledge development.

7. Integral nursing is applicable in any context, and its scope includes all aspects of human experience.

8. An integral nurse is an instrument in the healing process and facilitates healing through her or his knowing, doing, and being.

Source: Copyright © Barbara Dossey, 2007.

[intersubjective, cultural], and collective exterior [interobjective, systems/structures]); and (5) "all quadrants, all levels, all lines," that are adapted from Wilber.[49]

Content Component 1: Healing

The first content component in the Theory of Integral Nursing is healing, which is illustrated as a diamond shape and shown in **Figure 1-8a**. The Theory of Integral Nursing enfolds the central core concept of healing. It embraces the individual as an energy field that is connected with the energy fields of all humanity and the world. Healing is transformed when we consider four perspectives of reality in any moment: (1) the individual interior (personal/intentional), (2) individual exterior (physiology/behavioral), (3) collective interior (shared/cultural), and (4) collective exterior (systems/structures). Using our reflective integral lens of these four perspectives of reality assists us to grasp the complexity that emerges in healing.

Healing includes knowing, doing, and being and is a lifelong journey and process of bringing aspects of oneself at deeper levels into harmony and stages of inner knowing that lead to integration.[5] This healing process places us in a space to face our fears, to seek and express self in its fullness, and to learn to trust life, creativity, passion, and love. Each aspect of healing has equal importance and value and leads to more complex levels of understanding and meaning.

We are born with healing capacities. It is a process inherent in all living things. No one can take healing away from life, although we often get stuck in our healing or forget that we possess it because of life's continuous challenges and perceived barriers to wholeness. Healing can take place at all levels of human experience, but it may not occur simultaneously in every realm. In truth, healing most likely does not occur simultaneously or even in all realms, and yet, the person may still have a perception of healing having happened.[63,64] Healing is not predictable; it may occur with curing of symptoms, but it is not synonymous with curing. Curing may not always happen, but the potential for healing to occur is always present, even at one's last breath. Intention and intentionality are key factors in healing.[65] Intention is the conscious determination to do a specific action or to act in a specific manner; it is the mental state of being committed to, planning to, or trying to perform an action.[64,65] Intentionality is the quality of an intentionally performed action.

Content Component 2: Meta-Paradigm of Nursing Theory

The second content component in the Theory of Integral Nursing is the recognition of the meta-paradigm in a nurse theory—nurse, person, health, and environment (society), shown in **Figure 1-8b**. These concepts are important to the Theory of Integral Nursing because they are encompassed within the quadrants of human experience, as shown in content component 4. Starting with healing at the center, a Venn diagram surrounds healing and implies the interrelated and interdependent impact of these domains as each informs and influences the others; a change in one creates a degree of change in the others, thus affecting healing at many levels.

An integral nurse is defined as a 21st-century Nightingale engaged in social action and sacred activism, and as a "health diplomat" and "integral health coach" who is "coaching for integral health."[3,28] As nurses strive to be integrally informed, they are more likely to move to a deeper experience of a connection with the Divine or Infinite, however defined or identified. Integral nursing provides a comprehensive way to organize multiple phenomena of human experience in the four perspectives of reality. The nurse is an instrument in the healing process. She or he brings the whole self into relationship with the whole self of another or a group of significant

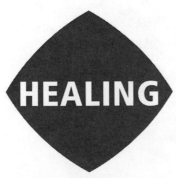

FIGURE 1-8a   Healing
Source: Copyright © Barbara Dossey, 2007.

others, and this reinforces the meaning and experience of oneness and unity.

A person is defined as an individual (patient/client, family member, significant other) who engages with a nurse in a manner that is respectful of a person's subjective experiences of health, health beliefs, values, sexual orientation, and personal preferences. A person also can be an individual nurse who interacts with a nursing colleague, other healthcare team members, or a group of community members or other groups.

Integral health is the process through which nurses reshape basic assumptions and worldviews about well-being and see death as a natural process of living. Integral health may be symbolically imagined as a jewel with many facets that is reflected as a "bright gem" or a "rough stone" depending on one's situation and stage of personal growth that influence states of health, health beliefs, and values.[63,64]

As described by Don Beck, this jewel may also be imagined as a spiral or a symbol of transformation to higher states of consciousness where we can more fully understand the essential nature of our beingness as energy fields and expressions of wholeness.[66] This includes evolving one's state of consciousness to higher levels of personal and collective understanding of one's physical, mental, emotional, social, and spiritual dimensions. This acknowledges the individual's interior and exterior experiences and the shared collective interior and exterior experiences where authentic power is recognized within each person. Disease and illness at the physical level may manifest for many reasons. It is important not to equate physical health with mental health or spiritual health because they are not the same. Each is a facet of the jewel of integral health.

An integral environment has both interior and exterior aspects. The interior environment includes the individual's feelings; meanings; mental, emotional, and spiritual dimensions; it also includes a person's brain stem, cortex, and other anatomic parts that are internal (inside) aspects of the exterior self. The interior environment also acknowledges the patterns that may not be understood but that may manifest related to various situations or relationships, such as those related to living and nonliving people and things, such as the memory of a deceased relative or animal, or a lost precious object stimulated by a current situation (for example, a touch may bring forth past memories of abuse or suffering). Insights gained through dreams and other reflective practices that reveal symbols, images, and other connections also influence one's interior environment. The exterior environment includes objects that can be seen and measured and that are related to the physical and social in any of the gross, subtle, and causal levels that are discussed in component 4.

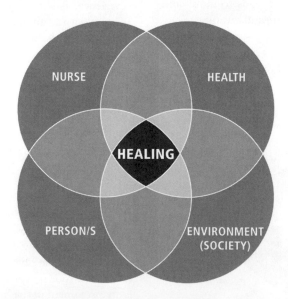

FIGURE 1-8b   Healing and Meta-Paradigm of Nursing Theory
Source: Copyright © Barbara Dossey, 2007.

Content Component 3: Patterns of Knowing

The third content component in the Theory of Integral Nursing is the recognition of the patterns of knowing in nursing, as shown in **Figure 1-8c**. These six patterns of knowing are personal, empirics, aesthetics, ethics, not knowing, and sociopolitical. As a way to organize nursing knowledge, Carper,[67] in her now classic 1978 article, identifies the four fundamental patterns of knowing (personal, empirics, ethics, aesthetics), which was followed by the introduction of the pattern of not knowing in 1993 by Munhall,[68] and the pattern of sociopolitical knowing by White in 1995.[69] All of these patterns continue to be refined and reframed with new applications and interpretations.[70-74] These patterns of knowing assist nurses in bringing themselves into the full expression of being present in the moment with self and others,[75-78] to integrate aesthetics with science, and to develop the flow of ethical experience with thinking and acting. (As all patterns of knowing in the Theory of Integral Nursing are superimposed on Wilber's four quadrants in Figure 1-8f, these patterns will primarily be positioned as shown; however, they may also appear in one, several, or all quadrants and inform all other quadrants.)

Personal knowing is the nurse's dynamic process and awareness of wholeness that focuses on the synthesis of perceptions and being with self.[79-81] It may be developed through art, meditation, dance, music, stories, and other expressions of the authentic and genuine self in daily life and nursing practice.

Empirical knowing is the science of nursing that focuses on formal expression, replication, and validation of scientific competence in nursing education and practice.[5,71] It is expressed in models and theories and can be integrated into evidence-based practice. Empirical indicators are accessed through the known senses and are subject to direct observation, measurement, and verification.

Aesthetic knowing is the art of nursing that focuses on how to explore experiences and meaning in life with self or another that includes authentic presence, the nurse as a facilitator of healing, and the artfulness of a healing environment.[64,79] It is the combination of knowledge, experience, instinct, and intuition that connects the nurse with a patient or client to explore the meaning of a situation about the human experiences of life, health, illness, and death. It calls forth resources and inner strengths from the nurse to be a facilitator in

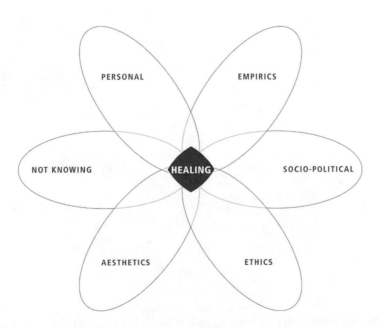

FIGURE 1-8c   Healing and Patterns of Knowing in Nursing
Source: Adapted from B. Carper (1978). Copyright © Barbara Dossey, 2007.

the healing process. It is the integration and expression of all the other patterns of knowing in nursing praxis.

Ethical knowing is the moral knowledge in nursing that focuses on behaviors, expressions, and dimensions of both morality and ethics.[67,71] It includes valuing and clarifying situations to create formal moral and ethical behaviors intersecting with legally prescribed duties. It emphasizes respect for the person, the family, and the community that encourages connectedness and relationships that enhance attentiveness, responsiveness, communication, and moral action.

Not knowing is the capacity to use healing presence, to be open spontaneously to the moment with no preconceived answers or goals to be obtained.[79,80] It engages authenticity, mindfulness, openness, receptivity, surprise, mystery, and discovery with self and others in the subjective space and the intersubjective space that allows for new solutions, possibilities, and insights to emerge.

Sociopolitical knowing addresses the important contextual variables of social, economic, geo-graphic, cultural, political, historical, and other key factors in theoretical, evidence-based practice and research.[69] This pattern includes informed critique and social justice for the voices of the underserved in all areas of society along with protocols to reduce health disparities.

Content Component 4: Quadrants

The fourth content component in the Theory of Integral Nursing, as shown in **Figure 1-8d**, examines four perspectives for all known aspects of reality, or expressed another way, it is how we look at and describe anything. The Theory of Integral Nursing core concept of healing is transformed by adapting Ken Wilber's integral model.[50-53]

Starting with healing at the center to represent our integral nursing philosophy, human capacities, and global mission, dotted horizontal and vertical lines are shown to illustrate that each quadrant can be understood as permeable and porous, with each quadrant experience integrally informing and empowering all other quadrant experiences. Within each quadrant we see "I," "We," "It," and "Its" to represent four

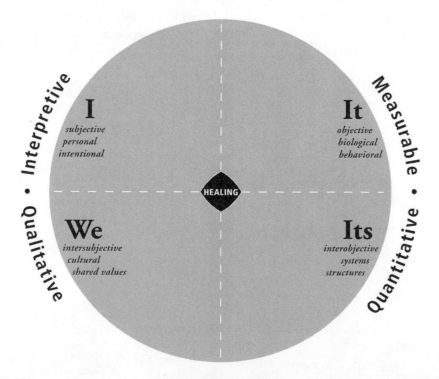

FIGURE 1-8d   Healing and the Four Quadrants (I, We, It, Its)
Source: Adapted with permission from Ken Wilber. http://www.kenwilber.com. Copyright © Barbara Dossey, 2007.

perspectives of realities that are already part of our everyday language and awareness. (When working with various cultures it is important to know that within many cultures the "I" comes last or is never verbalized or recognized because the focus is on the "we" and relationships. However, this development of the "I" and awareness of one's personal values are critical to a healthy nurse to decrease burnout and increase nurse renewal and nurse retention.)

Virtually all human languages use first-, second-, and third-person pronouns. First person is "the person who is speaking," which includes the pronouns *I*, *me*, *mine* in the singular and *we*, *us*, *ours* in the plural. Second person means "the person who is spoken to," which includes the pronouns *you* and *yours*. Third person is "the person or thing being spoken about," such as *she*, *her*, *hers*, *he*, *him*, *his*, or *they*, *it*, *their*, and *its*. For example, if I am speaking about my new car, "I" am first person, and "you" are second person, and the new car is third person. If you and I are communicating, the word *we* is used to indicate that we understand each other. *We* is technically first person plural, but if you and I are commu-

nicating, then your second person and my first person are part of this extraordinary *we*. We can simplify first, second, and third person as *I*, *we*, *it*, and *its*.[50,52]

These four quadrants show the four primary dimensions or perspectives of how we experience the world; these are represented graphically as the Upper-Left (UL), Upper-Right (UR), Lower-Left (LL), and Lower-Right (LR) quadrants. It is simply the inside and the outside of an individual and the inside and outside of the collective. It includes expanded states of consciousness where one feels a connection with the Divine and the vastness of the universe and the infinite that is beyond words. Integral nursing considers all of these areas in our personal development and any area of practice, education, research, and healthcare policy—local to global. Each quadrant, which is intricately linked and bound to each other, carries its own truths and language. The specifics of the quadrants are as follows and are shown in **Table 1-9**:

- *Upper-Left (UL):* In this "I" space (subjective; the inside of the individual) can be

---

TABLE 1-9   Integral Model and Quadrants

UPPER LEFT	UPPER RIGHT
INDIVIDUAL INTERIOR **(intentional/personal)**	**INDIVIDUAL EXTERIOR** **(behavioral/biological)**
"I" space includes self and consciousness (self-care, fears, feelings, beliefs, values, esteem, cognitive capacity, emotional maturity, moral development, spiritual maturity, personal communication skills, etc.)	"It" space that includes brain and organisms (physiology, pathophysiology [cells, molecules, limbic system, neurotransmitters, physical sensations], biochemistry, chemistry, physics, behaviors [skill development in health, nutrition, exercise, etc.])

- Subjective   I   IT   • Objective
- Interpretive   • Observable
- Qualitative   WE   ITS   • Quantitative

COLLECTIVE INTERIOR (cultural/shared)	COLLECTIVE EXTERIOR (systems/structures)
"We" space includes the relationship to each other and the culture and worldview (shared understanding, shared vision, shared meaning, shared leadership and other values, integral dialogues and communication/morale, etc.)	"Its" space includes the relation to social systems and environment, organizational structures and systems (in healthcare—financial and billing systems), educational systems, information technology, mechanical structures and transportation, regulatory structures (environmental and governmental policies, etc.)
LOWER LEFT	**LOWER RIGHT**

Source: Ken Wilber, *Integral Psychology: Consciousness, Spirit, Psychology, Therapy* (Boston: Shambhala, 2000). Table adapted with permission from Ken Wilber. http://www.kenwilber.com. Copyright © by Barbara M. Dossey, 2007.

found the world of the individual's interior experiences. These are the thoughts, emotions, memories, perceptions, immediate sensations, and states of mind (imagination, fears, feelings, beliefs, values, esteem, cognitive capacity, emotional maturity, moral development, and spiritual maturity). Integral nursing requires development of the "I."

- *Upper-Right (UR):* In this "It" (objective; the outside of the individual) space can be found the world of the individual's exterior. This includes the material body (physiology [cells, molecules, neurotransmitters, limbic system], biochemistry, chemistry, physics), integral patient care plans, skill development (health, fitness, exercise, nutrition, etc.), behaviors, leadership skills and integral life practices (see the section titled "Process"), and anything that we can touch or observe scientifically in time and space. Integral nursing with our nursing colleagues and healthcare team members includes the "It" of new behaviors, integral assessment and care plans, leadership, and skills development.

- *Lower-Left (LL):* In this "We" (intersubjective; the inside of the collective) space can be found the interior collective of how we can come together to share our cultural background, stories, values, meanings, vision, language, relationships, and how to form partnerships to achieve a healing mission. This can decrease our fragmentation and enhance collaborative practice and deep dialogue around things that really matter. Integral nursing is built upon "We."

- *Lower-Right (LR):* In this "Its" space (interobjective; the outside of the collective) can be found the world of the collective, exterior things. This includes social systems/structures, networks, organizational structures, and systems (including financial and billing systems in health care), information technology, regulatory structures (environmental and governmental policies, etc.), and any aspect of the technological environment and in Nature and the natural world. Integral nursing identifies the "Its" in the structure that can be enhanced to create more integral awareness and integral

partnerships to achieve health and healing—local to global.

On the outside of the Figure 1-8d, the left-hand quadrants (Upper-Left, Lower-Left) describe aspects of reality as interpretive and qualitative. In contrast, the right-hand quadrants (Upper-Right, Lower-Right) describe aspects of reality as measurable and quantitative. When we fail to consider these subjective, intersubjective, objective, and interobjective aspects of reality, our endeavors and initiatives are fragmented and narrow and we often fail to reach identified outcomes and goals. The four quadrants are a result of the differences and similarities in Wilber's investigation of the many aspects of identified reality.[49-54] The model describes the territory of our own awareness that is already present within us and an awareness of things outside of us. These quadrants help us connect the dots of the actual process to understand more deeply who we are and how we are related to others and all things.

Content Component 5: AQAL (All Quadrants, All Levels)

The fifth content component in the Theory of Integral Nursing is the exploration of Wilber's "all quadrants, all levels, all lines, all states, all types" or AQAL (pronounced ah-qwul), as shown in **Figure 1-8e**. These levels, lines, states, and types are important elements of any comprehensive map of reality. The integral model simply assists us in further articulating and connecting all areas, awarenesses, and depths in these four quadrants. Briefly, these levels, lines, states, and types are as follows:[49]

- *Levels:* Levels of development that become permanent with growth and maturity (e.g., cognitive, relational, psychosocial, physical, mental, emotional, spiritual) that represent increased organization or complexity. These levels are also referred to as waves and stages of development. Each individual possesses the masculine and feminine voice or energy. Neither masculine nor feminine is higher or better; they are two equivalent types at each level of consciousness and development.

- *Lines:* Developmental areas that are known as multiple intelligences: cognitive line

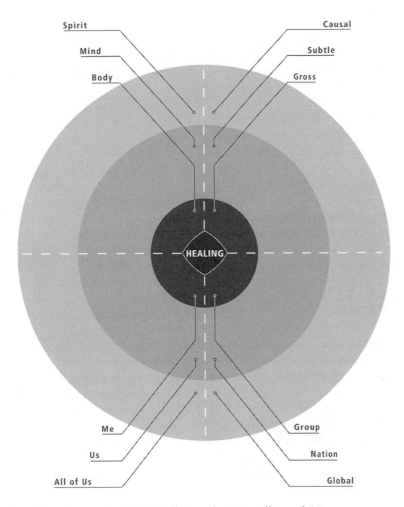

FIGURE 1-8e Healing and AQAL (All Quadrants, All Levels)
Source: Adapted with permission from Ken Wilber. http://www.kenwilber.com. Copyright © Barbara Dossey, 2007.

(awareness of what is); interpersonal line (how I relate socially to others); emotional/affective line (the full spectrum of emotions); moral line (awareness of what should be); needs line (Maslow's hierarchy of needs); aesthetics line (self-expression of art, beauty, and full meaning); self-identity line (who am I?); spiritual line (where spirit is viewed as its own line of unfolding, and not just as ground and highest state); and values line (what a person considers most important; studied by Clare Graves and brought forward by Don Beck[66] in his Spiral Dynamics Integral that is beyond the scope of this chapter).

- *States:* Temporary changing forms of awareness: waking, dreaming, deep sleep, altered meditative states (resulting from meditation, yoga, contemplative prayer, etc.), altered states (resulting from mood swings, physiology, and pathophysiology shifts with disease, illness, seizures, cardiac arrest, low or high oxygen saturation, or drugs), peak experiences (triggered by intense listening to music, walks in Nature, love making, mystical experiences such as hearing the voice of God or the voice of a deceased person, etc.).

- *Types:* Differences in personality and masculine and feminine expressions and development (e.g., cultural creative types, personality types, enneagram).

This part of the Theory of Integral Nursing, as shown in Figure 1-8e, starts with healing at the center surrounded by three increasing concentric circles with dotted lines of the four quadrants. This aspect of the integral theory moves to higher orders of complexity through personal growth, development, expanded stages of consciousness (permanent and actual milestones of growth and development), and evolution. These levels or stages of development can also be expressed as being self-absorbed (such as a child or infant), which evolves to ethnocentric (centers on group, community, tribes, nation), to worldcentric (care and concern for all peoples regardless of race, color, sex, gender, sexual orientation, creed), to the global level.

In the Upper Left, the "I" space, the emphasis is on the unfolding awareness from body to mind to spirit. Each increasing circle includes the lower as it moves to the higher level. This quadrant is further explained in the section on process.

The Upper Right, the "It" space, is the external of the individual. Every state of consciousness has a felt energetic component that is expressed from the wisdom traditions as three recognized bodies: gross, subtle, and causal.[49] We can think of these three bodies as the increasing capacities of a person toward higher levels of consciousness. Each level is a specific vehicle that provides the actual support for any state of awareness. The gross body is the individual physical, material, sensorimotor body that we experience in our daily activities. The subtle body manifests when we are not aware of the gross body of dense matter, but of a shift to light, energetic, emotional feelings and fluid and flowing images. Examples are a shift during a dream, during different types of body work, during walks in Nature, or during other experiences that move us to a profound state of bliss. The causal body is the body of the infinite that is beyond space and time. Causal also includes all aspects of Era III medicine and nonlocality where minds of individuals are not separate in space and time. When this is applied to consciousness, separate minds behave as if they are linked regardless of how far apart in space and time they may be. Nonlocal consciousness may underlie phenomena such as remote

healing, intercessory prayer, telepathy, premonitions, as well as so-called miracles. Nonlocality also implies that the soul does not die with the death of the physical body—hence, immortality forms some dimension of consciousness.[33,34] Nonlocality can also be both an upper- and lower-quadrant phenomenon.

The Lower Left, the "We" space, is the interior collective dimension of individuals who come together. The concentric circles from the center outward represent increasing levels of complexity of our relational aspect of shared cultural values. This is where teamwork and the interdisciplinary and transpersonal disciplinary development occur. The inner circle represents the individual labeled as *me*; the second circle represents a larger group labeled *us*; the third circle is labeled *all of us* to represent the largest group consciousness that expands to all people. These last two circles may include not only people, but animals, Nature, and nonliving things that are important to individuals.

The Lower Right, the "Its" space, the exterior social system and structures of the collective, is represented with concentric circles. An example within the inner circle might be a group of healthcare professionals in a hospital clinic or department or the complex hospital system and structure. The middle circle expands in increased complexity to include a nation; the third concentric circle represents even greater complexity to the global level where the health of all humanity and the world is considered. It is also helpful to emphasize that these groupings are the physical dynamics such as the working structure of a group of healthcare professionals versus the relational aspect that is a lower-left aspect, and the technical and informatics structure of a hospital or a clinic.

Integral nurses strive to integrate concepts and practices related to body, mind, and spirit (all levels) in self, culture, and Nature (all quadrants). The individual interior and exterior—"I" and "It"—as well as the collective interior and exterior—"We" and "Its"—must be developed, valued, and integrated into all aspects of culture and society. The AQAL integral approach suggests that we consciously touch all of these areas and do so in relation to self, to others, and the natural world. Yet to be integrally informed does not mean that we have to master all of these areas; we just need to be aware of them and choose to integrate integral awareness and integral practices. Because these areas are already part of our being-in-the-world and can't be imposed from the outside (they are part of our makeup from the inside), our challenge is to identify specific areas for development and find new ways to deepen our daily integral life practices.

Wilber uses the term *holon* to describe anything that is itself whole or part of some other whole that creates structures, from the very smallest to the largest, with increasing complexity.[49] The upper half of the model represents the individual holons, or the "micro world." The lower quadrants represent the social or communal holons, or the "macro world." These holons create a holarchy of natural evolutionary processes. As one progresses up a holarchy, the lower levels of holons are transcended and included and thus are foundational. All of the entities or holons in the right-hand quadrants possess simple location. These are things that are perceived with our senses such as rocks, villages, organisms, ecosystems, and planets. However, none of the entities or holons in the left-hand quadrants possess simple location. One cannot see feelings, concepts, states of consciousness, or interior illumination. They are complex experiences that exist in emotional space, conceptual space, spiritual space, and in our mutual understanding space. The development of one's individual consciousness as part of self-care is primary to the development of all other quadrants and integral thinking, application, and integration.

This aspect of the Theory of Integral Nursing helps us understand coherence and resilience.[78] *Coherence* is the quality of being logically integrated, consistent, and intelligible (as a coherent statement). It implies correlations, connectedness, consistency, efficient energy utilization, wholeness, and global order. A *coherent state* is an increase in physiologic efficiency, and alignment of the mental and emotional systems accumulates resilience (energy) across all four energetic domains. *Resilience* is related to self-management and efficient utilization of energy resources across four domains: physical, emotional, mental, and spiritual. High-level resilience helps us recover from challenging situations and prevents unnecessary stress reactions (frustration, impatience, anxiety) that deplete physical and psycho-

logical resources. *Physical resilience* is reflected in physical flexibility, endurance, and strength. *Mental resilience* is reflected in attention span, mental flexibility, optimistic worldview, and ability to integrate multiple points of view. *Emotional resilience* is related to one's ability to self-regulate the degree of emotional flexibility, positive emotions, and relationships. *Spiritual resilience* is related to commitment to core values, intuition, and tolerance of others' values and beliefs.

Structure

The structure of the Theory of Integral Nursing is shown in **Figure 1-8f**. All content components are overlaid to create a mandala to symbolize wholeness. Healing is placed at the center, and then the meta-paradigm of nursing (integral nurse, person, integral health, integral environment), the patterns of knowing (personal, empirics, aesthetics, ethics, not knowing, sociopolitical), the four quadrants (subjective, objective, intersubjective, interobjective), and all quadrants and all levels of growth, development, and evolution. (Note: Although the patterns of knowing are superimposed as they are in the various quadrants, they can also fit into other quadrants.)

Using the language of Ken Wilber[49] and Don Beck[66] and his Spiral Dynamics Integral, individuals move through primitive, infantile consciousness to an integrated language that is considered first-tier thinking. As they move up the spiral of growth, development, and evolution and expand their integral worldview and integral consciousness, they move into what is considered second-tier thinking and participation. This is a radical leap into holistic, systemic, and integral modes of consciousness. Wilber also expands to a third-tier stage of consciousness that addresses an even deeper level of transpersonal understanding that is beyond the scope of this chapter.[54]

Context

Context in a nursing theory is the environment in which nursing acts occur and the nature of the world of nursing. In an integral nursing environment, the nurse strives to be an integralist, which means that she or he strives to be integrally informed and is challenged to further develop an integral worldview, integral life

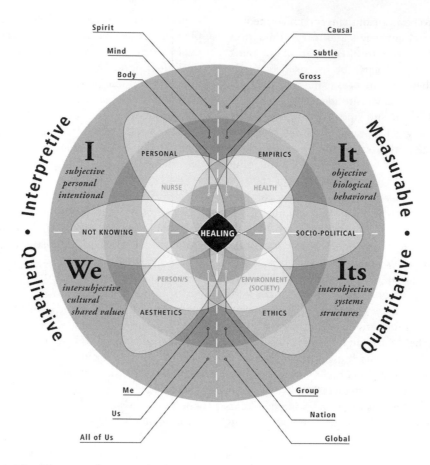

FIGURE 1-8f   Theory of Integral Nursing (Healing, Meta-Paradigm, Patterns of Knowing in Nursing, Four Quadrants, and AQAL)
Source: Adapted with permission from Ken Wilber. http://www.kenwilber.com. Copyright © Barbara Dossey, 2007.

practices, and integral capacities, behaviors, and skills. An integral nurse values, articulates, and models the integral process and integral worldview, as well as integral life practices and self-care in nursing practice, education, research, and healthcare policies. The term *nurse healer* is used to describe a nurse as an instrument in the healing process and a major part of the exterior healing environment of a patient, family, or another. Nurses assist and facilitate individuals with accessing their own healing process and potentials; the nurses do not do the actual healing. An integral nurse also recognizes self as part of the exterior healing environment interacting with a person, family, or colleague and enters

into a shared experience (or field of consciousness) that promotes healing potentials and an experience of well-being.

A key concept in an integral healing environment, both interior and exterior, is meaning, which addresses that which is indicated, referred to, or signified.[82] Philosophical meaning is related to one's view of reality and the symbolic connections that can be grasped by reason. Psychological meaning is related to one's consciousness, intuition, and insight. Spiritual meaning is related to how one deepens personal experience of a connection with the Divine, or whatever mechanism or modalities are used by an individual to feel a sense of oneness, belonging, and a feeling of connection in this human journey of life.

Process

Process in a nursing theory is the method by which the theory works. An integral healing process contains both nurse processes and patient, family, healthcare workers' processes (individual interior and individual exterior), and collective healing processes of individuals and of systems/structures (collective interior and exterior). This is the understanding of the unitary whole person interacting in mutual process with the environment.

There are many opportunities to increase our integral awareness, application, and understanding each day. Reflect on all that you do each day in your work and life—analyzing, communicating, listening, exchanging, surveying, involving, synthesizing, investigating, interviewing, mentoring, developing, creating, researching, teaching, and creating new schemes for what is possible. Before long you will realize how these four quadrants and realities fit together. You will also discover whether you are completely missing a quadrant, thus an important part of reality. As we address and value the individual interior and exterior, the "I" and "It," as well as the collective interior and exterior, the "We" and "Its," a new level of integral understanding emerges, and we may find that there is also more balance and harmony each day. By incorporating the integral nursing principles discussed next, we may assist others to discover their own healing path. The reader is referred to Figure 1-8f and Table 1-9 for specific components of each quadrant. **Figure 1-9** provides examples of Florence Nightingale's integral ideas as related to each integral nursing principle.

Integral Nursing Principle 1: Nursing Requires Development of the "I"

Integral nursing principle 1 recognizes the interior individual "I" (subjective) space. Each of us must value the importance of exploring one's health and well-being starting with our own personal exploration and development on many levels.[83–86]

Nightingale saw nursing first as a calling that was very individual and personal. Throughout her life and nursing career, she reflected carefully on her own thoughts, motives, and desires, as well as her own knowledge, skills, and conduct. In her 1888 address she wrote: "Nursing work must be quiet work—An individual work—Anything else is contrary to the whole realness of the work. Where am I, the individual, in my utmost soul? What am I, the inner woman [man], called 'I'?—That is the question."[87] This development of the individual "I" supports each nurse in deeply understanding one's interior as well as developing the qualities of nursing presence, the aesthetic knowing of nursing as art, and much more. As Nightingale wrote in 1868:

> Nursing is an art; and if it is to be made an art, it requires as exclusive a devotion, as hard a preparation, as any painter's or sculptor's work; for what is the having to do with dead canvas or cold marble, compared with having to do with the living spirit—the temple of God's spirit? It is one of the Fine Arts; I had almost said, the finest of the Fine Arts.[88]

As nurses continually address their stress, burnout, suffering, and soul pain, as discussed in the next principle, this can assist us to understand the necessity of personal healing and self-care directly related to nursing as art, where we develop qualities of nursing presence and inner reflection. Nurse presence is also a way of approaching a person that respects and honors the person's essence; it is relating in a way that reflects a quality of "being with" and "in collaboration with," as discussed in the next principle.[79] Our own inner work also helps us to hold deeply a conscious awareness of our own roles in creating a healthy world. We recognize the importance of addressing one's own shadow that, as described by Jung[89] is a composite of personal characteristics and potentials that have been denied expression in life and of which a person is unaware; the ego denies the characteristics because they are in conflict and incompatible with a person's chosen conscious attitude.

In this "I" space, integral self-care is valued, which means that integral reflective practices

[a]   **Nightingale's "Integral" Ideas**
                    from "Sick-Nursing and Health-Nursing" 1893

Subjective "I"   *Objective "It"*

"What is it to feel a calling for anything? Is it not to do our work in it to satisfy the high idea of what is right and best and not because we shall be found out if we don't do it?" [p.193]

She distinguished "calling" as the creation of a life of caring, that deep desire to serve with an involvement of one´s whole being – physically, emotionally, mentally and spiritually.

Florence Nightingale addressed her concerns for health by reminding her readers of their responsibilities as citizens. Speaking from her own long experience with informing the public about health issues, she asked her readers to join her: "You must form public opinion.... Officials will only do what you make them. You, the public, must make them do what you want." [p.191]

She called for an "espirit de corps" to forge new methods, collaborations and foster bridge-building in her time. She noted that "the health of the unity of is the health of the community. Unless you have the health of the unity, there is no community health." and called people together secure the best air, the best food, and all that makes life useful, healthy and happy." [p.197]

Her definition of health was "not only to be well, but to be able to use well every power we have." [p.186] She reminded her readers that nursing addressed such "stupendous issues as life and death, health and disease." [p.187] She noted that — as we address these issues, at both micro and macro levels — ultimately "health is [our] only capital." [p.191]

Intersubjective "We"   *Interobjective "Its"*

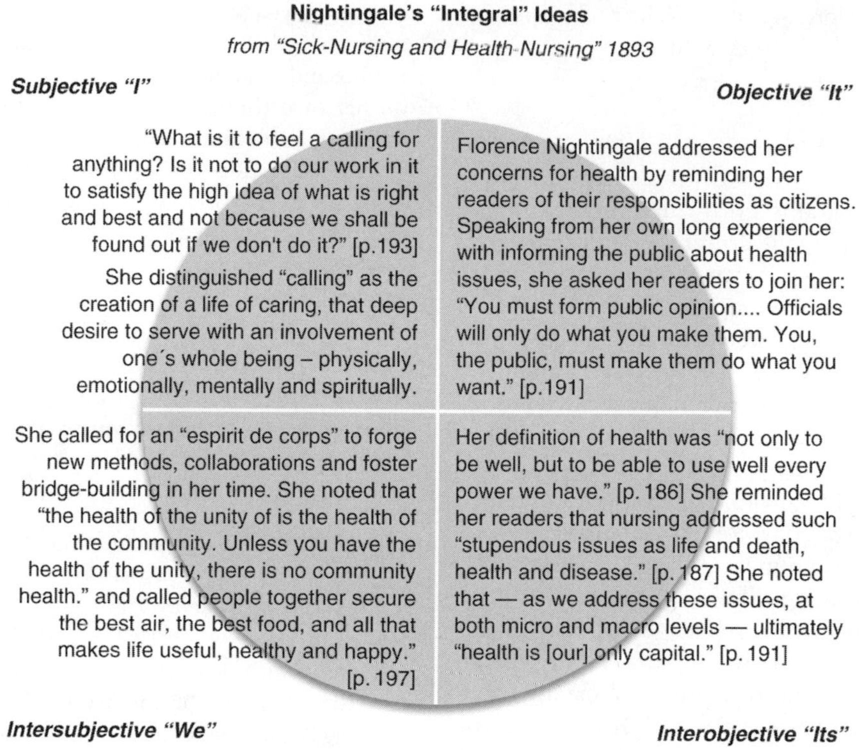

FIGURE 1-9   Florence Nightingale's integral ideas.
Source: Used with permission from the Nightingale Initiative for Global Health (NIGH), Ottawa, Ontario, Canada and Washington, DC and B. M. Dossey, L. C. Selanders, D. M. Beck, and A. Attewell, *Florence Nightingale Today: Healing, Leadership, Global Action* (Silver Spring, MD: Nursesbooks.org, 2005).

are integrated and can be transformative in our developmental process. We become more integrally conscious in our knowing, doing, and being and in all aspects of our personal and professional endeavors. Mindfulness is the practice of giving attention to what is happening in the present moment such as our thoughts, feelings, emotions, and sensations. To cultivate the capacity of mindfulness practices one may include mindfulness meditation, centering prayer, and other reflective practices such as journaling, dream interpretation, art, music, or poetry that leads to an experience of nonseparateness and love; it involves developing the qualities of stillness and being present for one's own suffering, which also allows for full presence when with another.

In our personal process, we recognize conscious dying where time and thought are given to contemplate one's own death. Through a reflective practice one rehearses and imagines one's final breath to practice preparing for one's own death. This integral practice prepares us to not be so attached to material things, not to spend so much time thinking about the future but living in this moment as often as we can, and to live fully until death comes. We are more likely to participate and fully engage with deeper compassion in the death process with others and ultimately with self. Death is seen as the mirror in which the entire meaning and mystery of life are reflected—the moment of liberation. Within an integral perspective the state of transparency, the understanding that there

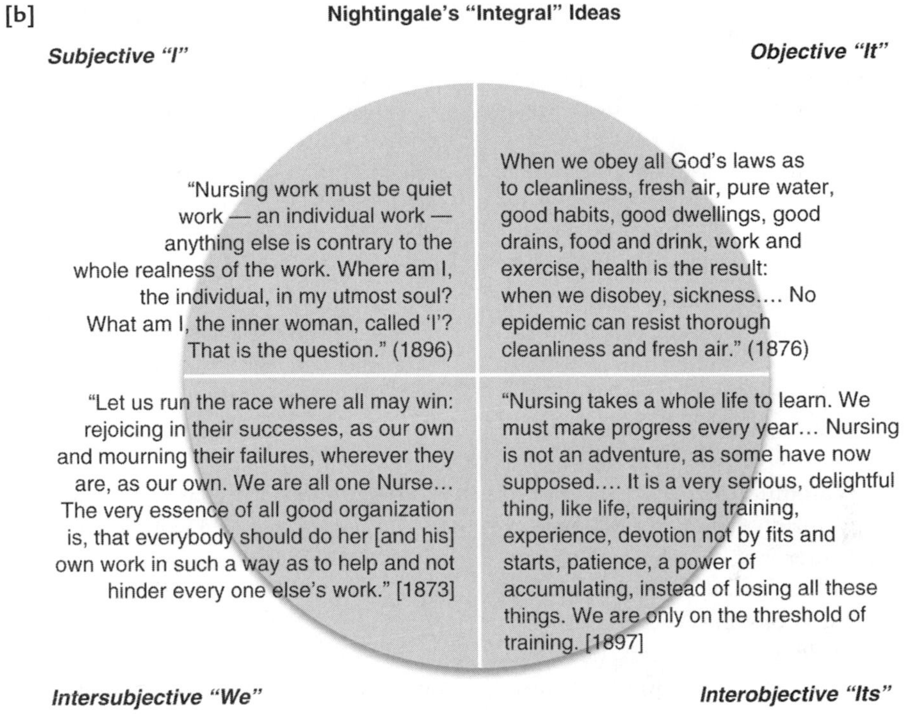

[b]

Nightingale's "Integral" Ideas

Subjective "I"   *Objective "It"*

"Nursing work must be quiet work — an individual work — anything else is contrary to the whole realness of the work. Where am I, the individual, in my utmost soul? What am I, the inner woman, called 'I'? That is the question." (1896)

When we obey all God's laws as to cleanliness, fresh air, pure water, good habits, good dwellings, good drains, food and drink, work and exercise, health is the result: when we disobey, sickness.... No epidemic can resist thorough cleanliness and fresh air." (1876)

"Let us run the race where all may win: rejoicing in their successes, as our own and mourning their failures, wherever they are, as our own. We are all one Nurse... The very essence of all good organization is, that everybody should do her [and his] own work in such a way as to help and not hinder every one else's work." [1873]

"Nursing takes a whole life to learn. We must make progress every year... Nursing is not an adventure, as some have now supposed.... It is a very serious, delightful thing, like life, requiring training, experience, devotion not by fits and starts, patience, a power of accumulating, instead of losing all these things. We are only on the threshold of training. [1897]

Intersubjective "We"   *Interobjective "Its"*

FIGURE 1-9   Florence Nightingale's integral ideas.
Source: Used with permission from the Nightingale Initiative for Global Health (NIGH), Ottawa, Ontario, Canada and Washington, DC and B. M. Dossey, L. C. Selanders, D. M. Beck, and A. Attewell, *Florence Nightingale Today: Healing, Leadership, Global Action* (Silver Spring, MD: Nursesbooks.org, 2005).

is no separation between our practice and our everyday life, is recognized.[79,80] This is a mature practice that is wise and empty of a separate self.

Integral Nursing Principle 2: Nursing Is Built on "We"

Integral nursing principle 2 recognizes the importance of the "We" (intersubjective) space where nurses come together and are conscious of sharing their worldviews, beliefs, priorities, and values related to enhancing integral self-care and integral health care. It includes being fully present and focused with intention to understand what another person (patient, family, colleague, or other) is expressing, or not expressing. Deep listening is valued. When we listen authentically to a client share her or his story, whether it is about illness or other life challenges that include

the person's cultural worldviews and rituals, we assist them to transform crisis into wisdom and helplessness into hope that increases body-mind-spirit healing.[90,91]

This focus begins an energy flow—by setting an intention for the healing of the client/patient—that moves from gross body (physical), to the subtle body (light, energy, emotional feelings), to the causal body (the infinite formless state) where realization of not being separate from others is experienced. This energy healing is used to describe the subtle flow of energy within and around a person—creating a field that is experienced by the individual. This is the ability to open one's heart, to be present for all levels of suffering, such that suffering may be transformed for others, as well as for self. This is bearing witness and being present for things as they are—a state achieved through reflective and contemplative practice that leads to an experience of nonseparateness.[80] It involves developing the qualities of stillness to be present for suffering and the sufferer.

Within nursing, health care, and society, there is much suffering, moral suffering, moral distress, and soul pain, as shown in **Table 1-10**.[81] We are often called on to "be with" these difficult human experiences and to use our nursing presence. Our sense of "We" supports us in recognizing the phases of suffering—"mute" suffering, "expressive" suffering, and "new identity" in suffering.[80,81] When we feel alone, as nurses, we experience mute suffering; this is an inability to articulate and communicate with others one's own suffering. Our challenge in nursing is to more skillfully enter into the phase of "expressive" suffering where sufferers seek language to express their frustrations and experiences such as in sharing stories in a group process. Outcomes of this experience often move toward new identity in suffering through new meaning-making where one makes new sense of the past, interprets new meaning in suffering, and can envision a new future. A shift in one's consciousness allows for a shift in one's capacity to be able to transform her or his suffering from causing distress to finding some new truth and meaning in it. As we create times for sharing and giving voice to our concerns, new levels of healing may happen.

Nightingale consistently realized the value of collaborating well with others, especially nursing colleagues. She focused on what "we" as nurses can do together as a team. She saw that sustainable nursing practice constantly requires strong nursing teamwork, as she expressed in 1883:

> Let us run the race where all may win, rejoicing in their successes, as our own, and mourning their failures, wherever they are as our own. . . . We are all one Nurse. The very essence of all good organizations is, that everybody should do her [or his] own work in such a way as to help and not hinder every one else's work.[92]

An integral nurse considers transpersonal dimensions. This means that interactions with others move from conversations to a deeper dialogue that goes beyond the individual ego; it includes the acknowledgment and appreciation for something greater that may be referred to as spirit, nonlocality, unity, or oneness.[32,35] Transpersonal dialogues contain an integral

---

TABLE 1-10   Suffering, Moral Suffering, Moral Distress, and Soul Pain

Suffering: An individual's story around pain where the signs of suffering may be physical, mental, emotional, social, behavioral, and/or spiritual; it is an anguish experienced—internal and external—as a threat to one's composure, integrity, and the fulfillment of intentions.

Moral suffering: Occurs when an individual experiences tensions or conflicts about what is the right thing to do in a particular situation; it often involves the struggle of finding a balance between competing interests or values.

Moral distress: Occurs when an individual is unable to translate moral choices into moral actions and when prevented by obstacles, either internal or external, from acting upon them.

Soul pain: The experience of an individual who has become disconnected and alienated from the deepest and most fundamental aspects of one's self.

Source: Used with permission. J. Halifax, B. M. Dossey, and C. H. Rushton, *Being With Dying: Compassionate End-of-Life Training Guide* (Santa Fe, NM: Prajna Mountain Press, 2007). Adapted from A. Jameston, *Nursing Practice: The Ethical Issues* (Englewood Cliffs, NJ: Prentice Hall, 1984), and M. Kearney, *Mortally Wounded* (New York: Scribner, 1996).

worldview and recognize the role of spirituality, which is the search for the sacred or holy that involves feelings, thoughts, experiences, rituals, meaning, value, direction, and purpose as valid aspects of the universe. Spirituality is a force that can unify a person with all that is—the essence of beingness and relatedness that permeates all of life and is manifested in one's knowing, doing, and being; it is usually, though not universally, considered the interconnectedness with self, others, Nature, and God/Life Force/Absolute/Transcendent. From an integral perspective, spiritual care is an interfaith perspective that takes into account dying as a developmental process and natural human process that emphasizes meaningfulness and human and spiritual values.[82] Religion is recognized as the codified and ritualized beliefs, behaviors, and rituals that take place in a community of like-minded individuals involved in spirituality.[82] Our challenge is to enter into deep dialogue to more fully understand religions different from our own so that we may be tolerant where there are differences.

In this "We" space, nurses come together and are conscious of sharing their worldviews, beliefs, priorities, and values related to working together in ways that enhance integral self-care and integral health care. Deep listening is valued; this is being present and focused with intention to understand what another person is expressing or not expressing. Bearing witness to others, the state achieved through reflective and mindfulness practices, is also valued.[80] Through mindfulness one can achieve states of equanimity, the stability of mind that allows us to be present with a good and impartial heart no matter how beneficial or difficult the conditions; it is being present for the sufferer and suffering just as it is while maintaining a spacious mindfulness in the midst of life's changing conditions. Compassion is bearing witness and loving kindness, which is manifest in the face of suffering. The realization of the self and another as not being separate is experienced; it is the ability to open one's heart and be present for all levels of suffering so that suffering may be transformed for others, as well as for the self. A useful phrase to consider is "I'm doing the best that I can."[80] Compassionate care assists us in living as well as being with the dying person, the family,

and others. We can touch the roots of pain and become aware of new meaning in the midst of pain, chaos, loss, and grief.

Integral action is the actual practice and process that creates the condition of trust where a plan of care is cocreated with the patient, and care can be given and received. Full attention and intention to the whole person, not merely the current presenting symptoms, illness, crisis, or tasks to be accomplished, reinforce the person's meaning and experience of community and unity. Engagement between an integral nurse and a patient, family member, or colleague is done in a respectful manner; each patient's subjective experience about health, health beliefs, and values are explored. We deeply care for others and recognize our own mortality and that of others.

The integral nurse uses intention, which is the conscious awareness of being in the present moment with self or another person, to help facilitate the healing process; it is a volitional act of love. The nurse is also aware of the role of intuition, which is the perceived knowing of events, insights, and things without a conscious use of logical, analytical processes; it may be informed by the senses to receive information. Intuition is a type of experience of sudden insight into a feeling, a solution, or problem where time and things fit together in a unified experience, such as understanding about pain and suffering, or a moment in time with another. This is an aspect within the pattern of unknowing. Integral nurses recognize love as the unconditional unity of self with others. This love generates lovingkindness, the open, gentle, and caring state of mindfulness that assist one's with nursing presence.

There is an awareness of integral communication that is a free flow of verbal and nonverbal interchange between and among people and pets and significant beings such as God/Life Force/Absolute/Transcendent. This type of sharing leads to explorations of meaning and ideas of mutual understanding and growth and loving kindness.

Integral Nursing Principle 3: "It" Is About Behavior and Skill Development

Integral nursing principle 3 recognizes the importance of the individual exterior "It" (objective) space. In this "It" space of the individual exterior, each person develops and integrates her or his integral self-care plan. This includes skills, behaviors, and action steps to achieve a fit body through strength training and stretching, as well as the conscious eating of healthy foods. It is also modeling integral life skills. For the integral nurse and patient, this is also the space where the "doing to" and "doing for" occur. However, the integral nurse also combines her or his nursing presence with nursing acts to assist the patient to access personal strengths, to release fear and anxiety, and to provide comfort and safety. There is the awareness of conscious dying to assist the dying patient who wishes to have minimal medication and treatment to stay as alert as possible while receiving comfort care until she or he makes the death transition.

Nightingale saw nursing as an integral and spiritual practice where each nurse blends knowledge with ongoing observations to develop and refine nursing practice—to continually combine the external observations of the body and behaviors and, thus, to develop new skills and behaviors. About this dynamic, Nightingale eloquently observed and wrote in 1876:

> When we obey all God's laws as to cleanliness, fresh air, pure water, good habits, good dwellings, good drains, food and drink, work and exercise, health is the result: when we disobey, sickness. 110,000 lives are needlessly sacrificed every year in this kingdom by our disobedience, and 22,000 people are needlessly sick all year round. And why? Because we will not know, will not obey God's simple health laws. No epidemic can resist thorough cleanliness and fresh air.[93]

Within this integral nursing principle, integral nurses with nursing colleagues and healthcare team members compile the data around physiologic and pathophysiologic assessment, nursing diagnosis, outcomes, and plans of care (including medications, technical procedures, monitoring, treatments, protocols, implementation, and evaluation). This is also the space that includes patient education and evaluation. Integral nurses cocreate plans of care with patients when possible, combining caring, healing interventions and modalities and integral life practices that can interface and enhance the success of traditional medical and surgical technology and treatment. Some common interventions are relaxation, music, imagery, massage, touch therapies, stories, poetry, healing environment, fresh air, sunlight, flowers, soothing and calming pictures, pet therapy, and more.

Integral Nursing Principle 4: "Its" Is Systems and Structures

Integral nursing principle 4 recognizes the importance of the exterior collective "Its" (interobjective) space. In this "Its" space, integral nurses and the healthcare team come together to examine their work, their priorities, use of technologies, and any aspect of the technological environment. They also create exterior healing environments that incorporate Nature and the natural world when possible such as with outdoor and indoor healing gardens, use of green materials with soothing colors, and sounds of music and Nature. Integral nurses identify how they might work together as an interdisciplinary team to deliver more effective patient care and coordination of care.

Nightingale saw nursing as a profession where continual progress with self and others required attention, and she wrote about this in 1897:

> Nursing takes a whole life to learn. We must make progress in it every year. . . . It has been recorded that the three principles which represent the deepest wants of human nature, both in the East and the West, are the principles of discipline, of religion (or the tie to God), of contentment. . . . Nursing is not an adventure, as some have now supposed: "Where fools rush in where angels fear to tread." It is a very serious, delightful thing, like life, requiring training, experience, devotion not by fits and starts, patience, a power of accumulating, instead of losing—all these things. We are only on the threshold of training.[94]

Application

This section offers examples of how to apply the Theory of Integral Nursing to practice, education, research, healthcare policy, and global nursing.

Practice

The Theory of Integral Nursing can be used in any clinical situation to explore aspects of integral awareness within all quadrants. The following example illustrates this point. Following a shopping trip with her husband and daughter, a woman had a seizure as she sat in her car. She lost consciousness but regained a conscious and alert state within several minutes. The husband immediately drove her to an emergency room. In this situation, which is more important? Is it the patient's brain (Upper Right—neural pathways and brain seizure focal areas) or the patient's and family's mind (Upper Left—emotions, meaning, thoughts, perceptions, fears)? Is it the nurse (Upper Left) or the nurse with the neurologist working together (Lower Left) or the emergency room (Lower Right)?

In an integral approach, the answer is that all of these questions are equally important to prevent this individual from further seizures and potential complications. When all quadrants are addressed a collaborative, integral treatment plan can be developed. It is also important to ensure that the patient and the family are kept aware of what is happening, and the patient flow in the emergency room is kept at a safe and effective pace. Each quadrant represents an equal quarter of reality, of the totality of our being and existence. This model helps us touch and link all aspects of reality, including the importance of the nurse addressing her or his own needs.

Another example of integral theory in clinical practice is from an empirical study that provides support for the use of story as a mechanism to promote well-being in nurses and to improve environments in which nurses work.[95] These nurses' stories reveal that data descriptors include dimensions of the individual interior and exterior and the collective interior and exterior. Nurses can communicate a common bond and connection through sharing stories about

the nursing profession that span generations, care settings, specialty, levels of education, training, and experience.

The Theory of Integral Nursing (TIN) provides a conceptual framework for nurses that is the integration of complementary and alternative therapies (CAT) into the routine care of patients receiving rehabilitation services. Juliann Perdue developed the Integrative Rehabilitation Model, shown in **Figure 1-10**, as a foundation for the integration of complementary and alternative therapies in integrative rehabilitation that occurs in a number of settings: general hospital, inpatient rehabilitation facility, outpatient rehabilitation clinic, and skilled nursing facilities or long-term care.[96]

The model also depicts the core aspects of rehabilitation nursing's research agenda, which includes: (1) nursing and nursing-led interdisciplinary interventions to promote function in people of all ages with disability and/or chronic health problems; (2) experience of disability and/or chronic health problems for individuals and families across the life span; (3) rehabilitation in the changing healthcare system; and (4) the rehabilitation nursing profession.

The Integrative Rehabilitation Model correlates well with the meta-paradigm of nursing and the four quadrants of reality. **Table 1-11** outlines the interconnectedness of the nurse, person, health, and environment with the realities of "I," "It," "We," and "Its." Through true presence and effective dialogue, the nurse establishes a safe environment for open communication regarding personal use and disclosure of CAT, as well as the sharing of knowledge and attitudes toward CAT.

The Theory of Integral Nursing with the Vulnerability Model (see Chapter 24) and the Integrative Functional Health Model (see Chapters 13 and 29) is one of the three major components of a 6-month Integrative Nurse Coach Certificate Program.[97] (See Chapter 9.) James Baye has also applied integral principles in his private coaching practice as well as in his global projects that have been implemented in more than 30 countries across six continents.[98] Linda Bark includes integral principles in her Bark Coaching Institute program.[99] Another use of

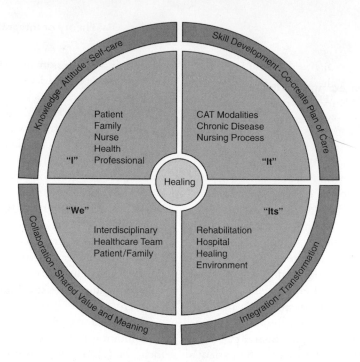

FIGURE 1-10 Integrative rehabilitation model.

Source: Used with permission. Copyright ©2011. Juliann S. Perdue, DNP, RN, FNP, Assistant Professor & Clinical Site Coordinator, California Baptist University, School of Nursing, Riverside, California.

		Meta-Paradigm of Nursing			
TABLE 1-11 Meta-Paradigm of Nursing and the Four Quadrants of Reality					
		Nurse	Person	Health	Environment
Quadrants of Reality	"I" Individual Exterior	Self	Patient Family Healthcare professional	Self-care	Knowledge Attitude Values & Beliefs
	"It" Individual Exterior	Nursing Process ▪ Assessment ▪ Diagnosis ▪ Outcomes ▪ Planning ▪ Implementation ▪ Evaluation	Chronic disease Disability	CATs Skill development Cocreate plan of care	Patient room/unit Therapeutic space
	"We" Collective Interior	Nursing profession ▪ CRRN*	Interdisciplinary team Patient/Family	Relationship-centered care	Collaboration Shared meaning
	"Its" Collective Exterior	Theory of Integral Nursing (TIN)	Rehab professionals Vision & Mission of organization CAT practitioners	Integral healthcare	Rehabilitation hospital Healing environment Transformational healthcare

Integrative Rehabilitation Model correlates well with the meta-paradigm of nursing and the four quadrants as modified from Barbara Dossey's Theory of Integral Nursing (2008).

Source: Used with permission. Copyright © 2011. Juliann S. Perdue, DNP, RN, FNP, Assistant Professor & Clinical Site Coordinator, California Baptist University, School of Nursing, Riverside, California.

integral theory is by Diane Pisanos in her health coaching practice with individuals and groups, as shown in **Figure 1-11**.[100]

Education

The Theory of Integral Nursing can assist educators to be aware of all quadrants while organizing and designing curricula, continuing education courses, health education presentations, teaching guides, and protocols. Most curricula focus minimally on the individual subjective "I" and the collective intersubjective "We"; the emphasis is on passing an examination or learning a new skill or procedure and, thus, the learner retains only small portions of what is taught. Before teaching any technical skills, the instructor might guide a student or patient in a relaxation and imagery rehearsal of the event to encourage the person to be in the present moment.

The reader is referred to Olga Jarrin, who explores integral theory and related definitions for nursing.[61,101] Cynthia Barrere and her nurse educator colleagues also use the Theory of Integral Nursing in their undergraduate curriculum.[102] (See Chapter 36.)

Darlene Hess uses the Theory of Integral Nursing in her Brown Mountain Visions business where she provides clinical, education, and consulting services.[103] She designed an RN-to-BSN curriculum based on the Theory of Integral Nursing (**Table 1-12**) that was adopted by Northern New Mexico College (NNMC) in Espanola, New Mexico. In May 2011, baccalaureate nursing degrees were awarded to the first graduates of the program. The program applied for accreditation from the Commission on Collegiate Nursing Education (CCNE) and completed the CCNE accreditation site visit in February 2011. The formal decision on accreditation status occurred in

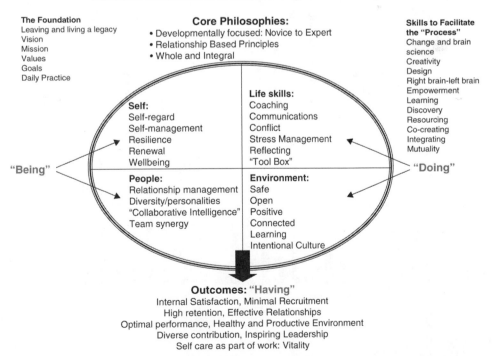

FIGURE 1-11   Integral coaching model.
Source: Used with permission. Copyright © 2001, 2009. Diane Pisanos, RNC, MS, AHN-BC, NNP, Integrative Health Care Consulting, Denver, CO. E-mail: dpisanos1@aol.com.

TABLE 1-12	Curriculum for RN-to-BSN Program Using the Theory of Integral Nursing		
Course Title	**Nursing in Transition (2 Cr)**	**An Integral Approach to Nursing (3 Cr)**	**Pathophysiology (6 Cr)**
Course Description	This course examines the expanded role of the baccalaureate-prepared nurse in today's health-care systems. Historic, contemporary, and future roles of the nurse are addressed. Skills in scholarly exposition and the use of technology are developed	This course examines the Theory of Integral Nursing. Holistic Nursing Theories are explored. The concept of praxis is introduced. Florence Nightingale's legacy and philosophical foundation are included. Students develop skills related to self-awareness, self-care, relationship-centered care, and reflective practice. The use of conscious intention is emphasized.	This two-part course addresses pathophysiological responses and adaptation of the physical body to an insult. Analysis of pathological alterations in health at the cellular and systems level and implications for nursing care are emphasized. Students focus on multisystem interaction of the body to an illness or injury. The pathophysiological basis of addictions and behavioral disorders is explored. Students are introduced to the biology of belief.
Course Topics	Role of baccalaureate-prepared nurse	Integral nursing/Integral health	Cellular biology
	Scholarly writing and use of scholarly resources	Holistic nursing	Genetic disease
	Critical thinking	Integrative nursing practice	Immunity
	Ethics	Healing	Inflammation
	Evolution of holistic nursing	Nursing meta-paradigm concepts	Stress and disease, Psychoneuroimmunology
	Principles of holistic nursing	Patterns of knowing	Neurologic system
	Standards of care	Relationship-centered care	Endocrine system
	Professional nursing organizations	Self-care	Reproductive system
	Working in groups	Reflective practice	Hematologic system
	Technology and informatics	Intention	Cardiovascular and lymphatic system
	Advanced nursing education	Florence Nightingale	Pulmonary system
	The nurse of the future	Spirituality	Renal and urologic system
		Therapeutic use of self	Digestive system
		Holistic nursing theories	Musculoskeletal system
		Self-confidence	Integumentary system
		Nurse as environment	Multiple organ dysfunction
		Holistic caring process	Pathophysiology of addictions
			Pathophysiology of behavioral disorders
			Biology of belief

TABLE 1-12   Curriculum for RN-to-BSN Program Using the Theory of Integral Nursing *(continued)*

	An Integral Approach to Health Assessment (4 Cr)	Community & Global Health I (4 Cr)	Community & Global Health II (4 Cr)
Course Title			
Course Description	This course emphasizes development of skills in health assessment of (allopathic) human systems. Alternative systems (i.e., ayurvedic, Native American, oriental medicine, intuitive) are introduced. Skills in interviewing, history taking, physical examination, and documentation and use of assessment data in planning care are developed. Laboratory and selected clinical settings are used to practice skill development. The Theory of Integral Nursing is explored as a model to frame data collection, organization, and synthesis into a cohesive whole.	This first of a 2-part course provides an overview of contemporary community health nursing practice. The influence of culture on healthcare beliefs and practices is emphasized. Health problems of selected populations within New Mexico are examined. Public Health Nursing Competencies are linked with the Theory of Integral Nursing to form the basis for student's learning experiences in community settings.	This second of a 2-part course examines global health issues in relationship to local, regional, and international nursing practice. In this course students select and focus upon a global health issue relevant to local community nursing practice. A service learning project based upon the selected issue provides the focus of clinical experience.
Course Topics	Presence Active listening, deep listening Centering Therapeutic interviewing Health history Nutritional assessment Spiritual assessment Cultural assessment Physical examination Mental status exam Documentation Synthesis of clinical information	Cultural diversity Cultural competence Spiritual diversity Community partnerships Community as client Population focused care Epidemiology Demographics Health promotion Health prevention "Upstream thinking" Communicable disease risk prevention Case management	Global warming Sustainability Immigration Bioterrorism Hazardous waste Pollution Aging Disaster management Vulnerable populations Poverty and homelessness Migrant health issues Mental health issues Violence Role of the nurse in community and global health

(continues)

TABLE 1-12   Curriculum for RN-to-BSN Program Using the Theory of Integral Nursing *(continued)*

	An Integral Approach to Evidence-Based Practice (4 Cr)	**Health Policy from an Integral Perspective (3 Cr)**	**Integral Communication and Teaching (2 Cr)**
Course Title			
Course Description	This course examines research methodologies utilized in nursing research. Emphasis is on utilization of research findings to establish evidence-based nursing interventions. Students analyze research findings aimed at selected health concerns. Students explore definitions of evidence-based practice and examine how worldviews influence research	This course emphasizes empowering students with knowledge, skills, and attitudes to effect change in health policy to improve healthcare delivery. Students analyze contemporary healthcare issues of concern to nursing and learn strategies for effective involvement in policy-making decisions and policy implementation. Students examine work environments and the impact of organizational systems on the quality of care. Students apply the Theory of Integral Nursing to a current health policy issue in a position paper expressed orally to a group.	This course examines communication techniques, counseling, coaching, and teaching strategies to enhance and facilitate cognitive and behavioral change. Students integrate principles of integral communication, integral health coaching, motivational interviewing, and Non-Violent Communication.
Course Topics	Historical evolution of nursing research	Current healthcare trends	Motivational Interviewing
	Quantitative research	Healthcare delivery systems	Educational theory
	Qualitative research	Healthcare financing	Fundamentals of Health Coaching
	Ethics in nursing research	Complexity and change theory	Helping others create healthy lifestyles
	Theory and research frameworks	Empowerment	Helping others navigate the healthcare system
	Outcomes research	Effective patient advocacy	Non-Violent Communication (NVC)
	Statistics	Navigating the legislative process	Presence
	Using research in an integral nursing practice	Healthcare reform	Learning styles
	Alternative philosophies of science	Communicating the essence of nursing/developing a nursing voice	Instructional design methods
			Counseling
			Ways of knowing

TABLE 1-12 Curriculum for RN-to-BSN Program Using the Theory of Integral Nursing *(continued)*

	Transformational Leadership in Nursing (3 Cr)	Integrating Complementary & Alternative Approaches to Nursing (4 Cr)	Integral Nursing Practice Senior Project (3 Cr)
Course Title			
Course Description	This course focuses on the principles of transformational leadership as applied to the nurse leader at the bedside, within an organization, in the community, and in the profession. The student is introduced to Complexity Science, Appreciative Inquiry, and Emotional Intelligence. Career advancement through lifelong learning is emphasized.	This course provides an introduction to evidence-based complementary and alternative approaches to health care. Students acquire knowledge related to alternative and complementary healing modalities that can be incorporated into professional nursing practice and self-care practices. Students experience and develop beginning skills in the provision of CAM modalities as they interact with practitioners in selected clinical settings.	This course provides the student an opportunity to critically examine in-depth a personally relevant topic in preparation for an expanded role as an integral nurse. Students develop learning objectives, a learning contract, and criteria for evaluation of project outcomes.
Course Topics	Transformational Model Leadership development Complexity Science Professional ethics Interdisciplinary leadership Appreciative Inquiry Emotional Intelligence Conflict resolution/Mediation Delegation Customer needs and expectations Visioning and strategic planning Managing care across the continuum Improving quality and performance Human resource management	NICAM Whole medical systems Mind-Body interventions Energy therapies Biologically based therapies Manipulative and body-based therapies Therapeutic environment Arts and healing	

Total Credit Hours: 42

Source: Used with permission. Copyright © 2007. Darlene Hess, PhD, RN, AHN-BC, PMHNP-BC, ACC, Brown Mountain Visions, Los Ranchos, NM 87101. http://www.brownmountainvisions.com

November 2011. The program expects to offer online classes in 2012. More information about the program is available at www.ncmc.edu.

The RN-to-BSN program based on the Theory of Integral Nursing prepares registered nurses to assume leadership roles as integral nurses at the bedside, within an organization, in the community, and in the profession. With an integrative care focus, the program prepares nurses to provide holistic, intentional, relationship-centered care that addresses individual and collective health. This holistic integrative model emphasizes self-care and personal development for the nursing student and for faculty who teach in the program. Program learning outcomes, course competencies, and assignments are linked to the Theory of Integral Nursing. Expected outcomes for the RN-to-BSN program are listed in **Table 1-13**. An example is provided in **Table 1-14** that shows how integral nursing principles are explicitly embedded in an assignment.

Research

Evidence-based practice (EBP) too often connotes a research-based approach to care, rather than the more complete definition of EBP that includes practitioner expertise and patient preferences.[104] Useful evidence is derived from many sources, and the utilization of research findings is but one aspect of delivering safe, accurate nursing care. An intentional approach to evaluating and using diverse evidence from varied sources supports holistic care. Knowing how to elicit patient preferences is an essential clinical skill.

The Theory of Integral Nursing can assist nurses to consider the importance of qualitative and quantitative research.[104,105] Often among scientists, researchers, and educators there are arguments as to whether qualitative or quantitative research is more important. Wilber often uses the term *flatland thinking and approaches* to describe the thinking of individuals who use a reductionistic perspective that can be situated in any quadrant or explanations of both the interior and exterior dimensions through only quantitative methodologies that focus on empirical data. Our challenges in integral nursing are to consider the findings from both qualitative and quantitative data and always consider triangulation of data when appropriate. We must always

---

TABLE 1-13   Expected Outcomes for RN-to-BSN Program Using Theory of Integral Nursing

1. Use the Theory of Integral Nursing and the American Holistic Nurses Association and the American Nurses Association *Holistic Nursing Scope and Standards of Practice* (2007) to provide integral and holistic nursing care in a variety of settings. (See Integral Principles #1–#4, pp. 37–43).

2. Demonstrate critical thinking skills from an "I," "It," "We," "Its" perspective.

3. Communicate effectively from a relationship-centered care perspective involving Patient-Practitioner, Community-Practitioner, and Practitioner-Practitioner relationships.

4. Conduct integral holistic health assessments in relation to client needs.

5. Apply concepts of integral nursing to a personal plan for holistic self-care.

6. Integrate and apply knowledge to support individual and collective health.

7. Analyze the links between and among individual, community, and global health issues from an integral worldview.

8. Analyze and utilize research findings to facilitate individual and collective health.

9. Demonstrate the role of the integral nurse as change agent in regards to current health policy issues.

10. Utilize integral coaching strategies in relation to client-centered goals.

11. Apply transformational leadership principles to professional nursing practice.

12. Integrate selected complementary/alternative health practices into professional nursing practice.

13. Demonstrate commitment to lifelong learning to facilitate personal and professional development.

Source: Used with permission. Copyright © 2011. Darlene R. Hess, PhD, AHN-BC, PMHNP-BC, ACC, Brown Mountain Visions, Los Ranchos, NM 87107, www.brownmountainvisions.com

value introspective, cultural, and interpretive experiences and expand our personal and collective capacities of consciousness and intentionality as evolutionary progression toward achieving our goals.[106] In other words, knowledge does emerge from all four quadrants. This helps us to understand more about the unitary paradigm of consciousness and intentionality, particularly with the World Wide Web and other technological advances.

Healthcare Policy

The Theory of Integral Nursing can guide us to consider many areas related to healthcare policy. Compelling evidence in all of the healthcare professions shows that the origins of health and illness cannot be understood by focusing only on the physical body. Only by expanding the equations of health, exemplified by an integral approach or an AQAL approach, to include our entire physical, mental, emotional, social, and spiritual dimensions and interrelationships can we account for a host of health events.[3,101] Some of these include, for example, the correlations between poor health and shortened life span; job dissatisfaction and acute myocardial infarction; social shame and severe illness; immune suppression and increased death rates during bereavement; improved health and longevity as spirituality and spiritual awareness increase.

Global Nursing

Our challenge as integral and holistic nurses is that we see global health imperatives as common concerns of humankind; they are not isolated problems in far-off countries. Like Nightingale, we must see prevention and prevention education as important to the health of humanity.[3]

We can explore all aspects of the Theory of Integral Nursing and apply them to our endeavors in underserved communities and populations. Often in the developed world of health care we believe that decent care is having access to technology, procedures, tests, or surgery when we need it and as quickly as we want. However, the majority of the world does not have access as do those in wealthy, developed nations. And this is still a limited view of what integral or even holistic health care is because primary prevention such as self-care is rarely given its just due in healthcare initiatives.

Consider the World Health Organization (WHO) call for "decent care" for HIV/AIDS patients and their families throughout the

---

TABLE 1-14   Example of Integral Nursing Principles Explicitly Embedded in a Course Assignment

Community Health Issue Scholarly Paper (See Integral Nursing Principles #1–#4, pp. 37–43).

Each student will select and define a community health issue to investigate. Identify your personal relationship to the issue (INP 1, 2) and why this issue is important to nursing (INP 2). Relate the issue to *Healthy People 2020 Goals* (http://www.healthypeople.gov/Document/tableofcontents.htm) (INP 4). Identify and evaluate relevant data pertinent to the issue from a variety of sources. Determine populations affected by this issue (INP 3). Include at least one nursing research article related to this issue. Summarize the information relevant to the issue and identify gaps in the information that is available. Determine if/how you will incorporate your learning about this issue into your self-care plan (INP 3).

Identify at least one agency or program that provides health promotion or health prevention services that address the selected issue (INP 4). State the mission and goals of the agency or program. Determine how the agency or program is funded. Describe the agency or program's emergency response plan (if it has one). Determine how the agency or program monitors and evaluates outcomes.

Compile the data into an organized and scholarly paper that will be discussed with your nurse classmates (INP 3). Solicit classmate perspectives regarding the selected issue, your findings, and their experiences (INP 1, 2).

Source: Used with permission. Copyright © 2007. Darlene R. Hess, PhD, AHN-BC, PMHNP-BC, ACC, Brown Mountain Visions, Los Ranchos, NM 87107, www.brownmountainvisions.com

world.[15] As you read this, reflect on the Theory of Integral Nursing and see how all aspects of this theory are covered in this WHO description of decent care. The primary objective is to delineate a new term within the taxonomy and politics of HIV/AIDS care—*decent care*—that repositions the individual as the focal point of the care cycle and agency that emphasizes not only what type or kind of care individuals receive, but also how that care is received. Decent care implies the comprehensive ideal that the medical, physiologic, psychological, and spiritual needs of others are addressed. This includes universal access to treatment with utilization and enforcement of universally accepted precautionary measures for healthcare practitioners, along with adequate supplies and equipment, safe food, free access to clean water, autoclaves, laundries, and safe methods for sterilizing and disposing of infected materials in incinerators.

An example of the Theory of Integral Nursing that has been applied to global nursing is the Nightingale Initiative for Global Health (NIGH).[3,16] This author is a founding NIGH board member and co-director. The NIGH is a catalytic grassroots-to-global movement, envisioned in 2000 and officially established in 2003, to honor and extend Florence Nightingale's timeless legacy. NIGH's twin purposes are, first, to increase global public awareness about the priority of health; and second, to empower nurses, nursing students, and concerned citizens to address the critical health issues of our time. Since the beginning of NIGH's development, these interrelated approaches have been developed intentionally, keeping Nightingale's deep and broad integral legacy in mind.

As NIGH's vision was articulated, we understood what Wilber[49] meant when he noted that omitting the focus of any one of the integral quadrants would cause "hemorrhaging" in attempts to achieve work represented by the other three integral quadrants. Without focusing on strengthening and sustaining individuals, groups of individuals cannot thrive (individual and collective interior). Without focusing on the worldviews underlying all situations in any society, the structures we live and work within cannot be properly understood and sustained (individual and collective exterior). Without first

populating an understanding of the nature of these worldviews—with real people in real groups with real needs in mind—structures can quickly become limited and worldviews irrelevant. Without understanding the value of envisioning and proposing structures from worldviews that can make a difference in the world, people and groups tend to drift away from purposeful efforts to actually ever make a difference.

By using the Theory of Integral Nursing, we realized how Wilber's integral modeling would help us to present NIGH's whole picture, as well as the pieces of the whole and—perhaps most important—the relationships among these pieces.[5] Using this jigsaw puzzle metaphor, NIGH's team has recently shaped a related series of NIGH Integral Models. **Figure 1-12** shows the NIGH Integral Models and the outcomes we are envisioning. The UL "I" quadrant is named "among Individuals"; the LL "We" quadrant is named "within Groups"; the UR "It" quadrant is named "at Grassroots Levels"; and the LR "Its" quadrant is named "at Global Levels."

We explored the complex dynamics within our NIGH project by considering Kreisberg's organization of first-, second-, and third-level complexity.[107] The first level of complexity is an individual (or individuals); the second level of complexity is community (groups); and the third level of complexity is the environment and structures and global systems. Thus, we placed individuals in the UL, groups in the LL, grassroots in the UR, and global systems in the LR. In Integral Theory, persons are individual holons whereas groups are social holons. (A full description of these distinctions is beyond this discussion.) From an Integral Theory/AQAL perspective, the individuals who we placed in the UL are really holons *of all four quadrants*. Individual commitments to the *Nightingale Declaration for a Healthy World* and individual nurses taking care of their own health are examples of behaviors—UR actions, rather than UL experiences. Yet, we know that UL experiences also continuously arise from these actions, and so forth. Nursing's first priority is devotion to human health—of individuals, of communities, and the world. An integral perspective can assist nurses who are educated and prepared—physically, emotionally, mentally, and spiritually—to

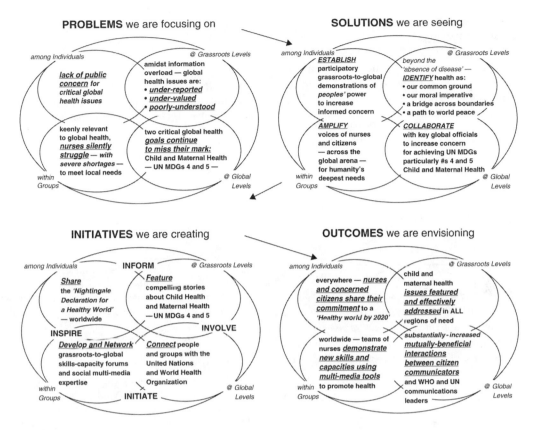

FIGURE 1-12   NIGH's 4 "Integral" Models
Source: Used with permission, Nightingale Initiative for Global Health (NIGH), http://www
.nightingaledeclaration.net

effectively accomplish the activities required for healthy people and healthy environments.[3]

■ CONCLUSION

The Theory of Integral Nursing addresses how we can increase our integral awareness, our wholeness, and healing and strengthen our personal and professional capacities to be more fully open to the mysteries of life's journey and the wondrous stages of self-discovery for ourselves and others. Our time demands a new paradigm and a new language where we integrate the best of what we know in the science and art of nursing that includes holistic and human caring theories and modalities. With an integral approach and worldview we are in a better position to share with others the depth of nurses' knowledge, expertise, critical-thinking capaci-

ties, and skills for assisting others in creating health and healing. Only by paying attention to the heart of nursing—*sacred* and *heart* reflect a common meaning—can we generate the vision, courage, and hope required to unite nursing in healing. This will help us as we engage in healthcare reform to address the challenges in these troubled times—local to global. This is not a matter of philosophy but of survival.

Directions for
FUTURE RESEARCH

1. Examine the components of relationship-centered care for clinical practice, education, research, and healthcare policy.
2. Analyze the Theory of Integral Nursing and its application in holistic nursing practice, education, research, and healthcare policy.

Nurse Healer
REFLECTIONS

After reading this chapter, the nurse healer will be able to answer or to begin a process of answering the following questions:

- How can I apply more of the components of relationship-centered care each day?
- In what ways can the Theory of Integral Nursing inform my personal and professional endeavors?
- What integral awareness and practices may I consider for development in my personal and professional life?

> *For a full suite of assignments and additional learning activities, use the access code located in the front of your book to visit this exclusive website: http://go.jblearning.com/dossey. If you do not have an access code, you can obtain one at the site.*

NOTES

1. F. Nightingale, "Sick-Nursing and Health-Nursing," in *Florence Nightingale Today: Healing, Leadership, Global Action*, ed. B. M. Dossey et al. (Silver Spring, MD: NurseBooks.org, 2005): 296–297.

2. Institute of Medicine, *The Future of Nursing: Leading Change, Advancing Health* (Washington, DC: IOM, October 5, 2010). http://www.iom.edu/Reports /2010/The-Future-of-Nursing-Leading-Change-Advancing-Health.aspx.

3. D. M. Beck, B. M. Dossey, and C. H. Rushton, "Integral Nursing and the Nightingale Initiative for Global Health (NIGH): Florence Nightingale's Integral Legacy for the 21st Century—Local to Global." *Journal of Integral Theory and Practice* 6, no. 4 (2011): 71–92.

4. B. M. Dossey, "Theory of Integral Nursing," *Advances in Nursing Science* 31, no. 1 (2008): E52–E73.

5. B. M Dossey, "Barbara Dossey's Theory of Integral Nursing," in *Nursing Theories and Nursing Practice*, 3rd ed., ed. M. E. Parker and M. C. Smith (Philadelphia, PA: F. A. Davis, 2010).

6. B. M. Dossey, *Integral Nursing: Practice, Education, Research, Policy* (in press).

7. American Holistic Nurses Association & the American Nurses Association, *Holistic Nursing Practice: Scope and Standards* (Silver Spring, MD: NurseBooks.org, 2007).

8. Consortium of Academic Health Centers for Integrative Medicine, "Definition of Integrative Medicine." http://www.imconsortium.org/about/home .html.

9. Interprofessional Education Collaborative Expert Panel, *Core Competencies for Interprofessional Collaborative Practice: Report of an Expert Panel* (Washington, DC: Interprofessional Education Collaborative, 2011).

10. D. M. Hess, B. M. Dossey, M. E. Southard, S. Luck, B. G. Schaub, and L. Bark, *Professional Nurse Coach Role: Defining Scope of Practice and Competencies* (in press).

11. B. M. Dossey et al., *Florence Nightingale Today: Healing, Leadership, Global Action* (Washington, DC: NurseBooks.org, 2005).

12. B. M. Dossey, D. M. Beck, and C. H. Rushton, "Nightingale's Vision for Collaboration," in *Nursing Without Borders: Values, Wisdom and Success Markers*, ed. S. Weinstein and A. M. Brooks (Indianapolis, IN: Sigma Theta Tau, 2008): 13–29.

13. N. R. Gantz, *101 Leadership Lessons for Nurses: Shared Legacies from Leaders and Their Mentors* (Indianapolis, IN: Sigma Theta Tau International, 2010).

14. L. O. Gostin, "Meeting the Survival Needs of the World's Least Healthy People," *Journal of American Medical Association* 298, no. 2 (2007): 225–227.

15. T. Karph, J. T. Ferguson, and R. Y. Swift, "Light Still Shines in the Darkness: Decent Care for All," *Journal of Holistic Nursing* 28, no. 4 (2010): 266–274.

16. Nightingale Initiative for Global Health, *Nightingale Declaration*. http://www.nightingaledeclaration.net.

17. D. M. Beck, B. M. Dossey, and C. H. Rushton, "Florence Nightingale: Connecting Her Legacy with Local-to-Global Health Today," *NurseWeek, Nursing Spectrum Nurse.com* (Hoffman Estates, IL: Gannett Healthcare Group, 2010): 104–109.

18. World Health Organization, *World Health Statistics Report 2009*. http://www.learningnurse.com /content/view/34/49/.

19. International Council of Nurses, *The Global Shortage of Registered Nurses: An Overview of Issues and Action* (Geneva, Switzerland: International Council of Nurses, 2004). http://www.icn.ch/images /stories/documents/publications/GNRI/Global_ Shortage_of_Registered_Nurses_Full_report.pdf

20. United Nations, *United Nations Millennium Development Goals* (New York, NY: United Nations, 2000). http://www.un.org/millenniumgoals/.

21. F. Nightingale, Letter to Sir Frederick Verney. 23 November 1892, Add. Mss. 68887 ff102–05.

22. B. M. Dossey, *Florence Nightingale: Mystic, Visionary, Healer*, Commemorative ed. (Philadelphia, PA: F. A. Davis, 2010).

23. B. M. Dossey, "Florence Nightingale: A 19th Century Mystic," *Journal of Holistic Nursing* 28, no. 1 (2010): 10–35.

24. B. M. Dossey, "Florence Nightingale: Her Crimean Fever and Chronic Illness," *Journal of Holistic Nursing* 28, no. 1 (2010): 38–53.

25. B. M. Dossey, "Florence Nightingale: Her Personality Type," *Journal of Holistic Nursing* 28, no. 1 (2010): 57–67.

26. L. McDonald, *The Collected Works of Florence Nightingale*, Vols. 1–16 (Waterloo, Ontario: Wilfreid Laurier Press, 2001–2012). http://www.uoguelph.ca/~cwfn/.

27. A. Harvey, *The Hope: A Guide to Sacred Activism* (Carlsbad, CA: Hay House Inc., 2009).

28. P. H. Walker, personal communication, May 15, 2007.

29. F. Nightingale, *Notes on Hospitals* (London, England: John W. Parker & Son, 1859).

30. F. Nightingale, *Notes on Nursing* (London, England: Harrison, 1860).

31. F. Nightingale, "Letter from Miss Nightingale to the Probationer-Nurses in the 'Nightingale Fund' at St. Thomas's Hospital, and the Nurses Who Were Formerly Trained There, 1888," in *Florence Nightingale Today: Healing, Leadership, Global Action*, ed. B. M. Dossey et al. (Silver Spring, MD: NurseBooks.org, 2005): 203–285.

32. L. Dossey, *Healing Words: The Power of Prayer and the Practice of Medicine* (San Francisco, CA: HarperSanFrancisco, 1993).

33. L. Dossey, *Recovering the Soul: Scientific and Spiritual Search* (New York, NY: Bantam, 1989).

34. L. Dossey, *Meaning and Medicine: A Doctor's Tales of Breakthrough and Healing* (New York, NY: Bantam Books, 1991).

35. L. Dossey, *Healing Beyond the Body: The Infinite Reaches of the Mind* (Boston, MA: Shambhala, 2000).

36. L. Dossey, *Premonition: How Knowing the Future Can Shape Our Lives* (New York, NY: Dutton, 2009).

37. C. Tresoli, *Pew-Fetzer Task Force on Advancing Psychosocial Health Education: Health Professions Education and Relationship-Centered Care* (San Francisco, CA: Commission at the Center for the Health Professions, University of California, 1994).

38. J. P. Belack and E. H. O'Neill, "Recreating Nursing Practice for a New Century: Recommendations and Implications of the Pew Health Professions Commission's Final Report," *Nursing Health Care Perspective* 21, no. 1 (2000): 14–21.

39. A. L. Suchman, D. J. Sluyter, and P. R. Williamson *Leading Change in Healthcare: Transforming Organizations Using Complexity, Positive Psychology, and Relationship-Centered Care* (London, England: Radcliffe Publishing, 2011).

40. R. M. Frankel, F. Eddins-Folensbee, and T. S. Irui, "Crossing the Patient-Centered Divide: Transforming Health Care Quality Through Enhanced Faculty Development," *Academy of Medicine* 86, no. 4 (2011): 445–452.

41. Samueli Institute of Information Biology, *Optimal Healing Environments*. http://www.siib.org/research/research-home/optimal-healing.html.

42. Planetree International, *Planetree Vision, Mission and Belief Statements*. http://planetree.org/?page_id=510

43. Penny George Institute for Health and Healing, *Penny George Center for Health and Healing Overview and Outcomes Report 2010*. http://abbottnorthwestern.com/ahs/anw.nsf/page/ANW_PGIHH_Outcomes_FNL-1.ForWeb.pdf/$FILE/ANW_PGIHH_Outcomes_FNL-1.ForWeb.pdf.

44. J. Crawford and L. Thornton, "Why Has Holistic Nursing Taken Off in the Last Five Years? What Has Changed?" *Alternative Therapies in Health and Medicine* 16, no. 3 (2010): 28–30.

45. M. Mittelman, "Nursing and Integrative Health Care," *Alternative Therapies* 16, no. 3 (2010): 84–94.

46. B. M. Dossey, S. Luck, and B. G. Schaub, *Integrative Nurse Coaching for Health and Wellness* (Huntington, NY: Florence Press, 2012).

47. Compilation of the Patient Protection and Affordable Care Act, May 2010. http://docs.house.gov/energycommerce/ppacacon.pdf

48. HHS Press Office, "Obama Administration releases National Prevention Strategy" (June 16, 2011). http://www.hhs.gov/news/press/2011pres/06/20110616a.html.

49. K. Wilber, *Integral Psychology* (Boston, MA: Shambhala, 2000).

50. K. Wilber, *The Collected Works of Ken Wilber*, Vols. 1–4 (Boston, MA: Shambhala, 1999).

51. K. Wilber, *The Collected Works of Ken Wilber*, Vols. 5–8 (Boston, MA: Shambhala, 2000).

52. K. Wilber, *Integral Operating System* (Louisville, CO: Sounds True, 2005).

53. K. Wilber, *Integral Life Practice* (Denver, CO: Integral Institute, 2005).

54. K. Wilber, *Integral Spirituality* (Boston, MA: Shambhala, 2006).

55. C. S. Clark, "An Integral Nursing Education: Exploration of the Wilber Quadrant Model," *International Journal of Human Caring* 10, no. 3 (2006): 22–29.

56. N. C. Frisch, "Nursing Theory in Holistic Nursing Practice," in *Holistic Nursing: A Handbook for Practice*, 6th ed., ed. B. M. Dossey and L. Keegan (Burlington, MA: Jones & Bartlett, 2012).

57. J. F. Quinn et al., "Research Guidelines for Assessing the Impact of the Healing Relationship in Clinical Nursing," *Alternative Therapies in Health and Medicine* 9, no. 3 (2003): A65–A79.

58. M. Mittelman, S. Y. Alperson, P. M. Arcari, G. F. Donnelly, L. C. Ford, M. Koithan, and M. J. Kreitzer, "Nursing and Integrative Health Care," *Alternative Therapies in Health and Medicine* 16, no. 5 (2010): 84–94.

59. R. Zahourek, "Holistic Nursing Research," in *Holistic Nursing: A Handbook for Practice*, 6th ed., ed. B. M. Dossey and L. Keegan (Burlington, MA: Jones & Bartlett, 2012).

60. J. Watson, *Caring Science as Sacred Science* (Philadelphia, PA: F. A. Davis, 2005).

61. O. Jarrin. "An Integral Philosophy and Definition of Nursing," *Journal of Integral Theory and Practice* 2, no. 4 (2007): 79–101.

62. B. S. Barnum, *Nursing Theory: Analysis, Application, Evaluation*, 6th ed. (Philadelphia, PA: Lippincott Williams & Wilkins, 2005).

63. H. L. Gaydos, "The Experience of Immobility Due to Trauma," *Holistic Nursing Practice* 19, no. 1 (2005): 40–43.

64. H. L. Gaydos, "The Co-Creative Aesthetic Process: A New Model for Aesthetics in Nursing," *International Journal of Human Caring* 7 (2004): 40–43.

65. R. Zahourek, "Intentionality Forms the Matrix of Healing: A Theory," *Alternative Therapies in Health and Medicine* 10, no. 6 (2004): 40–49.

66. D. Beck, *Spiral Dynamics Integral*. http://www.spiraldynamics.net.

67. B. A. Carper, "Fundamental Patterns of Knowing in Nursing," *Advances in Nursing Science* 1, no. 1 (1978): 13–23.

68. P. L. Munhall, "Unknowing: Toward Another Pattern of Knowing in Nursing," *Nursing Outlook* 41, no. 3 (1993): 125–128.

69. J. White, "Patterns of Knowing: Review, Critique, and Update," *Advances in Nursing Science* 17, no. 2 (1995): 73–86.

70. J. B. Averill and P. T. Clements, "Patterns of Knowing as a Foundation for Action-Sensitive Pedagogy," *Qualitative Health Research* 17, no. 3 (2007): 386–399.

71. P. L. Chinn and M. K. Kramer, *Theory and Nursing: Integrated Knowledge Development*, 6th ed. (St. Louis, MO: Mosby, 2004).

72. W. R. Cowling and E. Repede, "Unitary Appreciative Inquiry: Evolution and Refinement," *Advances in Nursing Science* 33, no. 1 (2010): 64–77.

73. M. E. Parker and M. C. Smith, "Nursing Theory and the Discipline of Nursing," eds M. E. Parker and M. C. Smith, *Nursing Theories and Nursing Practice*, 3rd ed. (Philadelphia, PA: F. A. Davis, 2010).

74. A. L. Meleis, *Theoretical Nursing: Development and Progress*, 5th ed. (Philadelphia, PA: Lippincott Williams & Wilkins, 2012).

75. M. A. Newman, "A World of No Boundaries," *Advances in Nursing Science* 26, no. 4 (2003): 240–245.

76. M. A. Burkhardt and M. G. Najai-Jacobson, "Spirituality and Health," in *Holistic Nursing: A Handbook for Practice*, 6th ed., ed. B. M. Dossey and L. Keegan (Burlington, MA: Jones & Bartlett, 2012).

77. D. McElligott "Self-Care," in *Holistic Nursing: A Handbook for Practice*, 6th ed., ed. B. M. Dossey and L. Keegan (Burlington, MA: Jones & Bartlett, 2012).

78. R. McCraty and D. Childre, "Coherence: Bridging Personal, Social, and Global Health," *Alternative Therapies in Health and Medicine* 16, no. 4 (2010): 10–24.

79. J. Koerner, *Healing: The Essence of Nursing* (New York, NY: Springer, 2011).

80. J. Halifax, B. M. Dossey, and C. H. Rushton, *Being With Dying: Compassionate End-of-Life Training Guide* (Santa Fe, NM: Prajna Mountain Press, 2007).

81. W. T. Reich, "Speaking of Suffering: A Moral Account," *Soundings* 72 (1989): 83–108.

82. L. Dossey, "Samueli Conference on Definitions and Standards in Healing Research: Working Definitions and Terms," *Alternative Therapies in Health and Medicine* 9, no. 3 (2003): A11.

83. C. Jackson, "Self-Regulate or Self-Medicate: We All Must Choose," *Holistic Nursing Practice* 24, no. 6 (2010): 317–321.

84. J. D. Levin and J. L. Reich, "Self-Reflection," in *Holistic Nursing: A Handbook for Practice*, 6th ed, eds. B. M. Dossey and L. Keegan, (Burlington, MA: Jones & Bartlett, 2012).

85. C. Jackson, "Using Loving Relationships to Transform Health Care: A Practical Approach," *Holistic Nursing Practice* 24, no. 4 (2010): 181–186.

86. D. McElligott, K. L. Capitulo, D. L. Morris, and E. R. Click, "The Effect of a Holistic Program on Health-Promoting Behaviors in Hospital Registered Nurses," *Journal of Holistic Nursing* 28, no. 3 (2010): 175–183.

87. F. Nightingale, "To the Probationer-Nurses in the Nightingale Fund School at St. Thomas's Hospital from Florence Nightingale, 16th May 1888 (Privately printed)," in *Florence Nightingale Today: Healing, Leadership, Global Action*, ed. B. M. Dossey et al. (Silver Spring, MD: NurseBooks.org, 2005): 274.

88. F. Nightingale, "Una and the Lion," Good Words, June (1868), 362, in *Florence Nightingale: Mystic, Visionary, Healer*, B. M. Dossey (Philadelphia, PA: Lippincott Williams & Wilkins, 2000): 294.

89. C. G. Jung, *The Archetypes and the Collective Unconscious*, 2nd ed., Vol. 9, Part I (Princeton, NJ: Bollingen, 1981).

90. D. Cameron, K. Leathers, and G. Schodde, *One Hill, Many Voices: Stories of Hope and Healing* (Centralia, WA: Gorham Printing, 2011).

91. J. Engebretson, "Clinically Applied Medical Ethnography: Relevance to Cultural Competence in Patient Care," *Nursing Clinics of North America* 46, no. 2 (2011): 145–154.

92. F. Nightingale, "To the Nurses and Probationers Trained Under the 'Nightingale Fund,' 1883,

Privately printed" (London: Spottiswoode), in *Florence Nightingale Today: Healing, Leadership, Global Action*, ed. B. M. Dossey et al. (Silver Spring, MD: NurseBooks.org, 2005): 267.

93. F. Nightingale, "Address from Miss Nightingale to the Probationer-Nurses in the 'Nightingale Fund' at St. Thomas's Hospital, and the Nurses Who Were Formerly Trained There, Privately Printed, 1876" (London: Spottiswoode), in *Florence Nightingale Today: Healing, Leadership, Global Action*, ed. B. M. Dossey et al. (Silver Spring, MD: NurseBooks.org, 2005): 251.

94. F. Nightingale, "To the Probationer-Nurses in the Nightingale Fund School at St. Thomas' Hospital from Florence Nightingale 16th May 1897, Privately printed," in *Florence Nightingale Today: Healing, Leadership, Global Action*, ed. B. M. Dossey et al. (Silver Spring, MD: NurseBooks.org, 2005): 283.

95. J. L. Reich, *The Anatomy of Story* (unpublished doctoral dissertation, University of Arizona College of Nursing, Tucson, AZ, 2011).

96. J. S. Perdue, *Integration of Complementary and Alternative Therapies in an Acute Rehabilitation Hospital, a Readiness Assessment* (unpublished doctoral dissertation, Western University of Health Sciences, Pomona, CA, 2011).

97. Integrative Nurse Coach Certificate Program. http://www.iNurseCoach.com

98. J. Baye, Wayfinder and Integral Life Coach. http://www.jamesbaye.com

99. L. Bark, "Holistic Coach Training for Health Practitioners," Bark Coaching Institute. http://www.barkcoaching.com/.

100. D. Pisanos, "Integral Coaching Model," personal communication, June 15, 2012.

101. O. Jarrin, "The Integrality of Situated Caring in Nursing and the Environment," *Advances in Nursing Science* 35 no. 1 (2012).

102. C. Barrere, "Teaching Future Holistic Nurses," in *Holistic Nursing: A Handbook for Practice*, 6th ed., ed. B. M. Dossey and L. Keegan (Burlington, MA: Jones & Bartlett, 2012).

103. D. R. Hess, "Curriculum for an RN to BSN Program Using the Theory of Integral Nursing," personal communication, September 20, 2012.

104. C. Jackson, "Evidence-Based Practice: Pushback from a Holistic Perspective," *Holistic Nursing Practice* 24, no. 3 (2010): 120–124.

105. S. Esbjorn-Hargens, "Integral Research: A Multi-Method Approach to Investigating Phenomena," *Constructivism in the Human Sciences* 11, no. 1 (2006): 79–107.

106. R. P. Zahourek and D. M. Larkin, "Consciousness, Intentionality, and Community," *Nursing Science Quarterly* 22, no. 1 (2009): 15–22.

107. J. Kreisberg, personal communication, August 25, 2011.

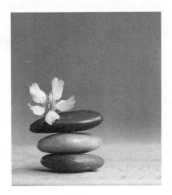

Holistic Nursing: Scope and Standards of Practice

Carla Mariano

Nurse Healer
OBJECTIVES

Theoretical

- Describe the scope of holistic nursing.
- Describe the standards of holistic nursing.
- Discuss the five core values of holistic nursing.

Clinical

- Integrate the principles of holistic nursing into practice.
- Identify how you implement the standards of holistic nursing in your practice.
- Discuss *Holistic Nursing: Scope and Standards of Practice* with colleagues.

Personal

- Reflect on your worldview and how it is similar to or different from the philosophy of holism.
- Explore how the concepts of holistic nursing apply to your personal life.

This chapter is derived from *Holistic Nursing: Scope and Standards of Practice* (2007), C. Mariano, primary contributor. Printed with permission of the American Holistic Nurses Association (AHNA) and American Nurses Association (ANA).

DEFINITIONS*

Allopathic/conventional therapies: Medical, surgical, pharmacological, and invasive and noninvasive diagnostic procedures; those interventions most commonly used in allopathic, Western medicine.

Complementary/alternative modalities (CAM): A broad set of healthcare practices, therapies, and modalities that address the whole person—body, mind, emotion, spirit, and environment, not just signs and symptoms—and that may replace or be used as complements to conventional Western medical, surgical, and pharmacological treatments.

Critical thinking: An active, purposeful, organized cognitive process involving creativity, reflection, problem solving, both rational and intuitive judgment, an attitude of inquiry, and a philosophical orientation toward thinking about thinking.

Cultural competence: The ability to deliver health care with knowledge of and sensitivity to cultural factors that influence the health behavior and the curing, healing, dying, and grieving processes of the person.

---

* Many of the definitions in this chapter were adapted from *Holistic Nursing: Scope and Standards of Practice*, 2007, with permission, and from Dossey & Keegan, 2009.

Environment: The context of habitat within which all living systems participate and interact, including the physical body and its physical habitat along with the cultural, psychological, social, and historical influences; includes both the external physical space and the person's internal physical, mental, emotional, social, and spiritual experience.

Evidence-based practice: The process by which integrative healthcare practitioners make clinical decisions using the best integrative philosophy and theories, research evidence, clinical expertise, and patient preferences within the context of available resources.

Healing: A lifelong journey into wholeness, seeking harmony and balance in one's own life and in family, community, and global relations. Healing involves those physical, mental, social, and spiritual processes of recovery, repair, renewal, and transformation that increase wholeness and often (though not invariably) order and coherence. Healing is an emergent process of the whole system bringing together aspects of one's self and the body, mind, emotion, spirit, and environment at deeper levels of inner knowing, leading toward integration and balance, with each aspect having equal importance and value. Healing can lead to more complex levels of personal understanding and meaning and may be synchronous but not synonymous with curing.

Healing process: A continual journey of change and the evolving of one's self through life that is characterized by the awareness of patterns that support or that are challenges or barriers to health and healing and that may be done alone or in a healing community.

Healing relationships: The quality and characteristics of interactions between one who facilitates healing and the person in the process of healing. Characteristics of such interactions involve empathy, caring, love, warmth, trust, confidence, credibility, competence, honesty, courtesy, respect, sharing expectations, and good communication.

Healing system: A true healthcare system in which people can receive adequate, non-toxic, and noninvasive assistance in maintaining wellness and healing for body, mind, emotion, and spirit, together with the most sophisticated, aggressive curing technologies available.

Health: An individually defined state or process in which the individual (nurse, client, family, group, or community) experiences a sense of well-being, harmony, and unity such that subjective experiences about health, health beliefs, and values are honored; a process of becoming an expanding consciousness.

Health promotion: Activities and preventive measures to promote health, increase well-being, and actualize the human potential of people, families, communities, society, and ecology; such activities and measures include immunizations, fitness and exercise programs, breast self-exam, appropriate nutrition, relaxation, stress management, social support, prayer, meditation, healing rituals, cultural practices, and promoting environmental health and safety.

Holistic communication: A free flow of verbal and nonverbal interchange between and among people and significant beings such as pets, nature, and God/Life Force/Absolute/Transcendent that explores meaning and ideas leading to mutual understanding and growth.

Holistic ethics: The basic underlying concept of the unity and integral wholeness of all people and of all nature, identified and pursued by finding unity and wholeness within the self and within humanity. In this framework, acts are not performed for the sake of law, precedent, or social norms, but rather from a desire to do good freely to witness, identify, and contribute to unity.

Holistic healing: A form of healing based on attention to all aspects of an individual—physical, mental, emotional, sexual, cultural, social, and spiritual.

Holistic nurse: A nurse who recognizes and integrates body-mind-emotion-spirit-environment principles and modalities in daily life and clinical practice, creates a caring healing space within herself or himself that allows the nurse to be an instrument of healing, shares authenticity of unconditional presence that helps to remove the barriers to the healing process, facilitates another person's growth (body-mind-emotion-spirit-energetic-environment connections), and assists with recovery from illness or transition to peaceful death.

Holistic nursing practice process: An iterative and integrative process that involves six steps that can occur simultaneously: (1) assessing; (2) diagnosing or identifying patterns, challenges, needs, and health issues; (3) identifying outcomes; (4) planning care; (5) implementing the plan of care; and (6) evaluating.

Honor: An act or intention indicating the holding of self or another in high respect, esteem, and dignity, including valuing and accepting the humanity of people with regard for the decisions and wishes of another.

Human caring: The moral ideal of nursing in which the nurse brings one's whole self into a relationship with the whole self of the person being cared for to protect that person's vulnerability, preserve her or his humanity and dignity, and reinforce the meaning and experience of oneness and unity.

Human health experience: That totality of human experience including each person's subjective experience about health, health beliefs, values, sexual orientation, and personal preferences that encompasses health-wellness-disease-illness-death.

Illness: A subjective experience of symptoms and suffering to which the individual ascribes meaning and significance; not synonymous with disease; a shift in the homeodynamic balance of the person.

Intention: The conscious awareness of being in the present moment to help facilitate the healing process; a volitional act of love.

Interdisciplinary: Conversation or collaboration across disciplines where knowledge is shared that informs learning, practice, education, and research; it includes individuals, families, community members, and various disciplines.

Meaning: That which is signified, indicated, referred to, or understood. More specifi-cally: Philosophical meaning is meaning that depends on the symbolic connections that are grasped by reason. Psychological meaning is meaning that depends on connections that are experienced through intuition or insight.

Patient-centered care: Care that is respectful of and responsive to individual patient preferences, needs, and values, and that ensures that patient values guide all clinical decisions. Patient-centered care encompasses identifying, respecting, and caring about patients' differences, values, preferences, and expressed needs; relieving pain and suffering; coordinating continuous care/listening to, clearly informing, communicating with, and educating patients; sharing decision making and management; and continuously advocating disease prevention, wellness, and promotion of healthy lifestyles, including a focus on population health.[1]

Person: An individual, client, patient, family member, support person, or community member who has the opportunity to engage in interaction with a holistic nurse.

Person-centered care: The human caring process in which the holistic nurse gives full attention and intention to the whole self of a person, not merely the current presenting symptoms, illness, crisis, or tasks to be accomplished, and that also includes reinforcing the person's meaning and experience of oneness and unity; the condition of trust that is created in which holistic care can be given and received.

Presence: The essential state or core of healing; approaching an individual in a way that respects and honors her or his essence; relating in a way that reflects a quality of being with and in collaboration with rather than doing to; entering into a shared experience (or field of consciousness) that promotes healing potential and an experience of well-being.

Relationship-centered care: A process model of caregiving that is based in a vision of community where three types of relationships are identified: (1) patient–practitioner relationship, (2) community–practitioner relationship, and (3) practitioner–practitioner relationship.

Each of these interrelated relationships is essential within a reformed integrative healthcare delivery system in a hospital, clinic, community, or in the home. Each component involves a unique set of responsibilities and tasks that addresses the three areas of knowledge, values, and skills.[2]

Spirituality: The feelings, thoughts, experiences, and behaviors that arise from a search for meaning; that which is generally considered sacred or holy; usually, though not universally, considered to involve a sense of connection with an absolute, imminent, or transcendent spiritual force, however named, as well as the conviction that meaning, value, direction, and purpose are valid aspects of the individual and universe; the essence of being and relatedness that permeates all of life and is manifested in one's knowing, doing, and being; the interconnectedness with self, others, nature, and God/Life Force/Absolute/Transcendent; not necessarily synonymous with religion.

Transpersonal: A personal understanding that is based on one's experiences of temporarily transcending or moving beyond one's usual identification with the limited biological, historical, cultural, and personal self at the deepest and most profound levels of experience possible; that which transcends the limits and boundaries of individual ego identities and possibilities to include acknowledgment and appreciation of something greater. From this perspective the ordinary, biological, historical, cultural, and personal self is seen as an important, but only a partial, manifestation or expression of this much greater something that is one's deeper origin and destination.

Wellness: Integrated, congruent functioning aimed toward reaching one's highest potential.

■ SCOPE AND STANDARDS OF HOLISTIC NURSING PRACTICE

Extraordinary changes have occurred in health care and nursing during the past decade. During this time, holistic nurses recognized that not only

were they practicing a unique specialty within nursing, but that they needed to develop and publish standards of practice to document and define that specialty practice. Holistic nursing was officially recognized as a distinct specialty within the discipline of Nursing by the American Nurses Association (ANA) in November 2006. The American Holistic Nurses Association (AHNA) *Holistic Nursing: Scope and Standards of Practice* (2007) was written to inform holistic nurses, the nursing profession, students and faculty, other healthcare providers and disciplines, employers, third-party payers, legislators, and the public about the unique scope of knowledge and the standards of practice and professional performance of a holistic nurse.[3] The current standards are an updated and substantive revision of previous standards disseminated through the AHNA.* See Appendix 2-1 for development of the original *Holistic Standards of Practice: Basic and Graduate*, and see Appendix 2-2 for select works of individuals and AHNA documents.

Function of the Scope of Practice Statement of Holistic Nursing

The scope of practice statement describes the who, what, where, when, why, and how of the practice of holistic nursing.[3,4] The answers to these questions provide a picture of that specialty nursing practice, its boundaries, and its membership.

Nursing: Scope and Standards of Practice, 2nd ed. (2010) applies to all professional registered nurses (RNs) engaged in practice, regardless of specialty, practice setting, or educational preparation.[4] With the *Guide to the Code of Ethics for Nurses: Interpretation and Application*[5] and *Nursing's Social Policy Statement: The Essence of the Profession*,[6] it forms the foundation of practice for all registered nurses. The scope of holistic nursing practice is specific to this specialty, but it builds on the scope of practice expected of all registered nurses.

---

* To obtain a complete copy of *Holistic Nursing: Scope and Standards of Practice* (2007) or most recent copy, contact the American Holistic Nurses Association (AHNA), 323 N. San Francisco Street, Suite 201, Flagstaff, AZ 86001; 1-800-278-2462 or 1-928-526-2196; www.ahna.org or www.info@ahna.org.

Function of the Standards of Holistic Nursing

"The Standards of Professional Nursing Practice are authoritative statements of the duties that all registered nurses, regardless of role, population, or specialty, are expected to perform competently."[4, p.2]

> Standards reflect the values and priorities of the profession. Standards provide direction for professional nursing practice and a framework for evaluation of this practice. Written in measurable terms, these standards define the nursing profession's accountability to the public and the outcomes for which registered nurses are responsible.[7, p.1]

The standards of holistic nursing practice are specific to this specialty but build on the standards of practice expected of all registered nurses. *Holistic Nursing: Scope and Standards of Practice* (2007) presents a differentiation between practice at the basic and advanced practice levels. The *Scope and Standards* are organized according to the criteria ANA uses in recognizing a nursing specialty area and build on nursing knowledge, skills, and competencies required for licensure.[8,9] *Holistic Nursing: Scope and Standards of Practice* (2007) provides a blueprint for holistic practice, education, and research. The standards guide clinicians, educators, researchers, nurse managers, and administrators in professional activities, knowledge, and performance that are relevant to holistic nursing basic and advanced practice, education, research, and management. Because holistic nursing emphasizes that human experiences are subjectively described and that health and illness are determined by the view of the individual, *Holistic Nursing: Scope and Standards of Practice* (2007) is derived from values that are central to the specialty and are consistent with the philosophies and theories of holism.

Evolution of Holistic Nursing

Holism in health care is a philosophy that emanates directly from Florence Nightingale, who believed in care that focused on unity, wellness, and the interrelationship of human beings, events, and environment. Even Hippocrates, the father of Western medicine, espoused a holistic orientation when he taught doctors to observe their patients' life circumstances and emotional states. Socrates stated, "Curing the soul; that is the first thing." In holism, symptoms are believed to be an expression of the body's wisdom as it reacts to cure its own imbalance or disease.

The root of the word *heal* comes from the Greek word *halos* and the Anglo-Saxon word *healan*, which means "to be or to become whole." The word *holy* also comes from the same source. Healing means "making whole"—or restoring balance and harmony. It is movement toward a sense of wholeness and completion. Healing, therefore, is the integration of the totality of the person in body, mind, emotion, spirit, and environment.

One of the driving forces behind the holistic nursing movement in the United States was the formation of the AHNA. In 1981, founder Charlotte McGuire and 75 founding members began the national organization in Houston, Texas. The national office is now located in Flagstaff, Arizona. The AHNA's mission is to advance the philosophy and practices of holistic nursing and unite nurses in healing with a focus on holistic principles of health, preventive education, and the integration of allopathic and complementary caring and healing modalities to facilitate care of the whole person and significant others. From its inception in 1981, the AHNA has been the leader in developing and advancing holistic principles, practices, and guidelines. The association predicted that holistic principles, caring and healing, and the integration of complementary and alternative therapies would emerge into mainstream health care.

The AHNA, the definitive voice for holistic nursing, has as its vision "a world in which nursing nurtures wholeness and inspires peace and healing." The mission of the AHNA is to advance holistic nursing through community building, advocacy, research, and education. It is committed to promoting wholeness and wellness in individuals, families, communities, nurses themselves, the nursing profession, and the environment. Through its various activities, AHNA provides vision, direction, and leadership in the advancement of holistic nursing; integrates the art and science of nursing in the profession; empowers holistic nursing through education, research, and standards; encourages nurses to be models of wellness; honors individual excellence in the advancement of holistic nursing; and influences policy to change the healthcare system to a more humanistic orientation.

The goals and endeavors of AHNA have continued to map conceptual frameworks and the blueprint for holistic nursing practice, education, and research, which is the most complete way to conceptualize and practice professional nursing. Beginning in 1993, AHNA undertook an organization development process that included the following areas:

- Identifying the steps toward national certification in 1993–1994.
- Revising the 1990 Standards of Holistic Nursing Practice, completed in 1995.
- Completing a role delineation study, the Inventory of Professional Activities and Knowledge Statements of a Holistic Nurse (also known as the IPAKHN Survey) in 1997.
- Developing a national holistic nursing certification examination, completed in 1997.
- Completing major revisions of the 1995 Standards of Holistic Nursing Practice in 1999, with additional editorial changes in January 2000 and 2005.
- Developing a core curriculum for basic holistic nursing based on the basic standards (1997).
- Approving and adopting Standards of Advanced Holistic Nursing Practice for Graduate-Prepared Nurses (2002, revised 2005).
- Developing a core curriculum for advanced holistic nursing based on the advanced standards (2003). The American Holistic Nurses Certification Corporation (AHNCC) then developed the Certification Exam for Advanced Holistic Nursing Practice first offered in 2005.
- Revising both the basic and advanced Standards of Holistic Nursing Practice to meet ANA criteria for recognition of holistic nursing as a specialty (2006, 2007).

■ SCOPE OF HOLISTIC NURSING

Holistic nursing is defined as "all nursing practice that has healing the whole person as its goal."[10] Holistic nursing is a specialty practice that draws on nursing knowledge, theories of nursing and wholeness, expertise and intuition to guide nurses in becoming therapeutic partners with people in strengthening human responses to facilitate the healing process and achieve wholeness. Holistic nursing focuses on protecting, promoting, and optimizing health and wellness; assisting healing; preventing illness and injury; alleviating suffering; and supporting people to find peace, comfort, harmony, and balance through the diagnosis and treatment of human response.

Holistic nursing care is healing oriented and centered on the relationship with the person in contrast to an orientation toward diseases and their cures. Holistic nursing emphasizes practices of self-care, intentionality, presence, mindfulness, and therapeutic use of self as pivotal for facilitation of healing and patterning of wellness in others. In some sense, all nursing practice can be comprehensive, that is, all nursing practice may have a biopsychosocial perspective. What makes holistic nursing practice a specialty is that there is a philosophy, a body of knowledge, and an advanced set of nursing skills applied to practice that recognize the totality of the human being and the interconnectedness of body, mind, emotion, spirit, energy, society, culture, relationships, context, and environment. Philosophically, holistic nursing is a worldview, a way of being in the world, not just a modality. This philosophy honors the unique humanness of all people regardless of who and what they are. Knowledge for holistic nursing practice derives not only from nursing, but from theories of wholeness, energy, and unity as well as from other healing systems and approaches. Holistic nurses incorporate both conventional nursing and complementary/alternative/integrative modalities (CAM) and interventions into practice.

Through unconditional presence and intention, holistic nurses create environments conducive to healing, using techniques that promote empowerment, peace, comfort, and a subjective sense of harmony and well-being for the person. The holistic nurse acts in partnership with the individual or family in providing options and alternatives regarding health and treatment. Additionally, the holistic nurse assists the person to find meaning in the health and illness experience.

Holistic nursing focuses on simultaneously integrating as an iterative process all of these realms: a philosophy of being and living, using theories of nursing and wholeness with related knowledge and skills, focusing on the unity and totality of humans, incorporating healing approaches, creating healing environments, partnering with and empowering individuals, and assisting in the exploration of meaning in the care of people. In holistic nursing, the nurse is the facilitator of healing, honoring that the person heals him- or herself. The holistic nurse assists individuals in identifying themselves as the healer and accessing their own innate healing capacities.

The practice of holistic nursing requires nurses to integrate self-care and self-responsibility into their own lives and to serve as role models for others. Holistic nurses strive for an awareness of the interconnectedness of individuals to the human and global community. Thus, holistic nurses also attend to the health of the ecosystem.

Holistic nurses are instruments of healing and facilitators in the healing process. They honor the individual's subjective experience of health, health beliefs, and values. To become therapeutic partners with individuals, families, communities, and populations, holistic nurses draw on nursing knowledge, theories, research, expertise, intuition, and creativity, incorporating the roles of clinician, educator, consultant, coach, partner, role model, and advocate. Holistic nursing

practice encourages peer review of professional practice in various clinical settings and provides care based on current professional standards, laws, and regulations that govern nursing practice. The major phenomena of concern to holistic nursing are listed in **Table 2-1**.

The Core Values of Holistic Nursing: Integrating and the Art and Science of Nursing

Holistic nursing emanates from five core values summarizing the ideals and principles of the specialty. These core values are listed here and then are discussed:

1. Philosophy, Theory, and Ethics
2. Holistic Caring Process
3. Holistic Communication, Therapeutic Environment, and Cultural Diversity
4. Holistic Education and Research
5. Holistic Nurse Self-Care

Core Value 1: Holistic Philosophy, Theory, and Ethics

Holistic nurses (HNs) recognize the human health experience as a complicated, dynamic relationship of health, illness, and wellness, and they value healing as the desired outcome of the practice of nursing. Their practice is based on scientific foundations (theory, research, evidence-based practice, critical thinking, reflection) and

---

TABLE 2-1   Phenomena of Concern to Holistic Nursing

- The caring–healing relationship
- The subjective experience of and meanings ascribed to health, illness, wellness, healing, birth, growth and development, and dying
- The cultural values and beliefs and folk practices of health, illness, and healing
- Spirituality in nursing care
- The evaluation of complementary/alternative modalities used in nursing practice
- Comprehensive health promotion and disease prevention
- Self-care processes
- Physical, mental, emotional, and spiritual comfort, discomfort, and pain
- Empowerment, decision making, and the ability to make informed choices
- Social and economic policies and their effects on the health of individuals, families, and communities
- Diverse and alternative healthcare systems and their relationships with access and quality of health care
- The environment and the prevention of disease

art (relationship, communication, creativity, presence, caring). Holistic nursing is grounded in nursing knowledge and skill and guided by nursing theory. Florence Nightingale's writings are often referenced as a significant precursor of the development of holistic nursing. Although each holistic nurse chooses which nursing theory to apply in any individual case, the nursing theories of Jean Watson (the Theory of Human Caring), Martha Rogers (the Science of Unitary Human Beings), Margaret Newman (Health as Expanding Consciousness), Madeleine Leininger (Theory of Cultural Care), Rosemarie Rizzo Parse (Theory of Human Becoming), Josephine Paterson and Loretta Zderad (Humanistic Nursing Theory), and Helen Erickson (Modeling and Role-Modeling) are most frequently used to support holistic nursing practice.

In addition to nursing theory, holistic nurses use other theories and perspectives of wholeness and healing to guide their practice. These scientific theories and philosophies present a worldview of connectedness. Examples include the following:

- Theories of Consciousness
- Energy Field Theory
- C. Pribram's Holographic Universe
- D. Bohm's Implicate/Explicate Order
- C. Pert's Psychoneuroimmunology
- K. Wilber's Integral Vision and Unified Field Theory of Consciousness
- Spirituality
- Alternative medical systems such as Traditional Oriental Medicine, Ayurveda, Native American, and indigenous healing
- Eastern contemplative orientations such as Zen Buddhism and Taoism

Holistic nurses further recognize and honor the ethic that the person is the authority on his or her own health experience. The holistic nurse is an "option giver" and helps the person develop an understanding of alternatives and implications of various health and treatment options. The holistic nurse first ascertains what the individual thinks or believes is happening to him/her, and then assists the person to identify what will help the situation. The assessment begins from where the individual is. The holistic nurse then discusses options, including the person's choices across a continuum and the possible effects and implications of each. For instance, if a person diagnosed with cancer is experiencing nausea caused by chemotherapy, the individual and nurse may discuss the choices and effects of pharmacologic agents, imagery, homeopathic remedies, and so on, or a combination of these. The holistic nurse acts as partner and coprescriber versus sole prescriber. The relationship is a copiloting of the individual's health experience where the nurse respects the person's decision about his or her own health. It is a process of engagement versus compliance.

Client narratives, whether they arise from individuals, families, or communities, provide the context of the experiences and are used as an important focus in understanding the person's situation. Holistic nurses hold the belief that people, through their inherent capacities, heal themselves. Therefore, the holistic nurse is not the healer but the guide and facilitator of the individual's own healing.

In the belief that all things are connected, the holistic perspective espouses that an individual's actions have a ripple effect throughout humanity. Holism places the greatest worth on individuals' developing higher levels of human awareness. This, in turn, elevates the whole of humanity. Holistic nurses believe in the sacredness of one's self and of all nature. One's inner self and the collective greater self have stewardship not only over one's body, mind, and spirit but also the planet. Holistic nurses focus on the meaning and quality of life deriving from their own character and from their relationship to the universe rather than that imposed from without.

Holistic nurses hold to a professional ethic of caring and healing that seeks to preserve the wholeness and dignity of the self and others. They support human dignity by advocating and adhering to the Patient Bill of Rights,[11] the *ANA Guide to the Code of Ethics for Nurses: Interpretation and Application*,[5] and the AHNA Position Statement on Holistic Nursing Ethics.[12]

Core Value 2: Caring Process

Holistic nurses provide care that recognizes the totality of the human being (the interconnectedness of body, mind, emotion, spirit, society, culture, relationships, context, and environment).

This is an integrated as well as comprehensive approach. Although physical symptoms are treated, holistic nurses also focus on how the individual cognitively perceives and emotionally deals with the illness; the illness's effect on the person's family, social relationships, and economic resources; the person's values and cultural and spiritual beliefs and preferences regarding treatment; and the meaning of this experience to the person's life. In addition, holistic nurses may also incorporate a number of modalities (e.g., cognitive restructuring, stress management, visualization, aromatherapy, therapeutic touch) with conventional nursing interventions. Holistic nurses focus on care interventions that promote healing, peace, comfort, and a subjective sense of well-being for the person.

The holistic caring process involves six often simultaneously occurring steps: assessment, diagnosis (pattern, problem, need identification), outcomes, therapeutic plan of care, implementation, and evaluation. Holistic nurses apply the holistic caring process in all settings with individuals and families across the life span, population groups, and communities.

Holistic nurses incorporate a variety of roles in their practice, including expert clinician and facilitator of healing; consultant, coach, and collaborator; educator and guide; administrator, leader, and change agent; researcher; and advocate. Holistic nurses strongly emphasize partnership with individuals throughout the entire decision-making process. Holistic assessments include not only physical, functional, psychosocial, mental, emotional, cultural, and sexual aspects, but also the spiritual, transpersonal, and energy field assessments of the whole person. Energy assessments are based on the concept that all beings are composed of energy. Congestion or stagnation of energy in any realm creates disharmony and disease. Spiritual assessments glean not only religious beliefs and practices but query a person's meaning and purpose in life and how these may have changed because of the present health experience. Spiritual assessments also include questions about an individual's sense of serenity and peace, what provides joy and fulfillment, and the source of strength and hope.

Holistic assessment data are interpreted into patterns, challenges, and needs from which meaning and understanding of the health and disease experience can be mutually identified with the person. Holistic nurses first ask an individual, "What do you think is going on (happening) with you?" and then, "What do you think would help?" Another important responsibility of the holistic nurse is to help the person identify risk factors such as lifestyle, habits, beliefs and values, personal and family health history, and age-related conditions that influence health, and then to find and use opportunities to increase well-being. The focus is on the individual's goals, not the nurse's.

Therapeutic plans of care respect the person's experience and the uniqueness of each healing journey. The same illness may have very different manifestations in different individuals. A major aspect of holistic nursing practice, in addition to competence, is intention. That is, the nurse intends for the wholeness, well-being, and highest good of the person in every encounter and intervention. This intention honors and reinforces the innate capacity of people to heal themselves. Therefore, holistic nurses respect that outcomes may not be those expected and may evolve differently based on the person's individual healing process and health choices. Holistic nurses endeavor to detach themselves from the outcomes. The nurse does not produce the outcomes; the individual's own healing process produces the outcomes, and the nurse facilitates this process. A significant focus of the holistic nurse is on guiding individuals and significant others to use their inner strength and resources through the course of healing.

Holistic nurses consistently provide appropriate and evidence-based information (including current knowledge, practice, and research) regarding the health condition and various treatments and therapies and their side effects. Holistic care always occurs within the scope and standards of practice of registered nursing and in accordance with state and federal laws and regulations.

Holistic nurses integrate complementary/alternative modalities (CAM) into clinical practice to treat people's physiologic, psychological, and spiritual needs. Doing so does not negate the validity of conventional medical therapies but serves to complement, broaden, and enrich the scope of nursing practice and to help individuals access their greatest healing potential. Holistic nurses advocate for integration rather than separation. The National Center for Complementary and Alternative Medicine has categorized CAM approaches and these are identified in **Table 2-2**.

Therapies frequently incorporated in holistic nursing practice include the following interventions: meditation; relaxation therapy; breath work; music, art, and aroma therapies; energy-based touch therapies such as therapeutic touch, healing touch, and Reiki; acupressure; massage; guided imagery; hypnotherapy; animal-assisted therapy; biofeedback; prayer; reflexology; diet;

TABLE 2-2   Categories of Complementary/Alternative Modalities (CAM) Therapies

In the context of this chapter, these descriptive categories encompass generally, but not exhaustively, those therapies described as alternative or complementary.

Natural products. This area includes substances found in nature such as a variety of herbal medicines (also known as botanicals), vitamins, minerals, whole diet therapies, and other "natural products." Many are sold over the counter as dietary supplements. (Some uses of dietary supplements—e.g., taking a multivitamin to meet minimum daily nutritional requirements or taking calcium to promote bone health—are not thought of as CAM.) CAM "natural products" also include probiotics—live microorganisms (usually bacteria) that are similar to microorganisms normally found in the human digestive tract and that may have beneficial effects. Probiotics are available in foods (e.g., yogurts) or as dietary supplements.

Mind–body medicine. Mind–body practices focus on the interactions among the brain, mind, body, and behavior, with the intent to use the mind to affect physical functioning and promote health. Many CAM practices embody this concept—in different ways. Some techniques that were considered CAM in the past have become mainstream (for example, patient support groups, psychotherapy, cognitive-behavioral therapy). Mind–body techniques include meditation, relaxation, imagery, hypnotherapy, yoga, biofeedback, and Tai Chi. Other therapies are autogenic training, spirituality, prayer, mental healing, and therapies that use creative outlets such as art, music, dance, or journaling. Acupuncture is considered to be a part of mind–body medicine, but it is also a component of energy medicine, manipulative and body-based practices, and traditional Chinese medicine.

Manipulative and body-based practices. Manipulative and body-based practices focus primarily on the structures and systems of the body, including the bones and joints, soft tissues, and circulatory and lymphatic systems. Two commonly used therapies fall within this category: spinal manipulation including Chiropractic or osteopathic manipulation, and massage.

Movement therapies. CAM also encompasses movement therapies—a broad range of Eastern and Western movement-based approaches used to promote physical, mental, emotional, and spiritual well-being. Examples include Feldenkrais method, Alexander technique, Pilates, Rolfing Structural Integration, and Trager psychophysical integration.

Practices of traditional healers. Traditional healers use methods based on indigenous theories, beliefs, and experiences handed down from generation to generation. Examples include Native American healer/medicine man, African, Middle Eastern, Tibetan, Central and South American, and Curanderismo.

Energy therapies. Some CAM practices involve manipulation of various energy fields to affect health. Such fields may be characterized as veritable (measurable) or putative (yet to be measured). Practices based on veritable forms of energy include those involving electromagnetic fields (e.g., magnet therapy, light therapy, or alternating-current or direct-current fields). Practices based on putative energy fields (also called biofields) generally reflect the concept that human beings are infused with subtle forms of energy. Some forms of energy therapy manipulate biofields by applying pressure, such as acupressure and manipulating the body by placing the hands in or through these fields. Examples include Gong, Reiki, therapeutic touch, and healing touch.

Whole medical systems. Complete systems of theory and practice that have evolved over time in different cultures and apart from conventional or Western medicine, may be considered CAM. Examples of ancient whole medical systems include Ayurvedic medicine and Traditional Chinese medicine. More modern systems that have developed in the past few centuries include Homeopathy and Naturopathy.

Source: National Center for Complementary and Alternative Medicine, National Institutes of Health (2011); http://nccam.nih.gov.

herbology; and homeopathy. Other interventions frequently employed in holistic nursing practice in addition to conventional nursing interventions include anxiety reduction and stress management, calming techniques, emotional support, exercise and nutrition promotion, smoking cessation, patient contracting, resiliency promotion, forgiveness facilitation, hope installation, presence, journaling, counseling, cognitive therapy, self-help, spiritual support, and environmental management.

Because many of today's healthcare problems are stress related, holistic nurses empower individuals by teaching them techniques to reduce their stress. Many interventions used in holistic nursing elicit the relaxation response (e.g., breath work, meditation, relaxation, imagery, aromatherapy and essential oils, and diet). People can learn these therapies and use them without the intervention of a healthcare provider. This allows people to take an active role in the management of their own health care. Holistic nurses also can teach families and caregivers to use these techniques for loved ones who may be ill (e.g., simple foot or hand massage for older clients with dementia). In addition, individuals are taught how to evaluate their own responses to these modalities.

Holistic nurses prescribe as legally authorized. They instruct individuals regarding drug, herbal, and homeopathic regimens, and, just as important, they consult on the side effects and interactions between medications and herbs. They consult, collaborate, and refer, as necessary, to both conventional allopathic providers and to holistic practitioners. They provide information and counseling to people about alternative, complementary, integrative, and conventional healthcare practices. Very important, holistic nurses facilitate negotiation of services as they guide individuals and families between conventional Western medicine and alternative systems. Holistic nurses, in partnership with the individual and others, evaluate whether care is effective and whether changes in the meaning of the health experience occur for the individual.

Core Value 3: Holistic Communication, Therapeutic Environment, and Cultural Diversity

The holistic nurse's communication ensures that each individual experiences the presence of the nurse as authentic, caring, compassionate, and sincere. This is more than offering therapeutic techniques such as responding, reflecting, summarizing, and so on. This is deep listening, or as some say "listening with the heart and not just the ears." It is done with conscious intention and without preconceptions, busy-ness, distractions, or analysis. It takes place in the "now" within an atmosphere of shared humanness—human being to human being. Through presence or "being with in the moment," holistic nurses provide each person with an interpersonal encounter that the individual can experience as a connection with one who is giving undivided attention to his or her needs and concerns. Using unconditional positive regard, holistic nurses convey to the individual receiving care the belief in his or her worth and value as a human being, not solely as a recipient of medical and nursing interventions.

The holistic nurse recognizes the importance of context in understanding the person's health experience. Space and time are allowed for exploration. Each person's health encounter is truly seen as unique and may be contrary to conventional knowledge and treatments. Therefore, the holistic nurse must be comfortable with ambiguity, paradox, and uncertainty. This requires a perspective that the nurse is not "the expert" regarding another's health and illness experience but is actually a "learner."

Holistic nurses have a knowledge base of the use and meanings of symbolic language and use interventions such as imagery, creation of sacred space and personal rituals, dream exploration, and aesthetic therapies such as music, visual arts, and dance. They encourage and support others in the use of prayer, meditation, and other spiritual and symbolic practices for healing purposes.

A cornerstone of holistic nursing practice is assisting individuals to find meaning in their experience. Regardless of the person's condition, the meaning that individuals ascribe to their situation can influence their response to it. Holistic nurses attend to the subjective world of the individual. They consider meanings such as the person's concerns in relation to health and family economics, as well as deeper meanings related to the person's purpose in life. Regardless of the technology or treatment, holistic nurses address the human spirit as a major force in healing. Each person's perception of meaning is related to all factors in health-wellness-disease-illness.

Holistic nurses realize that suffering, illness, and disease are natural components of the human condition and have the potential to teach us about ourselves, our relationships, and our universe. Every experience is valued for its meaning and lesson.

Holistic nurses have a particular obligation to create a therapeutic environment that values holism, caring, social support, and integration of conventional and CAM approaches to healing. They seek to create environments where individuals, both clients and staff, feel connected, supported, and respected. A particular perspective of holistic nursing is the nurse as the "healing environment" and "an instrument of healing." Holistic nurses shape the physical environment (e.g., light, fresh air, pleasant sounds or quiet, neatness and order, healing smells, earth elements). And they provide a relationship-focused environment by creating sacred space through presence and intention where another can feel safe, can unfold, and can explore the dimensions of self in healing.

Culture, beliefs, and values are inherent components of a holistic approach. Concepts of health and healing are based in culture and often influence people's actions to promote, maintain, and restore health. Culture also may provide an understanding of a person's concept of illness or disease and appropriate treatment. Holistic nurses possess knowledge and understanding of numerous cultural traditions and healthcare practices from various racial, ethnic, and social backgrounds. However, holistic nurses honor the individual's understanding and articulation of his or her own cultural values, beliefs, and health practices rather than relying on stereotypical cultural classifications and descriptions. The nurse then uses these understandings to provide culturally competent care that corresponds with the beliefs, values, traditions, and health practices of people. Holistic nurses ask individuals, "What do I need to know about you culturally in caring for you?"

Holistic healing is a collaborative approach. Holistic nurses take an active role in trying to remove the political and financial barriers to the inclusion of holistic care in the healthcare system. Of particular importance to holistic nurses is the human connection with the ecology.

Holistic nurses actively participate in building an ecosystem that sustains the well-being of all life. This includes raising the public's consciousness about environmental issues and stressors that affect not only the health of people but the health of the planet.

Core Value 4: Holistic Education and Research

Holistic nurses possess an understanding of a wide range of norms and healthcare practices, beliefs, and values concerning individuals, families, groups, and communities from a variety of racial, ethnic, spiritual, and social backgrounds. This rich knowledge base reflects their formal academic and continuing education preparation. Their knowledge also includes a wide diversity of practices and modalities outside of conventional Western medicine. Because of this, holistic nurses have a significant impact on people's understanding of healthcare options and alternatives, thus serving as both educators and advocates.

Additionally, holistic nurses provide much needed information to individuals on health promotion including such topics as healthy lifestyles, risk-reducing behaviors, preventive self-care, stress management, living with changes secondary to illness and treatment, and opportunities to enhance well-being.

Holistic nurses value all the ways of knowing and learning. They individualize learning and appreciate that science, intuition, introspection, creativity, aesthetics, and culture produce different bodies of knowledge and perspectives. They help others to know themselves and access their inner wisdom to enhance growth, wholeness, and well-being.

Holistic nurses often guide individuals and families in their healthcare decisions, especially regarding conventional allopathic and complementary/alternative practices. Therefore, holistic nurses must be knowledgeable about the best evidence available for both conventional and CAM therapies. In addition to developing evidence-based practice using research, practice guidelines, and expertise, holistic nurses strongly consider the person's values and healthcare practices and beliefs in practice decisions.

Holistic nurses look at alternative philosophies of science and research methods that are compatible with investigations of humanistic and holistic occurrences, that explore the context in which phenomena occur and the meaning of patterns that evolve, and that take into consideration the interactive nature of the body, mind, emotion, spirit, and environment.

Holistic nurses conduct and evaluate research in such diverse areas as follows:

- Outcome measures of holistic therapies such as therapeutic touch, prayer, and aromatherapy
- Instrument development to measure caring behaviors and dimensions; spirituality; self-transcendence; cultural competence, and so forth
- Client responses to holistic interventions in health and illness
- Explorations of clients' lived experiences with various health/illness phenomena
- Theory development in healing, caring, intentionality, cultural constructions, empowerment, and so forth

Further, research that advances the work of holistic nursing theories (Watson, Rogers, Newman, Parse, Erickson, and Leninger) helps to build the knowledge base of nursing and advance the nursing science of holism. The AHNA has incorporated an active research agenda by assisting and mentoring members in research endeavors, granting research awards, identifying and reporting on research that focuses on holistic healing phenomena and modalities, and applying research in practice.

Core Value 5: Holistic Nurse Self-Care

Self-care as well as personal awareness and continual focus on being an instrument of healing are significant requirements for holistic nurses. Holistic nurses value themselves and mobilize the necessary resources to care for themselves. They endeavor to integrate self-awareness, self-care, and self-healing into their lives by incorporating practices such as self-assessment, meditation, yoga, good nutrition, energy therapies, movement, art, support, and lifelong learning. Holistic nurses honor their unique patterns and the development of the body, the psychosocial and cultural self, the intellectual self, the energetic self, and the spiritual self. Nurses

cannot facilitate healing unless they are in the process of healing themselves. Through continuing education, practice, and self-work, holistic nurses develop the skills of authentic and deep self-reflection and introspection to understand themselves and their journey. It is seen as a lifelong process.

Holistic nurses strive to achieve harmony and balance in their own lives and assist others to do the same. They create healing environments for themselves by attending to their own well-being, letting go of self-destructive behaviors and attitudes, and practicing centering and stress-reduction techniques. By doing this, holistic nurses serve as role models to others, be they clients, colleagues, or personal relations.

■ STANDARDS OF HOLISTIC NURSING PRACTICE

Overarching Philosophical Principles of Holistic Nursing

Holistic nurses express, contribute to, and promote an understanding of the following: a philosophy of nursing that values healing as the desired outcome; the human health experience as a complex, dynamic relationship of health, illness, disease, and wellness; the scientific foundations of nursing practice; and nursing as an art. Holistic nursing is based on the following overarching philosophical tenets that are embedded in every standard of practice. The following principles underlie holistic nursing:

Person

- There is unity, totality, and connectedness of everyone and everything (body, mind, emotion, spirit, sexuality, age, environment, society, culture, belief systems, relationships, and context).
- Human beings are unique and inherently good.
- People are able to find meaning and purpose in their own lives, experiences, and illnesses.
- All people have an innate power and capacity for self-healing. Health and illness are subjectively described and determined by the view of the individual. Therefore, the person is honored in all phases of his or her

healing process regardless of expectations or outcomes.

- Various people are the recipients of holistic nursing services: clients, patients, families, significant others, populations, or communities. They may be ill and within the healthcare delivery system or well, moving toward personal betterment to enhance well-being.

Healing and Health

- Health and illness are natural and a part of life, learning, and movement toward change and development.
- Health is seen as balance, integration, harmony, right relationship, and the betterment of well-being, not just the absence of disease. Healing can take place without cure. The focus is on health promotion, disease prevention, health restoration, and lifestyle patterns and habits as well as symptom relief.
- Illness is considered a teacher and an opportunity for self-awareness and growth as part of the life process. Symptoms are respected as messages.
- As active partners in the healing process, people are empowered when they take some control of their own lives, health, and well-being including personal choices and relationships.
- Treatment is a process that considers the root of the problem and does not merely treat the obvious signs and symptoms.

Practice

- Practice is a science using critical thinking, reflection, evidence, research, theory; practice is also an art requiring intuition, creativity, presence, and self-knowledge.
- The values and ethic of holism, caring, moral insight, dignity, integrity, competence, responsibility, accountability, and legality underline holistic nursing practice.
- There are various philosophies and paradigms of health, illness, and healing and approaches and models for the delivery of health care both in the United States and in other countries that need to be understood and utilized.

- Older adults represent the predominant population served by nurses.
- Public policy and the healthcare delivery system influence the health and well-being of society and professional nursing.

Nursing Roles

- The nurse is part of the healing environment using warmth, compassion, caring, authenticity, respect, trust, and relationship as instruments of healing in and of themselves.
- The holistic nurse uses conventional nursing interventions as well as holistic, complementary, alternative, and integrative modalities that enhance the body-mind-emotion-spirit connectedness to foster the healing, health, wholeness, and well-being of people.
- The holistic nurse collaborates and partners with all constituencies in the health process including the person receiving care and his or her family, significant others, community, colleagues, and individuals from other disciplines; this is all accomplished using principles and skills of cooperation, alliance, and respect and honoring the contributions of all.
- The holistic nurse participates in the change process to develop more caring cultures in which to practice and learn.
- The holistic nurse assists nurses to nurture and heal themselves.
- The holistic nurse participates in activities that contribute to the improvement of communities, the environment, and the betterment of public health.
- The holistic nurse acts as an advocate for the rights of and equitable distribution and access to health care for all persons, especially vulnerable populations.
- The holistic nurse honors the ecosystem and our relationship with and need to preserve it.

Self-Care

- Holistic nurses' self-reflection and self-assessment, self-care, healing, and personal development are necessary for service to others and for growth/change in their own well-being and for understanding of their personal journey.

- Holistic nurses value themselves and their calling to holistic nursing as a life purpose.

Holistic nursing practice is guided by the holistic caring process, whether used with individuals, families, population groups, or communities. This process involves assessment, diagnosis, outcome identification, planning, implementation, and evaluation. It encompasses all significant actions taken in providing culturally competent, ethical, respectful, compassionate, and relevant holistic nursing care to all persons.

The Standards of Holistic Nursing Practice*

There are 15 standards in the *Holistic Nursing: Scope and Standards of Practice* (2007), 6 for practice and 9 for professional performance.[3] Each standard addresses measurement criteria (competencies) for both the registered nurse and the advanced practice registered nurse. Included here are only one or two examples of measurement criteria because each standard has numerous measurement criteria.

Standard 1. ASSESSMENT: The holistic nurse collects comprehensive data pertinent to the person's health or situation.

The holistic registered nurse:

1. Collects comprehensive data including but not limited to physical, functional, psychosocial, emotional, mental, sexual, cultural, age-related, environmental, spiritual, transpersonal, and energy field assessments in a systematic and ongoing process while honoring the uniqueness of the person.
2. Identifies areas such as the person's health and cultural practices, values, beliefs, preferences, meanings of health, illness, lifestyle patterns, family issues, and risk behaviors and context.

---

* The complete and comprehensive statement of standards of holistic nursing practice are contained in *Holistic Nursing: Scope and Standards of Practice* (2007), which can be obtained from the American Holistic Nurses Association (AHNA), 323 N. San Francisco Street, Suite 201, Flagstaff, AZ 86001; 1-800-278-2462 or 1-928-526-2196; www.ahna.org or info@ahna.org.

The holistic advanced practice registered nurse:

1. Initiates and interprets diagnostic procedures relevant to the person's current status.
2. Explores the meanings of the symbolic language expressing itself in areas such as dreams, images, symbols, sensations, or prayers that are a part of the individual's health experience.

Standard 2. DIAGNOSIS OR HEALTH ISSUES: The holistic nurse analyzes the assessment data to determine the diagnosis or issues expressed as actual or potential patterns/problems/needs that are related to health, wellness, disease, or illness.

The holistic registered nurse:

1. Derives the diagnosis or health issues based on holistic assessment data.
2. Assists the person to explore the meaning of the health/disease experience.

The holistic advanced practice registered nurse:

1. Utilizes complex data and information obtained during interview, examination, and diagnostic procedures in making the diagnosis.

Standard 3. OUTCOMES IDENTIFICATION: The holistic registered nurse identifies outcomes for a plan individualized to the person or the situation. The holistic nurse values the evolution and the process of healing as it unfolds. This implies that specific unfolding outcomes may not be evident immediately because of the non-linear nature of the healing process so that both expected, anticipated, and evolving outcomes are considered.

The holistic registered nurse:

1. Defines outcomes in terms of the person: the individual's values, beliefs, and preferences; age; spiritual practices; ethical considerations; environment; or situation. Consideration is given to associated risks, benefits and costs, and current scientific evidence.
2. Partners with the person to identify realistic goals based on the person's present and potential capabilities and quality of life.

The holistic advanced practice registered nurse:

1. Identifies outcomes that incorporate patient satisfaction, the person's understanding and meanings in their unique patterns and processes, quality of life, cost and clinical effectiveness, and continuity and consistency among providers.

Standard 4. PLANNING: The holistic registered nurse develops a plan that identifies strategies and alternatives to attain outcomes.

The holistic registered nurse:

1. Develops in partnership with the person an individualized plan considering the person's characteristics or situation including, but not limited to, values, beliefs, spiritual and health practices, preferences, choices, age and cultural appropriateness, and environmental sensitivity.
2. Develops the plan in conjunction with the person, family, and others, as appropriate.
3. Establishes practice settings and safe space and time for both the nurse and person, family, and significant others to explore suggested potential and alternative options.

The holistic advanced practice registered nurse:

1. Identifies assessments, diagnostic strategies, and therapeutic interventions within the plan, including therapeutic effects and side effects that reflect current evidence, data, research, literature, expert clinical knowledge, and the person's experiences.
2. Uses linguistic and symbolic language including but not limited to word associations, dreams, storytelling, and journals to explore possibilities and options with individuals.

Standard 5. IMPLEMENTATION: The holistic registered nurse implements in partnership with the person the identified plan.

The holistic registered nurse:

1. Partners with the person, family, significant others, and caregivers to implement the plan in a safe and timely manner while honoring the person's choices and unique healing journey.

The holistic advanced practice registered nurse:

1. Facilitates utilization of systems and community resources to implement the plan.
2. Incorporates new knowledge and strategies to initiate change in nursing care practices if desired outcomes are not achieved.

Standard 5A. COORDINATION OF CARE: The holistic registered nurse coordinates care delivery.

The holistic registered nurse:

1. Coordinates implementation of the plan.

The holistic advanced practice registered nurse:

1. Provides leadership in the coordination of multidisciplinary health care for integrated delivery of services.

Standard 5B. HEALTH TEACHING AND HEALTH PROMOTION: The holistic registered nurse employs strategies to promote holistic health, wellness, and a safe environment.

The holistic registered nurse:

1. Provides health teaching to individuals, families, and significant others or caregivers that enhances the mind–body and emotion–spirit connection.
2. Uses health promotion and health teaching methods appropriate to the situation and the individual's values, beliefs, health practices, age, learning needs, readiness and ability to learn, language preference, spirituality, culture, and socioeconomic status.
3. Assists others to access their own inner wisdom that may provide opportunities to enhance and support growth, development, and wholeness.

The holistic advanced practice registered nurse:

1. Synthesizes empirical evidence on risk behaviors, decision making about life choices, learning theories, behavioral change theories, motivational theories, epidemiology, and other related theories and frameworks when designing holistic health information and education.

Standard 5C. CONSULTATION: *The holistic advanced practice registered nurse provides consultation to influence the identified plan, enhance the abilities of others, and effect change.*

The holistic advanced practice registered nurse:

1. Facilitates the effectiveness of a consultation by involving all stakeholders including the individual in decision making and negotiating role responsibilities.

Standard 5D. PRESCRIPTIVE AUTHORITY AND TREATMENT: *The holistic advanced practice registered nurse uses prescriptive authority, procedures, referrals, treatments, and therapies in accordance with state and federal laws and regulations.*

The holistic advanced practice registered nurse:

1. Prescribes treatments, therapies, and procedures based on evidence, research, current knowledge, and practice considering the person's holistic healthcare needs and choices.
2. Uses advanced knowledge of pharmacology, psychoneuroimmunology, nutritional supplements, herbal and homeopathic remedies, and a variety of complementary and alternative therapies in prescribing.
3. Evaluates therapeutic and potential adverse effects of pharmacologic and non-pharmacologic treatments including but not limited to drug, herbal, and homeopathic regimens as well as their side effects and interactions.

Standard 6. EVALUATION: *The holistic registered nurse evaluates progress toward attainment of outcomes while recognizing and honoring the continuing holistic nature of the healing process.*

The holistic registered nurse:

1. Conducts a holistic, systematic, ongoing, and criterion-based evaluation of the outcomes in relation to the structures and processes prescribed by the plan and the indicated timeline.

2. Evaluates in partnership with the person the effectiveness of the planned strategies in relation to the person's responses and the attainment of the expected and unfolding outcomes.

The holistic advanced practice registered nurse:

1. Uses the results of the evaluation analyses to make or recommend process or structural changes, including policy and procedure or protocol documentation, as appropriate to improve holistic care.

Standard 7. QUALITY OF PRACTICE: *The holistic registered nurse systematically enhances the quality and effectiveness of holistic nursing practice.*

The holistic registered nurse:

1. Participates in quality improvement activities for holistic nursing practice.

The holistic advanced practice registered nurse:

1. Evaluates the practice environment and quality of holistic nursing care rendered in relation to existing evidence and feedback from individuals and significant others, identifying opportunities for the generation and use of research.

Standard 8. EDUCATION: *The holistic registered nurse attains knowledge and competency that reflects current nursing practice.*

The holistic registered nurse:

1. Seeks experiences and formal and independent learning activities to maintain and develop clinical and professional skills and knowledge and personal growth to provide holistic care.

The holistic advanced practice registered nurse:

1. Uses current healthcare research findings and other evidence to expand clinical knowledge, enhance role performance, and increase knowledge of professional issues and changes in national standards for practice and trends in holistic care.

Standard 9. *PROFESSIONAL PRACTICE EVALUATION: The holistic registered nurse evaluates one's own nursing practice in relation to professional practice standards and guidelines, relevant statutes, rules, and regulations. The holistic registered nurse's practice reflects the application of knowledge of current practice standards, guidelines, statutes, rules, and regulations.*

The holistic registered nurse:

1. Reflects on one's practice and how one's own personal, cultural, and spiritual beliefs; experiences; biases; education; and values can affect care given to individuals, families, and communities.
2. Engages in self-evaluation of practice on a regular basis, identifying areas of strength, as well as areas in which professional development and personal growth would be beneficial.

The holistic advanced practice registered nurse:

1. Engages in a formal process, seeking feedback regarding one's own practice from individuals receiving care, peers, professional colleagues, and others.

Standard 10. *COLLEGIALITY: The holistic registered nurse interacts with and contributes to the professional development of peers and colleagues.*

The holistic registered nurse:

1. Shares knowledge and skills with peers and colleagues as evidenced by such activities as patient care conferences or presentations at formal or informal meetings.
2. Promotes work environments conducive to support, understanding, respect, health, healing, caring, wholeness, and harmony.

The holistic advanced practice registered nurse:

1. Models expert holistic nursing practice to interdisciplinary team members and healthcare consumers.

Standard 11. *COLLABORATION: The holistic registered nurse collaborates with the person, family, and others in the conduct of holistic nursing practice.*

The holistic registered nurse:

1. Communicates with the person, family, significant others, caregivers, and interdisciplinary healthcare providers regarding the person's care and the holistic nurse's role in the provision of that care.

The holistic advanced practice registered nurse:

1. Facilitates the negotiation of holistic, complementary, integrative, and conventional healthcare services for continuity of care and program planning.

Standard 12. *ETHICS: The holistic registered nurse integrates ethical provisions in all areas of practice.*

The holistic registered nurse:

1. Uses the *Guide to the Code of Ethics for Nurses: Interpretation and Application*[5] and AHNA *Position Statement on Holistic Nursing Ethics* to guide practice and articulate the moral foundation of holistic nursing.
2. Advocates for the rights of vulnerable, repressed, or underserved populations.

The holistic advanced practice registered nurse:

1. Actively contributes to creating an ecosystem that supports well-being for all life.

Standard 13. *RESEARCH: The holistic registered nurse integrates research into practice.*

The holistic registered nurse:

1. Utilizes the best available evidence, including theories and research findings, to guide practice decisions.
2. Actively and ethically participates in research activities related to holistic health at various levels appropriate to the holistic nurse's level of education and position.

The holistic advanced practice registered nurse:

1. Contributes to nursing knowledge by conducting or synthesizing research that discovers, examines, and evaluates knowledge, theories, philosophies, context, criteria, and creative approaches to improve holistic healthcare practice.

2. Formally disseminates research findings through activities such as presentations, publications, consultations, and journal clubs for a variety of audiences including nursing, other disciplines, and the public to improve holistic care and further develop the foundation and practice of holistic nursing.

Standard 14. RESOURCE UTILIZATION: *The holistic registered nurse considers factors related to safety, effectiveness, cost, and impact on practice in the planning and delivery of nursing services.*

The holistic registered nurse:

1. Assists the person, family, and significant others or caregivers as appropriate in identifying and securing appropriate and available services to address health-related needs.
2. Identifies discriminatory healthcare practices as they affect the person and engages in effective nondiscriminatory practices.

The holistic advanced practice registered nurse:

1. Utilizes organizational and community resources to formulate multidisciplinary or interdisciplinary plans of care.

Standard 15. LEADERSHIP: *The holistic registered nurse provides leadership in the professional practice setting and the profession.*

The holistic registered nurse:

1. Displays the ability to define a clear vision, associated goals, and a plan to implement and measure progress toward holistic health care.
2. Promotes advancement of the profession through participation in professional organizations and by focusing on strategies that bring unity and healing to the nursing profession.

The holistic advanced practice registered nurse:

1. Works to influence decision-making bodies to improve holistic, integrated care.
2. Articulates the ideas underpinning holistic nursing philosophy, places these ideas in a historical, philosophical, and scientific context while projecting future trends in thinking.

■ EDUCATIONAL PREPARATION AND CERTIFICATION FOR HOLISTIC NURSING PRACTICE

Holistic nurses are registered nurses who are educationally prepared for practice from an approved school of nursing and are licensed to practice in their individual state, commonwealth, or territory. The holistic registered nurse's experience, education, knowledge, and abilities establish the level of competence. *Holistic Nursing: Scope and Standards of Practice* (2007) identifies the scope of practice of holistic nursing and the specific standards and associated measurement criteria of holistic nurses at both the basic and advanced levels.[3] Regardless of the level of practice, all holistic nurses integrate the previously identified five core values.

A registered nurse may prepare for the specialty of holistic nursing in a variety of ways. Educational offerings range from associate degree, baccalaureate, and graduate courses and programs, to continuing education programs with extensive contact hours.

Basic Practice Level

The education of all nursing students preparing for registered nurse (RN) licensure includes basic content on physiological, psychological, emotional, and some spiritual processes with populations across the life span and conventional nursing care practices within each of these domains. Additionally, basic nursing education incorporates experiences in a variety of clinical and practice settings from acute care to community. However, the educational focus is most frequently on specialties often emanating from the biomedical disease model and cure orientation. In holistic nursing, the individual across the life span is viewed in context as an integrated totality of body, mind, emotion, environment, society, energy, and spirit, with the emphasis on wholeness, well-being, health promotion, and healing using both conventional and complementary/alternative practices. Because of the lack of intentional focus on integration, unity, and healing, the educational exposure of most nursing students is not adequate preparation for assuming the specialty role of a holistic nurse.

A number of schools of nursing are beginning to incorporate holistic nursing content at the undergraduate level, whether it be as discrete courses such as therapeutic touch, relaxation, aromatherapy, and so on, or integrated in courses such as nursing therapeutics.

Advanced Practice Level

As with the basic level, there are a variety of ways through both academic and professional development that registered nurses can acquire the additional specialized knowledge and skills that prepare them for practice as an advanced practice holistic nurse. These nurses are expected to hold a master's or doctoral degree and demonstrate a greater depth and scope of knowledge, a greater integration of information, increased complexity of skills and interventions, and notable role autonomy. They provide leadership in practice, teaching, research, consultation, advocacy, and policy formation in advancing holistic nursing to improve the holistic health of people. Several schools of nursing that offer graduate programs in holistic nursing have a stable or growing number of applicants. Current advanced practice nurses are increasingly gaining specialized knowledge preparing them as holistic nurses through postmaster's programs, continuing education offerings in holistic nursing care, and certificate programs throughout the country that focus on specific modalities and on the essence of holism.

Continuing Education for Basic and Advanced Practice Levels

The AHNA is a provider and approver of continuing education and is recognized by the American Nurses Credentialing Center (ANCC). Continuing educational programs, workshops, and lectures in holistic nursing and CAM have been popular nationwide, with AHNA or other bodies granting continuing education units.

The AHNA endorses certificate programs in specific areas. These include Integrative Healing, Reflexology, Imagery, Aromatherapy, Healing Touch, Spirituality, Craniosacral Therapy, Holistic Stress Management, Integrative Healing Arts, Coaching, and Whole Health Education. It also approves continuing education offerings

in holistic nursing as well as giving the AHNA home study course, Foundation of Holistic Nursing. Other programs in distinct therapies such as acupuncture, Reiki, homeopathy, massage, imagery, healing arts, holistic health, Chinese Oriental Medicine, nutrition, Ayurveda, therapeutic touch, healing touch, herbology, Chiropractic, and so on, are given nationally as degrees, certificates, or continuing education programs by centers, specialty organizations, or schools.

Certification

Competency mechanisms for evaluating holistic nursing practice as a specialty exist through a national certification/recertification process overseen by the American Holistic Nurses Certification Corporation (AHNCC). AHNCC offers three Certifications: *Holistic Nurse, Board Certified* (HN-BC) which requires a minimum of a diploma or associate degree in nursing from an accredited school; *Holistic Baccalaureate Nurse, Board Certified* (HNB-BC) which requires a baccalaureate degree in nursing from an institution regionally accredited by the Association of Schools and Colleges (ASC); and *Advanced Holistic Nurse, Board Certified* (AHN-BC) which requires a master's degree in nursing from an institution regionally accredited by ASC. Further, the AHNCC provides endorsement for schools of nursing meeting the specifications put forth in *Holistic Nursing: Scope and Standards of Practice* (2007).[3] Additionally, holistic nurses often are certified in specific CAM modalities such as imagery, Reiki, aromatherapy, healing touch, biofeedback, and Reflexology.

■ SETTINGS FOR HOLISTIC NURSING PRACTICE

Holistic nurses practice in numerous settings, including but not limited to private practitioner offices; ambulatory, acute, long-term, and home care settings; complementary care centers; women's health centers; hospice and palliative care; psychiatric mental health facilities; schools; rehabilitation centers; community nursing organizations; student and employee health centers; managed care organizations; independent self-employed practice; correctional facilities; professional nursing and healthcare organizations; administration; staff development; and universities and colleges. There are increasing numbers of holistic nurses who hold leadership roles as clinicians, educators, authors, and researchers in university-based schools of nursing, practice environments, nursing, and other professional organizations. Holistic nursing practice also occurs when there is a request for consultation or when holistic nurses advocate for care that promotes health and prevents disease, illness, or disability for individuals, communities, or the environment. A holistic nurse may choose not to work in a critical care setting but provide consultation regarding self-care or stress management to nurses practicing in that area. Or holistic nurses may practice in preoperative and recovery rooms instituting a "Prepare for Surgery" program for individuals who are going to have surgery that teaches them meditation and positive affirmation techniques for both before and after surgery while incorporating a homeopathic regimen for trauma and cell healing. Employment or voluntary participation of holistic nurses also can influence civic activities and the regulatory and legislative arenas at the local, state, national, or international levels.

Because holistic nursing focuses on wellness, wholeness, and development of the whole person, holistic nurses also practice in health enhancement settings such as spas, gyms, and wellness centers. With all populations and in any setting, nurses can empower patients/clients/families by teaching them self-care practices for a healthier lifestyle. Because holistic nursing is a worldview, a way of being in the world, and not just a modality, holistic nurses can practice in any setting and with individuals throughout the life span. As the public increasingly requests holistic and CAM services, there will be a greater need for holistic nurses in a wider array of settings. Holistic nursing takes place wherever healing occurs.[13]

■ CONCLUSION

The specialty practice of holistic nursing is generally not well understood. Therefore, each holistic nurse must educate other nurses, healthcare providers and disciplines, and the public about the role, value, and benefits of holistic nursing, whether it be in direct practice, education, management, or research. Holistic nurses articu-

late the ideas underpinning the holistic paradigm and the philosophy of the caring–healing relationship. Jean Watson reminds us that society and the public are searching for something deeper in terms of realizing self-care, self-knowledge, and self-healing potentials. Nurses need to acknowledge the human aspects of practice—attending to people and their experience rather than just focusing on the medical orientation and disease. She concludes that "nurses have a covenant with the public to sustain caring. It is our collective responsibility to transform caring practices into the framework that identifies and gives distinction to nursing as a profession."[14] *Holistic Nursing: Scope and Standards of Practice* (2007) is a means through which holistic nurses are educating the profession and others about the values, principles, and practice requirements of the specialty.[3]

Directions for
FUTURE RESEARCH

1. Explore research modalities and approaches that are congruent with the holistic paradigm.
2. Examine how the standards of holistic nursing practice are being implemented in nursing settings.

Nurse Healer
REFLECTIONS

After reading this chapter, the holistic nurse will be able to answer or to begin a process of answering the following questions:

- What attributes do I have that reflect the core values of holistic nursing?
- What contributions can I make as a holistic nurse to the wholeness and betterment of humankind?

---

www *For a full suite of assignments and additional learning activities, use the access code located in the front of your book to visit this exclusive website: http://go.jblearning.com/dossey. If you do not have an access code, you can obtain one at the site.*

NOTES

1. Institute of Medicine, *Crossing the Quality Chasm: A New Health System for the 21st Century* (Washington, DC: National Academies Press, 2001).

2. C. Tresoli and Pew-Fetzer, Task Force on Advancing Psychosocial Health Education, *Health Professions Education and Relationship-Centered Care* (San Francisco: Commission at the Center for the Health Professions, University of California, 1994).

3. American Holistic Nurses Association & American Nurses Association, *Holistic Nursing: Scope and Standards of Practice* (Silver Spring, MD: NurseBooks.org, 2007).

4. American Nurses Association, *Nursing: Scope and Standards of Practice*, 2nd ed. (Silver Spring, MD: NurseBooks.org, 2010).

5. American Nurses Association, *Guide to the Code of Ethics for Nurses: Interpretation and Application* (Silver Spring, MD: NurseBooks.org, 2010).

6. American Nurses Association, *Nursing's Social Policy Statement: The Essence of the Profession* (Silver Spring, MD: NurseBooks.org, 2010).

7. American Nurses Association, Nursing: Scope and Standards of Practice (Silver Spring, MD: NurseBooks.org, 2004).

8. American Nurses Association, *Recognition of a Nursing Specialty, Approval of a Specialty Nursing Scope of Practice Statement and Acknowledgement of Specialty Nursing Standards of Practice* (Washington, DC: ANA, 2005).

9. C. Mariano, *Proposal for Recognition of Holistic Nursing as a Nursing Specialty* (New York: Unpublished document submitted to ANA, 2006).

10. American Holistic Nurses Association, *Description of Holistic Nursing* (Flagstaff, AZ: AHNA, 1998).

11. "Patient Bill of Rights," in *Accreditation Manual for Hospitals* (Oakbrook Terrace, IL: Joint Commission on Accreditation of Healthcare Organizations, 1992).

12. American Holistic Nurses Association, *American Holistic Nurses Association Position Statement on Holistic Ethics* (Flagstaff, AZ: AHNA, reapproved 2007).

13. C. Mariano, "Holistic Nursing: Every Nurse's Specialty," *Beginnings* 29, no. 4 (2009).

14. C. Mariano, "Caring for Our Future: An Interview with Jean Watson," *Beginnings* 25, no. 3, 12 (2005).

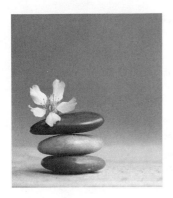

Development of the Original Holistic Nursing Standards of Practice: Basic and Advanced

BASIC STANDARDS DEVELOPMENT

The American Holistic Nurses Association (AHNA) first developed *Standards of Holistic Nursing Practice* in 1990; these were subsequently revised in 1995. Between 1994 and 1997, the AHNA conducted a 3-year role delineation study, the Inventory of Professional Activities and Knowledge of a Holistic Nurse (IPAKHN survey). In this practice analysis study the activities and knowledge basic to current holistic nursing practice were determined through administration of a structured inventory to a representative sample of holistic nurses.

This 3-year endeavor was successfully completed by a four-member AHNA task force and reviewed by the AHNA leadership council, select AHNA members, and other recognized holistic nurse members and nonmembers representing the diversity of holistic nurse representation from practice, education, research, and administration. An extensive five-step process was used to revise the 1995 AHNA *Standards of Holistic Nursing Practice* and to delineate core values.

Step 1: Literature Review, Inventory of Professional Activities and Knowledge of a Holistic Nurse (IPAKHN) Survey Data Analysis, and Expert Reviews

Step 2: Review Process

Following the first step, the AHNA Standards of Practice Task Force incorporated the suggestions and additional data from the literature review and the IPAKHN survey analysis that reflected the most recent holistic nursing professional activities, knowledge, and caring–healing modalities. Based on this review and the additional comments, deletions, modifications, and recommendations by expert nurses, six areas were further refined and developed including five core values.

Step 3: AHNA Standards of Practice Advisory Committee

Following the second step, the revised AHNA standards of practice were next sent to the 24-member advisory committee, who gave additional comments, modifications, and recommendations. Five subsequent revision rounds by the AHNA task force occurred until consensus was achieved, and then the standards were sent back to the advisory committee for additional comments, modifications, and recommendations, which were incorporated.

Step 4: AHNA Standards of Practice Review Committee

Next, the revised AHNA standards of practice were sent to the 24-member review committee, who gave additional comments, deletions, modifications, and recommendations, which were incorporated.

Step 5: AHNA Standards of Practice Leadership Council

In the fifth step of the standards development process, the final draft of the *Standards of Holistic*

Nursing Practice was submitted to the AHNA leadership council. After discussion, a final vote of approval accepted the *Standards of Holistic Nursing Practice*. These were then presented at the business meeting of the annual AHNA conference in June 1999 in Scottsdale, Arizona. The AHNA standards received a vote of approval by the AHNA membership. Minor editorial changes were approved by the AHNA leadership council in January 2000, with additional minor revisions in 2004 and 2005.*

■ ADVANCED STANDARDS DEVELOPMENT

In response to the growing number of graduate programs with a holistic nursing focus, the AHNA leadership council appointed a nine-member task force in January 2000 to develop standards for advanced practice. From that time until later autumn 2001, the task force worked to develop standards for advanced holistic nursing practice. The final draft was completed and accepted for submission to the council by the task force members in September 2001.

The task force used the core values as the foundation for developing the advanced practice standards. Regardless of the type of practice of the holistic nurse, these values should serve as the philosophical underpinning for practice. The *Essentials of Master's Education for Advanced Practice Nursing* (1996), published by the American Association of Colleges of Nursing, and ANA's *Scope and Standards of Advanced Practice Registered Nursing Practice* (1996) served as additional guides for the scope of practice that should be addressed by the standards because these documents are employed in the development of graduate nursing curricula.

The AHNA conducted an advanced practice standards review process similar to that used to create the basic practice standards. In addition to the task force, leaders in the field of holistic nursing and nursing education were asked to review the draft standards to establish content validity. The first draft was completed and circulated to task force members for review and comment in Spring 2000. The comments were then used to prepare the second draft for the task

force to review. A decision was made that the standards for advanced practice would apply to those nurses with a graduate degree even though there are nurses in practice with an expanded scope created not by graduate education but by certifications in particular specialties. These certifications were created before graduate education became the entry level for advanced practice. It was felt that the basic standards more than adequately address the scope of practice for all except graduate practice, and the need was to have standards to address holistic nursing practice by graduate-prepared nurses that would guide in the development of curricula for graduate education in holistic nursing.

The third draft was completed during the summer of 2000 and then circulated in the autumn to task force members. The fourth draft was prepared from the feedback of task force members and circulated to the responding and corresponding committees for review and comment. Comments on the fourth draft were received throughout the spring and summer of 2001. In September, these comments were collated into a final draft. This draft was reviewed and accepted for submission to the leadership council. The *Standards of Advanced Holistic Nursing Practice for Graduate-Prepared Nurses* were approved and adopted by the AHNA leadership council in January 2002, followed by a minor revision in 2005.

■ HOLISTIC NURSING: SCOPE AND STANDARDS OF PRACTICE

During the interval from 2004 until 2006 the original *Standards of Holistic Nursing Practice* (advanced and basic) were substantively revised to incorporate language and content required by ANA to support the application for formal recognition of holistic nursing as a nursing specialty. The leadership council of the AHNA reviewed and approved the preliminary draft statement of the standards in June 2005, and then the draft *Holistic Nursing: Scope and Standards of Practice* in March 2006. *Holistic Nursing: Scope and Standards of Practice* was approved by the ANA in November 2006. Holistic nursing was recognized as an official specialty within Nursing by the American Nurses Association that same month. *Holistic Nursing: Scope and Standards of Practice* was published jointly by AHNA and ANA in 2007.

---

* Adapted from N. C. Frisch et al., *AHNA Standards of Holistic Nursing Practice with Guidelines for Caring and Healing* (Gaithersburg, MD: Aspen, 2000).

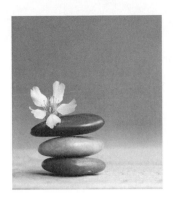

Select Works of Individuals and AHNA Documents

The foundation of *Holistic Nursing: Scope and Standards of Practice* (2007) is based on the works of a number of individuals and from AHNA documents, including the following:

American Holistic Nurses Association, *AHNA Standards of Holistic Nursing Practice* (Flagstaff, AZ: AHNA, 2004).

American Holistic Nurses Association, *AHNA Standards of Advanced Holistic Nursing Practice for Graduate-Prepared Nurses* (Flagstaff, AZ: AHNA, 2004).

American Holistic Nurses Association, *Description of Holistic Nursing* (Flagstaff, AZ: AHNA, 1998).

American Holistic Nurses Association, *AHNA Position Statement on the Role of Nurses in the Practice of Complementary and Alternative Therapies* (Flagstaff, AZ: AHNA, revised and reapproved, 2007).

American Holistic Nurses Association, *AHNA Position Statement on Nursing Research and Scholarship* (Flagstaff, AZ: AHNA, revised and reapproved, 2007).

American Holistic Nurses Association, *AHNA Position Statement on Holistic Ethics* (Flagstaff, AZ: AHNA, revised and reapproved, 2007).

American Holistic Nurses Association, *AHNA Position Statement on a Healthful Environment* (Flagstaff, AZ: AHNA, n.d.).

B. M. Dossey, ed., *Core Curriculum for Holistic Nursing* (Gaithersburg, MD: Aspen, 1997).

B. M. Dossey, L. Keegan, and C. E. Guzzetta, *Holistic Nursing: A Handbook for Practice*, 4th ed. (Sudbury, MA: Jones & Bartlett, 2005).

N. C. Frisch et al., *AHNA Standards of Holistic Nursing Practice with Guidelines for Caring and Healing* (Gaithersburg, MD: Aspen, 2000).

C. E. Guzzetta, *Essential Readings in Holistic Nursing* (Gaithersburg, MD: Aspen, 1998).

C. Mariano, *Proposal for Recognition of Holistic Nursing as a Nursing Specialty* (New York: Unpublished manuscript submitted to ANA, 2006).

C. Mariano, "An Overview of Holistic Nursing," *Imprint* 52, no. 2 (2005): 1148–1152.

C. Mariano, "Advanced Practice in Holistic Nursing," in *Nurse Practitioners: Evolution of Advanced Practice*, ed. M. Mezey, D. McGivern & E. Sullivan-Marx, 4th ed. (New York: Springer, 2003).

RESOURCE LIST

American Holistic Nurses Association (AHNA)
323 N. San Francisco Street
Suite 201
Flagstaff, AZ 86001
Phone: 1-800-278-2462
info@ahna.org
www.ahna.org

American Holistic Nurses Certification
    Corporation (AHNCC)
811 Linden Loop
Cedar Park, TX 78613
Phone: 1-877-284-0998
AHNCC@flash.net

National Center for Complementary and
    Alternative Medicine (NCCAM)
National Institutes of Health
P.O. Box 7923
Gaithersburg, MD 20898
Phone: 1-888-644-6226
http://nccam.nih.gov

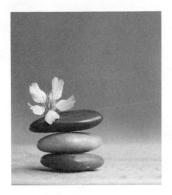

Chapter 3

Current Trends and Issues in Holistic Nursing

Carla Mariano

Nurse Healer
OBJECTIVES

Theoretical

- Describe the major issues in health care and holistic nursing today.
- Identify changes needed in health care to promote health, wellness, and healing.
- Discuss recommendations of the Institute of Medicine (IOM) report *The Future of Nursing.*

Clinical

- Evaluate how current trends in health care will affect clinical nursing practice.
- Discuss with other health professionals the unique and common contributions of each other's practice.

Personal

- Become a member of the American Holistic Nurses Association (AHNA) to participate in improving holistic health care for society.

The American public increasingly demands health care that is compassionate and respectful, provides options, is economically feasible, and is grounded in holistic ideals. A shift is occurring in health care where people desire to be more actively involved in health decision making. They have expressed their dissatisfaction with conventional (Western allopathic) medicine and are calling for a care system that encompasses health, quality of life, and a relationship with their providers. The National Center for Complementary and Alternative Medicine's *Strategic Plan for 2011–2015*[1] and *Healthy People 2020*[2] prioritize enhancing physical and mental health and wellness, preventing disease, and empowering the public to take responsibility for their health. The vision of *Healthy People 2020* is "A society in which all people live long, healthy lives" and its goals are as follows:

- Attain high-quality, longer lives free of preventable disease, disability, injury, and premature death.
- Achieve health equity, eliminate disparities, and improve the health of all groups.
- Create social and physical environments that promote good health for all.
- Promote quality of life, healthy development, and healthy behaviors across all life stages.[2]

■ HEALTH CARE IN THE UNITED STATES

Western medicine is proving ineffective, wholly or partially, for a significant proportion of common chronic diseases. Furthermore, highly technological health care is too expensive to be universally affordable. In a May 2011 poll, 55% of Americans indicated that the healthcare system has major problems, 50% indicated that the healthcare system needs fundamental changes, and 36% stated that there is so much wrong with the healthcare system that it needs to be completely rebuilt.[3]

> Although medical advances have saved and improved the lives of millions, much of medicine and health care have primarily focused on addressing immediate events of disease and injury, generally neglecting underlying socioeconomic factors, including employment, education, and income and behavioral risk factors. These factors, and others, impact health status, accentuate disparities, and can lead to costly, preventable diseases. Furthermore, the disease-driven approach to medicine and health care has resulted in a fragmented, specialized health system in which care is typically reactive and episodic, as well as often inefficient and impersonal.[4]

Chronic diseases—such as heart disease, cancer, hypertension, diabetes, depression—are the leading causes of death and disability in the United States. Chronic diseases account for 70% of all deaths in the United States, which is 1.7 million deaths each year. These diseases also cause major limitations in daily living for almost 1 out of 10 Americans, or about 25 million people.[5]

> Stress accounts for 80% of all healthcare issues in the United States. *Super Stress* "is a result of both the changing nature of our daily lives and our choices in lifestyle habits, as well as a series of unfortunate events. Extreme chronic stress . . . has silently become a pandemic that disturbs not only how we perceive our quality of life but also our health and mortality. . . . The APA [American Psychological Association] issued a report on stress, revealing that nearly half of all Americans were experiencing stress at a significantly higher level than the previous year and rated its level as extreme.[6]

Healthcare costs have been rising for several years. Expenditures in the United States for health care surpassed $2.3 trillion in 2008, more than three times the $714 billion spent in 1990, and more than eight times the $253 billion spent in 1980. Healthcare expenditures are projected to be $2.7 trillion in 2011 and $4.3 trillion by 2017.[7]

In 2008, U.S. healthcare spending was about $7,681 per resident and accounted for 16.2% of the nation's gross domestic product (GDP); this is among the highest of all industrialized countries. Total healthcare expenditures continue to outpace inflation and the growth in national income.[8] The U.S. healthcare system is the most expensive in the world, but it yields worse results than the systems in Britain, Canada, Germany, Australia, and New Zealand. U.S. residents with below-average incomes are more likely than their counterparts in other countries not to have received needed care because of cost. The Centers for Medicare and Medicaid Services (CMS) compare what healthcare costs per capita have been and will be over the next few years:[9]

1993:	$3,468.60
2004:	$6,321.90
2007:	$7,498.00
2011:	$9,525.00
2016:	$12,782.00

Healthcare cost for a family of four rose again in 2011, with employees paying a much larger share of the rising expense. The total cost of health care for a typical family of four is $19,393, an increase of 7.3% over 2010. This is double the cost families had to pay in 2002 ($9,235). As costs continue to grow, the cost for health care constitutes a larger and larger portion of the household budget.[8] And what are families paying for? The 2011 Milliman Medical Index indicates that physician costs represent 33% of the overall health costs; hospital inpatient costs account for 31%; outpatient costs, 17%; pharmacy, 15%; and other expenses such as medical equipment, about 4%.[10]

Additionally, workers paid 47% more in 2010 than they did in 2005 for the health coverage they get through their jobs, while their wages have increased only 18%. Employers, in contrast, pay 20% more toward their employees' health insurance than they did 5 years ago. Premiums for employer-sponsored health insurance have risen from $5,791 in 1999 to $13,375 in 2009, with the amount paid by workers rising by 128%.[11]

In addition to the rising costs, there is disparity in the numbers of Americans insured for health coverage. The U.S. Census Bureau cites the number of uninsured Americans at 50.7 million, 16.7% of the population, rising from 13.7% in 2000, or almost 1 in 6 U.S. residents.[12] The number of underinsured has grown 60% to 25 million over the past 4 years.[13] The reasons for the rise in both categories include workers losing their jobs in the recession, companies dropping employee health insurance benefits, and families going without coverage to cut costs—primarily as a result of the high costs of health care. Additionally, in 2009, an average of 7% of the population failed to obtain *needed* medical care because of costs, with the percentages of Hispanics and blacks and those 18 to 64 years of age being the largest.[14]

The Kaiser Family Foundation identifies the following forces driving healthcare costs:[8]

- *Technology and prescription drugs:* Because of development costs and generation of consumer demand for more intense, costly services even if they are not necessarily cost effective.
- *Chronic disease:* Chronic disease accounts for more than 75% of national healthcare expenditures and places tremendous demands on the system, particularly the increased need for treatment of ongoing illnesses and long-term services. One-quarter (25%) of Medicare spending is for costs incurred during the last year of life.
- *Aging of the population:* Health expenses rise with age. The baby boomers begin qualifying for Medicare in 2011 and many of their costs will shift to the public sector.
- *Administrative costs:* At least 7% of healthcare expenditures are for marketing, billing, and other administrative costs. Overhead costs and large profits are fueling healthcare spending.

The Kaiser Family Foundation also offers the following proposals to contain costs:[8]

- *Invest in information technology (IT).* Make greater use of technology such as electronic medical records (EMRs). This is a major component of the health reform plan.
- *Improve quality and efficiency.* Decrease unwarranted variation in medical practice and unnecessary care. Experts estimate that 30% of health care is unnecessary.
- *Adjust provider compensation and increase comparative effectiveness research (CER).* Ensure that fees paid to physicians reward value and health outcomes rather than volume of care, and determine which treatments are most effective for given conditions.
- *Increase government regulation in controlling per capita spending.*
- *Increase prevention efforts.* Provide financial incentives to workers to engage in wellness and to decrease the prevalence of chronic conditions. Improve disease management to streamline treatment for common chronic health conditions.
- *Increase consumer involvement in purchasing.* Encourage greater price transparency and use of health reimbursement accounts (HRAs).

Much has been written about the current healthcare crisis: the high cost of health care, the lack of universal access to health care and the resulting 51 million uninsured Americans, the insurance morass and that industry's control of healthcare spending, the disenchantment and disempowerment of healthcare providers, the frustration of clients/patients and healthcare consumers, the lack of incentive for practitioners or insurers to foster prevention and health promotion, and the startling lack of measures being taken for high-quality healthcare outcomes. Hyman states that the national healthcare dialogue omits discussions about the nature and quality of care:

> We speak of evidence-based medicine, not quality-based medicine. Although evidence is important, it is not enough, particularly when the evidence is limited mostly to what is funded by private interest or grounded in the pharmacologic treatment of disease. The fundamental flaw in our approach to the discussion about evidence-based medicine versus quality-based medicine is the lack of focus on prevention and wellness and the lack of funding and research on comparative approaches to chronic healthcare problems. Though

it is still a matter of public debate, there is ample evidence that lifestyle therapies equal or exceed the benefits of conventional therapies. Nutrition, exercise, and stress management no longer can be considered alternative medicine. They are essential medicine, and often the most effective and cost-effective therapies to treat chronic disease, which has replaced infectious and acute illnesses as the leading cause of death in the world, both in developed and developing countries. It is hoped then that the next 10 years will see a focus on not just the mechanisms of complementary and integrative therapies, but also on measuring their role in improving overall healthcare quality and reducing healthcare costs. It is hoped the discourse begun by the IOM report will spur policy makers to refocus federal efforts and funding on quality, disease prevention, and health promotion and will help us find the right medicine, regardless of its origin.[15]

Use of CAM in the United States

The American public has pursued alternative and complementary care at an ever-increasing rate. In 1993, David Eisenberg and colleagues published a now-classic study that indicated that one-third of (61 million) Americans were using some form of alternative or complementary medicine.[16] The researchers' ongoing study on the use of alternative/complementary care in 1998 indicated that the use of such modalities not only continued, but sharply increased to 42% (83 million Americans). The total number of visits to providers of complementary care increased by 47% from 427 million in 1990 to 629 million in 1997.[17] The out-of-pocket dollars the American public spent on CAM was $12.2 billion, which exceeded the out-of-pocket expenditures for all U.S. hospitalizations and compared with total out-of-pocket expenses for all physician services.

The most recent survey, the 2007 National Health Interview Survey,[18] indicates that 38.3% of adults in the United States aged 18 years and older (almost 4 of 10 adults) and nearly 12% of children aged 17 years and younger (1 in 9 children) used some form of CAM within the previous 12 months. Use among adults remained relatively constant from previous surveys. The 2007 survey provides the first population-based estimate of children's use of CAM. Americans spent $33.9 billion out-of-pocket on CAM during the 12 months prior to the survey. This accounts for approximately 1.5% of total U.S. healthcare expenditures and 11.2% of total out-of-pocket expenditures. Nearly two-thirds of the total out-of-pocket costs that adults spent on CAM were for self-care purchases of CAM products, classes, and materials ($22.0 billion), compared with about one-third spent on practitioner visits ($11.9 billion). Despite this emphasis on self-care therapies, 38.1 million adults made an estimated 354.2 million visits to practitioners of CAM.[19]

Barnes and colleagues found that people who use CAM approaches seek ways to improve their health and well-being, attempt to relieve symptoms associated with chronic or even terminal illnesses or the side effects of conventional treatments, have a holistic health philosophy or desire a transformational experience that changes their worldview, and want greater control over their health. The majority of individuals using CAM do so to complement conventional care rather than as an alternative to conventional care. Other findings include the following:[18]

- CAM therapies most commonly used by U.S. adults in the past 12 months were nonvitamin, nonmineral natural products (17.7%), deep breathing exercises (12.7%), meditation (9.4%), chiropractic or osteopathic manipulation (8.6%), massage (8.3%), and yoga (6.1%).
- CAM therapies with increased use between 2002 and 2007 were deep breathing exercises, meditation, yoga, acupuncture, massage therapy, and naturopathy.
- Adults used CAM most often to treat a variety of musculoskeletal problems, including back pain or problems (17.1%), neck pain or problems (5.9%), joint pain or stiffness or other joint condition (5.2%), arthritis (3.5%), and other musculoskeletal conditions (1.8%).

- CAM therapies used most often by children were for back or neck pain (6.7%), head or chest colds (6.6%), anxiety or stress (4.8%), other musculoskeletal problems (4.2%), and attention-deficit hyperactivity disorder or attention-deficit disorder (ADHD/ADD) (2.5%).
- CAM use was more prevalent among women, adults aged 30–69 years, adults with higher levels of education, adults who were not poor, adults living in the West, former smokers, and adults who were hospitalized in the last year.
- CAM usage was positively associated with number of health conditions and number of doctor visits in the past 12 months; however, about one-fifth of adults with no health conditions and one-quarter of adults with no doctor visits in the past 12 months used CAM therapies.
- In both 2002 and 2007, when worry about cost delayed the receipt of conventional medical care, adults were more likely to use CAM than when the cost of conventional care was not a worry. When unable to afford conventional medical care, adults were more likely to use CAM.

The survey of consumer use of CAM by the American Association of Retired Persons (AARP) and National Center for Complementary and Alternative Medicine (NCCAM) found that people 50 years of age and older tend to be high users of complementary and alternative medicine:[20]

- More than one-half (53%) of people 50 years and older reported using CAM at some point in their lives, and nearly as many (47%) reported using it in the past 12 months.
- Herbal products or dietary supplements were the type of CAM most commonly used, with just more than a third (37%) of respondents reporting their use, followed by massage therapy, chiropractic manipulation, and other bodywork (22%); mind–body practices (9%); and naturopathy, acupuncture, and homeopathy (5%).
- Women were more likely than men to report using any form of CAM.

- In most cases, the use of CAM increased with educational attainment.
- The most common reasons for using CAM were to prevent illness or for overall wellness (77%), to reduce pain or treat painful conditions (73%), to treat a specific health condition (59%), or to supplement conventional medicine (53%).

Chronically and terminally ill persons consume more healthcare resources than the rest of the population does. The great interest in CAM practices among those who are chronically ill, those with life-threatening conditions, and those at the end of their lives suggests that increased access to some services among these groups could have significant implications for the healthcare system. With the number of older Americans expected to increase dramatically over the next 20 years, alternative strategies for dealing with the elderly population and end-of-life processes will be increasingly important in public policy. If evaluations show that some uses of CAM can lessen the need for more expensive conventional care in these populations, the economic implications for Medicare and Medicaid could be significant. If safe and effective CAM practices become more available to the general population, special and vulnerable populations should also have access to these services, along with conventional health care. CAM would not be a replacement for conventional health care but would be part of the treatment options available. In some cases, CAM practices may be an equal or superior option. CAM offers the possibility of a new paradigm of integrated health care that could affect the affordability, accessibility, and delivery of healthcare services for millions of Americans.

A significant aspect of the AARP/NCCAM study was that respondents were asked if they had discussed CAM use with any of the healthcare providers they see regularly:

- More than two-thirds (67%) of respondents reported that they had not discussed CAM with any healthcare provider (HCP).
- If CAM was discussed at a medical appointment, it was brought up by the patient 55% of the time, by the healthcare provider 26% of the time, or by a relative/friend 14% of

the time. Respondents were twice as likely to say that they raised the topic rather than their healthcare provider.

- The main reasons that respondents and their healthcare providers do not discuss CAM are as follows: the provider never asks (42%), respondents did not know that they should bring up the topic (30%), there is not enough time during a visit (17%), the HCP would have been dismissive or told the respondent not to do it (12%), or the respondent did not feel comfortable discussing the topic with the HCP (11%).
- People aged 50 years and older who use CAM get their information about it from a variety of sources: from family or friends (26%), the Internet (14%), their physician (13%, or 21% for all healthcare providers), publications including magazines, newspapers, and books (13%) and radio or television (7%).

It is clear that people aged 50 years and older are likely to be using CAM. It is also clear that this population frequently uses prescription medications. Common use of CAM as a complement to conventional medicine—and the high use of multiple prescription drugs—further underscores the need for healthcare providers and clients, patients, and families to have an open dialogue to ensure safe and appropriate integrated medical care. The lack of this dialogue points to a need to educate both consumers and healthcare providers about the importance of discussing the use of CAM, how to begin that dialogue, and the implications of not doing so.

Nondisclosure raises important safety issues, such as the potential interactions of medications with herbs used as part of a CAM therapy. In addition, a majority of adults who use CAM therapies use more than one CAM modality and do so in combination with conventional medical care. In the literature, there are few data about the extent to which use of a CAM therapy may interfere with compliance in the use of conventional therapies. It is not known whether clients/patients use products as directed or even for the purpose recommended. Such information is important. Even if a therapy is efficacious, it may have little or no effect if it is taken or used incorrectly.

Furthermore, medicines and other CAM products and procedures may be the source of iatrogenic health problems if they are used incorrectly. Clients/patients who believe that herbal medicines are harmless may be more willing to self-regulate their medication in unsupervised ways.

Healthcare Reform and Integrative Health Care

On March 23, 2010, President Obama signed comprehensive health reform, the *Patient Protection and Affordable Healthcare Act (HR 3590)*, into law. This law and subsequent legislation focus on provisions to expand health coverage, control health costs, and improve the healthcare delivery system. Discussion of the specifics of this legislation is beyond the scope of this chapter; however, sections that will shape policy relative to integrative healthcare practices in the future are discussed here.[21]

1. *Inclusion of Licensed Practitioners Insurance Coverage* (SEC. 2706. NON-DISCRIMINATION IN HEALTH CARE). Providers: A group health plan and a health insurance issuer offering group or individual health insurance coverage shall not discriminate with respect to participation under the plan or coverage against any healthcare provider who is acting within the scope of that provider's license or certification under applicable state law.

2. *Inclusion of Licensed Complementary and Alternative Medicine Practitioners in Medical Homes* (SEC. 3502. ESTABLISHING COMMUNITY HEALTH TEAMS TO SUPPORT THE PATIENT-CENTERED MEDICAL HOME). The Secretary of Health and Human Services shall establish a program to provide grants to or enter into contracts with eligible entities to establish community-based interdisciplinary, interprofessional teams(referred to as 'health teams') to support primary care practices. Such teams may include medical specialists, nurses, pharmacists, nutritionists, dietitians, social workers, behavioral and mental health providers, doctors of chiropractic, licensed complementary and alternative medicine practitioners.

3. *Integrative Health Care and Integrative Practitioners in Prevention Strategies* (SEC. 4001. NATIONAL PREVENTION, HEALTH PROMOTION AND PUBLIC HEALTH COUNCIL). This council will provide coordination and leadership at the federal level, and among all federal departments and agencies, with respect to prevention, wellness and health promotion practices, the public health system, and integrative health care in the United States; develop a national prevention, health promotion, public health, and integrative healthcare strategy that incorporates the most effective and achievable means of improving the health status of Americans and reducing the incidence of preventable illness and disability in the United States; propose evidence-based models, policies, and innovative approaches for the promotion of transformative models of prevention, integrative health, and public health on individual and community levels across the United States.

4. *Dietary Supplements in Individualized Wellness Plans* (SEC. 4206. DEMONSTRATION PROJECT CONCERNING INDIVIDUALIZED WELLNESS PLAN). Establish a pilot program to test the impact of providing at-risk populations who utilize community health centers funded under this section an individualized wellness plan that is designed to reduce risk factors for preventable conditions. An individualized wellness plan prepared under the pilot program under this subsection may include one or more of the following as appropriate to the individual's identified risk factors:

   (i)   Nutritional counseling
   (ii) A physical activity plan
   (iii) Alcohol and smoking cessation counseling and services
   (iv) Stress management
   (v)   Dietary supplements that have health claims approved by the Secretary

5. *Licensed Complementary and Alternative Providers and Integrative Practitioners in Workforce Planning* (SEC. 5101. NATIONAL HEALTH CARE WORKFORCE COMMISSION). The term *healthcare workforce* includes all healthcare providers with direct patient care and support responsibilities, such as physicians, nurses, nurse practitioners, primary care providers, preventive medicine physicians, optometrists, ophthalmologists, physician assistants, pharmacists, dentists, dental hygienists, and other oral healthcare professionals, allied health professionals, doctors of chiropractic, community health workers, healthcare paraprofessionals, direct care workers, psychologists and other behavioral and mental health professionals, social workers, physical and occupational therapists, certified nurse midwives, podiatrists, the emergency medical services (EMS) workforce, licensed complementary and alternative medicine providers, integrative health practitioners, public health professionals.

6. *Experts in Integrative Health and State Licensed Integrative Health Practitioners in Comparative Effectiveness Research* (SEC. 6301. PATIENT-CENTERED OUTCOMES RESEARCH). Identify national priorities for research, taking into account factors of disease incidence, prevalence, and burden in the United States (with emphasis on chronic conditions); gaps in evidence in terms of clinical outcomes, practice variations and health disparities in terms of delivery and outcomes of care; the potential for new evidence to improve patient health, well-being, and the quality of care; the effect on national expenditures associated with a healthcare treatment, strategy, or health conditions, as well as patient needs, outcomes, and preferences; the relevance to patients and clinicians in making informed health decisions. Advisory panel consisting of practicing and research clinicians, patients, and experts in scientific and health services research, health services delivery, and evidence-based medicine who have experience in the relevant topic and, as appropriate, experts in integrative health and primary prevention strategies.

Trends

In addition to the data already cited, a number of trends affect and will continue to affect the health of society, delivery, and holistic practices.

Workplace Clinics

Interest has intensified in recent years (particularly with the newly enacted healthcare reform law) as employers move beyond traditional occupational health and convenience care to offering clinics that provide a full range of wellness, health promotion, and primary care services. This is seen as a tool to contain medical costs, such as specialist visits, nongeneric prescriptions, emergency department visits, and avoidable hospitalizations, boost productivity, reduce absenteeism, prevent disability claims and work-related injuries, and enhance companies' reputations as employers while attracting and retaining competitive workforces. Types of clinical services for new workplace programs can include traditional occupational health; acute care ranging from low-acuity episodic care to exacerbations of acute chronic conditions; preventive care including immunizations, lifestyle management, mind–body skills, screenings; wellness assessments and follow-up, health coaching, and education; and disease management for chronic conditions.[22]

Many of the nation's largest employers are focusing on prevention and disease management by adopting an integrative medicine approach. At present, the Corporate Health Improvement Program (CHIP) members include the Ford Motor Company, IBM, Corning, Kimberly Clark, Dow Chemical, Medstat, Nestlé, NASA, Canyon Ranch Resorts, and American Specialty Health. Walmart will open health clinics at approximately 400 U.S. stores over the next 3 years, and at 2,000 stores in the next 5 to 7 years. The clinics will offer preventive and routine care. More than half of the people visiting the existing workplace clinics lack health insurance, and 15% said they would have to go to an emergency department if the clinics were unavailable.

Primary Care

The Institute for Alternative Futures, funded by the Kresge Foundation, forecasts the following aspects of the future of primary care in 2025:[23]

- *Focus on primary prevention.* Primary prevention will be the major focus of primary care in 2025 and will be community focused.
- *Continuously improving health.* Health will be continually assessed and worked on along

multiple dimensions in 2025 so that the physical, medical, nutritional, behavioral, psychological, social, spiritual, and environmental conditions are measured and improved for all covered by primary care.

- *Patient–provider relationships.* Trusting relationships between providers and patients will be the basis of primary care's capacity for promoting health and managing disease. Health provider education will support this capacity. The primary care team members will work to instill caring, joy, love, faith, and hope into their relationship with each person. Once trust has been established, usually through in-person contact, effective communications using responsive and empathic email, phone calls, and avatar-based "cyber care" will reinforce this personal relationship.
- *Primary care team.* Primary care team members will include the patient, nurse practitioners, physicians, psychologist, pharmacist, a health information technician, and community health workers. "Visits" most often will be phone calls, televisits, or virtual visits, though in some cases the visit will be in the clinic. Besides a strong relationship among the patient and some of the primary care team members, most patients will have a relational agent or personal health avatar made available by (or enhanced by) their healthcare provider. This virtual agent will provide health education, coaching, and reinforcement, driven by the person's biomonitoring data and advanced care protocols.
- *Focus on behavioral change.* Primary care routinely will work with individuals to understand how to move choices from the limbic system of the brain that unconsciously controls emotionally directed behaviors to the frontal areas of the cognitive brain, which controls conscious behaviors.
- *Focus on quality and safety.* The chronic care model will evolve to the expanded care model and beyond. By 2025, quality in primary care will include the triple aims of excellent healthcare experience, lower per capita costs, and improved population health.
- *Genome and epigenetic data use.* By 2025, most individuals' genomes will be mapped

and documented in their electronic health record (EHR), with secure access available from anywhere according to established permissions.

- *Broadened vital signs.* The nature of vital signs and their collection will evolve to include a wider range of biophysical, mental/neurological, and place/environmental measures.
- *Personal and community vital signs.* In 2025, primary care will be nearly inseparable from community health. Providers will network with neighborhoods and share their data (with appropriate privacy and security protections) with public health officials who coordinate activities to improve population health.
- *Person-centered care.* In 2025, the individual or person involved in and receiving primary care will not be considered the "patient" except when he or she is in "inpatient care" or having care for acute episodes. Individuals will be doing enhanced self-care. Patient-centered primary care will have evolved to person- and family-centered primary care. The whole person will be the focus of care.
- *Integrative encounters in primary care.* Integrative encounters will address all dimensions of health by bringing the knowledge of conventional, unconventional, complementary, alternative, traditional, and integrative medicine disciplines to bear across the many different cultural traditions of persons cared for.
- *24/7 health care access.* By 2025, health care will be available anytime and everywhere. People seldom will need to be evaluated in the primary care clinic. People will have 24/7 access to their relational agent and access by phone, email, or televisit to some human member of the primary care team much of the time.

Health Care

PricewaterhouseCoopers identifies the following top healthcare issues of the day:[24]

1. Industry-wide, intense efforts to reduce healthcare costs by hospitals, physicians, other providers, payers, and employers.

2. Increased oversight, tax changes, coverage, and consumer demand.
3. Scrambling to adopt healthcare IT.
4. Greater emphasis on fraud and abuse recovery.
5. Technology and telecommunications sectors playing leading roles in health care.
6. Pharmaceutical and life sciences companies evolving from manufacturer and supplier to full partner as focus shifts from lab-based outcomes to promoting wellness and prevention and patient outcomes.
7. Physician groups joining health systems, with more and more hospitals employing physicians.
8. Alternative care delivery models emerging as traditional care delivery gives way to alternative models outside of physicians' offices and hospitals. There also will be an increase in numbers and scope of services by work sites, retail health clinics, home health services, and technology-enabled delivery, for example, email, telehealth, and remote monitoring.
9. Community health becoming a new social reality with a major boost in funding from the government.

Health Workforce

HealthLeaders Media projects that job growth will continue in the healthcare sector. The Bureau of Labor Statistics reports that with the healthcare reform bill mandating insurance for another 30 million Americans and the graying of the U.S. population at an unstoppable pace the healthcare sector will have a hiring resurgence. Census Bureau data show that the ambulatory services sector accounts for nearly one-half of new hires in health care and for the past 3 years has generated more revenues than hospitals have.[25]

Holistic Health

Holistic leader Bill Manahan offers "eight transitions that will bring light and balance to health-care."[26] These include the following transitions:

- From health care being a business to also being a calling
- From the Dominator Model ("what is good for me?") to the Partnership Model ("what is good for all of us?")

- From health care being a science to also being an art—from material, mechanistic, and scientific worldviews to consciousness, mindfulness, and spirit
- From a focus on individual health to a focus also on community health—a balance of these two paradigms
- From unrealistic expectations of the medical system to more realistic expectations—a true understanding of what medical care and pharmaceuticals can and cannot do for people
- From Type II medical malpractice (doing the wrong thing the right way) to no malpractice or only Type I medical malpractice (doing the right thing the wrong way) and decreasing the number of unnecessary and inappropriate procedures, tests, and treatments that are not evidence based
- From living in fear of illness and death to acceptance of illness and death as normal parts of life
- From single-causality mentality to an understanding and acceptance of the multiple causality of disease

The preceding driving forces will propel mainstream health care into the future. Access to healthcare providers who possess knowledge and skills in the promotion of healthful living and the integration of holistic/integrative modalities is a critical need for Americans. Holistic nurses are professionals who have knowledge of a wide range of complementary, alternative, and integrative modalities; health promotion and restoration and disease prevention strategies; and relationship-centered, caring ways of healing. They are in a prime position to meet this need and provide leadership in this national trend.

Recommendations

In 2002, the White House Commission on CAM Policy (WHCCAMP) *Final Report* stated that people have come to recognize that a healthy lifestyle can promote wellness and prevent illness and disease and that many individuals have used CAM modalities to attain this goal.[27] Wellness incorporates a broad array of activities and interventions that focus on the physical, mental, spiritual, and emotional aspects of one's life. The effectiveness of the healthcare delivery system in the future will depend on its ability to use all approaches and modalities to contribute to a sound base for promoting health. Early interventions that promote the development of good health habits and attitudes could help modify many of the negative behaviors and lifestyle choices that begin in adolescence and continue into old age. The report recommends the following items, which are equally if not more important today than when the report was first published:

- Include more evidence-based teaching about CAM approaches in the conventional health professions schools.
- Emphasize the importance of approaches to prevent disease and promote wellness for the long-term health of the American people.
- Increase in importance teaching the principles and practices of self-care and provide lifestyle counseling in professional schools so that health professionals can, in turn, provide this guidance to their patients as well as improve their own health.
- Provide those in the greatest need, including those with chronic illnesses and those with limited incomes, access to the most accurate, up-to-date information about which therapies and products may help and which may harm.
- Design the education and training of all practitioners to increase the availability of practitioners knowledgeable in both CAM and conventional practices. The report was based on the guiding principles shown in **Table 3-1.**

Similarly, the 2005 Institute of Medicine report titled *Complementary and Alternative Medicine in the United States* recommends the following, which necessitate attention in today's healthcare context:[28]

- Health professionals take into account a patient's individuality, emotional needs, values, and life issues; implement strategies for reaching those who do not ask for care on their own, including healthcare strategies that support the broader community; and enhance prevention and health promotion.

TABLE 3-1   The White House Commission on CAM Policy Guiding Principles

1. A wholeness orientation in healthcare delivery
2. Evidence of safety and efficacy
3. The healing capacity of the person
4. Respect for individuality
5. The right to choose treatment
6. An emphasis on health promotion and self-care
7. Partnerships as essential for integrated health care
8. Education as a fundamental healthcare service; education about prevention, healthful lifestyles, and the power of self-healing should be made an integral part of the curricula of all healthcare professionals and should be made available to the public at all ages
9. Dissemination of comprehensive and timely information
10. Integral public involvement; the input of informed consumers and other members of the public must be incorporated in setting priorities for health care, healthcare research, and in reaching policy decisions, including those related to CAM, within the public and private sectors

- Health professions schools (e.g., medicine, nursing, pharmacy, allied health) incorporate sufficient information about CAM into the standard curriculum at the undergraduate, graduate, and postgraduate levels to enable licensed professions to competently advise patients about CAM.

- National professional organizations of all CAM disciplines ensure the presence of training standards and develop practice guidelines. Healthcare professional licensing boards and crediting and certifying agencies (for both CAM and conventional medicine) should set competency standards in the appropriate use of both conventional medicine and CAM therapies, consistent with practitioners' scope of practice and standards of referral across health professions.

- Needed is a moral commitment of openness to diverse interpretations of health and healing, a commitment to finding innovative ways of obtaining evidence, and an expansion of the knowledge base relevant and appropriate to medical practice. One way to honor social pluralism is in the recognition of medical pluralism, meaning the broad differences in preferences and values expressed through the public's prevalent use of CAM modalities. Medical pluralism should be distinguished from the co-optation of CAM therapies by conventional medical practices. The hazard of integration is that certain CAM therapies may be delivered within the context of a conventional medical practice in ways that dissociate CAM modalities from the epistemological framework that guides the tailoring of the CAM practice. The proper attitude is one of skepticism about any claim that conventional biomedical research and practice exhaustively account for the human experiences of health and healing.

- Research aimed at answering questions about outcomes of care is crucial to ensuring that healthcare professionals provide evidence-based, comprehensive care that encourages a focus on healing, recognizes the importance of compassion and caring, emphasizes the centrality of relationship-based care, encourages patients to share in decision making about therapeutic options, and promotes choices in care that can include complementary and alternative medical therapies when appropriate.

- The National Institutes of Health (NIH) and other public and private agencies sponsor research to compare the outcomes and costs of combinations of CAM and conventional medical treatments and develop models that deliver such care.

- The U.S. Congress and federal agencies, in consultation with industry, research scientists, consumers, and other stakeholders, amend the current regulatory scheme for dietary supplements

A recent initiative, Wellness Initiative for the Nation (WIN),[29] was created to proactively prevent disease and illness, promote health and productivity, and create well-being and flourishing of the people of the United States. WIN also plays an important role in preventing the looming fiscal disaster in the healthcare system by addressing preventable chronic illness and creating a productive, self-care society. This may be the only long-term hope for changing a system that costs too much and is delivering less health and little care to fewer people. WIN, focusing on promotion of health through lifestyle change and integrative health practices, would be overseen by the White House, with a director and staff to guide relevant aspects of health reform. It would establish a network of Systems Wellness Advancements Teams (SWAT) with national and local leaders in health promotion and integrative practices; establish educational and practice standards for effective, comprehensive lifestyle and integrative healthcare delivery; create an advanced information tracking and feedback system for personalized wellness education; and create economic incentives for individuals, communities, and public and private sectors to create and deliver self-care training, wellness products, and preventive health practices. The components of human health behavior and productivity optimization identified by WIN include stress management and resilience, physical exercise and sleep, optimum nutrition and substance use, and social integration and the social environment.

In September 2010, the Surgeon General convened the National Prevention and Health Promotion Council to create the *National Prevention Strategy*.[30] The vision of this Strategy is working together (state, local and territorial governments, businesses, health care, education and community faith-based organizations) to improve the health and quality of life for individuals, families, and communities by moving the nation from a focus on sickness and disease to one based on wellness and prevention. The Strate-

gic Directions are Healthy and Safe Communities, Clinical and Community Preventive Services, Empowered People, and Elimination of Health Disparities. The goals are to create community environments that make the healthy choice the easy and affordable choice, to implement effective preventive practices by creating and recognizing communities that support prevention and wellness, to connect prevention-focused health care and community efforts to increase preventive services, to empower and educate individuals to make healthy choices, and to eliminate disparities in traditionally underserved populations. The Strategic Priorities (e.g., active lifestyles, countering alcohol/substance misuse, healthy eating, healthy physical and social environment, injury and violence-free living, reproductive and sexual health, mental and emotional well-being) are designed to address ways to prevent significant causes of death and disability by focusing on the factors that underlie their causes.

In February 2009, the Institute of Medicine (IOM) and the Bravewell Collaborative convened the Summit on Integrative Medicine and the Health of the Public that brought together more than 600 participants from numerous disciplines to examine the practice of integrative medicine/health care, its scientific basis, and its potential for improving health.[4] The Summit sessions covered overarching visions for integrative medicine/health care, models of care, workforce, research, health professions education needs, and economic and policy implications. Participants assessed the potential and the priorities and began to identify elements of an agenda to improve understanding, training, and practice to improve integrative medicine's contributions to better health and health care. Recurring themes of the Summit are identified in **Table 3-2**.

A number of considerations for healthcare reform were articulated:

- *The progression of many chronic diseases can be reversed and sometimes even completely healed through lifestyle modifications.* Lifestyle modifications programs have been proven not only to improve people's overall health and well-being but also to mitigate cardiac disease and prostate cancer, among other chronic conditions.

TABLE 3-2   Themes of the Summit on Integrative Medicine and the Health of the Public

- *Vision of optimal health:* Alignment of individuals and their health care for optimal health and healing across a full life span
- *Conceptually inclusive:* Seamless engagement of the full range of established health factors—physical, psychological, social, preventive, and therapeutic
- *Life span horizon:* Integration across the life span to include personal, predictive, preventive, and participatory care
- *Person-centered:* Integration around, and within, each person
- *Prevention-oriented:* Prevention and disease minimization as the foundation of integrative health care
- *Team-based:* Care as a team activity, with the patient as a central team member
- *Care integration:* Seamless integration of the care processes, across caregivers and institutions
- *Caring integration:* Person- and relationship-centered care
- *Science integration:* Integration across scientific disciplines, and scientific processes that cross domains
- *Integration of approach:* Integration across approaches to care—for example, conventional, traditional, alternative, complementary—as the evidence supports
- *Policy opportunities:* Emphasis on outcomes, elevation of patient insights, consideration of family and social factors, inclusion of team care and supportive follow-up, and contributions to the learning process

- *Genetics is not destiny.* Recent research shows that gene expression can be turned on or off by nutritional choices, levels of social support, stress reduction activities such as meditation, and exercise.
- *The environment influences health.* Mounting evidence suggests that the environment outside one's body rapidly becomes the environment inside the body.
- *Improving the primary care and chronic disease care systems is paramount.* The U.S. primary care system is in danger of collapse and we must retool how both primary and chronic disease care are delivered. The new system must focus on prevention and wellness and put the patient at the center of care.
- *The reimbursement system must be changed.* The current reimbursement system rewards procedures rather than outcomes, and changes are needed that incentivize healthcare providers to focus on the health outcomes of their patients/clients.
- *Changes in education will fuel changes in practice.* Implementation of an integrated approach to health care requires changes in health provider education. All healthcare practitioners should be educated in team

approaches and the importance of compassionate care that addresses the biopsychosocial dimensions of health, prevention, and well-being. Core competencies need to be redefined and new categories explored.
- *Evidence-based medicine/health care is the only acceptable standard.* Health care should be supported by evidence. Further research and testing to expand the evidence base for integrative models of care requires attention.
- *Research must better accommodate multifaceted and interacting factors.* Research must clarify the nature by which biological predispositions and responses interact with social and environmental influences. Projects are needed to identify effective integrated approaches that demonstrate value, sustainability, and scalability.
- *A large demonstration project is recommended.* Because funding for research on the effectiveness of specific models of care is difficult to obtain from standard grant channels, participants voiced support for pursuing a demonstration project funded by the government that would fully exhibit the effectiveness of the integrative approach to care.

■ ISSUES IN HOLISTIC NURSING

In December 2006, holistic nursing was officially recognized by the American Nurses Association (ANA) as a distinct nursing specialty with a defined scope and standards of practice, acknowledging holistic nursing's unique contribution to the health and healing of people and society. This recognition provides holistic nurses with clarity and a foundation for their practice and gives holistic nursing legitimacy and voice within the nursing profession and credibility in the eyes of the healthcare world and the public. *Holistic Nursing: Scope and Standards of Practice*[31] was published in 2007.

Yet a number of issues exist or will emerge in the future for holistic nursing. Acceptance of holistic nursing's influence and contribution, both within nursing as well as other disciplines, continues as one of the most pressing matters. Other concerns can be categorized into the areas of education, research, clinical practice, and policy. It is important to note that because holistic nursing as well as nursing in general and other disciplines face many of the same issues, an interdisciplinary approach is imperative for success in achieving the desired outcomes.

Education

There are several areas of educational challenge in the holistic arena. With increased use of complementary/alternative/integrative therapies by the American public, both students and faculty need knowledge of and skill in their use. One urgent priority is the integration of holistic, relationship-centered philosophies and integrative modalities into nursing curricula. Core content appropriate for both basic and advanced practice programs needs to be identified, and models for integration of both content and practical experiences into existing curricula are necessary. An elective course is not sufficient to imbue future practitioners of nursing with this knowledge.

On a positive note, in 2008, the AHNA worked with the American Association of Colleges of Nursing (AACN) in the revision of the *Essentials of Baccalaureate Education for Professional Nursing Practice*.[32] Included in these new *Essentials* is language on preparing the baccalaureate generalist graduate to practice from a holistic, caring framework; engage in self-care; develop an understanding of complementary and alternative modalities; and incorporate patient teaching and health promotion, spirituality, and caring, healing techniques into practice. Holistic nurses will need to continue to work with the accrediting bodies of academic degree programs to ensure that this content is included in educational programs.

Benner and associates note that the need for better nursing education in nursing, social and natural sciences, humanities, problem solving, teaching, and interpersonal capacities is even more acute than it was even 10 years ago. The 2010 Carnegie Foundation's report *Educating Nurses: A Call for Radical Transformation*[33] recommends the following:

- Broadening clinical experiences to community health care
- Promoting and supporting students' learning the skills of inquiry and research
- Teaching the ethics of care and responsibility, the ethos of self-care in the profession, skills of involvement and clinical reasoning and reflection
- Teaching strategies for organizational change, organizational development, policy making, leadership, and improvement of healthcare systems
- Incorporating evidence-based practice and critical reflection
- Assisting students to better understand the patient's context and how they can help patients improve their access and continuity of care
- Teaching relational skills of involvement and caring practices
- Teaching collegial and collaborative skills

The National Educational Dialogue, an outgrowth of the Integrated Healthcare Policy Consortium (IAHC), sought to identify a set of core values, knowledge, skills, and attitudes necessary for all healthcare professional students. The Task Force on Values, Knowledge, Skills, and Attitudes, chaired by Carla Mariano, identified the following core values:[34]

- Wholeness and healing—interconnectedness of all people and things with healing as an innate capacity of every individual
- Clients/patients/families as the center of practice

- Practice as a combined art and science
- Self-care of the practitioner and commitment to self-reflection, personal growth, and healing
- Interdisciplinary collaboration and integration embracing the breadth and depth of diverse healthcare systems and collaboration with all disciplines, clients, and families
- Responsibility to contribute to the improvement of the community, the environment, health promotion, healthcare access, and the betterment of public health
- Attitudes and behaviors of all participants in health care demonstrating respect for self and others, humility, and authentic, open, courageous communication

There is a definitive need for increased scholarship and financial aid to support training in all of these areas. Faculty development programs also are necessary to support faculty in understanding and integrating holistic philosophy, content and practices into curricula.

A major report by the IOM in 2010, *The Future of Nursing: Leading Change, Advancing Health*,[35] will have a significant effect on the nursing profession. The report recommends that *nurses should achieve higher levels of education and training through improved educational systems* by increasing the proportion of nurses with a baccalaureate degree to 80% by 2020, doubling the number of nurses with a doctorate by 2020, and ensuring that nurses engage in lifelong learning. Nurses need more education and preparation to adopt new roles quickly in response to rapidly changing healthcare settings and an evolving healthcare system. Competencies are especially needed in community, geriatrics, leadership, health policy, system improvement and change, research and evidence-based practice, and teamwork and collaboration.

To improve the competency of practitioners and the quality of services, holistic and CAM education and training needs to continue beyond basic and advanced academic education. Continuing education programs at national and regional specialty organizations and conferences may assist in meeting this need. Working with practitioners in other areas of nursing to increase their understanding of the philosophical and theoretical foundations of holistic nursing practices

(e.g., consciousness, intention, presence, centering) will also be a role of holistic nurses.

Research

Research in the area of holistic nursing will become increasingly important in the future. Three areas of research seem to be widely proposed: whole systems research, exploration of healing relationships, and outcomes of healing interventions, particularly in the areas of health promotion and prevention.

There is a great need for an evidence base to establish the effectiveness and efficacy of complementary/alternative/integrative therapies. Formidable tasks for nurses will be to identify and describe outcomes of CAM and holistic therapies such as healing, well-being, and harmony and to develop instruments to measure these outcomes. The IOM report on CAM in the United States recommends qualitative and quantitative research to examine the following:[28]

- The social and cultural dimensions of illness experiences, the processes and preferences of seeking health care, and practitioner–patient interactions
- How often users of CAM, including patients and providers, adhere to treatment instructions and guidelines
- The effects of CAM on wellness and disease prevention
- How the American public accesses and evaluates information about CAM modalities
- Adverse events associated with CAM therapies and interactions between CAM and conventional treatments
- Accessing information about CAM, such as follows:
  - Where the public goes to search for information about CAM modalities
  - What sources of information they commonly find and access
  - The effect of CAM advertising on the methods of seeking health care
  - What types of the information are deemed credible, marginal, and spurious
  - How risks and benefits are understood and how such perceptions inform decision making
  - What the public expects their providers to tell them

The current mission of the National Center for Complementary and Alternative Medicine (NCCAM) is developing evidence requiring support across the continuum of basic science (How does the therapy work?), translational research (Can it be studied in people?), efficacy studies (What are the specific effects?), and outcomes and effectiveness research (How well does the CAM practice work in the general population or healthcare settings?). The *NCCAM Third Strategic Plan Exploring the Science of Complementary and Alternative Medicine: 2011–2015*[1] identifies five strategic objectives:

- Advance research on mind and body interventions, practices, and disciplines.
- Advance research on natural products.
- Increase understanding of "real-world" patterns and outcomes of CAM use and its integration into health care and health promotion.
- Improve the capacity of the field to carry out rigorous research.
- Develop and disseminate objective, evidence-based information on CAM interventions.

These objectives address the three long-range goals of (1) advancing the science and practice of symptom management; (2) developing effective, practical, personalized strategies for promoting health and well-being; and (3) enabling better evidence-based decision making regarding CAM use and its integration into health care and health promotion.[1]

Presently, most outcome measures are based on physical or disease symptomatology. However, methodologies need to be expanded to capture the wholeness of the individual's experience because the philosophy of these therapies rests on a paradigm of wholeness.

> Integrative health care is *derived from lessons integrated across scientific disciplines, and it requires scientific processes that cross domains.* The most important influences on health, for individuals and society, are not the factors at play within any single domain—genetics, behavior, social or economic circumstances, physical environment, health care—but the dynamics and synergies across domains. Research tends to examine these influ-

ences in isolation, which can distort interpretation of the results and hinder application of results. The most value will come from broader, systems-level approaches and redesign of research strategies and methodologies.[4 p.7]

In 2010, the Patient Protection and Affordable Care Act created a Patient-Centered Outcomes Research Institute (PCORI) that will act as a nonprofit organization to assist patients, clinicians, purchasers, and policy makers in making informed health decisions by carrying out research projects that provide high-quality, relevant evidence on how diseases, disorders, and other health conditions can effectively and appropriately be prevented, diagnosed, treated, monitored, and managed. Patient Centered Outcomes Research (PCOR) helps people make informed healthcare decisions and allows their voice to be heard in assessing the value of healthcare options. This research answers patient-focused questions.[36]

1. "Given my personal characteristics, conditions and preferences, what should I expect will happen to me?"
2. "What are my options and what are the benefits and harms of those options?"
3. "What can I do to improve the outcomes that are most important to me?"
4. "How can the healthcare system improve my chances of achieving the outcomes I prefer?"

To answer these questions, PCOR:

- Assesses the benefits and harms of preventive, diagnostic, therapeutic, or health delivery system interventions to inform decision making, highlighting comparisons and outcomes that matter to people;
- Is inclusive of an individual's preferences, autonomy and needs, focusing on outcomes that people notice and care about such as survival, function, symptoms, and health-related quality of life;
- Incorporates a wide variety of settings and diversity of participants to address individual differences and barriers to implementation and dissemination; and
- Investigates (or may investigate) optimizing outcomes while addressing burden to

individuals, resources, and other stake-holder perspectives.[36]

The *Journal of Alternative and Complementary Medicine* collaborated with the International Society for Complementary Medicine Research (ISCMR) to sponsor a forum on the research issues for whole systems. Participants underscored the political and economic challenges of getting research funded and published if researchers look at the practices and processes that typify whole-person treatment. What is clear is that whole practices, whole systems, and related research need professional and organizational attention.

> Today researchers are being challenged to look at alternative philosophies of science and research methods that are compatible with investigations of humanistic and holistic occurrences. We also need to study phenomena by exploring the context in which they occur and the meaning of patterns that evolve. Also needed are approaches to interventions studies that are more holistic, taking into consideration the *interactive* nature of the body-mind-emotion-spirit-environment. Rather than isolating the effects of one part of an intervention, we need more comprehensive interventions and more sensitive instruments that measure the interactive nature of each client's biological, psychological, sociological, emotional, and spiritual patterns. In addition, comprehensive comparative outcome studies are needed to ascertain the usefulness, indications, and contraindications of integrative therapies. Further, researchers must evaluate these interventions for their usefulness in promoting wellness as well as preventing illness.[37]

Investigations into the concept and nature of the placebo effect also are needed because one-third of all medical healings are the result of the placebo effect.[38]

It will be imperative for nurses to address how to secure funding for their holistic research. They need to apply for funding from National Institutes of Health (NIH) centers and institutes in addition to the National Institute of Nursing Research and particularly the National Center for Complementary and Alternative Medicine. Hand in hand with this is the need for nurses to be represented in study sections and review panels to educate and convince the biomedical and NIH community about the value of nursing research; the need for models of research focusing on health promotion and disease prevention, wellness, and self-care instead of only the disease model; and the importance of a variety of designs and research methodologies including qualitative studies, rather than sole reliance on randomized controlled trials.

An area of responsibility for advanced practice holistic nurses is the dissemination of their research findings to various media sources (e.g., television, newsprint) and at nonnursing, interdisciplinary conferences. Publishing in nonnursing journals and serving on editorial boards of nonnursing journals also broadens the appreciation in other disciplines for nursing's role in setting the agenda and conducting research in the area of holism and CAM.

Clinical Practice

Clinical care models reflecting holistic assessment, treatment, health, healing, and caring are important in the development of holistic nursing practice. Implementing holistic and humanistic models in today's healthcare environment will require a paradigm shift for the many providers who subscribe to a disease model of care. Such an acceptance poses an enormous challenge. Holistic nurses, with their education and experience, are the logical leaders in integrative care and must advance that position.

Licensure and credentialing provide another challenge for holistic nursing. As complementary/alternative/integrative health care has gained national recognition, state boards of nursing began to attend to the regulation issues. The 2010 IOM report *The Future of Nursing*[35] notes that regulations defining scope-of-practice limitations vary widely by state. Some states have kept pace with the evolution of the healthcare system by changing their scope-of-practice regulations, but the majority of state laws lag behind in this regard. As a result, what nurse practitioners are able to do once they graduate can vary widely and is often not related to their ability, education or training, or safety concerns but to the political decisions of the state in which they work. The IOM recommends that *nurses should practice to the full extent of their education and training* and that *scope-of-practice barriers should be removed.* The IOM also recommends that *nurse residency programs should be implemented.*

In 2010, AHNA conducted a preliminary survey to ascertain the number of state boards of nursing that accepted and recognized holistic nursing and/or permitted holistic practices with its regulations and or the state's nurse practice act. Of the 39 states that responded, 8 states include holistic nursing in their nurse practice act. The findings from a review of actual state practice acts further revealed that 47 of 51 states/territories have some statements or positions that include holistic wording such as *self-care, spirituality, natural therapies,* and/or specific complementary/alternative therapies under the scope of practice.

It will be important in the future to monitor state boards of nursing for evidence of their recognition and support of holistic, integrative nursing practice and requirements that include CAM. Finally, holistic nursing has the challenge of working with the state boards to incorporate this content into the National Council Licensure Examination, thus ensuring the credibility of this practice knowledge.

Addressing the nursing shortage in this country is crucial to the health of our nation. Multiple surveys and studies confirm that the shortage of RNs influences the delivery of health care in the United States and negatively affects patient outcomes. According to the American Hospital Association, the United States is, by all accounts, in the midst of a significant shortage of registered nurses that is projected to last well into the future. Nationally, there is an average vacancy of approximately 116,000 RNs in hospitals. Although shortages of hospital staff nurses have received the greatest amount of national attention, shortages persist in other settings such as 19,400 RN vacancies in long-term-care settings, bringing the national RN vacancy rate to 8.1%.[39] Peter Buerhaus and coauthors found that the U.S. nursing shortage is projected to grow to 260,000 RNs by 2025, which would be twice as large as any nursing shortage experienced in this country since the mid-1960s. Because of the demand for RNs will increase as large numbers of RNs retire, a large and prolonged shortage of nurses is expected to hit the United States in the latter half of the next decade.[40]

According to the AACN's report *2010–2011 Enrollment and Graduations in Baccalaureate and Graduate Programs in Nursing,* in 2010 U.S. nursing schools turned away 67,563 qualified applicants from baccalaureate and graduate nursing programs because of insufficient number of faculty, clinical sites, classroom space, clinical preceptors, and budget constraints. Almost two-thirds of the nursing schools responding to the survey pointed to faculty shortages as a reason for not accepting all qualified applicants into their programs, thus constraining schools' ability to expand enrollment to alleviate the nursing shortage.[39]

Additionally, there are some distressing statistics: in the United States, 41% of nurses are dissatisfied with their present job. Nationally, nurses give themselves burnout scores of 30–40%, and 17% of nurses are not working in nursing. Moreover, 13% of newly licensed RNs had changed principal jobs after 1 year, and 37% reported that they felt ready to change jobs. Nurses often change jobs or leave the profession because of unhumanistic and chaotic work environments and professional and personal burnout. Research shows that reduction of perceived stress is related to job satisfaction. Holistic nurses, through their knowledge of self-care, resilience, caring cultures, healing environments, and stress management techniques, have an extraordinary opportunity to influence and improve the healthcare milieu, both for healthcare providers and for clients and patients[41]

Policy

Four major policy issues face holistic nursing in the future: leadership, reimbursement, regulation, and access. The IOM report *The Future of Nursing*[35] recommends that *nurses should be full partners with physicians and other health professionals in redesigning healthcare in the United States.* Nurses should be prepared and enabled to lead change in all roles—from the bedside to the boardroom—to advance health. Nurses should have a voice in health policy decision making and be engaged in implementation efforts related to healthcare reform, particularly regarding quality, access, value, and patient-centered care. Nurses must see policy as something they can shape rather than something that happens to them.

Public or private policies regarding coverage and reimbursement for healthcare services play a crucial role in shaping the healthcare system and will play a crucial role in deciding the future of wellness, health promotion, and CAM in the nation's healthcare system. According to the *2010 Complementary and Alternative Medicine Survey of Hospitals* conducted by the American Hospital Association and Samueli Institute, hospitals across the nation are responding to patient demand and integrating CAM services with conventional services. More than 42% of hospitals in the survey indicated they offer one or more CAM therapies, up from 37% in 2007 and 26.5% in 2005. Eighty-five percent of responding hospitals cited patient demand as the primary rationale in offering CAM services and 70% stated clinical effectiveness as their top reason.[42] Often, however, holistic modalities are offered as a supplemental benefit rather than as a core or basic benefit, and many third-party payers do not cover such services at all. In the 2010 CAM Survey of Hospitals, 69% of CAM services were paid for out of pocket by patients. Coverage and reimbursement for most CAM services depend on the provider's ability to legally furnish services within the scope of practice. The legal authority to practice is given by the state in which services are provided.

Reimbursement of advanced practice registered nurses also depends on appropriate credentials. Holistic nurses will need to work with Medicare and other third-party payers, insurance groups, boards of nursing, healthcare policymakers, legislators, and other professional nursing organizations to ensure that holistic nurses are appropriately reimbursed for services rendered. Another issue regarding reimbursement is the fact that the effectiveness of CAM is influenced by the holistic focus and integrative skill of the provider. Consequently, reimbursement must be included for the process of holistic and integrative care, not just for providing a specific modality.

There are many barriers to the use of holistic therapies by potential users, providing yet another challenge for holistic nurses. Barriers include lack of awareness of the therapies and their benefits, uncertainty about their effectiveness, inability to pay for them, and limited availability of qualified providers. Access is more difficult for rural populations; uninsured or underinsured populations; special populations, such as racial and ethnic minorities; and vulnerable populations, such as older adults and those with chronic or terminal illnesses.[27] Holistic nurses have a responsibility to educate the public more fully about health promotion, complementary/alternative modalities, and qualified practitioners and to assist people in making informed choices among the array of healthcare alternatives and individual providers. Holistic nurses also must actively participate in the political arena as leaders in this movement to ensure quality, an increased focus on wellness, and access and affordability for all.

By developing theoretical and empirical knowledge as well as caring and healing approaches, holistic nurses will advance holistic nursing practice and education and contribute significantly to the formalization and credibility of this work. They will lead the profession in research, the development of educational models, and the integration of a more holistic approach in nursing practice and health care.

■ CONCLUSION

In closing, I would like to share some thoughts and reflections of various leaders in the field of holistic health care and holistic nursing.

> We need to balance the acquisition of knowledge with a deepening in wisdom. That has to happen throughout the education of all healthcare professionals. There has to be a balance between wisdom and knowledge. And we've lost it. That depth has to do with knowing yourself as a human being as well as a practitioner and healer, being yourself and experiencing yourself and your own struggles and possibilities. There are four things: wisdom balancing knowledge, a community of healers, self-care as the heart of all health care, and health care as a right to which everyone is entitled. If we have these, then the whole health system changes, and all of us—our health and the way we look at the world—will change and improve.
>
> —James Gordon, MD[43]

The advancement of health care in general relies on the patience and professional contributions of people who are either trained across disciplines or are comfortable working across disciplines—people who are "bilingual" in their professional lives and comfortable in domains and professional cultures other than their own. Leadership is the ability to work across disciplines and facilitate collegiate relationships. Disciplines need to shake hands and admit that they don't speak the same language, but they share the same questions. That's how contributions are made and progress happens. That's how we will determine how this field [holistic health care] ends up. It will happen across disciplines and across international borders.

—David Eisenberg, MD[44]

Nurses are exceedingly well positioned to become leaders in integrative health. Nurses constitute the nation's largest group of health professionals [more than 3 million]. . . . Nightingale described the nurse's work as helping a patient attain the best possible condition so that nature can act and self-healing may occur. Nurses go beyond fixing or curing to ease the edges of patients' suffering. They help people return to day-to-day functioning, maintain health, live with chronic illness, and/or gracefully move through stages of dying into death. Nurses are experts in symptom management, care coordination, chronic disease management, and health promotion. In addition to caring for people from birth to death, nurses currently manage care for communities, conduct research, lead health systems, and address health policy issues.

—Mary Jo Kreitzer, PhD, RN, FAAN[45]

Our work—nursing—is a calling, not only to serve but to deepen our humanity. It is a spiritual practice. . . . The tasks of *Nursing* are the tasks of *Humanity*: healing and relationship with self,

others, the planet; developing a deeper understanding of human suffering; expanding and evolving an understanding of life itself; deepening an understanding of death and the sacred cycle. . . . We must revisit the foundations of our work. Caring is an ethic—it forces us to pay attention. Pause and realize that this one moment with this one person is the reason we are here at this time on this planet. When we touch their body, we touch their mind, heart, and soul. When we connect with another's humanity even for a brief moment, we have purpose in our life and work.

—Jean Watson, PhD, RN, AHN-BC, FAAN[46]

Directions for FUTURE RESEARCH

1. Identify the strengths and limitations of different research approaches to studying holistic phenomena.
2. Explore research findings on various CAM therapies.

Nurse Healer REFLECTIONS

After reading this chapter, the holistic nurse will be able to answer or to begin a process of answering the following questions:

- What is my vision of a caring, healing, holistic healthcare system?
- What are my beliefs, values, and assumptions about my contributions and other healthcare disciplines' contributions to the health of society?

 For a full suite of assignments and additional learning activities, use the access code located in the front of your book to visit this exclusive website: http://go.jblearning.com/dossey. If you do not have an access code, you can obtain one at the site.

NOTES

1. National Center for Complementary and Alternative Medicine, *Exploring the Science of Complementary and Alternative Medicine: Third Strategic Plan 2011–2015* (Washington, DC: U.S. Department of Health and Human Services, National Institutes of Health, 2011).

2. U.S. Department of Health and Human Services, *Healthy People 2020* (Washington, DC: USDHHS, 2010). http://www.healthypeople.gov.

3. Public Agenda, "Half of Americans Say the Health Care System Has Major Problems" (May 11, 2011). http://www.publicagenda.org/charts/half-americans-say-health-care-system-has-major-problems-and-most-say-it-needs-be-fundamentally-changed-or.

4. Institute of Medicine, *Summit on Integrative Medicine and the Health of the Public* (Washington, DC: National Academy of Sciences, 2009): 1–2.

5. Centers for Disease Control and Prevention, "Chronic Disease Prevention and Health Promotion" (May 11, 2011). http://www.cdc.gov/chronicdisease/index.htm.

6. R. Lee, "The New Pandemic: Superstress?" *Explore: The Journal of Science and Healing* 6, no. 1 (2010): 7–10.

7. U.S. Census Bureau, *Statistical Abstract of the United States: 2011* (Washington, DC: U.S. Centers for Medicare and Medicaid Services, Office of the Actuary, 2011). http://www.cms.hhs.gov/NationalHealthExpendData.

8. KaiserEdu.org, *U.S. Health Care Costs: Background Brief* (March 2010). http://www.kaiseredu.org/Issue-Modules/US-Health-Care-Costs.

9. J. Weeks, "Charting the Mainstream: Trends, Data and Action of Use to Efforts to Better Integrate Care," *Integrator Blog* (March 3, 2007). http://theintegratorblog.com/site/index.php?option=com_content&task=view&id=242&Itemid=189.

10. L. M. Milliman, "Milliman Medical Index Indicates Healthcare Costs for Typical American Family of Four Have Doubled in Fewer Than Nine Years," Press Release (May 11, 2011). http://www.milliman.com/news-events/press/pdfs/milliman-medical-index-indicates.pdf.

11. Henry J. Kaiser Family Foundation, "Kaiser Slides: Costs/Insurance" (September 2010). http://facts.kff.org/results.aspx?view=slides&topic=3.

12. R. Wolf, "Number of Uninsured Americans Rises to 50.7 Million," *USA Today*, September 16, 2010.

13. HealthCare Problems.org, "Health Care Statistics" (September 2011). http://www.healthcareproblems.org/health-care-statistics.htm.

14. Centers for Disease Control and Prevention, *Early Release of Selected Estimates Based on Data From the 2009 National Health Interview Survey: Obtaining Needed Medical Care* (June 2010). http://www.cdc.gov/nchs/data/nhis/earlyrelease/201006_03.pdf.

15. M. Hyman, "Quality in Health Care: Asking the Right Questions in Next Ten Years: The Role of CAM in the 'Quality Cure,'" *Alternative Therapies* 11, no. 3 (2005): 18–19.

16. D. Eisenberg et al., "Unconventional Medicine in the United States: Prevalence, Costs and Patterns of Use," *New England Journal of Medicine* 328, no. 4 (1993): 246–252.

17. D. Eisenberg et al., "Trends in Alternative Medicine Use in the United States, 1990–1997," *Journal of the American Medical Association* 280 (1998): 1569–1575.

18. P. M. Barnes, B. Bloom, and B. R. Nahin, "Complementary and Alternative Medicine Use Among Adults and Children: United States, 2007," *CDC National Health Statistics Reports* no. 12, (December 2008).

19. National Center for Complementary and Alternative Medicine, "Americans Spent $33.9 Billion Out-of-Pocket on Complementary and Alternative Medicine" (July 30, 2009). http://nccam.nih.gov/news/2009/073009.htm.

20. AARP/National Center for Complementary and Alternative Medicine, *Complementary and Alternative Medicine: What People Aged 50 and Older Discuss With Their Health Care Providers* (Washington, DC: USDHHS, April 2011).

21. J. Weeks, "Reference Guide: Language and Sections on CAM and Integrative Practice in HR 3590/Healthcare Overhaul," *Integrator Blog* (May 12, 2010). http://theintegratorblog.com/site/index.php?option=com_content&task=view&id=658&Itemid=2.

22. H. Tu, E. Boukus, and G. Cohen, "Workplace Clinics: A Sign of Growing Employer Interest in Wellness," *Health Systems Change*, HSC Research Brief no. 17 (2010).

23. C. Bezold, "Alert: Major Study on Future of Primary Care Seeks Input on IM Therapies and CAM Practitioners," *Integrator Blog* (April 25, 2011). http://theintegratorblog.com/index.php?option=com_content&task=view&id=744&Itemid=189.

24. D. Manos, "Healthcare IT among PricewaterhouseCoopers's (PWC) List of Top 10 Healthcare Issues for 2010," *HealthcareITNews.com* (December 17, 2009). http://www.healthcareitnews.com/news/healthcare-it-among-pwcs-list-top-10-healthcare-issues-2010.

25. J. Commins, "Eight Healthcare HR Trends for 2010," *HealthLeaders Media* (January 4, 2010). http://www.healthleadersmedia.com/content/HR-244371/Eight-Healthcare-HR-Trends-for-2010.html.

26. B. Manahan, "Revisioning Healthcare in 2009: Eight Transitions That Will Help Bring Light and Balance to Healthcare," *Integrator Blog* (January 14,

2009). http://theintegratorblog.com/site/index.php?option=com_content&task=view&id=519&Itemid=189.

27. White House Commission on Complementary and Alternative Medicine Policy (WHCCAMP), *Final Report* (Washington, DC: U.S. Government Printing Office, 2002).

28. Institute of Medicine, *Complementary and Alternative Medicine in the United States* (Washington, DC: National Academies Press, 2005).

29. Samueli Institute, *A Wellness Initiative for the Nation (WIN)* (2009). http://www.lifesciencefoundation.org/WellnessInitiative11feb09.pdf.

30. U.S. Office of the Surgeon General, *The National Prevention and Health Promotion Strategy (National Prevention Strategy)* (Washington, DC: U.S. Health and Human Services, 2011).

31. American Holistic Nurses Association & American Nurses Association, *Holistic Nursing: Scope and Standards of Practice* (Silver Spring, MD: NurseBooks.org, 2007).

32. American Association of Colleges of Nursing, *The Essentials of Baccalaureate Education for Professional Nursing Practice* (Washington, DC: AACN, 2008).

33. P. Benner, M. Sutphen, V. Leonard, and L. Day, *Educating Nurses: A Call for Radical Transformation*. (San Francisco: Jossey-Bass, 2010).

34. E. Goldblatt, P. Snider, S. Quinn, and J. Weeks, *Clinicians' and Educators' Desk Reference on the Licensed Complementary and Alternative Healthcare Professions* (Seattle, WA: ACCAHC, 2009).

35. Institute of Medicine, *The Future of Nursing: Leading Change, Advancing Health* (Washington, DC: National Academies Press, 2010). http://www.iom.edu/nursing.

36. J. Weeks, "Culture Change: Patient-Centered Outcomes at the Center of New $600-Million/Year Quasi-Governmental Research Institute (PCORI)," *Integrator Blog* (September 26, 2011).

37. C. Mariano, "Contributions to Holism Through Critique of Theory and Research," *Beginnings* 28, no. 2 (2008): 26.

38. C. Mariano, *Research in Holism: A Nursing Perspective*, Keynote Presentation, Lexington, KY (March 2011).

39. Colleges of Nursing, "Nursing Shortage" (AACN Fact Sheet, April, 2011). http://www.aacn.nche.edu/media/factsheets.

40. P. Buerhaus et al., "The Recent Surge in Nurse Employment: Causes and Implications," *Health Affairs* 28, no. 4 (2009): w657–w668.

41. C. Mariano, "The Nursing Shortages: Is Stress Management the Answer?" *Beginnings* 27, no. 1 (2007): 3.

42. Health Forum & Samueli Institute, *2010 Complementary and Alternative Medicine Survey of Hospitals Summary of Results* (Samueli Institute, 2011).

43. K. Gazella and S. Snyder, "James S. Gordon, MD: Connecting Mind, Body, and Beyond," *Alternative Therapies* 12, no. 2 (2006): 72–73.

44. K. Gazella and S. Snyder, "David Eisenberg, MD: Integrative Medicine Research Pioneer," *Alternative Therapies* 12, no. 1 (2006): 79.

45. M. Mittelman, S. Alperson, P. Arcari, G. Donnelly, L. Ford, M. Koithan, and M. J. Kreitzer, "Nursing and Integrative Health Care," *Alternative Therapies* 16, no. 5 (2010): 80.

46. J. Watson, *Human Caring and Holistic Healing: The Path of Heart and Spirit*, Keynote Presentation, AHNA Annual Conference, Colorado Springs, CO (2010).

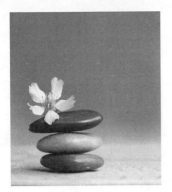

Chapter 4

Transpersonal Human Caring and Healing

Janet F. Quinn

Nurse Healer
OBJECTIVES

Theoretical

- Define transpersonal human caring.
- Define healing.
- Compare and contrast the processes of healing and curing.
- Discuss the nature of "right relationship" as it relates to healing.

Clinical

- Apply the elements of a "caring occasion" to facilitate healing.
- Describe examples of healing at the body, mind, and spirit levels of human experience that you have observed in practice.
- Begin to imagine how your own clinical practice setting might evolve to become a "Habitat for Healing."

Personal

- Imagine what right relationship would look like and feel like when applied to something you want to heal in yourself.
- Identify ways in which you can create your own healing environment.

Portions of this chapter have been published as: J. Quinn, "Healing: A Model for an Integrative Health Care System," *Advanced Practice Nursing Quarterly* 3, no. 1 (1997):1–7, by permission of Aspen Publishers.

DEFINITIONS

Habitats for Healing: Healthcare practice environments that provide a context of caring, for the purpose of healing, which may include curing.[1]

Healing: The emergence of right relationship at one or more levels of the bodymindspirit system.[2]

Healing system: A true healthcare system in which people can receive adequate, nontoxic, and noninvasive assistance in maintaining wellness and in healing for body, mind, and spirit, together with the most sophisticated, aggressive curing technologies available.

Human caring: The moral ideal of nursing in which the nurse brings his or her whole self into relationship with the whole self of the patient or client, to protect the vulnerability and preserve the humanity and dignity of the one caring and the one cared for.[3]

Right relationship: A process of connection among or between parts of the whole that increases energy, coherence, and creativity in the bodymindspirit system.

Transpersonal: That which transcends the limits and boundaries of individual ego identities and possibilities to include acknowledgment and appreciation of something greater. *Transpersonal* may refer to consciousness, intrapersonal dynamics, interpersonal relationships, and lived experiences of connection, unity, and oneness with the larger environment, cosmos, or Spirit.

■ THEORY AND RESEARCH

Within the discipline of nursing, there is widespread acceptance of the concept of caring as central to practice.[4,5] However, there is no widespread consensus as to what caring is. Morse and her colleagues, in their now classic paper, reported that five basic conceptualizations, or perspectives, on caring can be identified in the nursing literature: (1) caring as a human trait, (2) caring as a moral imperative or ideal, (3) caring as an affect, (4) caring as an interpersonal relationship, and (5) caring as a therapeutic intervention.[6]

The term *transpersonal human caring* is most often associated with Jean Watson's theory of nursing as the art and science of human caring.[7-9] Watson defines human caring as the moral ideal of nursing, in which the relationship between the whole self of the nurse and the whole self of the patient or client protects the vulnerability and preserves the humanity and dignity of the patient or client. This emphasis on the whole self—the whole person of both nurse and patient—requires the addition of the term *transpersonal* in Watson's framework and in the discussion of human caring as it relates to holistic nursing practice. Within a transpersonal perspective, people are more than the body physical and the mind as contained in that body. A transpersonal perspective acknowledges that all people are body, mind, and spirit or soul, and that interactions between people engage each of these aspects of the self. A nurse with a transpersonal perspective recognizes that this is a fact of human interaction, not an optional event. A holistic nurse recognizes, as Watson suggests, that there is something beyond the personal, separate selves of the nurse and the patient involved in the act of caring.

When nurses enter into caring–healing relationships with patients, bringing with them an acknowledgment and appreciation of the body, mind, and spirit dimensions of their own human existence, they are engaged in a transpersonal human caring process. In this type of relationship, they know themselves to be interconnected with the patient and with the larger environment and cosmos. They know that they are walking on sacred ground when they walk this path with their patients, and they recognize that neither one will be the same afterward. For that moment, they are joined with the other who is patient or client, and so become part of something larger than either alone. In this transpersonal healing process, they are each changed.[10]

Watson calls these healing encounters "caring occasions" and suggests that they actually transcend the bounds of space and time. The field of consciousness created in and through the caring–healing relationship has the potential to continue healing the patient long after the physical separation of nurse and patient. Moreover, the nurse, following engagement in a true caring occasion, will also continue to benefit from the mutual process. When nurses are able to engage their full, caring selves in the art of nursing, it is both energizing and satisfying.

It is often assumed that nurses burn out as a result of caring too much. However, today's nurses are far more likely to burn out for a different reason: the difficulty in finding the time to care for patients with their whole selves within healthcare systems that do not value caring.[11]

■ HEALING: THE GOAL OF HOLISTIC NURSING

Although caring is the context for holistic nursing, healing is the goal. The origin of the word *heal* is the Anglo-Saxon word *haelan*, which means to be or to become whole. Defining what it means to be or become whole is a challenging task. For example, is wholeness a goal, an end point that is something to work toward but is rarely achieved? Is wholeness a state of perfection of body, mind, and spirit? Is wholeness something that people either have or do not have, something that people can obtain and hold on to, or something that comes and goes? Is it a state or a process? Is wholeness dependent on the structure and functioning of the body? Can one ever be not whole; that is, can one ever be other than wholly who or what one is at any point in space and time? If one cannot be not whole, then how is it possible to talk about becoming whole? Each holistic nurse should spend some time thinking about what this means to her or him because a nurse's perspective on wholeness will influence everything that she or he does.

Healing as the Emergence of Right Relationship

Wholeness is frequently described as harmony of body, mind, and spirit, while harmony is defined as an ordered or aesthetically pleasing set of relationships among the elements of the whole. This simple definition illustrates the implications of associating harmony with healing. First, wholeness involves more than the intactness of physical structure and function, or the status of isolated parts of a person. Second, if healing is about harmony, it is necessary to expand the ways of knowing about healing to include the aesthetic as well as the scientific.

Synonyms for the word harmony include *unity, integrity, connection, reconciliation, congruence,* and *cohesion.* Taken together, these terms begin to suggest that wholeness is not necessarily a state of any kind, but a process that is fundamentally about relationship. Wholeness is about the relationship of the parts of a system to one another and to the larger systems of which they are a part. When the theoretical physicist David Bohm was asked, "How can anything become more whole if everything is already part of the indivisible wholeness of the implicit order of the universe?" he responded with one word. "Coherence," he said, creating no doubt that wholeness was not about adding and subtracting parts, but about how those parts related to each other.[12] Increasing the wholeness of a system is about establishing a pattern of relationships among its elements that is more and more coherent.

Healing, if it is a process of being or becoming whole, must be an emerging pattern of relationships among the elements of the whole person that leads to greater integrity, connection, and cohesion of the whole system. This pattern of relationships can be called right relationship. Thus, healing is the emergence of right relationship at or between or among any and all levels of the human experience. It is a process rather than a state. It is dynamic, and it always affects the whole person, no matter at what level the shift actually occurs. Key to an understanding of the effects of a shift into right relationship at any level are theories about how systems, particularly living systems, work.[13-16] The new sciences are "known collectively as the sciences of complexity, including general systems theory (Bertalanffy, Weiss), cybernetics (Wiener), nonequilibrium thermodynamics (Prigogine), cellular automata theory (von Neumann), catastrophe theory (Thom), autopoietic system theory (Maturana and Varela), dynamic systems theory (Shaw, Abraham), and chaos theories, among others."[17p14] Within a systems perspective, human beings are simultaneously autonomous wholes and parts of larger wholes. Each "holon" is embedded in an "irreversible hierarchy of increasing wholeness, increasing holism, increasing unity and integration."[18]

Several principles related to the nature of systems are fundamental to all these theories and have direct implications for the understanding of healing. The first and most basic is that a system is more than and different from the sum of its parts. It is "more than" its parts because the pattern of relationships among the parts of the whole gives the system its own unique identity. "A pattern of organization [is] a configuration of relationships characteristic of a particular system."[19p80]

A second principle is that a change in the part always leads to a change in the whole. Because human beings are living systems governed by these principles, any shift, no matter how small or at what level it appears, will always affect the whole bodymindspirit. Furthermore, because every person is simultaneously a part of the larger whole of family, society, the ecosystem, and the universe, a change in an individual bodymindspirit leads to a change in all of these as well. This awareness is, of course, part of the teaching of virtually every spiritual tradition, and it affirms that nurses' individual healing work matters to far more than just the nurses.

The third principle that relates directly to healing is that the nature of the change in the whole cannot be predicted by the nature of the change in the part. "The new state [of a system] is decided neither by initial conditions in the system nor by changes in the critical values of environmental parameters; when a dynamic system is fundamentally destabilized, it acts indeterminately."[20]

Human beings as living systems are self-organizing systems, capable of—indeed, striving toward—order, self-transcendence, and transformation.[21] "We are beginning to recognize the creative unfolding of life in forms of ever-increasing diversity and complexity as an inherent characteristic of all living systems."[19p222] Thus, the healing process itself is inherent within the person. This urge toward healing, toward right relationship, when manifested, may be thought of as the "haelan effect."[22]

In the context of these principles, right relationship is not a moral judgment, a statement about right and wrong, good or bad. Rather, it is a way of understanding a particular quality of pattern and organization. The inherent tendency of any living system, as part of the evolutionary process, is toward actualizing its "deep structure"[17p40] (i.e., an acorn "wants" to actualize its inherent tree nature). The consequence of not being in right relationship is the tendency toward "self-dissolution."[17p44] Right relationship may be thought of as any pattern of organization within the system that supports, encourages, allows, or generates actualization and self-transcendence—at any or all levels. Thus, consistent with the tendencies inherent in all living systems healing, the emergence of right relationship at any level of body, mind, or spirit:

- Increases coherence of the whole bodymindspirit
- Decreases disorder in the whole bodymindspirit
- Maximizes free energy in the whole bodymindspirit
- Maximizes freedom, autonomy, and choice in the whole
- Increases the capacity for creative unfolding of the whole bodymindspirit

Because of its inherently creative nature, true healing is always a process of emergence into something new, rather than a simple return to prior states of being.[23] Holistic nurses do not limit the focus of their care to recovery alone, but rather expand their focus to helping patients integrate their illness experience and transcend their former selves toward new patterns of self-actualization. This is the growth process of nature. Nightingale's statement that the goal is to put the patient in the best condition so that nature can act on him may refer to this natural, forward-moving tendency toward wholeness.[24]

Healing as the emergence of right relationship may occur at any level of the bodymindspirit. For example, when an organ is transplanted, the emergence of right relationship between the new organ and the surrounding cells and tissues of the recipient's bodymindspirit signals healing. If that right relationship does not occur, if the cells of the new organ do not become integrated into the existing bodymindspirit, if rejection rather than acceptance happens, then the patient may die from a lack of right relationship, and thus healing, at the cellular level. When broken bones knit together, or when the edges of a wound begin to approximate, right relationship is emerging at the physical level. Each of these emerging right relationships has an impact on the whole, as noted earlier.

The effects on the whole person of a shift toward right relationship at the emotional level are evident in a moment of forgiveness or a release of a long-held resentment. At such a time, the way in which a person stands in relationship to an event or a person from the past changes. The letting go of resentment carries with it an often overwhelming release of energy for new growth and an expanded consciousness. The bodymindspirit of one who is experiencing forgiveness moves toward integration and transcendence of previous patterns and forms. Forgiveness of one's self or another has profound effects at every level of being.

Sometimes right relationship emerges at the spiritual level before it manifests itself anywhere else. In moments of deep love—such as gratitude, or the sudden awareness that one is not alone but in fact connected to everything and everyone else in the cosmos—individuals have come into right relationship with the transcendent dimensions of life—God, the One, Ultimate Reality, the Ground of Being. The language is not as important as the recognition of change. Those who have this experience are more whole, more coherent, more free to become who they are most deeply meant to be, more healed.

Healing vs. Curing

Healing and curing are different processes. Curing is the elimination of the signs and symptoms of disease, which may or may not correspond to the end of the patient's disease or distress. The diagnosis and cure of disease provide the focus of the modern healthcare (sickness–cure) system. This is not a wrong focus, only an incomplete one. When it is estimated that 85% of health problems are either self-limiting or chronic, it becomes clear that something in addition to a focus on the curing of diseases is required. That something is healing, which is different from curing in several key ways.

Healing may occur without curing. The person dying of acquired immune deficiency syndrome (AIDS) who reconciles with his parents after a long separation is healing. The person who has become quadriplegic and uses this as an opportunity to recommit to living a life of meaning and service is healing. The mother of young children who consents to radical, invasive surgery for an otherwise incurable cancer is healing by coming into a new relationship with the disease and making choices based on her commitment to live for her children. The surgery may not cure her disease, but the choice to undergo the surgery is a healing choice. Curing is almost always focused on the person as a physical entity, a body. If the body cannot be fixed, if the physical disease state or state of disability cannot be cured, then there is "nothing more we can do for you." Healing is multidimensional. It can occur at the physical level, but it can also occur at each of the other levels of the human system—emotion, mind, and spirit.

Curing may or may not be possible, but healing is always possible. Many of the diseases of our time are, in fact, not curable, and people who are living with chronic illnesses of the immune system and cardiovascular systems make up a large percentage of the caseload of any primary care provider. In contrast, because healing is the emergence of right relationship at any or all levels of the human system, it can happen even when there is no possibility for physical cure. The potential for healing exists within every human being by the very fact that as humans, we have a multidimensional, self-reflective nature. Indeed, for some people, the very fact that they are facing an incurable disease or situation provides enough instability in the system to catalyze tremendous healing shifts, an "escape to a higher order" in the language of Prigogine's model of dissipative structures.[25]

Although curing follows a usual or predictable path, healing is always creative and unpredictable in both process and outcome. In textbooks on curing, the events that will be probable parts of recovery and the timeline are described, and the actual progress of the patient is measured against these referents. The misapplication of this information is increasingly apparent as patients in the modern sickness–cure system are being told exactly how many days of care they are permitted for cure to occur. The nature and the direction of a healing change cannot be predicted, however. Furthermore, because the direction of healing is always toward self-transcendence, something new is emerging, and the whole that was before becomes a part of the new, larger (or deeper) whole. This unidirectional unfolding toward increasing complexity and diversity is also, of course, a fundamental premise of the Science of Unitary Human Beings proposed by Rogers.[26] The end point of a healing process cannot be predicted ahead of time. It can only be observed as it emerges.

Death is seen as a failure in the sickness–cure system but as a natural process in the healing system. Death is seen as the enemy, that which is to be avoided at all costs, even at the expense of the humanity and personhood of the one being treated in the sickness–cure system. The increasingly widespread use of "living wills"—formal, legal documents that are required to allow death without the heroic battle waged in sickness–cure institutions—provides abundant evidence of this observation. Rather than being a failure, however, death is part of the natural unfolding of the life process. All living systems eventually die. In some spiritual traditions, death itself is viewed as the ultimate healing because it releases the eternal soul from the limitations, pain, and suffering of embodiment. This, of course, is a matter of individual belief.

■ THE HEALER

"It is often thought that medicine is the curative process. It is no such thing; medicine is the surgery of functions as surgery proper is that of limbs and organs. Neither can do anything but remove obstructions; neither can cure. Nature alone cures."[27] This same perspective applies to healing.

Healing is completely unique and creative and may not be coerced, manipulated, or controlled, even by the one healing. The nurse healer is a facilitator of this process, a sort of midwife, but is not the one doing the healing. Neither is the locus of the healing an isolated part of the patient (i.e., the mind or the spirit). All healing emerges from within the totality of the unique bodymindspirit of the patient, sometimes with the assistance of therapeutic interventions, but not because of them. Therapeutics (drugs, surgery, complementary therapies) may be necessary for the patient to be cured or healed, but they are not sufficient causes. Every nurse has cared for patients who "should have" gotten better but did not, as well as patients who "should have" died but went on to live long, healthy lives.

The assumption that the patient accomplishes all healing and curing does not mean that the patient controls all healing and curing. The causes of illness and cure are so complex and multifaceted that no simple statement of cause and effect is appropriate to describe either. Nurses can participate knowledgeably in the healing process, formulating a healing intention and doing what they believe is best in this situation, but the outcome of that process remains a mystery. At least part of the healing process will always be an unfolding mystery. Suggesting otherwise to patients may contribute to their sense of failure when they are unable to cure themselves of disease. True caring is a moral commitment to protect the vulnerability of another, not add to it.

■ A TRUE HEALING
   HEALTHCARE SYSTEM

As noted previously, the current healthcare system continues to focus almost exclusively on the curing process, thus making it more akin to a sickness–cure system, despite 2010 reforms, which were primarily about access to the existing system and not a fundamentally changed system. Although necessary and excellent in its own right, this system is incomplete. The use of new tools of care, including alternative, holistic, or complementary therapies, without a fundamental shift in the philosophy of care with which they are used will not transform the sickness–cure system

into a true, healing healthcare system, however. This error of confusing the tools of care with the philosophy of care may lead to serious consequences for both healthcare practitioners and their patients.

The fundamental orientation of a holistic practitioner is toward an appreciation of and attention to the wholeness and uniqueness of every person. Holistic nurses remember that, in effect, there is nothing that is not holistic. There is no intervention that does not affect the whole bodymindspirit of the patient because the bodymindspirit is integral and cannot be divided. There are natural and nonnatural modalities, for example, but both affect the whole bodymindspirit. There are invasive and noninvasive interventions, but both affect the whole bodymindspirit. There are interventions that start in the body (e.g., medications, surgery, exercise, movement therapy), the mind (e.g., autogenic training, hypnotherapy, guided imagery), or the spirit (e.g., meditation, prayer, gratitude practice, loving kindness). None of these interventions is inherently more holistic than the other, however, because all roads lead to the bodymindspirit; all interventions affect the whole.

For this reason, simply adding new tools of care will not transform the sickness–cure system. The way in which practitioners use the tools available, whether the tools are conventional or complementary, and their willingness to become a midwife to nature rather than the hero of success stories make the care holistic or integrative. The true healthcare system will emerge when both curing and healing processes are equally valued, sought after, and facilitated for all, and when the full range of curing, caring, and healing modalities is available to all. Holistic nurses have a key role to play in facilitating this level of change in the existing systems,[28-35] and in revisioning/re-creating hospitals and clinics, wellness centers and hospices, as *Habitats for Healing*, optimal healing environments in which nurses thrive and patients heal. Habitats for Healing are characterized by autonomy of the nursing staff; a holistic, caring/healing/relationship-centered framework that guides practice; and the integration of complementary and alternative healing modalities into regular nursing care.[1]

Integration of the Masculine and the Feminine

The Western sickness–care system is characterized almost exclusively by attributes usually ascribed to the masculine principle and usually carried by men. This is a natural consequence of the fact that men have been the principal creators of that system and continue to be the dominant culture of the system. These attributes are extremely useful in the treatment of acute injury and disease, but without the attributes usually ascribed to the feminine principle, they provide an incomplete foundation for a true, integrative healing healthcare system.

Table 4-1 suggests another perspective on these different attributes. A perspective that sees the goal as "getting the job done" can be associated with the sickness–cure model, while one that focuses on "holding sacred space" can facilitate healing of the whole bodymindspirit.[36]

Nurse as Healing Environment

One of the most powerful tools for healing is the presence of the nurse in the patient's environment. In fact, the nurse has the greatest impact of all the elements in the patient's environment. Simply by virtue of the role, a nurse has all the ritual power of the shaman of other cultures. The nurse is guardian of the patient's journey through illness and healing; the keeper and bestower of information, medicines, and treatments; the mediator of the system and the comings and goings of others in the system.

In a model of the universe that includes the nonlocal nature of consciousness[37] or the possibility for the existence of a human energy field that extends beyond the skin,[38] the nurse is not simply part of the patient's environment, but rather the nurse is the patient's environment.[36]

The healing environment of the patient may be optimized when the nurse intentionally shifts consciousness into a centered or meditative state. The interconnectedness of the energy fields of the nurse and the patient can facilitate relaxation, rest, or healing in the patient. When a nurse is centered in the present moment and has the intention to be a healing environment, he or she may carry this intention in the energy field and

---

TABLE 4-1   Ways of Being with People Seeking Help

"Getting the Job Done"	"Holding Sacred Space"
Authority vested in the external "expert"	Authority vested in the individual client(s)
Source of healing: what the expert provides	Source of healing: the body-mind-spirit of the client(s)
Gathering, collecting, taking in information	Receiving information
Problem solving/fixing	Life unfolding/facilitating
Making "something" happen, where "something" is	Allowing "something" to happen, where "something" is
▪ defined by the external "expert"	▪ defined mutually
▪ defined ahead of time	▪ defined in the moment
▪ meeting the goal	▪ emergence of mystery
Directing/taking over to make it happen	Guiding/helping to allow it to happen
Doing to or for	Being with
Leading	Walking with
Power over	Power with
Expert is accountable and responsible for outcome	Facilitator is accountable and responsible for competent practice
Failure is the nonachievement of predetermined outcome	Failure is giving up on the unfolding process

manifest it in the voice, the eyes, and the quality of touching. Nurses should ask themselves:

- Do patients hear in my voice that I care? That I have time for them? That they are safe with me?
- What is the quality of my facial expression? Of my eyes? Do they communicate care and compassion, or are they perfunctory and distant? Does the patient feel seen by me, or overlooked? If the eyes are the windows of the soul, what is my soul saying to the soul of my patient? What is the patient's soul saying?
- Am I focused on the task at hand and simply touching the patient to get the job done? Or does my touch convey care, support, nurture, and competence? Does my touch communicate that I know I am touching this person's spirit as I contact his or her skin, because where else is the spirit located but in the body? Do I speak of love and kindness and respect through my hands?

Learning how to shift consciousness into a healing state is a basic skill for the holistic nurse. Nurses are not simply separate selves "doing to" the patient, but an integral part of the patient's environment, "being with" them on the healing journey. The quality of the energy with which the patient is interacting is part of what nurses attend to, and this means attending to their own state of consciousness and well-being before, during, and after their interactions with patients. Thus, taking time for themselves to learn and practice relaxation, meditation, centering, or other self-care strategies becomes essential in this model and serves both nurses and patients.[39-41] Nurses are not being selfish by taking this time. They are recognizing that unless they are energized, relaxed, and centered, they will be trying to give what they do not have to give. This results in less than optimal care for the patients and burnout for the nurses.

■ CONCLUSION

Transpersonal human caring provides the context for holistic nurses to facilitate healing—the emergence of right relationship—in patients and

clients. Through the use of centering and intentionality, the holistic nurse may become a healing environment and participate in the creation of a true, healing healthcare system that integrates both masculine and feminine attributes. "Holding sacred space" for healing is an additional skill of the holistic nurse. This skill does not replace "getting the job (of curing) done," but it enhances it.

Directions for FUTURE RESEARCH

1. Collect personal stories and narratives that provide exemplars of "caring occasions."
2. Conduct interviews with patients who see themselves as healing, even in the absence of curing, to search for patterns that may facilitate this shift for other patients.
3. Explore the relationship between job satisfaction in nurses and the practice of centering and holding sacred space.
4. Explore the effects of caring–healing relationships on both nurses and patients.[42]

Nurse Healer REFLECTIONS

After reading this chapter, the holistic nurse will be able to answer or to begin a process of answering the following questions:

- How do I feel when I am engaged in a "caring occasion"?
- How do I know when healing is happening in my patients? In myself?
- What small changes could I make in my practice to begin to transform my work environment into a Habitat for Healing?

> www. *For a full suite of assignments and additional learning activities, use the access code located in the front of your book to visit this exclusive website: http://go.jblearning.com/dossey. If you do not have an access code, you can obtain one at the site.*

NOTES

1. J. F. Quinn, "Habitats for Healing: Healthy Environments for Health Care's Endangered Species," *Beginnings* 30, no. 2 (2010): 10–11.

2. J. F. Quinn, "Healing: A Model for an Integrative Health Care System," *Advanced Practice Nursing Quarterly* 3, no. 1 (1997): 1–7.

3. J. Watson, *Nursing: Human Science and Human Care* (New York: National League for Nursing Press, 1988): 54.

4. H. Covington, "Caring Presence. Delineation of a Concept for Holistic Nursing," *Journal of Holistic Nursing* 21, no. 3 (2003): 301–317.

5. W. R. Cowling and D. Taliaferro, "Emergence of a Caring-Healing Perspective: Contemporary Conceptual and Theoretical Directions," *Journal of Theory Construction and Testing* 8, no. 2 (2004): 54–59.

6. J. Morse et al., "Concepts of Caring and Caring as a Concept," *Advances in Nursing Science* 13, no. 1 (1990)· 1–14.

7. J. Watson, *Caring Science as Sacred Science* (Philadelphia: F. A. Davis, 2005).

8. J. Watson, "Theoretical Questions and Concerns: Response from a Caring Science Framework," *Nursing Science Quarterly* 20, no. 1 (2007): 13–15.

9. R. Foster, "Jean Watson Over the Years," *Nursing Science Quarterly* 20, no. 1 (2007): 7.

10. J. Ercums, "Nursing's Caring Paradigm: A Story of Mutuality and Transcendent Healing," *Alternative and Complementary Therapies* 4, no. 1 (1998): 68–72.

11. J. F. Quinn, "Revisioning the Nursing Shortage: A Call to Caring for Healing the Healthcare System," *Frontiers of Health Services Management* 19, no. 2 (2002): 3–21.

12. D. Bohm, response to a question raised at the International Transpersonal Association meeting, Prague, Czechoslovakia, 1992.

13. Lars Skyttner, *General Systems Theory* (River Edge, NJ: World Scientific Publishing Company, 2002).

14. E. Morin, *On Complexity: Advances in Systems Theory, Complexity, and the Human Sciences* (NY: Hampton Press, 2008).

15. C. Lindberg, S. Nash, and C. Lindberg, *On the Edge: Nursing in the Age of Complexity* (Bordentown, NJ: Plexus Press, 2008).

16. A. W. Davidson, M. A. Ray, and M. C. Turkel, *Nursing, Caring and Complexity Science* (New York: Springer, 2011).

17. K. Wilber, *Sex, Ecology and Spirituality: The Spirit of Evolution* (Boston: Shambhala, 1996).

18. K. Wilber, *The Marriage of Sense and Soul* (New York: Random House, 1998): 67.

19. F. Capra, *The Web of Life* (New York: Anchor Books, 1996).

20. E. Lazlo, *Evolution, the Grand Synthesis* (Boston: Shambhala, 1987): 36.

21. L. M. Holden, "Complex Adaptive Systems: Concept Analysis," *Journal of Advanced Nursing* 52, no. 6 (2005): 651–657.

22. J. F. Quinn, "On Healing, Wholeness and the Haelan Effect," *Nursing and Healthcare* 10, no. 10 (1989): 553.

23. D. McElligott, "Healing: The Journey from Concept to Nursing Practice," *Journal of Holistic Nursing* 28, No. 4 (2010): 251–259.

24. D. Wardell and J. Engebretson, "Professional Evolution," *Journal of Holistic Nursing* 16, no. 1 (1998): 64.

25. I. Prigogine, *Order Out of Chaos* (New York: Bantam Books, 1984).

26. M. E. Rogers, "The Science of Unitary Human Beings: Current Perspectives," *Nursing Science Quarterly* 7, no. 1 (1994): 33–35.

27. F. Nightingale, *Notes on Nursing: What It Is and What It Is Not* (New York: Dover Press, 1969): 133.

28. M. Tonuma and M. Winbolt, "From Rituals to Reason: Creating an Environment That Allows Nurses to Nurse," *International Journal of Nursing* 6, no. 4 (2000): 214–218.

29. M. Taylor and K. Keighron, "Healing Is Who We Are . . . and Who Are We?" *Nursing Administration Quarterly* 28, no. 4 (2004): 241–248.

30. J. Watson, "Caring Theory as an Ethical Guide to Administrative and Clinical Practices," *Nursing Administration Quarterly* 30, no. 1 (2006): 48–55.

31. S. I. McDonough-Means, M. J. Kreitzer, and I. R. Bell, "Fostering a Healing Presence and Investigating Its Mediators," *Journal of Alternative and Complementary Medicine* 10, suppl. 1 (2004): S25–S41.

32. L. Bernick, "Caring for Older Adults: Practice Guided by Watson's Caring-Healing Model," *Nursing Science Quarterly* 17, no. 2 (2004): 128–134.

33. J. F. Stichler, "Creating Healing Environments in Critical Care Units," *Critical Care Nursing Quarterly* 24, no. 3 (2001): 1–20.

34. T. Stickley and D. Freshwater, "The Art of Loving and the Therapeutic Relationship," *Nursing Inquiry* 9, no. 4 (2002): 250–256.

35. J. Watson and R. Foster, "The Attending Nurse Caring Model: Integrating Theory, Evidence and Advanced Caring-Healing Therapeutics for Transforming Professional Practice," *Journal of Clinical Nursing* 12, no. 3 (2003): 360–365.

36. J. Quinn, "Holding Sacred Space: The Nurse as Healing Environment," *Holistic Nursing Practice* 6, no. 4 (1992): 26–36.

37. L. Dossey, *Healing Words* (San Francisco: Harper San Francisco, 1993): 43.

38. M. Rogers, "Nursing: Science of Unitary, Irreducible, Human Beings: Update 1990," in *Visions of*

Rogers' Science-based Nursing, ed. E. A. M. Barrett (New York: National League for Nursing, 1990).

39. M. C. Turkel and M. A. Ray, "Creating a Caring Practice Environment Through Self-Renewal," *Nursing Administration Quarterly* 28, no. 4 (2004): 249–254.

40. J. D. Christianson, M. D. Finch, B. Findlay, W. B. Jonas, and C. G. Choate, *Reinventing the Patient Experience* (Chicago, IL: Health Administration Press, 2007).

41. A. Vitale, "Nurses' Lived Experience of Reiki for Self-Care," *Holistic Nursing Practice* 23, no. 3 (2009): 129–145.

42. J. F. Quinn et al., "Research Guidelines for Assessing the Impact of the Healing Relationship in Nursing," *Alternative Therapies in Health and Medicine* 9, no. 3 (2003): A65–A79, special supplement.

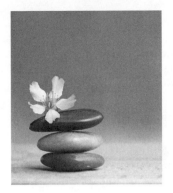

Chapter 5

Nursing Theory in Holistic Nursing Practice

Noreen Cavan Frisch

Nurse Healer
OBJECTIVES

Theoretical

- Describe the elements of holistic nursing and explain why the use of theory is one of the elements.
- Compare and contrast the following major nursing theories: Nightingale's Theory of Environmental Adaptation Model; the Modeling and Role-Modeling Theory, Watson's Theory of Transpersonal Caring; Rogers's Theory of Unitary Human Beings; Newman's Theory of Expanding Consciousness; and Parse's Theory of Human Becoming.
- Identify the use of midrange theories as supportive of nursing practice, particularly Kolcaba's Comfort Care Theory.
- Identify emerging theories that have attracted the attention of holistic nurses as applicable to their contemporary practice and the development of the Theory of Integral Nursing as a consequence of such examination and exploration of new ideas.

Clinical

- Apply the nursing theories discussed in the clinical setting.
- Determine how the perspective of each theory influences nursing care and the evaluation of that care.

Personal

- Select a nursing theory or theories that provide a framework and philosophy consistent with your own view.
- Use the theory or theories and evaluate their effect on your personal worldview.

DEFINITIONS

Concept: An abstract idea or notion.
Conceptual model: A group of interrelated concepts described to suggest relationships among them.
Framework: A basic structure; the context in which theory is developed; the structure that permits theory to be understood.
Grand theory: A theory that covers a broad area of the discipline's concerns.
Metaparadigm: Concepts that identify the domain of a discipline.
Metatheory: Theory about theory development; theory about theory.
Midrange theory: A focused theory for nursing that deals with a portion of nurses' concerns or that is oriented to patient outcomes.
Model: A representation of interactions between and among concepts.
Nursing theory: A framework; a set of interrelated concepts that are testable; a way of seeing the factors that contribute to nursing practice and nursing thought.
Worldview: A perspective; a way of viewing, perceiving, and interpreting one's experience.

■ THEORY AND RESEARCH

By definition and by history, nursing is a holistic practice. Nursing's work is concerned with the restoration and promotion of health, the prevention of disease, and the supports necessary to help the client gain a subjective sense of peace and harmony. As a profession, nursing has never focused solely on the physical body or the disease entity. Rather, taking into account the holistic nature of all persons, nursing is concerned with the client's experience of the condition. In addition, nurses attend to the environmental influences that promote recovery as well as the social and spiritual supports that promote a sense of well-being for clients. Nurses have found that nursing theories help to articulate the nature of nursing practice and guide nursing interventions to meet client needs.

Nursing Theory Defined

A nursing theory is a framework from which professional nurses can think about their work. Theory is a means of interpreting one's observations of the world and is an abstraction of reality. For example, most nurses have studied developmental theory, which provides a framework for viewing childhood behaviors expected with various ages and phases of child growth. Consequently, when nurses observe a toddler crying when his mother must leave him alone with nurses in the hospital, nurses interpret the child's crying as separation anxiety, an expected and predicted toddler behavior according to developmental theory. The theory provides a means of understanding behavior that otherwise might seem random and, therefore, is a framework from which to understand the child's actions. Thus, "a theory suggests a direction in how to view facts and events."[1]

In the past, four basic ideas (or concepts) were common to all nursing theories—the concepts of nursing, person, health, and environment. These concepts were thought to compose the core content of the discipline—the "metaparadigm" of nursing. As the discipline has matured, authors suggest that the four concepts are too restrictive for development of nursing knowledge,[2] and some suggest additions to the four. Full discussion of this debate is outside the scope of this chapter; however, it is important to recognize that there is an emerging view that other concepts may be equally important to the core of nursing.[3] For example, concepts such as caring, healing, energy fields, development, adaptation, consciousness, or nurse–client relationships may be as important to describing and understanding nursing as the concept of health.

When evaluating various theories, a nurse must understand that a concept will take on different meanings that are specific to the theoretical perspective. For example, one theory may define the environment in direct physical terms, while another theory may define the environment as an energy field. Each of these theories would certainly have a different perspective of the environmental impact on a client's health. The way that a nurse defines concepts basic to nursing care and the way that a nurse thinks about the relationship of these concepts affect the practice and, presumably, the outcome of nursing care.

Since the writings of Florence Nightingale,[4] who is considered to be the first nursing theorist and the founder of "modern secular nursing," nurses have had theories about how to practice nursing. Most of these theories, however, have been developed since the 1960s. Several nurses have put forth their ideas of what nursing is and how nursing care can be delivered to assist clients in achieving health. Many practicing nurses are unaware that the care they give is based on a specific theory. They have learned what nursing is by going to nursing school and working with a set of beliefs or assumptions about nursing and the outcomes of nursing care. Nursing curricula are based on nursing theories—in some schools, theory is taught as an assumption; in others, it is more explicitly taught as a theory. Nonetheless, all nurses have learned what nursing is from a viewpoint that includes definitions of the major concepts of nursing theory and have learned to practice nursing in a manner consistent with that viewpoint. When nurses study nursing theory, they have an opportunity to consider carefully the assumptions on which they base their practice. Knowledge of several theories gives nurses more choices in thinking about the situations in which they find themselves and their clients. Theory gives nurses tools to guide practice, and because nursing theory is grounded in research, theory provides a scientific basis for nursing care.

The Need for Theory

Whenever the topic of nursing theory comes up, some nurses ask, "Why do I need a theory? Isn't being holistic enough?" These are very important questions. Nurses committed to holism are kind and compassionate nurses who share a philosophy that emphasizes a balance between self-care and the ability to care for patients using the interconnectedness of body, mind, and spirit. Theory suggests—in fact demands—that nurses reflect on philosophy and consider how their practice is working (or not working) to achieve holistic ideals. One author writes that use of theory requires reflection and is a precondition for professional practice: "Theory is a purposeful form of abstract thinking essential to a discipline and, by definition, a characteristic of the professional nurse."[5]

The description of holistic nursing developed by the American Holistic Nurses Association (AHNA) states, "Holistic nursing practice draws on knowledge, theories, expertise, intuition, and creativity."[6] All five elements are necessary for the nurse to function in an ideal way: nursing knowledge is essential for the understanding of health and disease states and the various regimens required to achieve health. Theories enable one to reflect on practice and to consider carefully all alternatives of care. Expertise is necessary to perform nursing skills and for the ability to make accurate assessments and decisions about care. Intuition is needed to understand the client and to appreciate the subjective experiences of others. Creativity is helpful in solving care problems that seem insurmountable; it provides the nurse with novel ideas and ways of being with clients. Each one of these elements is as important as the others. Knowledge and theory are cognitive tools that help the nurse understand and reflect on practice. Expertise is an experiential tool that

comes from practice and a significant number of encounters in nurse–client situations. Intuition and creativity are affective tools that lead the nurse to feel, experience, and follow inner guidance when working with clients.

Professional practice requires that nurses use these five elements to achieve the best possible results. A holistic nurse can move back and forth between intuitive knowing and logical reasoning, between a creative approach to care and a standard care protocol, and between a hunch of what to do and a considered direction grounded in the predictions of a theory. All of the elements of practice come only by learning how to use them. **Table 5-1** presents a summary of the five elements of holistic nursing practice.

Theory in an Era of Evidenced-Based Practice

Holistic nurses entered the 21st century in a healthcare system committed to *evidence-based practice* as if evidence was new and all of healthcare quality issues could be remedied by a bit of attention to "evidence." That movement has progressed and, in acknowledgment of the fact that much of what holistic nurses do does not have clear evidence, the movement has been retitled *evidence-informed practice*. Certainly, basing practice decisions on sound knowledge, evidence, and reasoning is very positive. No educated nurse would dispute the need to know the current literature and make use of research findings as applied to practice decisions. Nonetheless, this movement seems to have decreased the emphasis on philosophy, theory, and interpretation. This writer has had experiences where nurses assert that they have little need for theory or for understanding of the caring or holistic aspects of the discipline simply because they believe they should

TABLE 5-1	Five Elements of Holistic Nursing Practice	

Element	Domain	Use in Practice
Knowledge	Cognitive	Understanding health and disease states; interpreting regimens of care
Theory	Cognitive	Reflection; considered judgments
Expertise	Experiential	Skilled performance
Intuition	Affective	Subjective knowing
Creativity	Affective	Spontaneity; solving problems or challenges

attend to evidence alone. Further, some current schools of nursing have dropped their courses or emphasis on nursing theory as something no longer required for professional practice. Such developments erode the fundamental nature of our professional practice because the essence of that practice is reflection on one's work. Once a nurse embraces the complexities of the lived experiences of clients and accepts ways of knowing that include aesthetics, personal and ethical knowledge as well as empirical knowledge, the nurse needs a means to assemble the ideas, concepts, thoughts, and feelings that originate from practice in a way that is coherent and personally meaningful. It is through the use of theory that one does just that. Theory provides the nurse with a framework from which to understand and make meaning out of complex experiences. Theory also provides guidance in practice—guidance to consider alternate explanations for what is observed and alternate ways of addressing concerns. At a time of evidence-informed practice, theory could never be more important. For the holistic nurse, practice ignoring theory is as unacceptable as practice ignoring evidence.

Theory Development

Theories develop over time as a theorist defines concepts, suggests relationships between concepts, tests and evaluates the relationships, and modifies the theory based on research findings. When the theorist provides definitions of the concepts and suggests possible relationships, the work is called a conceptual model. Some writers find the distinction between a theory and a conceptual model irrelevant,[7] and for purposes of this chapter, all works are called theories. It is important, however, for nurses to understand that theories develop and mature and that they pass through the following various stages serving increasingly complex purposes:

1. *Description:* The theory provides definitions of concepts, suggests a way of looking at the world, and provides a framework for describing the phenomena of nursing.
2. *Explanation:* The theory suggests relationships between and among various concepts and gives the nurse a means of explaining observed events.
3. *Prediction:* The theory has research findings that establish clear relationships between

aspects of nursing, and the nurse is able to predict outcomes.
4. *Prescription:* The theory is well developed and permits a nurse to prescribe nurse or client actions with confidence in the outcomes.

Most nursing theories are developed to the stage of description and explanation, and theorists and researchers are currently developing nursing theories to the stages of prediction and prescription. Concepts and relationships of a theory can be evaluated and tested through research. For example, if a theory states that a person is a human energy field and suggests that there is an exchange of energy between two persons, research can be designed to evaluate such an exchange. For a theory to reach the stages of prediction and prescription, a considerable body of research is needed.

■ SELECTED NURSING THEORIES

There are several recognized nursing theories; a current text on nursing theory covers 16 theories.[8] The following are the nursing theories most commonly used by holistic nurses. In addition, this chapter presents a section on emerging theories that are important for application to nursing and holistic work.

The Theory of Environmental Adaptation

Florence Nightingale gave nursing the first published theory by which to reflect on nursing. She presented views on concepts important to nursing and directed nurses in the provision of care. To Nightingale, the overarching goal of nursing care is putting patients in the best condition for nature to act on them. She believed that Nursing is a calling. Health is the "positive of which pathology is the negative."[4p74] Environment is emphasized in relation to healing properties of the physical environment, such as fresh air, light, warmth, and cleanliness. Person is described in relationship to the environment; the person is the recipient of nursing care. In relation to healing, Nightingale wrote, "Nature alone cures."[4p74]

For Nightingale, the focus of nursing care was the creation of an environment so that natural healing may take place. Cleanliness, fresh air, and order are emphasized, as are the patient's needs for nutrition. Although not stated as such in her writings, Nightingale and her nurses regularly provided emotional and interpersonal supports. The images of Nightingale with her lamp attending to patients' needs at night, writing letters for them, and being present as a caring nurse are as much a part of her theory of practice as preparing food and cleaning the sick room. Another important aspect of care for Nightingale is recognition of the spiritual nature of people. Deeply spiritual herself, Nightingale believed that nursing involves listening to God's instructions, moral ideals, and devotion to humanity.[9]

Although Nightingale did not develop her theory in the same sophisticated manner as our modern theories are developed, her work stands as a remarkable treatise on reflective and thoughtful practice. Nurses today often are surprised by the accuracy of her directions in guiding current practice. The theory has been studied and modernized by nurse scholars who have described it in terms of theory development used today. Selanders first noted that "the principle of environmental alteration has served as a framework for research studies."[10] Later, Selanders noted that Nightingale's work forms a model that is useful in practice as well as in the conceptualization of research studies.[11] Selanders's notions were validated by the work of a research team that recently documented the application of the basic principles of sunlight, fresh air, and cleanliness that led to healing when working with migrant workers who had foot infections.[12] Nightingale's theory is clearly a wonderful heritage for holistic nurses. A definitive statement on Nightingale's life and work is available in a biography prepared by Dossey.[13]

The Modeling and Role-Modeling Theory

In 1983, Helen Erickson and her colleagues published a theory and paradigm for nursing called the Modeling and Role-Modeling Theory.[14] The theory draws on work from many theoretical perspectives, including Maslow's Basic Needs, Erikson's Stages of Development, Piaget's Theory of Cognitive Development, and Selye's Stress Theory. The work of the psychiatrist Milton Erickson, the father-in-law of the theory's senior author, provided a perspective of the mind–body connection in health, healing, and disease. His work also supports the belief that the most important thing a professional can do is understand the world from the client's perspective.

According to this theory, Nursing is a process that demands an interpersonal and interactive relationship with the client. Facilitation, nurturance, and unconditional acceptance must characterize the nurse's caregiving. The human Person is seen as a holistic being with interacting subsystems (biological, psychological, social, and cognitive) and with an inherent genetic base and spiritual drive; the whole is greater than the sum of its parts. Health is a dynamic equilibrium between subsystems. Environment is seen as both internal and external; environment includes stressors as well as resources for adapting to them.

The client is seen as an individual with strengths that can and should be used to mobilize resources to adapt to stress. *Adaptive potential* is a theory-specific term used to describe conditions of adaptation-equilibrium (which can be adaptive or maladaptive), arousal, or impoverishment. The theory presents five aims of all nursing interventions: (1) to build trust, (2) to promote positive orientation, (3) to promote perceived control, (4) to promote strengths, and (5) to set mutual goals that are health directed. The nurse uses this theory by creating a model of the client's world (modeling) and using that model to plan interventions and to demonstrate and support health-producing behaviors from within the client's worldview (role modeling). Some of the research on the theory has focused on understanding the self-care actions and autonomy among specific populations of patients.[15,16] In her reflections, Erickson emphasizes that the client's self-knowledge should be the nurse's primary source of information. She writes, "People have an inherent ability to grow and become the most that they can be, but they sometimes need help discovering what they are not consciously aware of but already know at some level in their being."[17] Within this theory, our ability to trust in the client's self-care knowledge is where nursing begins.

In her most recent text on the theory, Erickson refers to nurses who believe they have a calling, nurses who want to help others and desire connections with their clients. Erickson writes that nurses who practice holistically need to discover "their gift to their clients—the gift of themselves."[18] She provides a foundation for self-nurturance, self-discovery, and self-growth as conditions of holistic nursing that becomes a way of living and provides meaning in life.

The Theory of Transpersonal Caring and Caring Science

First presented as a philosophy and science of caring in 1979,[19] Jean Watson's Theory of Transpersonal Caring emphasizes the humanist aspects of nursing combined with scientific knowledge. Within this framework, Nursing is mediated by "professional, personal, scientific, esthetic, and ethical human care transactions."[19] Person is seen holistically with the knowledge that the whole is greater than, and different from, the sum of the parts; every person is a valued individual to be cared for, cared about, and understood. Health is a subjective state that has to do with unity and harmony; illness can be understood as disharmony. Caring is achieved through the environment. Watson states that the environment provides social, cultural, and spiritual influences that may be perceived as caring.

In using the Theory of Transpersonal Caring, the foremost role of the nurse is to establish an intimate, caring relationship with the client. The nurse must be able to understand the client's subjective experiences and interact with the client in a meaningful relationship. For Watson, the "caring occasion" or the "caring moment" are situations where nurses and clients come together in unique ways such that there is a truly transformational encounter, leaving both the nurse and the client changed. Watson draws significant attention to the fact that the nurse must never "objectify" another human being (treat the client as an object) because every human being must be approached with unconditional acceptance and positive regard. The strength of the theory relies on the nurse's ability to provide high-quality, caring interactions with the client while simultaneously promoting health through nursing knowledge and interventions. Watson's theory gave rise to numerous qualitative research studies that documented the lived experiences of clients as they received care within a healthcare system. In later writings, Watson advocates a postmodern view of nursing, and of science, that comprises multiple truths, physical and nonphysical realities, and the relativity of time and space.[20] Postmodernism is characterized by ideas of balance, interconnectedness, and a holographic context that clearly brings nursing thought into a new dimension. Reflecting on the theory, one author notes that Watson's caring theory can be used in all settings because it transcends cultural and geographic boundaries because care is a universal phenomenon of the human experience.[21]

In current writings, Watson further describes the theory's development in terms of caring science. She writes that such science, having caring as a central feature, is a "foundational disciplinary framework for all caring–healing professions, moving beyond nursing."[22] The assumptions of caring science include "an expanding unitary, energetic worldview with a relational human caring ethic and ontology as its starting point."[22p28] Thus, the evolution of the theory brings one to the point where one understands caring sciences as a truly sacred call to care.

Work continues worldwide to apply, expand, and develop Watson's theory. Recent works include the application of the theory by an experienced nurse during that nurse's own life transitions[23] and applications to specific practice areas such as occupational health.[24] Nurse educators continue to apply concepts within the theory to educational processes including the ways in which faculty relate to one another.[25] Administrators are also using the theory to explore the conditions necessary for nurses' successful working lives.[26,27] A most interesting development of the theory is found in a new textbook related to curriculum and teaching coauthored by Watson and one of her colleagues.[28]

The Science of Unitary Human Beings

Martha Rogers was the first theorist to describe nursing in relation to the view that a person is an energy field. In addition, she believes that nursing is a "humanistic science dedicated to compassionate concern for maintaining and promoting health, preventing illness, and caring for and rehabilitating the sick and disabled."[29] Rogers's theory, which is an abstract system, is the basis for the Science of Unitary Human Beings. Within this theory, Nursing is the scientific study of human and environmental energy fields. A Person is a unified whole, defined as a human energy field; human beings evolve irreversibly and unidirectionally in space and time. Health is understood in terms of culture and, according to Rogers, is individually defined by the subjective values of each person. The Environment is the environmental energy field that is in constant interaction with the human energy field. There are no boundaries to the environmental or human energy fields. Over the years, many studies have tested concepts of this theory, and several authors have suggested research methodologies specifically appropriate to the Science of Unitary Human Beings. These include the Unitary Field Pattern Portrait Research Method described by Butcher,[30] rational hermeneutics described by Alligood and Fawcett,[31] and case study approaches described by Cowling.[32] One author comments on use of this theory by reflecting that "In caring for individuals and groups, we can achieve a greater understanding of reality and effectiveness in practice when we see humans and their environments as evolving through a mutual process."[33]

Current development of the theory is being carried out by a number of Rogerian scholars and perhaps most notably Howard Butcher. Butcher reminds us that Rogers understood that knowledge and practice were inseparable—thus at the theory's core is the praxis of nursing thought and action. Butcher presents a modern view of the theory depicted in a unitary pattern-based praxis model that links the cosmology (awareness and pandimensional nature of reality) and philosophy with science and practice.[34] He describes use of patterning strategies to promote harmony or health, which include techniques of creative suspension, guided imagery, and forging resolve, as well as activities that provide a source of enjoyment, concentration, and deep involvement.[34p23] Within his view of the theory, knowing refers to pattern manifestations, and data are a synthesis of the expressions, experiences, and perceptions of a situation. Voluntary mutual patterning describes a means of transferring the human and environmental field and facilitating the client's actualization. Butcher's work explores the depths of the theory, provides insightful syntheses of the ideas and concepts, and at the same time gives guidance to nursing care. He calls for continued innovations in research and methods to fully engage the capacity of this theory to address needed changes in nursing and human well-being.[35] The reader is referred to his writings and to other writings in *Visions, the Journal of Rogerian Nursing Science.*

The Theory of Expanding Consciousness

Margaret Newman included Rogers's concepts of energy patterns and unitary human beings in developing her own theory.[36] Newman viewed Nursing as a profession that is moving to an integrated role; nursing is caring, and caring is a moral imperative for nursing. The Person is seen as a dynamic energy field; humans are identified by their field patterns. Health is expanding consciousness that includes an individual's total pattern; pathologic conditions are manifestations of the individual's total pattern. Environment is the wholeness of the universe; there are no boundaries. For Newman, people are not separate entities, but instead are "open energy systems constantly interacting and evolving with each other."[37] Health and illness are paired as a unitary process of complementary forces of order and disorder that are essential in each person's continuing development. Newman notes that experiencing a significant illness often results in a turning point (a choice point) for a person where he or she sees him- or herself differently. Thus, a person can expand consciousness after transcending limitations of disease and other life events.

Research on Newman's theory has focused on the meaning and purpose of living with illness and the effects of disruptive processes on the patterns, change, and growth of the whole. From within this theory, research is praxis, "a method in which the researcher in relationship with the participant becomes part of the experience."[38] Jones reports that practice models based on this theory have promoted comfort and enriched nursing practice, as well as having increased nurse satisfaction.[38] Most current research on this theory involves application to varied practice populations, such as families with special needs children,[39] diabetic women,[40] and students who wish to quit smoking.[41]

The Theory of Human Becoming

Rosemarie Rizzo Parse further developed the idea of the person as a unitary whole and suggested that the person can be viewed only as a unity.[42] Nursing is seen as a scientific discipline, but the practice of nursing is an art in which nurses serve as guides to assist others in making choices affecting health. Person is a unified, whole being. Health is a process of becoming; it is a personal commitment, an unfolding, a process related to lived experiences. Environment is the universe. The human universe is inseparable and evolving as one.

Research on the theory of human becoming documented the importance of intersubjective dialogue in assisting clients to move toward different meanings and choices in their lives and has described the sense of caring that clients perceive from nurses guided by the theory.[43,44]

The concept of presence is critically important for this theory because the nurse offers authentic presence to each client in the process of becoming and living experiences. One author explored the meaning of lingering presence from within the theory and has identified meanings such as living within the familiar and unfamiliar while moving beyond, the surfacing of presence in the remembered moment, and the private experience of presence.[45] Reports of nurses who have used this model in practice document that theory-guided practice leads to critical evaluation of nurses' work and greater professionalism and satisfaction among nurses.[46] Further, recent work uses tenets of the theory to provide exploration of the ethical issues related to human dignity and nursing actions.[47]

■ DEFINITIONS OF PERSON

Since the emergence of Rogers's theory, the definition of person as a unitary whole has challenged nurses to reflect on the meaning of whole. Parse suggests that there are two worldviews in nursing: a summative paradigm in which the person is viewed as a combination of component parts (with the belief that the whole or the essence of the person is greater than the sum of the parts) and the simultaneity paradigm in which a person can be viewed only as a unity; that is, the person is a holistic energy field and cannot be broken into parts.[48] For Rogers, Newman, and Parse, the only appropriate definition of the person is in terms of the unitary whole. Adherents of their theories insist that it is impossible to think of persons as having component parts (e.g., biological, psychological, social, and spiritual components) and that any discussion of a "part" is improper. Other theorists (e.g., Erickson and Watson) have concluded that discussion of the "part" is helpful in considering the various ways in which a person functions, feels, and reacts to the environment.

Throughout the years of this debate, the AHNA has been asked to take a stand on the meaning of whole in holistic nursing practice.

The official AHNA description of holistic nursing states that holistic nursing is defined primarily as all nursing practice that has the enhancement of healing of the whole person as its goal.[49] The AHNA recognizes that there are two views of holism and has publicly stated that "Holistic nursing responds to both views, believing that the goals of nursing can be achieved within either framework."[49] The important aspect of nursing practice is that the nurse and the client believe that the care received is assisting the client to enhance healing and achieve a state of health. Any nurse who believes that a particular theory is helping to reach the goals mutually set between nurse and client should use the theory and reflect on how the theory's worldview changed and assisted nursing practice.

■ MIDRANGE THEORY

Over the years, many nurses have been interested in focused or midrange theories. These theories are focused because they deal with a portion of a nurse's concerns or, very often, are oriented to patient outcomes. In our complex world of work and the current emphasis on providing nurse-sensitive outcomes as part of our professional accountability, some of these midrange theories might prove very useful to practicing holistic nurses. Midrange theories deal with specific issues, for example: pain alleviation, postpartum depression, or maternal role attachment. Although all of the midrange theories could be useful to nurses addressing specific populations, there is one widely recognized midrange theory that lends itself well to the practice of holistic nursing: Kolcaba's Theory of Comfort. A brief review of the Theory of Comfort is provided here.

Theory of Comfort

Kolcaba first proposed comfort as a nurse-sensitive outcome in 1992, when she presented it as a holistic state that captures many of the simultaneous and interrelated aspects of positive human experience.[50] According to Kolcaba, comfort is not simply the absence of pain or distress; it is a positive subjective feeling reflecting a sense of holistic well-being.[51] The concept of comfort as a holistic phenomenon is manifested as feelings of relief, ease, and transcendence occurring "all at once." Kolcaba reminds us that many patients expect and hope to have their complex comfort needs addressed by the nurses from whom they receive care.[52] Holistic nurses resonate with the call for proving comfort as a nursing goal. This theory has been applied to nurses' work with many populations across the life span and across care environments. Also, several comfort measures make every effort to determine the client's response to nursing actions as a perceived state of comfort or a feeling of being comforted.[50,53,54] Attention to midrange theories such as Kolcaba's Theory of Comfort may provide helpful applications of theory to current work settings.

■ EMERGING THEORIES OF INTEREST

Existent nursing theories borrowed ideas from other disciplines and used theoretical concepts from authors such as Maslow, Erikson, Selye, von Bertalanffy, or Piaget to bring ideas into nursing to help those in practice understand the world in which they were living and working. Today, some developing theories have proved useful in thinking about the changing modern environment where a nurse can feel lost in the middle of fast-paced action, uninterpretable observations, and situations of great human need. Two of these modern theories have attracted attention of nurses and holistic practitioners alike because they each provide a new worldview and an additional means to understand human experiences. These two theories are Complex Adaptive Systems Theory or Complexity Science and Ken Wilber's Integral Theory. These are the next round of ideas and concepts that are being brought into nursing thought and have begun to make contributions to nursing theory development. For this reason, each is discussed briefly.

Complexity Science is defined as the study of complex adaptive systems.[55] This is a science that addresses diverse or multifaceted elements that are able to change, react, and adapt and that are interconnected in some way. As in Systems Theory, the elements studied from this theory adapt independently and affect the whole. However, Complexity Science focuses on systems that have a "densely connected web of interacting agents, each operating from its own schema,"[56] addressing structures that are self-organized, unpredictable, and ever changing. This theory is useful

when working within a structure that faces challenges of uncertainty, the need to act, the lack of a predictable outcome, and a level of complexity in which even complicated techniques such as model building and forecasting are inadequate to take into account all contingencies. Modern healthcare organizations are a perfect example of the type of system requiring a new way of thinking. Complexity Science suggests that, when organizations face uncertainty, managers can best operate by distributing (rather than centralizing) control and supporting individual parts (or people) of the organization who are trying to develop solutions.

Complexity Science postulates that, in an uncertain environment, freedom to innovate coupled with qualities of intelligence and resourcefulness will produce best outcomes. One author suggests that following the principles of Complexity Science permits order and creativity to emerge.[57] Complexity Science is undoubtedly useful to healthcare leaders and administrators and is perhaps especially helpful to holistic nurse managers who may already recognize the requirement to give over the control of actions and outcomes. The essence of applying Complexity Science is the ability to trust the process and the people to make the right choices and decisions, and to be accountable for their actions.

Wilber's Integral Theory draws on ideas, concepts, and theories from many traditions to integrate views that interpret world and life experiences from seemingly irreconcilable differences[58] (see discussion of integral and holistic nursing from a local to global perspective). Essentially, this theory divides "all that is" into four quadrants—the four corners of the universe—each quadrant representing a domain, a view of reality, or a dimension of "what is." The quadrants are the interior dimension of individuals (feelings, meanings, beliefs), the interior dimensions of the collective (cultural beliefs, shared worldviews), the exteriors of individuals (the body, its organs and tissues, behaviors), and the exteriors of the collective (social structures). Wilber embraces the notion that the domains of each quadrant represent four true realities, each that can be understood through differing methods of study, different sources of data, and different worldviews. Thus, to understand human experience, one must understand all four dimensions.

His theory can be easily applied to holistic health because it addresses the need for a comprehensive approach to treating illness and giving care to people.[58] Integral medicine treats the illness, the person, and the healthcare provider—going beyond the mind–body perspective and taking a panoramic look at all modes of inquiry. This theory can be considered a metatheory because it is so encompassing it can incorporate the perspectives of many of our existing nursing theories and other psychological theories in a framework of the quadrants identifying how each contributes to a panoramic whole.[59]

In addition, Integral Theory looks at a "chain of pathologies" that causes illness, rather than attempting to identify a singular cause. Holistic nurses understand the need for multiple modes of inquiry and multiple realities. Wilber's theory provides a scholarly framework from which to embrace new understandings of nursing's work. One author who has used the theory in her teaching explains that this model has helped students to care deeply for patients and to experience nursing's art as transformative.[60] In using the integral model as a framework to view the complexities of the healthcare system in which we work, one observes that the current system is dominated by thinking in the physical and social domains and requires attention in the individual and collective internal domains. The integral model calls for a more comprehensive understanding of the health–illness, caring–healing, mind–emotion–body, and individual–cultural group relationships than are accounted for in daily practices. Because holistic nurses are at the forefront of much of the scholarship related to the internal domains, the integral model applied to nursing practice and published in the literature provides a call for translating nursing knowledge beyond the profession of nursing.[61]

The Theory of Integral Nursing

In 2008, Barbara Dossey presented her work on the development of a grand theory of nursing that would incorporate Wilber's theory, particularly the use of the quadrants in understanding dimensions of how we perceive the world, coupled with Carper's theory of how we come to know what we know.[62] A grand theory is abstract and provides great stimulation for reflection and thought about a discipline. Dossey's Theory of Integral Nursing (TIN) is meant to address very broad areas of the discipline's concerns. The TIN is new and may also shift our paradigm in nursing to expand our notions of whom and what we are. The reader is referred to the discussion in this text of integral and holistic nursing, from local to global, for a description of the TIN theory and its application to nursing.

Dossey's work is a creative blending of worldviews that include how we define, know, experience, and react to our realities and how our new understandings of our realities can influence ourselves and our work. She provides a framework for application of integral principles with practice domains of direct care, education, and research. As scholars and practitioners take up this theory, there will be more learnings as a consequence of Dossey's expansion of our notions of nursing. Specific concepts within our nursing worldviews will be challenged, for example, Wilber's work includes concepts of human development in stages of growth that have been rejected by unitary nursing scholars who adhere to an evolutionary model of human change. Other issues will undoubtedly arise as nursing scholarship proceeds. The new TIN provides an exciting opportunity to move nursing's work and holistic nursing in entirely new directions that we do not yet fully understand.

■ CONCLUSION

A theory provides a means of interpreting and organizing information. Nursing theories give nurses tools to ensure that nursing assessments are comprehensive and systematic and that care is meaningful. Holistic nurses use several theories, and each nurse must decide which theory to use and when to use an alternative perspective. In selecting a theory, a nurse should ask two questions: What theory is most comfortable for me? and, What theory is most comfortable for my client? The perspective selected must be comfortable for both. Many clients, as well as nurses, have strong feelings and opinions about what nursing is and what type of care they wish to receive. If the theory's perspective is not comfortable for the client, the nurse is ethically obligated to change her or his perspective and adopt a framework that is compatible with the client's needs. Holistic nurses are challenged to continue the exploration in topics related to holistic nursing.[63]

Directions for
FUTURE RESEARCH

1. Holistic nurses should consider what is and is not known about any theory being applied to practice and evaluate the next steps needed to develop the theory in their own area of practice.
2. Evaluate theories related to the identification of specific outcomes of care.

Nurse Healer
REFLECTIONS

After reading this chapter, the holistic nurse will be able to answer or to begin a process of answering the following questions:

- What definition of the concept of person is a good fit with my view of myself and others?
- Which of the nursing theories described can I use in my practice?
- Which of the nursing theories would be uncomfortable for me to use? Can I openly explore why a particular theory or theories would be uncomfortable for me to use?
- How will I determine if the theory I am using is acceptable to my clients?
- In what ways am I able and willing to make a contribution to the use and development of nursing theory?
- What is my personal plan for studying new theories and learning to apply them to my professional work?

 For a full suite of assignments and additional learning activities, use the access code located in the front of your book to visit this exclusive website: http://go.jblearning.com/dossey. If you do not have an access code, you can obtain one at the site.

NOTES

1. J. S. Hickman, "An Introduction to Nursing Theory," in *Nursing Theories: A Base for Professional Practice*, 5th ed., ed. J. George (Upper Saddle River, NJ: Prentice Hall, 2002): 1–20.
2. V. M. Malinksi, "Response: Notes on Book Review of Analysis and Evaluation of Nursing Theories," *Nursing Science Quarterly* 8 (1995): 59.
3. M. E. Parker, *Nursing Theories and Nursing Practice*, 2nd ed. (Philadelphia: F. A. Davis, 2006).
4. F. Nightingale, *Notes on Nursing* (London: Harrison, 1860).
5. P. G. Reed and G. Rolfe, "Nursing Knowledge and Nurses' Knowledge: A Reply to Mitchell and Bournes," *Nursing Science Quarterly* 19 (2006): 121–123.
6. American Holistic Nurses Association & American Nurses Association, *Holistic Nursing Practice: Scope and Standards of Practice* (Silver Spring, MD: NurseBooks.org, 2007).
7. J. George, ed., *Nursing Theories: The Base for Professional Practice*, 5th ed. (Upper Saddle River, NJ: Prentice Hall, 2002).
8. M. R. Alligood and A. M. Tomey, *Nursing Theory, Utilization and Application* (St. Louis, MO: Mosby, 2006).
9. B. M. Dossey et al., *Florence Nightingale Today: Healing, Leadership, Global Action* (Silver Spring, MD: American Nurses Association, 2005).
10. L. C. Selanders, "The Power of Environmental Adaptation: Florence Nightingale's Original Theory for Nursing Practice," *Journal of Holistic Nursing* 16 (1998): 247–263.
11. L. C. Selanders, "The Power of Environmental Adaption," *Journal of Holistic Nursing* 28 (2010): 81–88.
12. M. Howett, A. Connor, and E. Downes, "Nightingale's Theory and Intentional Comfort Touch in Management of Tinea Pedis in Vulnerable Populations," *Journal of Holistic Nursing* 28 (2010): 244–250.
13. B. M. Dossey, *Florence Nightingale, Mystic, Visionary, Healer* (Springhouse, PA: Springhouse, 2000).
14. H. Erickson et al., *Modeling and Role-Modeling: A Theory and Paradigm for Nursing* (Lexington, KY: Pine Press, 1983).
15. J. E. Hertz and C. A. Anschutz, "Relationships Among Perceived Enactment of Autonomy, Self-Care, and Holistic Health in Community-Dwelling Older Adults," *Journal of Holistic Nursing* 20 (2002): 166–186.
16. C. W. Baldwin et al., "Self-Care as Defined by Members of the Amish Community Utilizing the Theory of Modeling and Role-Modeling," *Journal of Multicultural Nursing and Health* 8 (2002): 60–64.
17. H. L. Erickson, "Philosophy and Theory of Holism," *Nursing Clinics of North America* 42 (2007): 139–163.
18. H. L. Erickson, *Modeling and Role-Modeling: A View from the Client's World* (Cedar Park, TX: Unicorns Unlimited, 2006): 25.
19. J. Watson, *Human Science and Human Care* (New York: National League for Nursing, 1988).
20. J. Watson, *Postmodern Nursing* (London: Churchill Livingstone, 1999).
21. R. Rexroth and R. Davidbizar, "Caring: Utilizing the Watson Theory to Transcend Culture," *Health Care Manager* 22 (2003): 295–304.
22. J. Watson, *Caring Science as Sacred Science* (Philadelphia: F. A. Davis, 2006): 63.
23. M. Goldin and D. D. Kantz, "Applying Watson's Caring Theory and Caritas Processes to Ease Life

Transitions," *International Journal for Human Caring* 14 (2010): 11–14.

24. D. L. Noel, "Occupational Health Nursing Through the Humans Caring Lens," *AAOHN Journal* 58 (2010): 16–26.

25. S. K. Morby and A. Skalla, "A Human Care Approach to Peer Review," *Nursing Science Quarterly* 23 (2010): 297–300.

26. P. L. Burtson, "Nursing Work Environments and Nurse Caring," *Journal of Advanced Nursing* 66 (2010): 1819–1831.

27. S. Brousseau, M. Alerson, and C. Cara, "A Caring Environment for Foster Male Nurses' Quality of Work Life in Community Settings," *International Journal for Human Caring* 12 (2008): 33–43.

28. M. Hills and J. Watson, *Creating a Caring Science Curriculum* (New York: Springer, 2011).

29. M. Rogers, *The Theoretical Basis for Nursing* (Philadelphia: F. A. Davis, 1970): vii.

30. H. K. Butcher, "Crystallizing the Process of the Unitary Field Pattern Portrait Research Method," *Visions: The Journal of Rogerian Nursing Science* 6 (1998): 13–26.

31. M. E. Alligood and J. Fawcett, "Acceptance of the Invitation to Dialogue: Examination of an Interpretive Approach for the Science of Unitary Human Beings," *Visions: The Journal of Rogerian Nursing Science* 8 (1999): 5–13.

32. W. R. Cowling, "Unitary Case Inquiry," *Nursing Science Quarterly* 12 (1998): 139–141.

33. B. Wright, "Rogers' Science of Unitary Human Beings," *Nursing Science Quarterly* 19 (2006): 229–230.

34. H. K. Butcher, "Unitary Pattern-Based Praxis: A Nexus of Rogerian Cosmology, Philosophy, and Science," *Visions: The Journal of Rogerian Nursing Science* 14 (2006): 8–33.

35. H. K. Butcher, "Progress in the Explanatory Power of the Science of Unitary Human Beings: Frubes in a Lull or Surfing in the Barrel of the Wave," *Visions: The Journal of Rogerian Nursing Science* 15 (2008): 23–26.

36. M. Newman, *Health as Expanding Consciousness*, 2nd ed. (New York: National League for Nursing, 1994).

37. M. Newman, *Health as Expanding Consciousness*, 3rd ed. (Sudbury, MA: Jones & Bartlett, 1999): 25.

38. D. Jones, "Newman's Health as Expanding Consciousness," *Nursing Science Quarterly* 19 (2006): 330–331.

39. S. K. Falkenstern, S. H. Gueldner, and M. A. Newman, "Health as Expanding Consciousness with Families with a Child with Special Healthcare Needs," *Nursing Science Quarterly* 22 (2009): 262–279.

40. A. Yang, D. Xiong, E. Vang, and M. D. Pharris, "Hmong Women Living with Diabetes," *Journal of Nursing Scholarship* 41 (2009): 139–148.

41. E. Endo, M. Takaki, A. Nitta, K. Abe, and K. Terashim, "Identifying Patterns in Partnership with Students Who Want to Quit Smoking," *Journal of Holistic Nursing* 27 (2009): 256–265.

42. R. R. Parse, "Human Becoming: Parse's Theory of Nursing," *Nursing Science Quarterly* 5 (1992): 35–42.

43. S. Baumann, "Contrasting Two Approaches in a Community-Based Nursing Practice with Older Adults: The Medical Model and Parse's Nursing Theory," *Nursing Science Quarterly* 10 (1997): 124–130.

44. N. Janes and D. Wells, "Elderly Patients' Experiences with Nurses Guided by Parse's Theory of Human Becoming," *Clinical Nursing Research* 6 (1997): 205–222.

45. M. R. Ortiz, "Lingering Presence: A Study Using the Human Becoming Hermeneutic Method," *Nursing Science Quarterly* 16 (2003): 146–154.

46. D. A. Bournes, "Human Becoming–Guided Practice," *Nursing Science Quarterly* 19 (2006): 329–330.

47. C. L. Milton, "Human Dignity: Scenarios with Doing the Right Thing," *Nursing Science Quarterly* 24 (2011): 16–19.

48. R. R. Parse, *The Human Becoming School of Thought* (Thousand Oaks, CA: Sage, 1998).

49. American Holistic Nurses Association, *Description of Holistic Nursing* (Flagstaff, AZ: AHNA, 1998).

50. K. Kolcaba, "Holistic Comfort: Operationalizing the Construct as a Nurse-Sensitive Outcome," *Advances in Nursing Science* 15 (1992): 1–10.

51. K. Kolcaba, *Comfort Theory and Practice* (New York: Springer, 2003).

52. K. Kolcaba and R. Steiner, "Empirical Evidence for the Nature of Holistic Comfort," *Journal of Holistic Nursing* 19 (2000): 46–62.

53. K. Kolcaba, "A Theory of Comfort for Nursing," *Journal of Advanced Nursing* 19 (1994): 1178–1184.

54. K. Kolcaba, "Evolution of the Mid Range Theory of Comfort for Outcomes Research," *Nursing Outlook* 49 (2001): 86–92.

55. B. Zimmerman, "Complexity Science: A Route Through Hard Times and Uncertainty," *Health Forum Journal* (March/April 1999): 44–46, 69.

56. B. Penprase and D. Norris, "What Nurse Leaders Should Know About Complex Adaptive Systems Theory," *Nursing Leadership Forum* 9 (2005): 127–132.

57. J. A. Astin and F. Kelly, "Psychosocial Determinants of Health and Illness: Integrating Mind, Body, and Spirit," *Advances* 29 (2004): 14–21.

58. K. Wilber, online foreword to *Integral Medicine: A Noetic Reader* (Boston: Shambhala, 2007). http://wilber.shambhala.com/html/misc/integral-med-1.cfm.

59. O. Jarrin, "An Integral Philosophy and Definition of Nursing," *School of Nursing Scholarly Works* 47 (2007). http://digitalcommons.uconn.edu/son_articles/47/.

60. C. S. Clark, "An Integral Nursing Education: Exploration of the Wilber Quadrant Model," *International Journal for Human Caring* 10 (2006): 22–29.

61. K. Fiandt et al., "Integral Nursing: An Emerging Framework for Engaging the Evolution of the Profession," *Nursing Outlook* 51 (2003): 130–137, e52–e73.

62. B. M. Dossey, "Theory of Integral Nursing," *Advances in Nursing Science* 31, no. 1 (2008): e52–e73.

63. N. C. Frisch, ed., "Topics in Holistic Nursing," *Nursing Clinics of North America* (June 2007).

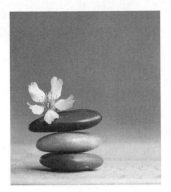

Chapter 6

Holistic Ethics

Margaret A. Burkhardt
and Lynn Keegan

Nurse Healer
OBJECTIVES

Theoretical

- Review the classic principles of ethics.
- Synthesize the basic tenets from the work of traditional ethical theorists.
- Explore the concept of holistic ethics.
- Discuss Earth ethics as an integral component of holistic ethics.

Clinical

- Relate ethical theory to clinical situations.
- Discuss nursing considerations related to advance directives and informed consent.
- Describe processes for ethical decision making in clinical situations.
- Discuss ethical imperatives for nurses involved in research.

Personal

- Discuss daily choices as opportunities to make a positive impact on the world.
- Clarify personal values and ideas.

DEFINITIONS

Being: The state of existing or living.

Consciousness: A state of knowing or awareness.

Earth ethics: A code of behavior that incorporates the understanding that the Earth community has core value in and of itself and includes ethical treatment of the nonhuman world and the Earth as a whole. This code influences the way that we individually and collectively interact with the environment and all beings of the Earth.

Ethical code: A written list of a profession's values and standards of conduct.

Ethics: The study or discipline concerned with judgments of approval and disapproval, right and wrong, good and bad, virtue and vice, and desirability and wisdom of actions, as well as dispositions, ends, objects, and states of affairs; disciplined reflection on the moral choices that people make.

Holistic: Concerned with the interrelationship of body, mind, and spirit in an ever-changing environment.

Holistic ethics: The basic underlying concept of the unity and integral wholeness of all people and of all nature, which is identified and pursued by finding unity and wholeness within one's self and within humanity. In this framework, acts are not performed for the sake of law, precedent, or social norms, but rather from a desire to do good freely, to witness, identify, and contribute to unity.

Informed consent: A process by which patients or participants in research studies are informed of the purpose, possible outcomes, alternatives, risks, and benefits of treatment or the research protocol; individuals are required to freely give their consent for the treatment or participation in the study.

Morals: Standards of right and wrong that are learned through socialization.

Nursing ethics: A code of values and behavior that influences the way nurses work with those in their care, with one another, and with society.

Personal ethics: An individual code of thought, values, and behavior that governs each person's actions.

Values: Concepts or ideals that give meaning to life and provide a framework for decisions and actions.

■ THE NATURE OF ETHICAL PROBLEMS

Because ethical issues reflect diverse values and perspectives, they are extremely complex. Ethical questions arise from all areas of life. The ramifications of life-sustaining technology, the population explosion, assisted suicide, euthanasia, genetic engineering, environmental degradation, and allocation of increasingly scarce resources are only a few examples of a host of controversial ethical issues. Ongoing developments in our society such as advances in medical technology, greater recognition of patients' rights, malpractice cases, court-ordered treatment, and end-of-life decisions call nurses to increase their ethical awareness. Another factor that becomes increasingly important in holistic ethics is the ethical treatment of the other than human world, indeed the Earth as a whole, the health of which is intricately connected to human health.

Unfortunately, ethical dilemmas are usually characterized by the fact that there is no right answer. There are often two or more unsatisfactory answers or conflicting responses. In addition, nurses often find that the expectations of employers, physicians, patients, or other nurses are sources of conflict.[1] Changes in the knowledge that forms the basis of our values and advances in health care are leading to new sources of ethical dilemmas. For example, technologies related to computers and communications have affected patient confidentiality. Life support technology may prolong living, but may also increase suffering and prolong the dying pro-

cess. In the midst of dealing with sophisticated technology, nurses often find that their focus is more on the machines than on the patient. Such advances have opened the doors to new possibilities for extending or prolonging life, but they also prompt a critical ethical question: Does having the technology always mean it should be used?

■ MORALS AND PRINCIPLES

Ethical principles serve as a guide for dealing with ethical issues. These principles are basic and obvious moral truths that offer guidance for both deliberation and action. Principles found in major ethical theories include autonomy, beneficence, nonmaleficence, veracity, confidentiality, justice, and fidelity. All of these ethical principles presuppose respect for persons. These principles represent many obligations: to respect the wishes of competent persons, to not harm others, to take actions that benefit others, to produce a net balance of benefits over harm, to distribute benefits and harms fairly, to keep promises and contracts, to be truthful, to disclose information, and to respect privacy and protect confidential information.[1,2]

Orentlicher, a physician, lawyer, and ethicist, thinks that there are, at root, only two ways to guide proper behavior: rules and precedents. He notes that rules are designed to support underlying values (e.g., speed limits are set to promote public safety). Rules are attractive because they provide seemingly clear lines of conduct that prevent metaphorical slippery slopes. They also can help to avoid the capriciousness of personal discretion and the obtrusiveness of governmental intrusion in decision making. However, Orentlicher is concerned with the unintended consequences of rules and cites, as an example, the case of mandating pregnant women to undergo certain medical procedures to prevent harm to their fetuses. Another moral concern is the political difficulty of having explicit rules where life-and-death decisions are being made, such as the allocation of scarce organs. Here, society tends to adopt a system of vague precedents that operate under the guise of rules. The appearance of objectivity, which is inherent to general rules, can hide the vagueness of the processes that actually are being used.[3]

Orentlicher argues that rules sometimes work to the detriment of the value that prompted implementation of the rule in the first place. In fact, this phenomenon is widely considered a kind of natural law: the law of unintended consequences. For example, a medicolegal question might ask whether pregnant women should be forced to undergo treatment to help their fetuses. If forced treatments were endorsed, then some women might avoid prenatal care, thus—and here is the unintended consequence—harming their fetuses. The answer might depend on whether forced treatment would help more fetuses than would be harmed by women who would be driven away from prenatal care. This is but one example of the complexity of ethical decision making.[3]

Within natural law ethics, the principle of double effect has special importance for nurses. Often, nurses are involved in actions that have untoward consequences. For example, administering a drug to relieve a cancer patient's pain may shorten the patient's life. In double effect situations, four conditions must be met before an act can be justified:

1. The act itself must be morally good, or at least indifferent.
2. The good effect must not be achieved by means of the bad effect.
3. Only the good effect must be intended, even though the bad effect is foreseen and known.
4. The good effect intended must be equal to or greater than the bad effect.[4]

Moral problems incorporate a mix of values, risks, benefits, and harms. They are as complex as they are important, include elements of uncertainty and conflict, and defy easy solutions. One must take care with moral decision making because many such decisions are irreversible. Ethics addresses different types of moral problems:

- Moral uncertainty (i.e., unsureness about moral principles or rules that may apply, or the nature of the ethical problem itself)
- Moral dilemma (i.e., conflict of moral principles that support different courses of action)
- Moral distress (i.e., inability to take the action known to be right because of external constraints)

- Practical dilemmas (i.e., a situation where moral claims compete with nonmoral claims)[1]

Ethical debate helps to relieve moral uncertainty by clarifying questions and illuminating the ethical features of a situation. Discussion and reflection help to clarify moral dilemmas by revealing general and specific obligations and values. Many factors contribute to the complexity of ethical problems:

- Context (i.e., a person's unique life circumstances)
- Uncertainty (i.e., a lack of predictability of the outcome of a given act)
- Multiple stakeholders with potentially strong and diverse preferences
- Power imbalance within the healthcare institution
- Variables outside of the direct patient care setting, such as institutional policies
- Urgency (i.e., situations in which a decision must be made before one has a chance to deliberate as much as one would like)[1]

Holistic nurses need to know the language of ethics and have the courage to participate fully in ethical decision making. This requires using principles and theory to deal with issues of relationships as well as healthcare concerns. A holistic approach to ethical problems incorporates both thinking and feeling as credible ways of knowing and recognizes a legitimate role for both in ethical decision making. Heart and mind, reason and emotion, need to be attended to when making ethical decisions, appreciating that what one feels in relation to the circumstances of the situation is as important as what one thinks is right or wrong.

■ TRADITIONAL ETHICAL THEORIES

Many nurse clinicians turn away in frustration when confronted with the details of ethical theories. Perhaps this is because in the past it has been difficult to see how these historical, philosophical theories relate to contemporary clinical situations. To make these theories meaningful to the work setting, it is helpful to think of situations in which they may apply to current clinical practice.

A number of ethical theories have played a role in Western civilization and have laid the foundation for the development of modern ethics. Aristotelian theory is based on the individual manifesting specific virtues and developing his or her own character. Aristotle (384–322 BCE) believed that an individual who practices the virtues of courage, temperance, integrity, justice, honesty, and truthfulness will know almost intuitively what to do in a particular situation or conflict.[5] The system of Immanuel Kant (1724–1804) formulated the historical Christian idea of the Golden Rule: "So act in such a way as your act becomes a universal for all mankind."[5p273] Kant was very much concerned with the "personhood" of human beings and persons as moral agents.

Other theories that are helpful in understanding a holistic approach to ethics include the Utilitarianism Theory of Jeremy Bentham (1748–1832) and John Stuart Mill (1806–1873), the Natural Rights Theory of John Locke (1632–1714), and the Contractarian Theory of Thomas Hobbes (1588–1679). Briefly stated, the consequentialist, or utilitarian, view of Bentham and Mill is that the consequences of our actions are the primary concern, the means justify the ends, and that every human being has a personal concept of good and bad. The Natural Rights Theory of Locke was the forerunner of the U.S. Declaration of Independence because it included the tenet that individuals have inalienable rights and that other individuals have an obligation to respect those rights. The Contractarian Theory of Hobbes contends that morality involves a social contract indicating what individuals can and cannot do.[5pp163–169]

Another way of viewing ethics is in terms of the two traditional forms: the deontologic style (from a Greek root meaning knowledge of that which is binding and proper) and the teleologic style (from a Greek root meaning knowledge of the ends). The former assigns duty or obligation based on the intrinsic aspects of an act rather than its outcome, meaning that action is morally defensible on the basis of its intrinsic nature. The latter assigns duty or obligation based on the consequences of the act, meaning that action is morally defensible on the basis of its extrinsic value or outcome.

■ THE DEVELOPMENT OF HOLISTIC ETHICS

Ethics is the study of the paths of practical wisdom. It is concerned with judgments of good and bad, and right and wrong, based on a philosophic view of the nature of the universe. The holistic view of reality reopens vistas of thought that were dominant in the pretechnologic era, when people were generally closer to their environment and the Earth. The allure of new science and technology sidetracked many of us into primarily linear, rational, unidirectional thought. Furthermore, although technology has provided conveniences and easy solutions, it has also contributed to a tendency to objectify the universe.

Holistic ethics is a philosophy that couples both reemerging and rapidly evolving concepts of holism and ethics. It involves a basic underlying concept of the unity and integral wholeness of all people, and of all nature, which is identified and pursued by finding unity and wholeness within one's self, within humanity, and within the larger Earth community. Within the framework of holistic ethics, acts are not performed solely for the sake of law, precedent, or social norms; they are performed from a desire to do good freely, to witness, identify, and contribute to unity of the self and of the universe, of which the individual is a part. Encompassing traditional ethical views, the holistic view is characterized by the balance and integration evident in the Eastern monad of the yin–yang mode and in the Western concept of masculine–feminine.

Holistic ethics originates in the individual's own character and in the individual's relationship to the universe. In some way, the universe is present totally in each individual; paradoxically, the person is just a small part of that same universe. Gregorios believed that wisdom is a condition in which the self and the world are in communion with each other, within the larger communion, and with the infinite totality of being in its integrity.[6] A holistic view takes into account the relationship of unity of all beings. Albert Einstein, in the course of a serious illness, was asked if he feared death. He replied, "I feel such a sense of solidarity with all living things that it does not matter to me where the individual begins and ends."[7]

Holistic ethics is grounded or judged not so much in the act performed or in the distant consequences of the act, as in the conscious evolution of an enlightened individual who performs the act. Understanding that all things are connected, the primary concern is the effect of the act on the individual and his or her larger self (i.e., that unity of which the individual is a part). Unethical acts are those that degrade or brutalize the individual who performs the act and that detract from his or her conscious evolution, which, in turn, degrades the whole. The effect of an unethical act is to make us aware of the deprivation of divinity within humanity and of humanity itself. The unethical act dissolves the unity of matter and takes away wholeness. Acts must be judged in this setting to determine whether they promote wholeness and integration of either an individual or the collective whole. As each of us evolves our own individual consciousness, we assess and direct the evolution of the consciousness of our species and contemplatively examine our relationship with the universal being.

An a priori belief for a holistic person is likely, "I believe in being," or even more simply, "I am." In this belief system, no act, principle, or person is independent, but all are interrelated; all are "I." Each and every action is a moral action, either contributing to the unity of being or diminishing it. It is the enlightened and completely expanded "I" that creates a holistic view of ethics.

Moral acts may be judged not solely in terms of their intrinsic nature nor solely in terms of their ends, but in both ways. The act may affect the nature of the person performing the act (the "I") and his or her relationships, as well as affect the object of the act and the object's relationships. In addition, it can be helpful to explore the relationship of the act to the present and future of humanity. Through this construct, holistic ethics is both deontologic and teleologic. Holistic ethics is specifically teleologic in questioning the meaning and quality of life.

As a philosophic design for living, holistic ethics is a system for the individual. It appeals to the emotions, senses, aesthetic appreciation, and the inner self as revealed by meditative techniques. Such techniques may be active (e.g., the body movements of tai chi or jogging), passive (e.g., a sitting, meditative posture), or traditional prayer.

The educative process of holistic ethics is not merely a matter of memorizing facts or historical perspectives, but is instead a process of developing an attitude of awareness of the sacredness of ourselves and all of nature. It is a process in which there is an expanded view that, for both internal and external transformation, our inner self and the collective greater self have stewardship not only of our bodies, minds, and spirits, but also of our planet and the total universe.

Based on this emergent ethical theory, the American Holistic Nurses Association (AHNA) has developed a position statement on holistic nursing ethics (**Exhibit 6-1**).

Holistic ethics embraces and strives for the fusion between self and others. In the process, it becomes a cosmic ecology, a flowing with the universal tide of events, and a cocreator of celestial harmony. All events and ethical decisions become part of the unfolding of a harmonious order and a realization of potentials. Even tragic events can be analyzed within this harmonious spectrum with full realization of the fusion of relationships. One's own actions can become courageous; full of truth, being, and beauty; assured; detached; and virtuous.

Earth Ethics

Ethical discussions and deliberations most often refer to principles and practices related to human experiences, values, and ways of being in the world. Such discussions seldom include consideration of ethical treatment of the nonhuman world. Our sense of relationship with the natural world flows from our worldview or cosmology. The worldview that underlies the Western scientific perspective holds that there is a radical distinction between humans as subjects and the natural world as object.[8] A sense that the human experience is separate from and in opposition to nature has engendered and permitted a destructive attitude toward Earth and a belief that all species and resources of the Earth have been put here primarily for human use. A shift, which began emerging in the 17th century, from an organic understanding of reality in which everything is alive, to a mechanistic view of reality, engendered the belief that humans have a right to do anything they want with nature. This attitude promotes little sense of ethical responsibility toward the

EXHIBIT 6-1   American Holistic Nurses Association Position Statement on Holistic Nursing Ethics

Code of Ethics for Holistic Nurses

We believe that the fundamental responsibilities of the nurse are to promote health, facilitate healing and alleviate suffering. The need for nursing is universal. Inherent in nursing is the respect for life, dignity and right of all persons. Nursing care is given in a context mindful of the holistic nature of humans, understanding the body-mind-spirit. Nursing care is unrestricted by considerations of nationality, race, creed, color, age, sex, sexual preferences, politics or social status. Given that nurses practice in culturally diverse settings, professional nurses must have an understanding of the cultural background of clients in order to provide culturally appropriate interventions.

Nurses render services to clients who can be individuals, families, groups or communities. The client is an active participant in health care and should be included in all nursing care planning decisions.

In order to provide services to others, each nurse has a responsibility toward him/herself. In addition, nurses have defined responsibilities towards the client, coworkers, nursing practice, the profession of nursing, society and the environment.

Nurses and Self

The nurse has a responsibility to model health behaviors. Holistic nurses strive to achieve harmony in their own lives and assist others striving to do the same.

Nurses and the Client

The nurse's primary responsibility is to the client needing nursing care. The nurse strives to see the client as a whole, and provides care that is professionally appropriate and culturally consonant. The nurse holds in confidence all information obtained in professional practice, and uses professional judgment in disclosing such information. The nurse enters into a relationship with the client that is guided by mutual respect and a desire for growth and development.

Nurses and Coworkers

The nurse maintains cooperative relationships with coworkers in nursing and other fields. Nurses have a responsibility to nurture each other, and to assist nurses to work as a team in the interest of client care. If a client's care is endangered by a coworker, the nurse must take appropriate action on behalf of the client.

Nurses and Nursing Practice

The nurse carries personal responsibility for practice and for maintaining continued competence. Nurses have the right to utilize all appropriate nursing interventions, and have the obligation to determine the efficacy and safety of all nursing actions. Wherever applicable, nurses utilize research findings in directing practice.

Nurses and the Profession

The nurse plays a role in determining and implementing desirable standards of nursing practice and education. Holistic nurses may assume a leadership position to guide the profession toward holism. Nurses support nursing research and the development of holistically oriented nursing theories. The nurse participates in establishing and maintaining equitable social and economic working conditions in nursing.

Nurses and Society

The nurse, along with other citizens, has responsibility for initiating and supporting actions to meet the health and social needs of the public.

Nurses and the Environment

The nurse strives to manipulate the client's environment to become one of peace, harmony, and nurturance so that healing may take place. The nurse considers the health of the ecosystem in relation to the need for health, safety and peace of all persons.

Source: Courtesy of the American Holistic Nurses Association, Flagstaff, AZ.

nonhuman world. Instead, it has allowed us to turn a blind eye to our complicity in the exploitation of the planet. After several centuries of demoting the natural world to a collection of material objects available for human exploitation, we are now realizing that this complete disregard for the realities of ecological systems and the limited capacity of the natural world to sustain this exploitation and destruction are contributing to the ill health of humans and to the planet itself.

There is an urgent need for holistic nurses and all of humanity to move beyond a human-centered focus in ethical concerns and begin to relate to all parts of the Earth community as having core value. We need to incorporate Earth ethics into our understanding and practice of holistic ethics. Remembering that we are part of the interconnected web of life, we recognize that what we do to the Earth we do to ourselves. Indigenous peoples, mystics of many traditions, and contemporary scholars teach us that the world is a seamless garment in which there is no separation between humans and nature, the sacred and the secular. We cannot have healthy minds or communities without healthy land and environment.[9,10] When we destroy the source of our life and sustenance, our health (physical, mental, emotional, and spiritual) suffers. When we understand that, as humans, we are only one part of the interconnected Earth community, and we recognize the interdependence and unity of all in the natural world, we appreciate that all species have an intrinsic right to exist. Within this understanding, our ethical principles must address the integrity and health of the entire community of life. The moral imperative of holistic ethics then directs us to apply principles of beneficence, nonmaleficence, and justice to our treatment of the whole Earth community, not only to its human members.

■ DEVELOPMENT OF PRINCIPLED BEHAVIOR

Healthcare providers with a holistic ethics perspective and high standards of principled behavior are best prepared to analyze clinical dilemmas. Nathaniel asserts that principled behavior flows from personal values that guide and inform one's responses, behaviors, and decisions in all areas of one's life.[11] Holistic nurses need to be aware of personal values and know how these values influence relationships with oneself, others, and the Earth community.

Values Clarification

Values develop over time and have cultural, familial, environmental, and educational components. Values clarification is a never-ending process in which an individual becomes increasingly aware of what is important and just—and why. Understanding and openly discussing different views in a given situation helps us to appreciate the truth inherent in the various perspectives. Values clarification within groups and organizations requires conscious identification of spoken and written (i.e., overt) values as well as those values that are unspoken or unwritten (i.e., covert) values. Identifying the underlying values of an organization enables us to determine whether our personal and professional values are congruent with those of the organization. This awareness serves as a basis for determining whether we can work in a particular environment or support a particular organization.

Often, patients must clarify their values to participate fully in ethical decision making. Holistic nurses can assist patients in this process in a variety of ways. One way is to listen carefully and reflect back what nurses hear patients say is personally important to them. Another might be to list several health behaviors or values such as happiness, good relationships with family, health, independence, and ask patients to rank them or to identify how they incorporate them into their lives.

Legal Aspects

Healthcare providers must adhere to the law. All nurses are responsible and accountable to comply with the Nursing Practice Act as well as the rules and regulations of the board of nurse examiners in the state where they are licensed and work. Standards of professional nursing practice require that each nurse practice to the level of his or her knowledge and skills. In this regard, holistic nurses need to be familiar with and adhere to the standards of practice for holistic nurses.[12] Whatever an individual nurse's personal ethic, he or she must still adhere to the standards of practice and to the law.

■ ETHICAL DECISION MAKING

Nurses are confronted daily with the need to make personal and professional ethical decisions, yet many of them feel unprepared to be equal participants in ethical decision making. Some decisions nurses face are minor, and others are fraught with long-term multifaceted ramifications. To make decisions appropriately, holistic nurses need to be grounded in an understanding of the integral wholeness of all beings and do their best to articulate and examine their core values and their relationship to nursing and institutional standards. Participation in decision-making groups necessitates that nurses become fluent in the language of nursing and bioethics and that they learn to appreciate the diverse moral perspectives of patients and colleagues. It is necessary as well that nurses operate from a set of principles and have facility with processes that help sort out and classify the elements of the problem. There are many well-established guidelines for analyzing individual cases in ethics that may be helpful to nurses. Two such processes are summarized here.

Burkhardt and Nathaniel[1] approach ethical decision making from a nursing problem-solving frame of reference that includes sensitivity to the human story. They suggest that, although the steps of an ethical problem-solving process may seem linear on paper, the process is nonlinear in practice. They note that the ethical decision-making process overlays other dynamic biological, psychological, and social processes—layer on layer. Because nothing in the human sphere is static, nurses need to appreciate that physical conditions and opinions change, knowledge evolves, and time passes. In light of the changing nature of human experience, these authors describe a decision-making process in which key facets are revisited from an evolving perspective as one moves toward a decision or resolution. They present a framework for entering a decision-making process that is spiral in nature. This process requires an ongoing evaluation and assimilation of information, with each step being revisited as often as is required and molded by the dynamics of changing facts, evolving beliefs, unexpected consequences, and participants who move in and out of the process. They have formed a five-step process of ethical decision making

with the following components: (1) articulating the problem, (2) gathering data and identifying conflicting moral claims, (3) exploring strategies, (4) implementing the strategy, and (5) evaluating outcomes of the action.

Articulating the Problem

Ethical decision making begins when there is concern that a moral problem exists. Clearly articulating and identifying the problem enables one to also clarify the goal because a problem consists of a discrepancy between the current situation and a desired state or goal. A goal must be identified before moving toward strategies, which is step 3 of this model.

Gathering Data and Identifying Conflicting Moral Claims

Clarify the issues by gathering information that provides evidence of conflicting goals, obligations, principles, duties, rights, loyalties, values, or beliefs. In this process, nurses must pay attention to societal, religious, and cultural values and beliefs of all involved. Data gathering should include information about facts as well as feelings that seem important, such as expectations, preferences, quality-of-life issues, understanding of the situation, relationships and supports, and projected outcomes of available options. Gaps in the information also need to be identified. Key participants (which include healthcare providers) need to be identified, including who is affected and how; who is legitimately empowered to make the decision; issues of conflict and agreement among participants and what is most important to each; the level of competence of the person most affected; and the rights, duties, authority, and capabilities of all participants. These data can help those involved to understand the ethical components, principles of concern, and the various perceptions of issues and principles of all involved in the situation.

Exploring Strategies

Through the assessment process, possible alternative strategies that address the desired outcomes begin to emerge. In consideration of legal and other consequences, participants need to determine which alternatives best meet the identified goals and fit their basic beliefs, lifestyles, and values. By reviewing options with both head and heart, participants need to eliminate unacceptable alternatives and begin the process of listing, weighing, prioritizing, and sensing the energy of those that are considered acceptable, recognizing that there is rarely a perfect solution. Once an option is chosen, the decision makers must be willing to act on the choice.

Implementing the Strategy

Although taking action is a major goal of the process, it can be one of the most difficult parts of the process. Emotions laced with both certainty and doubt about the rightness of the decision often emerge. Empowering patients and families to make difficult decisions requires special attention to the emotions that often manifest at this point of the process.

Evaluating Outcomes of Action

Once the action step is taken, participants begin a process of response and evaluation that sheds light on the effectiveness and validity of the process. In evaluating the action in terms of the effects on those involved, it is important to determine whether the original ethical problem has been effectively resolved and whether other problems have emerged related to the action. As new data emerge and the situation changes, participants may identify subsequent moral problems that require adjusting the course of action based on both new information and responses to the previous decision.

In developing the second method for analyzing individual cases in ethics, Jonsen and colleagues[13] divided the ethical case analysis process into four components: (1) medical indications, (2) patient preferences, (3) quality of life, and (4) contextual issues. Present in every clinical, ethical case, these four topics are necessary for a thorough analysis. The holistic approach adds relationship questions: Who am I? What is my relationship to others and to the whole? What other factors are contributing to my decisions? Am I wise and courageous enough to perceive and respect others' differences and honor them as I would honor my own beliefs?

Medical Indications

The underlying ethical principles in considering medical indications is beneficence—be of bene-fit—and do no harm. Discussion should focus on discerning the relationship between the pathophysiology and the diagnostic and therapeutic interventions (both conventional and integrative) available to remedy the patient's pathologic condition. Questions regarding the overall goal of the care are important considerations in this component. For example, for the patient who is terminally ill, there may be discussions about the time to switch from further medical treatment to palliative care.

Patient Preferences

In all interventions, the preferences of the patient are relevant. There are many questions to be asked: What does the patient want? Does the patient comprehend his or her choices? Is the patient being coerced? In some cases, there is no certainty because the patient is incapable of self-expression. Whenever possible, it is essential to ensure the patient's right to self-determination based on his or her personal values and evaluation of risks and benefits is honored. However, it is necessary to be clear about what is realistically feasible in relation to the patient's wishes.

In the case of a child, nurses must ask the questions: Do the parents understand the situation? Do the parents appear to have the best interests of the child at heart? Are the parents in agreement or discord?

Quality of Life

A patient enters a health crisis situation with an actual or potential reduction in quality of life, manifested by the signs and symptoms of the illness. The objective of healthcare interventions is to improve quality of life. In each case, multiple questions surround quality-of-life issues: What does quality of life mean, in general? In particular? How are others responding to their perceptions of it? How do particular levels of quality impose obligations, if any, on providers? This component may be a difficult part of the analysis of clinical problems, but it is indispensable.

Contextual Issues

Every case has a patient at its center. The patient exists in a social, psychological, spiritual, economic, and relational environment. To be relevant, all decisions must be considered in the light of this expanded conceptual and holistic view of personhood and personality. The major factors affected are psychological, emotional, financial, legal, scientific, educational, and spiritual.

ADVANCE DIRECTIVES

Many ethical dilemmas arise surrounding end-of-life care options and choices. Supporting a patient's right and ability to make choices is an essential element of holistic nursing practice and holistic ethics. The Patient Self-Determination Act, effective December 1, 1991, requires that all individuals receiving medical care also receive written information about their right to accept or refuse medical or surgical treatment and their right to initiate advance directives. Advance directives are instructions that indicate healthcare interventions to initiate or withhold, or that designate someone who will act as a surrogate in making such decisions in the event that decision-making capacity is lost. Advance directives support people in making decisions on their own behalf and help to ensure that patients have the kind of end-of-life care they want. Advance medical directives are of two types: treatment directives (often referred to as living wills), and appointment directives (often referred to as powers of attorney or health proxies). A living will specifies the medical treatment that a patient wishes to refuse in the event that he or she is terminally ill and cannot make those decisions. A durable power of attorney for health care appoints a proxy or surrogate, usually a relative or trusted friend, to make medical decisions on behalf of the patient if he or she can no longer make such decisions. It has broader applications than a living will and can apply to any illness or injury that causes the patient to lose decision-making capacity temporarily or long term. The authority of the surrogate is effective only for the duration of the loss of decision-making capacity.

An advance directive applies only if a patient is incapacitated. It may not apply if, in the opinion of two physicians, the patient can make decisions. Individuals can cancel advance directives at any time. An advance directive may be simple or complex. Individuals should give a copy of the advance directive to their family members and physician and should carry a copy if and when hospital admission is necessary.

As part of patient assessment, a nurse may consider asking the following questions:

- Have you discussed your end-of-life choices with your family and/or designated surrogate and healthcare team workers?
- Do you have basic information about advance medical directives, including living wills and durable powers of attorney?
- Do you wish to initiate an advance medical directive?
- If you have already prepared an advance medical directive, can you provide it now?

ETHICAL CONSIDERATIONS IN PRACTICE AND RESEARCH

Because nursing is inherently a moral endeavor, nurses may encounter challenges in making the right decisions and taking the right actions in both nursing research and nursing practice. An important consideration for nurses in ensuring legal and ethical protection of a patient's right to personal autonomy is the process of informed consent. Obtaining informed consent from patients is important both in relation to medical and other treatments and to participation in research studies. The process of informed consent for medical and other treatments provides the opportunity for the patient to choose a course of action regarding plans for health care, including the right to refuse medical recommendations and to choose from available therapeutic alternatives. An informed consent must include the following:

1. The nature of the health concern and prognosis if nothing is done
2. Description of all treatment options, even those that the healthcare provider does not favor or cannot provide
3. The benefits, risks, and consequences of the various treatment alternatives, including nonintervention

The issue of informed consent with complementary/alternative modalities (CAM) raises some important questions. Because listing alternative treatments is one of the elements of an informed consent, nurses must consider whether it is an ethical duty for practitioners of bioscientific medicine to include discussion of CAM in discussion of therapeutic alternatives. Nurses also need to ask whether practitioners of other healing modalities should ensure that their clients are aware of biomedical alternatives. Holistic nurses who offer CAM therapies should explain the intervention and discuss risks, expected effects and benefits, and treatment options prior to initiating therapy. Because CAM therapies may affect conventional interventions in varying ways, it is important to inform other health team members of the use of these therapies.

Research expands the unique body of knowledge of nursing and provides an organizing framework for nursing practice. Although participating in research is important and rewarding, it can also present dilemmas for the nurse and nurse researcher in both research institutions and clinical realms. Adding to nursing's knowledge and understanding is the expected motivation for conducting research. However, other motivating factors such as personal or institutional gains related to grant funding, prestige, or promoting a product may challenge principled behavior in regard to research.

The principles that underlie the ethical conduct of research include respect for human dignity (i.e., the rights to full disclosure and self-determination or autonomy), beneficence (i.e., the right to protection from harm and discomfort, as in balancing between the benefits and risks of a study), and justice (i.e., the rights of fair treatment and privacy, including anonymity and confidentiality). These principles provide the basis for informed consent related to participation in research studies.[14] Informed consent in research refers to freely choosing to participate in a research study after the research purpose, expected commitment, risks and benefits, any invasion of privacy, and ways that anonymity and confidentiality will be addressed have been explained. Nurses who work in clinical areas where research is being conducted must work to ensure that these principles are followed.

Nurses who assist with research or who work on units where research is being conducted need to be familiar with elements of informed consent and be attentive to ensuring informed consent is obtained from research participants. A particular area of concern is protection of human rights in research studies focused on vulnerable populations such as children; persons with disabilities; persons who are challenged, institutionalized, or incarcerated; older adults; pregnant women; and those who are dying. Nurses who are involved in research are accountable to professional standards for reporting research findings. An important consideration in this regard is the ethical treatment of data, which demonstrates the integrity of research protocols and honesty in reporting data.

■ CULTURAL DIVERSITY CONSIDERATIONS

Cultural values and beliefs guide our way of being in the world and our reaction to life experiences in patterned ways. Patterns influenced by culture that are significant in providing holistic health care include beliefs about health and practices related to health and healing. These beliefs and practices manifest in both direct and subtle ways, and sensitivity to them can affect patient outcomes and satisfaction with the care. The increasing cultural diversity in modern society may present challenges in transcultural ethical decision making for healthcare workers. Such transcultural issues arise when nurses, patients, and families are guided by different moral paradigms and hold differing views of what is important or necessary regarding health, recovery, illness, or the dying process. Ethical or legal dilemmas may arise from lack of understanding of language, procedures, expectations, and other elements of the culture that lead to miscommunication, unclear decisions, and a sense of powerlessness or lack of control. Dealing with transcultural issues requires self-awareness on the part of the nurse. A good starting point for becoming sensitive to the culture of another is to understand one's own culture and its influence on personal perceptions and behaviors. Similarly, incorporating cultural assessment into care with patients facilitates better understanding of sometimes overlooked factors that influence a patient's health behaviors and decisions. Nurses who are sensitive and knowledgeable about the cultural perspective of individual patients acknowledge an individual's cultural background and consider the characteristics of different cultures when planning the patient's care. This facilitates the process of ethical decision making.

Culture guides choices regarding when and where to go for health care, what kind of care to seek, and how long to participate in care. When considering definitions of health and values such as autonomy, beneficence, justice, or the right to self-determination, it is important to ask from whose perspective these values are understood—that of the nurse or that of the patient. For example, some cultures place a higher emphasis on loyalty to the group than on Western values of individual autonomy. Healthcare decisions in these cultures may require input and agreement from groups such as the family, community, or society, rather than relying primarily on the individual. Cultural assessment provides insight into the congruence, or lack thereof, between patients' and nurses' values and understandings of health.

Flowing from the concept of the unity and integral wholeness of all people, holistic ethics must encompass a global perspective. This perspective includes cultural competence and cultural humility that enable the nurse to acknowledge and respect multiple ethical paradigms. Nursing care and research require awareness of, respect for, and congruence with the culture and needs of individuals and the community that are the focus of services or research.[15] Broad principles and concepts that can guide holistic nursing practice and research with cultures other than one's own include respect for persons and for communities, honoring the unity and wholeness of all beings, beneficence, justice, respect for human rights, contextual caring, and fidelity to one's professional code of ethics.

■ CONCLUSION

The holistic view of reality reopens vistas of thought that were dominant in the pretechnologic era, when people were generally closer to their environment and the Earth. Holistic ethics is a philosophy that couples both reemerging and rapidly evolving concepts of holism and ethics. It involves a basic underlying concept of the unity and integral wholeness of all people, and of all nature, that is identified and pursued by finding unity and wholeness within the self, within humanity, and within the Earth community. The complexity of ethical issues relates to the diverse values and perspectives involved.

Skills in cultural assessment can help nurses to more effectively deal with ethical issues. Understanding the nature of ethical problems requires holistic nurses to be familiar with traditional ethical theories and concepts and aware of other ethical paradigms and to be able to integrate this knowledge with holistic theory and practice. An increasingly important factor in holistic ethics is the ethical treatment of the nonhuman world and the Earth as a whole, the health of which is intricately connected to human health. Awareness of personal values, beliefs, and understanding of health grounds the ability to deal effectively with ethical situations. The principles and processes of holistic ethics apply to research as well as to clinical practice situations. Holistic nurses need to know the language of ethics, be familiar with processes of ethical decision making, be attentive to cultural differences, and have the courage to participate fully in ethical decision making. This requires using principles, theory, and cultural competence and incorporates both thinking and feeling as credible ways of knowing in ethical decision making.

Directions for
FUTURE RESEARCH

1. Determine how and where the theory of holistic ethics fits into the continuum of emerging ethical theories.
2. Develop a process of clinical case analysis based on the process of holistic ethics.
3. Examine specific clinical situations and research protocols through a process of holistic ethics.
4. Analyze the application of holistic ethics to planetary ethical issues.

Nurse Healer
REFLECTIONS

After reading this chapter, the nurse healer will be able to answer or to begin a process of answering the following questions:

- What new insights do I have about the process of ethics?
- How do I incorporate ethics into my clinical practice?
- How am I involved in ethical decision making within my work setting?

- How do my ethical values influence my day-to-day personal life?
- Am I ready to look at planetary issues from a holistic ethical perspective?

 For a full suite of assignments and additional learning activities, use the access code located in the front of your book to visit this exclusive website: http://go.jblearning.com/dossey. If you do not have an access code, you can obtain one at the site.

NOTES

1. M. A. Burkhardt and A. K. Nathaniel, *Ethics and Issues in Contemporary Nursing*, 3rd ed. (Albany, NY: Delmar Publishers, 2008).

2. S. T. Fry, R. M. Veatch, and C. R. Taylor, *Case Studies in Nursing Ethics*, 4th ed. (Sudbury, MA: Jones & Bartlett Learning, 2011).

3. D. Orentlicher, *Matters of Life and Death: Making Moral Theory Work in Medicine and the Law* (Princeton, NJ: Princeton University Press, 2001).

4. A. McIntyre, "Doctrine of Double Effect," *Stanford Encyclopedia of Philosophy,* ed. E. N. Zalta (Fall 2011). http://plato.stanford.edu/entries/double-effect.

5. H. Sidgwick, *Ethics* (Boston: Beacon Press, 1960): 59-63.

6. P. M. Gregorios, *Science for Sane Societies* (New York: Paragon House, 1987).

7. M. Born, *Born–Einstein Letters* (New York: Walker, 1971).

8. C. Uhl, *Developing Ecological Consciousness: Path to a Sustainable World* (Lanham, MD: Rowman & Littlefield, 2004).

9. M. Nelson, "Stopping the War on Mother Earth," in *Ecological Medicine: Healing the Earth, Healing Ourselves*, ed. K. Ausubel (San Francisco, CA: Sierra Club Books, 2004): 228-230.

10. T. Berry and M. E. Tucker, *The Sacred Universe* (New York: Columbia University Press, 2009).

11. A. K. Nathaniel, "Moral Reckoning in Nursing," *Western Journal of Nursing Research* 28 (2006): 419-438.

12. American Holistic Nurses Association & American Nurses Association, *Holistic Nursing: Scope & Standards of Practice* (Silver Spring, MD: NurseBooks.org, 2007).

13. A. R. Jonsen et al., *Clinical Ethics: A Practical Approach to Ethical Decisions in Clinical Medicine*, 7th ed. (New York: McGraw Hill/Appleton Lange, 2010).

14. U.S. Department of Health and Human Services, Office for Human Research Protections (OHRP) home page (n.d.). http://www.hhs.gov/ohrp.

15. J. N. Harrowing et al., "Culture, Context, and Community: Ethical Considerations for Global Nursing," *International Nursing Review* 57, no 1 (2010): 70-77.

CORE VALUE 2

Holistic Caring Process

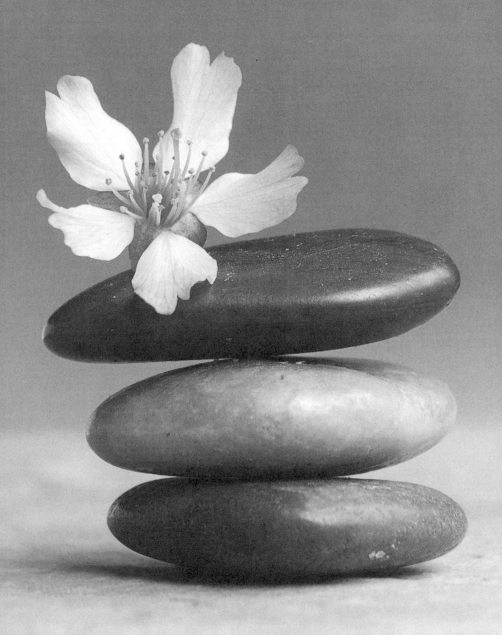

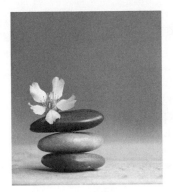

Chapter 7

The Holistic Caring Process

Pamela J. Potter and Noreen Cavan Frisch

Nurse Healer
OBJECTIVES

Theoretical

- Define the terms *nursing process* and *holistic caring process.*
- Outline the steps of the holistic caring process.
- Explore the ways in which conceptual models of nursing inform and guide the holistic caring process.
- Discuss the ways in which standards of holistic nursing practice are incorporated into the holistic caring process.

Clinical

- Analyze the assessment tool that you are using in clinical practice to determine whether the tool is consistent with a holistic nursing perspective.
- Explore the ways to document holistic nursing care in a computerized electronic health record (EHR) through use of standardized terms such as those found in nursing diagnostic taxonomies, the Nursing Interventions Classification, and the Nursing Outcomes Classification.
- Identify the nursing concerns and activities most relevant to your clients.
- Integrate prevention, health promotion, and wellness diagnoses into practice.

- Use the Trifocal Model as an organizing structure for a visual composite of the three levels of a person's health patterns in prioritizing and planning nursing interventions and patient outcomes within the nurse–person interaction.
- Implement the *Holistic Nursing: Scope and Standards of Practice* (2007) of the American Holistic Nurses Association (AHNA) and American Nurses Association (ANA) in your work and life.

Personal

- Observe the pattern appraisal and identification process in your everyday life as you walk into a new situation.
- Identify the four patterns of knowing (empirical, ethical, aesthetic, and personal knowledge) as they guide you within the nurse–person interaction.
- Develop and trust your intuitive thinking processes when assessing clients' conditions.
- Evaluate the impact of intuitive thinking in both your professional and personal lives.
- Explore your own beliefs and values regarding the concepts of holistic nursing.
- Write down specific examples of holistic nursing care while reflecting on your enactment of the holistic caring process.

DEFINITIONS

Electronic health record (EHR): A patient care record in digital format.

Holistic caring process: A circular process that involves six steps that may occur simultaneously. These steps are assessment, patterns/challenges/needs, outcomes, therapeutic care plan, implementation, and evaluation.

Holistic nursing: All nursing practice that has healing the whole person as its goal.

Intuition: The perceived knowing of things and events without the conscious use of rational processes; using all of the senses to receive information.

NANDA-I diagnosis: A multiaxial classification schema for the organization of nursing diagnoses based on functional domains and classes.[1]

Nursing diagnosis (NDx): "A clinical judgment about the individual, family, or community responses to actual and potential health problems or life processes. A nursing diagnosis is the basis for the selection of nursing interventions to achieve outcomes for which the nurse is accountable."[2]

Nursing Interventions Classification (NIC): A standardized comprehensive classification or taxonomy of treatments that nurses perform, including both independent and collaborative, as well as direct and indirect.[3]

Nursing Outcomes Classification (NOC): A standardized comprehensive taxonomy of frequently identified goals: measurable responses to nursing interventions.[4]

Nursing process: The original model describing the "work" of nursing, defined as steps used to fulfill the purposes of nursing, such as assessment, diagnosis, client outcomes, plans, intervention, and evaluation.

Paradigm: A model for conceptualizing information.

Patterns/challenges/needs: A person's actual and potential life processes related to health, wellness, disease, or illness, which may or may not facilitate well-being.

Person: An individual, client, patient, family member, support person, or community member who has the opportunity to engage in interaction with a holistic nurse.

Standards of practice: A group of statements describing the expected level of care by a holistic nurse.

Taxonomy of nursing practice (NDx/NIC/ NOC [NNN]): An atheoretical taxonomic framework that describes nursing practice by linking nursing diagnoses with nursing interventions and nursing outcomes.[1]

■ THEORY AND RESEARCH

Focused on establishing health and well-being, the holistic caring process represents the entire range of activities taking place within the nurse–person relationship. It is, quite simply, the process of nurse and client coming together in a professional interaction. The holistic caring process is not essentially different from the nursing process many nurses learned in school. However, the nursing process has come to represent something less than the whole encounter. Many think of the nursing process in terms of limited nursing care plans that focus on physiologic priorities of care and omit the important intangibles of practice, such as presence, hope, support, caring, and mutuality. Holistic nurses need to remember that the nursing process is a framework that gives us the means to reflect on the entire range of nursing activities. These activities are usually described as the following steps:

1. Assessment
2. Diagnosis, or identification of problems or needs, or pattern recognition
3. Plan of care
4. Implementation or intervention
5. Evaluation

The original concept of nursing process can be traced to the late 1950s and early 1960s when nurses in the United States sought to identify what they did as a distinct, autonomous profession within health care. In 1957, Kreuter first identified the nursing process formally as a conceptualization of an orderly approach used to conduct nursing activities.[5] Early on, proponents of the nursing process readily saw it as a tool to describe professional activities carried out by nurses that were unnoticed and unrecognized as having important contributions to care and recovery. For example, even very basic nursing activities such as those related to patient comfort (positioning, creating a calming atmosphere), nutrition (timing of meals and presentation of food and fluids), sleep (relaxation, back rubs), or skin integrity (massage, turning, and attention to bed linens) were carried out by nurses but often referred to as "common sense" rather than as professional responses to identified client needs. The concept of a nursing process allowed nurses to use a common language, systematize nursing practice and education, and enhance nursing autonomy.

There have been two definitions of the nursing process: one a linear process for solving problems, and the other a circular process for describing our understanding of our encounters with clients.[6] The linear process is a step-by-step depiction of nursing work and mirrors scientific problem solving. Here, the nurse gathers data and assesses the client situation; uses data to make clinical judgments, plan care and interventions; implements the plan of care; and evaluates the outcomes. The linear nursing process depicts nursing as if one step is always carried out before the next, as if the nurse attends to one client problem or concern at a time, and as if there is a conscious pattern of moving from one step to the other. Although experienced nurses know that the conditions of the linear nursing process are not met, the linear process was widely adopted in the 1980s as a foundation for education and practice. It made sense to guide novice nurses through one step at a time to assist them to grasp the connections between nursing assessments, judgments, and actions. Further, it made sense to think about nursing in a logical step-by-step fashion to document nursing as separate from medicine and to study outcomes of nursing care. Thus, the linear nursing process provided a framework that helped nurses identify their contributions to care.

In contrast, the circular nursing process is a way of thinking about nursing with a full understanding that every step of the nursing process may be happening all at once and that the nurse may be addressing multiple client needs simultaneously. The circular nursing process is more related to the subjective experience of "being a nurse" than is the linear model. A nurse may be assessing while she or he is intervening. A nurse may be evaluating while diagnosing, or she or he may be attending to comfort needs and gathering data related to spiritual needs at the same time. When a nurse walks into a client room, she or he begins the nurse–patient encounter with an intervention—the nursing presence. The circular model is readily understood by experienced nurses. Emphasizing holistic care, Erickson and colleagues supported the circular nursing process model and described the process as "the ongoing, interactive exchange of information, feelings, and behavior between nurse and client(s) wherein the nurse's goal is to nurture and support the client's self-care."[7] **Figure 7-1** presents a depiction of the two conceptualizations of the nursing process: the linear process as how nurses describe their work and the circular process as how nurses experience their work.

Today, the nursing process has its critics—those who believe that the nursing process is reductionistic and steeped in positivism emphasizing

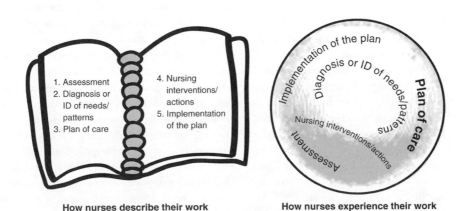

How nurses describe their work   **How nurses experience their work**

FIGURE 7-1   Two Conceptualizations of the Nursing Process
Source: © Noreen C. Frisch, 2007.

science and objectivity as the only source of knowing. Further, some believe that the nursing process serves the interests of the profession over the interests of the clients and are concerned with use of labels and jargon. The nursing process is atheoretical and is compatible with a variety of philosophical positions. The problem may not lie in the nursing process per se, but rather in the differing philosophic perspectives used to describe it.

The origins of the nursing process reside within the concept of pattern recognition, an innate tendency found among humans. Pattern recognition may be observed even in young infants who, early on, recognize and react to familiar as well as unfamiliar patterns (facial, vocal, and kinesthetic) in their caregivers. When nurses encounter a patient for the first time, they observe the state of the person's health. They notice the person's color (pale or cyanotic), affect and eye contact, respiration depth and rate, rate and volume of speech, body odor, scars, wounds, and more. Within 60 seconds, they notice if something is different from the expected and whether any nursing action is necessary. This is pattern appraisal and pattern recognition. Using all their nursing knowledge, nurses apply the patterns they observe to known patterns, make decisions about those patterns, and then act upon those decisions. After doing so, they reappraise and react based on the response of the person.

Further, this nursing process is culturally shaped, inseparable from the culture within which it is practiced.[8] Engebretson and Littleton describe the nursing process from an ecological perspective as one of cultural negotiation wherein the nurse and the person enter into a mutual partnership in which they exchange expert knowledge, collaborate on the analysis and interpretation of information, engage in joint decision making, implement mutually derived plans for action, and undertake an analytical appraisal of both process and expected outcomes. Key to the nursing process is the recognition that the reality of health and the healthcare environment is "constructed from selective observations and interpretations" by the culture within which it is situated.[8p224] An ecological approach to nursing process "is based in an understanding and negotiation of cultural and formal knowledge, experience, and unique individual factors that both client and nurse bring to this interaction."[8p230]

Because nursing cannot be conceptually separated from the cultural context within which it is practiced, the holistic nurse must consider this context when implementing theory-based practice. For example, although one's theoretical underpinnings for nursing may define nursing as "the practice of presence" within the nurse–person relationship, the culture and the patient may define nursing by activities carried out by the nurse on behalf of the patient. Holistic nurses who work within contemporary healthcare culture must balance formal knowledge and expertise gained from nursing education and practice with philosophies of health that may not yet be fully embraced by mainstream culture.

Reflective Practice

The holistic caring process is experienced within reflective practice. Insights derived from the four patterns of knowing identified by Carper guide the nurse's process within the nurse–person interaction.[9] Empirical or scientific knowledge is based on objective information measurable by the senses and by scientific instrumentation. Ethical knowledge flows from the "basic underlying concept of the unity and integral wholeness of all people and of all nature."[10] Aesthetic knowledge draws on a sense of form and structure and of beauty and creativity for discerning pattern and change. Personal knowledge incorporates the nurse's self-awareness and knowledge (emotional intelligence), as well as the intuitive perception of meanings based on personal experiences, and is demonstrated by the therapeutic use of self.

The Johns model of reflective practice within Carper's fundamental ways of knowing in nursing enables "the practitioner to access, understand, and learn through her or his lived experiences and, as a consequence, to take congruent action towards developing increasing effectiveness within the context of what is understood as desirable practice."[11] Within this structured reflection a set of cue questions challenges the nurse's unexamined norms and habitual practices, allows for interpreting the nurse's subjective experience, and facilitates projection of the effects of nursing actions on the observed outcomes (see **Exhibit 7-1**).

EXHIBIT 7-1   The Model for Structured Reflection

Reflective Cue	MSR Map*
Bring the mind home.	
Focus on a description of an experience that seems significant in some way.	Aesthetics
What particular issues seem significant to pay attention to?	Aesthetics
How were others feeling, and what made them feel that way?	Aesthetics
How was I feeling, and what made me feel that way?	Personal
What was I trying to achieve, and did I respond effectively?	Aesthetics
What were the consequences of my actions on the patient, others, and myself?	Aesthetics
What factors influenced the way I was feeling, thinking, or responding?	Personal
What knowledge did inform or might have informed me?	Empirics
To what extent did I act for the best and in tune with my values?	Ethics
How does this situation connect with previous experiences?	Personal Reflexivity*
How might I respond more effectively given this situation again?	Reflexivity
What would be the consequences of alternative actions for the patient, others, and myself?	Reflexivity
What factors might constrain me from responding in new ways?*	Personal*
How do I now feel about this experience?	Personal*
Am I more able to support myself and others better as a consequence?	Reflexivity
What insights have I gained from this reflection?	Reflexivity

Source: Christopher Johns, *Engaging Reflection in Practice: A Narrative Approach,* 15th ed. (Oxford: Blackwell Publishing, 2007).

Intuitive Thinking

The holistic caring process involves collection and evaluation of data not only from a rational, analytic, and verbal (or left brain) mode, but also from an intuitive, nonverbal (right brain) mode. Intuitive perception allows one to know something immediately without consciously using reason. Clinical intuition has been described as a "process by which we know something about a client that cannot be verbalized or is verbalized poorly or for which the source of the knowledge cannot be determined."[12] It is a "gut feeling" that something is wrong or that we should do something, even if there is no real evidence to support that feeling. Within the caring relationship between nurse and person, intuitive events emerge as the nurse is open and receptive to the person's subtle cues.

Effken describes this perception as the direct detection of environmental information.[13,14] Intuition, characterized as direct perception, occurs when the holistic nurse perceives in the environment higher-order variables that call for action. Framing intuition as direct perception offers an explanation for how experts who perceive complex higher-order variables cannot report with accuracy underlying lower-order properties, as well as how new information, outside of the nurse's previous experience, may be interpreted intuitively as an opportunity for action. Expert nurses, like "smart devices," sensitive to and capable of acting immediately upon higher-order information, directly apprehend environmental information as a whole—as a complex or composite variable. When characterized as direct perception, intuition becomes an "observable, lawful phenomenon that is measurable, potentially teachable, and appropriately part of nursing science."[13p252] Where Effken's definition could limit intuition to the objective, rational, cognitive realm of the expert nurse, the concept of emotional intelligence suggests that emotional intelligence facilitates interpretation of the nurse's perceptions.

Emotional Intelligence

Emotional intelligence informs the gut feeling dimension of intuition.[15] Described as an ability,[16] a set of traits and abilities,[17] or a combination of skills and personal competencies,[18,19] emotional intelligence is the assessment, expression, control, and use of emotions within the nursing intervention.[20] Emotional intelligence directs the emotional labor of the caring relationship associated with the holistic caring process. Emotional labor "is a process whereby nurses adopt a 'work persona' to express their autonomous, surface or deep emotions during patient encounters."[21p203]

Established on Goleman's[22] theoretical framework, Robertson[15] identifies four building blocks for cultivating emotional intelligence within the healthcare setting. Internal domains (intrapersonal) include Self-Awareness and Self-Management. Social Awareness and Relationship Management comprise external domains (interpersonal). Self-Awareness, the ability to recognize one's emotional response pattern to specific people and situations, is demonstrated through recognizing one's own emotions and their communication (facial expression, body language, word choice, and voice tone) to create congruence between intention and message sent. Self-Management, the ability to modulate one's emotional response, draws from emotional awareness to manage how those emotions are expressed. This response may be expressed through *surface acting*, in which the nurse changes the outward expression to display feelings appropriate to the situation, or through *deep acting*, in which the nurse changes the deeper feelings to those appropriate to the situation.[20] The purpose is to create safety for focusing on client-centered feelings and concerns. Social Awareness demonstrates the ability to accurately perceive and understand another's emotions even if they are expressed through a different cultural lens. Relationship Management consciously accesses Self-Awareness, Self-Management, and Social Awareness to support relationship enhancement and to avoid relationship-ending confrontations.

Essential to the holistic caring process emotional intelligence is a skill set with competencies that can be taught and learned through the use of journal prompts that guide nursing student reflection on the *emotion* components of nursing interactions.[23] Therapeutic use of self through the holistic caring process requires emotional intelligence. No longer encouraged to conceal emotions and maintain therapeutic distance, nurses in partnership with their patients manage their emotions as they express empathy and concern.[20] By distinguishing empathic concern from emotional contagion, they adopt emotionally intelligent strategies within the holistic caring process to support healing rather than enable stagnation.

Applications of Holistic Nursing Theory

Holistic nurses select a theory to guide their practice when they enact the nursing process. The theoretical context of the nurse, as well as the nursing institution, can work to enhance or constrain the practice. Nurses who contend that they work "without a theory" very likely base their practice unquestioningly on a rational, biochemical, mechanical, medical model. Applying holistic nursing philosophy to the nursing process helps to emphasize a holistic perspective and yet remains incomplete without a nursing theoretical framework compatible with holism. The theory the nurse uses to guide practice is identifiable in the application of the nursing process. (See Chapter 5 for a discussion of nursing theories.) Adaptation and expansion of the nursing process based on holistic nursing philosophy includes the person as a mutual participant in nursing care. The holistic caring process emphasizes the understanding that the person is primary in the nurse–person relationship. This has not always been the case. Historically, the disease or the problem was foremost. In today's managed care environment, sometimes the requirements of the insurance payer appear to take precedence over the person in the healthcare relationship.

The holistic caring process incorporates both the problem-solving components of natural science methodology and the caring dimension of the human science approach, which emphasizes the often unmeasurable human side of the traditional art of nursing.[24] It accommodates the whole person as a bio-psycho-social-spiritual being within the environmental context. Thus, the advantages of a holistic caring process parallel those delineated for the nursing process in general, with the addition of the whole-person perspective. The holistic framework is a person-centered process. This approach examines a person's reality, perceptions, and life meanings for insight into the lived experience of health and well-being. The holistic caring process is a relational process. Through mutual relationship, the nurse collaborates with the person to identify and pursue goals for health enhancement. As a synthesis of natural and human sciences, the holistic caring process reflects an equal valuing of qualitative and quantitative dimensions of the person's health patterns.

A systematic process for the practice of holistic nursing acts as a guiding structure for the novice and as an internalized ballast for the experienced nurse by unifying, standardizing, and directing nursing practice. Standardization of language about nurses' activities and responsibilities affords a unified structure for the application of nursing theory and subsequent nursing research. The holistic caring process lends itself to theory application. Within the holistic caring process, information relevant to the person's care is gathered and processed according to a theoretical model. Nurses must choose a theoretical practice model that is realistic, useful, and consistent with their professional values and philosophy. Patterns, desired outcomes, and nursing actions are identified through a synthesis of the theory base and information gathered from the person in mutual process with the nurse. Care is evaluated and documented in the language of the theory.

Taxonomies of Nursing Practice

As early as the 1970s, in efforts to acknowledge nursing as a distinct, autonomous healthcare profession nurses began developing standardized languages that would provide a way to name, label, and track those parts of nursing's work that nurses were licensed to perform. These initial efforts led to the nursing diagnosis movement and later to work that named and established common terms for nursing interventions and outcomes. The most well-known of the nursing diagnoses taxonomies are those nursing diagnoses (NDx) delineated by the NANDA International (NANDA-I). These diagnoses name and define patterns frequently appraised by nurses as indicating a need for care.[1] The Nurs-

ing Interventions Classification (NIC) is a list of activities performed by nurses for the purpose of achieving nurse–person care goals.[3] Frequently identified goals, observable and measurable throughout the course of care, are listed as the Nursing Outcomes Classification (NOC).[4]

Because the NDx/NIC/NOC (NNN) taxonomies are atheoretical, they can be used with a variety of nursing theories and a holistic perspective.[25] The linking of these languages provides a means of describing nursing activities and systematically evaluating outcomes of patient and person care for quality management, as well as for guiding nursing research questions. At one time, nurses reasoned that use of these taxonomies would result in a means of direct billing for nursing services, but that has not materialized. One group of authors suggests that direct billing for nursing services is considerably more complicated than direct billing for services such as physical therapy or radiology.[26] Nurses perform so many activities within a shift; it may in fact be more costly to track each activity and bill for every discrete action than to provide the "global" charge for nursing that we see today where nursing services are considered part of the room charge for hospital care. As it stands today, standardized nursing languages of nursing diagnoses, nursing interventions, and nursing outcomes exist as a means to organize, describe, and evaluate the data generated within the therapeutic nurse–person relationship. Use of standardized terms also permits documentation and retrieval of nursing information in an electronic health record (EHR) as will be described in the sections that follow related to documentation of the holistic caring process. An important issue for holistic nurses returns us to the original impetus for development of nursing standardized terms—the fact that much of what we do as nurses and as holistic nurses in particular remains invisible. There is opportunity to increase our visibility and to document the positive outcomes of the assessments and interventions we carry out daily if we document our care in such a way that what we do becomes coded as part of the permanent record. Currently, more than half of the nursing diagnoses and interventions listed in standard languages address the psycho-social-spiritual aspects of care; these certainly are of use to holistic nurses.

■ HOLISTIC CARING PROCESS

Nurses who adhere to the holistic caring process focus on the care of the whole unique person, respecting and advocating for the person's rights and choices. Based on a holistic assessment and identification of the person's health patterns, decisions about care flow from collaboration with the person, other healthcare providers, and significant others. The person assumes an active role in healthcare planning and decision making by seeking the professional expertise of the nurse via various nurse–person interactions. Facilitated by the nurse in the healing relationship, the person expresses health concerns and strengths—a unique health pattern—that the nurse identifies and documents in the healthcare record. The person is encouraged to participate as actively as possible, taking responsibility for personal health choices and decisions for self-care. The nurse must remember that the holistic caring process is merely a tool, a framework for ordering, documenting, and discussing the nurse–person interactions. Excessive reliance on structure and objectivity may reduce the person to a mere object. The holistic nursing caring process is presented here as a six-step process including holistic assessment, identification of patterns/problems/ needs, outcome identification, therapeutic plan of care, implementation, and evaluation. The following sections describe each phase and then discuss documentation of nursing's work.

Holistic Assessment

The holistic registered nurse collects comprehensive data pertinent to the person's health or situation.[27]

Assessment is the information-gathering phase in which the nurse and the person identify health patterns and prioritize the person's health concerns. A continuous process, assessment provides ongoing data for changes that occur over time. Each nurse–person encounter provides new information that helps to explain interrelationships and validates previously collected data and conclusions. A key to a holistic assessment is to appraise the overall pattern of the responses. The nurse gleans information about the person's patterns via interaction, observation, and measurement. Each pattern identification taps into the hologram of the person, contributing to the revelation of the whole.

Interpersonal interaction reveals perceptions, feelings, and thoughts about health patterns/ challenges/needs as identified by the person. Nursing observation relies on information perceived by the five senses and intuition, while measurement provides quantifiable information obtained from instruments. The client is the primary source and interpreter of the meaning of information obtained by the assessment process. Family, significant others, other healthcare professionals, and measurable data provide supplemental information. Within the cultural context of negotiation, the assessment phase may be seen as an "exchange of expert knowledge" wherein both the nurse and the person bring expertise to the exchange.[8]

During assessment of the person's bio-psycho-social-spiritual patterns, the holistic nurse looks for the overall pattern of interrelationships, uses appropriate scientific and intuitive approaches, assesses the state of the energy field, and identifies stages of change and readiness to learn. The nurse also collects pertinent data from previous client records and other members of the healthcare team, if appropriate. All pertinent data are documented in the person's record.

The holistic nurse views the person as a whole and listens for the meaning of the current health situation to the person within the environment. While acknowledging his or her own patterns and their potential influence on the healing relationship, the nurse reflects on the person's patterns recognized from the assessment. In response, the person validates the meanings of these identified health patterns. Assessment and documentation are continuous within the nurse–person interaction because changes in one pattern always influence the other dimensions. A lack of awareness about one's own personal beliefs and patterns may subtly influence the nurse–client interaction (e.g., communication barriers relative to culture, class, age, gender, sexual orientation, education, or physical limitation) and impede holistic assessment.

Identification of Patterns/Challenges/Needs

The holistic registered nurse analyzes the assessment data to determine the diagnosis or issues expressed as actual or potential patterns/problems/ needs that are related to health, wellness, disease, or illness.[27]

Within the second step of the holistic caring process, the nurse describes a person's patterns/ challenges/needs based on a standardized language that is understandable to nurses, other healthcare professionals, the managed care provider, and the person receiving nursing care. Nursing diagnoses (NDx) provide a universal descriptor language for common patterns identified by nurses giving care. A nursing diagnosis can be defined as a "clinical judgment about the individual, family, or community responses to actual and potential health problems and life processes. Nursing diagnoses provide the basis for selection of nursing interventions to achieve outcomes for which the nurse is accountable."[2] There are currently more than 130 approved diagnoses organized under 13 domains: health promotion, nutrition, elimination/exchange, activity/ rest, perception/cognition, self-perception, role relationship, sexuality, coping/stress tolerance, life principles, safety/protection, comfort, and growth/development.

The Diagnostic Statement

Nursing diagnoses describe human responses to health conditions and life processes in an individual, family, or community. The multiaxial structure of NANDA-I taxonomy delineates seven axes that may be incorporated explicitly or implicitly in every nursing diagnostic statement: the diagnostic concept, subject of the diagnosis (individual, family, community), judgment (impaired, ineffective), location (anatomic), age (infant, child, adult), time (chronic, acute, intermittent), and status of the diagnosis (actual, risk, wellness, health promotion).[1] Actual NDx exist as fact or reality in the present time. Risk NDx describe a vulnerability occurring in response to exposure to factors that intensify the possibility of injury or loss. Health promotion NDx reflect "behavior motivated by the desire to increase well-being and actualize human health potential."[1p44] Wellness NDx reflect "the quality or state of being healthy."[1p45] An NDx is constructed by combining the diagnostic concept (e.g., activity intolerance, elimination, energy field), subject of the diagnosis (individual, family, group, community), and a judgment (impaired, risk for, readiness for enhanced) where needed and adding values from the other axes for clarity. For example, for the

spiritual diagnostic concept, the judgment component of NDx is expressed through three different diagnoses: spiritual distress (impaired), risk for spiritual distress, and readiness for enhanced spiritual well-being.

Before making a specific NDx, the nurse compares assessment data with the defining characteristics of the diagnosis, which are those behaviors or signs and symptoms (observable cues and inferences) that cluster together as manifestations of the diagnosis. Defining characteristics serve to identify the diagnostic entity and differentiate between various nursing diagnoses. The list of diagnoses with defining characteristics and associated factors or risk factors, depending on the type of diagnosis, has been published and updated regularly to assist nurses in verifying a particular nursing diagnosis.[1p45] After assessing a client's condition and formulating the possible NDx, a nurse refers to the list of defining characteristics to determine if there are sufficient critical indicators to confirm the diagnosis. Although a particular diagnosis may have quite specific defining characteristics, nurses must use their knowledge, education, experience, and intuition to determine if the signs and symptoms observed during the nursing assessment are sufficient to confirm the existence of the particular health pattern/ challenge/need. After nursing diagnoses are identified and prioritized, they become the basis for the remaining steps of the nursing process.

Sometimes, when none of the available NDx appears to fit the person's circumstances, the nurse must develop a diagnosis. If such a diagnosis appears to recur in the nurse's practice, he or she may consider a formal submission of the diagnosis to NANDA-I. Although many diagnoses have not yet been identified, the current taxonomic structure facilitates the identification of gaps to be filled.

Nursing Language Across Levels of Prevention

There is a distinction between the concepts of illness prevention (or risk reduction), health maintenance, and health promotion. Illness prevention or risk reduction involves behaviors aimed at actively protecting against or reducing the chances of encountering disease, illness, or accidents. The risk NDx is directed toward prevention.

Nursing interventions associated with these diagnoses are actively selected to reduce or prevent the particular problem. Health maintenance focuses on sustaining a neutral state of health. For example, the NDx for people who are unable to identify, manage, or seek help to maintain health would be ineffective health maintenance. For these clients, nursing interventions would include activities not only to prevent illness, but also to protect health (e.g., eating a balanced diet, stopping smoking, having regular medical examinations, sleeping 6 to 8 hours per night).

Health promotion goes beyond illness prevention or health maintenance. Because it involves a personal responsibility for their health, individuals strive actively to improve their lifestyle to achieve high-level wellness. The diagnosis of health-seeking behaviors (i.e., health-promoting behaviors) is consistent with the concept of health promotion. Health-seeking behaviors may include such activities as requesting additional information and recipes to enhance a low-cholesterol, low-fat, low-salt, low-sugar, and high-fiber diet; practicing daily relaxation techniques; and participating in aerobic exercises three to five times per week. The categories of health promotion and wellness NDx use the qualifier of "readiness for enhanced," allowing the nurse to focus on wellness, facilitate responsibility for self-care, and promote healthy behaviors.

In 1995, Kelley, Frisch, and Avant developed a Trifocal Model for nursing diagnosis that orga-nized nursing needs and activities along a scale from illness to wellness, superimposed with a continuum representing three client states: (1) a health problem, (2) a risk for a health problem, and (3) an opportunity to enhance a well state.[28] Originally depicted as a pyramid with health problems at the base and wellness at the apex, the model has been updated by Frisch to give wellness equal attention as illness and to identify the client states as well as nursing activities. **Figure 7-2** pre-sents Trifocal 2: client states, nursing activities, and the illness–wellness continuum.

Nursing Diagnosis as a Descriptive Tool

Essential to the holistic caring process is the understanding that nursing diagnosis is a means for describing a person's health pattern mani-festation; nursing diagnoses are not the pattern. They are merely a descriptive tool for articulat-ing patterns identified in the nurse–person rela-tionship rather than a rigid, limiting diagnostic label that might constrict and stereotype care. The person's value system, not the nurse's, is the basis for holistic nursing decisions and diagnos-tic labeling. Setting aside preconceived notions about health enhancement for the person, the nurse chooses diagnoses that most accurately reflect the person's perceptions about his or her health patterns. Whenever possible, the nurse collaborates with the person to validate and prioritize nursing diagnoses. Impediments to a holistic nursing diagnosis result from neglecting

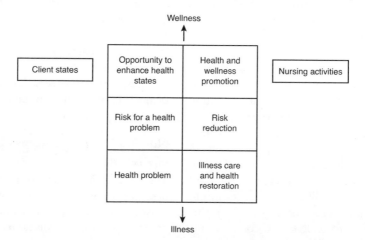

FIGURE 7-2   Trifocal 2: Client States, Nursing Activities, and the Illness-Wellness Continuum
Source: © Noreen C. Frisch, 2007.

to make the person the focus of the process and failing to have a continual, focused awareness of the person as a whole. Fitting the pattern of a dynamic, changing human being into an arbitrary diagnostic statement rather than reflecting the actual pattern of the person limits the effectiveness of the holistic caring process.

Use of a nursing theoretical framework in concert with a standardized language that describes nurses' phenomena of concern meets the cultural requirements of health care for a common language that demonstrates and documents the value of nursing care based on logic and predictive outcomes. This is essential for providing high-quality patient care as well as necessary for remuneration of nursing services. Frisch and Kelley suggest theory-oriented strategies that include "the use of theory-specific language in the 'related-to' clause of the diagnosis, writing narrative notes along with the standard classifications, and documenting impact of nursing activities on client conditions."[25] Such an approach meets system requirements and adds the possibility of evaluating theory-based practice outcomes. Further, theoretically derived nursing diagnoses and outcomes can be introduced to the standardized systems. For example, the diagnosis, readiness for enhanced power, wherein power is defined as "a pattern of participating knowingly in change that is sufficient for well-being and can be strengthened,"[1] appears to draw on Rogers's identification of power.[29] Holistic nursing is both the practice of presence and the implementation of process. Distinguishing nursing roles from other caregiver roles is essential for the profession—"a matter of extinction or distinction."[30] Frisch and Kelley observe, "The capacity to administer expert technical care in conjunction with expert human care constitutes the unique contribution of nursing."[25p61]

Outcome Identification

The holistic registered nurse identifies outcomes for a plan individualized to the person or the situation. The holistic nurse values the evolution and the process of healing as it unfolds. This implies that specific unfolding outcomes may not be evident immediately because of the nonlinear nature of the healing process so that both expected/anticipated and evolving outcomes are considered.[27]

An outcome is a direct statement of a goal identified through the nurse–person relationship that is to be achieved within a specific time frame; the person's significant others and other healthcare practitioners may participate in goal setting. An outcome indicates the maximum level of wellness that is reasonably attainable for the person in view of objective circumstances and the person's perceptions.

Outcome criteria outline the specific tools, tests, observations, or personal statements that determine whether the patient outcome has been achieved. They reflect the goals of the nurse–person intervention. The holistic nurse selects interventions on the basis of desired outcomes, discussing with the person possible ways for achieving these desired outcomes. The person helps to establish observable milestones for knowing whether desired changes have occurred and makes a commitment to move toward those desired changes. Client outcomes direct the plan of care.

Similar to the attempt to classify and codify nursing diagnoses, there has been major effort to standardize outcome measures. The Nursing Outcomes Classification (NOC) developed by the Iowa Outcomes Project at the University of Iowa provides a comprehensive taxonomy of 385 outcomes organized into 7 domains and 29 classes. Outcomes describe the expected effect or influence of the intervention on the person. Within this classification system a nursing-sensitive patient outcome is a measurable state, behavior, or perception that is responsive to nursing interventions.[4] Nursing outcomes are described along continuums that depict movement toward or away from desired goals. Using variable concepts allows for the measurement of change as positive, negative, or no change in the person's situation, behaviors, or perceptions. Each coded outcome is associated with a label, definition, set of indicators, a measurement scale, and supporting literature. Outcome measures can be used as indicators of individual change as well as for quantitative comparison with a greater population.

The seven NOC domains are functional health, physiologic health, psychosocial health, health knowledge and behavior, perceived health, family health, and community health. Classes under the domain of psychosocial health, for example, include psychological well-being, psychosocial adaptation, self-control, and social interaction. Measurable indicators of psychological well-being address outcomes describing an individual's emotional health. For example, self-esteem, an indicator of psychological well-being, is measured by a 20-item instrument that delineates observable qualities of self-esteem. As with the NDx taxonomy, NOC provides common nursing language for communicating about the effectiveness of nursing actions, a language that can be recognized by providers, payers, and other healthcare professionals.

If outcomes are to be achieved, the nurse must establish them with the assistance of the patient and family. The person must be motivated to establish healthy patterns of behavior. Assumptions made by the nurse concerning desired outcomes without collaboration with the person impede outcome achievement. Rigid adherence to specific outcomes by the person or the nurse may make it impossible to recognize the value of the journey with its myriad other paths and other possible outcomes.

Therapeutic Care Plan

The holistic registered nurse develops a plan that identifies strategies and alternatives to attain outcomes.[27]

During the planning stage, nurses who use the holistic caring process help the person identify ways to repattern her or his behaviors to achieve a healthier state. The planning process reveals interventions that will achieve outcomes. The plan outlines nursing interventions, which are the specific actions that the nurse performs to help the person solve problems and accomplish outcomes. Nursing interventions direct the implementation of care. A nursing intervention has been defined as "any treatment, based upon clinical judgment and knowledge that a nurse performs to enhance patient or client outcomes."[31]

The Iowa Intervention Project developed the Nursing Interventions Classification (NIC), which contains an alphabetic list of 542 interventions.[3] Each intervention is listed with a label, a definition, a set of related activities that describe the behaviors of the nurse who implements the intervention, and a brief list of background readings. The NIC includes all direct care

interventions, both independent and collaborative, that nurses perform for patients.

Holistic nurses frequently select complementary/alternative modalities and generally noninvasive nursing interventions to complement standard nursing care. Holistic nurses incorporate complementary modalities into their practice as interventions for treating the body (biofeedback, therapeutic massage), relieving the mind (humor, imagery, meditation), comforting the soul (prayer), and supporting significant interpersonal interaction (healing presence).[32] Therapies such as acupressure, meditation, guided imagery, and therapeutic touch are listed as nursing interventions in the taxonomy. Nurses should refer to the rules and regulations within their state of licensure to clarify the legal scope of practice within some jurisdictions.

The organization of the holistic care plan reflects the priority of identified opportunities to enhance the person's health. Priorities for intervention are based on an assessment of the urgency of the threat to the person's life and safety. The holistic nurse chooses interventions based on utility, relationship to the person's patterns/challenges/needs, effectiveness, feasibility, acceptability to the person, and nursing competency. Holistic nursing interventions reflect acceptance of the person's values, beliefs, culture, religion, and socioeconomic background. Any revision of the care plan reflects the person's current status or ongoing changes. This plan is documented in the person's record.

Implementation

The holistic registered nurse implements the identified plan in partnership with the person.[27]

Nurses who are guided by a holistic framework approach the implementation phase of care with an awareness that (1) people are active participants in their care; (2) nursing care must be performed with purposeful, focused intention; and (3) a person's humanness is an important factor in implementation. During this phase, the various persons deemed appropriate—the nurse, the person, the family, or another person or agency—implement the planned strategies.[8]

Within the holistic framework, anything that produces a physiologic change causes a corresponding psychological, social, and spiritual alteration. Conversely, anything that produces a psychological change causes a corresponding physiologic, social, and spiritual alteration. Thus, a nurse's encounter with a person, be it for the purpose of talking to the person, touching the person, or taking a blood pressure, produces psychophysiologic outcomes. The encounter changes the consciousness and the physiology of both the nurse and the person. Because human emotions can be translated into physiologic responses, the greatest tool or intervention for helping and healing clients is the therapeutic use of self.[33]

Evaluation

The holistic registered nurse evaluates progress toward attainment of outcomes while recognizing and honoring the continuing holistic nature of the healing process.[27]

Evaluation is a planned review of the nurse-person interaction to identify factors that facilitate or inhibit expected outcomes. Within the holistic caring process, evaluation is a mutual process between the nurse and the person receiving care. Data about the client's bio-psycho-social-spiritual status and responses are collected and recorded throughout the holistic caring process. The information is related to the person's patterns/challenges/needs, the outcome criteria, and the results of the nursing intervention. The nurse, in collaboration with the person during the course of care, may use measures from the NOC to document the effectiveness of the nursing interventions received.

The goal of evaluation is to determine if outcomes have been successful and, if so, to what extent. The nurse, person, family, and other members of the healthcare team all participate in the evaluation process. Together, they synthesize the data from the evaluation to identify successful repatterning behaviors toward wellness. During the evaluation, the person becomes more aware of previous patterns, develops insight into the interconnections of all dimensions of his or her life, and sees the benefits of repatterning behaviors. For example, does the person understand that his or her current job and level of stress have a direct impact on the current illness?

The evaluation of outcomes must be continuous because of the dynamic nature of human beings and the frequent changes that occur during illness and health. It may be necessary to develop new outcomes and revise the plan of care. Factors facilitating effective outcomes or preventing solutions to problems must also be explored. The failure to recognize that all measurable outcomes may not be immediate, but are in a process of becoming, is an impediment to evaluation.

Evaluation of the holistic caring process comes full circle with a self-aware appraisal of the entire nursing process by the nurse. From an ecological perspective, the evaluation of the holistic caring process extends beyond the level of the person to include the short- and long-term impact on the healthcare delivery system, the physical environment, and the greater social context. The holistic nurse must also reflect on the greater implications of the holistic caring process for professional practice standards and for health and environmental policy.

■ DOCUMENTING THE HOLISTIC CARING PROCESS

Most nurses are familiar with nursing care plans as tools to document all of the activities included in the nursing process. These care plans can be formal and lengthy such as those most students prepare in school to illustrate their thinking patterns for faculty preceptors or may be very brief identifications of needs and interventions on a computer system used in a busy acute care unit. The nursing care plan is a means to document that, based on nursing assessment data, a particular nursing concern (nursing diagnosis) was established and a plan (nursing orders) was prepared to address the concern. The expected outcome should be identified in the care plan so that an evaluation of outcome is possible. Thus, the care plan is a means to document and report nursing activities, to communicate nursing needs from one nurse to another, and to evaluate nursing care outcomes.

In contrast to the "traditional" nursing care plan, many nurses and nurse educators are now turning to concept maps as an alternative to the nursing care plan. A concept map is a diagrammatic representation of organized knowledge. In some regards, the concept map is an individual's interpretation of a real-life experience.[34] In a concept map, the professional nurse records assessment data and "maps" out the context of those data. A concept map presents an "all at once" view of the client's experiences and draws out connections between events so that they are not seen as unrelated parts. Arrows on the map indicate that one concept influences another. For example, a nurse may identify that a client is in physical pain, has sleep disturbances, and is anxious over not being at work. A concept map permits the nurse to illustrate that sleep disturbances affect anxiety, that anxiety affects both sleep and comfort, and that comfort affects sleep and anxiety. Thus, the nurse looking at the relationships will address comfort and pain as the first priority. In another example, the nurse may assess the following nursing diagnoses for a client who has recently moved to a new city: social isolation, feelings of sadness, anxiety over work performance, and sleep disturbances. **Figure 7-3** presents a concept map depicting the interrelationships of the diagnoses.

Mapping the concepts illustrates that social isolation and sleep disturbances are the first priorities of care because they affect the other problems of sadness and anxiety. Concept maps permit the nurse to view the situation as a whole and initiate care based on the contextual nature of the client's world.

Interest in nursing concept maps began in education as nurse educators drew on the expertise of faculty in scientific fields who reported that concept maps assist learners. Many in nursing have reported that students who use concept maps learn to think critically about care.[35-37] In relation to the holistic caring process,

nurses may find that concept mapping is more closely aligned with the circular nursing process, whereas the traditional nursing care plan is aligned with the linear nursing process.

It is important for the holistic nurse to recognize that nursing documentation of care is an essential part of professional practice and to realize that virtually all institutions require documentation in a traditional format. However, the concept map may assist all of us to see our professional work differently, and certainly a concept map helps us to select priorities of care.

Our modern practice world is moving rapidly to electronic documentation of care provided. The EHR is simply a clinical record in digital format. Electronic records have several advantages over paper ones: the records are readable, data are easily accessed and retrieved, and more than one user may be looking at parts of the record simultaneously. Additionally, electronic records can have features such as decision supports built in. For example, an electronic record system can include alerts related to allergies or drug interactions that help the clinician avoid error. These EHRs can also have care planning systems built in so that nurses can access an assessment form, collect and store data, and build a care plan based on those data. The most well-developed of such systems permit nurses to track client movement toward outcome goals and evaluate clients' readiness for discharge as well. Details of electronic documentation are outside of the scope of this chapter; however, holistic nurses need to understand that in an electronic system, only data entries that are codable by the computer system can be stored in

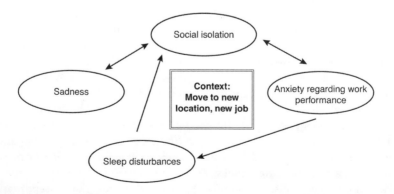

FIGURE 7-3   A Concept Map
Source: © Noreen C. Frisch, 2007.

a way that the data can be retrieved at a later date when one is conducting a chart review or audit or evaluating trends. This means that data entered according to one of the standardized language systems (NNN, for example) can be coded and retrieved later. Data entered in narrative form cannot be. Thus, it is in nursing's best interest for all nurses to use the standardized language systems while they document their work.

■ CONCLUSION

By definition, any nurse in any setting can practice holistic nursing. *Holistic Nursing: Scope and Standards of Practice*[27] (see Chapter 2) can be framed in the universal language of the holistic caring process and may easily be combined with other more physiologically based standards, such as those for cardiovascular and critical care nursing. Thus, *Holistic Nursing: Scope and Standards of Practice* can be incorporated into all subspecialty standards of care to ensure not only high-quality physiologic care, but also high-quality holistic nursing care to these specialty populations.

Holistic Nursing: Scope and Standards of Practice necessitates the application of a whole new lens to the nursing process. Although standardized language is beneficial for the acknowledgment and documentation of nursing expertise and practice, such labels do not always communicate adequately the person's health situation and need for care. Viewing standardized nursing diagnoses, interventions, and outcomes through a lens of *Holistic Nursing: Scope and Standards of Practice* gives nurses a means to refine and enhance their care as well as a means to describe and document the caring process of nursing.

Directions for
FUTURE RESEARCH

1. Evaluate each nursing diagnosis, nursing intervention, and nursing outcome for compatibility with holistic nursing practice standards.
2. Explore whether writing nursing diagnoses related to holistic nursing standards (e.g., readiness for enhanced nutrition) enhances outcomes.
3. Evaluate the effectiveness and nature of intuitive judgments used by holistic nurses.

4. Investigate whether incorporating the holistic caring process into practice positively affects subjective and objective client outcomes.
5. Determine the effects of incorporating the holistic caring process into practice on nurse work satisfaction and turnover.

Nurse Healer
REFLECTIONS

After reading this chapter, the nurse healer will be able to answer or to begin a process of answering the following questions:

- How am I guided in my everyday life and work by the holistic caring process?
- How do I reconcile what I know about health and healing with whatever beliefs and realities that might be held by the people to whom I give care and by my coworkers?
- How can I systematically begin to apply the holistic caring process in terms of standardized nursing taxonomies for diagnoses, interventions, and outcomes?
- How can I cultivate my intuitive processes?
- How do I react when clients indicate that they are not motivated to change health patterns and behavior?
- How do I feel when I incorporate the principles of holistic nursing into my nursing practice?

> *For a full suite of assignments and additional learning activities, use the access code located in the front of your book to visit this exclusive website: http://go.jblearning.com/dossey. If you do not have an access code, you can obtain one at the site.*

NOTES

1. NANDA International, *Nursing Diagnoses: Definitions and Classification, 2009–2011*, ed. T. H. Herdman (Oxford, England: Wiley-Blackwell, 2009).
2. NANDA International, *Nursing Diagnoses: Definitions and Classification, 2007–2008* (Philadelphia: Nanda-I, 2007): 332.

3. G. M. Bulechek, H. Butcher, and J. M. Dochterman, *Nursing Interventions Classification (NIC)*, 5th ed. (St. Louis: Mosby, 2008).

4. S. Moorhead, M. Johnson, M. Maas, and E. Swanson, *Nursing Outcomes Classification (NOC)*, 4th ed. (St Louis: Mosby, 2008).

5. F. R. Kreuter, "What Is Good Nursing Care?" *Nursing Outlook* 5 (1957): 302–304.

6. N. C. Frisch and L. E. Frisch, *Psychiatric Mental Health Nursing*, 4th ed. (Clifton Park, NY: Delmar Cengage Learning, 2011).

7. H. C. Erickson et al., *Modeling and Role-Modeling: A Theory and Paradigm for Nursing* (Englewood Cliffs, NJ: Prentice Hall, 1983): 103.

8. J. Engebretson and L. Y. Littleton, "Cultural Negotiation: A Constructivist-Based Model for Nursing Practice," *Nursing Outlook* 49 (2001): 223–230.

9. B. A. Carper, "Fundamental Patterns of Knowing in Nursing," *Advances in Nursing Science* 1, no. 1 (1978): 13–23.

10. American Holistic Nurses Association, *Position Statement on Holistic Nursing Ethics* (Flagstaff, AZ: AHNA/ANA, 2007).

11. C. Johns, "Framing Learning Through Reflection Within Carper's Fundamental Ways of Knowing in Nursing," *Journal of Advanced Nursing* 22 (1995): 227.

12. C. E. Young, "Intuition and Nursing Process," *Holistic Nursing Practice* 1, no. 3 (1987): 52.

13. J. A. Effken, "Information Basis for Expert Intuition," *Journal of Advanced Nursing* 34, no. 2 (2001): 246–254.

14. J. A. Effken, "The Informational Basis for Nursing Intuition: Philosophical Underpinnings," *Nursing Philosophy* 8, (2007): 187–200.

15. S. A. Robertson, "Got EQ? Increasing Cultural and Clinical Competence Through Emotional Intelligence," *Communication Disorders Quarterly* 29, no. 1 (2007): 14–19.

16. P. Salovey and J. D. Mayer, "Emotional Intelligence," *Imagination, Cognition and Personality* 9 no. 3 (1990): 185–211.

17. R. Bar-On, "The Bar-On Model of Emotional-Social Intelligence (ESI)," *Psichothema* 17, suppl. (2005): 1–28.

18. D. Goleman, *Working With Emotional Intelligence* (New York: Bantam, 1998).

19. K. B. Smith, J. Profetto-McGrath, and G. G. Cummings, "Emotional Intelligence and Nursing: An Integrative Literature Review," *International Journal of Nursing Studies* 46 no. 12 (2009): 1624–1636.

20. A. C. H. McQueen, "Emotional Intelligence in Nursing Work," *Journal of Advanced Nursing* 47, no. 1 (2004): 101–108.

21. T. Huynh, M. Alderson, and M. Thompson, "Emotional Labour Underlying Caring: An Evolutionary Concept Analysis," *Journal of Advanced Nursing* 64, no. 2 (2008): 195–208.

22. D. Goleman, A. McKee, and R. Boyatzis, *Primal Leadership: Realizing the Power of Emotional Intelligence* (Boston: Harvard Business School, 2002).

23. P. A. Harrison and J. L. Fopma-Loy, "Reflective Journal Prompts: A Vehicle for Stimulating Emotional Competence in Nursing," *Journal of Nursing Education* 49 no. 11 (2010): 644–652.

24. J. Watson, *Nursing: Human Science and Human Care* (Norwalk, CT: Appleton-Century-Crofts, 1985).

25. N. C. Frisch and J. H. Kelley, "Nursing Diagnosis and Nursing Theory: Exploration of Factors Inhibiting and Supporting Simultaneous Use," *Nursing Diagnosis* 13, no. 2 (2002): 53–61.

26. L. Unrul, S. B. Massmiller, and S. C. Reinhard, "The Importance and Challenge of Paying for Quality Nursing Care," *Policy, Politics and Nursing Practice* 9 (2008): 68–72.

27. American Holistic Nurses Association & American Nurses Association, *Holistic Nursing: Scope and Standards of Practice* (Silver Spring, MD: NurseBooks .org, 2007).

28. J. Kelley et al., "A Trifocal Model of Nursing Diagnosis: Wellness Reinforced," *Nursing Diagnosis* 6, no. 3 (1995): 123–128.

29. B. Wright, "Trust and Power in Adults: An Investigation Using Rogers' Science of Unitary Human Beings," *Nursing Science Quarterly* 17 (2004): 139–146.

30. L. Nagle, "A Matter of Extinction or Distinction," *Western Journal of Nursing Research* 21 (1999): 71–82.

31. J. Dochterman and G. M. Bulechek, *Classification of Nursing Interventions: Implications for Nursing Diagnoses* (St. Louis: Mosby, 2004): 3.

32. N. C. Frisch, "Standards for Holistic Nursing Practice: A Way to Think About Our Care That Includes Complementary and Alternative Modalities," *Online Journal for Issues in Nursing* 6, no. 2 (2001): Manuscript 4.

33. D. Krieger, *Foundation of Holistic Health Nursing Practice* (Philadelphia: J. B. Lippincott, 1981).

34. V. Johnson and N. Frisch, "Tools of Psychiatric Mental Health Nursing: Communication, Nursing Process and the Nurse–Client Relationship," in *Psychiatric Mental Health Nursing*, 4th ed., eds. N. Frisch and L. Frisch (Clifton Park, NY: Cengage Delmar Learning, 2011): 99–112.

35. D. Pesut and J. Herman, *Clinical Reasoning: The Art and Science of Critical and Creative Thinking* (Clifton Park, NY: Thompson Delmar Learning, 1999).

36. P. Schuster, *Concept Mapping: A Critical-Thinking Approach to Care Planning* (Philadelphia: F. A. Davis, 2002).

37. M. King and R. Shell, "Teaching and Evaluating Critical Thinking with Concept Maps," *Nurse Educator* 27, no. 5 (2002): 214–216.

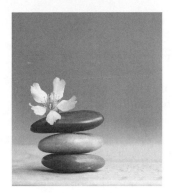

Self-Assessments

Barbara Montgomery Dossey, Susan Luck,
Bonney Gulino Schaub, and Lynn Keegan

Nurse Healer
OBJECTIVES

Theoretical

- Explore the *Healthy People 2020* initiative and its application for holistic nurses.
- Examine the Integrative Health and Wellness Assessment (IHWA) and the eight categories.

Clinical

- Use the IHWA with clients who wish to learn new healthcare behaviors.
- Incorporate the IHWA into clinical practice.

Personal

- Complete the IHWA.
- Identify your readiness to change related to your desired health goals.
- Create personal action plan goals that lead to new health behaviors.
- Increase your awareness of ways to gain access to your inner healing process.

DEFINITIONS

Healing: A process of understanding and integrating the many aspects of self, leading to a deep connection with inner wisdom and an experience of balance and wholeness.

Healing awareness: A person's conscious recognition of and focused attention on intuitions, subtle feelings, conditions, and circumstances relating to the needs of self or clients.

Health: An individual's (nurse, client, family, group, or community) subjective sense of well-being, harmony, and unity that is supported by the experience of health beliefs and values being honored; a process of opening and widening of awareness and consciousness.

Nurse healer: A professional nurse who supports and facilitates a person's process of growth and experience of wholeness through an integration of body, mind, and spirit and/or who assists in the recovery from illness or in the transition to peaceful death.

Process: The continual changing and evolution of one's self through life that includes reflecting on meaning and purpose in living.

Self-efficacy: The belief that one has the capability of initiating and sustaining desired behaviors with a sense of empowerment and ability to make healthful choices that lead to enduring change.

Transpersonal self: The self that transcends personal, individual identity and meaning and opens to connecting with purpose, meaning, values, unitive experiences and with universal principles.

Transpersonal view: The state that occurs during a person's life maturity whereby a sense of self expands.

Wellness: An integrated, congruent functioning toward reaching one's highest potential.

■ HOLISTIC NURSES, HEALTHY PEOPLE, AND A HEALTHY WORLD

Many 21st-century conversations and initiatives focus on health promotion, health maintenance, disease prevention, and prevention of the catastrophic impact of diseases. Currently, the United States is in an economic crisis and health promotion and cost-effective behavioral change strategies are needed. In 2010, the Institute of Medicine, in collaboration with Robert Wood Johnson Foundation (RWJF), published the *Future of Nursing* report, a landmark document that presents four key messages:[1]

- Nurses should practice to the full extent of their education and training.
- Nurses should achieve higher levels of education and training through an improved education system that promotes seamless academic progression.
- Nurses should be full partners, with physicians and other healthcare professionals, in redesigning health care in the United States.
- Effective workforce planning and policy making require better data collection and information infrastructure.

Holistic nurses are leaders practicing at the forefront of this initiative. As change agents, their objective is to increase the health of the nation, focusing on addressing the wellness and "health span" of people. They are sharing this information with nurses and other healthcare colleagues around the world. Their endeavors include using health and wellness assessments, assessing readiness to change, and implementing action plans for healthy lifestyle behaviors and approaches that lead to healthy people living in a healthy nation and on a healthy planet by 2020.

According to the Centers for Disease Control and Prevention, more than 133 million adults, or nearly half of all adults in the United States, are living with at least one chronic disease such as obesity, diabetes, and cardiovascular disease.[2] The cost of managing their care is an astounding $270 billion a year.[3] Seventy percent of today's healthcare costs are related to preventable, lifestyle-related diseases. There is an urgent need to develop initiatives to help shift the focus of health care by promoting

self-efficacy and empowering individuals to recognize their potential to engage in promoting their own health and well-being.

All diseases affect multiple systems of the body. Heart disease and stroke are the first and third causes of mortality, respectively, accounting for one-third of all deaths in the United States.[4] Cardiovascular problems include hypertension, dyslipidemia, heart failure, congenital heart disease, peripheral vascular disease, and peripheral arterial disease. If every form of cardiovascular disease was eliminated, Americans could add another 7 years to their life expectancy.[5] Risk factors that can be modified in cardiovascular disease include smoking, dyslipidemia, hypertension, physical inactivity, obesity, and diabetes. Although gender, age, and genetics are not modifiable, many lifestyle factors can be altered.

If the current "obesity epidemic" continues unchecked, 50% of the U.S. adult population will be obese, with body mass index values of 30 or higher, by 2030.[6] Using a simulation model and data from the National Health and Nutrition Examination Survey (NHANES) series from 1988 to 2008, it has been projected that, compared with 2010, there will be "as many as 65 million more obese adults" in the United States by that year. Obesity prevalence in both men and women in their 40s and 50s would approach 60%. Using this simulation modeling based on current obesity trends in the United States and United Kingdom, investigators estimate that up to 8.5 million additional cases of diabetes, 7.3 million more cases of cardiovascular disease and stroke, and 0.5 million more cancers will occur by 2030, with major increases in healthcare costs.

Many studies such as the European Prospective Investigation into Cancer and Nutrition (EPIC Study) are designed to investigate the relationships among diet, nutritional status, lifestyle and environmental factors, and the incidence of cancer and other chronic disease.[7] The EPIC Study is significant because it recruited more than half a million (520,000) people in 10 European countries: Denmark, France, Germany, Greece, Italy, The Netherlands, Norway, Spain, Sweden, and the United Kingdom. It studied the adherence of subjects to four simple behaviors: (1) not smoking; (2) exercising 3.5

hours a week; (3) eating a healthy diet of fruits, vegetables, beans, whole grains, nuts, seeds, and limited amounts of meat; and (4) maintaining a healthy weight (BMI <30). In those adhering to these behaviors, the following were prevented:

- 93% of diabetes
- 81% of heart attacks
- 50% of strokes
- 36% of all cancers

The EPIC Study is buttressed by another influential report from 2009 by the World Cancer Research Fund and the American Institute for Cancer Research that asserts that better eating habits and more physical activity will prevent one-third of all the cancers in the United States, and smoking cessation will prevent another third.[8] The next section discusses national initiatives that provide guidelines for healthcare transformation.

Healthcare Transformation

In the United States, actual solutions to health problems guide holistic nurses and healthcare professionals. The *Healthy People 2020* initiative continues the work started in 2000 with the *Healthy People 2010* initiative for improving the nation's health. *Healthy People 2020* is the result of a multiyear process that reflects input from a diverse group of individuals and organizations.[9] The leading health indicators are increased physical activity, reduce obesity, tobacco use, substance abuse, injury and violence, increased responsibility sexual behavior, improve mental health, environmental quality, immunizations, and access to health care. These health indicators were selected on the basis of their ability to motivate action, the availability of data to measure progress, and their importance as public health issues.

The *Healthy People 2010* vision, mission, and overarching goals provide structure and guidance for achieving the *Healthy People 2020* objectives. Although general in nature, they offer specific, important areas of emphasis where action must be taken if the United States is to achieve better health by the year 2020. Developed under the leadership of the Federal Interagency Workgroup (FIW), the *Healthy People 2020* framework is the product of an exhaustive

collaborative process among the U.S. Department of Health and Human Services (HHS) and other federal agencies, public stakeholders, and the advisory committee. The *Healthy People 2020* mission strives to accomplish the following:

- Identify nationwide health improvement priorities
- Increase public awareness and understanding of the determinants of health, disease, and disability and the opportunities for progress
- Provide measurable objectives and goals that are applicable at the national, state, and local levels
- Engage multiple sectors to take actions to strengthen policies and improve practices that are driven by the best available evidence and knowledge
- Identify critical research, evaluation, and data collection needs

The *Healthy People 2020* overall goals are to the following:

- Attain high-quality, longer lives free of preventable disease, disability, injury, and premature death
- Achieve health equity, eliminate disparities, and improve the health of all groups
- Create social and physical environments that promote good health for all
- Promote quality of life, healthy development, and healthy behaviors across all life stages

Other important endeavors in national health are the Patient Protection and Affordable Care Act[10] and the National Prevention Strategy.[11] (See Chapters 3 and 9 for details.) The following section addresses the use of the Integrative Health and Wellness Assessment (IHWA) in coaching clients to be active participants in increasing health-promoting behaviors, assessing readiness to change, and establishing action plans and goals.

■ INTEGRATIVE HEALTH AND WELLNESS ASSESSMENT (IHWA)

Holistic nurses use self-assessments and other strategies to assist individuals to learn how to prefer wellness to unhealthy habits. They are assuming a leadership role in the health-and-wellness coaching movement as "pioneers on the vast frontier of our nation's health care reform."[12]

The circle is an ancient symbol of wholeness. As shown in **Figure 8-1**, the Integrative Health and Wellness Assessment (IHWA) wheel has eight components: (1) Life Balance and Satisfaction, (2) Relationships, (3) Spirituality, (4) Mental, (5) Emotional, (6) Physical (Nutrition, Exercise, Weight Management), (7) Environmental, and (8) Health Responsibility. All are important components of the self that are interwoven and constantly interacting. The IHWA assists people in becoming aware of their human potentials in each of these categories, identifying strengths and weaknesses and considering and creating new health goals.

Individuals are complex feedback loops. As we learn about these feedback loops, we are able to understand our body-mind-spirit connections. Each individual body is in a constant state of change. Most of these internal energetic, hormonal, biochemical checks and balances occur outside of any conscious awareness of what is taking place in the body.

At an even more expansive, organic level, life is a *biodance*. We are participating in an endless exchange with all living things, with planet Earth, in which all living organisms participate, and at the energetic and cosmic levels as well. This energetic dance exists not only as we live, but also as we die. We do not wait until death to make an exchange with planet Earth, for we are constantly returning to the universe while alive. In every living moment, a portion of the atoms in our body returns to the world outside. This is another idea of wholeness, which explains why the notion of "boundary" begins to seem an arbitrary idea rather than a physical reality.[13] In the following sections, each of the eight IHWA components is explored.

The Integrative Health and Wellness Assessment is best used as a personal assessment by the nurse or as a coaching tool with clients.

The Integrative Health and Wellness Assessment (IHWA)[14] (Figure 8-2) was developed and is based on 35 years of the authors' holistic nursing clinical practices, education, and research with clients and patients in changing lifestyle behaviors, health promotion, health maintenance, and disease prevention.* This includes educat-

ing and supporting clients who are learning new self-management skills in living with an acute or chronic illness and/or symptoms. It is expanded from Self-Care Assessments.[15]

The IHWA is an effective coaching tool for holistic nurses and is designed to increase both nurse self-development (self-reflection, self-assessments, self-care) and client self-development. It is essential that holistic nurses deepen their personal exploration of self (see Chapters 1, 4, 9, 12, 32, and 37), examine their vulnerabilities (Chapters 9 and 24), and explore their wellness from a functional health perspective (Chapters 9 and 13). This also includes looking at their life balance and satisfaction, as well as recognizing which factors are contributing to imbalance(s) and how they affect well-being. Creating the time for nurse self-development through integrating body, mind, spirit skills, integrative health knowledge, and nutritional, psychological, and other integrative resources is essential for being an effective nurse coach.

In using the IHWA, the holistic nurse skillfully creates and holds sacred space in which the client feels trust, respect, listened to, and not being judged. Depending on the clinical situation, the tool can be given out at one time for the client to fill out in advance of a session or use one section at a time. It is a useful guide in assisting individuals to change health behaviors.

Life Balance and Satisfaction

Assessing our life balance and satisfaction (see the Life Balance and Satisfaction section in **Figure 8-2**) strengthens our capacities and human potentials. (See Chapters 12 and 37 for details.) It attunes us to our healing awareness that is the innate quality with which all people are born. Healing is recognizing our feelings, attitudes, and emotions, which are not isolated but which are literally translated into body changes. Images cause internal events through mind modulation that simultaneously affect the autonomic, endocrine, immune, and neuropeptide systems (see Chapter 31). Everyone has the capacity to, and can choose to, tap into this innate healing potential. Healing

---

* Disclaimer: The Integrative Health and Wellness Assessment (IHWA) is intended for informational purposes only. It is not a substitute for professional medical advice, diagnosis, or treatment.

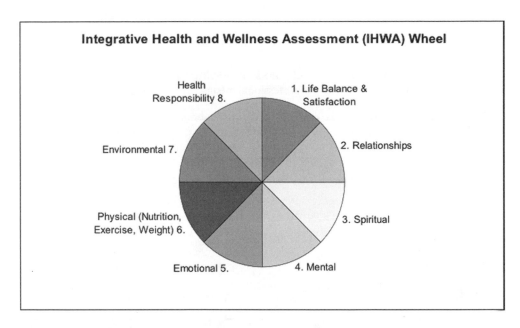

FIGURE 8-1   Integrative Health and Wellness Assessment (IHWA) Wheel
Source: Used with permission. Dossey, B. M., Luck, S., & Schaub, B. G. (2012). *Integrative Nurse Coaching for Health and Wellness.* Huntington, NY: Florence Press (www.iNurseCoach.com).

is more likely to occur on many levels when we attend to our life balance and satisfaction. During times of stress and crisis, focusing only on all the things that are wrong each day can block self-healing. Therefore, it is necessary for us to continually assess and reassess our wholeness, which includes attention to stress management, time management, and adequate sleep. Recognizing and celebrating the joys and good things in life add to experiencing life balance and satisfaction. Life is a journey. Willingness to be present for all this life journey brings, cultivating the ability to be fully in the moment with "what is," is a component of a transformative healing process.

Assessing our life balance and satisfaction acknowledges our capacity for both conscious and unconscious choices in our lives. Conscious choices involve awareness and skills such as self-reflection, self-care, discipline, persistence, goal setting, priority setting, action steps, discerning best options, and acknowledging and trusting perceptions. We can be active participants in daily living, not passive observers who hope that life will be good to us.

The unconscious also plays a major role in our choices.[16] Jung conceived of the uncon-scious as a series of layers. The layers closest to our awareness may become known; those farthest away are, in principle, inaccessible to our awareness and operate autonomously. Jung saw the unconscious as the home of timeless psychic forces that he called *archetypes*, which generally are invariant throughout all cultures and eras. He felt that every psychic force has its opposite in the unconsciousness—the force of light is always counterposed with that of darkness, good with evil, love with hate, and so on. Jung believed that any psychic energy can become unbalanced. Therefore, one of life's greatest challenges is to achieve a dynamic balance of the innate opposites and make this balancing process as conscious as possible.

Relationships

Healthy people live in intricate networks of relationships and are always in search of new, unifying concepts of the universe and social order. (See Chapter 26.) Learning how to understand and nurture our relationships (see the Relationships section in Figure 8-2) assists us in creating and sustaining meaningful relationships. A healthy person cannot live in isolation. In a

—— INTEGRATIVE HEALTH and WELLNESS ASSESSMENT™ ——

This **INTEGRATIVE HEALTH and WELLNESS ASSESSMENT** is intended for informational purposes only. It is not a substitute for professional medical advice, diagnosis or treatment.

DIRECTIONS: This questionnaire contains statements about your present way of life, feelings, and personal habits. Please respond to each item as accurately as possible, and try not to skip any item. Indicate the frequency with which you engage in each item by checking (✓) one of the following:

Never	Almost Never	Once in a While	Almost Always	Always

LIFE BALANCE and SATISFACTION	Never	Almost Never	Once in a While	Almost Always	Always
1. I have balance between my work, family, friends, and self.	❏	❏	❏	❏	❏
2. I appreciate who I am.	❏	❏	❏	❏	❏
3. I am satisfied with my occupation or profession.	❏	❏	❏	❏	❏
4. I feel joy and gratitude.	❏	❏	❏	❏	❏
5. I am hopeful about the future.	❏	❏	❏	❏	❏
6. I go to work feeling good about what I do.	❏	❏	❏	❏	❏
7. I give time and resources to people and causes I admire and respect.	❏	❏	❏	❏	❏
8. I experience healthy finances.	❏	❏	❏	❏	❏
9. I am coping well with life.	❏	❏	❏	❏	❏
10. I focus on my strengths.	❏	❏	❏	❏	❏
11. I get 6-8 hours of uninterrupted sleep each night.	❏	❏	❏	❏	❏
12. I wake up feeling rested and alert.	❏	❏	❏	❏	❏
13. I use strategies (breathing, stretching, relaxation, imagery, meditation) to manage stress daily.	❏	❏	❏	❏	❏
14. I use daily positive self-talk and affirmations.	❏	❏	❏	❏	❏
15. I set realistic goals.	❏	❏	❏	❏	❏
16. I can release anxiety, worry, and fear in a healthy way.	❏	❏	❏	❏	❏
17. I manage my time to meet my personal goals.	❏	❏	❏	❏	❏
18. I take time for leisure activities (gardening, hobbies).	❏	❏	❏	❏	❏
19. I take short breaks for play, laughter, and humor each day.	❏	❏	❏	❏	❏
20. I recognize negative thoughts and reframe them.	❏	❏	❏	❏	❏
21. I take on no more than I can manage.	❏	❏	❏	❏	❏

FIGURE 8-2   Integrative Health and Wellness Assessment

For items 22–24, check (✓) the response that most closely resembles how you feel about making changes or improvements to your **LIFE BALANCE** and **SATISFACTION.**

22. My readiness for change is

❑ Now   ❑ Within 2 weeks   ❑ Next month   ❑ In 6 months
❑ In a year or more

23. My priority for making change is

❑ Highest priority   ❑ Priority   ❑ Medium priority
❑ Very low priority   ❑ Never a priority

24. My confidence in my ability to make a positive change is

❑ Very confident   ❑ Confident   ❑ Somewhat confident
❑ Not very confident   ❑ Not at all confident

LIFE BALANCE and SATISFACTION ACTION PLAN. Please list 3 changes that you can implement into your current lifestyle over the next 3 months:

1. _____

2. _____

3. _____

Additional changes, comments, thoughts:

_____

RELATIONSHIPS	Never	Almost Never	Once in a While	Almost Always	Always
1. I create and participate in satisfying relationships.	❑	❑	❑	❑	❑
2. I have people in my life who I trust and can go to for support and guidance.	❑	❑	❑	❑	❑
3. I feel comfortable sharing my feelings/ opinions without needing approval from others.	❑	❑	❑	❑	❑
4. I am able to say no to others without feeling guilty.	❑	❑	❑	❑	❑
5. I clearly express my needs and desires.	❑	❑	❑	❑	❑
6. I am happy with the quality and quantity of nurturing physical contact (hugs, bodywork, partner yoga) that I have with others.	❑	❑	❑	❑	❑
7. I easily express love and concern to those I care about.	❑	❑	❑	❑	❑
8. I do my part in establishing and maintaining relationships.	❑	❑	❑	❑	❑
9. I feel comfortable with my sexuality.	❑	❑	❑	❑	❑

FIGURE 8-2   Integrative Health and Wellness Assessment *(continues)*

RELATIONSHIPS *(continued)*	Never	Almost Never	Once in a While	Almost Always	Always
10. I am happy with the quality and quantity of sexual intimacy in my life right now.	❏	❏	❏	❏	❏
11. I can talk about feelings related to death and other losses with friends and/or family.	❏	❏	❏	❏	❏
12. I have taken actions to ensure that my end of life care is as I would want it to be (Healthcare Proxy, Living Will, Power of Attorney).	❏	❏	❏	❏	❏

For items 13–15, check (✓) the response that most closely resembles how you feel about making changes or improvements to your RELATIONSHIPS.

13. My readiness for change is

❏ Now   ❏ Within 2 weeks   ❏ Next month   ❏ In 6 months
❏ In a year or more

14. My priority for making change is

❏ Highest priority   ❏ Priority   ❏ Medium priority
❏ Very low priority   ❏ Never a priority

15. My confidence in my ability to make a positive change is

❏ Very confident   ❏ Confident   ❏ Somewhat confident
❏ Not very confident   ❏ Not at all confident

RELATIONSHIPS ACTION PLAN. Please list 3 changes that you can implement into your current lifestyle over the next 3 months:

1. _____

2. _____

3. _____

Additional changes, comments, thoughts:
_____

SPIRITUAL	Never	Almost Never	Once in a While	Almost Always	Always
1. I feel that my life has meaning, value, and purpose.	❏	❏	❏	❏	❏
2. I feel connected to a force greater than myself.	❏	❏	❏	❏	❏
3. I follow a spiritual and/or religious practice.	❏	❏	❏	❏	❏

FIGURE 8-2 Integrative Health and Wellness Assessment *(continued)*

	Never	Almost Never	Once in a While	Almost Always	Always
SPIRITUAL *(continued)*					
4. I make time for reflective practice (affirmations, prayer, meditation).	❏	❏	❏	❏	❏
5. I feel that I am growing and changing in positive ways.	❏	❏	❏	❏	❏
6. I have a community that will be there for me in times of need (illness, crisis, death).	❏	❏	❏	❏	❏

For items 7–9, check (✓) the response that most closely resembles how you feel about making changes or improvements to your SPIRITUAL areas.

7. My readiness for change is
   ❏ Now   ❏ Within 2 weeks   ❏ Next month   ❏ In 6 months
   ❏ In a year or more

8. My priority for making change is
   ❏ Highest priority   ❏ Priority   ❏ Medium priority
   ❏ Very low priority   ❏ Never a priority

9. My confidence in my ability to make a positive change is

   ❏ Very confident   ❏ Confident   ❏ Somewhat confident
   ❏ Not very confident ❏ Not at all confident

SPIRITUAL ACTION PLAN. Please list 3 changes that you can implement into your current lifestyle over the next 3 months:

1. _____

2. _____

3. _____

Additional changes, comments, thoughts:

_____

MENTAL	Never	Almost Never	Once in a While	Almost Always	Always
1. I am open and receptive to new ideas and experiences.	❏	❏	❏	❏	❏
2. I use my imagination in considering new choices or possibilities.	❏	❏	❏	❏	❏
3. I am interested in and knowledgeable about many topics.	❏	❏	❏	❏	❏
4. I prioritize my work and set realistic goals.	❏	❏	❏	❏	❏
5. I enjoy developing new skills and talents.	❏	❏	❏	❏	❏

FIGURE 8-2   Integrative Health and Wellness Assessment *(continues)*

MENTAL *(continued)*	Never	Almost Never	Once in a While	Almost Always	Always
6. I can let go of unwanted thoughts.	❏	❏	❏	❏	❏
7. I am aware of the connection between my thoughts, emotions, and health.	❏	❏	❏	❏	❏
8. I ask for help/assistance as needed.	❏	❏	❏	❏	❏
9. I am committed and disciplined when I take on new projects.	❏	❏	❏	❏	❏
10. I follow through and work on decisions with clarity and action steps.	❏	❏	❏	❏	❏
11. I take important challenges as needed.	❏	❏	❏	❏	❏
12. I can accept circumstances and events that are beyond my control.	❏	❏	❏	❏	❏

For items 13–15, check (✓) the response that most closely resembles how you feel about making changes or improvements to your MENTAL areas.

13. My readiness for change is
  ❏ Now   ❏ Within 2 weeks   ❏ Next month   ❏ In 6 months
  ❏ In a year or more

14. My priority for making change is
  ❏ Highest priority   ❏ Priority   ❏ Medium priority
  ❏ Very low priority   ❏ Never a priority

15. My confidence in my ability to make a positive change is

  ❏ Very confident   ❏ Confident   ❏ Somewhat confident
  ❏ Not very confident   ❏ Not at all confident

MENTAL ACTION PLAN. Please list 3 changes that you can implement into your current lifestyle over the next 3 months:

1. _____

2. _____

3. _____

Additional changes, comments, thoughts:
_____

FIGURE 8-2   Integrative Health and Wellness Assessment *(continued)*

EMOTIONAL	Never	Almost Never	Once in a While	Almost Always	Always
1. I recognize my own feelings and emotions.	❏	❏	❏	❏	❏
2. I laugh freely and openly.	❏	❏	❏	❏	❏
3. I include my feelings when making decisions.	❏	❏	❏	❏	❏
4. I express my feelings in appropriate ways.	❏	❏	❏	❏	❏
5. I recognize my intuition.	❏	❏	❏	❏	❏
6. I can learn from my mistakes.	❏	❏	❏	❏	❏
7. I am compassionate with myself.	❏	❏	❏	❏	❏
8. I practice forgiveness.	❏	❏	❏	❏	❏
9. I am compassionate in my communication(s).	❏	❏	❏	❏	❏
10. I listen to and respect the feelings of others.	❏	❏	❏	❏	❏
11. I enjoy new challenges or experiences.	❏	❏	❏	❏	❏
12. I recognize and can deliberately try to shift negative emotions.	❏	❏	❏	❏	❏
13. I seek guidance when necessary.	❏	❏	❏	❏	❏

For items 14–16, check (✓) the response that most closely resembles how you feel about making changes or improvements to your EMOTIONAL areas.

14. My readiness for change is

❏ Now   ❏ Within 2 weeks   ❏ Next month   ❏ In 6 months
❏ In a year or more

15. My priority for making change is

❏ Highest priority   ❏ Priority   ❏ Medium priority
❏ Very low priority   ❏ Never a priority

16. My confidence in my ability to make a positive change is

❏ Very confident   ❏ Confident   ❏ Somewhat confident
❏ Not very confident   ❏ Not at all confident

EMOTIONAL ACTION PLAN. Please list 3 changes that you can implement into your current lifestyle over the next 3 months:

1. _____

2. _____

3. _____

Additional changes, comments, thoughts:

_____

FIGURE 8-2 Integrative Health and Wellness Assessment *(continues)*

PHYSICAL	Never	Almost Never	Once in a While	Almost Always	Always
NUTRITION					
1. I eat a nutritious breakfast daily.	❏	❏	❏	❏	❏
2. I eat at least 5 servings of vegetables & fruits daily.	❏	❏	❏	❏	❏
3. I eat whole foods (grains, beans, seeds and nuts).	❏	❏	❏	❏	❏
4. I eat low fat foods (fish, low fat dairy, beans, skinless chicken).	❏	❏	❏	❏	❏
5. I avoid red meat or eat it only a few times a week.	❏	❏	❏	❏	❏
6. I decrease high fat foods (hot dogs, steaks, cheese, ice cream, whole milk, cakes, sweets, fried foods, butter).	❏	❏	❏	❏	❏
7. I avoid sugar.	❏	❏	❏	❏	❏
8. I avoid junk food.	❏	❏	❏	❏	❏
9. I avoid regular soda drinks with sugar or diet drinks with artificial sweeteners.	❏	❏	❏	❏	❏
10. I drink 6-8 glasses of water daily.	❏	❏	❏	❏	❏
11. I read labels for ingredients.	❏	❏	❏	❏	❏
12. I avoid food colorings, flavoring, and additives in my foods.	❏	❏	❏	❏	❏
13. I avoid canned and processed foods.	❏	❏	❏	❏	❏
14. I eat organic and/or local produce.	❏	❏	❏	❏	❏
15. I eat my meals at home.	❏	❏	❏	❏	❏
16. I prepare my meals in an oven or on stove top burners.	❏	❏	❏	❏	❏
17. I have access to healthy food choices.	❏	❏	❏	❏	❏
18. I purchase healthy foods.	❏	❏	❏	❏	❏
19. I experience pain or inflammation in my body.	❏	❏	❏	❏	❏
20. I experience digestive discomfort.	❏	❏	❏	❏	❏
21. I am aware of foods that affect my digestion.	❏	❏	❏	❏	❏
22. I feel bloated after eating.	❏	❏	❏	❏	❏
23. I take medication for digestive reasons.	❏	❏	❏	❏	❏
24. I am aware of any food sensitivities or food allergies.	❏	❏	❏	❏	❏
25. I have a bowel movement daily.	❏	❏	❏	❏	❏
26. I chew my food thoroughly.	❏	❏	❏	❏	❏

FIGURE 8-2   Integrative Health and Wellness Assessment *(continued)*

NUTRITION *(continued)*	Never	Almost Never	Once in a While	Almost Always	Always
27. I eat mindfully (concentrate on my eating, not multi-tasking or eating in front of the television).	❑	❑	❑	❑	❑
28. I eat late at night.	❑	❑	❑	❑	❑
29. I crave sweets.	❑	❑	❑	❑	❑
30. I eat larger portions than I need.	❑	❑	❑	❑	❑
31. I feel energy after eating.	❑	❑	❑	❑	❑
32. I feel tired after eating.	❑	❑	❑	❑	❑

For items 33–35, check (✓) the response that most closely resembles how you feel about making changes or improvements to your NUTRITION.

33. My readiness for change is
   ❑ Now   ❑ Within 2 weeks   ❑ Next month   ❑ In 6 months
   ❑ In a year or more

34. My priority for making change is
   ❑ Highest priority   ❑ Priority   ❑ Medium priority
   ❑ Very low priority   ❑ Never a priority

35. My confidence in my ability to make a positive change is
   ❑ Very confident   ❑ Confident   ❑ Somewhat confident
   ❑ Not very confident   ❑ Not at all confident

NUTRITION ACTION PLAN. Please list 3 changes that you can implement into your current lifestyle over the next 3 months:

1. _____

2. _____

3. _____

Additional changes, comments, thoughts:

_____

EXERCISE (Know your limitations)	Never	Almost Never	Once in a While	Almost Always	Always
1. I do **aerobic exercise** (jogging, swimming, fitness walking using arms, aerobic dance, active sports) regularly. (*Vigorous intensity*—at least 20 minutes 3 or more days a week; *Moderate intensity*—at least 30 minutes per week)	❑	❑	❑	❑	❑
2. I do **strength exercises** (use strength-training equipment, sit-ups, push-ups) regularly.	❑	❑	❑	❑	❑
3. I do **stretching or flexibility exercises** (head, neck, shoulders, back, legs) for at least 5 minutes 3 days a week.	❑	❑	❑	❑	❑

FIGURE 8-2 Integrative Health and Wellness Assessment *(continues)*

EXERCISE *(continued)*

For items 4-6, check (✓) the response that most closely resembles how you feel about making changes or improvements to your EXERCISE.

4. My readiness for change is
   ❏ Now   ❏ Within 2 Weeks   ❏ Next month   ❏ In 6 Months
   ❏ In a year or more

5. My priority for making change is
   ❏ Highest Priority   ❏ Priority   ❏ Medium Priority
   ❏ Very low Priority   ❏ Never a priority

6. My confidence in my ability to make a positive change is
   ❏ Very Confident   ❏ Confident   ❏ Somewhat Confident
   ❏ Not very confident   ❏ Not at all confident

EXERCISE ACTION PLAN. Please list 3 changes that you can implement into your current lifestyle over the next 3 months:

1. _____

2. _____

3. _____

Additional changes, comments, thoughts:

_____

WEIGHT	Never	Almost Never	Once in a While	Almost Always	Always
1. I maintain my ideal weight.	❏	❏	❏	❏	❏
2. I have gained no more than 11 pounds in adulthood.	❏	❏	❏	❏	❏

For item 3-5, check (✓) the response that most closely resembles how you feel about making changes or improvements to your WEIGHT.

3. My readiness for change is
   ❏ Now   ❏ Within 2 Weeks   ❏ Next month   ❏ In 6 Months   ❏ In a year

4. My priority for making change is
   ❏ Highest priority   ❏ Priority   ❏ Medium priority
   ❏ Very low priority   ❏ Never a priority

5. My confidence in my ability to make a positive change is
   ❏ Very confident   ❏ Confident   ❏ Somewhat confident
   ❏ Not very confident   ❏ Not at all confident

WEIGHT MANAGEMENT ACTION PLAN. Please list 3 changes that you can implement into your current lifestyle over the next 3 months:

1. _____

2. _____

3. _____

Additional changes, comments, thoughts:

_____

FIGURE 8-2   Integrative Health and Wellness Assessment *(continued)*

ENVIRONMENT	Never	Almost Never	Once in a While	Almost Always	Always
1. I have a healthy, non-toxic home environment.	❑	❑	❑	❑	❑
2. I have a healthy, non-toxic work environment.	❑	❑	❑	❑	❑
3. I am aware of how my external environment affects my health and wellbeing.	❑	❑	❑	❑	❑
4. I share environmental awareness with others in my workplace and community.	❑	❑	❑	❑	❑
5. I make healthy environmental choices when I can.	❑	❑	❑	❑	❑
6. I notice allergies or other symptoms when I am in my home.	❑	❑	❑	❑	❑
7. I notice allergies or other symptoms when I am in my workplace.	❑	❑	❑	❑	❑
8. I check my home for mold.	❑	❑	❑	❑	❑
9. I change my filters in my air conditioner or heating unit at least twice a year.	❑	❑	❑	❑	❑
10. I use gas heat in my home or office with good ventilation (if applicable).	❑	❑	❑	❑	❑
11. I use a water filter in my home.	❑	❑	❑	❑	❑
12. I check my basement for radon (if applicable).	❑	❑	❑	❑	❑
13. I avoid pesticides in my home, garden, or lawn.	❑	❑	❑	❑	❑
14. I have hobbies that involve using chemicals (painting, stained glass, woodwork).	❑	❑	❑	❑	❑
15. I use a flea collar or other topical chemical treatments on my pets.	❑	❑	❑	❑	❑
16. I have a smoke-free environment.	❑	❑	❑	❑	❑
17. I am aware that what I apply to my skin absorbs into my body.	❑	❑	❑	❑	❑
18. I read labels and check ingredients for my personal care products.	❑	❑	❑	❑	❑
19. I choose non-toxic personal care products (shampoo, skin lotion, make-up, hair spray, perfume).	❑	❑	❑	❑	❑
20. I use environmentally friendly cleaning products in my home and/or workplace.	❑	❑	❑	❑	❑
21. I dry clean clothes and remove the plastic before hanging them in my closet.	❑	❑	❑	❑	❑
22. I use air fresheners or burn incense or scented candles in my home or office.	❑	❑	❑	❑	❑

FIGURE 8-2 Integrative Health and Wellness Assessment *(continues)*

ENVIRONMENT *(continued)*	Never	Almost Never	Once in a While	Almost Always	Always
23. I microwave my food in paper or glass and avoid plastic.	❏	❏	❏	❏	❏
24. I use my cell phone and hold it away from my ear or use an earpiece or headset.	❏	❏	❏	❏	❏
25. I purchase new products (shower curtain, carpeting, furniture) and ventilate the area or leave the product outside until the "off gas" smell disappears.	❏	❏	❏	❏	❏

For items 26–28, check (✓) the response that most closely resembles how you feel about making changes or improvements to your ENVIRONMENTAL areas.

26. My readiness for change is

   ❏ Now   ❏ Within 2 weeks   ❏ Next month   ❏ In 6 months
   ❏ In a year or more

27. My priority for making change is

   ❏ Highest priority   ❏ Priority   ❏ Medium priority
   ❏ Very low priority   ❏ Never a priority

28. My confidence in my ability to make a positive change is

   ❏ Very confident   ❏ Confident   ❏ Somewhat confident
   ❏ Not very confident   ❏ Not at all confident

ENVIRONMENTAL ACTION PLAN. Please list 3 changes that you can implement into your current lifestyle over the next 3 months:

1. _____

2. _____

3. _____

Additional changes, comments, thoughts:

_____

HEALTH RESPONSIBILITY	Never	Almost Never	Once in a While	Almost Always	Always
1. I believe that I am key to my wellbeing.	❏	❏	❏	❏	❏
2. My overall health is excellent.	❏	❏	❏	❏	❏
3. I receive yearly physical exams.	❏	❏	❏	❏	❏
4. I integrate self-care practices daily.	❏	❏	❏	❏	❏
5. I pay attention to my physical wellbeing and address symptoms as they arise.	❏	❏	❏	❏	❏

FIGURE 8-2   Integrative Health and Wellness Assessment *(continued)*

HEALTH RESPONSIBILITY *(continued)*	Never	Almost Never	Once in a While	Almost Always	Always
6. I am aware of any unusual weight loss, fever, etc., and seek the advice of my primary healthcare provider.	❑	❑	❑	❑	❑
7. I have had a baseline eye examination and get a regular eye examination as recommended for my age.	❑	❑	❑	❑	❑
8. I practice good oral hygiene (flossing, toothpicks, dental cleaning).	❑	❑	❑	❑	❑
9. I receive regular dental check ups.	❑	❑	❑	❑	❑
10. I check my skin for changing or suspicious moles.	❑	❑	❑	❑	❑
11. I recognize changes in bowel patterns and seek professional consultation.	❑	❑	❑	❑	❑
12. I know my blood pressure, cholesterol, triglycerides, and glucose levels.	❑	❑	❑	❑	❑
13. I avoid smoking or using smokeless tobacco.	❑	❑	❑	❑	❑
14. I can work and do regular activities of daily life.	❑	❑	❑	❑	❑
15. I buckle my seatbelt when driving or when riding as a passenger.	❑	❑	❑	❑	❑
16. I avoid talking on my cell phone when driving or doing critical tasks.	❑	❑	❑	❑	❑
17. I have been able to work free of pain or injury for the last 6 months.	❑	❑	❑	❑	❑
18. I worry that I am addicted to a substance or behavior (gambling, pornography, food, shopping, exercise, internet).	❑	❑	❑	❑	❑
19. I have family members and/or close friends who express concern about my alcohol or substance use.	❑	❑	❑	❑	❑
20. I have completed my personal Health Record.	❑	❑	❑	❑	❑

For items 21–23, check (✓) the response that most closely resembles how you feel about making changes or improvements to your HEALTH RESPONSIBILITY.

21. My readiness for change is

   ❑ Now   ❑ Within 2 weeks   ❑ Next month   ❑ In 6 months
   ❑ In a year or more

22. My priority for making change is

   ❑ Highest priority   ❑ Priority   ❑ Medium priority
   ❑ Very low priority   ❑ Never a priority

FIGURE 8-2 Integrative Health and Wellness Assessment *(continues)*

23. My confidence in my ability to make a positive change is

❏ Very confident ❏ Confident ❏ Somewhat confident
❏ Not very confident ❏ Not at all confident

HEALTH RESPONSIBILITY ACTION PLAN. Please list 3 changes that you can implement into your current lifestyle over the next 3 months:

1. _____

2. _____

3. _____

Additional changes, comments, thoughts:

_____

Source: Used with permission. Dossey, B. M., Luck, S., & Schaub, B. G. (2012). *Integrative Nurse Coaching for Health and Wellness.* Huntington, NY: INCA Publications (www.iNurseCoach.com). Adapted from Dossey, B. M., & Keegan, L. (2009). Self-Care Assessments. In Dossey, B. M., & Keegan, L. *Holistic Nursing: A Handbook for Practice* (5th ed.). Sudbury, MA: Jones & Bartlett Learning. Readiness for change section adapted from Moore, M. & Tschannen-Moran B. (2010). *Coaching Psychology Manual.* Philadelphia: PA. The IHWA format design for survey software available from Healthcare Environment (www.hcenvironment.com)

FIGURE 8-2 Integrative Health and Wellness Assessment *(continued)*

given day, we interact with many people: immediate family, extended family, colleagues at work, neighbors in the community, numerous people in organizations, and now, through the ever expanding web of electronic connection, friends, colleagues, and others around the world.

Relationships have different levels of meaning, from the superficial to the deeply connected. The challenges in relationships are multifaceted. First, we need to recognize what we personally are hoping for, and what we are bringing to the variety of relationships we engage in. How do we discern and decide when we feel willing to exchange feelings of honesty, trust, intimacy, compassion, openness, and harmony? Many, if not most, people spend at least half of their waking hours at work with colleagues. Within the context of a work environment we need to support and nourish these relationships as well.

Sharing life processes requires truthful and caring self-reflection and communication with others. This includes meaningful dialogues around end-of-life care. These conversations require deep, personal contemplation about what

is desired and hoped for. The dialogue may begin with the family and/or friends most intimately involved and may need to extend beyond to colleagues, clients, and the community at large.

It is essential that we identify both the cohesiveness and the disharmony in our relationships. We must be aware of the impact that we have on clients, family, and friends. Something always happens when people meet and spend time together, for life is never a neutral event. Our attitudes, healing awareness, and concern for self and others have a direct effect on the outcome of all our encounters. We also must extend our networks to include our immediate environment and consider that what we do locally has an impact on our larger community—the nation and planet Earth. (See Chapter 29.) Each of us can take an active role in developing local networks of relationships that can have a ripple effect on local to global health concerns.

Spiritual

Throughout history, there has been a quest to understand the purpose of the human life experience. Assessing aspects of our spiritual nature (see the Spiritual section in Figure 8-2) can be a profound learning opportunity. (See Chapters 32 and 37.) Spirit comes from our roots—it is a universal need to understand the human experience. It is a vital element and driving force in how we live our lives. It affects every aspect of our life balance and satisfaction and effects the degree to which we develop our human potentials. Usually, though not universally, spirituality is considered to involve a sense of connection with an absolute, imminent, or transcendent spiritual force, however named. It includes the conviction that ethical values, direction, meaning, and purpose are valid aspects of the individual and universe. It is the essence of being and relatedness that permeates all of life and is manifested in one's knowing, doing, and being. This interconnectedness with self, others, Nature, and God/Life Force/Absolute/Transcendent is not necessarily synonymous with religion. Religion is the codified and ritualized beliefs and behaviors of those involved in spirituality, usually taking place within a community of like-minded individuals.

Spirit involves the development of our higher self, also referred to as the transpersonal self. A transpersonal experience (i.e., transcendence) is described as a feeling of oneness, inner peace, harmony, wholeness, and connection with the universe. The meaning and joy that flow from developing this aspect of our human potential allow us to have a transpersonal view. Some of the ways we may come to know this transcendence are through prayer, meditation, organized religion, philosophy, science, poetry, music, inspired friends, and group work.

Our spiritual potential does not develop without some attention. Every day, with each of our experiences, we need to acknowledge that our spirit potential is essential to the development of a healthy value system. We shape our perception of the world through our value system, and our perceptions influence whether we have positive or negative experiences. Even through the pain of a negative experience (may be physical, mental, emotional, relational, spiritual), we have the ability to learn. Pain can be a great teacher. On the other side of the experi-ence we may find new wisdom, self-discovery, and the opportunity to make new choices based on freshly acquired knowledge.

Mental

Assessing our mental capacity (see the Mental section in Figure 8-2) helps us examine our belief systems. In our early life, we had role models who influenced our beliefs, thoughts, behaviors, and values. With maturity and as a result of life experiences we begin to recognize shifts that occur in regard to these same beliefs, thoughts, behaviors, and values. We may experience conflicts when we do not take the time to examine our changing perspectives, beliefs, and values.

Our challenge is to use our cognitive capacities to perceive the world with greater clarity. This includes recognizing, to the best of our ability, the variety of perspectives we are presented with both personally and in the world in general. (See Chapter 1 and the description of the Theory of Integral Nursing.) Through both logical and nonlogical mental processes, we become aware of a broad range of subjects that have the potential to enhance our full appreciation of the many great pleasures in life. We can also build our capacity to notice, process, and integrate both logical thought and intuitive awareness.

With interventions such as relaxation and imagery, we learn to be present in the moment. It is during these moments that we can notice and release the incessant, self-judging, critical inner voice that is constantly engaging in self-dialogue. These are the moments when we expand our mental knowing. We become more capable of focusing our attention away from fear-based, negative thought patterns and become more open and receptive to life-affirming information and patterns of thought. In this way, mental growth can occur. Every aspect of our life is a learning experience and becomes part of a lesson in change.

Emotional

Assessing our emotional potential (see the Emotional section in Figure 8-2) assists us in our willingness to acknowledge the presence of feelings, value them as important information to notice, and express them. (See Chapters

11, 12, 32, and 37.) Emotional health implies that we have the choice and freedom to process and/or express the full spectrum of emotions including love, joy, guilt, forgiveness, fear, and anger. The expression of these emotions can give us immediate feedback about our inner state, which may be crying out for a new way of being.

Emotions are responses to the events in our lives. We are living systems that are constantly exchanging with our environment. All life events affect our emotions and general well-being. We have the potential to lessen varying degrees of chronic anxiety, depression, worry, fear, guilt, anger, denial, failure, or repression, and experience true healing, when we are willing to confront our emotions.

As we start to live in a more balanced way, we allow our humanness to develop. We reach out and ask for human dialogue that is meaningful. Increasing emotional potential allows openness, creativity, and spontaneity to be experienced. This contributes to the emergence of a positive, healthy zest for living. We can learn to take responsibility for allowing this part of us, our spirit and intuition, to blossom and fully bloom.

Emotions are gifts. Frequently, a first step toward releasing a burden in a relationship is to share deep feelings with another. There is no such thing as a good or bad emotion; each is part of the human condition. Emotions exist as the light and shadow of the self; thus, we must acknowledge all of them. The only reason that we can identify the light is that we know its opposite, the shadow. When we recognize the value in both types of emotions, we are in a position of new insight and understanding, and we can make more effective choices. As we increase our attention to body-mind-spirit interrelationships, we can focus on the emotions that move us toward wholeness and inner understanding.

Physical

All humans share the common biological experiences of birth, gender, growth, aging, and death. When a person's basic biological needs for food,

shelter, and clothing have been met, there are many ways to seek wholeness of physical potential. Assessing our physical potential (see the Physical section in Figure 8-2) includes many elements with three major areas being nutrition (see Chapter 13), exercise (see Chapter 14), and weight management (see Chapter 22). Many people have become obsessed with these elements of the physical potential but have failed to recognize that it is not separate from—or more important than—the other potentials. Health is more than just physical and the absence of pain and symptoms, and it is present when there is balance. As we assess biological needs, we also must take into consideration our perceptions of these areas. Many illnesses have been documented as stress related because our consciousness plays a major role in health and physical potential.

Our body is a gift to nurture and respect. As we nurture ourselves, we increase our uniqueness in energy, sexuality, vitality, capacity for language, and connection with our other potentials. This nurturance strengthens our self-image, which in turn causes several things to happen. First, our body-mind-spirit responds in a positive and integrated fashion. Second, we become a role model with a positive influence on others. Finally, we actually enhance our general feeling of well-being, gaining strengths and becoming empowered. The resulting effect is a greater sense of balance and an openness to more fully realized potentials

Environmental

Assessing our environment (see the Environmental section in Figure 8-2) increases our awareness of its impact on our health and well-being. (See Chapter 29.) The environment is the context or habitat within which all living systems participate and interact. This includes the physical body and its physical habitat, and cultural, psychological, social, and historical influences; it includes both the external physical space and a person's internal space (physical, mental, emotional, social, and spiritual experiences). Healing environment includes everything that surrounds the nurse, healthcare practitioner, and student, the patient/client, family, community, and significant others as well as patterns not yet understood.

Florence Nightingale (1820-1910) was an environmentalist and wrote about the effects of polluted homes and environments and the importance of avoiding anything that makes one ill or might be considered toxic. Today this is recognized as the "precautionary principle"[17] that states that when an activity raises threats of harm to human health or the environment, precautionary measures shall be taken, even if some cause-and-effect relationships are not fully established scientifically, or "better safe than sorry." If there is a suspicion about a harmful environment or substance, even though all of the evidence is not in, remove the person from the situation or stop the use of suspected harmful substances. The emphasis is on *zero* contamination and pollution of our environments as acceptable, not minimal/moderate.

Health Responsibility

Health responsibility (see the Health Responsibility section in Figure 8-2) occurs when an individual takes an active role in making lifestyle choices to protect and improve his or her health. These actions and behaviors that enhance health and well-being are explored in the IHWA.

Health responsibility includes having physical examinations and eye examinations as recommended for one's age and health status by qualified healthcare practitioners. The Personal Health Record* (**Figure 8-3**) includes all baseline personal physiologic parameters, personal history, family history, and any current symptoms. In addition, all medications and supplements that are being taken should be

noted and evaluated in terms of any potential interactions of the pharmaceuticals with the supplements. Allergies, hospitalizations, surgeries, and other specific medical factors are also important to note.

In health care, we may hear that a client/patient is noncompliant with medical orders. This is often a misnomer because there are many reasons why an individual may not follow medical recommendations. The following are common reasons for this "noncompliance": too much information given at one time; lack of fully understanding the recommendations and having unanswered questions; language barriers or cognitive limitations; fear/s; denial; previous lack of commitment or lack of success (e.g., weight management, smoking cessation); side effects of medications; financial constraints; religious beliefs; disabilities; lack of support from significant others. In addition, there is usually an inadequate amount of time for effective patient education in clinics, doctors' offices, hospitals when providing discharge information, and other healthcare settings.

■ CONCLUSION

Use of the Integrative Health and Wellness Assessment and the Personal Health Record can engage both clients and nurses in self-development. Holistic nurses are challenged to learn new nurse coaching knowledge and skills to assist clients and self in new health behaviors and how to sustain them. If one IHWA category is not assessed or is left undeveloped, things do not seem to be as good as they could be. When one strives to develop in one or several areas, a sense of wholeness emerges, and one's self-worth increases, and action plans for healthier lifestyle behaviors and goals are actualized. Being alive becomes more exciting, rewarding, and fulfilling. By taking an active role in health promotion, health maintenance, and disease management, clients can integrate strengths, action plans, and affirmations and can continue on a creative journey of healing. By changing our perceptions and beliefs and empowering ourselves for effective change, we become healthier.

---

*Disclaimer: This Personal Health Record does not provide medical advice. It is intended for individual informational purposes only. It is not a substitute for professional medical advice, diagnosis, or treatment. Never ignore professional medical advice in seeking treatment. If you think you may have a medical emergency, immediately call your doctor or dial 911.

—— PERSONAL HEALTH RECORD (Age_____) ——

THIS PERSONAL HEALTH RECORD DOES NOT PROVIDE MEDICAL ADVICE. It is intended for informational purposes only. It is not a substitute for professional medical advice, diagnosis or treatment. Never ignore professional medical advice in seeking treatment. If you think you may have a medical emergency, immediately call your doctor or dial 911.

BLOOD PRESSURE
_____ Systolic (high number) (<120 desirable)
_____ Diastolic (low number) (<80 desirable)

BLOOD GLUCOSE (Fasting)
_____ Glucose (<100 desirable)
_____ If elevated, Hemoglobin A1c

BLOOD LIPIDS (Fasting)
_____ Total cholesterol (<200 desirable)
_____ HDL, good cholesterol (>50 women, >40 men desirable)
_____ LDL, bad cholesterol (<130 desirable)
_____ C-Reactive Protein (CRP)
_____ Homocysteine

HEIGHT in inches (without shoes) _____
Height at age 35 _____
Height at age 55 _____

WEIGHT in pounds (without shoes)
Current _____
1 year ago _____
3 years ago _____
5 years ago _____
10 years ago _____

BODY MASS INDEX (BMI)
Underweight = <18.5
Normal weight = 18.5–24.9
Overweight = 25.0–29.9
Obesity = >30
(Please see Body Mass Index tables on pp. 185–186.)

WAIST MEASUREMENT (in inches)
_____ (>35 for women or >40 for men indicates increased disease risk.)

WOMEN—Check all that apply:

❏ I discuss when to have a PAP smear with my primary healthcare provider.

❏ I discuss when to have a mammogram or thermogram with my primary healthcare provider.

❏ I discuss when to have a colonoscopy with my primary healthcare provider.

MEN—Check all that apply:

❏ I discuss when to have a prostate exam with my primary healthcare provider.

❏ I discuss when to do self-testicular exams with my primary healthcare provider.

❏ I discuss when to have a colonoscopy with my primary healthcare provider

I take the following daily supplements:
_____   _____
_____   _____

I take the following medications (including prescription, non-prescription medications for anxiety, mood, sleep or depression):
_____   _____
_____   _____
_____   _____

FIGURE 8-5 Personal Health Record

FAMILY HISTORY (in immediate family, alive or deceased)

Select one for each of the following:

Y = Yes and is not under control
C = Yes and is under control via treatment/medication
N = No or not applicable

Cancer   ❏ Y   ❏ C   ❏ N
Please specify type(s) _____

Cardiovascular Disease   ❏ Y   ❏ C   ❏ N
(heart attack, coronary heart disease, heart
surgery, congestive heart failure, stroke
before age 65 in women and age 55 in men)

Diabetes   ❏ Y   ❏ C   ❏ N

High Blood Pressure   ❏ Y   ❏ C   ❏ N

High Cholesterol   ❏ Y   ❏ C   ❏ N

Obesity   ❏ Y   ❏ C   ❏ N

Mental Illness   ❏ Y   ❏ C   ❏ N
Please specify type(s) _____

Alzheimer's Disease   ❏ Y   ❏ C   ❏ N

Suicide   ❏ Y   ❏ C   ❏ N

Other   ❏ Y   ❏ C   ❏ N
Please specify _____

PERSONAL HISTORY

I have been informed by my primary healthcare provider on the following health problems:

Arthritis   ❏ Y   ❏ C   ❏ N

Asthma   ❏ Y   ❏ C   ❏ N

Bowel Polyps   ❏ Y   ❏ C   ❏ N

Back Problems   ❏ Y   ❏ C   ❏ N
(sciatica, musculoskeletal)

Cancer (including skin cancer melanoma)   ❏ Y   ❏ C   ❏ N
Please specify type(s) _____

Chronic Bronchitis or Emphysema (COPD)   ❏ Y   ❏ C   ❏ N

Cardiovascular Disease   ❏ Y   ❏ C   ❏ N
(angina, heart attack, heart surgery,
congestive heart failure, stroke before
age 65 in women and age 55 in men)

Diabetes   ❏ Y   ❏ C   ❏ N

Chronic Bronchitis or Emphysema (COPD)   ❏ Y   ❏ C   ❏ N

High Blood Pressure (140/90 or higher)   ❏ Y   ❏ C   ❏ N

High Cholesterol (200 or higher)   ❏ Y   ❏ C   ❏ N

Mental Illness   ❏ Y   ❏ C   ❏ N
Please specify type(s) _____

FIGURE 8-3   Personal Health Record *(continues)*

CURRENT SYMPTOMS (within last month)

Heart flutters or frequent palpitations	❏ Y	❏ C	❏ N
Chest pain	❏ Y	❏ C	❏ N
Unusual shortness of breath	❏ Y	❏ C	❏ N
Dizziness or fainting	❏ Y	❏ C	❏ N
Temporal sensations of tingling, numbness, light-headedness	❏ Y	❏ C	❏ N
Restricted blood flow (to head, neck, legs)	❏ Y	❏ C	❏ N
Lower leg symptoms (calf muscle pain, tenderness, redness, swelling)	❏ Y	❏ C	❏ N
Trouble sleeping	❏ Y	❏ C	❏ N
Back pain or sciatica in last month	❏ Y	❏ C	❏ N
Frequent urination or unusual thirst	❏ Y	❏ C	❏ N
Vision problems	❏ Y	❏ C	❏ N
Memory loss	❏ Y	❏ C	❏ N
Increased fatigue	❏ Y	❏ C	❏ N
Digestive problems	❏ Y	❏ C	❏ N
Bowel changes	❏ Y	❏ C	❏ N
Hot flashes (hot flushes or night sweats)	❏ Y	❏ C	❏ N

FIGURE 8-3   Personal Health Record *(continued)*

Source: Used with permission. Dossey, B. M., Luck, S., & Schaub, B. G. (2012). *Integrative Nurse Coaching for Health and Wellness*. Huntington, NY: Florence Press (www.iNurseCoach.com).

BODY MASS INDEX (BMI) TABLES

Find the appropriate height in the left hand column. Label **Height**. Move across to a given weight (in pounds). The number at the top of the column is the **BMI** at that *height* and *weight*. Pounds have been rounded off. (http://www.nhlbi.nih.gov/guidelines/obesity/bmi_tbl.htm)

BMI Table

BMI	19	20	21	22	23	24	25	26	27	28	29	30	31	32	33	34	35
Height (inches)								Body Weight (pounds)									
58	91	96	100	105	110	115	119	124	129	134	138	143	148	153	158	162	167
59	94	99	104	109	114	119	124	128	133	138	143	148	153	158	163	168	173
60	97	102	107	112	118	123	128	133	138	143	148	153	158	163	168	174	179
61	100	106	111	116	122	127	132	137	143	148	153	158	164	169	174	180	185
62	104	109	115	120	126	131	136	142	147	153	158	164	169	175	180	186	191
63	107	113	118	124	130	135	141	146	152	158	163	169	175	180	186	191	197
64	110	116	122	128	134	140	145	151	157	163	169	174	180	186	192	197	204
65	114	120	126	132	138	144	150	156	162	168	174	180	186	192	198	204	210
66	118	124	130	136	142	148	155	161	167	173	179	186	192	198	204	210	216
67	121	127	134	140	146	153	159	166	172	178	185	191	198	204	211	217	223
68	125	131	138	144	151	158	164	171	177	184	190	197	203	210	216	223	230
69	128	135	142	149	155	162	169	176	182	189	196	203	209	216	223	230	236
70	132	139	146	153	160	167	174	181	188	195	202	209	216	222	229	236	243
71	136	143	150	157	165	172	179	186	193	200	208	215	222	229	236	243	250
72	140	147	154	162	169	177	184	191	199	206	213	221	228	235	242	250	258
73	144	151	159	166	174	182	189	197	204	212	219	227	235	242	250	257	265
74	148	155	163	171	179	186	194	202	210	218	225	233	241	249	256	264	272
75	152	160	168	176	184	192	200	208	216	224	232	240	248	256	264	272	279
76	156	164	172	180	189	197	205	213	221	230	238	246	254	263	271	279	287

(continues)

BODY MASS INDEX (BMI) TABLES *(continued)*

BMI Table

Body Weight (pounds)

BMI Height (inches)	36	37	38	39	40	41	42	43	44	45	46	47	48	49	50	51	52	53	54
58	172	177	181	186	191	196	201	205	210	215	220	224	229	234	239	244	248	253	258
59	178	183	188	193	198	203	208	212	217	222	227	232	237	242	247	252	257	262	267
60	184	189	194	199	204	209	215	220	225	230	235	240	245	250	255	261	266	271	276
61	190	195	201	206	211	217	222	227	232	238	243	248	254	259	264	269	275	280	285
62	196	202	207	213	218	224	229	235	240	246	251	256	262	267	273	278	284	289	295
63	203	208	214	220	225	231	237	242	248	254	259	265	270	278	282	287	293	299	304
64	209	215	221	227	232	238	244	250	256	262	267	273	279	285	291	296	302	308	314
65	216	222	228	234	240	246	252	258	264	270	276	282	288	294	300	306	312	318	324
66	223	229	235	241	247	253	260	266	272	278	284	291	297	303	309	315	322	328	334
67	230	236	242	249	255	261	268	274	280	287	293	299	306	312	319	325	331	338	344
68	236	243	249	256	262	269	276	282	289	295	302	308	315	322	328	335	341	348	354
69	243	250	257	263	270	277	284	291	297	304	311	318	324	331	338	345	351	358	365
70	250	257	264	271	278	285	292	299	306	313	320	327	334	341	348	355	362	369	376
71	257	265	272	279	286	293	301	308	315	322	329	338	343	351	358	365	372	379	386
72	265	272	279	287	294	302	309	316	324	331	338	346	353	361	368	375	383	390	397
73	272	280	288	295	303	311	318	325	333	340	348	355	363	371	378	386	393	401	408
74	280	287	295	303	311	319	326	334	342	350	358	365	373	381	389	396	404	412	420
75	287	295	303	311	319	327	335	343	351	359	367	375	383	391	399	407	415	423	431
76	295	304	312	320	328	336	344	353	361	369	377	385	394	402	410	418	426	435	443

Source: Retrieved from http://www.nhlbi.nih.gov/guidelines/obesity/bmi_tbl.htm

Directions for
FUTURE RESEARCH

1. Determine whether the percentage of desired client outcomes increases when the nurse uses the Integrative Health and Wellness Assessment (IHWA) as a coaching tool.
2. Determine whether the client's self-efficacy and self-esteem increase with use of the IHWA.
3. Evaluate changes in health behavior and perceived quality of life when assessing the IHWA eight categories.

Nurse Healer
REFLECTIONS

After reading this chapter, the nurse healer will be able to answer or to begin a process of answering the following questions:

- What is my process when I complete the Integrative Health and Wellness Assessment?
- Am I consciously aware of the daily opportunity to increase my health and well-being?
- What can I do to increase my conscious awareness of fully participating in my life?
- What do I experience when I acknowledge my healing potential?

> *For a full suite of assignments and additional learning activities, use the access code located in the front of your book to visit this exclusive website: http://go.jblearning.com/dossey. If you do not have an access code, you can obtain one at the site.*

NOTES

1. Institute of Medicine, *The Future of Nursing: Leading Change, Advancing Health* (2010). http://www.iom.edu/Reports/2010/The-Future-of-Nursing-Leading-Change-Advancing-Health.aspx.
2. Centers for Disease Control and Prevention, *Obesity Index.* http://www.cdc.gov/obesity/data/index.html.
3. R. Snyderman and M. Dinan, "Improving Health by Taking It Personally," *Journal of the American Medical Association* 303, no. 4 (2010): 363–364.
4. American Heart Association, *Heart Disease and Stroke Statistics—2009 Update.* (Dallas, TX: American Heart Association, 2009).
5. Centers for Disease Control and Prevention, "Heart Disease and Stroke Prevention: Addressing the Nation's Leading Killers: At a Glance 2011." http://www.cdc.gov/chronicdisease/resources/publications/AAG/dhdsp.htm.
6. Y. C. Wang, K. McPherson, T. Marsh, S. L. Gortmaker, and M. Brown, "Health and Economic Burden of the Projected Obesity Trends in the USA and the UK," *Lancet* 378, no. 9793 (2011): 815–825.
7. E. S. Ford, M. M. Bergmann, J. Kröger, A. Schienkiewitz, C. Weikert, and H. Boeing, "Healthy Living Is the Best Revenge: Findings from the European Prospective Investigation into Cancer and Nutrition—Potsdam Study," *Archives of Internal Medicine* 169, no. 15 (2009): 1355–1362.
8. World Cancer Research Fund and the American Institute for Cancer Research, *Policy and Action for Cancer Prevention* (February 2009). http://www.dietandcancerreport.org/policy_report/index.php.
9. U.S. Department of Health and Human Services, *Healthy People 2020* (Washington, DC: USDHHS, 2010). http://www.healthypeople.gov.
10. Compilation of the Patient Protection and Affordable Care Act (2010). http://docs.house.gov/energycommerce/ppacacon.pdf
11. U.S. Department of Health and Human Services, "Obama Administration Releases National Prevention Strategy" (June 16, 2011). http://www.hhs.gov/news/press/2011pres/06/20110616a.html.
12. S. Luck, "Changing the Health of Our Nation: The Role of Nurse Coaches," *Alternative Therapies in Health and Medicine* 16, no. 5 (2010): 78–80.
13. L. Dossey, *Space, Time and Medicine* (Boston, MA: Shambhala, 1982).
14. B. M. Dossey, S. Luck, and B. G. Schaub, *Integrative Nurse Coaching for Health and Wellness* (Huntington, NY: Florence Press, 2012).
15. L. Keegan and B. Dossey, *Self Care: A Program to Improve Your Life* (Port Angeles, WA: Holistic Nursing Consultants, 2007).
16. C. Jung, "The Archetypes and the Collective Unconscious," in *Collected Works of C. G. Jung,* Vol. 9, Part 1, trans. R. F. C. Hull (Princeton, NJ: Princeton University Press, 1980).
17. C. Raffensperger and J. Tickner, *Protecting Public Health and the Environment: Implementing the Precautionary Principle* (Washington, DC: Island Press, 1999).

18. S. Rollnick, W. R. Miller, and C.C. Butler, *Motivational Interviewing in Healthcare: Helping Patients Change Behavior* (New York, NY: Guilford Press, 2008).

19. Potter, P., and Frisch, N. C, (2009). The nursing process. In Dossey, B. M. & Keegan, L. *Holistic nursing: A handbook for practice* (5th ed) (141-156). Sudbury, MA: Jones & Bartlett.

20. J. Prochaska, J. C. Norcross, and C.C. DiClemente, *Changing for Good. A Revolutionary Six-Stage Program for Overcoming Bad Habits and Moving Your Life Positively Forward.* New York: Harper Collins, 1995).

21. M. Moore and B. Tschannen-Moran, *Coaching Psychology Manual* (Philadelphia: Lippincott, Williams & Wilkins, 2010).

22. M. A. Dart, *Motivational Interviewing in Nursing Practice.* (Sudbury, MA: Jones and Bartlett Publishers, 2011).

23. S. Roberts. *Communication for Health Promotion: Motivating Change,* 3rd ed. (Oakland, CA: Permanente Medical Group, 2005).

24. T. Stoltzfus. *Coaching Questions: A Coach's Guide to Powerful Asking Skills.* (Virginia Beach, VA: Coach 22, 2008).

25. J. Whitmore J. *Coaching for Performance: GROWing Human Potential and Purpose: The Principles and Practices of Coaching and Leadership, 4th ed.* (London: Nicholas Brealey Publishing, 2009).

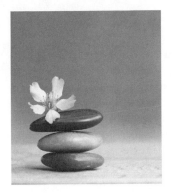

Chapter 9

Nurse Coaching

Barbara Montgomery Dossey, Susan Luck,
Bonney Gulino Schaub, and Darlene R. Hess

Nurse Healer
OBJECTIVES

Theoretical

- Review the history of coaching and nurse coaching.
- Define *professional nurse coach* and *nurse coaching*.
- Explore common belief structures for change.
- Examine the integral process and the four quadrants within a coaching session.

Clinical

- Analyze the middle of coaching conversations from an integral perspective.
- Explore the nurse coaching process and the nurse coaching core competencies.
- Increase use of deep listening skills.
- Use coaching questions to learn more from clients about goals.

Personal

- Engage in one or more reflective practices to deepen presence and intuition.
- Consider finding a nurse coach and entering into a coaching agreement to reach desired goals.

Note: The authors would like to acknowledge Mary Elaine Southard and Linda Bark for their collaborative work in the Professional Nurse Coaching Workgroup (PNCW) for *Professional Nurse Coach Role: Defining the Scope of Practice and Competencies* (Hess, Dossey, Southard, Luck, Schaub, and Bark, in press). This work is quoted in this chapter.

DEFINITIONS

Professional nurse coach: A registered nurse who incorporates coaching skills into his or her professional nursing practice and integrates a holistic perspective. This perspective, as applied to both self and client in a coaching interaction, emerges from an awareness that effective change evolves from within before it can be manifested and maintained externally. The professional nurse coach works with the whole person utilizing principles and modalities that integrate body-mind-emotion-spirit-environment.[1]

Professional nurse coaching: A skilled, purposeful, results-oriented, and structured relationship-centered interaction with clients provided by registered nurses for the purpose of promoting achievement of client goals.[1]

■ EVOLUTION OF THE FIELD OF HEALTH COACHING AND NURSE COACHING

Prior to the 1980s, the term *coach* was used to refer to a role in the field of human performance, specifically in the field of athletics. Coaches training athletes for the Olympic games began introducing relaxation, imagery rehearsal, and somatic awareness practices to enhance athletic performance. Winners of the Olympic games popularized these practices.

During the 1960s, with the beginning of the human potential movement, coaching moved outside of sports and into organizational settings. There was an increased demand for greater productivity and enhanced employee performance. This led to programs and coaching designed to promote employee self-development. Additionally, there was a desire to be able to measure and document the effectiveness of these initiatives in meaningful ways. New challenges emerged with the increase in technology, globalization, and multicultural teams located in different countries. Professional coaching and executive coaching became important factors in business. Formal coaching programs were still in their infancy.

By the 1990s, formal coaching programs, courses, and certifications emerged outside of the nursing profession. Most recently, many nurses have added coaching skills to their professional nursing practice. The time has arrived for nurse coaching to be recognized as embedded within the nursing profession and to be fully integrated into all nursing curricula. Criteria for training programs for professional nurse coaches need to be determined and a credentialing process must be developed.

The U.S. healthcare system is undergoing a transformation from a disease-focused system to one focused on wellness, health promotion, and disease prevention. In 2010, the Patient Protection and Affordable Care Act (PPACA) became law (HR 3590).[2] The language in Section 4001 includes partnerships with a diverse group of licensed health professionals including practitioners of integrative health, preventive medicine, health coaching, public education, and others. In 2011, the United States announced the release of the National Prevention and Health Promotion Strategy, a comprehensive plan that will help increase the number of Americans who are healthy at every stage of life.[3] Health coaches are emerging in the health professions and the lay community.

Nursing, recognizing the importance of this emerging role, is stepping forward and claiming its rightful position in this major shift from disease care to disease prevention, improved health, and enhanced well-being. Nurses constitute the largest group of healthcare providers and are uniquely situated for this role. Professional nursing practice is rooted in efforts to assist clients

to achieve optimal health. Nurses partner with clients to assess, strategize, and plan. Nurses utilize professional nursing knowledge and skills in their role as nurse coaches.

Professional nurse coaches are emerging as leaders who are informing governments, regulatory agencies, businesses, and organizations about the important part they play in achieving the goal of improving the health of the nation and health at a global level. For example, in 2009, the International Council of Nurses (ICN), a federation of more than 130 national nursing organizations representing millions of nurses worldwide, partnered with the Honor Society of Nursing, Sigma Theta Tau International (STTI) that represents more than 125,000 nurses worldwide, and published *Coaching in Nursing*.[4] Professional nurse coaches are taking the lead and engaging clients in self-care and management of healthcare practices and outcomes. Some examples of professional-led nurse coach programs and books are the Bark Coaching Institute,[5,6] the Integrative Nurse Coach Certificate Program (INCCP),[7,8] and the Watson Caring Science Institute Caritas Coach Education Program.[9]

■ PROFESSIONAL NURSE COACH SCOPE OF PRACTICE AND COMPETENCIES*

The first edition of *Professional Nurse Coach Role: Defining the Scope of Practice and Competencies* brings the nurse coach role in healthcare reform to the forefront.[1] It demonstrates nursing's proactive stance in healthcare transformation and clarifies nursing perspectives concerning the role of the nurse coach in four key ways: (1) it specifies the philosophy, beliefs, and values of the nurse coach and the nurse coach's scope of practice; (2) it articulates how *Professional Nurse Coach Role: Defining the Scope of Practice and Competencies* aligns with the American Nurses Association *Nursing: Scope and Standards of Practice,* 2nd edition;[10] (3) it provides the basis for continued interdisciplinary conversations related to professional health and wellness coaches and lay

---

* This section is used with permission and adapted from Hess et al.'s *Professional Nurse Coaching: Scope of Practice and Competencies.*

health and wellness coaches; and (4) it provides the foundation for an international certification process in professional nurse coaching.

Nurse coaches are guided in their thinking and decision making by four professional resources. The American Nurses Association (ANA) *Nursing: Scope and Standards of Practice*, 2nd edition, outlines the expectations of the professional role of registered nurses and the scope of practice and standards of professional nurse practice and their accompanying competencies.[10] The ANA *Code of Ethics for Nurses with Interpretive Statements* lists the nine provisions that establish the ethical framework for registered nurses across all roles, levels, and settings.[11] *Nursing's Social Policy Statement: The Essence of the Profession* conceptualizes nursing practice, describes the social context of nursing, and provides the definition of nursing.[12] *Holistic Nursing: Scope and Standards of Practice* from the American Holistic Nurses Association (AHNA) and ANA provides the philosophical underpinnings of a holistic nurse coaching practice.[13]

Description of Professional Nurse Coaching Practice

Nurse coaches work with individuals and groups and are found in all areas of nursing practice serving as staff nurses, ambulatory care nurses, case managers, advanced practice registered nurses, nursing faculty, nurse researchers, educators, administrators, nurse entrepreneurs, and nurse coaches in full-time private practice. For some, nurse coaching is their primary role. The depth and breadth to which registered nurses engage in the total scope of nurse coach practice depend on education, experience, role, and the population they serve.

Professional Nurse Coaching Scope of Practice

Professional Nurse Coaching: Scope of Practice and Competencies describes a competent level of nurse coaching practice and professional performance common to all nurse coaches.[1] Effective nurse coaching interactions involve the development of a coaching partnership, creation of a safe space, and sensitivity to client issues of trust and vulnerability as a basis for further exploration.[14] The nurse coach must be able to structure a coaching session, explore client readiness for

coaching, facilitate achievement of the client's desired goals, and co-create a means of determining and evaluating desired outcomes and goals.[1,15] Nurse coaching is grounded in the principles and core values of professional nursing.

Nurse Coaching Core Values

The following five professional nurse coaching core values are adapted from and congruent with the AHNA and ANA *Holistic Nursing: Scope and Standards of Practice*:[13]

1. Nurse coach philosophy, theories, and ethics
2. Nurse coach process
3. Nurse coach communication and coaching environment
4. Nurse coach education, research, and leadership
5. Nurse coach self-development (self-reflection, self assessments, self-evaluation, self-care)

Core value 5 is worded according to a nurse coaching model. These core values and the specific nurse coaching competencies (see the section titled "Nurse Coaching Process" later in this chapter) align with the second edition of *ANA Nursing: Scope and Standards of Practice*[10] and are the foundation for curriculum development and a credentialing process.[16] Nurse coaches understand that professional nurse coaching practice is defined by these core values and competencies. Professional nurse coaching capabilities enhance foundational professional nursing skills and are acquired by additional training.

The Science and Art of Nurse Coaching

Nurse coaches incorporate approaches to nursing practice that are holistic, integrative, and integral and that include the work of numerous nurse scholars. Coaching is a systematic and skilled process grounded in scholarly evidence-based professional nursing practice. All chapters in this text can be used in a nurse coaching practice.

At the heart of nurse coaching is support for the client's healing process as it manifests in bodymindspirit. Nurse coaches realize that by being open and curious and asking powerful questions they may guide the client in the healing process while at the same time providing the client choices in determining priorities for change.

The quality of human caring is central to the relationship between the nurse coach and client.

The nurse is fully present in the coaching relationship, honoring the wholeness of the patient/client. This allows clients a safe environment in which to express their goals, hopes, and dreams and a setting where their vulnerability can be spoken of and addressed. Nurse coaches utilize a full spectrum of coaching strategies as listed in **Exhibit 9-1** to engage the client in meeting desired goals.

The Transtheoretical Model of Behavioral Change (see Chapter 22) is very important in nurse coaching because it is necessary to determine which stage a client is in regarding readiness to make changes.[17] The challenge of change also includes the client's willingness to sustain new behaviors and ways of being. The five stages of change are (1) precontemplation, (2) contemplation, (3) preparation, (4) action, and (5) maintenance; each stage is predictable and identifiable. Motivational interviewing and appreciative inquiry (see Chapter 10) are essential skills the nurse coach can use to help clients recognize resistance, ambivalence, and change talk.[18,19]

■ NURSE COACHING AND CHANGE*

Nurse coaches work with people to help them improve their overall wellness and gain an enhanced sense of well-being, balance, and satisfaction in their lives. Nurse coaching helps clients to flourish by making healthful choices and adopting healthier behaviors. *Wellness* is integrated, congruent functioning aimed at reaching one's highest potential. *Human flourishing* is when an individual finds and creates meaning in life and identifies his or her purpose in life, however defined; it includes taking charge of one's own health. Nurse coaches see clients as whole beings, each with the capacity to connect deeply with her or his own inner wisdom and truth.

As described in the Theory of Integral Nursing (see Chapter 1), nurse coaches can use an integral perspective that is a comprehensive way to organize multiple phenomena of human experience and reality in four areas: the individual interior (personal/intentional), individual exterior (physiologic/behavioral), collective interior (shared/cultural), and collective exterior (systems/structures).[20,21] The nurse coach has insight into her or his own way of orienting in the world. This awareness extends to recognizing personal preferences and biases within each quadrant.

Self-development (self-reflection, self-assessments, self-evaluation, self-care) promotes the recognition of what is going right in life, allowing for the celebration of little successes each day. Coaching is an opportunity to promote and acknowledge success, however small, and then to build on that to achieve further success.

In coaching sessions, the client may also access vulnerable moments and share pain and suffering. *Pain* is a physical and/or emotional discomfort or experience; *suffering* is the story people create around pain.[22] Signs of suffering may be physical, mental, emotional, social, behavioral, and/or spiritual. This is why it is so important for nurse coaches to develop a reflective practice to strengthen their own capacity to sit with the pain and suffering clients express without trying to fix the discomfort. A useful saying is "soft front and strong back." This relates to the nurse coach's skill and capacity to bear witness and engage in inner stillness, to be with the suffering and the sufferer fully in the moment, bearing witness without judgment.

Clients seek professional coaching for many reasons, including to help them explore possibilities and new directions in life, to celebrate successes and identify opportunities for personal and professional development, to enhance quality of life, and to improve relationships. Clients who come for coaching for such reasons usually are not focused solely on problems to overcome or issues to manage but are seeking opportunities to enrich a current way of being.

Other clients come with specific problems and health challenges, seeking nurse coaching to improve management of acute or chronic conditions. Their challenges may be related to self-esteem and self-image, fear and self-confidence, and general adaptation to actual or perceived changes. Other clients seek coaching to learn to handle personal and workplace challenges and stressors or to learn new behaviors in relation to improving health through nutrition, exercise, weight management, enhanced sleep, or

---

* This section is used with permission and adapted from Dossey, B. M., Luck, S. and Schaub, B. G. *Integrative Nurse Coaching for Health and Wellness.* Huntington, NY: Florence Press, 2012.

EXHIBIT 9-1   Interventions Frequently Used in Nurse Coaching Practice

Affirmation	Holistic Self-Assessments	Prayer
Appreciative Inquiry	Humor and Laughter	Presence
Aromatherapy	Intention	Probing Questions
Art	Journaling	Reflection
Celebration	Meditation	Relaxation Modalities
Client Assessments	Mindfulness Practice	Ritual
Cognitive Reframing	Motivational Interviewing	Self-Care Interventions
Contracts	Movement	Self-Reflection
Deep Listening	Music and Sound	Silence
Exercise	Observation	Somatic Awareness
Goal Setting	Play	Stories
Guided Imagery	Powerful Questions	Visioning

Source: Used with permission. Copyright © 2012. *Professional Nurse Coach Role: Defining the Scope of Practice and Competencies.*

stress management. An important area for nurse coaching is in working with clients who are facing end-of-life issues, either their own or those of loved ones, as well as those clients who are living with loss and grief.

By using a patient-centered, relationship-centered process, the nurse coach accompanies the client through the change and discovery processes during coaching sessions. Held within this safe relationship and environment, the coaching journey can arrive at a successful conclusion.

With a four-quadrant approach, the nurse coach is more likely to coach in a way that helps the client approach change, new behaviors, and insights that can be embodied and sustained. Embodying a new capacity means that the individual starts with a new idea and then comes to understand its full meaning and implications. For example, a person becomes aware of using a focused breathing practice to become more present and to feel connected in the present moment. This self-awareness practice starts as an idea that then becomes an action that ends as a capacity that is integrated throughout the day.

The discussion that follows provides more information on the four quadrants.

Coaching and the Four Quadrants

There are many approaches to coaching. An integral approach to coaching assists clients to change and sustain changes. Joanne Hunt,[23] founder and master certified coach of Integral Coaching Canada, mapped the four quadrants

and the role of the coach in each quadrant.[24] She explores how various coaching schools think change occurs and how these views shape the role of the coach. This integral process and the four quadrants are described as follows:

Upper left quadrant (UL): A UL coaching approach considers change to occur through the process of bringing what is unconscious, what resides in the client's inner experience, into conscious awareness, where the client can learn to hear it, recognize it, understand it, and give it voice. The inherent knowledge and wisdom come from within the client.

Coach's role in the upper left quadrant: The coach's role is to hold the space and ask questions to open the client more fully to her or his inner world. This opening brings awareness of beliefs, fears, and obstacles as well as wisdom, inner truth, and intelligence. The coach listens attentively to learn the client's perspective and underlying beliefs at both the personal and existential levels. This coaching approach emphasizes the client's interiority—inner awareness, reflection, and wisdom, and the connections with possibilities beyond the self. With this approach, clients build cognitive capacities, increase their ability to choose and make changes, and broaden their emotional perspective and understanding. This alone does not always lead to translation and integration in daily life, however. The coach is encouraged to address the elements of all four quadrants to come closer to a full coaching process.

Upper right quadrant (UR): A UR coaching approach considers that change occurs through deliberate action and goal setting, breakthroughs, and completing projects.

Coach's role in the upper right quadrant: The nurse coach's role is to help the client set behavior goals and design an action plan. The nurse coach works with clients as they begin to implement their plan. As clients accomplish goals, demonstrate new skills, and achieve new results, they build self-confidence and self-esteem. Clients may rely on a coach's skills and encouragement to sustain change.

Lower left quadrant (LL): The LL coaching approach to change is sparked through inter-action and shared meaning making between individuals. This intersubjective sharing gives rise to new ideas and perspectives that would not be fully available in isolation.

Coach's role in the lower left quadrant: The coach's role is as the client's conversational partner, with the client acting as the "thinking partner." It is the voice of the coach as "other" that helps expand and shift the client's perspective. This process occurs as the nurse coach remains fully present, staying attuned to the story line and following threads that may spontaneously arise. This allows for the possibility of deeper intimacy and insight witnessed and understood. Although the client accesses much information and new insights, if other quadrants are not addressed, the client may not be able to sustain change because coaching is insufficient and partial.

Lower right quadrant (LR): An LR coaching approach to change involves optimizing the function and fit of the client within the overall system (family, work, community). For example, in a work setting, the client may explore ways to improve skills, evaluate roles, recognize expectations, or consider other issues rel-evant to the work environment. The question then may arise as to how the client can align with, adapt to, contribute to, or influence the system or move to another position or job where there is a better fit. If the system being explored is the family, it becomes imperative for the client and coach to examine how new behaviors will affect the family.

Coach's role in the lower right quadrant: The coach's role requires a systems view and understanding of work and group interactions. The elements at play may include team structure, operating principles, organizational procedures, personal and professional relationships, and other factors that affect a system. The coach works with the client to determine the dynamics and how to interact at the desired level in the system. The coach helps the client determine the extent to which she or he can influence the system or discover whether another system is a better fit. This also applies to coaching around family structure. A focus on only this quadrant without connecting to the other quadrants is incomplete and partial.

The Four Quadrants and Coaching Approach Summary

Creating the conditions for sustainable change requires an exploration of the individual's inner space of interiority (UL); the outer space of actions, goals, and timelines (UR); shared space of relationships (LL); and outer space of systems/structures (LR). To neglect any quadrant leaves a client with insights and actions but no way to fully understand the challenges and succeed in integrating and sustaining the desired changes.

Coaching Conversations

Coaching conversations have a beginning (reasons for seeking coaching, a greeting, quick update), a middle (where the majority of time is spent), and an end (agreeing on next session date, reviewing action plan and other possibilities, completion of coaching sessions). After the client determines the topic for the coaching session, the nurse coach uses presence, intention, intuition, and deep listening to determine the most powerful questions to ask the client.

Following the intake process in the initial coaching session, and during all other coaching sessions, the coach becomes aware of how the client orients in the world. Does the person come from a place of reflection (UL)? Is the client focused on actions and accomplishing a project or assignment (UR)? Does the client need to engage with another to explore meaning and understanding (LL)? Does the client seek to know the big picture within a system/structure (LR)?

Use of silence, often referred to as the "power of the pause," throughout a coaching session allows time for both the client and the nurse coach to reflect on the process of discovery and insight. Further possibilities also emerge in the conversation, and the integrative nurse coach may rephrase what the client shares, leading to an opportunity to go deeper into the client's story.

As the coach listens to the client's responses to questions or insights, it is important for the coach to remember that moments of insight and "Ah-ha" moments are often examples of the mind grasping something new.[24] This insight is often just transitory and not yet embodied as a lived experience. This is where the coaching agreement and coaching sessions evolve to guide the client to desired skill building and commitments to specific actions.

Not all coaching leads to action. Insights can be very useful in understanding barriers to change. They may result in identifying thoughts that get in the way of achieving goals. In this way, they are extremely beneficial. Assisting a person in the recognition of the need for an adjustment in attitude or in challenging a belief may, in and of itself, be the catalyst for change.

The nurse coach is aware that although clients may be very expressive and make many connections, this does not indicate embodiment of insights, goals, and actions. For a change to become embodied a practice must be repeated over and over again. This leads to the creation of new capacities and competencies. Clients learning how to use self-awareness and self-observation throughout the day become able to understand and recognize thoughts, actions, behaviors, body sensations, and postures in the moment when they occur and how they relate to the desired changes.

Coaching, change and the four quadrants, and coaching conversations are foundational components of the Integrative Nurse Coach Certificate Program (INCCP).[7,8] **Figure 9-1** illustrates the common belief structures for change in the INCCP. **Figure 9-2** illustrates the INCCP approach to change. **Figure 9-3** illustrates the INCCP understanding of the middle of coaching conversations with possible questions.

Change and the Integrative Nurse Coach Method and Process

The Integrative Nurse Coach (INC) Method includes the following three components that are fully integrated and have equal value within a client coaching session: (1) Theory of Integral Nursing (TIN); (2) Vulnerability Model (VM); (3) Integrative Functional Health Model (IFHM).[8] The INC methodology is grounded in clinical knowledge and practice in the full spirit of the coaching movement as a human service.

Theory of Integral Nursing

The primary purpose of the Theory of Integral Nursing[20,21] (see Chapter 1) in the INC Method is as a nurse coaching framework to explore the client's inner space of interiority (UL); the outer space of actions, goals, and timelines (UR); the shared space of relationships (LL); and the outer space of systems/structures (LR). The application and understanding of the perspective inherent in these four quadrants allow for translation, new insight(s), and integration of the client's behaviors into daily life. The increase in self-efficacy—the belief that one has the capability of initiating and sustaining a desired behavior—leads to enduring change. Asking the client questions and weaving perspectives from these four quadrants throughout a coaching session reflect wholeness. The primary use of the TIN within the INC Method and process is to listen to the client's narrative along the dimensions of I/WE/IT:

- *I* refers to the client's subjective truth, awareness, and insight (internal) of her or his narrative of the current self (CS).
- *WE* refers to the client–nurse coach relationship and how this relationship can foster and support a process of change.
- IT refers to the facts and actions (external) that will move the client from her or his current self toward the desired goals of the

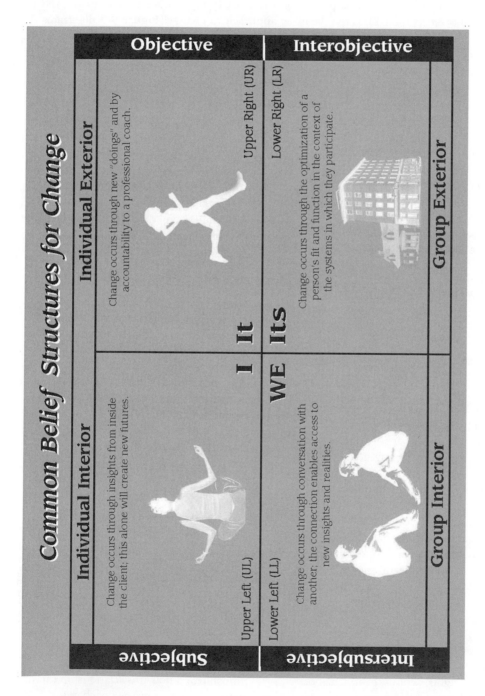

FIGURE 9-1   Common Belief Structures for Change

Source: Copyright © 2010. Integrative Nurse Coach Certificate Program (INCCP). www.iNurseCoach.com. Used with permission from Dossey, B. M., Luck, S. and Schaub, B. G. *Integrative Nurse Coaching for Health and Wellness*. Huntington, NY: Florence Press, 2012. Adapted with permission from Joanne Hunt, "Transcending and Including our Current Way of Being," *Journal of Integral Theory and Practice*, Spring, 4, no. 1 (2009): 1-20 and Integral Coaching Institute Canada, Inc. www.integralcoachingcanada.com.

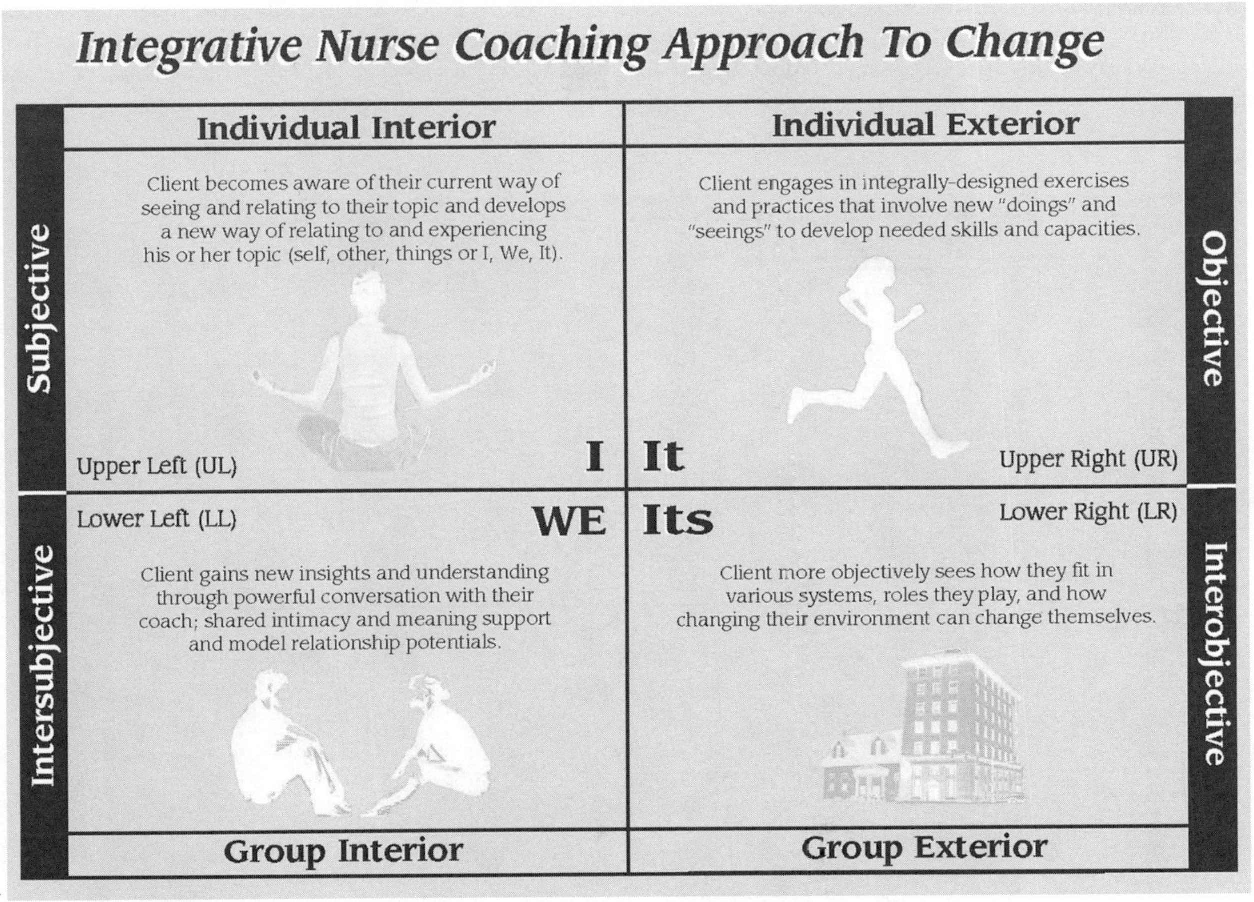

Integrative Nurse Coaching Approach To Change

	Objective	Interobjective
Individual Interior	**Individual Exterior**	
Client becomes aware of their current way of seeing and relating to their topic and develops a new way of relating to and experiencing his or her topic (self, other, things or I, We, It).	Client engages in integrally-designed exercises and practices that involve new "doings" and "seeings" to develop needed skills and capacities.	
I Upper Left (UL)	**It** Upper Right (UR)	
WE Lower Left (LL)	**Its** Lower Right (LR)	
Client gains new insights and understanding through powerful conversation with their coach; shared intimacy and meaning support and model relationship potentials.	Client more objectively sees how they fit in various systems, roles they play, and how changing their environment can change themselves.	
Subjective	**Group Interior**	**Group Exterior**
Intersubjective		

FIGURE 9-2 Integrative Nurse Coaching Approach to Change

Source: Copyright © 2010. Integrative Nurse Coach Certificate Program (INCCP). www.iNurseCoach.com. Used with permission from Dossey, B. M., Luck, S. and Schaub, B. G. *Integrative Nurse Coaching for Health and Wellness.* Huntington, NY: Florence Press, 2012. Adapted with permission from Joanne Hunt, "Transcending and Including our Current Way of Being," *Journal of Integral Theory and Practice,* Spring, 4, no. 1 (2009): 1-20 and Integral Coaching Institute Canada, Inc. www.integralcoachingcanada.com.

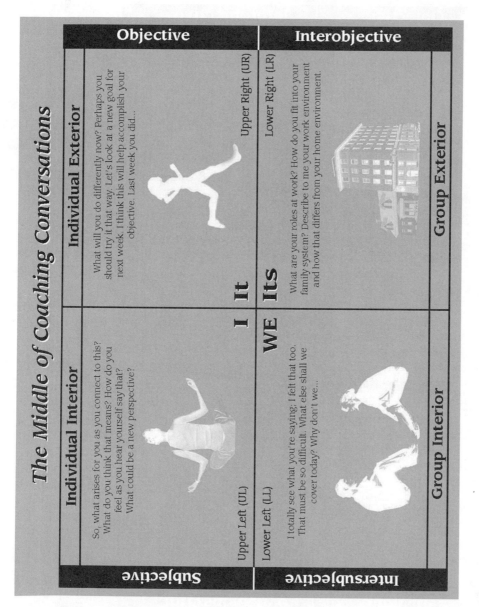

FIGURE 9-3 Middle of Four Different Coaching Conversations

Source: Copyright © 2010. Integrative Nurse Coach Certificate Program (INCCP). www.iNurseCoach.com. Used with permission from Dossey, B. M., Luck, S. and Schaub, B. G. *Integrative Nurse Coaching for Health and Wellness*. Huntington, NY: Florence Press, 2012. Adapted with permission from Joanne Hunt, "Transcending and Including our Current Way of Being," *Journal of Integral Theory and Practice*, Spring, 4, no. 1 (2009): 1–20 and Integral Coaching Institute Canada, Inc. www.integralcoachingcanada.com.

individual's transforming self (TS). See the section titled "Change and the Integrative Nurse Coach Five-Step Process" that follows for details.

Vulnerability Model

The purpose of the Vulnerability Model (VM)[8,25] is to aid the client–nurse coach relationship—the WE—to recognize the patterns of vulnerability, reactivity, and resistance that block clients from achieving their stated coaching goals. (See Chapter 24 for more on Vulnerability Model and willfulness, will-lessness, and willingness.) The INC Method also uses the VM for nurse coach self-knowledge to identify reactions to the client that can interfere with the shared environment of the WE.

Integrative Functional Health Model

The primary use of the Integrative Functional Health Model (IFHM)[26-28] in the INC Method is for the coach to listen to and explore the client's story and view the client's patterns of vulnerability, reactivity, and resistance as nonpathologic manifestations of imbalance in one or more dimensions of the client's essential wholeness—

his or her bio-psycho-social-environmental-spiritual nature. (For more information on the Integrative Functional Health Model, see Chapter 13 on nutrition and Chapter 29 on environment.) The IFHM then addresses how the imbalance(s) affect well-being through the INC's mind–body skills, integrative health knowledge, and the expanded, collaborative model that includes nutritional, psychological, and other integrative resources.

The IFHM embraces the Theory of Integral Nursing and Vulnerability Model and acknowledges the influences of the client's beliefs, lifestyle, culture, and community in guiding actions, goals, and plans for transforming self. By addressing the underlying imbalances and healing the client's internal and external environments, the client's desired change(s) are more likely to occur and be sustained.

Change and the Integrative Nurse Coach Five-Step Process

The Integrative Nurse Coach Five-Step Process (**Figure 9-4**) actualizes and integrates the three components of the Integrative Nurse Coach

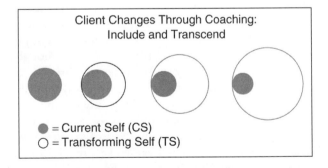

FIGURE 9-4   Client Changes Through Coaching

Legend. Clients bring to coaching their current self (CS) and life story. Through coaching, the client's current self (CS) opens to new opportunities, potentials, and change. The current self begins to shift and a transforming self (TS) emerges, with the outer circle going from black (CS) to gray. With the widening of awareness, transformation (TS) occurs, allowing desired goals and changes to be realized.

Source: Copyright © 2012. Integrative Nurse Coach Certificate Program (INCCP). Used with permission from Dossey, B. M., Luck, S. and Schaub, B. G. *Integrative Nurse Coaching for Health and Wellness.* Huntington, NY: Florence Press, 2012. www.iNurseCoach.com

Method (TIN, VM, and IFHM) just discussed. The five process steps are as follows:

Process 1: Connecting to the story (CS)

Process 2: Deep listening and skillful questioning

Process 3: Inviting opportunities, potentials, and change

Process 4: Practicing, integrating, and embodying change

Process 5: Guiding and supporting the transforming self (TS)

Process 1: Connecting to the Story

Before the coaching session begins, the nurse coach becomes fully present, centered, and grounded. This allows the nurse coach to be fully attentive to the client's topic and the elements of the story. This includes noticing both the affective and energetic state of the client, as well as the content of what the person presents in the initial meeting.

As a starting point, the client may bring a topic or specific intention or goal to the coaching session. If the client cannot identify clearly a topic to work on, the nurse coach, through skillful questioning and/or introducing awareness practices, can assist the client to identify what he or she is hoping for. The nurse coach conveys curiosity about what the client brings to the coaching session. The client provides the subject and direction of the coaching conversation. The nurse coach is open and attentive to what the coaching client presents.

Topics for exploration may be generated by the client's responses and reactions to such tools such as the Integrative Health and Wellness Assessment (IHWA) and Action Plan (see Chapter 8) or aspects of the Theory of Integral Nursing's four quadrants, the Vulnerability Model (VM), or the Integrative Functional Health Model (IFHM).

Nurse coaches align their intentions with clients' goals and attend to clients' subjective experiences and internal frames of reference. This builds trust and respect. The nurse coach's belief in the client's capacity to connect with inner resources, wisdom, and potentials supports the client's current self in the journey toward desired changes and goals. Being present with the client's process of discovery helps the nurse coach to step back from the nurse expert role, remem-

bering the wisdom of "less is more" in the coaching conversation.

Process 2: Deep Listening and Skillful Questioning

The nurse coach lets go of trying to fix a client. The session is conducted through deep listening and skillful questioning. If and when the client moves into vulnerable moments, bearing witness to the client's narrative is essential. *Bearing witness* to a story means being present with patience and respect for things just as they are. This includes learning to be with the client's joys and successes as well as giving full permission for the client to express pain and suffering. *Being curious and open* is attending to the present moment, allowing whatever emerges to come forth. By bringing awareness to her or his own inner wisdom, wealth of experience, and intuition, the nurse coach draws from inner resources to guide the direction of the questioning.

Cultivating a connection with the client that communicates safety and respect creates the opportunity for the client to explore vulnerability, doubts, and challenges as well as strengths, potentials, and successes. Skillful questions move the client toward goals by identifying attitudes, behaviors, and beliefs that have led to past successes and accomplishments. They also help identify blocks and obstacles, both internal and external, which have created limitations. Skillful questioning supports the client in identifying habits of thought and feeling that are self-defeating. Bringing awareness to these patterns provides the client with the possibility of making different choices.

When issues arise in coaching that are outside the scope of the nurse coach's expertise, the coach can make referrals. It is essential that the nurse coach be knowledgeable about and have information and referral sources for professional colleagues and the spectrum of community resources.

Process 3: Inviting Opportunities, Potentials, and Changes

The nurse coach recognizes and respects the client's subjective experiences, perceptions, learning style, and culture (e.g., beliefs, values, and customs). Additionally, the coach continually exhibits authenticity through honesty, sincerity, personal integrity, and maintenance of professional ethics.

Nurse coaching includes planning and negotiating clear actions and agreements as part of the coaching conversation. Following up on agreements and reevaluating their effectiveness or appropriateness are parts of the process, as is altering or creating new action plans when appropriate.

Before any coaching occurs, the nurse coach enters into a coaching agreement with the client. In returning sessions, the coach explores with the client what plans have been kept and reexamines the plans that have not been realized. Periodically reviewing the coaching plan with the client stimulates engagement and helps to identify barriers to change. Holding the person accountable for planned actions, results, and related time frames allows progress to continue as a result of the dynamics in the trusting relationship.

A client's new ideas, behaviors, and actions may feel uncomfortable or even risky as old patterns and habits are challenged. Fear of failure is often an issue. The nurse coach offers ongoing support. When unrealistic or unmanageable goals are established, the nurse coach suggests the client apply the 50% rule, cutting a goal in half to maximize the potential for an initial success.

Process 4: Practicing, Integrating, and Embodying Change

Employing deep listening and powerful questioning, the nurse coach focuses more completely on what the client is communicating. Changing behavior means practicing, integrating, and embodying change and bringing this awareness to day-to-day activities. This awareness opens the opportunity for the client to choose to take new actions and create new ways of thinking and being. This helps in planning ahead, rather than engaging in mindless, habituated behavior. This embodied change brings the possibility of being liberated from self-defeating patterns and thoughts with the spirit of engagement in new health behaviors and choices.

Encouraging and supporting the client in experimenting and applying what has been learned from the coaching interaction leads to new behaviors and sustained change. The nurse coach is an ally and support in this relationship. Being mindful of the power inherent in the coaching relationship, the nurse coach offers encouragement and feedback that is nonjudgmental, respectful, and appropriate. This allows the client to feel free to express strong feelings without fear of judgment.

When assessing the client's communication process, the nurse coach attends to the person's breath pattern, facial expressions, body language, vocal quality, and energy. In Skype or phone coaching conversations, the nurse can observe breathing patterns, vocal quality, and energy. When clients acknowledge that change is hard, they can identify their resistance and ambivalence to change. Clients who understand their own patterns of resistance gain an opportunity for self-awareness and growth.

Process 5: Guiding and Supporting the Transforming Self

The integral perspective honors the fact that every individual is always negotiating her or his experience at many levels. People observe their present interaction at the same time they are affected by, and shaped by, past experiences, some remembered and some forgotten. Individuals function in a bio-psycho-social-environmental-spiritual reality. Both challenges and opportunities can present themselves in any of these aspects of being.

Skillfully, the nurse coach assists clients in exploring and navigating the narrative of their life stories. Profound changes can occur in this coaching journey when clients are introduced to the power of their imagination. Introducing clients to meditative and imagery awareness practices may offer them an opportunity to identify metaphors, images, or words that resonate with their story. The intimate, personally meaningful quality of these experiences can help in keeping clients aligned with envisioned hopes and intentions. These images, metaphors, and other creative aspects of the coaching experience become useful resources that may be referred to frequently in coaching sessions. These symbols and stories are not static. They become part of a transformative process that can release or reconcile parts of clients' stories that no longer serve them. This coaching discovery process inspires clients to be open to broader perspectives and new ways of being.

As shown in Figure 9-4, the client current self (CS) includes the person's current reality. As changes are made, the old story remains but also opens into another way of being and transcends into the changing and transforming self (TS). The nurse coach recognizes this new way of being and acknowledges the changed behaviors and new commitments.

This process assists the client in recognizing what worked in moving forward. Clarity in what works provides the client with a strong foundation on which to build in the future when other challenges occur. This recognition also provides more insights and elicits opportunities for new commitments or actions. The client's old world-view and assumptions have been challenged. The transforming self becomes integrated into the broadened sense of self, leading to increased self-efficacy, self-esteem, and confidence.

■ NURSE COACHING PROCESS*

The nursing process involves six focal areas: assessment, diagnosis, outcomes, plan, intervention, and evaluation. These six areas are conceptualized as bidirectional feedback loops from each component.[10] The nurse coach uses the holistic caring process,[29] (see Chapter 7) with a shift in terminology and meaning to understand and incorporate the client's subjective experience: from *assessment* to establishing the relationship and identifying readiness for change; from *diagnosis* to identifying opportunities, issues and concerns; from *outcomes to* establishing client-centered goals; from *plan* to creating the structure of the coaching interaction; from *intervention* to empowering clients to reach goals; from *evaluation* to assisting the client to determine the extent to which goals were achieved. The nurse coach understands that growth and improved health, wholeness, and well-being are the result of an ongoing journey that is ever expanding and transformative.

Establishing Relationship and Identifying Readiness for Change (Assessment)

Professional Nurse Coach Role

In a coaching model, the foundation for coaching is laid during the assessment phase of the coaching interaction and establishes the relationship and identifies readiness for change. The nurse

coach begins with becoming fully present with self and client before initiating the coaching interaction. The session proceeds with an assessment, establishing the relationship with the client and listening to the client's subjective experience/story. The nurse coach helps the client assess readiness for change. Assessment is dynamic and ongoing. The nurse coach then determines if the client's concerns are appropriate for coaching or the client would be better served through a referral to psychotherapy or other services and resources.

Identifying Opportunities, Issues, and Concerns (Diagnosis)

Professional Nurse Coach Role

The nurse coach and the client together explore assessment data to determine areas for change. There is no attempt or need to assign labels or to establish a diagnosis. Instead, the nurse coach is open to multiple and fluid interpretations of an unfolding interaction in partnership with the client. This process identifies opportunities and issues related to growth, overall health, wholeness, and well-being. Opportunities for celebrating well-being are explored. The nurse coach understands that acknowledgment promotes and reinforces previous successes and serves to enhance further achievements.

Establishing Client-Centered Goals (Outcomes)

Professional Nurse Coach Role

The nurse coach assists the client in identifying goals that will lead to the desired change. The nurse coach values the evolution and the process of change as it unfolds. The nurse coach employs an overall approach to each coaching interaction that is designed to facilitate achievement of client goals.

Creating the Structure of the Coaching Interaction (Plan)

Professional Nurse Coach Role

The nurse coach with the client develops a coaching plan that identifies strategies to attain goals. The nurse coach structures the coaching interaction with a coaching agreement that identifies specific parameters of the coaching relationship, including coach and client responsibilities.

---

* This section is used with permission and adapted from Hess et al.'s *Professional Nurse Coaching: Scope of Practice and Competencies.* The reader is referred to this text for specific nurse coaching details and competencies.

Empowering Clients to Reach Goals (Implementation)

Professional Nurse Coach Role

The nurse coach supports the client's coaching plan while simultaneously remaining open to emerging goals based on new insights, learning, and achievements. The nurse coach supports the client in reaching for new and expanded goals using a variety of specific communication skills to facilitate learning and growth.

As key components of the coaching interaction the nurse coach employs effective communication skills such as motivational interviewing, appreciative inquiry, deep listening, and powerful questioning. In partnership with the client, the nurse coach facilitates learning and results by cocreating awareness, designing actions, setting goals, and planning and addressing progress and accountability. The nurse coach chooses interventions based on the client's statements and actions and interacts with intention and curiosity in a manner that assists the client to achieve the client's goals. The nurse coach effectively utilizes her or his nursing knowledge and a variety of skills acquired with additional coach training.

Assisting Client to Determine the Extent to Which Goals Were Achieved (Evaluation)

Professional Nurse Coach Role

The nurse coach partners with the client to evaluate progress toward attainment of goals. The nurse coach is aware that the evaluation of coaching (the nursing intervention) is done primarily by the client, not the nurse, and is based on the client's perception of success and achievement of client-centered goals.

CASE STUDY

Various chapters in this text include case studies related to nurse coaching.

Chapter 10: Brief case studies and coaching interactions using motivational interviewing and appreciative inquiry

Chapter 13: Nutrition and specific nurse coaching interactions

Chapter 22: Weight management and five stages of change details

Chapter 29: Environment and specific nurse coaching interactions

■ CONCLUSION

Nurse coaches are uniquely positioned to coach and engage individuals in the process of meaningful and health-promoting behavioral change. With a renewed focus on prevention and wellness in healthcare reform, now is an important time for the nursing profession to expand its visibility in the emerging coaching paradigm. Professional nurse coaching promotes opportunities for nurses to practice to the full extent of their education and experience in a way that leads to healthy people living in a healthy nation on a healthy planet.

Directions for FUTURE RESEARCH

1. Develop a qualitative research study to identify themes in nurse coach self-development and in coaching skills mastery.
2. Identify the most effective ways to incorporate nurse coaching in acute care settings.
3. Evaluate the effectiveness of nurse coaching in your institution and analyze themes.
4. Determine whether nurse coaching in the clinical setting increases job satisfaction and nurse retention.
5. Develop nurse coaching worksite wellness program and evaluate the long-term effects on finances, retention, quality indicators, and patient experiences.

Nurse Healer REFLECTIONS

After reading this chapter, the nurse healer will be able to answer or to begin a process of answering the following questions:

- How do I describe the role of nurse coach and nurse coaching to colleagues and others?
- What new understanding and insight do I have about my own capacity to change a behavior(s) considering an integral perspective and the four quadrants?
- In what ways have I become more aware of phrasing questions to clients/patients and others?
- Do I slow down to listen more deeply?

For a full suite of assignments and additional learning activities, use the access code located in the front of your book to visit this exclusive website: http://go.jblearning.com/dossey. If you do not have an access code, you can obtain one at the site.

NOTES

1. D. Hess, B. M. Dossey, M. E. Southard, S. Luck, B. G. Schaub, and L. Bark, *Professional Nurse Coach Role: Defining the Scope of Practice and Competencies* (in press).
2. Compilation of the Patient Protection and Affordable Care Act, May 2010 http://docs.house.gov/energycommerce/ppacacon.pdf
3. U.S. Department of Health and Human Services, "News Release: Obama Administration Releases National Prevention Strategy" (Washington, DC: USDHHS, June 16, 2011). http://www.hhs.gov/news/press/2011pres/06/20110616a.html.
4. G. Donner and M. Wheeler, *Coaching in Nursing: An Introduction.* (Indianapolis, IN: International Council of Nurses & Sigma Theta Tau, 2009). http://www.icn.ch/pillarsprograms/coaching-in-nursing-an-introduction/coaching-in-nursing-an-introduction.html.
5. Bark Coaching Institute, homepage. http://www.barkcoaching.com.
6. L. Bark, *The Wisdom of the Whole: Coaching for Joy, Health, and Success* (San Francisco, CA: Create Space, 2011).
7. Integrative Nurse Coach Certificate Program. http://www.iNurseCoach.com
8. B. M. Dossey, S. Luck, and B. G. Schaub, *Integrative Nurse Coaching for Health and Wellness* (Huntington, NY: Florence Press, 2012).
9. Watson Caring Science Institute, "Caritas Coaching Education Program (CCEP)." (n.d.). http://www.watsoncaringscience.org/index.cfm/category/3/caritas-coach-education-program-ccep.cfm.
10. American Nurses Association, *Nursing: Scope and Standards of Practice,* 2nd ed. (Silver Spring, MD: NurseBooks.org, 2010).
11. American Nurses Association, *Code of Ethics for Nurses with Interpretive Statements* (Washington, DC: NurseBooks.org, 2001).
12. American Nurses Association, *Nursing's Social Policy Statement: The Essence of the Profession* (Silver Spring, MD: NurseBooks.org, 2010).
13. American Holistic Nurses Association & American Nurses Association, *Holistic Nursing: Scope and Standards of Practice,* 2nd ed. (Silver Spring, MD: NurseBooks.org, 2012).
14. R. Schaub and B. G. Schaub, *The End of Fear: A Spiritual Path for Realists* (Carlsbad, CA: Hay House, 2009).
15. D. Hess, L. Bark, and M. E. Southard, *White Paper: Holistic Nurse Coaching,* paper presented to National Credentialing Team for Professional Coaches in Healthcare at the Summit on Standards and Credentialing of Professional Coaches in Healthcare and Wellness, Boston, MA, September 2010. http://www.wellcoach.com/images/WhitePaperHolisticNurseCoaching.pdf.
16. American Holistic Nurses Certification Corporation, "Certification Process" (n.d.). http://www.ahncc.org/certificationprocess.html.
17. J. Prochaska, J. C. Norcross, and C.C. Di Clemente, *Changing for Good. A Revolutionary Six-Stage Program for Overcoming Bad Habits and Moving Your Life Positively Forward* (New York, NY: Harper Collins, 1995).
18. M. A. Dart, *Motivational Interviewing in Nursing Practice* (Sudbury, MA: Jones & Bartlett, 2011).
19. M. E. Southard, L. Bark, and D. Hess, "Motivational Interviewing and Appreciative Inquiry," in *Holistic Nursing: A Handbook for Practice,* 6th ed., ed. B. M. Dossey and L. Keegan (Burlington, MA: Jones & Bartlett Learning, 2013).
20. B. M. Dossey, "Integral Nursing," in *Integrative Nurse Coaching for Health and Wellness,* ed. B. M. Dossey, S. Luck, and B. G. Schaub (Huntington, NY: Florence Press, 2012).
21. B. M. Dossey, "Integral and Holistic Nursing: Local to Global," in *Holistic Nursing: A Handbook for Practice,* 6th ed., ed. B. M. Dossey and L. Keegan (Sudbury, MA: Jones & Bartlett, 2012).
22. J. Halifax, B. M. Dossey, and C. H. Rushton, *Being With Dying: Compassionate End-of-Life Care Training Guide* (Santa Fe, NM: Prajna Mountain Press, 2007).
23. Integral Coaching Canada, Inc. http://www.integralcoachingcanada.com.
24. J. Hunt, "Transcending and Including Our Current Way of Being," *Journal of Integral Theory and Practice* 4, no. 1 (2009): 1–20.
25. B. G. Schaub and M. Burt, "Addictions and Recovery," in *Holistic Nursing: A Handbook for Practice,* 6th ed., ed. B. M. Dossey and L. Keegan (Burlington, MA: Jones & Bartlett Learning, 2013).
26. S. Luck, "Integrative Functional Health Model," in *Integrative Nurse Coaching in Health and Wellness,* ed. B. M. Dossey, S. Luck, and B. G. Schaub (Huntington, NY: Florence Press, 2012).
27. S. Luck, "Nutrition," in *Holistic Nursing: A Handbook for Practice,* 6th ed., ed. B. M. Dossey and L. Keegan (Burlington, MA: Jones & Bartlett Learning, 2013).
28. S. Luck, "Environment," in *Holistic Nursing: A Handbook for Practice,* 6th ed., ed. B. M. Dossey and L. Keegan (Burlington, MA: Jones & Bartlett Learning, 2013).
29. P. Potter and N. C. Frisch, "The Holistic Caring Process," in *Holistic Nursing: A Handbook for Practice,* 6th ed., ed. B. M. Dossey and L. Keegan (Burlington, MA: Jones & Bartlett Learning, 2013).

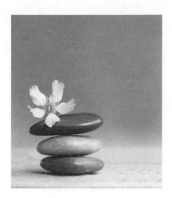

Chapter 10

Facilitating Change: Motivational Interviewing and Appreciative Inquiry

Mary Elaine Southard, Linda Bark, and Darlene R. Hess

Nurse Healer
OBJECTIVES

Theoretical

- Describe each of the four guiding principles of motivational interviewing (MI).
- Identify eight foundational assumptions of appreciative inquiry (AI).
- Describe the 4-D cycle of appreciative inquiry.

Clinical

- Describe the use of appreciative inquiry in a patient-centered exchange.
- Describe the use of motivational interviewing in a patient-centered exchange.

Personal

- Discuss how empathy is an essential component of a helping/caring relationship.
- Explore the importance of a healing presence.
- Describe how active listening enhances nurse–patient interactions.

DEFINITIONS

Appreciative inquiry: Appreciative inquiry (AI) is both a philosophy and a methodology for change. Appreciative inquiry is the study and exploration of strengths as a way to help patients and organizations function at their best. Instead of solving problems, AI is a process in which positive change is facilitated through identifying creative possibilities.

Empathy: An ability to "sense the patient's private world"; an essential component in understanding another person. Human sensitivity is developed by perceiving others and experiencing an awareness of the situation of the other.

Motivational interviewing: Motivational interviewing (MI) is an intervention strategy for changing behavior. The central purpose of MI is to help patients explore and eventually resolve ambivalence in reference to a current health behavior. MI emphasizes client choice and responsibility and can be used in a variety of clinical settings.

Nurse coaching: Holistic nurse coaching is skilled, purposeful, results-oriented, and structured relationship-centered interactions with clients provided by registered nurses for the purpose of promoting the health and well-being of the whole person. Nurse coaching is grounded in the principles and core values of holistic nursing. Effective nurse coaching interactions involve the ability to create a coaching partnership, build a safe space, and be sensitive to client issues of trust and vulnerability as a basic foundation for further exploration.[1] Nurse coaches are able to structure a coaching session, explore client readiness for coaching, facilitate achievement of the client's desired goals, and cocreate a means of determining and evaluating desired outcomes and goals.[2]

Therapeutic presence: Therapeutic presence is the conscious intention to be fully present for another person as a way to promote health, healing, wholeness, and well-being. Presence is generally defined as a multidimensional state of being available in a situation or exchange with another, acknowledging the sacred quality and interconnectedness of each person. Presence involves letting go of past or future concerns, resulting in the creation of an opening or opportunity to reveal what is needed in the moment.[3] Presence requires awareness, authenticity, and an appreciation of being in the moment.

Transtheoretical Stages of Change Model (Transtheoretical Model): The Transtheoretical Stages of Change Model is a model of behavioral change developed by Prochaska and DiClemente in 1984.[4] The five stages of the model are precontemplation, contemplation, preparation, action, and maintenance. Interventions designed to promote behavioral change are tailored to the individual's readiness for change. Relapses and recycling through the stages frequently occur. Relapse provides valuable information to assist in further change and is not viewed as a failure.

■ INTRODUCTION

This chapter concerns two holistic interventions nurses can learn and use in professional nursing practice to support client behavior change to enhance client health and well-being. Nurses have always been involved in health promotion and disease prevention. As healthcare systems developed over the past 50 years, nurses have witnessed the redirection of funding from health promotion efforts, primarily delivered through public health departments, to disease care delivered increasingly by private institutions and funded by complex payment mechanisms. Nurses have advocated for increased attention to the role that nurses play in assisting clients to adopt healthier lifestyles and change unhealthy health behaviors. Now policy makers, health pro-

fessionals, and the general public are awakening to the fact that unless significant changes are made, our nation will become increasingly burdened by runaway healthcare costs for treatment of conditions that could be eliminated or significantly ameliorated by behavioral changes. A report by the Kaiser Family Foundation (2010) indicates that workers are paying a notably larger share of health insurance expenses.[5] The cost of the average annual premium for a family policy increased 114% in the past decade and worker contributions accelerated 147%. More than a quarter of insured workers—up from 10% in 2006—now have a deductible of at least $1,000 for single coverage alone. Experts forecast that out-of-pocket expenses will continue to go up.

As a result of these huge healthcare cost increases, employers and insurance companies are looking for ways to lessen disease progression and promote policies and create systems that lead to improved health. Health professionals are looking for effective and cost-efficient ways to help clients make health behavior changes. Hospitals are exploring and developing coordinated systems to decrease hospitalizations, to reduce use of medications and other costly treatments, and to enhance the effectiveness of the care provided by health professionals. Health promotion and disease management programs now offer incentives to promote self-management. Unfortunately, many of these programs do not produce the desired results.

New approaches are needed to assist patients to achieve lasting behavior change. "Health professionals cannot assume that the only path to improving healthy lifestyles is looking for clients' problems in compliance and solving them."[6pS72] Ever-increasing numbers of nurses are learning evidence-based ways to assist clients to make the behavioral changes that can lead to improved health and well-being. Holistic nurse coaches are taking the lead in establishing models of coaching that are designed to engage clients in self-care and management of healthcare practices and outcomes.[2] Although there are many holistic strategies and approaches for assisting patients to reach their full potential, two accepted approaches used by many nurses are motivational interviewing and appreciative inquiry. Motivational interviewing is used when someone is ambivalent about change. Appreciative inquiry uncovers and expands what is working in a situation rather than focusing on what is not working.

■ MOTIVATIONAL INTERVIEWING

Motivational interviewing (MI) is a well-known, research-based method of interacting with patients that was developed in the 1980s to improve outcomes associated with substance abuse.[7] MI is a skillful interaction for eliciting motivation for change. The fundamental premise of MI is that patients are often ambivalent to change, and ambivalence affects a patient's motivation and readiness to alter behavior.[8]

The Transtheoretical Model created by DiClemente and Prochaska guides MI.[7] DiClemente and Prochaska noticed that people frequently do not succeed in changing behavior on the first attempt and often experience numerous attempts before successfully changing. There are multiple stages, progression, and relapses. Underlying the progressions are the patients' prior experiences with change and how they view the pros and cons of change. Patients consider whether or not they have the skills or resources to make a change.

MI is used in all aspects of behavior change. Motivational interviewing has been identified as an effective tool to improve medication adherence.[9] Adult patients with asthma who participated in a single session of education plus motivational interviewing were more likely to show an increased level of readiness to adhere to medication regimens compared with patients receiving education alone.[10] Patients with schizophrenia who participated in eight motivational interviewing sessions experienced significant improvement in overall psychotic symptoms and attitudes toward and satisfaction with medication compared with usual treatment.[11]

The application of motivational interviewing in addition to a comprehensive behavioral weight loss program has been shown to aid weight loss by increasing motivation. When MI was incorporated into a behavioral weight loss program, participants lost significantly more weight and engaged in significantly greater physical activity than did those in the program who did not receive motivational interviewing.[12]

Numerous studies have been published indicating that the use of MI is an effective intervention to reduce smoking.[13] MI has been shown to be more effective with a variety of medical problems than traditional clinical advice giving. MI can help people reduce alcohol consumption, lose weight, and lower blood pressure.[14]

Guiding Principles of Motivational Interviewing

Motivational interviewing is based on four guiding principles known by the acronym RULE:[15]

- *Resist the righting reflex.* The "righting reflex" is the natural tendency of the nurse to fix a patient's problems by imposing solutions.[16] The nurse must set aside any desire to correct the course and direction of the client. If the nurse is pushing for change and the client is resisting, the nurse is in the wrong role; it is the client who should be voicing the arguments for change. The nurse must suppress what may seem like the right thing to do and instead allow the client to determine what to do.
- *Understand and explore the client's motivation.* It is the client's reasons for change, and not the nurse's, that are likely to trigger change. The nurse explores the client's concerns, perceptions, and motivations. Allowing patients to tell their story and encouraging them to discuss not only their reason for change but also how they might see themselves make those changes is the core of the partnership.
- *Listen with empathy.* Answers lie within the client, and finding them requires listening. Good listening is a complex skill; it is more than asking questions and keeping quiet long enough to hear the reply. Empathy has been defined as a complex, multidimensional phenomenon[16] but is typically understood as the ability to identify with the client's difficulties or feelings. The ability to express empathy enhances the ability to engage patients in making necessary health changes and is a key component of MI.
- *Empower and encourage hope and optimism.* The nurse helps the client discover *how* change can happen. The nurse views the client as the expert consultant as ideas and resources for change are explored. Providing ongoing encouragement to foster the belief that the goals are achievable can help the patient carry out a plan to change behavior.

Partnering with Clients

By honoring client autonomy and effectively creating a collaborative partnership between patient and provider, nurses enable patients to become involved in identifying goals and determining how best to achieve them. Individuals are naturally motivated to improve their own well-being, and their willingness to become involved in managing their own care is closely tied to their ability to set goals and to their hopes for the future.[17] Accessing a client's hope for improved outcomes is a vital component of effective coaching for change.[18] The nurse applying an MI strategy seeks to evoke client strengths and to activate client motivation and resources for change.

MI is a refined form of guiding and includes skillful informing. The process of listening and guiding patients is a quite different stance from telling patients what they "should" be doing in terms of positive healthcare practices. For example, telling a patient she needs to cut down on calories or providing her with a dietary referral may be a misstep or lost opportunity to engage in meaningful dialogue that uncovers information that can enhance outcomes.

In motivational interviewing, the goal of the nurse coach is not to point out discrepancies between goals and behavior but to incrementally guide the patient to self-discovery. Self-efficacy is supported when the patient realizes that behavior and goals are not congruent and makes a conscious decision to make necessary changes. Nurses who utilize MI understand that it is not the nurse's job to fix the patient or the patient's problems. To attempt to do so places responsibility on the nurse and promotes either dependency on the nurse or leads to "difficult" patients who do not listen to the information or advice provided by the nurse.[19] Nurses using MI learn to go down the patient's path rather than create the path and expect the patient to follow.

Communication Skills

To negotiate behavior change successfully, nurses must build on basic communication skills and establish a therapeutic environment. Holistic nurses understand that sacred presence is invaluable in setting the stage for exploring the change process. Coaching clients to achieve their desired goals involves developing and honing specific communication techniques such as reflective listening, asking open-ended questions, and using clarifying statements. Using active/reflective listening ensures that the nurse understands the patient and his or her readiness to initiate change. Open-ended questions foster dialogue and the ability to gauge deficits/strengths in relation to desired changes. Inquiring about what the patient already knows and asking if the person would like additional information show respect.

Self-awareness is a necessary component of effective partnering with clients to effect change. Communication is facilitated when the nurse is aware of his or her voice inflections, posturing, or self-talk when interacting with a patient.

Practitioner time constraints and the perception by the client of a hurried approach can be a challenge and a barrier to empathic active listening. This can lead to unintended results and patient dissatisfaction. Increased use of technology has created streamlined documentation and time-saving record keeping processes while unfortunately often creating barriers to being fully present. However, motivational interviewing can be a time-saver by identifying the patient's goals, concerns, and ideas before proceeding with potentially ineffective interventions.

Application of Motivational Interviewing in the Clinical Setting

MI can be used in a variety of clinical settings. The following case study illustrates how MI can be used to assist a patient to stop smoking.

MOTIVATIONAL INTERVIEWING CASE STUDY

Setting: Clinic

Patient: J. V., a 64-year-old woman with a history of severe chronic obstructive pulmonary disease (COPD)

Patterns/challenges/needs: Wants to stop smoking

J. V. has been diagnosed with severe COPD, has had several hospitalizations over the last 4 years, and continues to smoke heavily. Last year, she was in the precontemplation stage of smoking cessation with denial statements that ranged from "I don't have a problem" to "I don't have any willpower and I could never stop smoking." However, following her most recent hospitalization, she moved into the contemplation stage of change, realized she did have a problem and wanted to do something about it, but still she believed she couldn't stop smoking.

A clinic nurse decided to use motivational interviewing to structure her conversation with J. V. In the left column of the following dialogue is the conversation between the patient and the nurse. In the right column are some guidelines for motivational interviewing.

Patient and Nurse Conversation	Motivational Interviewing Guidelines
Nurse: Good afternoon, Mrs. V. It is good to see you again.	
J. V.: Thanks. I like seeing you, too. It's nice when I get to see the same person.	
Nurse: It's nice for me, too. It allows me to follow up with patients, and I know that last time after your hospitalization you described the pros and cons of quitting smoking.	Motivational interviewing is especially designed to deal with people who are ambivalent about making health changes.
J. V.: Oh, I hate even talking about that. I just have no idea how I would ever give up that habit. You know I have been smoking since I was 16.	
Nurse: I can understand why you feel that way, but last time you did have some interest in thinking about reducing your smoking.	Validate the patient's feelings and experiences.
J. V.: Yes, you're right. Being in the hospital was really awful, and the doctor showed me some pictures of my lungs and how my smoking makes them worse.	
Nurse: So, you actually saw with your own eyes how smoking hurts your lungs?	Reinforce reasons for change and repeat in simple, direct statements about the effects of patient's choices.
J. V.: Yes, it was quite obvious.	
Nurse: How has your decreased lung capacity affected your life?	Explore potential concerns.
J. V.: Well, it does really limit my activity. I have a grandchild who is now 2 years old and I can't keep up with him at all. I can see that my capacity to be with him is getting worse. And, of course, just shopping and other activities are limited. My family is after me all the time to quit smoking. Even my older grandchildren are starting on me.	
Nurse: It is hard to change something in your life when others are pressuring you. It's up to you to make this decision about when and if you want to make a change in this behavior. Thanks for even talking to me about this. I know it is hard for you.	Acknowledge the patient's control of the decision.
J. V.: Yes, it is, and it's nice that you know that.	
Nurse: I remember that we talked about your interest in smoking before, and using a 1 to 10 scale, you said you were at a 5. What is the number today?	Explore interest in change.
J. V.: Hum. Let me see. I guess it has moved up to a 6.	
Nurse: What does that number mean to you and how would you define it in words?	Explore meaning about change.

Patient and Nurse Conversation	Motivational Interviewing Guidelines
J. V.: Well, I guess it means that I want to stop smoking more than I don't want to. Maybe I have fallen off the fence this time, but you know I can always get back on the fence.	
Nurse: Of course, using your control to change is always your decision.	Reinforce the fact that the patient has control.
J. V.: Yes, you're right.	
Nurse: Tell me why you chose a 6 today?	Explore how things have changed.
J. V.: I just keep thinking about how my breathing limits my life and it makes me want to stop.	
Nurse: I understand how your life would be different if you changed your smoking habit.	Reinforce concerns and the benefits of changing behaviors.
J. V.: I think about stopping, but then I get really scared and think I can't do it.	
Nurse: So, you have an interest, desire, reasons, and a need to change, but you are worried about your ability? If we were to rate your ability to change on that 1 to 10 scale, what would your number be?	Assess interest, desire, reasons, needs, ability, and commitment as appropriate.
J. V.: Now *that* is the real question. I think it is a zero. If it were higher, all those other numbers would go up too.	
Nurse: So, your belief that you can do it is really what is holding you back now. What would move you from zero to one?	Explore what would need to change for movement toward behavior change.
J. V.: Well when you ask that question, it doesn't seem too hard, but I still don't know. I really don't know what would work for me to go from zero to one.	
Nurse: Almost every person who quits smoking starts being concerned about their ability to change their smoking habit. If it is okay, I would like to tell you some things that have helped other people.	Reframe concern about inability to change.
J. V.: Okay.	
Nurse: One of the patients who talked with me this morning began by cutting out one cigarette a day. Yesterday, a man decided not to smoke in one room of his house. Last week, a woman decided she would not smoke from 10 AM to 11 AM just to see if she could get some control of her habit.	Offer suggestions that are beginning steps for change.
J. V.: I can see how that might work for them, and something like that might work for me. Now I am almost at a 1.	
Nurse: That is great to see change in your belief about your ability to quit smoking. I see that our time is moving to a close here. What kind of change, if any, do you want to make this next week?	Reinforce change.
J. V.: Well, I guess I could say that I won't smoke between 10 AM and 11 AM. I don't think I smoke much then anyway, so I think it will be easy. I kind of feel good about some kind of beginning.	

Patient and Nurse Conversation	Motivational Interviewing Guidelines
Nurse: So, the initial goal is to limit smoking during that hour. On that old 1 to 10 scale, how committed are you to follow through on that goal?	Encourage small, initial steps. Assess commitment.
J. V.: I don't exactly know. I suppose I am pretty high . . . maybe an 8 and don't ask me how to get to a 9. I am happy with an 8.	
Nurse: An 8 is great! I am very happy for you and really look forward to talking with you about this experiment at your next appointment. Congratulations on your progress today.	Encourage small, steady steps.
J. V.: Well, to tell you the truth, it feels good to me, too. I never thought I could take this first step. And even though I asked you not to ask me about what would get me to a 9, when you called my not smoking for an hour a day an experiment, that made it sound more doable and not so scary.	

In the next session, J. V. reported that she was able to limit smoking during that hour on all the weekdays. She found the weekends harder because she had more free time. Even though she didn't meet her goal of 1 hour every day, she did begin to feel that she had some beginning control of smoking. The nurse continued to work with her on her ability, and the patient enrolled her family for support. The patient's road to smoking cessation was long and somewhat bumpy, but after 9 months she did stop smoking and was very proud of herself. The empowerment she gained from changing that very long-standing habit allowed her to address other areas of her lifestyle with positive results.

■ APPRECIATIVE INQUIRY

Appreciative inquiry (AI) is another increasingly popular change method that originated from organizational systems development. *To appreciate* is to see the best in a situation or another person, while *to inquire* is to explore and discover. Thus, AI is a way of asking questions that creates relationships based on the basic goodness in a person, situation, or organization. Nurses can utilize AI principles and processes to assist patients to build on their inherent strengths as a way to design and create their desired future. The main precept of appreciative inquiry is that individuals in relationships with one another can cocreate an effective future that inspires new possibilities.[20]

AI differs from other change processes by focusing on transformational change—change that transforms and energizes a person, situation, or organization. AI is explicitly contrasted with problem solving, which the originators of AI describe as a deficit-based approach to change.[21] Although Cooperrider, Whitney, and Stavros describe the use of AI to effect organizational change, their discovery is that momentum for change and long-term sustainability increased the more they abandoned "delivery" ideas of action planning, monitoring progress, and building implementation strategies.[22] Such strategies are not grounded in transformational change patterns. Organizations that have utilized AI as a change strategy have achieved notable successes. Appreciative inquiry promotes a united approach to change,[23] fosters collaboration,[24,25] and serves to build trust among workers.[26]

Rather than focusing on problems that need solving, AI focuses on imagining the best or highest outcome for the organization or client. The traditional model of disease management, for example, is in direct contrast to AI. In the disease management model, the focus is on diagnosing the problem, generating and selecting change options, and then suggesting strategies to implement the change. However, with AI, "problems" are seen as opportunities to be embraced, and the inquiry is directed toward the exploration of possibilities and the creation of a new future based on what is already working—on what is good—on what is best about the situation.

As a method of inquiry, AI has the potential to inspire patients to consider a situation previously seen as hopeless as one that can evolve to something much better. AI can lead to recognition of limiting patterns of behavior so that new behaviors can be adopted. The focus is one in which the nurse holds the space for the client to see with a "new lens of perception." AI provides a way to address the discouragement felt by patients when their successes and achievements are overlooked and the focus is instead on the dire consequences of their diagnosis or on things that have not gone well.

Appreciative inquiry is based on the belief that change begins the moment a question is asked. Thus, the seeds of change are implicit in the very first questions asked by the nurse. The idea is that clients will move in the direction of the questions that are asked. Holistic nurse coaches who use AI pay close attention to the exact wording and the provocative potential of the questions. They know that the words they choose have an impact far beyond the words themselves. They understand that words create worlds and positive questions lead to positive changes. They attend carefully to the client's story, noting how language is used to convey sentiments, meanings, worldviews, and images. As they tune in to the client's reality, they ask questions that invoke new images and that serve to refashion that reality so that a new future can be brought into the present. AI is based on the conviction that successful change begins with images of the future, and images of the future affect present-day performance. Hopeful and positive images lead to positive actions.

Foundational Assumptions of Appreciative Inquiry

Hammond proposes eight assumptions about AI that are useful in understanding the AI process as a vehicle for change:[27]

1. In every society, organization, or group, something works.
2. What we focus on becomes our reality.
3. Reality is created in the moment, and there are multiple realities.
4. The act of asking questions of an organization or group influences the group in some way.

5. People have more confidence and comfort to journey to the future (the unknown) when they carry forward parts of the past (the known).
6. If we carry parts of the past forward, they should be what is best about the past.
7. It is important to value differences.
8. The language we use creates our reality.

4-D Cycle of Appreciative Inquiry

The main intervention model that has come to be associated with appreciative inquiry is the 4-D Cycle.[22] The model consists of four components: discovery (inquiry), dream (imagining what could be), design (how to), and destiny (what will be) (**Figure 10-1**). The aim of the 4-D AI Cycle is transformational change that originates in collaborative inquiry with participants. Use of the 4-D Cycle creates a method to achieve an organic, collaborative way of working for positive and sustainable learning and change.[28]

The 4-D process enables individuals to discover their foundation of strengths—their positive core. By doing this before envisioning the future (dream), articulating designs for change (design), and establishing a path forward (destiny), they create confidence and hope for the future.[29] They experience pride and recognition as they share their unique stories of success and weave them into dreams for the future. When people engage with others in conversations about what works well, they learn about capabilities and they gain confidence in their capacity for achievement. The 4-D Cycle evokes and supports a life-affirming consciousness that leads to the realization of desired results. Whitney concludes that the implicit spiritual nature of AI and the 4-D Cycle of inquiry has emerged as a key success factor.[29]

Discovery involves the identification of opportunities for improvement that build on previous accomplishments. The focus is on appreciating the best that the current situation has to offer. The nurse coach might ask questions such as: "What helps you to feel happy, positive, or motivated?" "What has been most helpful to you in this situation?" "What do you do well concerning this situation?" "Based on what you already know about this condition, what else do you want to learn?"

The *dream* phase involves creatively imagining the future. In this phase, the focus is on merging

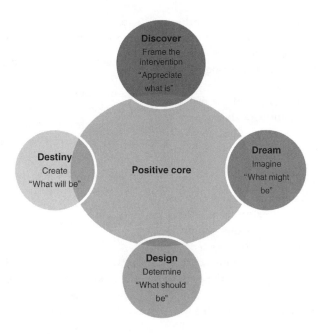

FIGURE 10-1   4-D Cycle Model

the best of what is with a vision of what could be. In this phase, the client's story, insights, and viewpoint are put to constructive use to come up with a vision of how things could be better. The nurse coach might ask questions such as: "What challenges do you anticipate and how might you meet them?" "Imagine a time when you felt healthy and energetic. What was significant to you when you felt this way?" "What possibilities do you see for yourself?"

In the *design* phase, the focus is on determining the structure for the envisioned future. Typically, choices must be made. The nurse coach might ask questions such as: "Of all the things you have imagined for your future, what is the one area you would like to focus on before our next visit?" "What would it take for you to make that change?" "How will you achieve that goal?" "How can you make your dream a reality for you?"

The *destiny* phase is when the nurse helps the client focus on the new future that is being created. The emphasis is on empowerment of the client and sustaining the learning that has occurred. The nurse might ask questions such as: "Now that you have achieved that goal, what do you think is the most important thing you have learned?" "What will you do to celebrate now that you have accomplished your goal? "If it's

okay with you, may we talk about how you will continue to manage your diabetes?"

Application of Appreciative Inquiry in the Clinical Setting

AI can be applied in numerous ways. The following case studies illustrate how AI can be applied in a variety of situations. Case study 1 illustrates the use of AI to assist unit staff to develop improved collaboration. Case study 2 concerns the application of AI as a means to enhance self-care. Case study 3 is about using AI to assist a patient with diabetes.

CASE STUDY 1

Setting: Medical-surgical unit in a hospital

Client: Unit staff

Patterns/challenges/needs: Improved collaboration

During a staff meeting, several nurses explained that they believed that the staff did not work together well. The nurse manager decided to use appreciative inquiry as a method to address this issue. She discussed this with her supervisor who thought it would be a good idea and was interested in how it might work in this situation.

If it was successful, it could be applied to other units. She thought it could be a pilot project but said the nurse manager would need to do this project within her regular work day. The nurse manager agreed.

First, the nurse manager initiated the discovery part of appreciative inquiry, or the "appreciate the best of what is" phase, by interviewing several of the nurses who spoke in the staff meeting as well as others who did not mention the issue. The short 5- to 10-minute interviews were designed to focus on and make explicit what was working in regard to collaboration. The nurse manager explained that she was using appreciative inquiry to address the item raised by the staff and that it is based on the idea that a group grows in the direction of what the group is focused on. She wanted to focus on what is going well. She further made it clear that she was not ignoring the issue: Quite the opposite, she was addressing the situation with an approach that might really benefit the staff.

The staff nurses seemed puzzled about the approach and wanted to talk about "the problem." Many said that they had never heard of looking at what was working when they were trying to solve a problem. A few thought it was an interesting idea, and most were able to mention some team situations that were effective. Several were surprised that they could come up with some positive examples and said that they had a little hope that perhaps things could change. One nurse, especially, was intrigued with this approach and came to the nurse manager several days after her interview with two more examples of things that were working. She said that she was beginning to see what the nurse manager meant about focusing on what was working because now she was more aware of positive communication and effective teamwork herself. The nurse manager was pleased with the first phase of her appreciative inquiry process because she knew this phase was more than just gathering facts: It was laying the foundation for a new way of thinking, facilitating hope about change, and building relationships and champions to maintain a positive approach.

During the next staff meeting, the nurse manager moved into the dreaming part of the appreciative inquiry process, or the "imagine what could be" part. She led 2 minutes of a relaxation meditation, and then the following guided imagery:

> Imagine a time when you felt that collaboration was really working well on our unit or on some other unit that you worked in the past. Staff was supporting each other easily and things were done well with even a sense of fun and joy. Even though some things happened that could have been a problem, the team took the situations in stride and moved through them quickly, which intensified the positive spirit of the team.

She waited a couple of minutes while the staff was thinking of this image.

Then, she asked each staff member to think about the following questions and write down their answers on a piece of paper: "What was significant in having this happen? How did it happen? Who was involved? What kept it going? If you could change things to your way of thinking, how would you like to see teamwork function on this unit?"

After the group had a few minutes to write down their answers, she gave them the following directions: "Now imagine it is 3 years from now, and our ability to collaborate has grown by 50 or even 100 times our current capacity. Imagine that your fondest wishes for excellent communication and teamwork have flourished. We are featured in an article in our hospital newsletter and then in a prominent nursing journal. What would the article say was happening on the unit each shift and each day? What would be described?"

After this dreaming period, the nurse manager asked people to share their insights and she wrote down the staff's answers on a flip chart. In this designing phase, or the "determine what should be" phase, the group looked for themes concerning the ways it should be. One of the topics brought up in many different ways was communication. Everyone realized that to have good teamwork, all the team members needed the appropriate information so that they could function well as part of the team. Another issue that emerged from the discussion was the need for each team member to know exactly what was expected and when it was needed for the team to function smoothly. One of the nurses brought up the concept of unit culture. In her imagery, everyone really respected one another and she realized that was the expected group norm. The last major trend that was relayed from the exercise had to do with positive acknowledgment. Team members not only felt appreciation for one another, but they demonstrated it often during their time together.

Because it was almost time for the staff meeting to end, the nurse manager asked the staff to select one of the three major themes that had emerged (communication, role clarification, and appreciation) so that they could move into the fourth phase of appreciative inquiry, which is destiny, or the "create what will be" part of the process. Then, she requested they identify one action step. The group came up with the idea of putting sticky notes up in the breakroom to acknowledge a team member who was working well as a good team member. A group of three staff members volunteered to create the process, manage it, and then report on the results at the next staff meeting. The nurse manager said the next staff meeting would be dedicated to planning how all insights could be turned into action steps and asked each staff member to be thinking and dreaming in the meantime for ideas. She ended the meeting by asking each member to state a "takeaway." She realized that about 90% of the comments were based on hope and promise for positive changes.

During the next staff meeting working in the destiny phase of appreciative inquiry, or the "create what will be" part of the process, the Sticky Note Committee reported on the results and said they believed that it worked some of the time but not all of the time. When it worked and staff put them up, people reported that it really felt good. Some staff reported that the more specific it was, the better it felt to them, although others said, "Great Team Member" felt good too and made their day. They thought it was a good beginning but perhaps not really manageable over time. They decided the idea could be used for short periods each month. Then, the group came up with what they called an "Appreciation Week" each month when staff would make it a priority to tell their fellow workers something they really did like about them and the way they worked with

the group. Even though it was only 25% of the time, they felt it would build some good habits.

Over the next year of staff meetings, three groups took over plans to design and implement the three major themes:

- **Communication:** This group developed bullet points and general scripts for shift change, handovers for break relief, and new patient admissions.

- **Role clarification:** The group that addressed this theme realized staff already knew their clinical role. So, they developed a team agreement that spoke to how they treated each other. It included the following:
  - Being respectful to each other
  - Upholding identified values such as honesty, trust, compassion
  - If a conflict came up between two staff members, people agreeing to talk directly to the other person rather than involve others in the disagreement
  - Supporting direct communication for all types of communication rather than gossiping about one another
  - Having some inservice training on how to identify and express needs
  - Arriving on time
  - Helping one another complete work assignments

- **Appreciation:** This group created a variety of ways to acknowledge appreciation for one another:
  - Two-minute team huddles spontaneously during the day and at the end of shift to acknowledge each other and what worked for building team collaboration
  - Appreciation Week
  - Appreciation circles during staff meetings, where each person says something he or she appreciates about each team member
  - Appreciation log where staff and management could write down comments about good teamwork

The appreciative inquiry process was helpful in improving the teamwork of the unit, and the culture of the unit became more positive. Some of the dreaming is coming into fruition. The nurse manager has been asked to share her experience with other managers, and an article in the hospital newsletter is coming out soon about the results of this appreciative inquiry process.

CASE STUDY 2

Setting: Medical-surgical unit

Client: Staff nurse

Patterns/challenges/needs: Self-care

C. B. is a nurse on the unit that is using appreciative inquiry to improve collaboration. She has been surprised by the improvements on the unit and enjoys the changes. She decided to use the appreciative inquiry method to look at her own self-care.

She began with the discovery phase by exploring the part of her exercise program that was working, but she found it hard to come up with much. All she could see was how she wasn't getting exercise in her day, but then she realized that she did take the stairs instead of the elevator and that gave her a glimmer of hope and encouragement that at least she was doing something. It was a choice she made several times a day and she did feel good about herself when she was on the stairs.

Next, she took some time on her weekend off to do the dreaming part of the process. She went into the "imagine what could be" and remembered years ago when she was trying out for a ski team and worked very hard to get in shape and build strength. She recalled how vital she felt and how people commented on her health. Even though she didn't ski for very long because she ended up moving away, the way she felt was anchored in her memory. She remembered another time on a vacation when she did some hiking that involved some steep climbing. When she reached the top of the mountain, she felt very alive. She began to imagine how her life would be if she had more of those experiences. Then, she realized that she could be that healthy. She became clear about the effect that would have on both her professional and personal life. She knew she would lose some weight, which would be wonderful, and she could fit into some old clothes she saved for the time when she would be a size smaller. A shopping trip could

be part of her future when she would be able to purchase some new clothes. Most of her delight in doing this imagery, though, was realizing how she would feel: alive, strong, and positive.

She began the design part of the process and determined what should be in terms of her exercise program. From her past ski training phase she knew that she needed four parts to her program: cardiovascular, core building, strength, and flexibility.

Suddenly, she became excited and really felt motivated as she moved into the destiny part of the appreciative inquiry process. She had received a coupon for a free week at a neighborhood gym just days before her exploration of this issue. So, she thought that could provide the cardiovascular training, strengthening exercises, and maybe the core building as well. A friend had been asking her to attend a yoga class and she realized that would help her with flexibility and reinforce the strengthening of her core and her muscles. She wanted to do it all but told herself to be careful and not take on more than she could complete. Her calendar was full with work and family commitments. She wanted to take slow and steady steps so that she would really make lasting changes. She put together a plan for the month that involved continuing to take the stairs and trying out the neighborhood gym. After a month, she decided that the gym really wasn't successful because it was not open at times that were convenient. During the times she did manage to get to the gym, she had hints of feeling alive and more vital. She knew she was on the right track.

The next month she went with her friend to the yoga studio to start a beginner's class. This didn't work out well because, with her busy schedule and her friend's busy schedule, they were not able to attend the classes together. However, at the studio she found a class that had music and dancing and she loved it. She did not spend the whole time counting the minutes until the class was over. Time flew by and she felt so alive and vital. She had found something that really worked and she made a commitment to it. It was the foundation for increasing her exercise and she realized that many errands or chores could be an excuse for another type of workout that strengthened her core, had her cardiovascular system working hard, and increased her flexibility and strength. At various times she used the four-step appreciative inquiry method to rediscover what was working, to dream of new goals, and to redesign her new destiny. She was delighted with the results.

CASE STUDY 3

Setting: Clinic

Patient: J. W., a 56-year-old man who had recently been diagnosed with type II diabetes

Patterns/challenges/needs: Improved health and well-being

J. W. came in for his routine annual physical for work. Because of his lab results, he was diagnosed with diabetes. He attended a diabetic course that included one individual session after the second of four classes. His nurse inquired into his progress in dealing with his diabetes and learned that J. W. was feeling quite defeated. He felt as if he was not making any progress and he was overwhelmed with the number of changes his doctor and the nutritionists wanted him to make. His nurse believed that using the appreciative inquiry process would be helpful at this point, so she started by seeing what was working—the discovery phase of appreciative inquiry. J. W. began to realize when he and the nurse reviewed the course outline that even if he wasn't where he wanted to be, he had learned a great deal about his disease. He had even made some behavior changes such as eating dessert 50% less often.

Next, the nurse helped him to imagine what his goal might be. When he said he was not where he wanted to be, she asked what he meant by that. What would that look like? How would he be living his life? He described a life that had some limits in terms of what he could eat, but he began to see that not eating so much sugar would probably help him be healthier in the long run. He also began to think that he wanted to increase his exercise program because he used to be a runner when he was younger and really found that to be a great stress reliever. The dreaming phase of this process continued as he wondered whether he could even return to a normal blood sugar level if he really made some significant changes.

J. W. knew that he should address his weight problem and realized that if he was really serious about this challenge, his new diet could help him. He and the nurse explored some of the other changes that would help him move toward a healthier life in the design phase of appreciative inquiry.

Then, their conversation moved to the destiny stage, or the "create what will be" phase, and he put together a plan that included some simple diet changes along with a beginning walking/running program. His nurse helped him set realistic goals so that he would not become overwhelmed and feel discouraged. She set up some time in each of the remaining diabetes education classes so that he, along with other patients, could report on progress with his diet and exercise plan. By the end of his course, he was running three times a week, and although he was not feeling like his diabetes diagnosis was a positive situation in his life, he realized that he was making the best of it and was making progress toward a higher level of health and well-being.

■ THE FUTURE

Current trends in healthcare innovations require obtaining data to support interventions that improve healthcare outcomes. Moore and Charvat pose questions regarding the use of AI with dyads, groups, or with families.[6] Research studies are needed that addresses the influence of MI and AI on patients' behavior over longer lengths of time. Qualitative and quantitative studies that compare the two interventional approaches could perhaps maximize the effects of MI and AI. Studies that evaluate the long-term effectiveness of combining such interventions as MI and AI in promoting healthy behavior change would be useful.

A common concern for nurses and others is how to document and bill for nurse services. Motivational interviewing and appreciative inquiry are dynamic processes and are utilized in multiple encounters with the patient. Depending on personal style and time constraints, nurses will choose to integrate MI/AI techniques into a routine encounter or have the patient schedule specific counseling/coaching sessions. Clear documentation of length of time of visit and topics discussed will enhance future learning and reimbursement.

Because these interventions involve a philosophical approach to care that is different from customary practice in many settings, caution should be taken to adhere to the particular framework of each. Clinicians should not just insert positive questions into the traditional problem-solving mode of diagnosing and treating clients and believe they are using these processes as they are meant to be used.[6]

The use of MI and AI to promote health and well-being for clients provides an opportunity for nurses to deliver care in a manner that is compatible with holistic nursing principles and core values.[30] By doing so, nurses may play a significant role in the transformation of healthcare delivery while simultaneously improving the effectiveness of care and reducing healthcare costs.

■ CONCLUSION

Motivational interviewing and appreciative inquiry are effective strategies for assisting clients to achieve health goals. Each is based on the ability to establish positive relationships, envision possibilities, communicate clearly, and listen attentively. The interpersonal process between each nurse and each client is a key component of MI and AI. The use of MI and AI can support a holistic model of nursing practice that incorporates creative, evidence-based approaches to facilitate change.

Directions for
FUTURE RESEARCH

1. Determine the effectiveness of MI and AI with dyads, families, and groups to sustain behavioral changes over longer periods of time.
2. Conduct qualitative and quantitative studies that compare the effects of MI and AI.
3. Evaluate the effectiveness of combining MI and AI in a coaching experience.
4. Explore the most effective ways for nurses to acquire change facilitation skills.
5. Identify ways to incorporate MI and AI into professional nursing practice.

Nurse Healer
REFLECTIONS

After reading this chapter, the holistic nurse will be able to answer or to begin a process of answering the following questions:

- Am I motivated to acquire the skills necessary to become an effective practitioner of motivational interviewing or appreciative inquiry?
- How can I begin incorporating the guiding principles of motivational interviewing or appreciative inquiry into my current nursing practice?
- What specific communication skills can I further develop to enhance my ability to assist clients to change behavior?

 For a full suite of assignments and additional learning activities, use the access code located in the front of your book to visit this exclusive website: http://go.jblearning.com/dossey. If you do not have an access code, you can obtain one at the site.

NOTES

1. R. Schaub and B. G. Schaub, *The End of Fear: A Spiritual Path for Realists* (Carlsbad, CA: Hay House, 2009).
2. D. Hess, L. Bark, and M. E. Southard, *White Paper: Holistic Nurse Coaching*, paper presented to the National Credentialing Team for Professional Coaches in Healthcare at the Summit on Standards and Credentialing of Professional Coaches in Healthcare and Wellness, Boston, MA, September 2010. http://www.wellcoach.com/images/WhitePaperHolisticNurseCoaching.pdf.
3. M. McKivergin, "The Nurse as an Instrument of Healing," in *Holistic Nursing: A Handbook for Practice*, 5th ed., ed. B. M. Dossey and L. Keegan (Sudbury, MA: Jones & Bartlett, 2009): 721–737.
4. S. K. Leddy, *Integrative Health Promotion: Conceptual Basis for Nursing Practice*, 2nd ed. (Sudbury, MA: Jones & Bartlett, 2006).
5. G. Claxton, B. DiJulio, H. Whitmore, J. D. Pickreigh, M. McHugh, A. Osei-Anto, and B. Finder, "Health Benefits in 2010; Premiums Rise Modestly, Workers Pay More Toward Coverage," *Health Affairs 29,* no. 10 (2010): 1942–1950. http://www.ncbi.nlm.nih.gov/pubmed/20813853.

6. S. M. Moore and J. Charvat, "Promoting Health Behavior Change Using Appreciative Inquiry: Moving from Deficit Models to Affirmation Models of Care," *Family and Community Health/Supplement* 30, suppl. 1 (2007): S64–S74.

7. W. R. Miller and S. Rollnick, *Motivational Interviewing: Preparing People for Change*, 2nd ed. (New York, NY: Guilford Press, 2002).

8. B. Berger, "Motivational Interviewing Helps Patients Confront Change," *US Pharmacology* 24 (1999): 88–95.

9. H. P. McDonald, A. X. Garg, and R. B. Haynes, "Interventions to Enhance Patient Adherence to Medication Prescriptions," *Journal of the American Medical Association* 288, no. 22 (2002): 2868–2679.

10. K. Schmaling, A. Blume, and N. Afari, "A Randomized Controlled Pilot Study for Motivational Interviewing to Change Attitudes About Adherence to Medications for Asthma," *Journal Clinical Psychology Medical Settings* 8, no. 30 (2001): 167–172.

11. S. Maneesakom, D. Robson, K. Gournay, and R. Gray, "An RCT of Adherence Therapy for People with Schizophrenia in Chiang Mai, Thailand," *Journal of Clinical Nursing* 16, no. 7 (2007): 1302–1312.

12. R. A. Carels, L. Darby, H. M. Cacciapaglia, K. Konrad, C. Coit, J. Harper, M. E. Kaplar, K. Young, C. A. Baylen, and A. Versland, "Using Motivational Interviewing as a Supplement to Obesity Treatment: A Stepped-Care Approach," *Health Psychology* 26, no. 3 (2007): 369–374.

13. J. E. Hettema and P. S. Hendricks, "Motivational Interviewing for Smoking Cessation: A Meta-analytic Review," *Journal of Consulting & Clinical Psychology* 78, no. 6 (2010): 868–884. doi: 10.1037/a0021498

14. Harvard Medical School, "Motivating Behavior Change," *Mental Health Letter* 27, no. 8 (2011): 1–8.

15. S. Rollnick, W. R. Miller, and C. C. Butler, *Motivational Interviewing in Healthcare: Helping Patients Change Behavior* (New York, NY: Guilford Press, 2008).

16. Levensky, E. R., Forcehimes, A., O'Donohue, W. T., & Beitz, K. (2007): Motivational interviewing: An evidence-based approach to counseling helps patients follow treatment recommendations. *American Journal of Nursing, 19*(9), 37–44.

17. P. McCarley, "Patient Empowerment and Motivational Interviewing: Engaging Patients to Self-Manage Their Own Care," *Nephrology Nursing Journal* 36, no. 4 (2009): 409–413.

18. K. Hammer, O. Mogensen, and E. Hall, "The Meaning of Hope in Nursing Research: A Meta-synthesis," *Scandinavian Journal of Caring Sciences* 23, no. 3 (2009): 549–557.

19. M. A. Dart, *Motivational Interviewing in Nursing Practice* (Sudbury, MA: Jones & Bartlett Learning, 2011).

20. M. A. Finegold, B. M. Holland, and T. Linghan, "Appreciative Inquiry and Public Dialogue: An Approach to Community Change," *Public Organizational Review* 2, no. 3 (2002): 235–252.

21. D. L. Cooperrider and D. Whitney, *Appreciative Inquiry: A Positive Revolution in Change* (San Francisco, CA: Berrett-Koehler, 2005).

22. D. L. Cooperrider, D. Whitney, and J. M. Stavros, *Appreciative Inquiry Handbook* (Brunswick, OH: Crown Custom Publishing, 2005).

23. T. Lavendar and J. Chapple, "An Exploration of Midwives' Views of the Current System of Maternity Care in England," *Midwifery* 20, no. 4 (2004): 324–334.

24. A. K. Meda, "Tendercare, Inc: A Case Study Using Appreciative Inquiry," *Organizational Development Journal* 21, no. 4 (2003): 81–86.

25. Reed, J., Pearson, P., Douglas, B., Swinburne, S., & Wilding, H. (2002). Going home from hospital—an appreciative inquiry study. *Health and Social Care in the Community, 10*(1), 36–45.

26. V. George, M. Farrell, and G. Brukwitzki, "Performance Competencies of the Chief Executive in an Organized Delivery System," *Nursing Administration Quarterly* 26, no. 93 (2002): 34–43.

27. S. A. Hammond, *The Thin Book of Appreciative Inquiry,* 2nd ed. (Plano, TX: Thin Book Publishing, 1998).

28. P. Seebohm, J. Barnes, S. Yasmeen, M. Langridge, and C. Moreton-Prichard, "Using Appreciative Inquiry to Promote Choice for Older People and Their Carers," *Mental Health and Social Inclusion* 14, no. 4 (2010): 13–21.

29. D. Whitney, "Appreciative Inquiry: Creating Spiritual Resonance in the Workplace," *Journal of Management, Spirituality, & Religion* 7, no. 1 (2010): 73–88.

30. American Holistic Nurses Association & American Nurses Association, *Holistic Nursing: Scope and Standards of Practice* (Silver Spring, MD: Nurse Books.org, 2007).

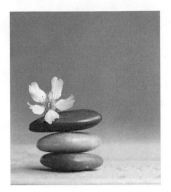

Chapter 11

Cognitive Behavioral Therapy

Eileen M. Stuart-Shor,
Carol L. Wells-Federman,
and Esther Seibold

Nurse Healer
OBJECTIVES

Theoretical

- Define cognitive behavioral therapy.
- Identify the three main principles of cognitive behavioral therapy.
- Discuss the connection between cognition(s), health, and illness.
- Identify four major contributors to the development of cognitive behavioral therapy.
- Compare and contrast potential bio-psycho-social-spiritual-behavioral responses to stress and their effects on health and illness.
- Discuss the roles of contracting and goal setting in cognitive restructuring.

Clinical

- Discuss the major diagnoses and health problems that respond favorably to cognitive behavioral therapy.
- Describe ways to facilitate cognitive restructuring.
- Identify stress warning signals.
- Describe and identify automatic thoughts.
- Describe and identify cognitive distortions and irrational beliefs.
- Describe a simple model for cognitive restructuring.

- Outline the guidelines for organizing a cognitive behavioral therapy session.
- Explore different practice settings in which cognitive restructuring can be used.

Personal

- Identify stress warning signals.
- In response to stress, stop, take a breath, reflect on the cause of the stress, and choose a more healthy response.
- Develop a list of meaningful personal rewards.
- Begin a healthy lifestyles and healthy pleasures journal.

DEFINITIONS

Cognition: The act or process of knowing.

Cognitive: Of or relating to consciousness, or being conscious; pertaining to intellectual activities (such as thinking, reasoning, imagining).

Cognitive behavioral therapy: A therapeutic approach that addresses the relationships among thoughts, feelings, behaviors, and physiology.

Cognitive distortions: Inaccurate, irrational thoughts; mistakes in thinking.

Cognitive restructuring: Examining and reframing one's interpretation of the meaning of an event.

■ THEORY AND RESEARCH

Historically, cognitive behavioral therapy is rooted in the treatment of anxiety and depression; however, in the last 10 years its application has broadened greatly. This chapter explores the application of cognitive behavioral therapy in the context of nursing practice along the wellness-illness continuum and the bio-psycho-social-spiritual domains. Cognitive behavioral therapy is integrated into expert nursing practice in myriad ways that are discussed throughout this chapter. In addition, the unique perspective that nurse healers bring to the application of cognitive behavioral therapy is addressed.

Cognitive behavioral therapy is based on the premise that stress and suffering are influenced by perception, or the way people think, and postulates that the thoughts that create stress are often illogical, negative, and distorted. These distorted negative thoughts can affect emotions, behaviors, and physiology and can influence the individual's beliefs. By changing negative illogical thoughts, specifically those that trigger and perpetuate distress, the individual can change physical and emotional states.

In this chapter, to illustrate the relationship between illogical thoughts that trigger and perpetuate stress and changes in physical and emotional states we draw from the biopsychosocial model.[1] The dimension of spirituality has been added to Engel's existing model.[2] In this eclectic bio-psycho-social-spiritual model, there is a tacit understanding that stress, or the perception of threat, can lead to changes in physical, emotional, behavioral, and spiritual states. If we accept that stress causes changes in physical and emotional states and is influenced by perception, and if we accept that perception is influenced by distorted thinking patterns (negative thoughts), then we have created a link between cognitive behavioral therapy, which restructures distorted, negative thinking patterns, and mind–body interactions, which influence health and illness. This link has implications for health promotion, symptom reduction, and disease management. Because understanding the dynamic interaction of cognitive behavioral therapy and the psychophysiology of mind–body connections is fundamental to the application of cognitive behavioral therapy in nursing, it is explored in greater detail later in this chapter.

Cognitive behavioral therapy was first used for depression and anxiety, as a short-term treatment that focused on helping people to recognize and change automatic, distorted thoughts that trigger and perpetuate distress.[3] It is now being applied successfully to reduce health-risking behaviors, physical symptoms, and the emotional sequelae of a variety of illnesses to which stress is an important causative or contributing factor.[4] Cognitive behavioral therapy is also useful in value clarification, which is the first step in establishing meaningful health goals.[4] Cognitive behavioral therapy has ancient origins. A millennium ago, the Greek philosopher Epictetus described how people most often are disturbed not by the things that happen to them but by the opinions they have about those things. Theorists including Beck,[5,6] Ellis,[7,8] Meichenbaum,[9] and Burns[10,11] have advanced the modern interpretation of cognitive therapy. In the late 1960s, Beck conceptualized cognitive theory as a model to treat depression and anxiety and developed effective intervention strategies to restructure cognitive distortions and successfully mitigate the symptoms of depression and anxiety. Ellis developed the approach known as rational emotive therapy to recognize and challenge distorted thinking. He was particularly interested in uncovering those beliefs and assumptions that people hold as absolutes and that provide the lens (or filter of life experience) that causes distortions. Meichenbaum and Burns further enhanced the theory and practice of cognitive behavioral therapy through research and clinical experience.

Research on cognitive behavioral therapy continues to provide evidence of its broad application to both psychological and physical health problems. Beck, in a 40-year retrospective review of the current state of cognitive behavioral therapy, affirmed the utility of cognitive behavioral therapy (often referred to as cognitive therapy) in treating an array of psychological disorders and medical symptoms.[12] A significant contributor to this extensive review, Butler and colleagues analyzed the current literature on outcomes of cognitive behavioral therapy (CBT).[13] They provided a comprehensive assessment of 16 methodologically rigorous meta-analyses and focused on effect sizes that contrast outcomes for CBT with outcomes for various control groups for each disorder. Large effect sizes were found for unipolar depression, generalized anxiety disorder, panic disorder with or without agoraphobia, social phobia, posttraumatic stress disorder, and childhood depressive and anxiety disorders. Effect sizes for CBT of marital distress, anger, childhood somatic disorders, and chronic pain were in the moderate range. CBT was somewhat superior to antidepressants in the treatment of adult depression. CBT was equally effective as behavior therapy in the treatment of adult depression and obsessive-compulsive disorder.

A recent meta-analysis of cognitive behavioral therapy,[14] which compared CBT to other forms of psychotherapy, showed that CBT was superior to psychodynamic therapy among patients with anxiety or depressive disorders at both treatment and follow-up. No significant difference was identified between CBT and interpersonal or supportive therapies; however, the results suggest that CBT should be a first line of treatment for patients with anxiety and depressive disorders. An expert panel of mental health and public health researchers and practitioners has recommended CBT as an effective modality for treating depression in community-based older adults.[15] This recommendation was made based on both the strength of evidence as well as feasibility and appropriateness for community-based delivery. A review and meta-analysis of five randomized controlled trials of individuals treated within 3 months of trauma indicated that early trauma-focused CBT is more effective than supportive counseling in preventing chronic post-traumatic stress disorder.[16]

Evidence continues to grow in support of the application of cognitive behavioral therapy to treat a wide variety of physical symptoms. Authors have reported its effective use in the treatment of chronic low back pain,[17] diabetes,[18-22] insomnia,[23,24] posttraumatic stress disorder,[25] sleep–wake disturbance in cancer patients,[26] chronic pain,[27,28] fibromyalgia,[29,30] migraine headache,[31] spinal cord injuries,[32] postconcussion syndrome,[33] and chronic fatigue syndrome.[34] In addition, it is found to be efficacious in the treatment of smoking in pregnant adolescents,[35] alcohol abuse,[36] binge eating,[37] tinnitus,[38] and teen cigarette smoking.[39]

Effects of Cognition on Health and Illness

Stress (the perception of a threat to one's well-being, and the perception that one cannot cope) can cause physical, psychological, behavioral, and spiritual changes. Both cognition (the way one thinks) and perception (the way one views, interprets, or experiences someone or something) are important to an understanding of cognitive restructuring. If individuals change the way they think (cognition), they may change their perception of the situation. And if they change their perception of a situation so that they no longer view that situation as threatening, they may not experience stress. Thus, changing thoughts and perceptions can influence physiologic, psychological, behavioral, and spiritual processes. The following paragraphs delineate the effects of stress on physical, psychological, social, behavioral, and spiritual pathways.

Physiologic Effects of Stress

In response to a perceived threat (stress), the body gears up to meet the challenge. This perception of threat (stress) stimulates a cascade of biochemical events initiated by the central nervous system (**Figure 11-1**).[40] Termed the fight-or-flight response[41] and later the stress response,[42] this heightened state of sympathetic arousal prepares the body for vigorous physical activity. Repeated exposure to daily hassles or prolonged stress activates the musculoskeletal system, increasing muscle tension. Concurrently, the autonomic nervous system, via the sympathetic branch, produces a generalized arousal that includes increased heart rate, blood pressure, and respiratory rate. In addition, there is a heightened awareness of the environment, shifting of blood from the visceral organs to the large muscle groups, altered lipid metabolism, and increased platelet aggregability.[43] The neuroendocrine system, in response to stimulation of the hypothalamic-pituitary-adrenal axis and the secretion of corticosteroids and mineralocorticoids, increases glucose levels, influences sodium retention, and increases the anti-inflammatory response in the acute phase. Over time, however, immune function decreases.[40,44] In addition, there is evidence that levels of other hormones regulated by the neuroendocrine system, such as

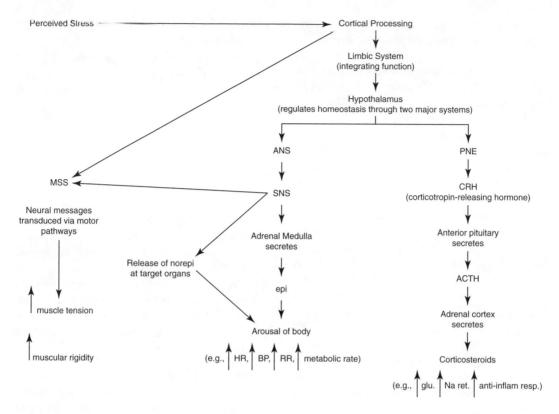

FIGURE 11-1   Stress Response. ACTH 5 adrenocorticotropic hormone; ANS 5 autonomic nervous system; BP 5 blood pressure; epi 5 epinephrine; glu. 5 blood glucose level; HR 5 heart rate; MSS 5 musculoskeletal system; Na ret. 5 sodium retention; norepi 5 norepinephrine; PNE 5 pituitary-neuroendocrine system; RR 5 respiratory rate; SNS 5 sympathetic nervous system.

Source: Reprinted with permission from C. L. Wells-Federman et al., *Clinical Nurse Specialist,* Vol. 9, No. 1, p. 60, © 1995, Williams & Wilkins.

reproductive and growth hormones, endorphins, and encephalins, can be affected.[40]

More recently, chronic inflammation has been identified as one likely mechanism through which stress affects disease risk.[45] For example, C-reactive protein (CRP), an inflammatory marker, is emerging as a predictor of cardiovascular disease. McDade and colleagues investigated the contribution of behavioral and psychosocial factors to variation in CRP concentrations in a population-based sample of middle-aged and older adults.[46] They found that psychosocial stresses, as well as health behaviors such as smoking, waist circumference, and latency to sleep, were important predictors of an increased concentration of CRP.

Prolonged or repeated exposure to stress has been shown to cause or exacerbate disease or symptoms of diseases such as angina, cardiac dysrhythmias, pain, tension headaches, insomnia, and gastrointestinal complaints. This influence is documented in extensive experimental and clinical literature.[40] Stress has been found to influence the development of coronary artery disease in women[47–49] and to influence pain perception in older adults.[44]

Psychological Effects of Stress

The psychological effects of stress are manifested by negative mood states such as anxiety, depression, hostility, and anger. These emotions (mood states) can in turn negatively influence a person's ability to concentrate and effectively problem solve. In addition, a growing body of research demonstrates the correlation between prolonged negative mood states and increased morbidity and mortality in several diseases.[44,49-51] Doering and colleagues found that after bypass surgery, depressive symptoms were associated with an increase in infections, impaired wound healing, and poor emotional and physical recovery.[49] Also, hostility has been found to play a role in a chronic cycle of inflammation among older adults and can dramatically affect their health.[44]

Concurrently, a growing body of research supports the importance of managing stress in the treatment of many diseases. Cancer[52-55] and other diseases of the immune system have been shown to respond to interventions that reduce the stress response, as have arthritis,[56,57] chronic pain,[58] tension headaches,[59,60] hypertension and heart disease,[61-68] asthma,[69] insomnia,[70] premenstrual syndrome, infertility,[71-73] and the symptoms of chronic diseases.[74-76]

The benefits of developing a positive attitude and an optimistic explanatory style have been well documented. The link between optimism and health was made by researchers tracking the lives of a group of Harvard alumni who graduated in 1945. They found that individuals who were optimistic in college were healthier in later life, whereas those who were pessimistic were less healthy. By middle age, the pessimists experienced more health problems. A more recent study found that a pessimistic explanatory style was significantly associated with a self-report of poorer physical and mental functioning 30 years later.[77] It is theorized that a pessimistic explanatory style or attitude, in addition to adversely affecting behavior, may weaken the immune system through a prolonged increase in sympathetic arousal. In addition, pessimists have more health-risking behaviors such as smoking, alcohol misuse, and sedentary lifestyle. Recognizing the influence of explanatory style on health and well-being furthers the understanding of how thoughts, feelings, behaviors, and physiology interact.

Social and Behavioral Effects of Stress

In response to stress, people often revert to less healthy behaviors.[78,79] The social and behavioral pathway is best illustrated by appreciating the effect of behavior patterns on the incidence and progression of disease. How and what people eat, drink, and smoke, as well as how they take prescribed or illegal drugs, influence health. For many, stressful events can increase behaviors such as overeating or excessive intake of alcohol. As stress increases, self-control decreases. Lapsing to behaviors that provide immediate gratification is more likely when stress is high. This inability to control health-risking behaviors as a result of increased stress is called the stress-disinhibition effect.[80]

Behaviors such as social isolation that may be influenced by stress and negative thinking patterns have been shown to be associated with higher morbidity and mortality in the first year after myocardial infarction.[81] Conversely, social support has been found to have a positive effect on health outcomes in medical settings. A report by Frasure-Smith and Prince revealed that among patients hospitalized for myocardial infarction, those receiving social support through nurses' visits after discharge had a significantly lower risk of a second event compared with those in a control group.[82] The authors theorized that positive changes in the emotional state of patients in the experimental group modulated the stress response.

Positive health outcomes in labor and delivery appear to be affected by emotional support as well. The most common surgical procedure performed in the United States is cesarean section (c-section). Delivery by c-section increases the risk of complications for mother and child, as well as extends the length of their hospital stay. The presence of a supportive woman during labor and delivery has been shown to reduce the need for c-section, shorten labor and delivery time, and reduce prenatal problems.[83] Interestingly, greater benefits are realized when the provider is not a member of the hospital staff but rather a lay volunteer such as a female friend or family member taught supportive techniques.[84] This implies obvious cost benefits and continues to underscore the implications of social support to both the patient's health and the healthcare system.

Recent research on programs that influence behavior change have shown positive modification of some of the most widespread diseases. Lifestyle behavior change has been demonstrated to influence regression of coronary artery disease and reduce cardiac risk factors.[64,85] These are only a few of the hundreds of studies that provide continuing evidence of the multidirectional relationships among thoughts, feelings, beliefs, behaviors, and physiology.

Spiritual Effects of Stress

In response to stress, people can become disconnected from their life's meaning and purpose. In *Man's Search for Meaning*, Frankl draws a parallel between connection with life's meaning and survival.[86] He describes the survivors of the World War II concentration camps as being those individuals who were able to retain their sense of meaning and purpose and were able to draw meaning and purpose from this experience. A feeling of disconnection, however, in addition to being an effect of stress, can also be a precursor to stress. Several studies have examined the effects of spirituality, defined as connection with life's meaning and purpose, on health. Increased scores on measures of spirituality correlated with increased incidence of health-promoting behaviors.[87] Other studies have explored the association between religious affiliation and health and have found a positive correlation.[88-90] This area of study is of considerable interest in the scientific literature today.

■ COGNITIVE BEHAVIORAL THERAPY

In the preceding pages, a foundation has been established for how cognitions, which are exquisitely sensitive to perception, can influence physiologic, psychological, social and behavioral, and spiritual processes. Because of this influence, cognitive behavioral therapy is an important intervention in optimizing the positive links between mind, body, and spirit and in minimizing the negative consequences of adverse interactions. Cognitive behavioral therapy helps individuals reappraise or reevaluate their thinking. It is often referred to as cognitive restructuring because the intent of the intervention is to change or restructure the distortions in thinking patterns that cause stress. The basic principles of cognitive behavioral therapy are the following:[11, 91,92]

- Our thoughts, not external events, create our moods.
- The thoughts that create stress are usually unrealistic, distorted, and negative.

- Distorted, illogical thoughts and self-defeating beliefs lead to physiologic changes and painful feelings, such as depression, anxiety, and anger.
- By changing maladaptive, unrealistic, distorted thoughts, individuals can change how they feel (physically and emotionally).

The goals of cognitive behavioral therapy include training clients to do the following:

- Pinpoint the negative automatic thoughts and silent assumptions that trigger and perpetuate their emotional upsets.
- Identify the distortions, irrational beliefs, or cognitive errors.
- Substitute more realistic, self-enhancing thoughts, which will reduce the stress, symptoms, and painful feelings.
- Replace self-defeating silent assumptions with more reasonable belief systems.
- Develop improved social skills, as well as coping, communication, and empathic skills.[91]

The Process of Cognitive Behavioral Therapy

Cognitive behavioral therapy is a short-term intervention used to help modify habits of thinking that may be distorted, negative, or irrational. In the context of cognitive behavioral therapy, cognitive restructuring is an approach or series of strategies that helps people assess their thoughts, challenge them, and replace them with more rational responses. Importantly, cognitive restructuring does not deny affliction, suffering, misfortune, or negative feelings. There are many experiences in life where it is appropriate to feel angry, sad, depressed, or anxious. The technique of cognitive restructuring is used to help people experience a broad range of feelings when they become "stuck" in powerful negative mood states.

The nurse provider serves as a guide in the process of cognitive behavioral therapy. Unlike in biomedical interventions, the provider cannot perform this intervention to or for the client but guides the individual to do it for him- or herself. There is no way to predict what will surface during the therapy or what meaning it will have to the individual. The nurse must honor the premise that each individual can best interpret his or her own experience(s), belief(s), and distortion(s).

Step 1: Awareness

Developing awareness is the first step in a systematic approach to guide clients to a restructuring of their cognitive distortions. Clients are asked to bring to their conscious awareness two things. First is an awareness of how habits of distorted, negative thinking and silent assumptions influence them physically, emotionally, behaviorally, and spiritually. Second is awareness that a habit pattern (silent assumptions, irrational beliefs, and cognitive distortions) underlies these automatic negative thoughts. To facilitate development of this awareness, a four-step approach is used to explore a stressful situation systematically. Clients are asked to stop (break the cycle of "awfulizing," escalating thoughts—become aware that a stress has taken place); take a breath (release physical tension, promote relaxation—become aware of physical changes that have occurred in response to stress); reflect (realize what is going on—become aware of automatic thoughts, distortions, beliefs, assumptions); and choose (decide how to respond—become aware of choices in responding).[93]

Clients are first asked to identify their warning signals of stress. **Exhibit 11-1** is a sample form for identifying and recording this information. These cues (or signals) can be physical, emotional, behavioral, or spiritual. When asked to monitor responses to a particular event, clients become more consciously aware of these cues. **Exhibit 11-2** is an example of a format for

EXHIBIT 11-1   Stress Warning Signals

Physical Symptoms	Behavioral Symptoms	Emotional Symptoms	Cognitive Symptoms
❏ Headaches	❏ Excess smoking	❏ Crying	❏ Trouble thinking
❏ Indigestion	❏ Bossiness	❏ Nervousness, anxiety	clearly
❏ Stomachaches	❏ Compulsive gum	❏ Boredom—no	❏ Forgetfulness
❏ Sweaty palms	chewing	meaning to things	❏ Lack of creativity
❏ Sleep difficulties	❏ Attitude critical	❏ Edginess—ready	❏ Memory loss
❏ Dizziness	of others	to explode	❏ Inability to
❏ Back pain	❏ Grinding of teeth	❏ Feeling powerless	make decisions
❏ Tight neck,	at night	to change things	❏ Thoughts of
shoulders	❏ Overuse of alcohol	❏ Overwhelming	running away
❏ Racing heart	❏ Compulsive eating	sense of pressure	❏ Constant worry
❏ Restlessness	❏ Inability to get	❏ Anger	❏ Loss of sense
❏ Tiredness	things done	❏ Loneliness	of humor
❏ Ringing in ears		❏ Unhappiness for	
		no reason	
		❏ Easily upset	

Do any seem familiar to you?

Check the ones you experience when under stress. These are your stress warning signs.

Are there any additional stress warning signals that you experience that are not listed? If so, add them here.

_____

_____

_____

_____

_____

Source: Reprinted with permission from H. Benson and E. M. Stuart, *The Wellness Book,* p. 182, © 1992, Carol Publishing.

EXHIBIT 11-2   Challenging Stress and Winning—Stop, Take a Breath, Reflect, Choose

Situation	Physical Response	Automatic Thoughts	Moods and Emotions
Briefly describe a situation that caused you stress this week.	Describe how you felt physically in this situation.	Write your automatic thoughts in this situation.	Describe how you felt emotionally in this situation.
Exaggerated Beliefs	**Behavior**	**More Effective Response**	**Potential Outcome**
Write down the exaggerated beliefs behind your automatic thoughts.	Describe how you behaved during or immediately after the situation.	Describe how you might think or act differently that would help you cope more effectively.	Describe how this might make you feel and behave.

Source: Reprinted with permission from H. Benson and E. M. Stuart, *The Wellness Book*, p. 245, © 1992, Carol Publishing.

recording this information. Although it may initially increase an individual's perception of physical pain or emotional discomfort, conscious awareness is a necessary first step in recognizing the relationship of thoughts, feelings, behavior, and biology to distorted thinking patterns.

Often, clients have long ignored the cues their minds or bodies give them. Consider the client with disabling headaches who may ignore the shoulder and neck tension that precedes his headaches. Had he attended to his early stress warning signs (neck and shoulder tension), he might have avoided the headache. Becoming aware of these stress warning signs is the first step. Attending to the cues is the next. Once they make this connection, clients can more easily develop skills to reduce negative mood states, unhealthy behaviors, and physical symptoms. To continue with the preceding example, it is easier to stop a tension headache when the client notices shoulder tension and stops, takes a few deep diaphragmatic breaths, and gently stretches the area than it is to wait for the headache to become incapacitating before acting.

EXERCISE

Ask the client to identify his or her stress warning signals. Then, have the client identify a stressful experience and the physical or emotional reaction to this particular experience. For example, after being instructed to stop, take a breath, and notice the physical and emotional response to a stressful situation, one client related the following:

On my way home from work yesterday I sat in traffic. I noticed that my hands were gripping the steering wheel, my neck and shoulders were tight, and my jaw was clenched. I felt angry and frustrated because I wanted to be home.

Becoming aware of stress warning signals is an important first step. Although this seems very straightforward, the average person is often quite unaware of the effects of stress on the body-mind. Once the client is aware of the effects of stress, he or she may be able to release tension more easily. Clients build on this awareness as they proceed through cognitive restructuring.

Step 2: Automatic Thoughts

Once the client has been able to identify a stress or a stressful situation and identify the changes in the body–mind that accompany this stress, the next step is to identify the automatic thoughts. These thoughts usually occur automatically in response to a situation. Because these thoughts occur automatically and often are not in the conscious awareness of the individual, they are described as knee-jerk responses. Clients are taught a systematic approach to identifying these self-defeating automatic thoughts.

Automatic thoughts have the following characteristics in common:

- Reflex or knee-jerk responses to a perceived stressor
- Usually negative
- Quick, fleeting, a kind of shorthand (e.g., *should, ought, never, always*)
- Usually not in our conscious awareness
- Frequently unrealistic, illogical, and distorted

Because these thoughts form so quickly, it is often difficult to notice that they have occurred. Typically, people attribute the stress they experience or the feeling they have to the person or situation that is causing the stress. By stopping, taking a breath, and asking the question, "What is going on here?" clients gradually become aware that their stress does not always come from an outside event or situation but may come from the way they interpret these events. Automatic thoughts can be viewed as habits of thinking, inner dialogue, or perceptions, which in turn create the experience and influence the individual's physiology, emotions, and behaviors.

EXAMPLE

A very popular and successful teacher was reviewing the evaluations at the end of the semester. He read 20 very positive reviews. Then, he read one that contained some criticism of his teaching style. Instantly, he felt a tense sensation in his stomach and chest.

After stopping and taking a breath, he was able to identify the following automatic thoughts: "There's always one in a crowd . . . ought to have done [*whatever*] . . . never could teach that concept well . . . should have included the new material I saw in the library . . . I always come up short."

Notice that the teacher had an instant reaction to this stress (perception of threat) and that his automatic thoughts were quick, fleeting, negative, and probably not in his conscious awareness. (Does he really believe he always comes up short?) Identifying automatic thoughts is an important step in allowing clients to look realistically at their automatic reaction to a stressor and put it into perspective.

One of the most important and difficult tasks in cognitive restructuring is developing an awareness that these automatic thoughts occur. One reason that these reflex, knee-jerk responses are so pervasive is that the body does not know the difference between things that are imagined and things that are actually experienced. Another reason is that people are always talking to themselves, and after they say something to themselves often enough, they begin to believe it. A third reason is that people rarely stop to question their thoughts or emotions. For these reasons, clients need to be taught a structured way of exploring stress and uncovering these automatic thoughts.

Here is an exercise to uncover automatic thoughts, feelings, and physical responses (see also Exhibit 11-2):

EXERCISE

Stop (break the cycle of escalating, awfulizing thoughts).

Take a breath (release physical tension, promote relaxation).

Reflect:

- Physically, how do I feel?
- Emotionally, how do I feel?
- What are my automatic thoughts (e.g., *should, always, ought, never*)?

Step 3: Cognitive Distortions

Once clients have learned to identify stressful situations; their physical, emotional, and behavioral responses to stress; and the automatic thoughts that precipitate the experience, the next step in the process is to teach clients to identify distortions in thinking. Cognitive distortions are illogical ways of thinking that lead to adverse body-mind-spirit states. The problem is not that these thoughts are wrong or bad, but that people hold the beliefs so strongly. Cognitive distortions are based on beliefs or underlying assumptions that are generally out of proportion to the situation. These beliefs or assumptions are usually long held, are based on life experience, and often are not in one's conscious awareness.

Through years of research and clinical experience, Burns identified the following 10 general categories of cognitive distortions that lead to negative emotional states:[94]

- *All-or-nothing thinking:* Viewing things in black or white; considering oneself as a total failure when a performance falls short of perfection. (Think back to the example of the teacher. In the face of 20 excellent evaluations, and 1 constructive criticism, the teacher immediately focused all his attention on the imperfection and felt anxious and upset. "I should have taught the course all differently." "I never get a good review.")
- *Overgeneralization:* Viewing a single negative event as a never-ending pattern. "Fixing my car cost twice what they said it would. All mechanics are dishonest and always will be."
- *Mental filtering:* Picking out a negative detail and dwelling on it exclusively, "catastrophizing," or "awfulizing." "I got a lousy grade on that test. I'll probably have to drop out of school. I won't be able to find a decent job and will have to move back in with my parents."
- *Disqualifying the positive:* Rejecting positive experiences as if they don't count. "It was nothing." Being unable to accept praise. "You're just saying that because you have to."
- *Jumping to conclusions:* Reading the minds of others or predicting negative outcomes without sufficient evidence. "He went off

to bed without saying anything. He's angry with me for working late again."
- *Magnification:* Exaggerating the importance of mistakes or inappropriately minimizing the significance of one's own assets. "My performance tonight was horrible—I'll never get the lead part."
- *Emotional reasoning:* Assuming that one's emotions reflect the way things are. "I feel worthless—I must be worthless."
- *"Should" statements:* Trying to motivate oneself with shoulds and shouldn'ts. "Good employees should always get to the office early and be willing to stay late."
- *Labeling:* Name calling; labeling oneself "a loser" if a mistake is made; making an illogical leap from one characteristic to a category. "She's blond. What do you expect? She's an airhead."
- *Personalization:* Blaming oneself inappropriately as the cause of a negative event; seeing events only in relation to oneself. "It's my fault that my child didn't do well in school because I work."

Exaggerated, unrealistic, illogical, and distorted automatic thoughts are a result of deeply held silent assumptions and beliefs that are usually not in one's conscious awareness. A client is more likely to experience stress in any given situation if he or she holds these beliefs as absolutes. Situations that are encountered are far more likely to precipitate stress if the world is viewed in terms of black or white (e.g., all good or all bad) than if there is room for shades of gray. An important understanding for the clinician is that it is not the belief that needs to be examined, it is the degree to which the belief is held. All clients are entitled to their individual sets of beliefs. Assigning any value, right or wrong, to their beliefs is not in the nurse's purview. The nurse is simply inviting clients to examine their beliefs in the context of their stress and to assess whether the degree to which they hold these beliefs serves them well or contributes to stress. Clients can very easily be alienated if they feel the nurse is making value judgments about their beliefs. The core concept here is not to examine beliefs to decide whether they are right or wrong, but to decide whether they are practical or impractical. Some commonly held assumptions and beliefs are:[95]

- If I treat others fairly, then I can expect them to treat me fairly.
- I must always have the love and approval of family, friends, and peers to be worthwhile.
- I must be unfailingly competent and perfect in all that I do.
- My worth as a human being depends on my achievements (or intelligence or status or attractiveness).

Everyone has a right to his or her beliefs and opinions. Problems develop only when these beliefs are held as absolutes and therefore provide no room for flexibility in an imperfect world.

EXAMPLE

Reflect back on the previous example of the teacher reading course evaluations who had a strong reaction to criticism.

After taking a breath, interrupting his automatic response, and identifying his automatic thoughts, he was able to identify his cognitive distortions and irrational beliefs. They included all-or-nothing thinking (must be perfect all the time), overgeneralization (never will get it right), disqualifying the positive (20 excellent reviews wiped out by 1 negative review), and the belief that "I must be unfailingly competent and perfect in all I do to be loved and respected by family, friends, and peers."

Following is an extension to the exercise to uncover cognitive distortions:

EXERCISE

Stop (break the cycle of escalating, awfulizing thoughts).

Take a breath (release physical tension, promote relaxation).

Reflect:

- Physically, how do I feel?
- Emotionally, how do I feel?
- What are my automatic thoughts (e.g., should, always, ought, never)?

- What is going on here?
- Is it really true?
- Am I jumping to conclusions?
- Am I catastrophizing, awfulizing, getting things out of perspective?
- Is it really a crisis?
- Is it as bad as it seems?
- Is there another way to look at the situation?
- What is the worst that can happen?

Because these strongly held assumptions and beliefs are mostly silent or not in people's conscious awareness, it is a challenge to discover their existence and, consequently, their influence on people's thoughts, emotions, and behaviors. In addition to the systematic approach described here to explore a stressful situation (stop, take a breath, reflect, and choose), another technique that is helpful in discovering underlying assumptions and beliefs is the vertical arrow technique developed by Burns.[11]

VERTICAL ARROW EXERCISE

Ask the client to identify a stressful situation and to challenge the underlying assumptions in this stress. The client can challenge the assumption by asking the question, "If that is true, why is it so upsetting?"

For example, a nursing school student had severe panic that kept her from speaking up in class. Class participation was 50% of the grade, so she wanted to change this behavior. When she was asked why it was stressful to ask a question, the following sequence of thoughts emerged.

"If I speak up, I may say something stupid."
↓
If this is true, why is it so upsetting?
↓
"They will think I'm stupid."
↓
If this is true, why is it so upsetting?
↓

"The smart students won't invite me to join their study group."

↓

If this is true, why is it so upsetting?

↓

"I won't pass unless I'm in a good study group."

↓

If this is true, why is it so upsetting?

↓

"I'll flunk out of school."

↓

If this is true, why is it so upsetting?

↓

"My family and friends will be embarrassed."

↓

If this is true, why is it so upsetting?

↓

"They won't love me."

↓

If this is true, why is it so upsetting?

↓

"I'm unlovable."

Using this vertical arrow technique allowed the student to see how out of perspective her automatic thoughts were. She could clearly see that her stress was influenced by the exaggerated belief that to make a mistake would make her less than perfect and to be less than perfect was bad and would make people cease to love her. The awareness of this pattern of thinking allowed her to put the situation in perspective and helped her to get past her fear of asking a question.

Once a fear is recognized, it can be approached like any other stressor. If it is irrational, it can be challenged through cognitive restructuring. If it is rational, then appropriate problem-solving and coping strategies are required.

Identifying Emotions

The way people feel emotionally is an important part of health. Feelings of vigor, vitality, and general well-being are important correlates of health; conversely, feelings of anger, hostility, anxiety, or depression can contribute to ill health. Many people find their emotions troubling, either because they are out of touch with them or because they feel overwhelmed by them.

Family and cultural influences have a great deal to do with the way emotions are experienced. Many families and cultures do not encourage the expression of emotions, and individuals learn to ignore this aspect of their lives. As individuals become aware of their body-mind-spirit responses to stress by identifying their emotional stress warning signals, they become aware of their feelings and emotions, and the connection between these feelings and emotions and stress.

Feelings of depression, anger, fear, and guilt are all part of the human experience; however, individuals may need to be encouraged to acknowledge and honor these emotions. Emotions are genuine, and people are entitled to the way they feel. On the other hand, emotions, particularly exaggerated emotions, can interfere with effective problem solving. Individuals need to be guided through the process of recognizing their emotions and the thoughts that underlie these feelings. For example, anger is often perpetuated by thoughts of unfair treatment. Frustration is often the result of unmet expectations. Thoughts related to loss contribute to the feeling of depression, and perception of a loss of control often causes anxiety. It is important to distinguish healthy fear from neurotic anxiety. Thoughts underlying healthy fear are realistic, keep one alert, and warn one of dangers. Neurotic anxiety is related to thoughts that are distorted and unrealistic and often contain "what ifs": "What if I don't get the job?" "What if I don't find a partner?" A great deal of time and energy are wasted on events that may never take place. The nurse must guide the client in discovering the thoughts that are behind the emotion. In this way, the nurse can facilitate a process of challenging the thoughts and dealing with the emotions.

When feelings are ignored, denied, or suppressed, they often become intertwined with stress. In this case, clients sometimes have difficulty identifying either the emotion or the automatic thoughts related to the emotion. Cognitive restructuring allows individuals to become aware of the emotions, the automatic thoughts related to a particular emotion, and the connection with stress. Reflecting on these underlying themes often helps individuals to explain why they feel as they do and, in turn, to choose a more effective coping mechanism.

Another danger in denying feelings is that individuals can become trapped in one of these emotional states so that the mind becomes a filter, letting into conscious awareness only material that confirms or reinforces their mood. For example, when people are depressed, they notice and experience only things that depress them more; nothing that would bring joy and pleasure is allowed into their awareness. Through cognitive restructuring, they can learn to reduce the frequency, length, and intensity of these feelings.

This variation of the exercise uncovers the relationship of thoughts and feelings:

EXERCISE

Stop (break the cycle of escalating, awfulizing thoughts).

Take a breath (release physical tension, promote relaxation).

Reflect (What am I feeling? What am I thinking? Is there a theme that underlies my stress triggers?).

Feeling	Thoughts related to
Anger	Being treated unfairly
Frustration	Unmet expectations
Depression	Loss
Anxiety	Loss of control, fear of the unknown

As an example, consider the situation of a person who is laid off from his or her job. An angry person often views situations through the lens of his or her standard of fairness. In response to being laid off, such a person might be angry and think, "Why me? I've worked hard all these years, never complaining, doing more than I was asked, and this is how they reward me?" A depressed individual often responds with distortions such as all-or-nothing thinking, personalization, and overgeneralization. In response to being laid off, such a person might become depressed and think, "This shows what a complete failure I am. I'll never amount to anything." In the same situation, an anxious person might experience an entirely different set of distortions. This person

might predict dire consequences (jump to conclusions) and take them as facts. An anxious person who just got laid off might think, "What if I never get a job again. I'll be broke, on the street, and living on welfare in a matter of months."

The nurse helps the client become aware of the relationship of these emotional themes to stress triggers and cognitive distortions. When the nurse guides the client through a stress awareness exercise, if the client identifies his or her emotional response as anger, the nurse helps the client to make the connection with automatic thoughts related to being treated unfairly (e.g., "This shouldn't have happened to me," or "Why me? This is so unfair").

Because clients have often spent so many years ignoring their emotional cues, they sometimes have difficulty recognizing either the thoughts or the emotions that are related to stressful situations. Keeping a diary or journal reflecting thoughts and feelings about stressful events has been found to be a valuable tool clients can use to identify automatic thoughts and underlying emotions. This method is explained further in the following section on coping. In addition to understanding stressors and common themes that trigger stress, acknowledging and honoring emotions is important to a healthy sense of self. Healthy self-esteem, in turn, is an important ingredient in stress hardiness or the ability to greet stressful events as challenges to be met rather than as threats to be feared.

Step 4: Choosing Effective Coping

The final step in the process of cognitive behavioral therapy is to help the client restructure or reframe distortions and beliefs and choose a more effective way of responding or coping. To accomplish this, one must recognize that stressful situations have two components, which Ells termed the practical problem and the emotional hook. The practical problem is the situation at hand, or the problem that needs to be addressed. The emotional hook is the client's opinion about the problem or the individual(s) who have caused the problem. Quite often people respond to situations as if they can solve the problem by addressing the emotional hook. In the following example, note the difference in these two elements of the stress.

EXAMPLE

John related that he became very upset when he was late for an appointment and, while he was in line at the grocery store, someone cut in front of him.

To cope effectively with this situation, John needed to separate the practical problem (getting through the line) from the emotional hook (his opinion about people who cut in line and his "right" to be treated fairly). When asked to stop, take a breath, and reflect, he was able to uncover his physical response (tense, tight jaw), his emotional response (anger), his automatic thoughts ("This always happens to me," "People ought not to cut in line," "Late"), and silent assumptions underlying the distorted thinking ("I treat others fairly, and I expect to be treated fairly").

This example shows that the process of solving the practical problem is different from the process of addressing the emotional hook. If John were to expend his energy in convincing the person who cut in front of him of the error of his ways regarding behavior in line, John would be unlikely to solve his problem (he was late and needed to get through the line efficiently). Moreover, in practical terms, John had no control over this other person. How likely was it that John could influence this person's behavior in future situations? Automatic thoughts—shoulds, nevers, always, musts, and oughts—often interfere with finding practical solutions to the problem. The emotional hook robs individuals of their ability to see the options for responding. This failure can make it impossible for clients to recognize when they have no control over a situation and need to concentrate on the practical problem rather than the emotional hook.

In this example, once John recognized how his underlying beliefs and assumptions were influencing his choices, he could take steps to stop the escalation of emotional upset and choose the best solution for the problem. Doing so involved making a decision about how to respond from conscious awareness and without continued emotional arousal. He might see several options. For example, he might choose to change lines or to calmly ask the person who cut in front of him to go to the end of the line (direct action). Or he might choose just to let it go because, although it is important to be treated fairly, in this instance he was in a hurry, he didn't have the time or desire to deal with this individual, and, because this didn't always happen to him, it wasn't worth getting upset about (acceptance, reframing). Whatever the decision, it could be made with awareness and choice, not in reaction to a deeply held belief about how people ought to behave, and without further escalating emotional distress.

EXERCISE: REFRAMING AND PROBLEM SOLVING

Stop: Train a client to stop each time a stress is encountered, before thoughts escalate into the worst possible scenario. The simple act of thinking "Stop" can help break a pattern of automatic response.

Breathe: Teach the client to breathe deeply and release physical tension. Physically taking a deep, diaphragmatic breath can be important because during times of stress, most people hold their breath. Taking a deep breath can elicit the physiologic changes of the relaxation response, the opposite of the stress response. This practice facilitates awareness of stress warning signals and the interaction between stress and bodymindspirit changes.

Reflect: Teach clients to ask themselves several questions about the automatic thoughts and underlying beliefs. Is this thought true? Is this thought helpful? (This is the process of developing awareness of automatic thoughts and cognitive distortions and challenging these distorted thoughts, beliefs, and assumptions.)

Choose: Train clients to select the most effective way to cope or solve the problem. Instruct the client to ask a series of questions:

- What is the practical problem?
- What is the emotional hook?

- How can I substitute more realistic, self-enhancing thoughts to reduce the painful feelings?
- How can I replace self-defeating silent assumptions (e.g., by substituting "I'm doing the best I can" for "I can't cope with this")?
- What do I need?
- What can I do?
- What do I want?
- What is possible?
- Do I have the time, skills, and personal investment to achieve a practical solution? Is the practical problem within my control to solve?
- Is it possible to deal with the practical problem (i.e., is it within my control)?
- Do I need to temper my emotional response before I can act responsibly, practically, and appropriately?
- Am I avoiding the best solution because it will be difficult for me?

Many techniques can be used to help clients effectively problem solve and cope with stressors. Effective coping requires that one attend to both the practical problem and the emotional hook. This sometimes requires two different approaches. Careful thought must be given to each stressful situation to choose the most effective coping strategy. The following list suggests a few ways to cope.[11]

Distraction: Worry about resolving a stress can be put off until the time is right. For example, the client receives a letter from the manager of the bank asking to speak with the client as soon as possible, but it is after closing hours. Distraction involves putting this worry aside until the bank opens the next day, at which time the client can deal directly with the situation. This is quite different from procrastination or denial because it is a necessary delay as opposed to avoidance.

Direct action: The problem can be dealt with directly to resolve it.

Relaxation: Using relaxation techniques to reduce emotional arousal is a way of cop-

ing with a stress that cannot be changed or avoided. Techniques to elicit the relaxation response include meditation, yoga, mindfulness, and tai chi, as well as many others. Relaxation techniques are covered in Chapter 16.

Reframing: Looking at a situation differently can help individuals cope. A glass filled halfway can be labeled either half full or half empty. This label changes the experience greatly. Illness, for example, can be viewed as catastrophic and life shattering or as an opportunity for reconnection with what is meaningful in one's life.

Affirmations: Positive thoughts can be used to recondition one's thinking. For example, individuals frequently tell themselves they cannot do something, and the statement becomes a self-fulfilling prophecy. Affirmations are a way of countering self-defeating silent assumptions. An affirmation is simply a positive thought, a short phrase, or a saying that has meaning for the individual. Clients can be coached to create an affirmation as a way of reframing or choosing a more helpful, reasonable belief system.

EXERCISE

Developing an affirmation: Ask the client to choose an aspect of life that is causing stress, such as work, family, or health. Have the client decide what he or she would want to have happen or how he or she would want to feel in the situation. Formulate the goal as a first-person statement, in the present, and in the positive (e.g., "I am confident in my work," "I can handle it," "I am peaceful," or "I am becoming healthy and strong"). Have the client repeat the affirmation often during the day, perhaps before or after eliciting the relaxation response or as part of a breathing exercise.

In a short time, affirmations can become second nature and help to enhance self-esteem and reduce stress.

Spirituality: A sense of connection to the universe, God, or a higher power, or connecting with what is important and meaningful in our life, can aid in coping with stress. Connection with life's meaning and purpose is addressed in greater detail in Chapter 32.

Catharsis: Emotional catharsis, either laughing or crying, can be very effective in relieving emotional distress.

Journal writing: Using a journal to write about thoughts, feelings, and experiences is often helpful in processing emotions. Pennebaker and colleagues found that writing to get in touch with one's deepest thoughts and feelings can measurably improve physical and mental health.[96] Suggest to clients that they get a special notebook and colorful pens for their journal. Chapter 12 contains more detailed information on journal writing.

Social support: Having supportive family, friends, and coworkers is important to effective coping and has been shown to contribute to stress hardiness. Talking out problems is often helpful to obtain good advice or uncritical support. Social support has been found to reduce the incidence of heart disease as well as other health problems. In the social support literature, it has been noted that both the number of supporters and the quality of the relationships are important.

Assertive communication: Communication is an important skill to help in solving problems and reducing conflicts and stress. Communication (also addressed in Chapter 28) is considered in some detail in the subsection titled "Developing Communication Skills" that follows because it is an important coping and problem-solving skill that can be adversely affected by deeply held beliefs and silent assumptions. Cognitive restructuring can influence the ability to communicate effectively and, in turn, improve coping.

Empathy: Empathy is the ability to take into consideration the other person's perspective. It is an effective coping technique because it facilitates communication. It helps clients become better listeners. Empathy is described in more detail in the exercise below.

Developing Communication Skills

People who have problems with communication usually experience the following challenges:[97]

- Disparity between what they say (statement) and what they want (intent).

- Confusion about or resistance to stating clearly how they feel, what they want, or what they need (assertiveness), there is either a tendency to deny their own feelings (passiveness) or to be indifferent toward the feelings of others (aggressiveness).
- Inability to listen.

The importance of matching the statement with the intention is illustrated by the following example.

EXAMPLE

After spending a long day at work and stopping to pick up some groceries at the store, Jill arrives home to find her husband Jack at his desk in his office going over some bills. Coming in the door, she remarks, "Wow, busy day. I just picked up some groceries." She begins bringing the bags of groceries into the kitchen, walking past him. Following each trip to the garage, she shuts the door a little more forcefully and sets each bag down a little more loudly as Jack continues to sit at his desk.

When he finally says, "Anything wrong?" Jill answers, "Nothing!" and storms out of the room, feeling that, if he loved her, he would know what she needed and wanted.

The first principle of effective communication is to be clear about what one wants and needs (intent) in statements to others. Although it would be wonderful if spouses, friends, and others were mind readers, assuming that they are does not help with communication. Matching statements with intentions is an art and a skill. It requires that individuals recognize their automatic thoughts, emotions, and cognitive distortions and take responsibility for their part of the conversation.

Consider the preceding example. If Jill's intention was for her husband to help bring the groceries into the house, then her statement should have reflected this. She might have said, "Wow, what a busy day. I just picked up some groceries. Could you help me bring them into the house?" Clients must understand that the other person is not obligated to respond as they would wish. However, what they are asking for will be a lot clearer to others if the statement reflects the intent.

The next principle of effective communication is to be assertive. In most cases, assertive communication is the most effective way to communicate. An assertive statement expresses one's feelings and opinions and reaffirms one's identity and rights. It is not judgmental. The general format of an assertive statement is "I feel [*label the emotion*] when you [*label the behavior*] because [*provide an explanation*]." The formula requires that all three elements be included. Cognitive restructuring facilitates assertive communication because it requires clients to identify their thoughts and feelings. In the example, Jill would

- **Stop** (break the cycle of escalating, awfulizing thoughts).
- **Take a breath** (release physical tension, promote relaxation).
- **Reflect:**
  - Emotionally how do I feel? (frustrated)
  - What are my automatic thoughts? ("If he loved me, he would get up and help me! He never helps me with the house. He always expects me to do everything around here. He doesn't care about me. He's never going to change.")

Recognizing her thoughts and feelings would help Jill to formulate an assertive statement when her husband asks, "Anything wrong?" She could then say, "I feel frustrated [*emotion*] when you don't help me bring in the groceries [*behavior*] because if you cared for me you would help me more with the chores around the house [*explanation*]." In this way, she would both have made her feelings clear and have explained why she felt that way. This, in turn, would have provided a better opportunity to work on problem solving. If clients cannot articulate both their feelings and their needs, they leave it up to others to figure them out. When others fail to do so correctly, the clients feel let down and blame others for not understanding. The nurse can help clients to recognize that they have a right to speak up and a responsibility to do so in an assertive rather than passive or aggressive way. The nurse can guide clients in matching their emotions with the explanation (e.g., frustration = unmet expectation) by reviewing the exercise on matching thoughts and emotions as in the preceding example. Clients should be reminded that this technique will feel awkward and uncomfortable at first. They may have to practice it many times before communications improve. Other people need time to adjust to the changes they are trying to make. Effective communication takes practice as well as patience with oneself and with others.

Developing Empathy Skills

Here is an exercise nurses can introduce to clients to help them develop skills in empathy:

EXERCISE: PROMOTING EMPATHY

Empathy can be facilitated through active listening. This technique requires conscious, nonjudgmental awareness. It helps to clarify the issues involved and can deescalate many emotional exchanges. Consider a situation in which the mother announces, "I can't stand this room any more. It's a mess." The response to this statement may be critical to resolving the issues without contributing to further miscommunication and escalating the problem. Instead of becoming hooked by a defensive emotional reaction, clients can learn to operate from empathy using the four-step approach.

Stop (break the cycle of escalating, awfulizing thoughts).

Take a breath (release physical tension, promote relaxation).

Reflect:
- Emotionally. how do I feel? (hurt, angry)
- What are my automatic thoughts? ("How could she say that? I work hard too. I'm always being blamed for how things are around here. No one understands kids.")
- What are the thoughts and emotions being expressed by the other person? (The simple practice of asking this question provides a very different perspective as the client begins to formulate a response.)

Choose:
- My feelings are hurt, but I choose not to react defensively.
- I choose to listen actively to the other person's response and will try to

understand that person's perspective, using this phrase: "You sound [*emotion*] about [*situation*]."

Rogers suggested using this last phrase as a way to facilitate communication and gain awareness of another person's perspective.[98] In the preceding scenario, the teenage child might say, "You sound upset about the messy house." Possible responses might include: "It's not just the room, everything seems to be in a mess, here and at the office. I can't seem to get anything done." Or the mother might say, "You're right about that. I hate coming home to a messy house after a busy day."

When a client uses the skill of active listening, the other person often feels heard, which may help to defuse further emotional arousal and defensive behavior. In addition, he or she now has an opportunity to clarify any misunderstanding. Also, active listening allows the client to buy time to obtain a better perspective on what the other person is thinking and feeling. Clients can then choose how they want to respond. This may be a time to use assertive communication or problem solving, or a time to step away from the interaction until emotions and defenses have settled. Active listening allows reflective, empathic, objective, and nonjudgmental communication. Coaching clients to use cognitive restructuring skills that include active listening techniques facilitates effective communication, in turn reducing conflict and stress.

Acceptance: Acceptance is facing the fact that some situations or people cannot be changed or avoided and letting go of resentment. Forgiveness is often a part of acceptance. Coping successfully means gaining the wisdom to achieve the delicate balance between acceptance and action, between letting go and taking control. It is the art of choosing the right strategy at the right time.

When clients feel that they can cope effectively, the harmful effects of stress are buffered. The situation is perceived not as a threat but as a challenge. This subtle difference has profound physiologic, psychological, behavioral, and spiritual effects. It is what allows people facing great adversity (such as illness) to see the opportunity the situation presents. Above all, as noted earlier, clients need to recognize that coping is the art of finding a balance between acceptance and action, between letting go and taking control. Cognitive restructuring helps clients distinguish these differences by providing a format for observing or objectifying their experiences. In so doing, they gain a sense of control that minimizes or buffers the harmful effects of stress.

Cognitive Behavioral Therapy in Children and Adolescents

Cognitive behavioral therapy is an effective treatment modality for children and adolescents, but it is modified to take into consideration the unique developmental needs of this population. The same basic principles discussed above are applied; however, factors such as cognitive, social, and emotional maturity are taken into consideration. Whereas adults can reflect on their thought processes, identify their responses to stressful situations and develop alternative strategies, children often do not have the capacity for this type of mental activity. An individualized treatment plan can be developed based on assessment of these factors. Families and school personnel should also be included in the treatment plan, to promote continuity and support across the environments where children spend most of their time.[99] Involvement of family members in cognitive behavioral therapy interventions has been demonstrated to show higher response rates than cognitive behavioral therapy for children alone, both after intervention and at 1-year follow-up. By the 6-year follow-up assessment, the two groups showed similar numbers of diagnosis-free individuals.[100] In addition, children and youth are less likely to identify a need for treatment; therefore, a critical factor in implementing cognitive behavioral therapy is engaging them in treatment. Interventions should be fun and build on specific interests and strengths of the child or youth, rather than following a standardized approach.

A review of cognitive behavioral therapy for anxiety and phobic disorders in children and adolescents discusses application of this treatment for generalized and separation anxiety disorders, social phobia, specific phobias, and school refusal.[100] In this group of individuals, therapy might be conducted either individually or in a group. Group intervention has the added value of providing both peer modeling and a built-in opportunity for social exposure. School-based cognitive intervention is also described and has been shown to be successful. A discussion of CBT intervention for children with depression addresses the importance of school-based interventions for reducing depressive symptomatology.[101] This review of 25 studies emphasizes that interventions for children and youth address both cognitions and behavior and include self-instruction retraining, problem-solving training, attribution retraining, and cognitive restructuring approaches. Techniques such as modeling, role playing, and positive role playing are effective techniques for working with young people. The evidence points to a strong role for school mental health practitioners such as school psychologists, nurses, school counselors, and special educators.

Techniques for working with the younger child:[99]

- To help children identify the somatic manifestations of anxiety, have them trace their body shape on a large piece of paper and then color the areas where they might feel different when they are anxious.
- Read children's books that discuss different emotions.
- Create a reward list based on the child's interests and developmental level. These can be tangible or social rewards.
- Actively include family members in the treatment plan so that they can gradually integrate strategies into the family's routine.

Techniques for working with adolescents:

- Making a collage from teen magazines with images that display different emotional states.
- Invite the youth to participate by using examples from the teen's life, for example, an interest in a particular sport or other activity.
- Provide age-appropriate rewards.

> ### *EXAMPLE*
>
> School refusal: An 8-year-old child refuses to go to school every morning and displays symptoms of separation anxiety. Treatment might include phased-in exposure to the school setting, application of social and other reinforcements, and training of parents and teachers about the various aspects of the intervention, such as coping skills training, holding the child responsible for his or her behavior, and fostering self-efficacy.[100]

Application of the General Principles of Cognitive Behavioral Therapy

Cognitive behavioral therapy is most useful for individuals, not for relationship problems or interpersonal conflict.[10] The nurse must be imaginative and tenacious. Cognitive behavioral therapy requires constant shifting between technique and process. The therapy combines problem resolution using cognitive and behavioral techniques with empathic focus on the client's feelings. The process requires the skills of presence, intention, and communication. Several attempts and several different ways of looking at a situation may be required before a client recognizes the automatic thoughts and underlying beliefs involved.

Cognitive behavioral therapy can be used in both inpatient and outpatient settings, but the goals and process are different in these settings. The goal of cognitive behavioral therapy in the outpatient setting is generally to restructure cognitive distortions to enhance a variety of self-management skills and healthy lifestyle behaviors, which in turn help to promote health, reduce symptoms, or manage illness. Outpatient cognitive behavioral therapy can be provided either individually or in a group. The majority of this chapter has been written for this application.

The goal of cognitive behavioral therapy in the inpatient setting is typically confined to assisting the patient to cope more effectively with those stresses that arise during hospitalization for an acute illness. In this context, the nurse must remember that he or she is viewing the patient from a cross-sectional perspective (through one episode in the continuum of the patient's life). Patients bring to this hospital experience a reliance on long-standing coping styles—some adaptive, some maladaptive, and many influenced by cognitive distortions. In view of the short hospital stay and critical needs during this time, long-standing maladaptive coping patterns are best left to be addressed after discharge from the hospital.

In the hospital, cognitive behavioral therapy can be integrated effectively into the many nurse–patient communications that occur each day. Each interaction can be an occasion to assist patients in identifying the relationship of thoughts, feelings, and behaviors to biology as it applies to their current symptoms and illness. The nurse can utilize the structure of cognitive behavioral therapy to assist the patient in identifying distorted thinking patterns and realistically appraising the situation as well as in seeing opportunity in adversity. Thus, the patient can often choose a more realistic and less stressful way to view the situation. This, in turn, can decrease physical and emotional symptoms.

Hospitalization can be a time of opportunity despite its difficulties. Because hospitalization usually occurs when individuals are in need or crisis, they often feel vulnerable and may be more open to exploring different ways of thinking. In addition, they may be more open to discussing the role that negative thoughts, pessimism, and stress play in their illness, or the role that enhanced self-management skills would play in promoting wellness. For this reason, the inpatient stay offers multiple opportunities for the nurse to integrate cognitive behavioral therapy. Such integration can help establish a plan of care that is congruent with the patient's core values and beliefs. In one study, patients reported that the social support offered by nursing staff (organized around cognitive restructuring) was an important factor in their ability to successfully modify adverse lifestyle behaviors.[102]

Therapeutic Care Plan and Interventions

Together the holistic nurse and client develop a plan to attend to the identified concerns and mutually established goals. The holistic nurse's

careful planning will effect the success of this interaction. The following are guidelines for developing a therapeutic care plan and intervention."

Before the session:
- Establish a therapeutic relationship by creating a space in which both you and the client feel physically and emotionally safe and comfortable.
- Provide materials for recording cognitive distortions and alternative rational thoughts and statements (e.g., paper and pen, blackboard, preprinted forms).
- Center yourself; clear your mind of personal or professional issues to be fully present.
- Establish the long-term goals (outcome) of therapy with the client.

At the beginning of the session:
- Assess the client's level of mood, discomfort, or relaxation.
- Review homework from the previous session, if appropriate. Ask the client to describe any changes that have occurred since the previous session.

During the session:
- Determine, with the client, which issues need to be addressed and set short-term goals for the session.
- Listen and guide with focused intention. Provide appropriate feedback, clarification, support, or interpretation.

At the end of the session:
- Have the client identify and verbalize changes that have occurred during the session. Assess progress toward goals.
- Assign homework to be done for the next session.
- Schedule a follow-up session.

CASE STUDY

The same process that has been discussed throughout this chapter can also be used for inpatients, but the nurse would typically guide the patient through the process at the time of the stress. The following example considers the situation of a patient newly admitted to the coronary care unit who experiences chest pain. As the nurse responds to this potentially urgent clinical situation, he or she can gently guide the patient through the following exercise.

- **Stop:** Break the cycle of escalating, awfulizing, negative automatic thoughts. "I need you to stop and focus on letting go of the worry cycle. If we work together, we will get the best outcome. We have things under control, and I want you to let me worry about the technical things that need to be done. I want you to . . ."
- **Breathe:** Release physical tensions. "Focus on your breathing and leave the rest to me. Take nice, slow breaths, in and out. Concentrate on letting go of tension in your hands, jaw, and feet. Put all of your effort into feeling your fingers and toes, and let the jaw be relaxed and easy. Do you still feel tension somewhere in your body? If so, begin to relax that area. With each breath in, breathe in relaxation; with each breath out, breathe out tension. Now, begin to think about a favorite place and, as you breathe in, feel the peace of that place fill you; as you breathe out, let the worries and tension of the moment flow out."

The nurse guides the person through this relaxation/distraction exercise as he or she proceeds to treat the patient's chest pain. Obviously, it is not in the client's best interest for the nurse to stop what he or she is doing; rather, this skill needs to be such an integral part of the nurse's practice that it can be done while technologic tasks are performed. Empathic communication, presence, and touch enhance the process.

The next steps occur after the acute situation is over. "Tidying up" might be useful as a metaphor for dealing with the feelings that probably emerged in the patient. To continue with the chest pain example: The nurse guides the patient through the remainder of the cognitive restructuring steps.

- **Reflect:** Think back on what happened during the chest pain.
  - "Physically, how did you feel? Were there any areas you felt were particularly tense? Were you able to release physical tension? What works for you to release tension?" The nurse discusses the effect of

relaxation on ischemia and mental stress. The nurse empowers the patient with a specific skill that can be called on to help treat his or her myocardial ischemia.
  - "Emotionally, how did you feel?" The nurse invites the patient to talk about his or her feelings during this episode (e.g., worry, fear, anger, sadness). Using the concepts of awareness, automatic thoughts, and cognitive distortions, the nurse guides the patient through the process of realistic appraisal. Giving the patient permission to discuss his or her emotions and stress may help avoid all-or-nothing thinking, overgeneralization, jumping to conclusions, mental filtering, disqualification of the positive, and magnification. The patient is allowed to talk. The patient is gently encouraged to reveal any fears. The nurse helps the patient make an association between the emotional reaction to pain and the cycle of escalating pain this can create. Drawing a picture or writing in a journal can be useful if the person is reluctant to talk. The person's ability to identify his or her emotions needs to be accepted in a nonjudgmental way. Using a real-life, real-time, stressful experience provides a rich opportunity for dialogue and for teaching concrete self-management skills.
  - Is there another way to look at the situation? Are there opportunities here? An opportunity to reconnect with what is important in life? An opportunity to learn self-management skills that can treat the underlying pathophysiology? An opportunity to break the cycle of stress-worry-chest pain-stress-worry-chest pain? This is also an opportunity for the nurse to praise the patient for doing the best he or she could in a very stressful situation.
- **Choose:** Replace maladaptive, unrealistic, distorted thinking patterns with a more effective and realistic response. At this stage of illness, it is most helpful to focus on a plan that replaces the anxiety and tension response to chest pain with focused relaxation and affirmation. Additional coping

mechanisms can be addressed later in the hospital stay or in the outpatient setting.

Evaluation

Client outcomes that were established prior to initiating cognitive behavioral therapy and the client's subjective experiences are used to evaluate progress toward long-term goals. To evaluate progress toward short-term goals, client outcomes that were established prior to starting the session and the client's subjective experiences are used. Revising and updating goals are a part of each session.

Recognizing self-defeating automatic thoughts and silent assumptions in addition to changing long-standing health-risking behaviors is often challenging and frustrating to clients. With careful choice of interventions, honest and thoughtful feedback, and continuing support, the nurse can help clients gain significant health-affirming benefits. In turn, the nurse can realize the value of enhancing the client's autonomy and self-confidence in healthy behavior change and self-regulation.

■ CONCLUSION

Understanding and applying the principles of cognitive behavioral therapy provides an important tool for nurses to understand and address their own reactions to stress as well as to assist clients to optimize health and/or illness across the lifespan. Integrating cognitive behavioral therapy into nursing practice requires an appreciation for the effect of cognition on health and illness. Simple skills such as developing an awareness of stress warning signals, automatic thoughts and cognitive distortions, coupled with skills to choose a more effective coping strategy can enhance the health and illness experience. Although these skills are low-tech and inexpensive, mastery of these skills requires a skilled nurse and a committed client. It is a subtle process. Several attempts and several different ways of looking at a situation may be required before a client can recognize the automatic thoughts and underlying beliefs involved. Once they have this insight however the principles can be applied broadly and the effect is powerful.

Directions for FUTURE RESEARCH

1. Continue to evaluate the effectiveness of using the four-step approach of cognitive restructuring in helping clients change health-risking behaviors such as smoking, alcohol misuse, or overeating.
2. Continue to evaluate whether there are differences in the application of cognitive behavioral therapy among different gender, age, or cultural groups.
3. Continue to investigate cognitive distortions in children. Do the distortions change or intensify as children grow? Do children with similar distortions develop similar health issues as they mature?

Nurse Healer REFLECTIONS

After reading this chapter, the nurse healer will be able to answer or to begin the process of answering the following questions:

- What are my stress warning signals?
- What are the current stressors in my life?
- Can I pinpoint my negative automatic thoughts and silent assumptions that trigger and perpetuate my emotional upset?
- Can I use the four-step approach to help reduce my distress and effectively solve problems?
- Is there an affirmation I can create to help me counter self-defeating automatic thoughts and silent assumptions?

> **www** *For a full suite of assignments and additional learning activities, use the access code located in the front of your book to visit this exclusive website: http://go.jblearning.com/dossey. If you do not have an access code, you can obtain one at the site.*

NOTES

www.

1. G. Engel, "The Clinical Application of the Biopsychosocial Model," *American Journal of Psychiatry* 137 (1980): 535–544.

2. E. M. Stuart, "Spirituality in Health and Healing: A Clinical Program," *Holistic Nursing Practice* 3 (1989): 35–36.

3. A. T. Beck, "A Systematic Investigation of Depression," *Comprehensive Psychiatry* 2 (1961): 163–170.

4. H. Benson and E. M. Stuart, *The Wellness Book: A Comprehensive Guide to Maintaining Health and Treating Stress-related Illness* (New York: Fireside, Simon & Schuster, 1993).

5. A. T. Beck, *Cognitive Therapy* (New York: New American Library, 1979).

6. A. Beck, *Prisoners of Hate: The Cognitive Basis of Anger, Hostility and Violence* (New York: Harper Collins, 2000).

7. A. Ellis, *Reason and Emotion in Psychotherapy* (New York: Lyle Stuart, 1962).

8. A. Ellis, "A Critique of the Theoretical Contributions of Nondirective Therapy," *Journal of Clinical Psychology* 56 (2000): 897–905. Previously published in *Journal of Clinical Psychology* 4 (1948): 248–255.

9. D. Meichenbaum, *Cognitive Behavior Modification: An Integrative Approach* (New York: Plenum Press, 1977).

10. D. D. Burns, *Ten Days to Self-Esteem* (New York: William Morrow, 1993).

11. D. D. Burns, *The New Mood Therapy* (New York: William Morrow Paperbacks, 1999).

12. A. T. Beck, "The Current State of Cognitive Therapy: A 40-Year Retrospective," *Archives of General Psychiatry* 62 (2005): 953–959.

13. A. C. Butler, J. E. Chapman, E. M. Forman, and A. T. Beck, "The Empirical Status of Cognitive-Behavioral Therapy: A Review of Meta-analyses," *Clinical Psychology Review* 26 (2006): 17–31.

14. D. F. Tolin, "Is Cognitive-Behavioral Therapy More Effective Than Other Therapies? A Meta-analytic Review," *Clinical Psychology Review* 30 (2010): 710–720.

15. L. E. Steinman, J. T. Frederick, T. Prochaska, et al., "Recommendations for Treating Depression in Community-Based Older Adults," *American Journal of Preventive Medicine* 22 (2007): 175–181.

16. H. Kornor, D. Winje, O. Ekeberg, et al., "Early Trauma-Focused Cognitive-Behavioural Therapy to Prevent Chronic Post-Traumatic Stress Disorder and Related Symptoms: A Systematic Review and Meta-analysis," *BMC Psychiatry* 8 (2008): 81.

17. J. Fairbank, H. Frost, J. Wilson-MacDonald, L. M. Yu, K. Barker, and R. Collins, "Randomised Controlled Trial to Compare Surgical Stabilisation of the Lumbar Spine with an Intensive Rehabilitation Programme for Patients with Chronic Low Back Pain: The MRC Spine Stabilisation Trial," *British Medical Journal* 3330 (2005): 1233.

18. N. C. van der Ven, C. H. Lubach, M. H. Hogenelst, et al., "Cognitive Behavioural Group Training (CBGT) for Patients with Type 1 Diabetes in Persistent Poor Glycaemic Control: Who Do We Reach?" *Patient Education and Counseling* 56 (2005): 313–322.

19. N. C. van der Ven, M. H. Hogenelst, A. M. Tromp-Wever, et al., "Short-Term Effects of Cognitive Behavioural Group Training (CBGT) in Adult Type 1 Diabetes Patients in Prolonged Poor Glycaemic Control. A Randomized Controlled Trial," *Diabetic Medicine* 22 (2005): 1619–1623.

20. G. Forlani, C. Lorusso, S. Moscatiello, et al., "Are Behavioural Approaches Feasible and Effective in the Treatment of Type 2 Diabetes? A Propensity Score Analysis vs. Prescriptive Diet," *Nutrition, Metabolism, and Cardiovascular Diseases* 19 (2009): 313–320.

21. L. E. Egede and M. A. Hernandez-Tejada, "Type I Diabetes: Motivational Enhancement Therapy Delivered with CBT by Nurse Therapists to People with Type I Diabetes Leads to Lowering of HbA1C Values," *Evidence-Based Mental Health* 14 (2010): 19.

22. K. Ismail, E. Maissi, S. Thomas, et al., "A Randomised Controlled Trial of Cognitive Behaviour Therapy and Motivational Interviewing for People with Type 1 Diabetes Mellitus with Persistent Sub-optimal Glycaemic Control: A Diabetes and Psychological Therapies (ADaPT) Study," *Health Technology Assessment* 14, no. 1 (2010): 1–101, iii–iv.

23. M. Y. Wang, S. Y. Wang, and P. S. Tsai, "Cognitive Behavioural Therapy for Primary Insomnia: A Systematic Review," *Journal of Advanced Nursing* 50 (2005): 553–564.

24. C. M. Morin, R. R. Bootzin, D. J. Buysse, J. D. Edinger, C. A. Espie, and K. L. Lichstein, "Psychological and Behavioral Treatment of Insomnia: Update of the Recent Evidence (1998–2004)," *Sleep* 29 (2006): 1398–1414.

25. M. Sijbrandij, M. Olff, J. B. Reitsma, I. V. Carlier, M. H. de Vries, and B. P. Gersons, "Treatment of Acute Posttraumatic Stress Disorder with Brief Cognitive Behavioral Therapy: A Randomized Controlled Trial," *American Journal of Psychiatry* 164 (2007): 82–90.

26. M. S. Page, A. M. Berger, and L. B. Johnson, "Putting Evidence into Practice: Evidence-Based Interventions for Sleep–Wake Disturbances," *Clinical Journal of Oncology Nursing* 10 (2006): 753–767.

27. C. Wells-Federman, P. Arnstein, and M. Caudill, "Nurse-Led Pain Management Program: Effect

on Self-Efficacy, Pain Intensity, Pain-Related Disability, and Depressive Symptoms in Chronic Pain Patients," *Pain Management Nursing* 3 (2002): 131–140.

28. K. L. Kirsh and S. M. Fishman, "Multimodal Approaches to Optimize Outcomes of Chronic Opioid Therapy in the Management of Chronic Pain," *Pain Medicine* 12, suppl. 1 (2011): S1–11.

29. K. Bernardy, N. Fuber, V. Kollner, and W. Hauser, "Efficacy of Cognitive-Behavioral Therapies in Fibromyalgia Syndrome—a Systematic Review and Meta-analysis of Randomized Controlled Trials," *Journal of Rheumatology* 37 (2010): 1991–2005.

30. J. A. Glombiewski, A. T. Sawyer, J. Gutermann, K. Koenig, W. Rief, and S. G. Hofmann, "Psychological Treatments for Fibromyalgia: A Meta-analysis," *Pain* 151 (2010): 280–295.

31. R. E. Goslin, R. N. Gray, D. C. McCrory, D. Penzien, J. Rains, and V. Hasselblad, *Behavioral and Physical Treatments for Migraine Headache* (Rockville, MD: Agency for Healthcare Research and Quality, February 1999).

32. D. Dorstyn, J. Mathias, and L. Denson, "Efficacy of Cognitive Behavior Therapy for the Management of Psychological Outcomes Following Spinal Cord Injury: A Meta-analysis," *Journal of Health Psychology* 16 (2011): 374–391.

33. A. Al Sayegh, D. Sandford, and A. J. Carson, "Psychological Approaches to Treatment of Postconcussion Syndrome: A Systematic Review," *Journal of Neurology, Neurosurgery, and Psychiatry* 81 (2010): 1128–1134.

34. A. J. Wearden, L. Riste, C. Dowrick, et al., "Fatigue Intervention by Nurses Evaluation—the FINE Trial. A Randomised Controlled Trial of Nurse Led Self-Help Treatment for Patients in Primary Care with Chronic Fatigue Syndrome: Study Protocol" [ISRCTN74156610]. *BMC Medicine* 4 (2006): 9.

35. S. A. Albrecht, D. Caruthers, T. Patrick, et al., "A Randomized Controlled Trial of a Smoking Cessation Intervention for Pregnant Adolescents," *Nursing Research* 55 (2006): 402–410.

36. R. D. Weiss and K. D. Kueppenbender, "Combining Psychosocial Treatment with Pharmacotherapy for Alcohol Dependence," *Journal of Clinical Psychopharmacology* 26 (2006): S37–S42.

37. S. Munsch, E. Biedert, A. Meyer, et al., "A Randomized Comparison of Cognitive Behavioral Therapy and Behavioral Weight Loss Treatment for Overweight Individuals with Binge Eating Disorder," *International Journal of Eating Disorders* 40, no. 2 (2007): 102–113.

38. H. Hesser, C. Weise, V. Z. Westin, and G. Andersson, "A Systematic Review and Meta-analysis of Randomized Controlled Trials of Cognitive-Behavioral Therapy for Tinnitus Distress," *Clinical Psychology Review* 31 (2011): 545–553.

39. S. Sussman, P. Sun, and C. W. Dent, "A Meta-analysis of Teen Cigarette Smoking Cessation," *Health Psychology* 25 (2006): 549–557.

40. G. M. Bartol and N. F. Courts, "The Psychophysiology of Bodymind Healing," in *Holistic Nursing: A Handbook for Practice*, ed. B. Dossey, C. Guzetta, and L. Keegan (Sudbury MA: Jones & Bartlett, 2005): 111–133.

41. W. B. Cannon, "The Emergency Function of the Adrenal Medulla in Pain and the Major Emotions," *American Journal of Physiology* 33 (1914): 356–372.

42. H. Selye, "Handbook of Stress: Theoretical and Clinical Aspects," in *History and Present Status of Stress Concept*, ed. L. Goldberger and S. Breznitz (New York: Free Press, 1982): 7–20.

43. J. Shelby and K. L. McCance, "Stress and Disease," in *Pathophysiology: The Biologic Basis for Disease in Adults and Children*, ed. K. L. McCance and S. E. Heuther (St. Louis, MO: Mosby, 1998).

44. J. E. Graham, T. F. Robles, J. K. Kiecolt-Glaser, W. B. Malarkey, M. G. Bissell, and R. Glaser, "Hostility and Pain Are Related to Inflammation in Older Adults," *Brain, Behavior, and Immunity* 20 (2006): 389–400.

45. N. Ranjit, A. V. Diez-Roux, S. Shea, et al., "Psychosocial Factors and Inflammation in the Multi-ethnic Study of Atherosclerosis," *Archives of Internal Medicine* 167 (2007): 174–181.

46. T. W. McDade, L. C. Hawkley, and J. T. Cacioppo, "Psychosocial and Behavioral Predictors of Inflammation in Middle-Aged and Older Adults: The Chicago Health, Aging, and Social Relations Study," *Psychosomatic Medicine* 68 (2006): 376–381.

47. M. B. Olson, D. S. Krantz, S. F. Kelsey, et al., "Hostility Scores Are Associated with Increased Risk of Cardiovascular Events in Women Undergoing Coronary Angiography: A Report from the NHLBI-Sponsored WISE Study," *Psychosomatic Medicine* 67 (2005): 546–552.

48. D. S. Krantz, M. B. Olson, J. L. Francis, et al., "Anger, Hostility, and Cardiac Symptoms in Women with Suspected Coronary Artery Disease: The Women's Ischemia Syndrome Evaluation (WISE) Study," *Journal of Women's Health* 15 (2006): 1214–1223.

49. L. V. Doering, D. K. Moser, W. Lemankiewicz, C. Luper, and S. Khan, "Depression, Healing, and Recovery from Coronary Artery Bypass Surgery," *American Journal of Critical Care* 14 (2005): 316–324.

50. G. S. Alexopoulos, I. R. Katz, C. F. Reynolds III, D. Carpenter, and J. P. Docherty, "The Expert Consensus Guideline Series. Pharmacotherapy of

Depressive Disorders in Older Patients," special issue, *Postgraduate Medicine* (2001): 1–86.

51. S. Vocks, T. Legenbauer, A. Wachter, M. Wucherer, and J. Kosfelder, "What Happens in the Course of Body Exposure? Emotional, Cognitive, and Physiological Reactions to Mirror Confrontation in Eating Disorders," *Journal of Psychosomatic Research* 62 (2007): 231–239.

52. F. I. Fawzy, N. W. Fawzy, C. S. Hyun, et al., "Malignant Melanoma. Effects of an Early Structured Psychiatric Intervention, Coping, and Affective State on Recurrence and Survival 6 Years Later," *Archives of General Psychiatry* 50 (1993): 681–689.

53. D. Spiegel, J. R. Bloom, H. C. Kraemer, and E. Gottheil, "Effect of Psychosocial Treatment on Survival of Patients with Metastatic Breast Cancer," *Lancet* 2 (1989): 888–891.

54. A. Mehnert, A. Scherwath, L. Schirmer, et al., "The Association Between Neuropsychological Impairment, Self-Perceived Cognitive Deficits, Fatigue and Health Related Quality of Life in Breast Cancer Survivors Following Standard Adjuvant Versus High-Dose Chemotherapy," *Patient Education and Counseling* 66 (2007): 108–118.

55. P. Sherwood, B. A. Given, C. W. Given, et al., "A Cognitive Behavioral Intervention for Symptom Management in Patients with Advanced Cancer," *Oncology Nursing Forum* 32 (2005): 1190–1198.

56. R. Curtis, A. Groarke, R. Coughlan, and A. Gsel, "Psychological Stress as a Predictor of Psychological Adjustment and Health Status in Patients with Rheumatoid Arthritis," *Patient Education and Counseling* 59 (2005): 192–198.

57. R. K. Dissanayake and J. V. Bertouch, "Psychosocial Interventions as Adjunct Therapy for Patients with Rheumatoid Arthritis: A Systematic Review," *International Journal of Rheumatic Disorders* 13 (2010): 324–334.

58. J. A. Turner, S. Holtzman, and L. Mancl, "Mediators, Moderators, and Predictors of Therapeutic Change in Cognitive-Behavioral Therapy for Chronic Pain," *Pain* 127 (2007): 276–286.

59. J. C. Rains, G. L. Lipchik, and D. B. Penzien, "Behavioral Facilitation of Medical Treatment for Headache—Part I: Review of Headache Treatment Compliance," *Headache* 46 (2006): 1387–1394.

60. J. C. Rains, D. B. Penzien, and G. L. Lipchik, "Behavioral Facilitation of Medical Treatment for Headache—Part II: Theoretical Models and Behavioral Strategies for Improving Adherence," *Headache* 46 (2006): 1395–1403.

61. E. A. Kuhl, S. F. Sears, and J. B. Conti, "Internet-Based Behavioral Change and Psychosocial Care for Patients with Cardiovascular Disease: A Review of Cardiac Disease-Specific Applications," *Heart & Lung* 35 (2006): 374–382.

62. C. F. Mendes de Leon, S. M. Czajkowski, K. E. Freedland, et al., "The Effect of a Psychosocial Intervention and Quality of Life After Acute Myocardial Infarction: The Enhancing Recovery in Coronary Heart Disease (ENRICHD) Clinical Trial," *Journal of Cardiopulmonary Rehabilitation* 26 (2006): 9–13, quiz 4-5.

63. S. F. Sears, Jr., L. A. Stutts, J. M. Aranda, Jr., E. M. Handberg, and J. B. Conti, "Managing Congestive Heart Failure Patient Factors in the Device Era," *Congestive Heart Failure* 12 (2006): 335–340.

64. Writing Group of the PREMIER Collaborative Research Group, "Effects of Comprehensive Lifestyle Modification on Blood Pressure Control: Main Results of the Premier Clinical Trial," *Journal of the American Medical Association* 289 (2003): 2083–2093.

65. R. Sethness, M. Rauschhuber, A. Etnyre, I. Gilliland, J. Lowry, and M. E. Jones, "Cardiac Health: Relationships Among Hostility, Spirituality, and Health Risk," *Journal of Nursing Care Quality* 20 (2005): 81–89.

66. P. van Andel, R. A. Erdman, P. A. Karsdorp, A. Appels, and R. W. Trijsburg, "Group Cohesion and Working Alliance: Prediction of Treatment Outcome in Cardiac Patients Receiving Cognitive Behavioral Group Psychotherapy," *Psychotherapy and Psychosomatics* 72 (2003): 141–149.

67. L. L. Yan, K. Liu, K. A. Matthews, M. L. Daviglus, T. F. Ferguson, and C. I. Kiefe, "Psychosocial Factors and Risk of Hypertension: The Coronary Artery Risk Development in Young Adults (CARDIA) Study," *Journal of the American Medical Association* 290 (2003): 2138–2148.

68. M. Gulliksson, G. Burell, B. Vessby, L. Lundin, H. Toss, and K. Svardsudd, "Randomized Controlled Trial of Cognitive Behavioral Therapy vs Standard Treatment to Prevent Recurrent Cardiovascular Events in Patients with Coronary Heart Disease: Secondary Prevention in Uppsala Primary Health Care Project (SUPRIM)," *Archives of Internal Medicine* 171 (2011): 134–140.

69. V. M. Deshmukh, B. G. Toelle, T. Usherwood, B. O'Grady, and C. R. Jenkins, "Anxiety, Panic and Adult Asthma: A Cognitive-Behavioral Perspective," *Respiratory Medicine* 101 (2007): 194–202.

70. G. D. Jacobs, E. F. Pace-Schott, R. Stickgold, and M. W. Otto, "Cognitive Behavior Therapy and Pharmacotherapy for Insomnia: A Randomized Controlled Trial and Direct Comparison," *Archives of Internal Medicine* 164 (2004): 1888–1896.

71. S. L. Berga and T. L. Loucks, "Use of Cognitive Behavior Therapy for Functional Hypothalamic Amenorrhea," *Annals of the New York Academy of Science* 1092 (2006): 114–129.

72. A. D. Domar, "The Impact of Group Psychological Interventions on Distress in Fertile Women," *Health Psychology* 1 (2000): 568–575.

73. T. M. Cousineau and A. D. Domar, "Psychological Impact of Infertility," *Best Practice and Research Clinical Obstetrics and Gynaecology* 21 (2007): 293–308.

74. K. R. Lorig, D. S. Sobel, A. L. Stewart, et al., "Evidence Suggesting That a Chronic Disease Self-Management Program Can Improve Health Status While Reducing Hospitalization: A Randomized Trial," *Medical Care* 37 (1999): 5–14.

75. C. L. Bockting, A. H. Schene, P. Spinhoven, et al., "Preventing Relapse/Recurrence in Recurrent Depression with Cognitive Therapy: A Randomized Controlled Trial," *Journal of Consulting and Clinical Psychology* 73 (2005): 647–657.

76. M. Tazaki and K. Landlaw, "Behavioural Mechanisms and Cognitive-Behavioural Interventions of Somatoform Disorders," *International Review of Psychiatry* 18 (2006): 67–73.

77. T. Maruta, R. C. Colligan, M. Malinchoc, and K. P. Offord, "Optimism-Pessimism Assessed in the 1960s and Self-Reported Health Status 30 Years Later," *Mayo Clinic Proceedings* 77 (2002): 748–753.

78. A. Steptoe, C. Wright, S. R. Kunz-Ebrecht, and S. Iliffe, "Dispositional Optimism and Health Behaviour in Community-Dwelling Older People: Associations with Healthy Ageing," *British Journal of Health Psychology* 11 (2006): 71–84.

79. A. Steptoe, J. Wardle, T. M. Pollard, L. Canaan, and G. J. Davies, "Stress, Social Support and Health-Related Behavior: A Study of Smoking, Alcohol Consumption and Physical Exercise," *Journal of Psychosomatic Research* 41 (1996): 171–180.

80. G. Marlatt, "Relapse Prevention: Theoretical Rationale and Overview of the Mode," in *Relapse Prevention*, ed. G. Marlatt and J. Gordon (New York: Guilford, 1985, pp. 280–350).

81. F. Lesperance and N. Frasure-Smith, "Depression and Heart Disease," *Cleveland Clinic Journal of Medicine* 74, Suppl. 1 (2007): S63–S66.

82. N. Frasure-Smith and R. Prince, "Long-Term Follow-up of the Ischemic Heart Disease Life Stress Monitoring Program," *Psychosomatic Medicine* 47 (1989): 485–513.

83. E. D. Hodnett, S. Gates, G. J. Hofmeyr, and C. Sakala, "Continuous Support for Women During Childbirth," *Cochrane Database of Systematic Reviews* 2, Art. No. CD003766 (2003).

84. D. A. Campbell, M. F. Lake, M. Falk, and J. R. Backstrand, "A Randomized Control Trial of Continuous Support in Labor by a Lay Doula," *Journal of Obstetric, Gynecologic, and Neonatal Nursing* 35 (2006): 456–464.

85. D. Ornish, "Intensive Lifestyle Changes for Reversal of Coronary Heart Disease," *Journal of the American Medical Association* 280 (1998): 2001–2007.

86. V. Frankl, *Man's Search for Meaning* (Boston: Beacon Press, 1963).

87. I. S. Harvey and M. Silverman, "The Role of Spirituality in the Self-Management of Chronic Illness Among Older Africans and Whites," *Journal of Cross-Cultural Gerontology* 22 (2007): 205–220.

88. K. S. Masters and G. I. Spielmans, "Prayer and Health: Review, Meta-Analysis, and Research Agenda," *Journal of Behavioral Medicine, 30*(4), 329–338 (2007).

89. F. A. Curlin, S. A. Sellergren, J. D. Lantos, and M. H. Chin, "Physicians' Observations and Interpretations of the Influence of Religion and Spirituality on Health," *Archives of Internal Medicine* 167 (2007): 649–654.

90. E. J. Yuen, "Spirituality, Religion, and Health," *American Journal of Medical Quality* 22 (2007): 77–79.

91. A. R. Childress and D. D. Burns, "The Basics of Cognitive Therapy," *Psychosomatics* 22 (1981): 1017–1027.

92. A. Webster, "How Thoughts Affect Health," in *The Wellness Book*, ed. H. Benson and E. Stuart (New York: Fireside, Simon & Schuster, 1993).

93. E. Stuart et al., "Coping and Problem Solving," in *The Wellness Book*, ed. H. Benson and E. Stuart (New York: Fireside, Simon & Schuster, 1993).

94. D. Burns, *The Feeling Good Handbook: Using the New Mood Therapy in Everyday Life* (New York: William Morrow, 1989).

95. A. Ellis, *How to Make Yourself Happy and Remarkably Less Disturbable* (Lafayette, CO: Impact Publishers, 1999).

96. J. Pennebaker, *Opening Up: The Healing Power of Confiding in Others* (New York: William Morrow, 1990).

97. M. A. Caudill, *Managing Pain Before It Manages You*, 3rd ed. (New York: Guilford Press, 2008).

98. C. Rogers, *Client-Centered Therapy* (Boston: Houghton Mifflin, 1951).

99. J. N. Kingery, T. L. Roblek, C. Suveg, R. L. Grover, J. T. Sherrill, and R. L. Bergman, "They're Not Just 'Little Adults': Developmental Considerations for Implementing Cognitive-Behavioral Therapy with Anxious Youth," *Journal of Cognitive Psychotherapy: An International Quarterly* 20 (2006): 263–273.

100. N. J. King, D. Heyne, and T. H. Ollendick, "Cognitive-Behavioral Treatments for Anxiety and Phobic Disorders in Children and Adolescents: A Review," *Behavioral Disorders* 20 (2005): 241–257.

101. J. W. Maag and S. M. Swearer, "Cognitive-Behavioral Interventions for Depression: Review and Implications for School Personnel," *Behavioral Disorders* 30 (2005): 259–276.

102. C. J. Medich, E. Stuart, and S. K. Chase, "Healing Through Integration: Promoting Wellness in Cardiac Rehabilitation," *Journal of Cardiovascular Nursing* 11 (1997): 66–79.

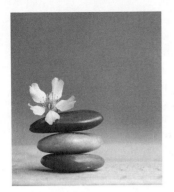

Self-Reflection

Jackie D. Levin and Jennifer L. Reich

Nurse Healer
OBJECTIVES

Theoretical

- Define the concept of self-reflection.
- Define reflective practice.
- Discuss theories integral to self-reflection: Newman, Rogers, Barrett, Watson, Dossey, and Smith and Liehr as they relate to the concept of self-reflection.

Clinical

- Identify specific ways that self-reflection strategies affect clinical practice.
- Identify ways to facilitate the integration of self-reflection strategies with clients.

Personal

- Identify one or more self-reflection strategies to use as part of your self-care practice.
- Explore one or more self-reflection strategies that are unfamiliar to you as a nurse healer.

DEFINITIONS

Consciousness: Information in the form of pattern and meaning.

Deliberative mutual patterning: Coparticipative process of nurse with client patterning and/or repatterning the unified human-environmental fields to promote health and inner coherence as the client defines it.

Habitual patterning: Automatic noncritical responses to thoughts, feelings, situations, and ideas.

Inner coherence: Internal harmony, synchronization, and order in a system.

Intention: Focusing attention from a place of conscious awareness.

Mind-body-spirit complex: Integrated unified aspects of being human.

Pattern appraisal/appreciation: Continuous process of recognizing the manifestation of the human and environmental fields as they are expressed.

Reflective practice: Continuous mutual process of inner awareness/self-reflection of internal and external pattern manifestation as it is occurring.

Self: A principle that underlies and organizes subjective experience.

Self-centering: Practice of coming into balance, aware of the forces that are pulling us one way and then the other.

Self-reflection: Inner awareness of our thoughts, feelings, judgments, beliefs, and perceptions.

Unknowing: A state of being that is open to not-knowing.

■ THEORY AND RESEARCH

> When we enlarge our worldview to face the depth of our humanity and to look into the face of the other, both literally and metaphorically, we establish a primordial basis for our caring and our shared humanity.
>
> —J. Watson, "Social Justice and Human Caring: A Model of Caring Science as a Hopeful Paradigm for Moral Justice for Humanity"

Self-reflection is both a self-care and a therapeutic clinical practice that integrates the critical thinking mind with the intelligent compassion of the heart.[1-3] It is a skill that requires focus and practice to develop inner awareness of one's thoughts, feelings, sensations, judgments, and perceptions. As a practice it requires the holistic nurse to face his or her inner self with honesty, compassion, curiosity, and humor; for without this practice, we may become captive to our own and others' habitual perceptions and automatic responses.

Self-reflection occurs in multiple realms and provides access to a number of ways of knowing. Carper first described *personal knowing, empirical knowing, aesthetic knowing,* and *ethical knowing* as four possible ways of knowing.[4] Munhall introduced *unknowing* as a way of knowing.[5] Unknowing, in particular, facilitates new insights and reduces the fears and anxieties that arise with questions, silence, and our inability to explain the unexplainable.[6] "It is a thinking process focused not on achievement of the answers, but on achievement of a coherence of understanding within the context of a situation."[2p211] Siegel describes self-reflection as a tripod. The three legs, openness, objectivity, and observation, create stability of the mind. "From this stabilization we gain all the gifts of acuity: keenness, insight, perception, and, ultimately, wisdom."[3p31]

Self-reflection is specifically addressed in the *Holistic Nursing: Scope and Standards of Practice* under *Practice Standards* and *Self-Care Standards.*[7] As such, it demonstrates that not only is self-reflection for personal awareness, but for clinical awareness as well.

To appreciate one's own pattern manifestations as well as those with whom we work, self-reflection engages a part of ourselves that often escapes our attention during the business of our workday. To dive more deeply into the source of our patterns, thoughts, and beliefs, a formal practice of setting aside time for quiet reflection facilitates awareness and insight. However, holistic nursing is more than awareness. It is awareness in practice, something that is both highly attentive and present to the moment. A *reflective practice*, therefore, is self-reflection in action. It is a coparticipative, mutual, and continuous process of awareness. It occurs in real time, fully engaging in our own and that of our patients'/clients' pattern appraisal.[8-9]

Rolfe describes the reflective practitioner as operating at a sixth level of nursing,[8] which is beyond Benner's five levels of novice to expert.[10] He writes:

> The reflexive practitioner, in contrast, requires a particular sort of mindfulness which involves an intense concentration on the task at hand. Even with very simple tasks such as wound dressing, the difference is striking: the expert nurse would perform the required actions swiftly and deftly and without conscious thought, whereas the reflexive practitioner would think about every move, every decision, relating them to this patient in this situation. . . . Reflection-in-action therefore serves to focus the attention of nurses on the here-and-now and on the uniqueness of their individual relationships with each of their patients, and reduces the possibility of the boredom and burn out that comes from over-familiarity with the tasks to be performed.[8p96]

Finally, self-reflection is an act of service. The time spent observing one's thoughts and beliefs prepares the nurse for the safe and deep relationship to self and others. Thich Nhat Hanh, a Vietnamese Buddhist monk, poet, and scholar, has written that the practices of compassionate listening and caring speech arise from a meditative reflective practice.[11] Watson notes that in a caring occasion with another individual we learn to identify our self within the other and the other within our self. Thus, we learn self-knowledge and our connection to the universal human self.[12]

> ### REFLECTION BREAK:
> ### UNKNOWING
>
> Find a space where you can sit quietly for 5 or 10 minutes undisturbed. What events or situations have motivated you to self-reflect? Begin to consider what relevance self-reflection has in your nursing practice.

Nursing Theory Related to Self-Reflection

Nursing theory, integral to self-reflection, is incorporated in theories at all levels on the ladder of abstraction. Examples of grand theories in which self-reflection is inherent are Rogers' Science of Unitary Human Beings (SUHB), Barrett's Power Theory, Dossey's Theory of Integral Nursing (TIN), Watson's Caring Science, and Newman's Theory of Health as Expanding Consciousness (HEC). Smith and Liehr's Story Theory is an example of self-reflection embedded in a middle-range theory.

Barrett's Power Theory formulates that "power is the capacity to participate knowingly in change."[13p48] It also consists of appraising "four inseparable dimensions—awareness, choices, freedom to act intentionally, and involvement in creating change."[13p49] Knowing participation on the part of the nurse and client/patient within a reflective practice is more than knowing what tests are to be performed and performing one's clinical skills with expertise. Knowing participation means the nurse and the patient are both aware to the degree possible (the nurse) and as much as desired (the patient) of her or his field patterning. Without this awareness, neither the nurse nor the patient can act intentionally.

Dossey developed her Theory of Integral Nursing (TIN) as praxis, theory in action.[14] (See Chapter 1.) One component of TIN is represented in a model with four quadrants. Each of the quadrants, the "I" individual interior (personal/intentional), the "IT" individual exterior (objective, behavioral), the "WE" (collective interior), and the "ITS" (collective exterior), formulate how we view and describe our reality. Dossey explains that the development of the "I," or self-awareness, is critical to becoming a healthy nurse. When the nurse engages in self-reflection, she or he develops insight into patterns and behaviors and is able to create a new future. In the WE space, the nurse engages with the client in a coparticipatory process. Key to this process, the nurse acts with intention, which arises from self-reflection.[14]

Intention

We can tap into our healing source
Without force or will
Or by taking a pill
For when we are still
We know
That all movement
Flows
From within
And begins
With intention[15]

> ### REFLECTION BREAK:
> ### INTENTION
>
> Take a moment to pause and reflect on what intention means to your practice as a nurse. What patterns do you notice connecting the way you care for self and the way you care for others?

Newman's Theory of Health as Expanding Consciousness (HEC) defines "consciousness as the *information* of the system: The capacity of the [human] system to interact with the environment [system]."[16p33] HEC is a coparticipatory consciousness, where one's experience and the meaning derived from it expands beyond the physical self into the greater consciousness of the unified field of awareness, which includes one's self, the environment, patients, and families. Health is not defined by the presence or the absence of disease, but rather by the transformation through chaos to a higher order of complexity and understanding. Chaos brings uncertainty, which is a component of unknowing pattern appreciation essential to the practice of self-reflection in action. The more comfortable the nurse becomes with uncertainty, the greater the possibilities for transformation, both for the nurse and the client/patient.[17] Without self-reflection, chaos remains chaos. The nurse, then, through the practice of self-reflection and reflective practice, facilitates increasing coherence and expanded consciousness.

Watson expresses that a caring science perspective is rooted in a relational ontology of being-in-relation, with unity and connectedness composing the worldview. She explains that caring science embraces multiple approaches to inquiry and is open to exploring other ways of knowing such as aesthetic, poetic, personal, intuitive, and spiritual among others.[18] Self-reflection as a process can assist the holistic nurse to access these realms.

Rogers' Science of Unitary Human Beings (SUHB) describes several important concepts essential to self-reflection. The concepts of wholeness and openness regard the person as an "irreducible, indivisible, multidimensional (now called pandimensionality) energy field identified by pattern and manifesting characteristics that are specific to the whole and which cannot be predicted from the knowledge of its parts."[19p7] The heart of the Rogerian ontology is the fundamental unity of the universe and that the universe is more than and different from the sum of its parts.[20] Pattern recognition is what identifies the nurse and client in their inherent uniqueness as well as their wholeness. Pandimensionality is a nonlinear domain with time and space as nonlocal and nontemporal. The self-reflective practitioner attunes to the pandimensional field, allowing the process of unfolding to occur, creating new patterning as desired.

Smith and Liehr's Story Theory holds assumptions consistent with unitary and neomodernist perspectives and is at the middle range level of abstraction.[21,22] Story Theory is built on the foundations of three concepts: intentional dialogue, connecting with self-in-relation, and creating ease. The concept of connecting with self-in-relation comprises personal history and reflective awareness.[22] The individual's personal history is described as his or her unique story that he or she uncovers through reflection on his or her life. Reflective awareness is explained

as a person's ability to be in touch with his or her experiences, thoughts, and feelings in the present moment. Intentional dialogue between nurse–person is what engages the human story and affords the nurse the ability to connect with self-in-relation to create ease.[22]

REFLECTION BREAK: WORLDVIEW

Take a moment to consider the theories mentioned here. How does your worldview align with these theories? How does it differ? Develop a statement of your worldview of nursing.

Research

Research on self-reflection and reflective practice can be found in a number of disciplines in the health and social sciences. Numerous self-reflection research studies evaluate the effect of self-reflection both on learning and on improvements in clinical practice.[1,2,9,23-26] There is a general belief that self-reflection does enhance the learner's ability to learn from experience and apply this learning to new situations; however, the research to date is inconclusive, diverse, and inconsistent.[2,9,23,24]

It is commonly agreed that self-reflection is part of being a professional in practice.[9] The challenge noted in the research is the lack of clarity of what exactly is being measured. Hays and Gay ask the following questions regarding the study of self-reflection:

> There is an urgent need to determine what it is we are trying to foster and to measure. Is reflective practice a single, stable construct? Is it a skill set that can be taught? Is it measurable, such that reflective practice can be assessed along the lines of other components of competence in medicine [and nursing]? How can insight and the taking of responsibility be taught and assessed? Is reflection something that should be assessed other than in writing, such as through verbal discussion?[24p117]

Self-reflection itself may be a challenge to measure; however, the manifestation of various self-reflective strategies can be observed. For example, Forneris and Peden-McAlpine's research on a small cohort of nursing students used a case-based approach to study self-reflection's impact on critical thinking. "Critical thinking is defined as a process of reflective thinking . . . focused not on achievement of the answers, but on achievement of a coherence of understanding within the context of a situation."[2p411] The study took place over three time periods using narrative reflective journaling, individual interviews, preceptor coaching, and leader-facilitated discussion groups. The results showed the novice nurse moved through anxiety (time period 1), to questioning in a linear format (time period 2), to the beginnings of the nurse as an "intentional critical thinker" (time period 3).

Neuroscience research is forging new territory exploring the changes the brain makes (neuroplasticity) when using self-reflective processes.[27] Siegel and Huther describe self-reflection as part of the natural neuronal wiring.[3,28] Self-reflection and reflective practice utilize the neuronal pathways that travel through the insula and inform and expand the brain's capacity for empathy and resonating with others.[3,28] Sensing and attuning to our internal states open up these pathways, and not only do we expand our consciousness this way, we also find resonance with those we reflect with and upon.[3]

Mindfulness meditation, a practice of moment-to-moment awareness, is also the subject of self-reflection research. Raffone and Srinivasan's review of several studies on meditation describes how meditation improved self-regulatory and metacognitive skills as well as increased self-awareness and empathy.[27] Carmody and Baer's research on an 8-week mindfulness-based stress reduction program resulted in less stress and a greater sense of well-being.[29] Matousek and Dobkin reported participants experienced a greater sense of coherence after an 8-week mindfulness-based stress awareness program.[30] Stress is a limiting factor in self-reflection, activating the fight-or-flight sympathetic system, whereas relaxation engages the parasympathetic system, allowing for more choices in awareness.

■ HOLISTIC CARING PROCESS

The holistic caring process (HCP) is a paradigm shift from the traditional nursing process. The HCP is exploratory, open to unknowing, and coparticipative rather than diagnostic, explanatory, and paternal. The following chart outlines both processes. Self-reflection and reflective practice are integral within the HCP.

Holistic Caring Process	Traditional Nursing Process
Holistic pattern knowing and appreciation	Assessment
Pattern recognition: coherence and incoherence	Identification of patterns/challenges/needs
Mutual pattern reflection	
Mutual health patterning process	Outcome identification therapeutic care plan and interventions

Holistic Pattern Appreciation

Holistic pattern knowing and appreciation (HPKA) is a process of observing the manifested aspects of the person with the awareness that these visible patterns are only part of the person's underlying, unseen, unitary self. Pattern appreciation of the human being's mind-body-spirit complex can be related to observing an iceberg. The manifested tip of the iceberg rises above the surface as a pattern of the mass of the iceberg that lies beneath the surface, unseen. In relating this metaphor to HCP and pattern knowing and appreciation, we come to realize that the hidden parts are potentially more significant and a force to be honored.

HPKA is a manifestation of our self-reflection practice and is demonstrated with open-ended questions, a curious attitude, and a presence of unitary coherence.[27,31,32] Newman writes, "Embrace the unfolding pattern of the whole whatever it is and grow with it."[17p93]

Nurses come into contact with patients/clients when they are in a state of change, chaos, or with a desire for improved health and well-being. The disorder in their system causes distress and disease and a rich opportunity for clients to engage in their own pattern knowing and appreciation. Reflective practice requires listening immersed in nonjudging attention to the clients' phrasing, metaphor, timing of speech, as well as to the silences. This is in contrast to the traditional medical and nursing models of asking a series of questions, often interrupting the patient/client several times. Consider the following familiar fairy tale as an example from Meyer:

> **Patient:** Once upon a time, there was a little girl who loved her grandmother very much, and her grandmother loved her. Her grandmother gave her a red velvet hood that the little girl wore all the time.
> **Clinician:** Was there a reason that she wore the hood all the time?
> **Patient:** No, she just liked it.
> **Clinician:** Did she have headaches or was she losing hair?
> **Patient:** No.
> **Clinician:** Did she have cold intolerance and need to keep her head warm?
> **Patient:** No, uh, maybe I could continue with my story. . . .[33]

Without self-reflection, we do not have the capacity for the self-monitoring needed to still ourselves from filling in the gaps created by silences and pauses in the patient's story or by the need to have our questions answered. In other words, we steal the story away from the patient and make it fit our own. Taking the time to be quiet, first with oneself, and then with patients/clients as they tell their story is when pattern knowing and appreciation occurs. Meyer concludes, "If we never let our patients' stories unfold with them as narrator and with us as listener, we'll never get to the wolf."[33]

Unfolding

When I walk with you I am amazed
For in this phase upon your journey
I feel greatness in your being
And what I'm seeing is not external
It's the eternal spirit you reflect
So as we connect in sacred space
There is not a trace of fear-
For here and now we meet as friends
In a time and space that never ends
And though we've had our twists and bends
We unfold along the way[34]

> ### REFLECTION BREAK: UNFOLDING
>
> What does it mean to unfold? Reflect on your own unfolding and enfolding. What have you or others missed in understanding you when overlooking what lies beneath the surface?

Pattern Recognition: Coherence and Incoherence

All of us have aspects of ourselves that are coherent and those that are incoherent. We experience coherence when our lived experience maintains a sense of harmony, purpose, and "rightness." Pattern incoherence is a person's experience of disharmony, disregulation, chaos, or a sense of "wrongness." A person may experience incoherence regarding cognitive patterning: ability to focus, orientation to time and space. The person may say things like, "I don't recognize myself and I'd like to have my life back." The person may be experiencing pain, shortness of breath, or other distressing symptoms. These experiences are often labeled from a list of nursing diagnoses. In pattern recognition, the nurse and patient engage in a mutual process dialogue with the patient identifying what is most distressing and possible self-reflective approaches to a deeper understanding of the pattern. By being present to another's distress without trying to "fix" the person, the reflective practitioner engages in self-centering, an awareness practice acknowledging the forces that pull us one way and then the other, maintaining or regaining our harmony.

Mutual Patterning Reflection

> In the causal, physical, material worldview, power says: "If I do this, then that will happen." In the acausal, unitary, spiritual worldview, power says: "If I do this, I will see what happens."
>
> —E. Barrett, "Power as Knowing Participation in Change: What's New and What's Next"

Mutual patterning reflection (MPR) may seem antithetical to the current climate of most healthcare settings such as busy hospital units, crowded emergency departments, overflowing primary care and specialty clinics, and under-staffed nursing home facilities. With this in mind, in MPR the reflective practitioner becomes the therapeutic milieu her- or himself. The nurse patterns openness, coherence, and spaciousness during the mutual reflective patterning time together, whether it is a moment or several min-utes. In this way, the client/patient can increase his or her openness to an increasingly coherent field patterning.

A reflective practice moment with a patient/client can occur amid one's nursing activities; for example, when hanging an IV, taking vitals, changing a dressing, or inserting a catheter. It can also be a distinct time that is mutually set aside for engaging in a specific self-reflection health patterning process.

EXAMPLE: REFLECTIVE PRACTICE IN ACTION

Before entering the room, take three breaths.

Align your intention and attention on the person with whom you will be engaging.

Be open to the pandimensional field and all its possibilities (Rogers).

Greet the person, and ask an open-ended question(s).

Listen deeply into the literal, physical, metaphorical, metaphysical, and spiritual realms for meanings.

Reflect on your personal feelings, thoughts, and perceptions and pattern manifestations.

Facilitate in mutual process reflection the patient/client's pattern expression.

Observe patterns and reflect on the pa-tient's expressed and symbolic language and experiences that hold coherence and/or incoherence.

Offer a time, now or in the future, when you can guide the patient into self-reflection for-mally or informally through conversation/dialogue.

■ SELF-REFLECTION STRATEGIES

The following self-reflection strategies facilitate access to the mind-body-spirit complex. Many themes such as metaphors, symbols, silence, acceptance, and listening to the deeper meanings repeat throughout these approaches. Nurses must be gentle and respectful of their inner guid-ance with the arising sensations, thoughts, and emotions as they engage and immerse them-selves. It is helpful for the nurse to become familiar with a self-reflection strategy through personal experience before introducing it to the patient/client.

Dreams

Dreams are filled with symbols, metaphors, pre-monitions, and insights delivered each night from the realms of our unconscious as well as the metaphysical world.[35-37] These nightly visi-tations come as bizarre, strange, or scary tales. They involve those we know and those we do not, places we've never been or a familiar home, and are speckled with animals, insects, parties, weddings, birth, and death. These images are to inform, serve, and expand our consciousness. Often, dreams represent parts of ourselves that are still hidden and their messages cryptic. Jung calls this unknown or repressed aspect "the shadow."[37,38] The way one makes heads or tails of these stories created while we sleep is to develop an understanding of one's personal iconogra-phy. Thus to make sense of the messages from one's dreams, we can view the images, the literal words, and the symbolic language as all parts of a puzzle. Jung also states that dreams make more sense when we connect them to personal events and issues in the dreamer's life.[38] Each dream is specific to the dreamer, as if sent by a mysterious source hoping to illuminate the person's intui-tive mind. Over time and with the practice of writing and reflecting on dreams, the dreamer develops skill in interpreting his or her own met-aphorical dream language. Also, archetypal pat-terns and generalities can be utilized, but these then are related to the individual dreamer and his or her life particulars. Dream work helps to bring our inner world (dream world) and outer world (awake world) into alignment.

For example, a client dreamed the follow-ing: "I was meeting an elderly man at a nuclear reactor. We got onto the elevator and he took me down to the core." One might connect literally to current events regarding the Japanese nuclear power plant meltdowns of 2011. Metaphorically, however, one might wonder about *nuclear* as an energy source; or *nucleus* as meaning center, heart, basis; and *core* as the core of oneself. The older man may represent the higher self–teacher. Reflecting on current events in his life, the client is contemplating changing careers and is yet to get to the core of what this will look like. We considered phrasing the dream events this way, "My higher self wants me to get to the core of an issue or what are the particulars for the core of my work?"

Try This: Dream Exploration

Keep a journal or notebook by your bed. Upon awaking, remain in the same position to remember your dream. This engages your "body memory." Then, write down the dream or parts of the dream that you remember. Circle specific words, phrases, and numbers that stick out as well as images, animals, the location, the cast of characters, and the overall feeling you get from the dream. See how these images may relate to your current life, issues at hand, or events from your past. Notice in the days to come whether the events in the dream coincide with events in one's physical life or the pandimensional environment. Move the pieces of the puzzle around, play with the different meanings that emerge. In this way, the dream itself becomes a guide and bridge from the metaphysical to the physical. Ask yourself, "Why was this dream sent to me? What does it want me to reflect on?"

Exercise and Physical Activity

Exercise can be a pathway to self-reflection. Individuals who regularly engage in physical activity often speak to the insight that they receive during a walk, run, swim, or other form of exercise. In addition to the numerous physiologic benefits of physical activity, exercise has positive mental health benefits, such as reduced incidence of depression.[39] Some practices such as yoga, tai chi, and qi gong combine breath-work, meditation, and physical movement to deepen awareness of the present moment. Some individuals keep exercise logs, noting not only their activity and time/distance, but also insights and feelings that arise during the session.

Try This: Physical Activity

Explore exercise as a self-reflective practice. Keep a reflective journal of your experience with a familiar or new form of activity. Reflect on how your body felt before, during, and after the session. How did you feel mentally? Did you experience any "aha" moments? Note any changes in mood during these time periods. Did you enjoy this activity? What other forms of physical activity might you like to try to enhance your self-reflective practice?

Reflective Writing

Writing for self-reflection can take many forms. Some individuals feel drawn to creative forms of writing such as poetry and story writing to reflect on their conscious experiences. Others use a daily journal for ongoing thoughts, brainstorming creative ideas, and recording insights. Journaling has also been cited in the literature as a tool to help nursing students reflect on their clinical experiences and understand the links between theory and practice.[26] With advances in technology over the past decade, blogging has become an alternative to traditional journaling for self-reflection. Whether traditional or high-tech, journal writing reveals to us our unique inner world while also connecting us to the shared experience of being human.

Try This: Journaling

Gather a notebook and pen or have your computer nearby. Set a timer for 10 to 20 minutes. Sit in quiet meditation for a few minutes, paying attention to the breath flowing in and out of your body. Then, begin to write. Allow whatever wants to be expressed to take form on the page. Write until the buzzer goes off or beyond, *without* editing. The writing may take any number of forms: a poem, narrative, lists, pictures, and doodles. Use this writing as a guide for reflection throughout the day.

Storytelling

Sturm explains that listening to stories can lead to changes in the experience of reality. He calls this the storytelling trance. As the story takes on a new dimension, Sturm describes how listeners transcend normal waking consciousness to experience the story with "remarkable immediacy," becoming part of the characters and plot of the story.[40] In listening to stories, we are drawn to archetypes. Marlaine Smith expresses that human beings have always used stories as a means to receive information as well as create structure around it. She explains that we are meaning seekers and makers and create symbolic stories that exemplify the universality of our experiences.[41]

Try This: Storytelling and Story Sharing

1. Take yourself to a professional storytelling performance. As you listen, notice where you find yourself in the story. Did you find yourself entering the storytelling trance?

2. Read the story of Diane and her colleagues in the section titled "Case Example 1: Diane's Story" later in this chapter. Reflect on your feelings as you witness Diane's experience. Is there an opportunity for you to participate in a story sharing circle in your nursing community?

Listening, Metaphors, and Images

Listening occurs on multiple depths simultaneously. The first depth of listening is to a person's words and interpreting the meaning through your own lens of life experiences and beliefs. The second depth is listening deeply to the words without judgment; allowing a fuller understanding of the patient's experience. The third depth of listening includes listening to the greater environmental field of language and messages beyond the words. This is tuning into body language, tone, pace, and the metaphoric and symbolic language as well as to synchronistic events occurring in the environment.[42]

A metaphor is the use of one image, word, or phrase to represent something else. For example, when describing a neck pain, the patient describes, "It feels like a tight knot." When exploring this knot, the nurse asks for the knot to be described in detail. "It's a thick, coarse rope and very heavy." Metaphors enrich our understanding and take us deeper into the underlying patterns. The nurse might venture further asking, "Does anything else in your life right now feel like it's tied up in a knot?" Smith writes,

"Metaphor is the product of an intuitive grasp of a unity of meaning; in it a familiar image used in an unfamiliar context fosters a holistic insight in a moment."[41p48] This then can become a source of information (expanding consciousness) for the person and, with the use of imagery, can begin to "untie the knot."[43]

This level of listening requires the holistic nurse to entrain herself to the unity of experience in the mutual process of pattern appreciation and pattern recognition.

Try This: Listening Beneath the Words

When entering into pattern appreciation with the patient/client, take three breaths, and set your intention to listen to the patient/client's story uninterrupted. To begin the connection ask the patient one of the following or another open-ended question:

- "Can you tell me what is most distressing for you right now?"
- "Can you describe to me what is most important to you right now?"
- "What has occurred over the last few days, weeks, or months that has led up to this [event or situation]?" Listen to the meaning beneath the words, listen to the messages hidden in metaphors and symbolic language, notice if events occur in the environmental field that would give greater significance or understanding to the patient's situation.* Engage in unknowing and allow the unfolding to occur.

The Medicine Walk

The medicine walk is an indigenous practice of going into nature with a question or intention for insight into a problem or personal dynamic. Indigenous peoples teach that the natural world is both teacher and mirror reflecting clearly one's unique gifts, strengths, and limiting patterns; it is a doorway to greater insight and transformation through the metaphorical and symbolic messages.[42,44,45] Domestic and wild animals, insects, birds, and reptiles cross our paths in both the natural and human-made worlds.

---

*A bird flies at the window, rain starts to fall, a car honks just when a significant insight occurs.

Most often these are not thought of as bringing a message for self-reflection. However, Sams and Carson in *Medicine Cards* and Andrews in *Animal-Speak* describe how these creatures can teach us about aspects of our own nature that may need greater attention or activation.[46,47] Deeper meanings and patterns emerge from many other messages from nature, such as sounds, smells, rocks, trees, vegetation, bodies of water, when the contact is reflected on.

The medicine walk involves three phases: (1) preparation, (2) solo time, and (3) returning to community. *Preparation* readies the individual for the coming journey within the context of a supportive community. The individual sits with a trusted friend or group or uses a journal to practice reflective listening to issues and concerns. *Solo time* involves going out on the medicine walk. The individual takes a walk by him- or herself with a particular focus, intention, or question. This practice can be done in the wilderness, one's own home or backyard, neighborhood park, the busy streets of a city, or the hallways of a clinical practice setting. *Returning to community* is done through sharing the story of the walk. The story, witnessed by trusted others or through journaling, can be told in first or third person. "I/she started out by heading down the street. It was crowded and colorful. I/she then noticed a person looking confused and asked if she needed help? . . ." When the story is complete, the person and the nurse reflect on and mirror it. Mirroring is an advanced level of listening and reflecting back, not simply repeating what was said. To continue with the preceding example, the one acting as mirror might suggest to the journeyer, "I hear the story of a woman who notices the vibrancy of her surroundings (life?) and who knows how to help people find their way." Upon hearing his or her story mirrored (reflected back), the journeyer can consciously integrate the deeper meanings and new insights into nursing practice and/or self-directed care. This practice can develop and refine the advanced skills of reflective listening.

Try This: Mini Medicine Walk

- Reflect on a conflict or question.
- Frame the issue in your mind in an open manner. For example, "I'd like to gain insight into my conflict, illness, relationship, or work choices." Let go of preconceived ideas of any outcome.
- Create a "threshold" separating your ordinary time into sacred reflective time. Use a doorway, gate, stick or imaginary line.
- Step through this threshold into timeless time and begin your walk, allowing an inner freedom to be your guide. Notice what path you take, who or what crosses your path, and any thoughts and feelings you experience.
- Write down the story of your medicine walk in the third person. Reflect on and self-mirror this story, noticing metaphors and symbols. Glean any new insights and understandings

Mindfulness Meditation

Mindfulness is moment-to-moment awareness, and mindfulness meditation is the practice of being awake and aware of one's breath, thoughts, feelings, and sensations as they occur. Kabat-Zinn identifies seven aspects of mindfulness: nonjudging, patience, beginner's mind, trust, nonstriving, acceptance, and letting go, with the object of the practice to see oneself more clearly and with compassion.[48] Imagine looking into a still pool of water at your reflection. A soft wind blows and now there are ripples distorting the image; a leaf floats by, blocking the image even more; and then, the rain comes and your image disappears beneath the heavy drops. A reflection is only as good as the mirror's clarity. Our mind is the wind, leaf, and rain. It distorts the clarity of our inner realms and uses distractions, preventing us from learning what is genuinely beneath the surface. Mindfulness practices can be sitting in a chair or on a cushion or lying down. It also can be through a form of movement such as walking, yoga, tai chi, qi gong, or walking a labyrinth. A patient with cancer describes dancing the tango with his wife as a form of mindfulness meditation. Mindfulness meditation is a self-reflection focused-attention strategy to help still the mind with the intention of dropping into your authentic self.

Try This: Formal Practice

Find a comfortable place and position to be in for several minutes. (You decide how long. A beginner can start with 5–20 minutes.) Take a few initial breaths to settle into your position, adjusting your posture so that the neck and spine are aligned, long and soft. Close your eyes or keep them slightly open and begin to bring your awareness to your breath. One breath in. One breath out. Bring awareness to the place where you experience the breath the most. Perhaps this is at your chest as it rises and falls or at the tip of your nose where the breath comes and leaves. As you notice thoughts, feelings, and sensations, observe them, neither grasping nor pushing away, as if they are a big cloud passing over the big blue sky. Each time you sit in formal mindfulness meditation will be unique. Journal any thoughts, feelings, and sensations you have and reflect on the experience.

Try This: Informal Practice

Take the sitting practice of observation to a daily activity; for example, when washing dishes, be fully present to washing the dishes, feeling the temperature of the water, the sensation of soap and sponge, the thoughts and feelings as they arise. Translate this into your clinical area; engage mindfulness moment when washing your hands.

■ BEGINNING AND EXPANDING SELF-REFLECTION AND REFLECTIVE PRACTICE

Starting a self-reflection practice and reflective practice is like training a puppy to heel, sit, stay, and come. When left to its own devices without training, the puppy gets into the garbage, digs holes, and is distracted by the many smells, sounds, and creatures in its environment. So, too, do our minds distract easily from reflective practice by outside activities, memories, and future anticipations. Self-reflection practice is the time we purposely set aside to go into our deeper selves and become aware of our thoughts, feelings, judgments, beliefs, and perceptions. Reflective practice is self-reflection in the context of daily activities; reaping the new awareness gleaned from self-reflection practice and sowing these into one's daily clinical practice and personal life. With a lived experience in both areas, these two dimensions of reflection merge: the self-reflective practitioner listening deeply to all realms of communication occurring within while simultaneously listening and being present with others and the environmental fields.

■ CASE EXAMPLES

CASE EXAMPLE 1: DIANE'S STORY

A small group of nurses gather to share stories, stories of practice, personal stories, and/or stories about what brought them to this gathering. They share snacks and informal conversation before coming together in a circle. They establish ground rules such as maintaining confidentiality, as well as the intention to create a sacred space for healing. The apartment host offers a talking stick* to start the sharing. One nurse, Diane, reaches for the talking stick and begins to tell a story of how she is starving herself, and then overeats since having repeated conflicts with her manager. She is afraid to leave her unit and often goes her whole shift without eating. On her way home, she picks up large amounts of food and binges. The group waits until she has completely finished. Diane places the talking stick on the coffee table. There is no judgment. There are several moments of silence. Someone picks up the talking stick and reflects on Diane's situation, asking her if she remembers a time in her past when this same pattern occurred? Surprised, Diane reflects back to the first time she engaged in bingeing to ease her stress. She shares with the group how her father would come home intoxicated and made disparaging remarks about her, especially about her body. In dialogue with the group, Diane begins to think about the connection between this earlier experience and her present situation. With this new awareness, she recognizes patterning and begins to transform the situation and reshape her current story. The group pauses for self-reflection on their own patterning. There is a feeling of shared lived experience.

In this example, we see how story from an integral nursing perspective has a purpose. In this face-to-face sharing of story, connections are formed as the teller and listeners find their own

---

* Talking stick is a tool used by the Native Americans when sitting in council. The one holding the stick is the speaker; the others are the listeners.

and each other's meanings in the stories. Time and space are not relevant, and we see the potential for transformation of the past and future into a present moment of caring and compassion; story as personal knowing. As Diane and the others leave the story space, each one of them has the opportunity to reflect on the patterns in his or her own stories.

CASE EXAMPLE 2: JACKIE'S MINI MEDICINE WALK

In the fall of 2008, I participated in a women's leadership retreat to explore myself as a leader. I began with a basic question: Who am I leading and where am I leading them?

I took these questions out with me on an early morning walk along the rim of a high desert mesa in northeastern Arizona. It was quiet except for some birds singing their dawn songs in the trees below. Leaning against a boulder, I surrendered my mind to the stillness around me and felt at peace. Then, a deerfly started buzzing in my face. I swatted it with my baseball cap, annoyed. My serenity dissipated into the air around me.

Later, in the growing heat of the day, I took a second walk asking for another message from nature. At that moment, I became aware of a falcon flying gracefully on the air currents overhead. I knew what appeared effortless took a particular kind of wisdom and elegance to work with the force of the winds and not against them.

Reflecting on both of these encounters with nature and using nature's wisdom as a metaphor for my own emerging leadership, I asked myself, "How often do I spend my energy swatting at small nuisances when I would be better off reading and navigating the larger currents?"

My quick annoyance at the irritating buzz in my outer world had mirrored to me how easily I allow my mind to become diverted by the buzz of all sorts of minor occurrences beyond my control. The fluidity of the falcon using the wind currents to soar effortlessly reflected the innate grace that is available to me when I take the time to balance mind with body, heart, and spirit.

I realized that my guiding question wasn't "who am I leading?" but rather, "who do I want to be as a leader?"[49]

■ IMPROVING PRACTICE THROUGH RESEARCH

Research on self-reflection can make known how self-reflection works as a transformational process for the individual nurse's growth and guide the way for interventions based on self-reflection. To demonstrate its relevance and importance to nursing in particular and health care in general, holistic nurses can engage and promote research in the power and benefits of self-reflection in practice.

Directions for FUTURE RESEARCH

1. Are nurses who learn self-reflection practices in nursing educational programs more likely to use self-reflection practices for self-learning and growth?
2. Does a reflective nursing practice improve the quality of patient care?
3. Does a reflective nursing practice affect patient self-reflection?
4. Do nurses who practice self-reflection together experience more unity with colleagues?
5. Does self-reflection enhance communication between and among different healthcare professionals?
6. Does self-reflection enhance the integration of theory with practice?

Nurse Healer REFLECTIONS

After reading this chapter, the nurse healer will be able to answer or to begin the process of answering the following questions:

- What are self-reflection and reflective practice?
- How do holistic nursing theories relate to the concept of self-reflection?
- How do self-reflection strategies affect clinical practice?
- How can self-reflection strategies be used in personal practice and with clients?
- What self-reflection strategies do you currently practice, and what new strategy might you try in the future for your own inner growth?

For a full suite of assignments and additional learning activities, use the access code located in the front of your book to visit this exclusive website: http://go.jblearning.com/dossey. If you do not have an access code, you can obtain one at the site.

NOTES

1. M. E. Asselin, "Reflective Narrative: A Tool for Learning Through Practice," *Journal for Nurses in Staff Development* 27, no. 1 (2011): 2–6.

2. S. G. Forniers and C. Peden-McAlpine, "Evaluation of a Reflective Learning Intervention to Improve Critical Thinking in Novice Nurses," *Journal of Advanced Nursing* 57, no. 4 (2007): 410–421.

3. D. Siegel, *Mindsight: The New Science of Personal Transformation* (New York: Bantam Books, 2010).

4. B. A. Carper, "Fundamental Patterns in Knowing," *Advances in Nursing Science* 1 (1978): 13–28.

5. P. Munhall, "Unknowing: Toward Another Pattern of Knowing," *Nursing Outlook* 41, no. 3 (1993): 125–128.

6. J. Levin, "Unitary Transformative Nursing: Using Metaphor and Imagery for Self-Reflection and Theory Informed Practice," *Visions: The Journal of Rogerian Nursing Science* 14, no. 1 (2006): 27–35.

7. American Holistic Nurses Association & American Nurses Association, *Holistic Nursing: Scope and Standards of Practice* (Silver Spring, MD: NurseBooks.org, 2007).

8. G. Rolfe, "Beyond Expertise: Theory, Practice and the Reflexive Practitioner," *Journal of Clinical Nursing* 6, no. 2 (1997): 93–97.

9. K. Mann, J. Gordon, and A. MacLeod, "Reflection and Reflective Practice in Health Professions Education: A Systematic Review," *Advances in Health Sciences Education* 14, no. 4 (2009): 595–621.

10. P. Benner, *From Novice to Expert: Excellence and Power in Clinical Nursing Practice* (Menlo Park, CA: Addison-Wesley, 1984).

11. T. Nhat Hanh, *Keeping the Peace: Mindfulness and Public Service* (Berkeley, CA: Parallax Press, 2005).

12. J. Watson, *Nursing: Human Science and Human Care: A Theory of Nursing* (Sudbury, MA: Jones & Bartlett, 1988).

13. E. Barrett, "Power as Knowing Participation in Change: What's New and What's Next," *Nursing Science Quarterly* 23, no. 1 (2010): 47–54.

14. B. M. Dossey, "Integral and Holistic Nursing," in *Holistic Nursing: A Handbook for Practice*, 5th ed., ed.

B. M. Dossey and L. Keegan (Sudbury, MA: Jones & Bartlett, 2009): 3–46.

15. Reich, J. L. (2010). Intention. Unpublished poem.

16. M. A. Newman, *Health as Expanding Consciousness* (New York: National League for Nursing Press, 1994).

17. M. A. Newman, *Transforming Presence: The Difference That Nursing Makes* (Philadelphia: F. A. Davis, 2008).

18. J. Watson, "Caring Science: Ten Caritas Processes," Watson Caring Science Institute. http://www.watsoncaringscience.org/index.cfm/category/61/10-caritas-processes.cfm.

19. Rogers, M. (1992). Nursing Science and the Space Age. *Nursing Science Quarterly* 5(1), 34.

20. H. K. Butcher, ed., *The Science of Unitary Human Beings: Theoretical Basis for Nursing* (2011). http://rogeriannursingscience.wikispaces.com/.

21. M. J. Smith and P. R. Liehr, "Story Theory: Advancing Nursing Practice Scholarship," *Holistic Nursing Practice* 19, no. 6 (2005): 272–276.

22. M. J. Smith and P. R. Liehr, "Story Theory," in *Middle Range Theory for Nursing*, 2nd ed. (New York: Springer, 2008): 205–224.

23. M. Cirocco, "How Reflective Practice Improves Nurses' Critical Thinking Ability," *Gastroenterology Nursing* 30, no. 6 (2007): 405–413.

24. R. Hays and S. Gay, "Reflection or 'Pre-Reflection': What Are We Actually Measuring in Reflective Practice?" *Medical Education* 45, no. 2 (2011): 116–118.

25. H. S. Kim, L. M. Lauzon Clabo, P. Burbank, M. Leveillee, and D. Martins, "Application of Critical Reflective Inquiry in Nursing Education," in *Handbook of Reflective Inquiry*, ed. N. Lyons (New York: Springer, 2010): 159–172.

26. R. Van Horn and S. Freed, "Journaling and Dialogue Pairs to Promote Reflection in Clinical Nursing Education," *Nursing Education Research* 29, no. 4 (2008): 220–225.

27. A. Raffone and N. Srinivasan, "The Exploration of Meditation in the Neuroscience of Attention and Consciousness," *Cognitive Process* 11 (2010): 1–7.

28. G. Huther, *The Compassionate Brain: How Empathy Creates Intelligence*, trans. M. H. Kohn (Boston: Trumpeter Books, 2006).

29. J. Carmody and R. A. Baer, "Relationships Between Mindfulness Practice and Levels of Mindfulness, Medical and Psychological Symptoms and Well-Being in a Mindfulness-Based Stress Reduction Program," *Journal of Behavioral Medicine* 31, no. 1 (2008): 23–33.

30. R. H. Matousek and P. L. Dobkin, "Weathering Storms: A Cohort Study of How Participation in a Mindfulness-Based Stress Reduction Program Benefits Women After Breast Cancer Treatment," *Current Oncology* 17, no. 4 (2010): 62–70.

31. R. McCraty and D. Childre, "Coherence: Bridging Personal, Social and Global Health," *Alternative Therapies in Health & Medicine* 16, no. 4 (2010): 10–24.

32. S. Rollnick, W. R. Miller, and C. C. Butler, *Motivational Interviewing in Health Care: Helping Patients Change Behavior* (New York: Guilford Press, 2008).

33. C. Meyer, (2007). "Editor's Note: The Inside Story," Minnesota Medical Association. http://www.minnesotamedicine.com/PastIssues/PastIssues2007/July2007/EditorsNoteJuly2007/tabid/1960/Default.aspx.

34. Reich, J. L. (2011). Unfolding. Unpublished poem.

35. R. Kamenetz, *The History of Last Night's Dream: Discovering the Hidden Path to the Seat of the Soul* (New York: HarperCollins, 2007).

36. S. Krippner, F. Bogzaran, and A. P. De Carvalho, *Extraordinary Dreams and How to Work with Them* (Albany: State University of New York Press, 2002).

37. C. Jung, *On the Nature of Dreams*, ed. R. Soulard, Jr., and K. Kramer (Seattle, WA: Scriptor Press, 1945).

38. C. Jung, *Dreams*, trans. R. F. C. Hull, ed. W. McGuire, H. Read, M. Fordham, and G. Adler (Princeton, NJ: Princeton University Press, 1974).

39. U.S. Department of Health and Human Services, Centers for Disease Control and Prevention, National Center for Health Statistics, *Healthy People 2020: Physical Activity*, HealthyPeople.gov (2010). http://healthypeople.gov/2020/topicsobjectives2020/overview.aspx?topicid=33.

40. B. Sturm, "The Enchanted Imagination: Storytelling's Power to Entrance Listeners," *School Library Media Research 2* (1999). http://www.ala.org/ala/mgrps/divs/aasl/aaslpubsandjournals/slmrb/slmrcontents/volume21999/vol2sturm.cfm.

41. M. C. Smith, "Metaphor in Nursing Theory," *Nursing Science Quarterly* 5, no. 2 (1992): 48–49.

42. J. Levin and S. Maida, *Four Shields of Leadership*, self-published course materials (2008).

43. J. Levin, *Imagery for Pattern Appreciation*, self-published course material (2008).

44. S. Foster and M. Little, *The Four Shields: The Initiatory Seasons of Human Nature* (Big Pine, CA: Lost Borders Press, 1998).

45. J. Levin, abstract of *The Medicine Walk: Integrating Indigenous Wisdom into Pain Management Nursing*, American Society of Pain Management Nursing Conference, September 9, 2011.

46. J. Sams and D. Carson, *Medicine Cards: The Discovery of Power Through the Ways of Animals* (New York: St. Martin's Press, 1999).

47. T. Andrews, *Animal-Speak: The Spiritual and Magical Power of Creatures Great and Small* (St. Paul, MN: Llewellyn Publications, 2001).

48. J. Kabat-Zinn, *Full Catastrophe Living: Using the Wisdom of Your Body and Mind to Face Stress, Pain and Illness* (New York: Delta, 1990).

49. J. Levin, (2009) "Transformational Nurse Leadership—Cultivating Leaders Through Personal Encounters with Nature" (2009). http://EzineArticles.com/2285978.

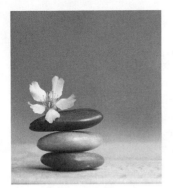

Chapter 13

Nutrition

Susan Luck

Nurse Healer
OBJECTIVES

Theoretical

- Learn the definitions of terms in this chapter.
- Differentiate between the Recommended Daily Allowance (RDA) and the optimal daily allowance (ODA).
- Develop a plan that combines good nutrition with a healthy lifestyle.
- Learn the benefits of healthy eating for wellness promotion and disease prevention.
- Explore the nurse's role as coach in behavioral and dietary change.

Clinical

- Observe the meaning of foods in different cultural traditions.
- Listen to the client/patient story around health and nutrition.
- Identify nutritional foods that support the client/patient healing process.
- Use open-ended questions to learn more from clients about eating habits and health behaviors.
- Increase knowledge of current nutrition research.

Personal

- Assess the quality of your food intake and note how it increases or decreases your energy level at work.

- Heighten your awareness of the way in which what you eat affects how you feel.
- Examine your eating patterns and the meaning of food in your life.
- Explore new foods and food preparation to support your health and well-being.
- Plan a day's menu, asking yourself, "What does my body need to enhance my wellness?"
- Explore mindful eating practices.
- Prepare foods to bring to your workplace to support your health goals.
- Find a nurse coach and enter into a coaching agreement to reach desired nutrition goals.
- Employ strategies to improve nutrition in your workplace.

DEFINITIONS

Antioxidants: Substances that limit free radical formation and damage by stabilizing or deactivating free radicals before they attack cells.

Diabesity: A popular term for the common clinical association of type 2 diabetes mellitus and obesity.

Epigenetics: The study of changes produced in gene expression caused by mechanisms other than changes in the underlying DNA sequence.

Free radicals: Electrically charged molecules with an unpaired electron capable of attacking healthy cells in the body, causing them to lose their structure and function.

Glycemic index: An index that classifies carbohydrate foods according to their glycemic response (effect on blood glucose levels), which varies with fiber content, starch structure, food processing, and presence of proteins and fats.

HDL: High-density lipoprotein form of cholesterol associated with reduced risk of atherosclerosis.

Homocysteine: An amino acid found in the blood and intermediate product of methionine metabolism.

Leptin: A peptide hormone neurotransmitter produced by fat cells and involved in the regulation of appetite.

LDL: Low-density lipoprotein form of cholesterol strongly associated with increased risk of atherosclerosis.

Metabolic syndrome: A collection of heart disease risk factors that increase the chance of developing heart disease, stroke, and diabetes. The condition is also known by other names including Syndrome X, cardiometabolic and insulin resistance syndrome.

Mineral: An inorganic trace element or compound that works in synergy with other compounds and is essential for human life.

Nutrigenomics: The study of the effects of foods and food constituents on gene expression. It is about how our DNA is transcribed into mRNA and then to proteins and provides a basis for understanding the biological activity of food components.

Nutraceuticals: Food, or parts of food, that provide medical or health benefits, including the prevention and treatment of disease.

Obesogens: Identifiable industrial pollutants contributing to the obesity epidemic by increasing fat cells in the body and altering metabolism and feelings of hunger and fullness.

Optimal nutrition: Adequate intake of nutrients for health promotion and disease prevention.

Organic food: Food from plants and animals that have been grown without the use of synthetic fertilizers or pesticides, and without antibiotics, growth hormones, and feed additives.

Phytochemicals: Biologically active compounds found in foods and plants.

Phytoestrogens: Family of compounds found in plants that have some estrogenic or anti-estrogenic activity.

Probiotic: Formulation containing beneficial living microorganisms that maintain health as part of the internal ecology of the digestive tract.

Vitamin: An organic substance necessary for normal growth, metabolism, and development of the body; acts as a catalyst and coenzyme, assisting in many chemical reactions while nourishing the body.

Xenoestrogens: Synthetic, environmental, hormone-mimicking compounds found in many pesticides, drugs, plastics, and personal care products.

■ CURRENT NUTRITION THEORY AND RESEARCH

Nutrition is integral to maintaining health throughout the life cycle and has a profound influence on disease prevention, health maintenance, and the aging process. Dietary habits play a central role in almost all health problems seen today including inflammation and pain, digestive and gastrointestinal disturbances, allergies and food sensitivities, fatigue, mood disorders, and immune dysfunction. Food and nutrients are no longer viewed merely as providing substances whose absence would produce disease, but as having a positive impact on an individual's overall health including physical performance, aging process, cognitive function, energy levels, and daily quality of life.

It is common knowledge that foods produced today are processed and denatured, depleted of nutrients, and often contain toxic chemicals including additives, preservatives, pesticides, hormones, antibiotics, and many other residues. The changes to our food supply contribute to a rising number of chronic health issues including learning disabilities, obesity, diabetes, atherosclerosis, heart disease, hypertension, immune and autoimmune diseases, and various cancers.[1]

According to several recently published studies, evidence-based guidelines regarding recommendations on lifestyle and healthy nutrition as a primary preventive intervention demonstrate consistent results. Furthermore, the cost-effectiveness of primary prevention services is proven. Health promotion and disease prevention are emerging as a national strategy and nurses in all healthcare settings are in a key position to use their professional skills to coach and educate individuals and communities in nutrition and lifestyle changes that affect long-term health goals and health policy. Integrating nurse coaching into clinical practice is a new direction for nurses in a patient-centered care model.

The evidence-based science of nutrition and lifestyle interventions for preventing or treating chronic disease demonstrates the powerful, cost-effective, and critical role nutrition plays in the promotion and restoration of health. Current research supports healthful dietary patterns, such as the Mediterranean diet, which includes whole grains, legumes, nuts, vegetables, fruits, olive oil, and fish and is associated with a decrease in chronic disease and death from all causes. The harmful effects of trans and certain saturated fats, refined carbohydrates, high-fructose corn syrup, and many food additives are well documented in the medical literature.[2]

Current Health Crisis

According to a recent American Heart Association report completed in conjunction with the Centers for Disease Control and Prevention (CDC) and the National Institutes of Health, in 2009 the economic costs of cardiovascular disease and stroke in the United States were estimated at $475.3 billion. In this report, nutrition and dietary intake and their relationship to the chronic disease patterns burdening the nation's health and healthcare system, including metabolic syndrome, obesity, and diabetes, are highlighted.[3]

Since 1980, obesity prevalence among children and adolescents has almost tripled. It is estimated that 66% of adults in the United States, 48 million Americans, are overweight, and 50 million are now classified as obese.

Obesity and metabolic syndrome have the potential to impact the incidence and severity of cardiovascular pathologies, with grave implications for worldwide healthcare systems. The metabolic syndrome is characterized by visceral obesity, insulin resistance, hypertension, chronic inflammation, and thrombotic disorders contributing to endothelial dysfunction and, subsequently, to accelerated atherosclerosis. Obesity is a key component in development of the metabolic

syndrome and it is becoming increasingly clear that a central factor in this is the production by adipose cells of bioactive substances that directly influence insulin sensitivity and vascular injury

According to the CDC, *overweight* and *obese* are labels for ranges of weight that are greater than what is generally considered healthy for a given height. For adults, overweight and obesity ranges are determined by using weight and height to calculate a number called the body mass index (BMI). It can also be defined as weighing in excess of 40 pounds more than ideal body weight. The national prevalence of overweight and obesity is monitored using data from the National Health and Nutrition Examination Survey (NHANES). According to the most recent survey, 17% of (or 12.5 million) children and adolescents aged 2 to 19 years are obese. *Healthy People 2010* identified overweight and obesity as leading health indicators and as indicators of future health risks and called for a reduction in the proportion of children and adolescents who are overweight or obese.[4] Obesity reduces life expectancy while increasing the risk of illness and death from a range of other diseases. It is now so common in adults and children that the World Health Organization characterizes this condition as a global epidemic.

Type 2 diabetes mellitus is a preventable disease and a growing public health problem. Epidemiologic and interventional studies suggest that weight loss is the main driving force to reduce diabetes risk. Landmark clinical trials of lifestyle changes in subjects with prediabetes have shown that diet and exercise leading to weight loss consistently reduce the incidence of diabetes.[5]

Energy imbalance is the immediate cause of obesity: a combination of excess dietary calories and a lack of physical activity. A study published in the *Journal of the American Medical Association* in April 2010 concludes that sugar intake significantly contributes to ill health and specifically increases triglycerides and cholesterol levels. Hypertriglyceridemia is a common lipid abnormality in persons with visceral obesity, metabolic syndrome and type 2 diabetes

Researchers at Emory University and the Centers for Disease Control and Prevention examined the added sugar intake and blood fat levels in more than 6,100 adults. Participants consumed an average of 21.4 teaspoons of added sugars a day, or more than 320 calories a day from these sources.[5] According to the report, type 2 diabetes and obesity hold long-term health implications for the U.S. population: "Obesity is a contributing cause of many health problems, including heart disease stroke, diabetes, and some types of cancer." Statistically, these are some of the leading causes of death in the United States.

Other symptoms and health risks attributed to obesity include sleep apnea, asthma and breathing problems, limited mobility, inflammation, and early deterioration of joints leading to arthritis, and osteoporosis and hip fractures. Obesity can cause problems during pregnancy and indicates a higher risk for obesity in children of obese parents.[6]

Emerging Research in the Study of Obesity

Recent research focuses on how environmental toxins, described as *obesogens,* are stored in fat tissue and can influence and interfere with healthy fat cell signaling and fat metabolism and how overeating can interfere with cell signaling messengers that control feelings of satiety after eating. For healthy fat metabolism, leptin, an adipocyte-derived hormone, plays an essential role in the maintenance of normal body weight and energy expenditure, as well as glucose homeostasis. Leptin resistance occurs in those who are chronically overweight. The role of leptin in the fat cells is to reduce appetite and stimulate fat burning. The relationship between leptin and perceived hunger, and on the eating behavior of leptin-deficient individuals appears to be blocked in chronically overweight individuals as they develop leptin resistance, making losing weight increasingly difficult, if not impossible.[7]

Fat also regulates the processes by which the body burns fuel for energy, especially in muscle. Adiponectin, another hormone-like chemical, plays a central role in the biology of fat and is normally produced to curb appetite and spark the burning of fat. But unlike leptin, which remains present but stops functioning, chronically overweight individuals have an adiponectin deficiency. Many adipokines are also mediators of inflammation and promote and encourage the inflammatory response, which further affects fat metabolism and homeostasis.[8] Weight loss is associated with reduced inflammation systemically.[9]

Routine exposures to human-made chemicals may also increase an individual's risk of obesity. The obesogen hypothesis proposes that perturbations in metabolic signaling that result from exposure to environmental chemicals known as endocrine disruptors, and stored in the body's adipose tissue, may further exacerbate the effects of imbalances, resulting in an increased susceptibility to obesity and obesity-related disorders.[10] These markers indicate the potential for nutritional coaching for behavioral change to improve metabolism, cellular communication, and promote long-term health.

Obesity is on the minds of health policy analysts and healthcare providers, nationally and globally. According to the CDC report, "Obesity is a complex problem that requires both personal and community action." The report goes on to mandate that people in all communities should be able to make healthy choices.

> As part of a health strategy and health care policy to promote lifestyle behavioral change, nurses as coaches are in a prime position to guide and motivate individuals toward healthy behaviors. Effective health promotion programs include awareness practices, exercise, behavioral motivation for change, and nutrition education. Comprehensive effective nutrition programs integrate coaching skills for the patient/client to set attainable goals. This process is a gradual and highly individualized process for reversing patterns that can eventually lead to chronic disease.
>
> Effective therapeutic nutritional guidelines honor the totality of the individual. An individual's metabolism, environment, genetics, emotional health, social networks, and life stressors must be considered in evaluating nutritional needs and nutritional goals. Beliefs, attitudes, eating patterns, food choices and culinary styles are deeply embedded in one's cultural, physiological, psychological, emotional, spiritual, and socioeconomic needs and must be considered for whole person healing. Listening to an individual's story is central to guiding behavioral change around food.[11]

From an evolutionary and cultural perspective, our modern-day food supply has been dramatically altered, although our biological nutrient needs have not. The human diet remained constant for thousands of years but has radically changed in the past few decades. It now becomes painfully clear that our modern dietary habits influence our health and well-being. For example, we know that food composition and macronutrient content are essential for biochemical processes, working synergistically to produce energy on a cellular level. Without proper nutrient synergy and healthy cellular communication, the end result is diminished function that often results in decreased energy output, inflammation, and lowered immune response. Essential macronutrients and micronutrients include carbohydrates, proteins, fats, vitamins, and minerals, and essential fatty acids.[11]

Food as Energy

The body is an energy flow system and cells must live in harmony in the extracellular matrix. Over time, nutritional deficiencies create disharmony within the cellular structure and diminish energy exchange within cells, essential for healthy cell signaling and healthy cell function. Overt symptoms of nutrient deficiency are the result of a long chain of reactions in the body. When an individual consumes a nutrient-deficient diet, the initial reactions occur on a molecular level. First, enzymes that are dependent on the deficient nutrients become depleted. This depletion brings about changes within cells. The deficiencies may continue for many years until the body can no longer carry out its normal functions. Eventually, overt signs and symptoms appear, even though the deficiency may still be considered subclinical because routine laboratory tests do not necessarily uncover nutritional deficiencies. Nevertheless, these unseen deficiencies can lead to a broad range of nonspecific conditions that can diminish an individual's overall quality of life. Undiagnosed, nutrient deficiencies over many years leave the body more vulnerable to illnesses to which the individual may be genetically predisposed and to immune system compromise. Yet, as resilient beings, even when health is compromised, we can reprogram our cells and create an internal and external healing environment to restore health and balance.

Debate continues over the most efficient "diet" for weight loss and overall health. Advocates of high-fat, low-carbohydrate diets including the Atkins Diet are challenged by vegan-type diets consisting of high amounts of complex carbohydrates and high intake of fruits and vegetables. A study of more than 100,000 people over more than 20 years, the Nurses' Health Study, concludes that a low-carbohydrate diet high in vegetables and with a larger proportion of proteins and oils coming mostly from plant sources decreases mortality. In contrast, a low-carbohydrate diet with largely animal sources of protein and fat increases mortality.[13]

An Integrative Functional Health Model

In a nutritional coaching model, the client moves beyond the concept of a "diet" to set attainable goals leading to a healthier lifestyle, new behaviors, and improved health outcomes. As nutrition research and information reach the public and the existing healthcare model, there is a hunger for a new paradigm that explores and examines the underlying causes of disease. Functional medicine is an emerging field in medicine with a special emphasis on nutrition and lifestyle interventions. For holistic nurses, in a patient centered care, model health is viewed as a positive vitality, representing more than the absence of disease. Through maintaining balance of a complex web of physiologic, cognitive/emotional, and physical processes, health and well-being are achieved

Adapted from Functional Medicine, an Integrative Functional Health Model (IFHM) is congruent and compatible with holistic nursing philosophy and practice.

The IFHM is a unique nursing model that expands on the functional medicine model, integrating the art and science of nursing and nursing theories, and builds on the holistic nursing process. The IFHM views health and balance as a dynamic interaction and interconnectedness between the individual and his or her environment. In this model, the nurse coach is a partner, understanding the therapeutic use of self in relationship-centered care to promote health and well-being. Coaching strategies for a healthy lifestyle integrate nutritional knowledge and nutritional coaching; they are opportunities for nurses to bring new skills and tools to the art and science of nursing. This model moves nurses beyond understanding a client's chemistry, diagnosis, and ailments from a medical construct and helps them view health, energy, and balance through an expanded, holistic, integrative perspective. The physical, integral, and social environment in which symptoms occur; the dietary habits of the person (present and past); the environment in which the person lives; his or her beliefs about health, illness, and diagnosis; and the combined impact of these factors on social, physical, and psychological function are all interconnected to one's lifestyle choices and influence health outcomes. Discovery of the factors that aggravate or ameliorate symptoms and that predispose the client to illness or facilitate recovery provides for the possibilities of co-creating lifestyle and behavioral changes and establishing an integrative care plan. The nurse coach's collaborative relationship recognizes and acknowledges the individual's experience of health or illness and explores the totality of the individual.

Within this larger context of the whole person, nurses increase their knowledge, understand the current nutrition science and research, and stay informed so as to evaluate and educate clients and patients. Increasing awareness, assessing the client's relationship to nutrition and food, evaluating the client's eating patterns and nutritional needs, assisting in developing a personalized nutrition plan and goals, and implementing effective nutritional guidelines and strategies for enhancing wellness are all part of the role of nurse coaches.

Foundations of a Nurse-Based Functional Health Model

- *Interconnectedness:* Includes the mind, body, and spiritual dimensions of physiologic factors. An abundance of research now supports the view that the human body functions as an orchestrated network of interconnected systems rather than as individual systems that function autonomously and without effect on each other.
- *Energy field principles and dynamics:* An understanding of how thoughts, stress, toxic environments, and a nutrient-deficient diet can disrupt human energy fields, impair optimal functioning, and contribute to disease.

- *Patient-centeredness:* Honors and emphasizes the individual's unique history, beliefs, and story rather than a medical diagnosis and disease orientation.
- *Biochemical individuality:* Recognizes the importance of variations in metabolic function that derive from unique genetic and environmental vulnerabilities and strengths among individuals.
- *Health on a wellness continuum:* Views health as a dynamic balance on multiple levels and seeks to identify, restore, and support delete our innate reserve as the means to enhance well-being and healing throughout the life cycle.
- *Optimization of our internal and external healing environments:* Holds the worldview that human health is the microcosm of the macrocosm in the web of life.

© 2010 Integrative Nurse Coach Certificate Program (INCCP)

Overview of Clinical Nutrition

Changes to the U.S. food supply contribute to a rising number of health problems including atherosclerosis, heart disease, hypertension, diabetes, and various cancers—diseases virtually unknown a hundred years ago. Basic essential nutrient requirements are unavailable for healthy cell signaling and to meet the demands and needs of people throughout the various stages of life, beginning with prenatal development and continuing into old age.

Can we get all of our nutritional needs met from the foods available today?

The Standard American Diet

Nutrient deficiencies most often result from a high intake of processed and refined foods. According to the 2009 American Heart Association report, it is estimated that the average American adult consumes 22 teaspoons of sugar a day; teens eat 34 teaspoons of refined sugar and high-fructose corn syrup each day. High-fructose corn syrup is produced by chemically converting the starch in corn to a substance that is about 90% fructose, a sugar that is sweeter than the glucose that fuels body cells and that is processed differently by the body. Fructose is metabolized primarily in the liver, which favors the formation of fats and results in elevated triglycerides, one of the markers for increased risk of metabolic syndrome. Sweeteners permeate the food supply and are used to sweeten soft drinks, juices, jams, yogurts, and breakfast cereals, to name a few. In addition, it is estimated that more than 28% of calories in the standard American diet (SAD) consist of refined products such as white bread and white rice, deficient in 28 essential nutrients including essential vitamins (in particular the B vitamins), minerals, protein, and fiber, all contained in the whole grain prior to processing.

As the field of nutrition evolves, understandings and traditional guidelines are changing. In 2010, the U.S. Department of Agriculture released the new *Dietary Guidelines for Americans* to "promote health, reduce the risk of chronic diseases, and reduce the prevalence of overweight and obesity through improved nutrition and physical activity." With more than one-third of children and more than two-thirds of adults in the United States overweight or obese, the seventh edition of *Dietary Guidelines for Americans* places stronger emphasis on reducing calorie consumption and increasing physical activity.

For the first time in more than 40 years, the U.S. Department of Agriculture has reissued its guidelines for nutrient needs, originally defined as the Recommended Daily Allowances (RDAs) by the U.S. Food and Nutrition Board. The RDA guidelines specified the levels of nutrients required to prevent overt symptoms of deficiency. Since their inception, the RDA guidelines have been periodically reevaluated and updated based on continuing analysis of science advances in the field. In 2010, to meet the growing healthcare crisis, the new guidelines known as Dietary Reference Intakes, or DRIs, address the questions that have been asked by experts in the field.[14]

Clinical Nutrition Research

As nurses expand their knowledge about nutrition, nutraceuticals and medical foods currently prescribed in conjunction with pharmaceuticals, they can assist clients in their decision-making process. including lifestyle and nutritional choices. Nurses are becoming increasingly aware of what Americans spend out of pocket on nutrition-related products: an estimated $22 billion a year, according to the National Health

Statistics report in 2009. The introduction of pharmaceutical-grade omega-3 essential fatty acids (EFAs) is an example of a nutraceutical recently recommended by the American Heart Association. An extensive body of research supports the fact that by taking Omega 3 essential fatty acids, deficient in the modern food supply, they may prevent heart disease and stroke and lower triglycerides. Omega-3 EFAs have also been well researched in the treatment of arthritis, diabetes, obesity, cancer, immune and autoimmune disorders, cognitive function, and a variety of women's health problems.[16]

Many epidemiologic studies report strong correlations between Western diseases and dietary habits. Mortality rates for certain cancers, as well as the incidence of cardiovascular disease, are higher among those who consume the standard American diet than among those who consume Asian, Scandinavian, or Mediterranean diets.[17] (The Mediterranean diet pyramid is shown in **Figure 13-1**.)

Tests for elevated levels of homocysteine are routine diagnostics for assessing increased risk for cardiovascular disease and stroke. A growing body of research indicates that elevated homocysteine levels result from subclinical deficiencies of the B vitamins, including folic acid, vitamin B_6, and vitamin B_{12}. Knowledge about nutrient deficiencies and their potentially life-threatening consequences is slowly being integrated into routine physical examinations and health assessments. Two articles in the *New England Journal of Medicine* report that "high plasma homocysteine concentrations and low concentrations of folate and vitamin B_6 play roles in homocysteine metabolism, inflammation, and cardiovascular health." Deficiencies in many of these nutrients, especially vitamin B_6 (pyridoxine), are also associated with diabetes, heart disease, depression, anxiety, and premenstrual syndrome.[18]

Cardiovascular disease and cancer are the two leading causes of death among women in the United States. Heart disease is responsible for 45% of all deaths among women, and nearly 40% of all females are expected to develop cancer at some point in their lifetime. Research suggests that both heart disease and cancer are strongly related to dietary habits and nutrient status. Helping women make healthy dietary and

EXHIBIT 13-1   Hypoglycemic Diet Plan

This diet plan assists in weight loss, blood glucose regulation, energy maintenance, nutrient needs, and satiation. The following are guidelines for a low-fat, low–refined carbohydrates, and high-protein diet.

- Eliminate caffeine, soda, fruit juice, white sugar, white flour, white rice, artificial sweeteners, and white bread.
- Limit fruits—two per day and divide into four portions. Avoid grapes and bananas (high in sugar).
- Throughout the day, consume several small meals consisting of protein with vegetables, and complex carbohydrate if needed.
- Vegetables—unlimited—raw or cooked depending on your preference (and digestion); limit beets, peas, and carrots.

SAMPLE MENU PLAN

Protein

Fish	Wild Alaskan salmon (or canned); sardines; broiled, baked, steamed fish
Chicken	Baked, broiled; remove skin; white meat preferred
Turkey	Fresh turkey, white meat
Beans*	Lentils, soy (tofu), black beans, red beans, garbanzo beans, hummus, tempeh
Whole grains*	Brown rice, oatmeal, quinoa, millet, buckwheat (kasha), barley, whole wheat, spelt, amaranth
Seeds and nuts*	Almonds, sunflower seeds, walnuts, pumpkin seeds, nut butters (almond, sesame; raw, unsalted)
Eggs	Boiled, poached
Dairy	Low-fat plain yogurt, or skim-milk ricotta or mozzarella cheese, goat feta, yogurt (plain)

Vegetables 5-7 servings daily

Salads

Steamed vegetables; fresh or frozen; avoid canned

Whole Grains + Beans= Complete Protein (represents complex carbohydrates)

- Salad with grilled chicken or fish
- Hummus and vegetables in whole-wheat pita
- Lentil soup with gluten free rice crackers or whole grains (millet, brown rice, quinoa, whole wheat pita)
- Grilled skinless chicken breast with 0.5 cup brown rice or quinoa and steamed vegetables
- Tofu or black beans with brown rice and steamed vegetables
- Grilled fish with half baked sweet potato and salad

Snacks: Small meals to have between meals, midmorning and midafternoon

- Low-fat plain yogurt with 0.5 cup fresh fruit, whole-wheat or rice crackers with tuna salad, hummus with whole-wheat pita or vegetables
- 1-2 tablespoons almonds or sunflower seeds, or nut butter (almond or sesame tahini) on whole-wheat or rice crackers, leftover lunch portion
- Protein Shake (Whey, Rice, Hemp, Pea, or Soy protein)

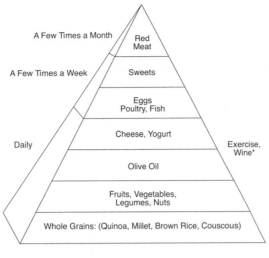

A Few Times a Month — Red Meat

A Few Times a Week — Sweets

Eggs Poultry, Fish

Cheese, Yogurt

Daily — Exercise, Wine*

Olive Oil

Fruits, Vegetables, Legumes, Nuts

Whole Grains: (Quinoa, Millet, Brown Rice, Couscous)

*Daily, wine in moderation

FIGURE 13-1   Mediterranean Diet Pyramid

lifestyle choices can have a significant, positive impact on their health. Recent research demonstrates the cardioprotective effects of several dietary nutrients, including fiber (both soluble and insoluble), antioxidants (vitamins C and E, beta-carotene, selenium, coenzyme Q10), folic acid, and omega-3 essential fatty acids. According to several recent studies, women can lower their risk of heart disease and heart attacks by improving their blood lipid and fatty acid profiles by consuming a combination of essential fatty acids including eicosapentaenoic acid (EPA), docosahexaenoic acid (DHA), and gamma-linolenic acid (GLA) derived from fish oils and certain vegetable oils. Researchers estimate this combination produces a 43% risk reduction over a 10-year period.[19]

Review of Nutrient Sources

Carbohydrates

Carbohydrates provide the main source of energy for all body functions, aiding in digestion, assimilation, and metabolism of proteins and fats. Carbohydrates are classified as simple and complex. Simple carbohydrates include refined white flour products, white rice, white table sugar (dextrose), honey, fruit sugars (fructose), and milk sugars (lactose). Complex carbohydrates are found in whole grains, legumes, and vegetables and contain protein, vitamins, minerals, and fiber. Through-

out human history foods that contain complex carbohydrates have been important diet staples in diverse cultures. Complex carbohydrates supply the body with essential nutrients and protein amino acids and provide longer-lasting energy than do simple carbohydrates.[20] All animal proteins are complete, including red meat, poultry, seafood, eggs, and dairy. Complete proteins can also be obtained through plant foods including soy, lentils, amaranth, buckwheat, and quinoa. Foods can be combined to make complete proteins like pairing beans with brown rice.

Fiber

Dietary fiber is plant material that is left undigested after passing through the body's digestive system. Fiber contains polysaccharides and can be subdivided into insoluble fiber and soluble fiber, each with a different mixture of compounds. Food sources of dietary fiber are often classified according to whether they contain predominantly soluble or insoluble fiber. Plant foods usually contain a combination of both types of fiber in varying degrees, according to the plant's characteristics. Insoluble fiber includes pectin and cellulose, hemicellulose, and lignins.[21] Insoluble fiber is present in fruits, leafy vegetables, whole grains and brans, and beans. Soluble fiber is a gelatin-like substance, such as the mucilage found in oatmeal and legumes.

Research clearly documents that the modern Western diet with its low fiber content has led to an increase in digestive problems, including diverticulitis, constipation, colon cancer, gallstone formation, and other gastrointestinal disturbances. Although dietary fiber is not digested, it increases fecal bulk and weight, making the passage of waste products more efficient and assisting in carrying toxins and metabolic byproducts through the intestines to be eliminated quickly from the system. Fiber also is important in modulating insulin response and thereby stabilizing blood glucose levels. In recent years, research into the benefits of dietary fiber has led many practitioners to recommend a low-fat, high-fiber diet for prevention of heart disease, diabetes, obesity, digestive disorders, and cancer.

According to Seymour Handler of the North Memorial Medical Center in Minneapolis, Minnesota, most of the serious diseases of the colon, including appendicitis and diverticular disease, can be linked etiologically to high levels of saturated fat and low levels of fiber in the Western diet. A diet high in saturated animal fat and low in fiber increases the risk of colon cancer. Guidelines for minimizing risk of colon cancer include reducing consumption of saturated fats and increasing consumption of fiber. Complex-carbohydrate foods offer fiber and are also good sources of protein, vitamins, and minerals.[22] Fiber-rich diets help lower blood cholesterol levels and stabilize blood glucose levels and are considered heart healthy by multiple research studies. According to *Dietary Guidelines for Americans 2010*, at least half of all grains consumed daily should be whole and unrefined. The goal for fiber is 25 grams per day for women and 28 grams per day for men. Achieving these goals may reduce a person's risk of dying from heart disease, infections, and respiratory diseases, according to a new study published in the *Archives of Internal Medicine*.[23]

Protein

Protein is the second most plentiful substance in the body (after water) and constitutes approximately one-fifth of the body's weight. Protein is the basic building block of the body and makes up the rigid structures such as bone, solid organs, and blood vessels. It is essential for the growth and maintenance of all body tissues, including muscle, skin, hair, nails, and eyes. Hormones, chemicals such as antibodies, and enzymes are composed of protein. Protein molecules, essentially composed of amino acids, form long chains and branched structures. Amino acids contain nitrogen, carbon, hydrogen, and sometimes sulfur. Twenty-two amino acids are required to build protein; half of these are produced in the body when adequate nutrients are available, and eight are considered essential.

Excessive protein consumption taxes the kidneys and digestive system. Because the majority of Americans consume most of their protein through animal products—a source of saturated fat as well—consumption of a large quantity of animal protein is associated with increased risk of cardiovascular disease and breast, colon, and prostate cancers. Plant foods such as whole grains, legumes, seeds, and nuts provide excellent protein, but this protein is incomplete, and these foods must be combined with others to provide all of the essential amino acids. Protein requirements depend on an individual's activity level, energy requirements, age, and digestive health. The recommended protein allowance for health maintenance in the United States is 0.8 grams per kilogram of body weight per day. Men and women who body build require up to 1.2 grams per kilogram of body weight per day.[24]

Lipids

Lipids are a group of fats and fatlike substances, including essential fatty acids, that account for more than 10% of body weight in most adults. The principal function of fats is to serve as a source of energy. Stored fats also act as a thermal blanket, insulating the body and providing a protective cushion for many tissues and organs. According to the third National Health and Nutrition Examination Survey, Americans are eating less fat than they were 10 years ago. Americans now average 34% of their total daily calories (82 grams) from fat, with approximately 12% (29 grams) from saturated fats. Current dietary recommendations call for 20% of total calories from fat and less than 10% from saturated fats. The RDA for dietary fat suggested by the National Academy of Sciences to ensure the intake of essential fatty acids is 25 grams. Unsaturated fats are usually liquid at room temperature and are derived from vegetables, nuts and seeds, soybeans, and olives. Saturated fats—found in animal products, including meat and dairy products—are generally associated with increased risk of cancer and cardiovascular disease. Foods often contain a mixture of saturated and unsaturated fatty acids. Fats are calorie rich and contain approximately 9 calories per gram, almost twice the calories of carbohydrates and proteins.

Essential fatty acids are found in both monosaturated and polyunsaturated fats. Monosaturated fats include olive, peanut, avocado, and canola oils. Polyunsaturated fats (PUFAs) are found in safflower, sunflower, corn, sesame, and soy oils. Fats can be further divided into two main classes: omega-3 fatty acids and omega-6 fatty acids. Essential fatty acids form a structural part of all cell membranes. They hold proteins in the membrane, maintain fluidity of the membrane, and create electrical potentials across the membrane, facilitating the generation of bioelectrical currents that transmit messages. Certain essential fatty acids substantially shorten the time required for the recovery of fatigued muscles after exercise by facilitating the conversion of lactic acid to water and carbon dioxide.[25] Essential fatty acids act as precursors

for a family of hormone-like substances called prostaglandins, which regulate many functions in the body, including inflammatory processes and immune responses. Omega-3 essential fatty acids are immune enhancing and are often deficient in the modern diet. They contain high concentrations of linoleic acid and are necessary for normal growth and development throughout the life cycle. Omega-3 essential fatty acids are found in high concentrations in fish, fish oils, flax seeds, and walnuts. Research has shown that these essential fatty acids can lower blood pressure, lower cholesterol and triglyceride levels, and reduce the risk of heart disease and stroke. High concentrations of DHA are found in the brain, and a deficiency of this omega-3 essential fatty acid component can lead to impaired learning and decreased cognitive function. Other EFA deficiency symptoms include poor immune response, dry skin and hair, behavioral changes, menstrual irregularities, and arthritic and inflammatory conditions. **Table 13-1** serves as a guide for general dietary goals and recommendations.[26]

Vitamins

Vitamins are nutrients essential to life. They contribute to good health by regulating the

---

TABLE 13-1   Dietary Goals and Recommendations

Dietary Goals

Reduce or eliminate:

- Saturated fats—fried and greasy foods
- Refined sugars—soft drinks, pastries, white sugar, corn syrup solids
- Refined carbohydrates and processed foods—white rice, white bread, pasta
- Sodium—table salt, monosodium glutamate (MSG)
- Caffeine—substitute with herbal teas, natural coffee substitutes
- Alcohol
- Chemicals in foods—choose organic or local produce

Dietary Recommendations

Increase:

- Complex carbohydrates—beans and whole grains including lentils, tofu, brown rice, quinoa, oats, whole-grain breads, fiber cereals
- Fruits and vegetables (5–7 servings daily)
- Water—6–8 glasses daily

Remember to read ingredients on labels.

metabolism and assisting in biochemical processes that release energy from digested food. Vitamins function mostly as coenzymes that activate the chemical reactions continually occurring in the body. Vitamins are the foundation for all aspects of body function, from nervous system transmission to proper composition of bodily fluids. Vitamins are divided into two major groups: water soluble and fat soluble. Water-soluble vitamins must be taken into the body daily and are excreted within 1 to 4 days. They include vitamin C and the B-complex vitamins. Because excessive quantities are excreted rather than stored, water-soluble vitamins are seldom associated with toxicity problems. Fat-soluble vitamins are absorbed into the blood along with dietary fats. Because they are insoluble in water, they are transported via the lymphatic vessels and are stored in the body's adipose tissue and in the liver. Fat-soluble vitamins include vitamins A, D, E, and K.[27]

Table 13-2 provides more information about vitamins and their food sources.

Minerals

Minerals are naturally occurring elements or compounds found in the Earth. Minerals are essential components of all cells and function as coenzymes. They are necessary for proper composition of body fluids, formation of blood and bone, and maintenance of healthy nerve function. Once a mineral is absorbed, it must be carried from the blood to the cells, and then must be transported across the cell membrane in a form that can be utilized by the cell. Minerals, like vitamins, work in combination with other nutrients and have both synergistic and antagonistic effects. Some minerals compete with one another for absorption, while others enhance the absorption of other minerals. For example, too much calcium can decrease the absorption of magnesium; therefore, these minerals should be consumed in the proper ratio to maintain balance.

Minerals are classified as either major minerals or trace minerals; however, this classification does not reflect their importance. A deficiency of either type of mineral can have a deleterious impact on health. To be classified as a major mineral, the mineral must make up no less than 0.01% of body weight. Major minerals include calcium, magnesium, phosphorus, potassium, sodium, and

chloride. Trace minerals include arsenic, boron, chromium, cobalt, copper, fluoride, iodine, iron, manganese, molybdenum, nickel, selenium, silicon, tin, vanadium, and zinc.[28]

Although normal dietary intake of trace nutrients poses no threat to human health, long-term therapeutic doses of one or more minerals at the expense of other minerals might result in secondary deficiencies that could impair immunological or antioxidant processes. Even borderline levels of certain minerals can suppress a variety of immune responses. Cell-mediated immunity, antibody response, and other immune responses may be impaired by marginal deficiencies in trace minerals. For example, borderline zinc deficiency is associated with depletion of lymphocytes and lymphoid tissue atrophy. Excessive long-term consumption of competing minerals, such as iron, might suppress immune response by producing a secondary deficiency of zinc.

Bioavailability and supplementation are some of the most controversial areas in nutrition research and practice. Nutrient intake through food consumption depends on many factors, including the quality of the soil in which the foods were grown, use of fertilizers, and genetic engineering of foods, to name a few. Consumption of a wide variety of fresh fruits and vegetables and unprocessed whole foods, locally grown and organic whenever possible, is recommended. **Table 13-3** provides further information on minerals and their food sources.

Antioxidants

Some vitamins and minerals function as antioxidants. These include vitamins C and E, beta-carotene (a precursor of vitamin A), coenzyme Q10, alpha lipoic acid, Vitamin D, and the trace mineral selenium. Antioxidants protect the body from the formation of free radicals. Free radicals are electrically charged molecules that have an unpaired electron. Free radicals can damage healthy cells. They can also stress the immune system and suppress its ability to defend the host adequately against organisms, toxins, and metabolic by-products, all of which can lead to degenerative or infectious disease states. Antioxidants can stabilize or deactivate free radicals before the latter attack cells. Antioxidants are absolutely critical for maintaining optimal cellular and systemic health and well-being.[29]

TABLE 13-2   Fat-Soluble and Water-Soluble Vitamins

Vitamin	Function	Food Source
Fat-Soluble Vitamins		
Vitamin A (retinol)	Antioxidant. Aids in maintenance and repair of mucous membranes and epithelial tissue. Assists in growth and development of bones.	All orange and yellow fruits and vegetables: sweet potatoes, squash, yams, carrots, pumpkin, parsley, mango, apricots. Dark leafy greens: kale, spinach, broccoli, salmon, fish oils.
Carotenoids (carotenes, lycopenes)	Antioxidant. Enhances cell communication and immune competence.	Orange, yellow, and dark green fruits and vegetables.
Vitamin D	Aids in transport of calcium. Promotes intestinal and renal absorption of phosphorus. Aids in growth of bones and teeth and neuromuscular function. Immunoprotective.	Liver, oils, egg yolk, alfalfa, dairy products, fish, especially fatty fish such as halibut, salmon, sardines.
Vitamin E	Antioxidant. Promotes wound healing. Protects cell membranes against lipid perioxidation and destruction. Improves circulation.	Cold-pressed vegetable oils, whole grains, dark leafy green vegetables, nuts, seeds, legumes, wheat germ, oatmeal.
Vitamin K	Aids in blood clotting. Promotes formation and maintenance of healthy bone.	Green leafy vegetables, egg yolks.
Water-Soluble Vitamins		
Vitamin B$_1$ (thiamine)	Coenzyme in oxidation of glucose. Assists in production of hydrochloric acid.	Dried beans, brown rice, egg yolks, fish, chicken, peanuts.
Vitamin B$_2$ (riboflavin)	Assists in red blood cell formation. Aids in metabolism of carbohydrates, fats, and proteins.	Beans, eggs, fish, poultry, meat, spinach, yogurt, asparagus, avocado.
Vitamin B$_3$ (niacin)	Promotes healthy skin and nervous system. Lowers cholesterol, improves circulation.	Fish, eggs, beef, cheese, potatoes, whole wheat.
Vitamin B$_5$ (pantothenic acid)	"Antistress" vitamin. Aids in production of adrenal hormones. Assists in formation of antibodies and protein metabolism.	Beans, beef, eggs, mother's milk, fresh vegetables, whole wheat, pork, saltwater fish.
Vitamin B$_6$ (pyridoxine)	Acts as coenzyme in metabolism of amino acids and essential fatty acids necessary for production of serotonin and other neurotransmitters. Essential for healthy nervous system. Assists in converting iron to hemoglobin.	Eggs, fish, spinach, peas, meat, nuts, carrots, poultry, soybeans, bananas, avocado, whole grain cereals, prunes.
Vitamin B$_{12}$ (cobalamin)	Aids in synthesis of red blood cells. Required for proper digestion and absorption of foods. Prevents nerve damage	Beef, herring, cheese, sardines, salmon, tempeh, miso, tofu, eggs, dairy products.
Folic acid	Participates in amino acid conversion, manufacture of neurotransmitters. Cardioprotective.	Dark green vegetables, kidney beans, asparagus, broccoli, whole grains, cereals.
Vitamin C (ascorbic acid)	Antioxidant. Aids in collagen formation, absorption of iron, interferon production. Promotes capillary integrity. Aids in release of stress hormones.	Citrus fruits, papaya, parsley, watercress, berries, tomatoes, broccoli, brussels sprouts.

TABLE 13-3   Major Minerals and Trace Elements

Mineral	Function	Food Source
Calcium	Formation of strong bones, transmission of nerve impulses, muscle growth and movement. Blood clotting. Prevention of hypertension.	Dairy products, salmon, sardines, green leafy vegetables, seeds and nuts, tofu, blackstrap molasses, seaweed.
Chromium	Metabolism of glucose. Stabilization of blood sugar levels. Synthesis of cholesterol, fats, and proteins.	Brewer's yeast, brown rice, cheese, whole grains, beans, mushrooms, potatoes.
Copper	Formation of bone, hemoglobin, red blood cells. Healing process.	Whole grains, avocado, oyster, lobster, dandelion greens, mushrooms, blackstrap molasses, nuts, seeds, soybeans.
Iodine	Energy production. Body temperature regulation, thyroid gland health.	Seaweed, iodized salt, dairy products, seafood, saltwater fish, garlic, Swiss chard, summer squash.
Iron	Hemoglobin production. Stress and disease resistance. Energy production. Immune system health.	Eggs, fish, poultry, dark leafy greens, blackstrap molasses, almonds, seaweed.
Magnesium	Formation of bone. Carbohydrate and mineral metabolism. Maintenance of proper pH balance. Immune function.	Dairy products, fish, seafood, blackstrap molasses, garlic, whole grains, seeds, tofu, green leafy vegetables, nuts.
Manganese	Enzyme activation. Sex hormone production. Nerve health. Energy production.	Avocados, nuts, seeds, seaweed, whole grains.
Phosphorus	Bone and teeth formation. Cell growth. Contraction of heart muscle. Kidney function.	Asparagus, brewer's yeast, fish, dried fruits, garlic, legumes, seeds and nuts.
Potassium	Healthy nervous system. Regulation of body fluids with sodium. pH balance.	Apricots, bananas, potatoes, sunflower seeds, blackstrap molasses, sprouts, broccoli.
Selenium	Antioxidant function. Immune system protection, cancer prevention.	Brazil nuts, brewer's yeast, brown rice, dairy products, garlic, onions, whole grains.
Sodium	With potassium, regulation of body fluids necessary for nerve and muscle function.	Table salt, seaweed.
Zinc	Burn and wound healing. Carbohydrate digestion. Prostate gland function, reproductive organ growth and development. Immune system health, production of antibodies.	Sardines and other fish, legumes, poultry, meat, egg yolks, beans, pumpkin seeds, sunflower seeds.

The body can manufacture its own antioxidant, glutathione. Glutathione is a powerful antioxidant composed of the amino acids cysteine, glycine, and glutamic acid. It is potentized and recycled by other antioxidants, including vitamin C, selenium, alpha lipoic acid, and coenzyme Q10. It is synthesized and most concentrated in the liver, where it is involved in detoxification pathways and protects against free radical damage. Glutathione helps to recycle other antioxidants.[30] Glutathione is involved in the synthesis and repair of DNA. Decline in glutathione concentrations in intracellular fluids correlates directly with indicators of immunological function and longevity. Liver stores of glutathione can be depleted by disease processes, malnutrition, and poor-quality nutrient intake. Dietary amino acids are essential to glutathione synthesis. Lifestyle factors that affect efficient utilization of glutathione include stress, alcohol, cigarette smoking, excessive pharmaceutical use, drug abuse, and aging.[31]

Phytonutrients

Plant-based chemicals and nutrients have been used throughout human evolution to benefit health. Many phytochemicals contain protective, disease-preventing compounds and their discovery has been the basis for many pharmaceuticals in use today. Although phytochemicals are not yet classified as nutrients, "substances necessary for sustaining life," they have been identified as having properties that support health. Plant nutrients and their bioactive components have been studied for the treatment of cancer, diabetes, cardiovascular disease, and hypertension. They have been shown to exhibit potent antioxidant properties and modulate many processes including cellular protection, healthy cell signaling, cancer cell replication and apoptosis (cancer cell death), and they can decrease cholesterol levels.[32]

One of the interesting observations in nature has been the role these chemical components play in providing built-in protection from disease, injuries, insects, drought, excessive heat, ultraviolet rays, and poisons or pollutants in the air or soil. They appear to form part of plants' immune system. Current research explores the mechanisms of these compounds to affect immunological and epigenetic changes in humans, an emerging field in cancer research and in the application of novel chemotherapeutic interventions,[33] as well as the potential synergistic effects of phytochemicals used in combination with current chemotherapy.[34]

To ensure adequate amounts of nutrients and phytochemicals are obtained from fruits and vegetables, it is recommended that people eat a minimum of five to seven portions daily of a variety of foods from the following color groups:

Red: Beets, red cabbage, cherries, cranberries, pink grapefruit, red grapes, red peppers, pomegranates, red potatoes, radishes, raspberries, rhubarb, strawberries, tomatoes, watermelon

Orange: Apricots, butternut squash, cantaloupe, carrots, mangoes, nectarines, oranges, papayas, peaches, persimmons, pumpkin, tangerines

Yellow-green: Green apples, artichokes, asparagus, avocados, green beans, broccoli, brussels sprouts, green cabbage, cucumbers, green grapes, honeydew melon, kiwi, lettuce, lemons, limes, green onions, peas, green pepper, spinach, zucchini

Blue-purple: Purple kale, purple cabbage, purple potatoes, eggplant, purple grapes, blueberries, blackberries, boysenberries, raspberries, raisins, figs, plums

Sample a variety of flavors. By consuming small amounts of nature's diverse foods and flavors, you can enhance taste and pleasure while benefiting from phytochemicals that support your health.

Digestion, Absorption, Assimilation

Assessing nutrition includes not only examining what people eat but how they digest, absorb, assimilate, and eliminate foods—all essential for good health. Diet is the food we eat. Nutrition is the study of what happens after we eat it.

Optimal absorption of nutrients depends on the integrity of the digestive system. Good health requires proper digestion and absorption. Digestion is the mechanical and chemical breakdown of the food we eat. Digestion is initiated when we chew food and begin to break it down with digestive enzymes. As food is digested, it needs to be absorbed. Absorption is the process of bringing the nutrients from the gastrointestinal tract to the rest of the body's tissues. The entire gastrointestinal tract is lined with mucosal tissue that secretes enzymes and multiple protective antibodies, an essential part of our immune defense. The gastrointestinal tract also contains billions of friendly microflora. These microorganisms assist in metabolic processes while maintaining the integrity of the mucosal lining.[35]

Digestion in the stomach occurs as food is churned and mixed with hydrochloric acid and various enzymes, which prepares it for entry into the small intestine via the duodenum. In the small intestine, digestive enzymes from the liver, gallbladder, and pancreas are added to the partially digested food. The pancreas secretes amylase, lipase, protease, and chymotrypsin, while the liver and gallbladder secrete bile to aid in the digestion of fats and the absorption of essential fatty acids and fat-soluble vitamins. Food spends 1 to 4 hours in the small intestine, which is approximately 25 feet long. As food is digested, it is absorbed into small blood vessels in the lining of the intestine. Toxins and waste products enter the large intestine to be excreted as fecal matter. The large intestine processes primarily fiber and water. The proper absorption and utilization of nutrients depends on a complex orchestration of processes in the digestive tract, and therefore it is essential to maintain the health and balance of this system.[36]

The friendly bacteria that live in the gastrointestinal tract, including strains of *Lactobacillus* and acidophilus, have many beneficial effects on health. They assist in synthesizing B vitamins, digesting proteins, balancing intestinal pH, reducing serum cholesterol, strengthening the immune system in the gut, preventing parasites and overgrowth of yeast, and maintaining bowel regularity. The most common reason for the destruction of friendly bacteria in the gastrointestinal tract is from the use of antibiotics and from ingestion through consumption of antibiotic-treated animal products. Leaky gut syndrome can occur with the loss of integrity of the mucosal lining tissue. Studies indicate that beneficial bacteria must be replaced by probiotic supplementation following antibiotic therapy to prevent symptoms of dysbiosis and leaky gut syndrome that manifest as fatigue, bloating, gas, diarrhea, constipation, food allergies, inflammatory disorders, migraine headache, yeast overgrowth, and weight gain.[37]

Improving digestion includes dietary modification, such as the elimination of fried foods, sugars, and any foods that stress an individual's digestive system. Keeping a food journal and then following an elimination diet is helpful in identifying foods that may trigger digestive disorders, food allergies, and autoimmune responses. Removing "triggers" from the diet for a minimum of 21 days can be an important dietary intervention for those with food sensitivities. Wheat, gluten, lactose, and casein products are the most common foods to eliminate and often can relieve many common gastrointestinal problems including constipation, bloating after consuming, and irritable bowel syndrome.[38] The

individual can slowly reintroduce the food item and observe whether symptoms return. Each person has a unique relationship with food and its chemical properties, and therefore nutritional assessment and dietary recommendations are based on biochemical individuality. As nutrition is integrated into clinical care, assessing the unique needs of each individual and offering health education and self-care tools can affect the health and well-being of the individual over time.

Nutrition offers a holistic approach and takes into account the individual's physiologic, psychological, social, genetic, cultural, religious, economic, and environmental needs. The individual's eating patterns, food preferences, motivation, attitudes, and beliefs are all part of nutrition coaching, counseling, and education.

■ EATING TO PROMOTE HEALTH

Increasing awareness of how diet can affect health and well-being is an essential component in nutrition coaching and education. Nurses can use the following questions as a guideline.

Sit down in a quiet place and plan a day's menu by asking yourself these questions:

- What does my body need to enhance wellness?
- What are my past eating patterns? Which do I want to keep? Which do I want to change?
- What are my activity levels, and how should I include foods that meet my needs?
- How do I need to plan for psychological factors?
- What factors, unique to me, influence my food planning?

Stress and Nutrient Needs

The consequences of stress in our lives and its impact on our health can be mediated through increasing nutrient intake to support normalization of stress-induced biochemical changes, increased nutrient needs, and natural resistance to stress responses. Research increasingly supports the critical role in disease played by stress-induced hormones, including elevated cortisol levels, which induces inflammation, sleep disturbances, and obesity. Inflammation is part of the body's natural response to infection, injury, allergens, and other foreign substances in the body including chemicals in the environment. Removing inflammatory triggers is an important intervention to calm the inflammatory chemicals and cytokines produced. Chronic inflammation plays a role in diabetes, osteoporosis, hypertension, cardiovascular disease, infectious disease, gastric ulcer, cancer, immune system disturbances, and gastrointestinal, skin, endocrine, and neurologic disorders. Chronic stress has been shown to affect behavior and has been linked to anxiety states and depression. The vulnerability of a particular bodily system to stress varies from one individual to another, is determined by genetic makeup and constitution, and may be influenced by nutritional and environmental factors. A healthy diet rich in whole foods that contain antioxidants, B vitamins, essential fatty acids, and trace minerals can mediate the stress response and support overall health and well-being throughout life.

Eco Nutrition

Breast cancer is the second most common cause of cancer-related deaths in women in the United States. Research indicates that poor nutrient intake, chronic stress, inflammatory processes, and obesity are all risk factors. Mounting evidence shows that chemical exposure to xenotoxins is another risk factor for breast cancer.[39] Environmental xenoestrogens—synthetic hormone-mimicking compounds found in certain pesticides, drugs, and plastics, and occupational exposures—may play a role in the etiology of breast cancer.[40] Xenoestrogens accumulate in the fatty tissues of the body and may interact with estrogen receptor sites in the breast, enhancing breast cell proliferation. Also, women with breast cancer often have higher concentrations of pesticides in their blood and fatty tissues than do healthy women.[41]

Fat intake and obesity appear to be primary risk factors associated with cardiovascular disease, diabetes, and cancer in women. Many epidemiologic studies associate a high-fat, low-fiber diet with an increased risk of developing cancer of the colon, prostate, and breast. A review of the literature also suggests an inverse relationship between the quantity of fresh fruits and vegetables consumed and the incidence of cancer. Weight loss plans that support a low-fat, high-fiber whole foods diet, stress reduction, and exercise are part of a comprehensive health approach for the prevention of cardiovascular disease and breast cancer in women.

Fruits and vegetables are rich in fiber, antioxidants, and other plant-derived substances, or phytonutrients, believed to contain cancer-protective properties. Fiber is thought to influence hormone levels by facilitating the fecal excretion of estrogen metabolites, which at high levels can pose a risk for many women.[42] Other ingredients that contain potential anti-cancer compounds include cruciferous vegetables (watercress, broccoli, cauliflower, brussels sprouts), which contain isothiocynates, such as sulforophane, and are rich in indoles. These substances may help in liver detoxification, aid in the removal of carcinogens and environmental toxins, and play a role in cancer prevention.[43,44] Soy products that contain natural plant phytoestrogens (genistein and daidzen) called isoflavones may play a significant role in the prevention, and possibly the treatment, of some hormone-related diseases, although this remains controversial in the literature.[45] Curcumin and resveratrol, phytonutrients that demonstrate both antioxidant and anti-inflammatory properties, appear to be immunoprotective and chemopreventive. These phytonutrients appear to be protective against both breast cancer and prostate cancer.[46]

Cancer Prevention Tips

- Choose a predominantly plant-based diet rich in a variety of vegetables and fruits.
- Avoid being underweight or overweight, and limit weight gain in adulthood to less than 11 pounds.
- Eat eight or more servings per day of cereals and grains (e.g., brown rice, whole-grain breads), legumes (e.g., lentils, soy), tubers (e.g., potatoes), and roots (e.g., beets).
- Eat five or more servings per day of other fruits and vegetables.
- Limit consumption of white sugar.
- Limit alcoholic drinks.
- Limit intake of red meat to less than 3 ounces a day, if it is eaten at all. In place of red meat, eat fish, poultry, or soy products.
- Limit consumption of fatty foods, particularly those of animal origin.
- Limit consumption of salted foods. Use herbs and spices to season foods.

- Avoid eating charred foods.
- Avoid smoking or chewing tobacco.

© 2010 Integrative Nurse Coach Certificate Program (INCCP)

The following guidelines ensure optimal digestion, absorption, and elimination and promote optimal health and well-being. This approach offers a hypoallergenic and anti-inflammatory response to optimize cellular energy.

Whole Food Nutrition Plan

- *Plant-based diet:* Whole, unprocessed, predominately plant-based diet
- *Low glycemic load:* High in foods that slow the speed at which the blood glucose level is raised
- *Proper fatty acid composition:* High level of healthy omega-3 essential fatty acids including walnuts, flax seeds, and fish oils
- *High phytonutrient density:* High level of phytonutrients and antioxidants
- *Healthy protein:* Lean, healthy, predominately plant-based proteins, or pasture-raised, chemical-free animal products
- *High micronutrient density:* High amounts of vitamins and minerals
- *Low allergenic burden:* Low in foods that are highly allergenic (based on individual)
- *Elimination diet:* Gluten- and casein-free diet for a minimum of 3 weeks
- *Low toxic burden:* Minimizes toxic burden of food: no added hormones, pesticides, antibiotics, or any other artificial additives or preservatives
- *Organic fruits, vegetables, and animal products:* Whenever possible, high in organic products; local produce is the next best choice
- *Healthy pH balance:* Provides proper balance between acidity and alkalinity
- *High fiber content:* High in fiber to help slow the insulin response and optimize digestive health, detoxification
- *Optimized elimination pathways.*

© 2010 Integrative Nurse Coach Certificate Program (INCCP)

Osteoporosis

The best treatment for osteoporosis is prevention. Along with lack of exercise, osteoporosis often is the result of deficiencies of several key nutrients,

of which calcium is but one. Research indicates that other essential nutrients, including vitamin D_3, vitamin K, magnesium, boron, and other trace minerals must be available in the proper balance to facilitate calcium resorption and uptake into the bone. In multiple studies, supplementation has been shown to be effective in preventing fractures in both men and women.[47]

Beyond maintaining healthy bones (and preventing rickets), research on the role of vitamin D in maintaining health has exploded in recent years. Vitamin D is not only a vitamin but a pro-hormone that has hundreds of receptor sites on every cell. Emerging nutritional science is rethinking the need for vitamin D_3 and reexamining optimal levels needed for supporting immune health, cognitive function, and cancer prevention.[48] Vitamin D deficiency in adults is reported to exacerbate osteopenia, osteoporosis, muscle weakness, fractures, common cancers including prostate and breast,[49] autoimmune diseases, infectious diseases, cognitive impairment and Alzheimer's disease,[50] and cardiovascular disease. The vitamin may reduce the incidence of several types of cancer and type 1 diabetes.[51] Recent research published in the *Journal of the American Medical Association* and *Lancet* explores vitamin D_3 deficiency and the increased risk of multiple sclerosis.[52]

Common Dietary Risk Factors for Osteoporosis

- Low intake of vitamin D, calcium, magnesium, and trace minerals (note that vitamin D is now first in this list)
- High intake of animal protein
- High intake of caffeine
- Excessive intake of carbonated beverages
- High intake of sodium
- High intake of refined sugar
- Lack of exercise
- Lack of sunlight exposure
- Excessive intake of alcohol
- Hypochlorhydria (low HCl) that can occur with aging and with intake of antacids

Guidelines for Healthy Bones

- Increase consumption of calcium-rich foods, including green leafy vegetables, whole grains, beans, tofu, dairy products, nuts, and seeds.

- Increase weight-bearing exercise, such as walking.
- Decrease consumption of soda, caffeine, and alcohol.
- Check vitamin D levels (25-hydroxyvitamin D).
- Spend at least 15 minutes a day exposed to direct sunlight.

Supplement Recommendations for Healthy Bones

The current RDA for calcium is 800–1,200 milligrams per day of elemental calcium. Magnesium and calcium function in balance. The recommended ratio of calcium to magnesium is usually 2:1; thus, the recommended dosage of magnesium is 400–600 milligrams per day. According to new research, the daily amount of vitamin D, taken in as vitamin D_3, depends on exposure to sunlight, genetics, skin pigmentation, geographical location, and individual physiologic requirements. Testing 25-hydroxyvitamin D levels is recommended prior to and during supplementation. Compelling research suggests that vitamin D levels be maintained above 40 and supplementation is recommended to achieve this level. Other nutrients that help maintain bone mass include vitamin K, boron, vitamin B_6, manganese, folic acid, vitamin C, and zinc.[53]

Nutrition and Healthy Aging

According to the U.S. Census Bureau, by the year 2025, with the aging of the baby boomers, there will be more people older than 60 years than younger than 25 years for the first time in this nation's history.

Nutrition practices play a fundamental role in and greatly influence the aging process. Research reveals the health benefits of improving nutrition anywhere in the life cycle including in the older years, which can affect and prevent much of the decline associated with aging. Older adults are vulnerable to the cumulative health impact of inadequate nutrition. The National Health and Nutrition Surveys conducted by the Department of Health and Human Services reveal that the nation's older citizens remain at high risk of macronutrient and micronutrient deficiencies.

Inadequate nutrition and protein deficiencies, for example, can lead to increased muscle loss, cognitive decline, fatigue, and immune system impairment. Medical foods such as whey protein powder, high in glutamine and other amino acids, have been shown to improve protein stores and rebuild muscle mass.[54] Untreated and often undiagnosed deficiencies take a heavy toll on older people, resulting in accelerated aging. Research over the past decade clearly shows that many of the ailments previously thought to be an inevitable result of old age can be prevented by aggressive detection and treatment of subclinical nutrient deficits.[55]

Oxidative stress without adequate repair mechanisms may contribute to the onset of Alzheimer's disease, and the risk of Alzheimer's disease may be reduced by intake of antioxidants that counteract the detrimental effects of oxidative stress.[56] Regardless of a person's age, calcium, vitamin D_3, and trace nutrients are essential for maintaining bone mass and overall good health. Recent research indicates that vitamin D may be involved in neuroprotection, control of pro-inflammatory cytokine-induced cognitive dysfunction, and synthesis of calcium-binding proteins.[57] The role of vitamin D receptors in the pathophysiology of cognitive decline, incidence of Alzheimer's disease, and vascular dementia and/or cognitive decline with respect to previous plasma 25-hydroxyvitamin D concentration has been observed in several studies.[58]

Although elderly individuals must be evaluated individually, many psychosocial factors need to be considered when addressing nutrition needs and goals, including economics, ability to shop and prepare meals, and social support networks. Many older adults suffer from vitamin B_{12} deficiency as a result of impaired absorption of micronutrients. Other issues that interfere with nutrient intake include chewing difficulties, impaired cognitive function and forgetting to eat, social isolation and apathy in food preparation, and inability to shop or carry packages. Impaired memory in elderly people often is related to the effect of B vitamins, vitamin D, antioxidant, and essential fatty acid deficiencies.

Undetected hypochlorhydria, a deficiency of hydrochloric acid in the stomach, leads to bacterial overgrowth in the small bowel and results in impaired digestion and absorption of essential nutrients, including vitamins B_6 and B_{12}.[59] Americans older than age 65 years consume 30% of the over-the-counter drugs sold in the United States. Many of these medications are known to impair absorption, and metabolism of nutrients and act as nutrient antagonists. The most commonly used over-the-counter drugs among older adults are laxatives, which can impair the status of the fat-soluble vitamins A, E, D, and K. Vitamin deficiencies remain subclinical in older adults and are the result of inadequate nutrient stores over many years. One of the hallmarks of biologic aging is altered glucose metabolism, which affects many age-related diseases, including heart disease, inflammatory disorders, dementia, and diabetes. Establishing a reservoir of nutrients throughout the life cycle is key for healthy aging.

Successful weight loss and improvements in health are achieved and maintained with a regular exercise program, psychological support, and a personal commitment to wellness. Working with a coach supports goals and plans to achieve desired results. Healthy food choices along with caloric restriction promote healthy aging and longevity.[31,60,61]

Weight Management Guidelines

- Recognize management of obesity as a lifelong commitment that requires lifestyle changes.
- Set realistic goals for weight loss.
- Implement meal planning with daily menus.
- Serve smaller portions (use smaller plates).
- Avoid keeping ready-to-eat snack food around the house.
- Prepare grocery shopping from a list and not on an empty stomach.
- Do all eating in one room and focus on eating without distractions.
- Increase intake of vegetables ("free" foods).
- Leave a small amount of food on the plate.
- Increase activity level.
- Avoid skipping meals.
- Avoid late-night eating.
- Drink at least six glasses of water daily.
- Try a food allergy elimination diet.
- Eliminate all junk foods (processed, refined foods) from the diet.

Eating with Awareness

Taking time for the eating experience can help to reduce cravings, control portion sizes, enhance the eating experience, improve digestion and overall health, and engender a sense of well-being. Nurse coaches can recommend the following guidelines to their clients:

1. *Eat in a setting where you feel relaxed.* This practice helps with the digestive process including absorption to assimilation of nutrients. Create healing environments at home and in the workplace.
2. *Chew thoroughly.* The process of digestion begins in the mouth where enzymes are secreted in saliva to break down food. Explore the texture in your mouth. If we do not properly chew and make our food morsels smaller, indigestion and other digestive problems can occur. The act of eating allows us to be mindful, and in the moment, of the exchange of energy in the food.
3. *Eat mindfully.* Become increasingly aware of how what you eat nurtures your body-mind. At the end of each meal, leave a small amount of food on your plate. Take time to feel your satiety. Step away from the table. Observe your physical sensations. With gratitude and a sense of abundance, know you have nurtured and cared for yourself.
4. *Choose foods to support your health and well-being.* Avoid processed, packaged, fast, and prepared foods. Broil, steam, bake to avoid fried foods. Fresh is always best. Choose organic or local produce whenever possible.

© 2010 Integrative Nurse Coach Certificate Program (INCCP)

■ HEALTHY NUTRITION CHOICES

High-Fiber Diet

- *Whole grains:* Oatmeal, brown rice, quinoa, buckwheat (kasha), millet, whole wheat, enriched pasta
- *Beans:* Lentils, tofu, split peas, garbanzo beans, black beans, tempeh
- *Vegetables:* Green, yellow, orange—steamed, raw, or stir-fried
- *Nuts and seeds:* Sunflower seeds, Brazil nuts, almonds, sesame seeds, pumpkin seeds, nut butters, walnuts
- *Fruits:* Local and in season, such as papaya, melon, mango, grapefruit, berries

Note: Grains + beans = complete protein.

Low-Fat Diet

- Limit meats.
- Eliminate sandwich meats (ham, salami, bacon, sausage).
- Increase fish, chicken, turkey (white meat).
- Use cold-pressed, unprocessed oils—olive, canola, sesame.
- Avoid fried and greasy food.
- Use low-fat dairy products.
- Bake, broil, steam, or poach food.

Foods to Avoid

- *Sugars:* Cookies, soda, candy, jelly, syrup, corn syrup.
- *Processed foods:* Additives, preservatives, artificial colorings, flavorings, artificial sugars including aspartame (Equal, diet sodas).
- *Canned foods:* Fresh is best, frozen is next best.
- *Refined hydrogenated oils:* Crisco, palm oil, cottonseed oil.
- *Fast foods and junk foods.*

Nutrition Guidelines for Maintaining Healthy Cholesterol Levels

1. *Oatmeal, oat bran, and high-fiber foods:* Oatmeal contains soluble fiber, which reduces low-density lipoprotein (LDL). Soluble fiber is also found in such foods as kidney beans, apples, pears, barley, and prunes. Five to 10 grams or more of soluble fiber a day decreases LDL cholesterol. Eating 1.5 cups of cooked oatmeal provides 6 grams of fiber.

2. *Fish and omega-3 fatty acids:* Eating fatty fish can be heart healthy with its high levels of omega-3 fatty acids. In people with a history of heart attacks, fish oil or omega-3 fatty acids reduce the risk of sudden death. The highest levels of omega-3 fatty acids are in the following types of fish:
   - Mackerel
   - Lake trout
   - Herring
   - Sardines
   - Wild salmon
   - Halibut

   Bake or grill to avoid adding unhealthy fats or heated oils. Most farm-raised fished fish are high in chemicals including hormones and antibiotics. Other Plant sources of omega-3 EFAs are walnuts and ground flaxseeds.

3. *Walnuts, almonds, and other nuts:* Walnuts, almonds, and other nuts can reduce blood cholesterol. Rich in polyunsaturated fatty acids, walnuts also help keep blood vessels healthy. According to the Food and Drug Administration, eating about a handful (1.5 ounces, or 42.5 grams) a day of most nuts, such as almonds, hazelnuts, peanuts, pecans, some pine nuts, pistachio nuts, and walnuts, may reduce the risk of heart disease. Nuts should be raw if possible and without additional oils added. All nuts are high in calories, so a handful will do. Replace foods high in saturated fat with nuts.

4. *Olive oil:* Olive oil contains a potent mix of antioxidants that can lower "bad" (LDL) cholesterol but leave "good" (HDL) cholesterol untouched. Evidence from epidemiologic studies also suggests that a higher proportion of monounsaturated fats (MUFAs) in the diet is linked to a reduction in the risk of coronary heart disease. This is significant because olive oil is considerably rich in monounsaturated fats, most notably oleic acid.

   Olive oil contains a wide variety of valuable antioxidants that are not found in other oils. Hydroxytyrosol is thought to be the main antioxidant compound in olives and is believed to play a significant role in the many health benefits attributed to olive oil.

   The Food and Drug Administration recommends using about 2 tablespoons (23 grams) of olive oil a day in place of other fats to receive heart-healthy benefits. To add olive oil to your diet, you can sauté vegetables in it, add it to a marinade, or mix it with vinegar as a salad dressing. The cholesterol-lowering effects of olive oil are even greater in cold-pressed extra-virgin olive oil, meaning the oil is less processed and contains more heart-healthy antioxidants, than in other types of olive oils that are processed differently.[62] For example, "light" olive oils are usually more processed than is extra-virgin or virgin olive oils and are lighter in color but not in fat or calories.

Other Important Health-Promoting Tips

- Drink four to six glasses of liquid daily—spring or filtered water or herbal teas.
- Cook and prepare food in cast-iron or stainless steel cookware (avoid aluminum).
- Chew foods slowly and thoroughly.
- Eat smaller, simpler meals.
- Include fiber with each meal.
- Exercise daily—walk, bicycle, jog, dance, swim, stretch.
- Reduce stress through yoga, meditation, deep breathing, relaxation practice, and visualization.
- Avoid alcohol, caffeine, smoking, recreational drugs, and over-the-counter drugs.
- Get sufficient rest and sleep.

■ HOLISTIC CARING PROCESS

The nurse as coach restores balance and improves overall health and well-being by managing complex, chronic illnesses and facilitating and deepening awareness of the relationship between nutrition, wellness, disease, and mind-body health. The nurse as coach:

- Explores the totality of the individual
- Explores the beliefs and meaning, relationship, and behaviors around food
- Assesses the client/patient's nutritional patterns including food choices, food preparation, meal planning, food budget, and accessibility
- Evaluates the client's nutritional needs
- Guides client in developing a personalized nutrition food plan
- Increases understanding of effective nutritional guidelines for enhancing wellness
- Increases awareness of environmental factors that influence health
- Offers information, handouts, and guidelines in the role of the nurse coach/expert

© 2010 Integrative Nurse Coach Certificate Program (INCCP)

Holistic Assessment

Nurse Coaching in Behavioral and Lifestyle Change

In preparing to use nutrition interventions, the nurse assesses the following parameters:

- The client's relationship to nutrition and diet: biochemical, genetic, cultural, social, emotional, religious/spiritual, economic, environmental, and physiologic components
- The client's eating habits, food preferences, and nutritional needs
- The client's motivation and ability to make the necessary dietary and lifestyle changes
- The client's understanding that changing food and eating patterns is part of a wellness process

Identification of Patterns/Challenges/Needs

Patterns/challenges/needs (see Chapter 7) compatible with nutrition interventions are as follows:

- Altered nutrition
- Altered circulation
- Altered oxygenation
- Altered energy
- Altered coping
- Altered physical mobility
- Sleep pattern disturbances
- Altered patterns of daily living
- Disturbance in body image
- Disturbance in self-esteem
- Potential hopelessness
- Potential powerlessness
- Knowledge deficit
- Pain
- Anxiety
- Grieving
- Depression
- Fear

Outcomes Identification

Exhibit 13-2 guides the nurse in client outcomes, nurse coaching, and evaluation of changes in awareness, eating patterns, relationship to food, healthier food choices, and overall health using standard evaluations including weight, BMI, bioelectrical impedance analysis (BIA), and laboratory testing. Integrating nurse coaching with nutrition education is an effective nursing intervention.

Therapeutic Care Plan and Interventions

The nurse coach can implement the following activities over one session or several sessions.

Before the session:
- Prepare self to be fully present with client.
- Create an environment in which the client feels comfortable discussing beliefs about

EXHIBIT 13-2   Nursing Interventions: Nutrition

Client Outcomes	Nursing Prescriptions	Evaluation
The client will be motivated to improve nutrition.	Assist the client in a personal self-assessment.	The client completed a self-assessment form.
	Encourage the client to participate with the nurse to develop goals and action plans.	The client participated with the nurse to develop a personalized program.
	Prepare the client to follow through with the nurse on evaluation and formulation of new goals.	The client met with the nurse for program evaluation.
The client will demonstrate knowledge of healthful nutrition.	Motivate the client to contribute to discussions about his or her program.	The client participated in the session discussion.
	Encourage the client to learn more about healthful behaviors as he or she works with the nurse.	The client demonstrated new knowledge.

health and exploring his or her relationship to food.

- Listen deeply to the client's story.
- Prepare assessment tools.
- Focus on the client's nutritional and physical needs.
- Prepare educational materials.

At the beginning of the session:

- Introduce relaxation and centering techniques.
- Take and record the necessary physical assessment data (e.g., weight, skin-fold thickness measurements).
- Guide the client to disclose past habits and patterns that affect eating behaviors.
- Engage the client in sharing his or her association between food and feelings of well-being or distress.
- Ask the client to describe food intake in a typical day.
- Assist the client in creating a sample menu or food plan.
- Encourage the client to participate in setting nutritional goals and action plans.
- Present specific nutritional guidelines for the client to follow.
- Direct the client to keep a food journal to present at a follow-up session.

During the session:

- Serve as a coach, guiding the process.
- Emphasize the connection between nutrition and whole-person health.
- Guide the client to develop strategies for changing nutrition habits, nutrient intake, and eating patterns and behaviors.
- Assist the client in optimizing diet and nutrition by doing the following:
  - Creating an image for food as a healing medicine
  - Reframing the nutrition process into a positive action
  - Reframing nutrition and food as an empowerment tool
  - Illustrating how external nutrition changes promote internal healing responses
  - Reinforcing the client's positive changes in nutrition as part of the healing process
  - Ending sessions with images of the desired state of well-being.

At the end of the session:

- Client identifies the options presented that best fit with his or her lifestyle.
- Invite the client to create an action plan with an attainable goal.
- Work together with the client to write down goals and target dates.

- Encourage the client to create specific affirmations to support these goals.
- Give the client handout materials to reinforce the teaching.
- Reinforce the client's plan and positive outcomes that were established before each session (see Exhibit 13-2) and listen to the client's subjective experiences (see **Exhibit 13-3**) to evaluate the session and deepen the process.
- Schedule a follow-up session.

Possible Supportive Interventions for Optimal Nutrition

To optimize nutrient intake, the nurse as coach supports the client in the following interventions for optimal nutrition:

- Offers guidelines for a mindfulness eating practice
- Encourages keeping a food journal for 1 week to increase awareness of food choices, patterns, and behaviors and observe emotional and stress triggers
- Reinforces benefits of adhering to the recommended healthy food plan and of the client observing changes, challenges, and benefits
- Offers relaxation techniques to integrate into daily practice
- Includes exercise plan following evaluation by a trained professional

In the role as health educator, nurses can share information and research data on health benefits of phytonutrients, antioxidants, and food components known to assist balancing the body in supporting the healing process.

When developing a new menu plan to fit the client's particular needs, the following is part of a whole-person assessment:

- Daily activity status
- Current health status
- Physical limitations
- Economic considerations
- Social and cultural influences
- Emotional state of being
- Individual differences, including food preferences and religious dietary customs

To motivate and assist the client, the nurse coach can do the following:

- Encourage the client to write a food journal daily.
- Develop mindful eating practices.
- Demonstrate the daily practice of asking the body what it needs to be healthy.
- Create daily menus using healthy choices that are mutually agreed upon.
- Explore health goals
- Establish attainable goals
- Guide the client to self-assess health changes that occur with dietary interventions.
- Encourage the client who is currently using nutritional supplementation to organize a routine to optimize compliance and benefits.

The nurse coach can use open-ended questions, images, journal writing, drawing, and other creative strategies to integrate nutrition into the client's daily life to close the session.

EXHIBIT 13-3   Evaluation of the Client's Subjective Experience with Nutrition

1. Is this the first time you have considered the effects of healing nutrition from a holistic perspective?
2. Have you discovered ways you can eat for increased vitality and vibrant living?
3. Do you believe there are any links between your food choices and development of health-related concerns or current symptoms?
4. Is your life filled with healing foods? Do you want it to be?
5. What support systems would help you develop and adhere to a lifestyle that includes healing foods?
6. Can you think of anything else that would help you to maintain a routine that includes healing nutrition?
7. What is your next step (or your plan) to integrate these experiences on a daily basis?

CASE STUDY

Setting: An integrative medicine/wellness center

Client: B. V., a 40-year-old married woman who seeks counseling for weight loss

Patterns/Challenges/Needs:

1. Altered nutrition (more than body requirements) related to improper eating and lack of exercise
2. Altered self-esteem related to obesity
3. Ineffective reversal/prevention of coronary artery disease risk factors (hypertension, hypercholesterolemia, obesity) related to stress and low self-esteem

B. V. came to the wellness center after having a physical examination by her primary care physician and being told for the sixth straight year that she needs to lose weight. Her total cholesterol is 340 milligrams per deciliter, blood pressure is 180/100 mm Hg, height is 5'7", and weight is 220 pounds. She is a nurse and seeks help from a nurse colleague at the wellness center because her elevated cholesterol level has finally motivated her to lose weight. Her husband has been encouraging this for years, but she just cannot seem to make it happen.

During the initial session, the nurse takes a food intake history and does a nutrition assessment (see **Figure 13-2**). Like most self-referrals for weight loss, B. V. is knowledgeable about various diet programs and has tried different plans for several years. She has a pattern of losing and then regaining up to 50 pounds on each attempt. At this point, she is willing to try anything. The nurse discovers during the interview that B. V. has been on numerous antihypertensive drugs for 10 years without attaining consistent control. The assessment shows that, in general, B. V. is physically out of shape and emotionally depressed and discouraged.

After establishing 6-week and 6-month goals, B. V. and the nurse schedule weekly sessions. At the next session, B. V. reviews what she has discovered about her eating patterns and food choices and reflects on changes as compared to the initial nutrition assessment. Rather than be given a standard weekly diet, the nurse as coach encourages B. V. to explore the steps to reach her desired outcome and her challenges to reaching her goals. B. V. discusses her desire to begin to exercise and how her emotions affect her activities and her food choices. The nurse asks her to write down everything she eats, as well as the feeling that she has before, during, and after eating, for the week leading up to her follow-up visit.

In the second session, B. V. and the nurse review her eating/feeling diary and discuss what she has observed and where significant relationships between feelings and eating are observed. During this and subsequent sessions, it is important to explore and acknowledge B. V.'s feelings that are closely tied to her eating behaviors. In addition, the nurse records the physical parameters of weight, and body fat calibration measurements for B. V.

Goals that are too difficult to achieve can discourage the client altogether. Therefore, during each session, B. V. sets several small attainable goals for the following week. Exercise is one of her goals and she chooses to begin with taking the stairs in her apartment building. At the next session, she reports feeling more energy and that she is using the stairs daily. She also reports that she is controlling her portion size, and she notes that her eating patterns are shifting for the first time in years. She states that she is feeling more in control.

B. V. meets with the nurse coach on a regular basis for 6 months. During that time, she joins a gym and works out in a regular aerobic exercise program three to four times a week. She reports an interest in nutrition and has begun reading nutrition books, increasing her knowledge and interest in healthful food consumption. At the end of this period, she has reduced her weight to 160 pounds (approximately 10 lbs monthly). B. V. shares that with a new self-image she has begun to look for a new job that will allow her time to care for herself. At her 6-month medical checkup, her labs are normal and she is taken off of her blood pressure and cholesterol-lowering medications. B. V. and her nurse coach agree to move to monthly visits for the next three sessions and plan for termination of the appointments at that time, with the knowledge that B. V. can return for a "check-in" as needed.

—— INTEGRATIVE HEALTH and WELLNESS ASSESSMENT™ ——

This **INTEGRATIVE HEALTH and WELLNESS ASSESSMENT** is intended for informational purposes only. It is not a substitute for professional medical advice, diagnosis, or treatment.

DIRECTIONS: This questionnaire contains statements about your present way of life, feelings, and personal habits. Please respond to each item as accurately as possible, and try not to skip any item. Indicate the frequency with which you engage in each item by checking (✓) one of the following:

Never   Almost Never   Once in a While   Almost Always   Always

	Never	Almost Never	Once in a While	Almost Always	Always
PHYSICAL					
1. I eat a nutritious breakfast daily.	❏	❏	❏	❏	❏
NUTRITION					
2. I eat at least 5 servings of vegetables & fruits daily.	❏	❏	❏	❏	❏
3. I eat whole foods (grains, beans, seeds, and nuts).	❏	❏	❏	❏	❏
4. I eat low fat foods (fish, low fat dairy, beans, skinless chicken).	❏	❏	❏	❏	❏
5. I avoid red meat or eat it only a few times a week.	❏	❏	❏	❏	❏
6. I decrease high fat foods (hot dogs, steaks, cheese, ice cream, whole milk, cakes, sweets, fried foods, butter).	❏	❏	❏	❏	❏
7. I avoid sugar.	❏	❏	❏	❏	❏
8. I avoid junk food.	❏	❏	❏	❏	❏
9. I avoid regular soda drinks with sugar or diet drinks with artificial sweeteners.	❏	❏	❏	❏	❏
10. I drink 6-8 glasses of water daily.	❏	❏	❏	❏	❏
11. I read labels for ingredients.	❏	❏	❏	❏	❏
12. I avoid food colorings, flavoring, and additives in my foods.	❏	❏	❏	❏	❏
13. I avoid canned and processed foods.	❏	❏	❏	❏	❏
14. I eat organic and/or local produce.	❏	❏	❏	❏	❏
15. I eat my meals at home.	❏	❏	❏	❏	❏
16. I prepare my meals in an oven or on stove top burners.	❏	❏	❏	❏	❏
17. I have access to healthy food choices.	❏	❏	❏	❏	❏
18. I purchase healthy foods.	❏	❏	❏	❏	❏
19. I experience pain or inflammation in my body.	❏	❏	❏	❏	❏

FIGURE 13-2   Nutrition Assessment

NUTRITION (continued)	Never	Almost Never	Once in a While	Almost Always	Always
20. I experience digestive discomfort.	❏	❏	❏	❏	❏
21. I am aware of foods that affect my digestion.	❏	❏	❏	❏	❏
22. I feel bloated after eating.	❏	❏	❏	❏	❏
23. I take medication for digestive reasons.	❏	❏	❏	❏	❏
24. I am aware of any food sensitivities or food allergies.	❏	❏	❏	❏	❏
25. I have a bowel movement daily.	❏	❏	❏	❏	❏
26. I chew my food thoroughly.	❏	❏	❏	❏	❏
27. I eat mindfully (concentrate on my eating, not multitasking or eating in front of the television).	❏	❏	❏	❏	❏
28. I eat late at night.	❏	❏	❏	❏	❏
29. I crave sweets.	❏	❏	❏	❏	❏
30. I eat larger portions than I need.	❏	❏	❏	❏	❏
31. I feel energy after eating.	❏	❏	❏	❏	❏
32. I feel tired after eating.	❏	❏	❏	❏	❏

For items 33–35, check (✓) the response that most closely resembles how you feel about making changes or improvements to your NUTRITION.

33. My readiness for change is

❏ Now   ❏ Within 2 weeks   ❏ Next month   ❏ In 6 months
❏ In a year or more

34. My priority for making change is

❏ Highest priority   ❏ Priority   ❏ Medium priority
❏ Very low priority   ❏ Never a priority

35. My confidence in my ability to make a positive change is

❏ Very confident   ❏ Confident   ❏ Somewhat confident
❏ Not very confident   ❏ Not at all confident

NUTRITION ACTION PLAN. Please list 3 changes that you can implement into your current lifestyle over the next 3 months:

1. _____

2. _____

3. _____

Additional changes, comments, thoughts:

_____

FIGURE 13-2   Nutrition Assessment (continued)

EXERCISE (Know your limitations)	Never	Almost Never	Once in a While	Almost Always	Always
1. I do **aerobic exercise** (jogging, swimming, fitness walking using arms, aerobic dance, active sports) regularly. (*Vigorous intensity*—at least 20 minutes 3 or more days a week; *Moderate intensity*—at least 30 minutes per week)	❑	❑	❑	❑	❑
2. I do **strength exercises** (use strength-training equipment, sit-ups, push-ups) regularly.	❑	❑	❑	❑	❑
3. I do **stretching or flexibility exercises** (head, neck, shoulders, back, legs) for at least 5 minutes 3 days a week.	❑	❑	❑	❑	❑

For items 4-6, check (✓) the response that most closely resembles how you feel about making changes or improvements to your EXERCISE.

4. My readiness for change is
   ❑ Now   ❑ Within 2 weeks   ❑ Next month   ❑ In 6 months
   ❑ In a year or more

5. My priority for making change is
   ❑ Highest priority   ❑ Priority   ❑ Medium priority
   ❑ Very low priority   ❑ Never a priority

6. My confidence in my ability to make a positive change is
   ❑ Very confident   ❑ Confident   ❑ Somewhat confident
   ❑ Not very confident   ❑ Not at all confident

EXERCISE ACTION PLAN. Please list 3 changes that you can implement into your current lifestyle over the next 3 months:

1. _____

2. _____

3. _____

Additional changes, comments, thoughts:
_____

WEIGHT	Never	Almost Never	Once in a While	Almost Always	Always
1. I maintain my ideal weight.	❑	❑	❑	❑	❑
2. I have gained no more than 11 pounds in adulthood.	❑	❑	❑	❑	❑

For item 3-5, check (✓) the response that most closely resembles how you feel about making changes or improvements to your WEIGHT.

3. My readiness for change is
   ❑ Now   ❑ Within 2 weeks   ❑ Next month   ❑ In 6 months   ❑ In a year

FIGURE 13-2   Nutrition Assessment *(continued)*

4. My priority for making change is
   ❑ Highest priority   ❑ Priority   ❑ Medium priority
   ❑ Very low priority   ❑ Never a priority
5. My confidence in my ability to make a positive change is
   ❑ Very confident   ❑ Confident   ❑ Somewhat confident
   ❑ Not very confident   ❑ Not at all confident

WEIGHT MANAGEMENT ACTION PLAN. Please list 3 changes that you can implement into your current lifestyle over the next 3 months:

1. _____

2. _____

3. _____

Additional changes, comments, thoughts:

_____

Source: © 2011. Dossey, B. M., Luck, S., & Schaub, B. G. *Nurse Coaching for Health and Wellness.* (2012). Huntington, NY: International Nurse Coach Association. (www.intergrativenursecoach.com). Adapted from Dossey, B. M., & Keegan, L. (2008). Self-Care Assessments. In Dossey, B. M., and Keegan, L. *Holistic Nursing: A Handbook for Practice* (5th ed.). Sudbury, MA: Jones & Bartlett Learning. The format is designed for survey software of Healthcare Environment (www.hcenvironment.com).

FIGURE 13-2   Nutrition Assessment *(continued)*

Evaluation

In a patient-centered model, the client and the nurse as coach and educator develop a nutrition program based on the client establishing goals and action steps. This process in the nurse coach model establishes SMART goals, integrative goals that are specific, measurable, action based, realistic, have a timeline and that are attainable and sustainable.

A client decides on the next step in moving closer to the desired health goals that he or she has established through using a series of tools, practices, and processes for increasing awareness, implementing change (Exhibit 13-2), and achieving goals. To evaluate the session further, the nurse may again explore with the client the subjective effects of the experience using the evaluation questions in Exhibit 13-3.

Nurses always chart all information they share with the client, as well as an evaluation of the session. When the nurse works in an inpatient facility, other staff need to be informed of the program and its progress. Nurses who work in wellness centers, in centers using integrative models, and

in private practice also keep records for each client and need to include nursing diagnosis, coaching tools employed, educational and counseling interventions, and the effectiveness of each session along with the overall plan, goals, and next steps. Embedded within the holistic nursing and integrative nurse coach process is the implementation of self-care practices including developing nutrition goals and plans for health and wellness.

Directions for FUTURE RESEARCH

1. Investigate the hypothesis that those who eat a nutritionally balanced diet live longer.
2. Continue the investigation on how a healthy diet and lifestyle affect a person's sense of well-being and quality of life.
3. Study the role of the nurse coach in guiding nutritional changes and eating behaviors and the impact on health outcomes.
4. Investigate the role of vitamin and mineral supplementation in disease prevention and health promotion.

5. Analyze the qualities of effective nutrition programs in diverse cultural and ethnic groups in a community setting.

6. Study and analyze health outcomes and cost savings for patients receiving Integrative Nurse Coaching sessions.

Nurse Healer
REFLECTIONS

After reading this chapter, the nurse healer will be able to answer or to begin the process of answering the following questions:

- What sensations accompany physical well-being because of my improved nutrition?
- What composes healthy eating for me and my clients?
- How can I model healthy nutrition practices?
- What are my next steps in coaching myself to create nutritional goals and an action plan?

> **www** *For a full suite of assignments and additional learning activities, use the access code located in the front of your book to visit this exclusive website: http://go.jblearning.com/dossey. If you do not have an access code, you can obtain one at the site.*

NOTES

1. M. Miller, N. J. Stone, C. Ballantyne, et al., "Triglycerides and Cardiovascular Disease: A Scientific Statement from the American Heart Association," American Heart Association Clinical Lipidology, Thrombosis, and Prevention Committee of the Council on Nutrition, Physical Activity, and Metabolism; Council on Arteriosclerosis, Thrombosis, and Vascular Biology; Council on Cardiovascular Nursing; Council on the Kidney in Cardiovascular Disease, *Circulation* 123, no. 20 (2011): 2292–333.

2. R. Solá, M. Fitó, R. Estruch, et al., "Effect of a Traditional Mediterranean Diet on Apolipoproteins B, A-I, and Their Ratio: A Randomized, Controlled Trial," *Atherosclerosis* 218, no. 1 (September 2011): 174–180.

3. A. T. Merchant, H. Vatanparast, S. Barlas, et al., "Carbohydrate Intake and Overweight and Obesity Among Healthy Adults," *Journal of the American Dietetic Association* 109, no. 7 (July 2009): 1165–1172.

4. C. Ogden and M. Carroll, "Prevalence of Obesity Among Children and Adolescents: United States, Trends 1963–1965 Through 2007–2008," *Health E-Stat.* http://www.cdc.gov/nchs/data/hestat/obesity_child_07_08/obesity_child_07_08.pdf.

5. D. L. Jones, R. Adams, et al., "Heart Disease and Stroke Statistics, 2009 Update: A Report from the American Heart Association Statistics Committee," *Circulation: Journal of the AHA* 119 (January 27, 2009): e21–e181.

6. Office of Disease Prevention and Health Promotion, U.S. Department of Health and Human Services, *Healthy People 2010*. http://www.healthypeople.gov/2010.

7. T. Fung, R. Van Dam, S. Hankinson, M. Stampfer, W. Willett, and F. Hu, "Low-Carbohydrate Diets and All-Cause and Cause-Specific Mortality: Two Cohort Studies," *Annals of Internal Medicine* 153, no. 5 (2010): 289–298.

8. J. Levi, S. L. Gray, M. Speck, et al., "Acute Disruption of Leptin Signaling in Vivo Leads to Increased Insulin Levels and Insulin Resistance," *Endocrinology* 152, no. 9 (2011): 3385–3395.

9. O. K. Basoglu, F. Sarac, S. Sarac, and H. Uluer, "Metabolic Syndrome, Insulin Resistance, Fibrinogen, Homocysteine, Leptin, and C-Reactive Protein in Obese Patients with Obstructive Sleep Apnea Syndrome," *Annals of Thoracic Medicine* 6, no. 3 (2011): 120–125.

10. F. Grün and B. Blumberg, "Minireview: The Case for Obesogens," *Molecular Endocrinology* 23, no. 8 (2009): 1127–1134.

11. L. Capuron, C. Poitou, D. Machaux-Tholliez, V. Frochot , J. L. Bouillot, A. Basdevant, S. Layé, and K. Clément, "Weight Loss: Relationship Between Adiposity, Emotional Status and Eating Behaviour in Obese Women: Role of Inflammation," *Endocrinology* 12 (July 2011).

12. M. C. de Oliveira Otto, A. Alonso, D. H. Lee, et al., "Dietary Micronutrient Intakes Are Associated with Markers of Inflammation but Not with Markers of Subclinical Atherosclerosis," *Journal of Nutrition* 141, no. 8 (2011): 1508–1515.

13. J. L. Jones, M. Comperatore, et al., "A Mediterranean-Style, Low-Glycemic-Load Diet Decreases Atherogenic Lipoproteins and Reduces Lipoprotein (a) and Oxidized Low-Density Lipoprotein in Women with Metabolic Syndrome," *Metabolism*, September 22, 2011 [Epub ahead of print]. A. P. Simopoulos, "Evolutionary Aspects of Diet, the Omega-6/Omega-3 Ratio and Genetic Variation: Nutritional Implications for Chronic Diseases," *Biomedicine and Pharmacotherapy* 60, no. 9 (2006): 502–507.

14. National Research Council, *Recommended Daily Allowance*, 10th ed. (Washington, DC: National Academy Press, 1989).

15. M. A. Pereira and V. L. Fulgoni, "Consumption of 100% Fruit Juice and Risk of Obesity and Metabolic Syndrome: Findings from the National Health and Nutrition Examination Survey 1999–2004," *Journal of the American College of Nutrition* 29, no. 6 (2010): 625–629.

16. J. Salas-Salvado, M. Bullo, N. Babio, et al., "Reduction in the Incidence of Type 2 Diabetes with the Mediterranean Diet," *Diabetes Care* 34 (2011): 14–19.

17. J. L. Jones, M. L. Fernandez, M. S. McIntosh, et al., "Mediterranean-Style Low-Glycemic-Load Diet Improves Variables of Metabolic Syndrome in Women, and Addition of a Phytochemical-Rich Medical Food Enhances Benefits on Lipoprotein Metabolism," *Journal of Clinical Lipidology* 5, no. 3 (2011): 188–196.

18. R. Clarke, Y. Smulders, B. Fowler, and C. D. Stehouwer, "Homocysteine, B Vitamins, and the Risk of Cardiovascular Disease," *Seminars in Vascular Medicine* 5, no. 2 (2005): 75–76.

19. C. Galli and P. Risé, "Fish Consumption, Omega 3 Fatty Acids and Cardiovascular Disease: Science and the Clinical Trials," *Nutrition and Health* 20, no. 1 (2009): 11–20.

20. P. J. Boyle and J. Zrebiec, "Management of Diabetes-Related Hypoglycemia," *Southern Medical Journal* 100, no. 2 (2007): 183–194.

21. A. Mente, L. de Koning, H. S. Shannon, and S. S. Anand, "A Systematic Review of the Evidence Supporting a Causal Link Between Dietary Factors and Coronary Heart Disease," *Archives of Internal Medicine* 169, no. 7 (2009): 659–669.

22. M. S. Touillaud et al., "Dietary Lignan Intake and Postmenopausal Breast Cancer Risk by Estrogen and Progesterone Receptor Status," *Journal of the National Cancer Institute* 99, no. 6 (2007): 475–486.

23. Y. Park, A. F. Subar, A. Hollenbeck, and A. Schatzkin, "Dietary Fiber Intake and Mortality in the NIH-AARP Diet and Health Study," *Archives of Internal Medicine* 171, no. 12 (2011): 1061–1068.

24. R. Deminice, G. V. Portari, J. S. Marchini, H. Vannucchi, and A. A. Jordao, "Effects of a Low-Protein Diet on Plasma Amino Acid and Homocysteine Levels and Oxidative Status in Rats," *Annals of Nutrition and Metabolism* 54, no. 3 (2009): 202–207.

25. M. Fotuhi, P. Mohassel, and K. Yaffe, "Fish Consumption, Long-Chain Omega-3 Fatty Acids and Risk of Cognitive Decline or Alzheimer Disease: A Complex Association," *Nature Clinical Practice Neurology* 5, no. 3 (2009): 140–152.

26. P. Barberger-Gateau, C. Samieri, et al., "Dietary Omega 3 Polyunsaturated Fatty Acids and Alzheimer's Disease: Interaction with Apolipoprotein E Genotype," *Current Alzheimer Research* 8, no. 5 (May 23, 2011): 479–491.

27. B. N. Ames, "Optimal Micronutrients Delay Mitochondrial Decay and Age-Associated Diseases," *Mechanisms of Ageing and Development* 131, no. 7–8 (2010): 473–479

28. J. Thompson, "Vitamins, Minerals and Supplements: Overview of Vitamin C (5)," *Community Practice* 80, no. 1 (2007): 35–36.

29. J. Dusting and C. Triggle, "Are We Overoxidized? Oxidative Stress, Cardiovascular Disease, and the Future of Intervention Studies with Antioxidants," *Vascular Health Risk Management* 1, no. 2 (2005): 93–97.

30. P. Chen, J. Stone, G. Sullivan, J. A. Drisko, and Q. Chen, "Anti-Cancer Effect of Pharmacologic Ascorbate and Its Interaction with Supplementary Parenteral Glutathione in Preclinical Cancer Models," *Free Radical Biology and Medicine* 51, no. 3 (2011): 681–687.

31. M. Meydani, S. Das, M. Band, S. Epstein, and S. Roberts, "The Effect of Caloric Restriction and Glycemic Load on Measures of Oxidative Stress and Antioxidants in Humans: Results from the CALERIE Trial of Human Caloric Restriction," *Journal of Nutrition and Healthy Aging* 15, no. 6 (2011): 456–460.

32. C. Martin, E. Butelli, K. Petroni, and C. Toneli, "How Can Research on Plants Contribute to Promoting Human Health?" *Plant Cell* 23, no. 5 (2011): 1685–1699.

33. S. Reuter, S. C. Gupta, B. Park, A. Goel, and B. B. Aggarwal, "Epigenetic Changes Induced by Curcumin and Other Natural Compounds," *Genes and Nutrition* 6, no. 2 (2011): 93–108.

34. A. Malhotra, P. Nair, and D. K. Dhawan, "Curcumin and Resveratrol Synergistically Stimulate p21 and Regulate cox-2 by Maintaining Adequate Zinc Levels During Lung Carcinogenesis," *European Journal of Cancer Prevention* 20, no. 5 ((2011): 411–416.

35. T. C. Wallace, F. Guarner, K. Madsen, M. D. Cabana, G. Gibson, E. Hentges, and M. E. Sanders, "Human Gut Microbiota and Its Relationship to Health and Disease," *Nutrition Review* 69, no. 7 (2011): 392–403. doi:10.111 1/j.1753-4887.2011.00402

36. W. Deechakawan, K. C. Cain, M. E. Jarrett, R. L. Burr, and M. M. Heitkemper, "Effect of Self-Management Intervention on Cortisol and Daily Stress Levels in Irritable Bowel Syndrome," *Biological Research for Nursing* (July 15, 2011). http://www.ncbi.nlm.nih.gov/pubmed/21765120.

37. R. A. Rudel, S. E. Fenton, J. M. Ackerman, S. Y. Euling, and S. L. Makris, "Environmental Exposures and Mammary Gland Development: State of the Science, Public Health Implications, and

Research Recommendations," *Environmental Health Perspectives* 119, no. 8 (2011).

38. S. Guandalini and C. Newland, "Differentiating Food Allergies from Food Intolerances," *Current Gastroenterology Reports* 13, no. 5 (2011): 426–434.

39. Z. Nahleh, "Breast Cancer, Obesity and Hormonal Imbalance: A Worrisome Trend," *Expert Review of Anticancer Therapy* 11, no. 6 (2011): 817–819.

40. F. Labrèche, M. S. Goldberg, M. F. Valois, and L. Nadon, "Postmenopausal Breast Cancer and Occupational Exposures," *Occupational and Environmental Medicine* 67, no. 4 (2010): 263–269.

41. S. L. Teitelbaum et al., "Reported Residential Pesticide Use and Breast Cancer Risk on Long Island, New York," *American Journal of Epidemiology* 165, no. 6 (2007): 643.

42. E. Sonestedt, B. Gullberg, and E. Wirfalt, "Both Food Habit Change in the Past and Obesity Status May Influence the Association Between Dietary Factors and Postmenopausal Breast Cancer," *Public Health and Nutrition* 5 (2007): 1–11.

43. V. Hanf and U. Gonder, "Nutrition and Primary Prevention of Breast Cancer: Foods, Nutrients and Breast Cancer Risk," *European Journal of Obstetrics, Gynecology and Reproductive Biology* 123, no. 2 (2005): 139–149.

44. American Institute for Cancer Research, homepage.

45. H. B. Patisaul and W. Jefferson, "The Pros and Cons of Phytoestrogens," *Frontiers in Neuroendocrinology* 31, no. 4 (2010): 400–419.

46. L. Nonn, D. Duong, and D. M. Peehl, "Chemopreventive Anti-Inflammatory Activities of Curcumin and Other Phytochemicals Mediated by MAP Kinase Phosphatase-5 in Prostate Cells," *Carcinogenesis* 28, no. 6 (2007): 1188–1196.

47. E. Warensjö, L. Byberg, H. Melhus, R. Gedeborg, H. Mallmin, A. Wolk, and K. Michaëlsson, "Dietary Calcium Intake and Risk of Fracture and Osteoporosis: Prospective Longitudinal Cohort Study," *British Medical Journal* 342 (2011): d1473. doi:10.1136/bmj.d1473.

48. R. Scragg, "Vitamin D and Public Health: An Overview of Recent Research on Common Diseases and Mortality in Adulthood," *Public Health Nutrition* 14, no. 9 (2011): 1–18.

49. J. Welsh, "Vitamin D Metabolism in Mammary Gland and Breast Cancer," *American Journal of Clinical Nutrition* 90, no. 4 (2009): 889–907.

50. T. Constans, K. Mondon, C. Annweiler, and C. Hommet, "Vitamin D and Cognition in the Elderly," *Gériatrie et Psychologie Neuropsychiatrie du Vieillissement* 8, no. 4 (2010): 255–262.

51. N. Binkley, "Low Vitamin D Status Despite Abundant Sun Exposure," *Journal of Clinical Endocrinology and Metabolism* 92 (2007): 2130.

52. A. Ascherio, K. L. Munger, and K. C. Simon, "Vitamin D and Multiple Sclerosis," *Lancet Neurology* 9, no. 6 (2010): 599–612.

53. K. Barnard and C. Colón-Emeric, "Extraskeletal Effects of Vitamin D in Older Adults: Cardiovascular Disease, Mortality, Mood, and Cognition," *American Journal of Geriatric Pharmacotherapy* 8, no. 1 (2010): 4–33.

54. C. S. Katsanos, D. L. Chinkes, D. Paddon-Jones, X. Zhang, A. Aarsland, and R. R. Wolfe, "Whey Protein Ingestion in Elderly Results in Greater Muscle Protein Accrual Than Ingestion of Its Constituent Essential Amino Acid Content," *Nutrition Research* 28, no. 10 (2008): 651–658.

55. G. Buhr and C. W. Bales, "Nutritional Supplements for Older Adults: Review and Recommendations—Part I," *Journal of Nutrition for the Elderly* 28, no. 1 (2009): 5–29.

56. M. S. Wellan, "Prevention, Prevention, Prevention: Nutrition for Successful Aging," *Journal of the American Dietetic Association* 107, no. 5 (2007): 741–743.

57. Q. Liu et al., "Prevention and Treatment of Alzheimer's Disease and Aging: Antioxidants," *Mini Reviews in Medicinal Chemistry* 7, no. 2 (2007): 171–180.

58. L. M. Donini et al., "Nutritional Status Determinants and Cognition in the Elderly," *Archives of Gerontology and Geriatrics* 44, suppl. 1 (2007): 143–153.

59. M. S. Morris et al., "Folate and Vitamin B-12 Status in Relation to Anemia, Macrocytosis, and Cognitive Impairment in Older Americans," *American Journal of Clinical Nutrition* 85, no. 1 (2007): 193–200.

60. C. Mason, L. Xiao, I. Imayama, et al., "Effects of Weight Loss on Serum Vitamin D in Postmenopausal Women," *American Journal of Clinical Nutrition* 94, no. 1 (2011): 95–103

61. L. Fontana and S. Klein, "Aging, Adiposity, and Calorie Restriction," *Journal of the American Medical Association* 297, no. 9 (2007): 986–994.

62. M. I. Covas, V. Konstantinidou, and M. Fitó, "Olive Oil and Cardiovascular Health," *Journal of Cardiovascular Pharmacology* 54, no. 6 (2009): 477–482.

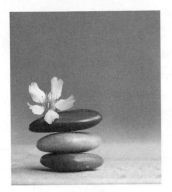

Chapter 14

Exercise and Movement

Francie Halderman and
Christina Jackson

Nurse Healer
OBJECTIVES

Theoretical

- Differentiate among exercise, fitness, and movement.
- Discuss the benefits of exercise and movement both in illness and in health.
- Understand psychological, environmental, and other types of barriers to starting a personal fitness program.
- Define mindful movement practices.
- Identify recommended amounts of exercise for various age groups.
- Review special considerations related to various populations and disease states.
- Discern between a compliance or achievement model of fitness and a holistic model of engagement and adherence based on enjoyable activity.

Clinical

- Assess exercise and movement when working with individuals across the life span.
- Involve clients in self-assessment of their movement and exercise patterns as a routine part of health promotion and as a strategy for management and recovery from illness.
- Seek current clinical research regarding special health concerns and the recommen-

dations for therapeutic exercise and movement, and make the information available to clients.
- Learn about a wide variety of exercise and movement modalities and their efficacies and provide education to clients that will expand their options for activity.
- Collaborate with clients to develop an individualized fitness plan that combines mindful movement and exercise.
- Become aware of community-based health programs that support exercise and movement for various populations and age groups and disseminate this information as appropriate.
- Act as a role model for daily movement and exercise.

Personal

- Assess your activities and patterns related to both exercise and movement.
- Experiment with new modalities of exercise and movement.
- Practice mindful exercise and movement to increase self-awareness.
- Practice centering techniques to become fully present when working with clients.
- Cultivate equanimity and respect for every individual's innate wisdom and timing of their unique process related to physical activity.

DEFINITIONS

Aerobic exercise: Sustained muscle activity within the target heart rate range that challenges the cardiovascular system to meet the muscles' needs for oxygen.

Endurance: The period of time the body can sustain exercise or movement.

Fitness: The ability to carry out daily tasks with vigor and alertness, without undue fatigue, and with ample reserve to enjoy leisure pursuits. It is the ability to respond to physical and emotional stress without an excessive increase in heart rate and blood pressure. Fitness comprises flexibility, endurance, strength, and balance.

Flexibility: The ability to use a joint throughout its full range of motion and to maintain some degree of elasticity of major muscle groups.

Kinesthetic: The felt sense that detects bodily position, weight, or movement of the body.

Maximal heart rate: The rate of the heart when the body is engaged in intense physical activity.

Mindful movement: Movement with intention to notice present moment sensations, thoughts, feelings, and emotions with a nonjudgmental and compassionate attitude. A focus on full, rhythmic breathing is incorporated to enhance mindful awareness.

Moderate-intensity activity: That which induces an intermediate change in breathing and heart rate.

Posture: Pose or placement of parts of the body in spatial relationships.

Resistance training: The use of weights or opposing forces to strengthen muscle groups.

Resting heart rate: The heart's rate when the body is at rest.

Strength: The power of muscle groups.

Target heart rate: The safe rate for the heart during exercise that produces health benefits.

Training: Repetitive bouts of exercise over a period of time with the intention of developing fitness.

Vigorous-intensity activity: That which induces large changes in breathing and heart rate.

■ THEORY AND RESEARCH

Exercise and Movement

Exercise and movement are the physical expression of the whole person. They reflect patterns of energy expenditure that are intertwined with a person's bodymindspirit. Exercise plays an integral role not only in disease prevention but also in health promotion and well-being. Physical activity can release endorphins resulting in a sense of well-being and can elevate mood and promote a positive outlook.[1] The benefits of exercise on well-being have been repeatedly documented for more than two decades. A meta-analysis of 11 studies of exercise for depression concludes that clinicians should integrate exercise as an intervention into their practice because of its high efficacy.[2] Recent research confirms that moderate exercise improves immunity and protects against upper-respiratory illness, the most prevalent infectious disease worldwide. It also lowers the risk of chronic disease by exerting anti-inflammatory influences that prevent diabetes, cardiovascular disease, arthritis, osteoporosis, chronic obstructive pulmonary disease, several types of cancer, and premature mortality.[3] Exercise and movement positively affect both physical and mental health and are effective interventions to promote wellness and prevent illness.

Fitness Paradigms for Exercise and Movement

A new paradigm of fitness is emerging. Its orientation is broader and it focuses more on enjoyment, engagement, and adherence. **Table 14-1** depicts the old and new fitness paradigms.

The primary purpose of exercise is to produce fitness. The following are the four basic components of fitness:

1. Flexibility is the ability to use a joint throughout its full range of motion and to maintain some degree of elasticity of major muscle groups. It is important for the following reasons:
   - It provides increased resistance to muscle and joint injury.
   - It helps prevent mild muscle soreness if flexibility exercises are done before and after vigorous activity.

TABLE 14-1   Fitness Paradigms for Exercise and Movement

Old Fitness Paradigm	New Fitness Paradigm
Compliance Model	Engagement and Adherence Model
Sense of obligation or dread	Enjoyable and fun
Rigorous and punitive	Mindful and reflective
Competitive with comparison to others	Self-aware with goal for personal best
Body focused and achievement oriented	Integration of bodymindspirit
Lacking in focus on breathing	Awareness of using the breath to energize and calm the body-mind throughout movement
Regimented routines with little variety	Encompassing many types of activities including interactive video games, aerobic and nonaerobic, group and individual practices
Compartmentalized time of the day or week dedicated to fitness: "all or nothing" view	Awareness of cumulative effects of activities throughout the week: "some better than none"

2. Muscle strength is the contracting power of a muscle. It is important for the following reasons:
   - Daily activities become less strenuous as muscles become stronger.
   - Strong abdominal and lower back muscles help prevent lower back problems.
   - Appearance improves as muscles become firmer.
3. Cardiorespiratory endurance is the ability of the circulatory and respiratory systems to maintain blood and oxygen delivery to the exercising muscles. It is important for the following reasons:
   - It increases resistance to cardiovascular diseases.
   - It improves the ability to maintain activity levels (endurance).
   - It allows for a high-energy return from daily activities.
4. Postural stability is the body's ability to balance and stay balanced during dynamic action. This ability declines naturally with age. Exercise and movement practices such as yoga, standing Pilates, and tai chi assist with fall prevention through integration of neuromuscular and sensory responses.

Flexibility, strength, endurance, and balance refer not only to the physical body but to the whole person and bodymindspirit. Movement practices from Eastern traditions have embraced this understanding for several thousand years and in this sense the paradigm is not new. However, adaptations of these traditions have developed as the practices came to the West. There are many styles of yoga that range from meditative and restorative to athletic and achievement-oriented practice. Research is currently under way to evaluate the particular benefits of various types of yoga. In general, styles with pacing of movements and postures that are slow, flowing, meditative, and mindful may be more conducive to relaxation and positive parasympathetic response while promoting endurance, balance, strength, and flexibility.[4]

Movement Modalities

Movement practices promote health, wellness, and disease prevention. Modalities from Eastern traditions such as yoga, tai chi, and qi gong have become increasingly available and help cultivate mindfulness in movement. These practices employ rhythmic patterns and sequences of movement and/or holding postures or poses along with mindful breathing. They help enhance present moment awareness of what is happening in one's interior environment of sensations, thoughts, emotions, feelings, and energy flow, as well as awareness in the exterior environment. A greater sense of connection with oneself can be cultivated as well as a sense of being part of a greater unity and flow of life.

A comparison review of 81 scientific and nursing journal articles found that yoga was as effective or better than other forms of exercise in improving various health metrics such as glucose regulation, reduction of depression, pain, and fatigue, improved balance and flexibility, and stress reduction.[4] Movement that involves slow rhythmic patterns, breathwork, and holding postures may regulate the body's hormonal response to stress and improve health outcomes in ways equal to or better than exercise in populations with and without disease.[4] However, aerobic exercise and movement that is more physically active such as dancing are more effective in improving cardiorespiratory fitness. A routine that integrates aerobic exercise, strength training, and mindful movement practices can provide variety and enjoyment that leads to sustained behavior change over time.

Recommendations for Physical Activity

In 2008, the U.S. Department of Health and Human Services (DHHS) released the Physical Activity Guidelines for Americans (PAG) that serve as the first ever national guidelines for exercise and movement.[5] **Table 14-2** illustrates weekly recommendations of aerobic activity and muscle strengthening activity according to age group.

In addition to these guidelines, research supports a new trend in cardiovascular fitness called peak interval training (PIT). PIT has been shown to be a highly effective and efficient means to achieve aerobic fitness. By intermittently taking the body up to peak heart rate and respiratory rate for short bursts of 1–3 minutes, and then allowing an interval of reduced effort, true aerobic metabolism is achieved. Typically, one will go through eight cycles of brief peak effort followed by several minutes of reduced effort. In this way, one can experience a complete and productive aerobic workout in 20 minutes. The cyclic intensity of PIT has been shown to improve aerobic ability and quality of life in people with heart failure after myocardial infarctions.[6] In the absence of contraindications, PIT is a recommended method for all populations to achieve maximum health benefits in a minimal amount of time.

Adherence

Fewer than 20% of adult Americans meet the U.S. Physical Activity Guidelines for both aerobic and muscle-strengthening activities.[7] Individual barriers to physical activity may vary but often include "lack of time." The benefits of exercise

---

TABLE 14-2   National Physical Activity Guidelines (PAG) for Americans

Age	Weekly Aerobic Exercise Recommendations	Weekly Muscle Strengthening Recommendations
Children (aged 6–17 years)	Moderate intensity: 60 minutes 4 days per week AND Vigorous activity: 60 minutes 3 days per week or more	3 days per week of muscle and bone strengthening activity (biking, running, jumping rope)
Adults (aged 18–64 years)	Moderate intensity: 2 hours and 30 minutes a week OR Vigorous intensity: 1 hour and 15 minutes a week	2 or more days per week Include all major muscle groups: legs, hips, back, chest, stomach, shoulders, arms Repeat 8–12 times per session
Older Adults (65 years and older)	Follow adult guidelines: adjust as appropriate to abilities.	Choose activities that maintain or improve balance if they are at risk of falling.

Source: Adapted from U.S. Department of Health and Human Services, Office of Disease Prevention and Health Promotion, *2008 Physical Activity Guidelines for Americans,* ODPHP Publication No. U0036. http://www.health.gov/paguidelines/pdf/paguide.pdf.

are cumulative, and just 10 minutes of sustained vigorous activity can be beneficial and count cumulatively toward the weekly guideline totals.

The nurse can use motivational interviewing techniques to assess the person's phase of readiness and level of intrinsic motivation (see Chapter 10). It is important to understand the common factors that *enhance* adherence for many people, as well as learn the unique motivations of each individual. Multiple studies show that exercise adherence in adults is greatly enhanced by the following: enjoyment derived from using a variety of activities; ability to self-select the level, intensity, and type of exercise; and establishing a regular routine.[8] The holistic nurse can empower the person to explore types and levels of activity that are uniquely appealing to him or her and find creative ways to implement them. This individualized approach will increase likelihood of engagement and adherence over time.

Cultural and Socioeconomic Considerations

A person's cultural background includes his or her beliefs, practices, values, and preferences.

The meaning and purpose of exercise may be culturally and economically influenced. The preference to play a team sport, for example, may come from the desire for community and connection with others and/or may be a result of limited access to health facilities.[9] Conversely, an individual working out in a health club may be purposefully working toward health maintenance and has the financial means to do so. When working with clients, the holistic nurse discusses relevant cultural and economic factors that may affect choice of activities. Where economic disparities exist, the nurse finds creative ways to meet clients' needs. Community centers and churches may offer free programs for those who are motivated to exercise in groups. Public television and basic cable channels frequently offer yoga and cardiovascular workout shows for those who are motivated to exercise individually or who may otherwise need to work out at home. Libraries frequently offer free DVD rentals including those for health and fitness. High-quality exercise and movement classes can be easily found online as well as support groups and blogs that foster community and virtual connections with others. As with any exercise class, online classes (such as YouTube videos) should be evaluated for quality of instruction and safety of movements.

Healthy People 2020 identifies the most common factors that positively and negatively affect adult exercise adherence. (See **Table 14-3**). *Healthy People 2020* has several new objectives that reflect a multidisciplinary approach to

TABLE 14-3   Adherence Factors

Factors That Positively Impact Exercise Adherence in Adults	Factors That Negatively Impact Exercise Adherence in Adults
Education beyond high school	Advancing age
Higher income	Low income
Enjoyment of exercise	Lack of time
Expectation of benefits	Low motivation
Belief in ability to exercise	Rural residency
History of activity in adulthood	Belief that great effort needed to exercise
Social support from peers, family, or spouse	Overweight or obese
Access to acceptable facilities	Perception of poor health
Pleasant scenery in environment	Disability
Safe neighborhood	

Source: Adapted from U.S. Department of Health and Human Services, Office of Disease Prevention and Health Promotion, *2008 Physical Activity Guidelines for Americans,* ODPHP Publication No. U0036. http://www.health.gov/paguidelines/pdf/paguide.pdf.

promote exercise for all. They also address the underlying disparities regarding access to environments that support physical activity including the availability of parks, sidewalks, and the presence of policies in the worksite, schools, and communities that promote fitness.[7]

Nurses can advocate for justice to reduce disparities in access to healthy environments and resources for exercise and movement.

Special Considerations

Aging Populations

According to the 2007 Centers for Disease Control and Prevention's Behavioral Risk Factor Surveillance Survey (BRFSS), less than one-third of older Americans meet the guidelines for physical activity[10] despite the risk reduction that exercise provides for diabetes, falls and fractures, osteoporosis, cardiovascular disease, and some forms of cancer.[8]

According to data from multiple interventional studies, older patients who practiced aerobic exercise also had improved cognitive function.[11] Patients who are told by their doctor to exercise are more likely to start a fitness program. However, there is consistent evidence that health providers *fail to recommend* exercise and movement to older patients on a routine basis.[12]

Studies show that older populations have better exercise adherence when supervised by medical professionals and when the program is tailored to their needs.[8] One randomized controlled study with frail elderly males found that exercise counseling over the phone improved exercise adherence and reduced frailty status. Because the care for frail older adults is triple the cost of caring for nonfrail older adults, telephonic supervision and exercise support could provide cost-effective care and improve functional capacity in this population.[13] Because of the mental, physical, and cognitive benefits of exercise and movement in older populations, every health encounter with older patients should include some discussion on starting, maintaining, and/or evaluating a fitness plan whenever possible.

Cardiovascular Disease

Currently, one in three Americans have some form of cardiovascular disease. Heart disease and stroke are, respectively, the first and third leading causes of death in the United States.[14] Strong evidence exists that regular exercise lowers the risk of coronary heart disease, stroke, and high blood pressure and also offers benefits after an event. A randomized clinical trial of more than 18,800 patients from 41 countries found that people who had an initial cardiac event had a 50% lower risk for recurrence *of all major cardiac events* with adherence to exercise and diet. The risk reduction for death may be even more influenced by exercise, and benefits for all outcomes were seen as early as 6 months.[15] The benefits from lifestyle recommendations for exercise as well as diet and smoking cessation are additive and should begin immediately after the cardiac event. Early behavioral interventions including exercise counseling should be given as high a priority as medications and secondary invasive procedures.

Depression and Anxiety

A systematic review of 17 studies found that yoga is effective in reducing depression and anxiety in populations with and without existing disease. Yoga lowers stimulation of the sympathetic nervous system and promotes stress reduction. It has been widely shown that lower-intensity exercise reduces cortisol levels while sustained high-intensity exercise increases cortisol release as if the body were responding to stress.[4] Multiple randomized controlled studies have repeatedly shown that moderate exercise alone was as effective at reducing major depressive disorder (MMD) as antidepressant medication.[16] A meta-analysis of 11 studies of exercise for depression concludes that clinicians should integrate exercise as an intervention into their practice because of its high efficacy.[2]

Diabetes

People with type 2 diabetes have more health risks than the general population. Exercise improves glycemic control, yet this population remains sedentary despite well-established research that exercise reduces diabetic complications and premature death. Studies show that 69% of people with type 2 diabetes reported doing less than the recommended levels of exercise or no exercise at all.[17] A longitudinal randomized control study of 175 people with type 2 diabetes found that patients moved from preaction stage (without exercise) to maintenance phase of an ongoing exercise program for 6 months by linking exercise with enjoyment and achieving their life goals. Furthermore, as the patients exercised over time their motivation changed from extrinsic to intrinsic, which led to more sustained behavioral change. Intrinsic or self-determined motivation improved not only exercise adherence over time, but also improved *overall* self-management of diabetes.[18] Nurses can engage clients with type 2 diabetes to discuss exercise by identifying their goals and pleasurable activities, encouraging them to stay the course, and informing them that initial adherence can generate even stronger motivation over time.

Eating Disorders

Of all mental disorders, anorexia nervosa has the highest mortality rate.[19] Both anorexia nervosa and bulimia nervosa can commonly involve a type of dysfunctional and excessive exercise called exercise dependence.[20] Vigorous and compulsive exercise is used as a compensatory mechanism to control weight or shape. Missing a workout can cause extreme guilt and anxiety, and excessive exercise can interfere with important life activities. People with bulimia nervosa may have body weights in the normal or overweight range whereas signs of malnutrition may be present with anorexia nervosa. Further inquiry into eating habits, body image, and other physical or emotional symptoms may be warranted for someone who demonstrates exercise dependence. Excessive exercise should *not* be reinforced for people with known eating disorders and follow-up with a mental health specialist is important because of the serious nature of these conditions.

Musculoskeletal Pain

Clients with osteoarthritis and rheumatoid arthritis can benefit from modified aerobic and strengthening exercises.[21] During episodes of joint inflammation, the intensity of activity can be decreased to avoid joint damage and decrease pain. Movement modalities can be particularly helpful for several types of musculoskeletal pain because the slow, rhythmic movement and postures promote balance, strength, and endurance without harsh impact on the joints or muscle fibers. In a randomized controlled trial, tai chi reduced pain and improved function for people older than age 65 years with knee osteoarthritis. Additionally, the experimental group also had improved depression and self-efficacy correlated with the tai chi practice.[22] Another randomized controlled study comparing yoga and exercise for chronic low back pain found that after 7 days of practice in a residential setting, yoga reduced pain, increased functional ability, and improved flexibility more effectively than physical exercise led by a physiatrist in the same setting and time frame.[23]

Osteoporosis

Osteoporosis can lead to fractures of the vertebrae and hips, which can cause loss of function, disability, and death.[24] Exercise is widely acknowledged as an essential preventative strategy to avoid osteoporosis. A meta-analysis of randomized controlled trials found that exercise can significantly increase bone strength in children but not adults.[25] Therefore, exercise in childhood is essential for prevention later in life. However, exercise in older adults can prevent rapid loss of bone and improve muscle strength, flexibility, and mobility, thereby reducing the risk of falls and fractures.[24] Movement modalities are useful interventions in conjunction with exercise for those who have osteoporosis.

Trauma

Avoidance of exercise and movement may be the result of past physical or emotional trauma. As the landmark book *Waking the Tiger: Healing Trauma* describes, the body's immediate response to trauma may include the fight, flight, or freeze response. When unable to fight or run away, a person may freeze or become immobilized as a survival mechanism. If there is no way to release the bound tension in the nervous system after the event is over, the immobility can become chronic. Significant immobility and lack of exercise may be presenting symptoms of the fear response from trauma.[26] Movement and exercise can play an integral role in unwinding the tension held in the nervous system in conjunction with support from a trauma-informed mental health professional.

■ HOLISTIC CARING PROCESS

Holistic Assessment

In preparing to use exercise and movement interventions, the nurse assesses the following parameters:

- The client's motivation, phase of readiness, and ability to make the necessary lifestyle changes in the areas of exercise and movement (see Chapter 10)
- The client's history of exercise and movement, any positive associations and past enjoyment of activities, and any modalities about which the client might be curious
- Perception of barriers to perform exercise and movement
- Cultural, socioeconomic, and environmental factors
- Support systems that may enhance adherence

Identification of Patterns/Challenges/Needs

The following are patterns/challenges/needs (see Chapter 7) compatible with exercise and movement interventions:

- Altered nutrition
- Altered circulation
- Altered oxygenation
- Altered coping
- Altered physical mobility
- Sleep pattern disturbance
- Altered activities of daily living
- Disturbance in body image
- Disturbance in self-esteem
- Potential hopelessness
- Potential powerlessness
- Pain
- Anxiety

Outcome Identification

Figure 14-1 guides the nurse in client outcomes, nursing prescriptions, and evaluation for the use of exercise and movement as nursing interventions.

Therapeutic Care Plan and Interventions

Before the session:

- Create a safe environment in which the client feels comfortable discussing the needs of his or her physical body from a physical movement perspective.
- Clear your mind of other client or personal encounters to be fully present when meeting with the client.
- Bring intention for wholeness and highest good of the person to the session and respect for his or her healing process and choice.

Client Outcomes	Nursing Prescriptions	Evaluation
The client will demonstrate knowledge of healthful exercise and movement programs and resources.	Engage the client to discuss his or her program.	The client participated in the session discussions.
The client will develop a personal plan for fitness.	Assist the client in identifying resources for healthful exercise and movement.	The client demonstrated content knowledge and resource acquisition for using new behaviors in exercise.
The client will engage in exercise and movement practice and meet with the nurse for evaluation of goals.	Assist the client in a personal self-assessment.	The client completed a self-assessment.
	Encourage the client to participate with the nurse to develop goals and action plans.	The client participated with the nurse to develop a personalized program of exercise and movement.
	Prepare the client to start his or her personal fitness plan and establish follow-up meeting.	The client started his or her fitness plan and met with the nurse to discuss outcomes and follow-up.

FIGURE 14-1   Nursing Interventions: Exercise and Movement

At the beginning of the session:
- Take and record any necessary physical assessment data (e.g., height, weight, skin-fold thickness measurements, hip–waist ratio, blood pressure, data on range of motion and mobility limitations).
- Guide the client as he or she discloses past habit patterns that affect exercise behavior.
- Assess the client's phase of readiness and level of motivation.

During the session:
- Ascertain the client's current weekly exercise pattern and practice.
- Be alert to psychological clues that may relate to exercise behavior or extremes (i.e., completely sedentary or excessive exercise dependence).
- Help the client identify any barriers that prevent starting or maintaining a program. Guide his or her exploration of creative solutions and available resources.
- Assist the client to explore multiple types of activities that are enjoyable and cumulative throughout the week.
- Discuss rhythmic breathing and awareness of full breathing during movement to increase attention to mindful movement practice.
- Support the client to develop an individualized exercise and movement program.
- Ensure that the teaching is at the client's cognitive and emotional levels.

At the end of the session:
- Have the client identify the options presented that best fit his or her lifestyle.
- Work with the client to establish written attainable goals and target dates.
- Give the client specific affirmations to use to support these goals.
- Give the client handout material or refer to pertinent resources to reinforce the teaching.
- Use the client outcomes that were established before the session (see Figure 14-1) and the client's subjective experiences (see **Figure 14-2**) to evaluate the session.
- Schedule a follow-up session.

Getting Started

Beginning the fitness regimen in a disciplined manner increases the chances of maintaining the program. Thus, before beginning an exercise program, an individual should be encouraged to follow these basic guidelines:

- Learn about the different types of exercise and movement programs available in the area.
- Consult a physician or exercise authority. If you are older than 35 years, have never seriously exercised, have a disability or chronic illness, or are pregnant, obtain guidance to avoid injuries or complications.
- Warm up and cool down. Stretching exercises are essential before and after each activity or period of exercise.

---

1. How has your fitness program been going in general?
2. Do you have any concerns or questions about the program or your response to it?
3. Has your vitality increased since beginning regular exercise?
4. Does exercise give you a sense of reduced stress in your life?
5. Do you find time during your normal day to integrate mindful movement and breathing techniques?
6. Would you like to learn more ways to incorporate movement into your work environment?
7. What support systems have you discovered that assist you with maintaining and developing your exercise regimen?
8. Is there some other support that you need to assist you in adhering to your new exercise regimen?
9. What is your next step for integrating exercise and therapeutic movement into your daily life?
10. Do you need help in obtaining more resources for this final step?

FIGURE 14-2   Evaluation of the Client's Subjective Experience with Exercise and Movement Interventions

- Wear shoes with proper support for the activity and choose proper ground surfaces for activities.
- Establish an exercise routine.
- Evaluate your program periodically. Determine if you are making progress. If you want to go further, set new goals.
- Create competition for yourself only if it benefits you. If you have allowed too much competition, exercise may become more of a burden than a joy.

Many rewards of exercise and physical activity do begin immediately. Mental and spiritual improvements include beneficial changes in the following areas:

- Mental attitude and outlook on life
- Ability to cope with stress
- Ability to avoid or control mild depression
- Sleep patterns
- Strength and endurance
- Eating habits
- Appearance and vitality
- Posture
- Physical stamina as you age

To reduce risks associated with exercise, clients must know not only how often and how long to exercise but also how vigorously to exercise. Although the target pulse range allows for a heart rate within 60–80% of maximal capacity, the American Heart Association guidelines state that regular exercise of a moderate level, or from 50–75% of maximal capacity, appears to be sufficient. Maintaining the target pulse rate during physical exercise for 15–30 minutes three to five times per week reduces the risk of overexertion, enhances enjoyment, and results in cardiovascular fitness. Each person can discern whether activity is vigorous or moderate based on his or her body's response. If one can talk but not sing while exercising, that person has reached moderate intensity. If one can say only a few words and then needs to catch his or her breath while exercising, that person has reached vigorous intensity.

Because uncontrolled exercising may result in injury, it is wise to follow these guidelines:

- Always warm up for at least 5 to 10 minutes.
- If you are tired, stop.
- If something hurts, stop.
- If you feel dizzy or nauseated, stop.
- Take your pulse at regular intervals.
- Cool down after exercising.

To ease your heart rate into the training range, clients should begin with 10 minutes of low-intensity, warm-up exercise. To cool down, they should do 10 minutes of the same slow activity.

CASE STUDY

Setting: School of nursing

Client: J. C. is a 32-year-old BSN student who is a single mother of an active toddler

Patterns/Challenges/Needs:

1. Altered physical mobility (less than body requirements) related to lifestyle changes
2. Altered nutrition (more than body requirements) related to excessive intake and improper eating patterns
3. Sleep pattern disturbance related to self-care deficit

J. C. is a 32-year-old BSN student who is a single mother of an active toddler. Her general health is sound, but recently she's experiencing high levels of stress related to the demands of nursing school and single parenting. With little time, her nutritional and exercise behaviors have become a lower priority. Her food consumption is mostly of packaged processed food for convenience. She has become sedentary from studying and gained 15 pounds over the past 6 months. After growing concerned about her weight gain, she began to run for several weeks but failed to do proper warm-up stretching or use proper shoe support and developed extremely sore feet and then stopped. Concerned about her health and fitness, she met with the university health services nurse for guidance, relating, "I'm pulled in so many different directions and don't feel like I'm doing anything well." She is interested in becoming more physically active but doesn't believe she can adjust her diet right now. Recently, she began to have trouble falling asleep and states she feels it is related to not having any time to herself. The nurse listened with open presence, and then helped her explore a self-assessment and self-care plan. It was identified that her physical and social aspects are most in need of attention.

The interview revealed that J. C. loved to dance but has not been able to since her daughter was born. Since starting nursing school a year ago, she has lost contact with other friends who are mothers of young children like herself. J. C. states she feels guilty about relying on the television to entertain her daughter and wished she felt more present with her. She describes a decreased ability to focus while studying and a general sense of feeling overwhelmed. At night when trying to sleep she feels a sense of loneliness and disconnection.

The nurse helped J. C. begin to explore ways of adding movement and exercise that would support her bodymindspirit by incorporating activities she loves to meet her unique needs. Together they found a 20-minute mother–child dance cardio DVD that she could play three times per week that would utilize her exercise time as a means to also connect with her daughter. She has been wanting to try yoga and a biweekly class was discovered at a nearby YMCA that also offers affordable child care. They reviewed how to stretch before exercising and how to incorporate warm-up and cool-down periods. The nurse identified the free resource of the university gym at J. C.'s school of nursing and a plan was made for her to attend twice a week (right before her nursing classes) and work out with weights for strength training, as well as park in the farthest parking lot to promote walking and take stairs at all times. She believed other nursing students in her cohort might want to join her for both the yoga class and the weight training and a plan was made to invite them. The nurse suggested that J. C. create a written self-care contract that includes the steps discussed and share with another person to enhance accountability. J. C. wanted to lose 8 pounds in the next 4 weeks, and a follow-up visit was planned for 1 month to review the status of the exercise and movement plan.

J. C. returned to the health services department for her follow-up visit and had a 5-pound weight loss over the past month. She reported that she is feeling "so much more upbeat and clear" since starting a yoga class and playing with her daughter while exercising together with the cardio DVD. She found two nursing cohort friends who have joined her for a community yoga class and strength training at the university gym before classes, and she exchanged a self-care contract with one of them. She is feeling motivated to eat differently and desires to improve her nutritional intake, as well as her daughter's. She describes being better able to concentrate on her studies as well as being more present for her daughter. Her sleep has improved and she reports that the feeling of overwhelm and loneliness has significantly decreased. The stretching has eased the soreness in her feet and she feels motivated to step up her fitness program.

Together they discussed strategies to obtain additional videos for her and her daughter to avoid boredom and ways to include outdoor activity such as bicycling instead of just going for walks to maximize aerobic conditioning. J. C. established a new goal to lose the remaining 10 pounds and the nurse provided J. C. with a link to a free Internet video that reviews peak interval training. The nurse will also begin focused nutritional counseling with J. C. (see Chapter 13).

Evaluation

The nurse determines with the client whether the client outcomes for exercise and movement (Figure 14-1) were successfully achieved. To evaluate the session further, the nurse may again explore the subjective effects of the experience with the client using the evaluation questions in Figure 14-2.

Nurses should chart the information they impart to the client as well as the evaluation of the session. When the nurse works in an inpatient facility, other staff must be apprised of the program and the client's progress. Nurses who work in wellness centers, independent practices, or other areas in which counseling sessions are the primary care modality should keep records for each client that state the nursing diagnosis, type of counseling employed, and effectiveness of each session. Whenever possible, every healthcare encounter with all populations should include discussions and documentation about exercise and movement for health promotion and disease prevention.

Directions for
FUTURE RESEARCH

1. Further investigate the benefit of various types of movement modalities for specific disease states.
2. Continue investigating ways in which the lifestyle behaviors of exercise and movement affect a person's well-being and optimal health as well as act as an intervention for disease.
3. Study the specific factors that are important in tailoring exercise programs to ethnic and cultural groups as well as aging populations.
4. Identify the most effective means to shift nursing practice so that all populations receive teaching on exercise and movement at every possible healthcare encounter.

Nurse Healer
REFLECTIONS

After reading this chapter, the nurse healer will be able to answer or to begin the process of answering the following questions:

- How would I describe the meaning and practice of exercise and movement in my life today?
- Do I meet or exceed the recommended weekly Physical Activity Guidelines?
- Are there any barriers that interfere with my own practice of exercise and movement?
- What exercise and movement changes can I incorporate that will improve my fitness and bring pleasure and enjoyment into my life?
- How does fitness affect my experience of bodymindspirit, sense of self, and others?
- Do I view myself and others as whole, with an innate ability to heal, throughout all the stages of readiness regarding exercise?
- How can I best learn, practice, and model healthy exercise and movement?

 For a full suite of assignments and additional learning activities, use the access code located in the front of your book to visit this exclusive website: http://go.jblearning.com/dossey. If you do not have an access code, you can obtain one at the site.

NOTES

1. R. K. Dishman and P. J. O'Connor, "Lessons in Exercise Neurobiology: The Case of Endorphins," *Mental Health and Physical Activity* 2, no. 1 (2009): 4–9.
2. G. Stathopoulou et al., "Exercise Interventions for Mental Health: A Quantitative and Qualitative Review," *Clinical Psychology: Science and Practice* 13, no. 2 (2006): 179–193.
3. D. Nieman, "Moderate Exercise Improves Immunity and Decreases Illness Rates," *American Journal of Lifestyle Medicine* (2007): 1–8. http://ajl.sagepub.com/content/early/2011/04/26/1559827610392876.
4. A. Ross and S. Thomas, "The Health Benefits of Yoga and Exercise: A Review of Comparison Studies," *Journal of Alternative and Complementary Medicine* 16, no. 1 (2010): 3–12.
5. U.S. Department of Health and Human Services, Office of Disease Prevention and Health Promotion, *2008 Physical Activity Guidelines for Americans,* ODPHP Publication No. U0036. http://www.health.gov/paguidelines/pdf/paguide.pdf.
6. U. Wisloff et al., "Superior Cardiovascular Effect of Aerobic Interval Training Versus Moderate Continuous Training in Heart Failure Patients," *Circulation* 115 (2007): 3086–3094.
7. U.S. Department of Health and Human Services, "*Healthy People 2020*: Physical Activity: Overview," *HealthyPeople.gov*. http://healthypeople.gov/2020/topicsobjectives2020/overview.aspx?topicid=33.
8. J. S. Larson and M. Winn, "Health Policy and Exercise: A Brief BRFSS Study and Recommendations," *Health Promotion Practice* 11, no. 2 (2010): 268–274.
9. J. M. Saint Onge and P. M. Krueger, "Education and Racial-Ethnic Differences in Types of Exercise in the United States," *Journal of Health and Social Behavior* 52, no. 2 (2011): 197–211. http://hsb.sagepub.com/content/52/2/197.abstract.

10. B. Resnick et al., "The Exercise Assessment and Screening for You (EASY) Tool: Application in the Oldest Population," *American Journal of Lifestyle Medicine* 2, no. 5 (2008): 432–440.

11. R. F. Zoeller, Jr., "Exercise and Cognitive Function: Can Working Out Train the Brain Too?" *American Journal of Lifestyle Medicine* 4, no. 5 (September/October 2010): 397–409.

12. J. A. Dauenhauer, C. A. Podgorski, and J. Karuza, "Prescribing Exercise for Older Adults: A Needs Assessment Comparing Primary Care Physicians, Nurse Practitioners, and Physician Assistants," *Gerontology and Geriatrics Education* 26 (2006): 81–99.

13. M. J. Peterson et al., "Effect of Telephone Exercise Counseling on Frailty in Older Veterans: Project LIFE," *American Journal of Men's Health* 1, no. 4 (December 2007): 326–334.

14. U.S. Department of Health and Human Services, "*Healthy People 2020*: Heart Disease and Stroke," *HealthyPeople.gov*. http://healthypeople.gov/2020/topicsobjectives2020/overview.aspx?topicid=21.

15. C. K. Chow et al., "Association of Diet, Exercise, and Smoking Modification of Early Cardiovascular Events After Acute Coronary Syndromes," *Circulation* 121 (2010): 750–758.

16. J. Blumenthal et al., "Exercise and Pharmacotherapy in the Treatment of Major Depressive Disorder," *Psychosomatic Medicine* 69 (2007): 587–596.

17. American Association of Diabetes Educators Position Statement, "Diabetes and Exercise," *Diabetes Educator* 34, no. 1 (January/February 2008): 37–40.

18. M. S. Fortier et al., "Self-Determination and Exercise Stages of Change: Results from the Diabetes Aerobic and Resistance Exercise Trial," *Journal of Health Psychology* (2011): 1–13. doi:10.1177/1359105311408948

19. C. A. Miller and H. H. Golden, "An Introduction to Eating Disorders: Clinical Presentation, Epidemiology, and Prognosis," *Nutrition in Clinical Practice* 25, no. 2 (April 2010): 110–115.

20. B. J. Cook and H. A. Hausenblas, "The Role of Exercise Dependence for the Relationship Between Exercise Behavior and Eating Pathology: Mediator or Moderator?" *Journal of Health Psychology* 13, no. 4 (2008): 495–502.

21. W. G. Herbert, R. Humphrey, and J. N. Myers, eds., *ACSM's Resources for Clinical Exercise Physiology: Musculoskeletal, Neuromuscular, Neoplastic, Immunologic, and Hematologic Conditions,* 2nd ed. (Baltimore, MD: Lippincott Williams & Wilkins, 2010).

22. C. Wang et al., "Tai Chi Is Effective in Treating Knee Osteoarthritis: A Randomized Controlled Trial," *Arthritis Care & Research* 61, no. 11 (November 2009): 1545–1553.

23. P. Tekur, C. Singphow, H. R. Nagendra, and N. Raghuram, "Effect of a Short-Term Intensive Yoga Program on Pain, Functional Disability and Spinal Flexibility in Chronic Low Back Pain: A Randomized Control Study," *Journal of Alternative and Complementary Medicine* 14, no. 6 (2008): 637–644.

24. S. Tuzun, I. Aktas, U. Akarirmak, S. Sipahi, and F. Tuzun, "Yoga Might Be an Alternative Training for the Quality of Life and Balance in Postmenopausal Osteoporosis," *European Journal of Physical and Rehabilitation Medicine* 46, no. 1 (2010): 69–72.

25. R. Nikander et al., "Targeted Exercise Against Osteoporosis: A Systemic Review and Meta-Analysis for Optimising Bone Strength Throughout Life," *BMC Medicine* 8, no. 47 (2010). http://www.biomedcentral.com/1741-7015/8/47.

26. P. A. Levine, *Waking the Tiger* (Berkeley, CA: North Atlantic Books, 1997).

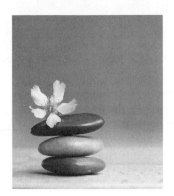

Chapter 15

Humor, Laughter, and Play

Patty Wooten

Nurse Healer

OBJECTIVES

Theoretical

- Define humor, laughter, and play, and explain how they interrelate.
- Describe the psychosocial and physiologic benefits of laughter and play.
- Explain how humor, laughter, and play can aid in stress reduction.

Clinical

- Organize and integrate playful activities into your clinical practice.
- Document the psychophysiologic changes that occur in clients as they allow themselves to laugh and engage in playful activities.
- Develop a collection of humorous books, cartoons, games, and comedy DVDs, videos, and audiocassettes that are appropriate for use in your area of nursing practice.

Personal

- Describe strategies for integrating a humorous perspective and playful activities into each day.
- Clarify and expand awareness of your personal humor preferences and favorite playful activities.
- Develop a heightened awareness of opportunities to insert humor and encourage playfulness.

DEFINITIONS

Humor: A quality of perception and attitude toward life that enables an individual to experience joy even when facing adversity; a perception of the absurdity or incongruity of a situation.

Laughter: A physical behavior that occurs in response to something that is perceived as humorous, amusing, or surprising. This behavior engages most of the muscle groups and organ systems in the body. Laughter is often preceded by physical, emotional, or cognitive tension.

Play: A spontaneous or recreational activity that is performed for sheer enjoyment rather than to reach a goal or produce a product. Playfulness is a mood or attitude that infuses the individual with a sense of joy and positive emotions.

■ THEORY AND RESEARCH

Humor is a complex phenomenon that is an essential part of human nature. Anthropologists have never found a culture or society at any time in history that was completely devoid of humor. A sense of humor is both a perspective on life—a way of perceiving the world—and a behavior that expresses that perspective. As Moshe Waldoks declared, "A sense of humor can help you overlook the unattractive, tolerate the unpleasant, cope with the unexpected, and smile through the unbearable."[1]

Humor is a word of many meanings. It is derived from the Latin word *umor*, meaning liquid or fluid. In the Middle Ages, humor referred to an energy that was thought to interact with a body fluid and an emotional state. This energy was believed to influence health and disposition (e.g., "he's in a bad humor"). A sanguine humor was cheerful and associated with blood. A choleric humor was angry and associated with bile. A phlegmatic humor was apathetic and allied with mucus. A melancholic humor was depressed and related to black bile. This belief system was an early recognition of the energy links between the mind and the body.

One of the earliest and most extensive reviews of humor and its use by health professionals was compiled in the early 1970s by nurse–educator Vera Robinson as part of her doctoral thesis.[2] First published in 1977, her work was updated and released again in 1991. Today, more than 30 years later, it continues to be one of the most comprehensive studies of humor and its importance in nursing practice. Her review of the theories of humor is both comprehensive and concise. Her findings are summarized here.

Humor from Different Perspectives

The humanities and the literature of the world, from the time of the ancient Greeks to the present, have been concerned with the nature of comedy and laughter. Comedy reveals people's imperfections, gives them courage to face life, and leaves them more tolerant. Tragedy is idealistic and expresses "the pity of it," while comedy tends to be more skeptical and expresses "the absurdity of it."[3]

Early philosophers were concerned with the nature of humor in relation to the issues of good and evil and the nature of humans. Both Plato and Aristotle felt that laughter arose from enjoyment of the misfortunes of others and that comedy was an imitation of people at their worst. Other philosophers viewed laughter as a valuable asset in correcting the minor follies of society.

According to the psychoanalytic view of humor set forth by Sigmund Freud, civilization has led to repression of many basic impulses, and joking is a socially acceptable way of satisfying these repressed needs. Freud described four major types of jokes: the sexual joke, the aggressive and hostile joke, the blasphemous joke, and the skeptical joke. This joking activity serves to preserve psychic energy. Freud differentiated between wit, the comic effect, and humor. The pleasure of wit comes from an economy of inhibition; the pleasure of the comic, from an economy of thought; and the pleasure of humor, from an economy of feelings.[4]

Psychologists go beyond Freud's interpretation to assert that humor is not simply determined by the present stimulus situation but also depends on recollections of the past and anticipation of the future. A collective process is important in generating the pleasure of humor. Humor is cognitively based and involves information-processing and problem-solving abilities. Psychologist Harvey Mindess proposed the liberation theory of humor. He views humor and laughter as the agents of psychological liberation. They free us from the constraints and restrictive forces of daily living and, in doing so, make us joyful.[5]

Anthropologists have described the use of humor within various cultures or ethnic groups. They have identified a joking relationship that is a kind of "permitted disrespect," in which one person is required to tease or make fun of another, who is in turn required to take no offense. This kind of social relationship is widespread in different societies and provides a basis for comparative studies of social structures.[6] One of the first cross-cultural studies of humor found that humor is the result of cultural perceptions, both individual and collective; it is a cognitive experience that must have a cultural niche and cannot occur in a vacuum.[7] Humor is universal, but the culture, society, or ethnic group in which it occurs influences the style and content of humor and the situations in which humor is used and is considered appropriate.

Many sociological studies have explored exactly how humor is used within society. Humor is a social relationship and occurs in a social environment. Research has shown that it promotes group cohesion, initiates relationships, relieves tension during social conflict, and can be a means of expressing approval or disapproval of social action. Joking relationships within organizations serve to minimize stress and release antagonism.[8–10]

The three major theories of humor are (1) the superiority theory, (2) the incongruity theory, and (3) the release theory. The superiority theory asserts that people laugh at the inferiority, stupidity, or misfortunes of others so that they may feel superior to them. This type of laughter can be cruel and scornful or can reflect warmth and empathy. For example, people watch the foolish actions of beloved comics such as Lucille Ball or Charlie Chaplin and feel smart and dignified compared to them. Essentially, people are laughing at themselves, at their own imperfections. For the moment, they feel superior. What they are laughing at did not happen to them, but it could have. This type of comedy demonstrates that "man is durable, even though he may be weak, stupid, and undignified."[11] In the superiority theory, humor can be viewed as a continuum: from laughing at no one (nonsense jokes), to laughing at a specific person or group (jokes about morons or ethnic groups), to laughing with others in general at people's foibles (Charlie Chaplin's humor), to laughing at oneself, the most therapeutic of all.

The incongruity theory of humor holds that a sudden shock or unexpectedness, an incongruity, ambivalence, or conflict of ideas or emotions, is necessary to produce the absurdity provoking a burst of laughter.

The relief or release theory of humor proposes that humor and laughter provide a release of tension. The relief can be cognitive—an escape from reality, from seriousness, from reason. The relief can be an emotional release of anxiety, fear, anger, or embarrassment from social conflict. It also can be a release of nervous energy and physical tension.

Many of these theories and perspectives on humor obviously overlap. Some describe the nature of humor, while others describe the function of humor. However, this diversity of perspectives shows that humor, laughter, and play are very complex phenomena that serve people in many ways. The possibilities for the study of humor are endless. The importance and influence of humor have been examined from the perspectives of anthropology, psychology, literature, sociology, linguistics, religion, and so on. More information about the influence of humor in people's lives can be obtained from the International Society for Humor Studies.

A discussion of the therapeutic value of humor and its beneficial influence on the body, mind, and spirit follows.

Therapeutic Humor

Modern dictionaries define humor as the quality of being laughable or comical, or as a state of mind, mood, and spirit. Our sense of humor gives us the ability to find delight and experience joy even when facing adversity. Humor, then, is a flowing energy, involving and connecting the body, mind, and spirit.

Humor can take many forms: jokes, cartoons, amusing stories, outrageous sight gags, funny songs, whimsical signs, bloopers, "daffynitions," and physical slapstick antics. These humorous techniques stimulate the auditory, visual, or kinesthetic senses.

Therapeutic humor can be divided into three basic categories: hoping humor, coping humor, and gallows humor. Hoping humor gives the individual the courage to face challenges. Coping humor offers a release for physical and emotional tension. Gallows humor provides protection from the emotional impact of witnessing tragedy, death, and disfigurement. Sharing humor and laughter with clients and colleagues can have profound healing potential. Finding a humorous perspective on one's problems, or experiencing the relaxing effects of laughter, can be an effective stress management technique that helps one stay healthy.

The term *to heal* comes from the Anglo-Saxon word *haelen*, which means to bring together and make whole. Bringing together the body, mind, and spirit can be healing. Humor, laughter, and the resulting emotion, mirth, unite the body, mind, and spirit. Humor is a cognitive activity engaging the mind. Laughter is a physical activity involving the body. Mirth is an emotional state that lifts the spirit.[12]

Hoping Humor: The Courage to Face Challenges

The ability to hope for something better enables human beings to cope with difficult situations. Hoping humor laughs in spite of the overwhelming circumstances.[13] It reflects an acceptance of life with all its dichotomies, contradictions, and incongruities. This type of humor is usually warm and gentle and accepts the reality of the situation. Consider the following example of hoping humor.

Janet Henry had breast cancer. After her mastectomy, she received chemotherapy. First she lost her breast, and then she lost her hair, but Janet never lost her sense of humor. She wrote a little poem to describe her ritual as she prepared for bed each night.

The Nightly Ritual

> I prop my wig up on the dresser
> And tuck my prosthesis beneath
> And I thank God
> I still go to bed
> With my man and my very own teeth.

With whimsy and gratitude, Janet remembered the blessings in her life despite her losses.[14]

Hoping humor can also be used to sustain the spirit during the shock and trauma of natural disasters. People create humor to literally laugh in the face of their loss. Both disaster victims and those who offer professional assistance use humor to provide hope and courage as they deal with the overwhelming task of recovery. As Charlie Chaplin once noted, "To truly laugh, you must be able to take your pain and play with it."[15-17]

Sandy Ritz, a nurse from Hawaii, completed her doctoral thesis in public health on the topic of humor and disaster recovery.[18] Her research showed how humor changed as the stages of recovery progressed. After the devastating floods in the Midwest during 1997, a large billboard announced: "Concerned about the weather? Call 1-800-NOAH." After a tornado destroyed a house in Texas, the family moved across town to live with relatives. They placed a sign on their front lawn: "Gone with the wind." After an earthquake in Los Angeles, one house that had completely collapsed had this sign in front: "House for Rent. Some assembly required."

Nurses and other professional caregivers use hoping humor to acknowledge their own reality and to laugh in spite of the pressure and demands. For example:

How You Know It's Going to Be a Long Shift

1. You step off the elevator and emergency room gurneys are lined up in the hall.
2. The crash cart is not in its usual location.
3. There are too many people in the nursing station.
4. There is nobody in the nursing station.
5. Housekeeping is scrubbing a large area of the floor.
6. You get two admissions during report.[19]

Coping Humor: A Release for Tension

Illness and trauma cause stress and suffering. They disrupt our ability to function smoothly and present many challenges. Coping describes what people do to minimize this disruption and attempt to regain some control. To cope effectively, people must change how they think and how they behave. Humor often is used as a coping tool to change perspective, release tension, and regain a sense of control. As Freud noted, "Humor has a liberating element, it is the triumph of narcissism. It is the ego's victorious assertion of its invulnerability. It refuses to suffer the slings and arrows of reality."[4] Clients use coping humor to laugh about uncomfortable and embarrassing moments. Although they may not always be able to control their external reality, they can use humor to control how they perceive their situation and use their ability to laugh about it to provide some sense of empowerment,[20-22] as shown by the following example.

> The nurse was caring for Barbara during her weeklong hospitalization for chemotherapy. The drugs were powerful, with many uncomfortable side effects. Fortunately, the nurse had been successful in managing Barbara's nausea with antiemetic medications. However, when the nurse entered the patient's room on Thursday, she found her bending over the toilet bowl vomiting profusely. The nurse was surprised and, without thinking, blurted out, "What are you doing?" Barbara wiped her chin, looked up at the nurse, and said, "Well, I had a tuna sandwich for lunch and I began feeling sorry for the tuna, so I thought I'd return it to its natural habitat."

Barbara used humor to redefine her uncomfortable situation, took control of her perceptual process, and changed her attitude about the event.[23]

Coping humor often expresses anxiety or frustration about things that are out of one's control. Consider the following:

Handy Exercises You Can Do to Prepare for Hospitalization

1. Lie naked on the front lawn, covered with a napkin, and ask people to poke you as they go by.
2. Practice inserting your hand in a running garbage disposal and smile, saying, "Mild discomfort."
3. Set your alarm to go off every 10 minutes between 11 p.m. and 7 a.m., at which times you will awaken and stab yourself with a screwdriver.
4. Learn to urinate into an empty lipstick tube.[24]

Caregivers also create humor to help release feelings of hostility or frustration created by patients or other professionals.[25] Sometimes nurses enjoy making jokes about physicians. For example:

What do you call two orthopedic surgeons reading an electrocardiogram?

A double-blind study.

Why is a neurosurgeon just like a sperm?

One in 200,000 becomes a human.

What does it mean when a physician writes WNL on the History and Physical?

We Never Looked.

Sometimes, caring for patients who are noncompliant, combative, demanding, or ungrateful can be frustrating. These patients are sometimes referred to as gomers, an acronym created by Samuel Shem, a physician writing about his internship experience. GOMER stands for Get Out of My Emergency Room. Over the years, several versions and additions to the gomer criteria list have evolved.

You know your patient is a gomer if:

1. His old chart weighs more than 5 pounds.
2. His previous address was the VA hospital.
3. He keeps tying his pajama strings in with the Foley catheter.
4. He can have a seizure and never drop his cigarette.

5. He asks for a cigarette in the middle of his pulmonary function test.
6. His blood urea nitrogen level is higher than his IQ.

Coping humor is a socially acceptable form of expressing hostility, but it should be used with caution. It can be viewed as disrespectful and hurtful if overheard by someone who either identifies with the person being laughed at or feels that this type of humor is offensive and inappropriate for health professionals. Sharing any form of humor is always a risky venture because people vary greatly in what they find funny and which topics they consider too serious to laugh about. What is funny to one person may be viewed as offensive by another.[26-27] **Exhibit 15-1** shows guidelines for appropriate use of humor.

Gallows Humor: Protection from Pain

Gallows humor often is used by professionals who work in situations that are horrifying or tragic. Every day these people cope with the reality and horror of illness, suffering, and death. In this group are doctors, nurses, police officers, newspaper journalists, social workers, hospice workers, and many others. These professionals, because of their caring and compassion, are more likely to feel the impact of the suffering they witness. Caregivers often use humor as a means of maintaining some distance from the suffering to protect themselves from empathic pain.[28-29] Gallows humor acknowledges the disgusting or intolerable aspects of a situation and then attempts to transform it into something lighthearted and amusing. People's ability to laugh in this type of situation provides them with a momentary release from the intensity of what might otherwise be overwhelming. They are able to maintain their balance and professional composure so that they may continue to offer their therapeutic skills.

Consider the following example: One night, in the emergency room at a county hospital, an ambulance brought in a homeless person who had been found unconscious in an alley. The man was filthy, his breath reeked of alcohol, and he had lice crawling on his body. It took two nurses more than an hour just to clean the man up enough for admission. It was difficult work, and the nurses' senses were overwhelmed with

EXHIBIT 15-1   Concerns and Cautions About Using Humor in Healthcare Settings

Concerns

- Will clients or colleagues consider the use of humor unprofessional?

  Offer a brief explanation of the health benefits of humor to counter this. You can maintain your professionalism and still adopt a lighter style of interaction with patients and staff.

- Will I be seen as incompetent?

  Establish your competence first (especially among other staff), and then let your sense of humor emerge. Clients usually welcome a lighter style of interaction.

- Will clients misinterpret humor as indifference about their condition?

  Shared humor does not replace concern, care, and respect. It makes those qualities more personal and believable.

- What should I do if I really don't think the client's humor is funny?

  Don't laugh, but smile and acknowledge the joke.

- What should I do if the client's humor is offensive?

  Be honest and tell the client that you really don't enjoy that kind of humor. Be flexible, open, and supportive of the client's humor generally. There are limits to joking as with any other behavior.

Cautions

- Be sensitive to whether the client is responding positively or negatively to humor. Don't force your humor on the client if the client is not receptive. Think of humor as a medication. You must administer the right medicine, in the right dosage, at the right time for a therapeutic benefit to occur. Two clients with the same symptoms do not always get the same medication. Some clients have allergic reactions. Be sensitive to the client's humor allergies.

- Remember that clients may not respond to humor until they have come to accept the reality of their disease. Do not try to use humor to subdue their depression or anger. The time may come, however, when humor can help them turn the corner of acceptance.

- Remember that sometimes clients don't feel like laughing. They may be nauseated, in pain, or just not in the mood.

- Remember that many clients have no history of using humor under stress. It may be unrealistic to expect them to react favorably to humor when their health is threatened. People generally use the same coping mechanisms in the hospital that they have used in other stressful situations. This may include becoming angry, depressed, withdrawn, anxious, assertive, or demanding. Each of these coping styles is compatible with humor once you know the client well. Always be sensitive to how the client is responding to your playful style.

- Remember that some clients may have religious convictions that emphasize reverence for the seriously ill. This may be incompatible with any form of humor or light-hearted interaction.

- Humor is inappropriate under the following conditions:

  - The patient needs time to cry.
  - The patient needs quiet time to rest, contemplate, or pray.
  - The patient is trying to come to grips with any emotional crisis.
  - The patient is trying to communicate something important to you.
  - The person in the adjacent bed is very sick or dying.

- Avoid humor that has the following characteristics:

  - Ethnic, sarcastic, mocking
  - At the expense of another person (laugh with, not at)
  - Joking about any client or that client's condition

unpleasant sights and smells. One of the nurses read the intern's admission note on the way up in the elevator. It said, "Patient carried into emergency room by army of body lice, who were chanting, 'Save our host. Save our host.'" The nurse laughed heartily at this amusing picture. Suddenly the struggles of the last hours were put into a humorous perspective, and she felt a lot less anger and a lot more compassion.

One study of the use of humor among hospital staff in emergency rooms and critical care units described how gallows humor was used as a coping tool:

> There is a goodness of fit between how the provision of care induces stress in the emergency care environment and how the use of humor intervenes in that process. Emergency personnel experience a wide spectrum of serious events—trauma, life-threatening illness, chaotic emotional situations—often all at the same time. There is no time to emotionally prepare for these events, and little time to ventilate afterwards or "decompress." The spontaneous way in which humor can be produced in almost any situation, and its instantaneous stress-reducing effects, are well suited to the emergency care experience.[30]

It is important to note that gallows humor, so therapeutic for staff, may not be appreciated by clients or their families. One group of nurses hung the following sign in the visitor waiting room to reassure visitors that the staff's use of humor actually helped them provide better care for their loved ones:

> *You may occasionally see us laughing,*
> *Or even take note of some jest.*
> *Know that we are giving your loved one*
> *Our care at its very best.*
> *There are times when the tension is highest.*
> *There are times when our systems are stressed.*
> *We've discovered humor a factor*
> *In keeping our sanity blessed.*
> *So, if you're a patient in waiting,*
> *Or a relative, or a friend of one seeing,*
> *Don't hold our smiling against us,*
> *It's the way we keep from screaming.*[31]

Cathartic Laughter

Laughter is a smile that engages the entire body. At first, the corners of the mouth turn up slightly. Then, the muscles around the eyes engage and a twinkling can be seen in the eyes. Next the person begins to make noises, ranging from controlled snickers, escaped chortles, and spontaneous giggles to ridiculous cackles, noisy hoots, and uproarious guffaws. The chest and abdominal muscles become activated. As the noises get louder, the person begins to bend the body back and forth, sometimes slapping the knees, stomping the feet on the floor, or elbowing another person nearby. As laughter reaches its peak, tears flow freely. All of this continues until the person feels so weak and exhausted that he or she must sit down or fall down. Very strange behavior!

Of course, not everyone experiences such intense laughter every time they are amused. For example, people may struggle to contain themselves if they are concerned about how others might judge this behavior; if they are concerned with maintaining a dignified image; if they feel others might be offended by their robust laughter; or if the culture places strong taboos on such behavior.

Sounds of Laughter

If we listen to the sound of someone laughing, we hear that the laughter has different tones and rhythms, almost as if the laughter were coming from different parts of the body. These sounds can give us a clue as to why the person is laughing. A "tee hee" laugh is often a high-pitched titter that seems to come from the top of the head. This laugh arises when a person is very nervous and tries to disguise his or her anxiety with laughter. Like the valve atop a pressure cooker, this laughter acts as a safety valve and allows the person to release a little steam before he or she explodes from built-up pressure. A "heh heh" laugh is a shallow, almost hollow sound that comes from the throat area. This laugh occurs when a person feels socially obligated to laugh at a joke that is not really considered funny. A "ha ha" laugh emanates from the heart space with a warm resonance and palpable sincerity. This laugh occurs when someone is truly amused or delighted by the humorous stimuli. It is also the kind of laugh that occurs during deep insight or peaceful, joy-filled moments, such as during meditation. A "ho ho" laugh is the deep belly laugh, the kind in which a person really begins to let go of control and surrender to the experience of deep joy and amusement. The whole body is engaged in movement, which usually continues until exhaustion. The person must put down whatever is being held and must sit down to avoid falling down. Sometimes the laughter is so deep and so prolonged that the person is left gasping for air and exhausted from the activity. After the laughter, as the person becomes quiet, a warm glow fills his or her body. The person feels lighter, almost buoyant, and his or her mind is clear of worry, fear, and anger. His or her body feels energized yet relaxed. Usually, the person is no longer aware of any pain that was previously felt. If this laughter was shared with others, the person feels a sense of connection and trust. During these moments one's problems do not feel oppressive; one feels safe and at peace with the world. The body is listening to this emotional weather report and making subtle, or sometimes profound, changes at a molecular level. These changes have a powerful impact on the immune system and can enhance the ability to heal. As Barry Sultanoff, a holistic physician, explained:

> Laughing together can be a time of intimacy and communion, a time when we come forward, fully present and touch into each other's humanness and vulnerability. By joining in humor and acknowledging our oneness, we can have a profound experience of unity and cooperation. That in itself may be one of the most profound expressions of healing energy of which we are capable.[32]

What is this healing energy? Where does it come from? What does it do? For thousands of years we have extolled that "laughter is the best medicine." In many cultures, religions, and societies, people speak of the healing power of humor. The Old Testament says, "A merry heart does good like a medicine, but a broken spirit dries the bones" (Proverbs 17:22). This universally accepted truth is just now being explained by scientific research. Norman Cousins enlightened the medical com-

munity about the healing potential of laughter in his book *Anatomy of an Illness*. In 1968, Cousins was diagnosed with ankylosing spondylitis, a potentially life-threatening, degenerative disease involving the connective tissue of the body, which is essential in holding together the cells and larger structures of the body. Cousin's case was so extreme that he soon experienced great difficulty and pain in moving his joints. He was told that his prospect for recovery was very bleak. Because of discomfort and fatigue, he was unable to travel or play tennis, activities that brought him great joy and satisfaction.

Cousins refused to accept his grim prognosis and decided to take charge of his own treatment, working in partnership with his physician. He remembered reading about the adverse consequences of negative emotional states on the chemical balance of the body. He reasoned that, if negative emotions had played any part in predisposing him to illness, then perhaps positive emotions could aid in his recovery. He sought activities that increased his positive emotions, such as faith, hope, festivity, determination, confidence, joy, and a strong will to live. He knew that laughter helped create positive emotions. With this in mind, Cousins watched films of the Marx brothers and Candid Camera. He had nurses read to him from humorous books. He played practical jokes and told jokes. He began feeling better. Blood tests showed that his sedimentation rate (an index of the degree of infection or inflammation in the body) decreased after his laughter sessions, and they continued to fall as he gradually recovered.

After several months of this "humor therapy," his illness resolved and never returned. One could argue that Cousins would have recovered anyway, even without the laughter. Or one could comment that the results are not scientifically significant and represent the observations of a single case. However, Cousins continued his quest to understand just how his healing occurred.

Cousins spent the remaining 12 years of his life as an adjunct professor at the University of California at Los Angeles Medical School, where he established a "humor task force" to coordinate and support clinical research into laughter. Today, 25 years after Cousins's self-healing experience with laughter, there is scientific research providing evidence for the specific physiologic changes that his individual story suggested.[33] Cousins declared:

> Each human being possesses a beautiful system for fighting disease. This system provides the body with cancer-fighting cells—cells that can crush cancer cells or poison them one by one with the body's own chemotherapy. This system works better when the patient is relatively free of depression, which is what a strong will to live and a blazing determination can help to do. When we add these inner resources to the resources of medical science, we're reaching out for the best.[34]

Physiologic Response to Laughter

One of the first research teams to join Norman Cousins's humor task force was Lee Berk, a psychoneuroimmunologist, and Stanley Tan, an endocrinologist from Loma Linda University Medical Center. Their research shows that mirthful laughter can have the following effects:

- Increase the number and activity of natural killer cells, which attack viral-infected cells and some types of cancer cells
- Increase the number of activated T cells; these cells are "turned on and ready to go"
- Increase the level of the antibody IgA, which fights upper respiratory tract infections
- Increase the levels of gamma interferon, a lymphokine that activates many immune components
- Increase levels of complement 3, which helps antibodies to pierce infected cells
- Decrease levels of stress hormones (cortisol, dopamine, epinephrine) that weaken the immune response[35-37]

This research helps us to better understand the mind–body connection. The emotions and moods we experience directly affect our immune system. If we have a well-developed sense of humor, we are more likely to appreciate the amusing incongruities of life and experience more moments of joy and delight. These positive emotions can create neurochemical changes that buffer the immunosuppressive effects of stress.[38-43]

Even before Norman Cousins's experience, physician William Fry, Jr., professor emeritus of medicine at Stanford University, began his research into the physical effects of laughter in the 1950s.[44] He found that laughter caused the heart rate to elevate, sometimes reaching rates of above 120 beats per minute; respiratory rate and depth and minute volume also increased while the residual volume decreased. Coughing often occurs during laughter, dislodging mucus plugs. Peripheral vascular flow is increased as a result of vasodilatation. Systolic blood pressure is elevated during vigorous laughter but falls below resting levels after the laughter.

As the research surrounding the therapeutic effects of humor and laughter continues to grow, most studies focus on the ability of laughter, humor, and play to modulate our emotional experience. Extensive research shows that some emotions can create a toxic environment within the body (rage, depression, anxiety) where illnesses such as coronary artery disease, hypertension, and slower wound healing result.[45,46] These toxic emotional states have been shown to increase the production of proinflammatory cytokines that may lead to arthritis, osteoporosis, cardiovascular disease, and type 2 diabetes.[47-49]

More than 30 years of research in psychoneuroimmunology shows that the body's own healing system responds favorably to positive attitudes, thoughts, moods, and especially to emotions (e.g., love, hope, optimism, caring, intimacy, joy, laughter, and humor) and negatively to negative ones (hate, hopelessness, pessimism, indifference, anxiety, depression, loneliness, etc.).[50] Psychoneuroimmunology is the discipline that explores the connections and communication patterns linking the nervous, endocrine, and immune systems.

Candace Pert, one of the most respected researchers in the area of mind–body medicine, notes that emotions, which are registered and stored in the body in the form of chemical messages, are the most influential connection between the mind and the body. The emotions one experiences in connection with one's thoughts and daily attitudes—and, more specifically, the neurochemical changes that accompany these emotions—have the power to influence health.[51,52] In a 15-year prospective study, Kubzansky and Thurston show that individuals with higher levels of positive emotion reduced their risk of coronary artery disease.[53]

Recent research by Michael Miller, a cardiologist from University of Maryland, looked at the cardioprotective effects of laughter. He studied 300 people, half with documented coronary disease and half with healthy hearts. He found that those with heart disease were 40% less likely to laugh than those with healthy hearts, and the more people laughed the lower their scores were for anger and hostility. Miller's second study measured how humor may increase the ability of the endothelium of the brachial artery to relax and perhaps decrease blood pressure. This may also reflect humor's ability to decrease the intra-arterial inflammatory response.[54]

Tan and Berk also studied how a daily humor experience may influence the recurrence of myocardial infarction. They followed 48 newly postmyocardial infarction (MI) patients in a cardiac rehab program for longer than a year. One group was told to view 30 minutes of self-selected comedy each day. The researchers measured serum and urinary catecholamines, cardiac arrhythmias, and nitroglycerine use for each group. They found that the laughter group had fewer arrhythmias, lower catecholamine levels, and less use of nitroglycerine for chest pain. Their data show that only 8.3% of the laughter group had a recurrence of heart attack, while the control group had a 42% recurrence. Both Miller's and Tan and Berk's research perhaps clarifies the truth that "a merry heart does good like a medicine."[54,55]

Nurse–researcher Jaqueline Dowling studied children with cancer and found that children with high scores for sense of humor had better psychosocial adjustment to cancer stressors (fatigue, pain, nausea) than those with lower scores. She also noted that as cancer stressors increased, those children with high humor scores had fewer incidents of infection.[56]

Physicians Margaret Stuber and Lonnie Zeltzer, researchers at David Geffen UCLA School of Medicine, have found that pediatric patients who watch certain funny videos during treatment for a painful procedure are better able to tolerate the painful procedure with less anxiety and stress. The full report of this research was published in 2007 in an international journal.[57]

In March 2007, Sven Svebak, professor from Norwegian University of Science and Tech-

nology, presented his research findings at the American Psychosomatic Society meeting. He studied 54,000 Norwegians over a 7 year period and found that those who were able to find more humor in life were more likely to survive. In a subgroup of more than 2,000 cancer patients, he found that those with a high ability to find humor in life were 70% more likely to survive. Perhaps this proves that "he who laughs, lasts."[58]

In 2008, Swiss scientists published research showing that ventilation capacity improved in people with chronic obstructive pulmonary disease after they watched a funny clown performance.[59] The researchers found that the usual amount of "trapped air" that prevents adequate ventilation was reduced after the laughter and improved the movement of air into and out of the lungs.

Humor and laughter are effective methods to modulate our emotional experience probably because of humor's ability to trigger the experience of joy (a strong positive emotion) even in the midst of negative emotion.[60] Studies are showing that almost any program that reduces chronic negative emotion and/or increases daily positive emotion can be expected to support better health.

A new question is now being asked in the field of psychoneuroimmunology research: Can one's emotional state influence the expression of genes. Preliminary research in the field of epigenetics indicates this is possible. Several studies from Japan focus on the effect of humor and laughter on diabetes. Hayashi discovered that the expression of the prorenin receptor gene was less expressed in diabetic patients than in nondiabetic subjects. The decreased expression of this gene among diabetics contributes to increased levels of prorenin concentrations that lead to the release of angiotensin, which triggers vasoconstriction and microvascular problems.

Researchers also found that this prorenin receptor gene was up-regulated significantly after watching a comedy show, thus contributing to a lower level of prorenin and angiotension and perhaps the vasoconstriction they cause.[61] This same research team analyzed 41,000 genes and found that 39 of them were up-regulated for at least 90 minutes after watching a comedy video. Four hours after the comedy, 27 genes were still up-regulated and 14 of these genes were related to natural killer cell activity.[62,63] These studies support the findings of Berk and Tan in 1989 when they measured increased numbers and activity of natural killer cells.[64]

Some of the most exciting clinical research exploring the therapeutic possibilities of humor and laughter will soon be published in the journal of *Oncology Nursing*. Palliative care nurse Hob Osterlund at Queen's Medical Center in Honolulu together with the University of Hawaii designed a study to compare changes in symptoms related to cancer and chemotherapy, immune function, and emotional stress levels in two groups of patients who view a humorous or nonhumorous DVD. Subjects were recruited from the outpatient oncology clinic and were randomly assigned to view a 45-minute humorous DVD or nonhumorous DVD. Measurements were obtained before and after patients viewed the DVD. The results of this research will be in print soon. Because of copyright protection, I can share only a quote from one of the primary researchers, Hob Osterlund:

> Our research results showed that patients who watched the comedy film felt better on many levels. Statistical analysis showed that this change was significant over those who watched the noncomedy film. Measurements of immune function also improved though not as statistically significant.

You can find a reference to the article on Osterlund's website: www.ChuckleChannel.com. Chuckle Channel is a video resource company that provides hospitals with site-licensed wholesome comedy clips for patient viewing when broadcast through an in-house video programming system. More than 50 hospitals in the United States use this service.

The Power of Playfulness

The key to improving our sense of humor is the rediscovery of the playfulness we had as children. The joyous laughter that accompanies children's play leaves no doubt that they are happy. When we become more playful, we automatically become more spontaneous and enjoy whatever we are doing more than we otherwise

would. The dictionary defines *play* as activities that are amusing, fun, or otherwise enjoyable in their own right. When we truly play, we seek to impress no one, and we produce no product—we just enjoy being in the moment. Playing is as old as humankind, as evidenced by the remains of toys found in the ancient ruins of Egyptian, Babylonian, Chinese, and Aztec civilizations. When children play, they use their imagination to invent a reality that meets their needs. If we allow ourselves to be children and distort or exaggerate a situation to its most absurd limits, we create an opportunity for laughter. As we grow older, our ability to open ourselves to moments of playfulness becomes constrained. Serious attention to the business at hand may replace a willingness to laugh and play, subsequently reducing our health-promoting behaviors. Sometimes it is difficult to incorporate play into our lives again because it does not always fit our image of what is necessary and proper for an adult. Erickson noted that through the ages, some adults have been inclined to judge play to be neither serious nor useful, and thus unrelated to the center of human tasks and motives, from which the adult, in fact, seeks escape when he or she plays.[65]

Yet recent research on animals shows that play makes a crucial contribution to brain development. Natalie Angier summarized this research as follows:

> An animal plays most vigorously at precisely the time when its brain cells are frenetically forming synaptic connections, creating a dense array of neural connections that can pass an electrochemical message from one neighborhood of the brain to the next. . . . Scientists believe that the intense sensory and physical stimulation that comes from playing is critical to the growth of these cerebral synapses and thus to proper motor development.[66]

Play, then, is essential for survival in the animal world. Early childhood play is one way that humans practice socialization skills and mimic cultural rituals. It is a way that people create connections with others and build trust. Creative people are playful, experimental, and willing to take risks. Therefore, in serious situations such as illness or injury, which may require a change in lifestyle or other adaptation, creative problem solving can be a great help. Creative solutions seldom emerge when people are concentrating on something in a solemn, practical mood; they are more likely to come when people are in a relaxed, even playful mood.

Humor and Stress Management

If play serves to build up skills that are essential to effective adaptation as an adult, how then does humor help one adapt? Why does humor exist? One of the main reasons humor exists may be that it helps people adapt to the stresses in their lives. It is because of human beings' superior intellectual capacities that they have such high stress in their lives. As Hans Selye noted, stress is not the event, but rather our perception of the event. In other words, it is people's interpretation of events that causes stress, not the events themselves.[63] A sense of humor helps people to view difficult circumstances in a less stressful way.

Because different people respond differently to the same environmental stimuli, some people seem to cope with stress better than others.[64] Sociologist Suzanne Kobassa defined three "hardiness factors" that can increase a person's resilience to stress and prevent burnout: commitment, control, and challenge. If one has a strong commitment to oneself and one's work, if one believes that one is in control of the choices in one's life (internal locus of control), and if one views change as challenging rather than as threatening, then one is more likely to cope successfully with stress. A theme that is becoming more prominent in the literature is the idea that a sense of powerlessness is a causative factor in burnout.[67]

A recent study in the Midwest looked at the impact of a purposeful aerobic laughter intervention on employees' sense of self-efficacy in the workplace. Employees demonstrated a significant increase in several different aspects of self-efficacy, including self-regulation, optimism, positive emotions, and social identification. They concluded that purposeful laughter is a realistic and sustainable intervention that enhances employees' morale, resilience, and personal efficacy beliefs.[68-70]

In this context, humor can be an empowerment tool. Humor gives people a different per-

spective on their problems, and with an attitude of detachment, they feel a sense of self-protection and control in their environment. As comedian Bill Cosby is fond of saying, "If you can laugh at it, you can survive it." It is reasonable to assume that, if the locus of control is strongly internal, a person will feel a greater sense of power and thus be more likely to avoid burnout.

Humor and Locus of Control

This author's research, presented in 1990 at the Eighth International Conference on Humor Studies in England, documented changes in locus of control and appreciation of humor related to a humor training course. Using the Adult Nowicki-Strickland Scale, which has proven reliability and validity, the research team assessed the locus of control in 231 nurses in Pennsylvania, Kentucky, and California. The team then separated the nurses into two groups and administered Svebak's Sense of Humor Questionnaire, using only the subscales that have proven to be reliable and valid. The experimental group completed a 6-hour humor training course, in which they were given permission and techniques for appropriate use of humor with patients and coworkers. The control group had no such humor training. The same survey tools were readministered to each group 6 weeks later to determine changes in locus of control and appreciation of humor.

Using the Wilcoxon Matched Pairs Signed-Ranks Test, the team found that there was a significant decrease in the score for external locus of control in the experimental group ($P < .0063$, two-tailed). Using the same analysis for the control group, the team found no significant change. No significant differences were found in the initial locus of control scores for the experimental and the control groups when tested using the Mann-Whitney U and Kolmogorov-Smirnov tests. This study indicates that, if people are encouraged and guided in using humor, they can gain a sense of control in their lives. The use of humor represents what Kobassa calls cognitive control. We cannot control events in our external world, but we can control how we view these events and our emotional response to them.[68] Further research is needed to determine how long these effects persist.[70]

Ho Ho Holistic Health

Humor, laughter, and play contribute to our health and well-being in many ways. Each touches our body, mind, and spirit in its own way. Humor, as a cognitive process, is primarily a mental activity. The behavior of laughter affects the whole body, from cells to entire organ systems. Play and a playful spirit fill us with joy, connect us with others, and keep us focused on the present moment. The interaction of body, mind, and spirit with humor, laughter, and play forms the "Aha, Ha Ha, Ahhhh" continuum. The mind says, "Aha! I get the joke." The body says, "Ha Ha!" And the spirit says, "Ahhhh, everything feels much better now."

■ HOLISTIC CARING PROCESS

Holistic Assessment

In preparing to use humor, laughter, and play interventions, the nurse assesses the following parameters:

- The client's ability and willingness to smile and laugh
- The client's attitude toward using laughter and play in the current situation
- The client's history of using humor, laughter, and play in other circumstances
- The client's visual, auditory, cognitive, and physical limitations
- The client's preferred style of humor (i.e., jokes, cartoons, stories, comedy movies, animated cartoons, stand-up comedy, funny songs)
- The client's favorite comedy artists—performers, writers, cartoonists, and so on
- The client's feelings about previous experiences with humor and play
- The client's preferred playful activities

Identification of Patterns/Challenges/Needs

The patterns/challenges/needs (see Chapter 8) compatible with interventions for humor, laughter, and play are as follows:

- Altered parenting, actual or potential
- Social isolation
- Ineffective individual and family coping
- Activity intolerance, actual or potential
- Deficit in diversion activity
- Impaired physical mobility
- Powerlessness
- Disturbance in self-concept: altered self-esteem, role performance, personal identity
- Altered sensation or perception: visual, auditory, kinesthetic, gustatory, tactile, olfactory
- Altered thought processes
- Anxiety
- Pain
- Fear
- Potential for violence: self-directed or directed at others

Outcome Identification

Exhibit 15-2 guides the nurse in outcomes, nursing prescriptions, and evaluation for the use of humor, laughter, and play as a nursing intervention.

Therapeutic Care Plan and Interventions

Before the session:

- Assess your own ease and comfort with using humor and play as a therapeutic intervention.
- Practice smiling in front of a mirror: first scowl, and then smile. Feel the difference.
- Evaluate your ability to respond to humor or engage in playful activity for your own personal pleasure.
- Increase awareness of your own preferred humor style, artist, writer, performer.
- Allow yourself to laugh with abandon at things you find funny.
- Become familiar with the content and variety of humorous items and playful activities that are available for you to use.
- Ensure that all supplies and equipment are in working condition.
- Improve your ability to tell a good joke. Remember these tips: Keep it short—less than 2 minutes. Be sure you can remember the whole joke before you start. Let your body, face, and voice become animated as you tell the joke. Pause occasionally as you deliver the material; create a brief and concise setup for the punch line; pause before delivering the punch line; speak the punch line clearly and with punch!
- Review the client's chart or consult with others to assess changes in the client's situation since you last met.
- Sense your own needs and stress level. Give yourself permission to be silly and playful.

EXHIBIT 15-2   Nursing Interventions: Play and Laughter

Client Outcomes	Nursing Prescriptions	Evaluation
The client will smile or laugh in response to humorous stimuli.	Introduce the client to the concept that humor, laughter, and play benefit health. Guide the client in identifying his or her own preferred humor style. Help the client to clarify any blocks to using humor, laughter, or play.	The client requested some humor resources from family or friends. The client laughed in response to a selected humorous intervention. The client laughed at a joke, story, or cartoon provided by the nurse. The client shared a joke or story with the nurse or family. The client sees some absurdity in a personal incident and shares with staff or family.
The client will engage in playful activities.	Guide the client to select a playful activity that matches his or her preference and ability.	The client was observed amusing self with toy. The client plays game with family during visiting hours. The client wears amusing item to greet staff or family.
The client will experience decrease in subjective severity of target symptom as a result of humor or playful intervention.	Guide the client in grading the severity of a symptom on a scale of 1 to 10 before and after intervention.	Patient rated pain at 6 before humor intervention and graded pain at 3 after intervention.

At the beginning of the session:
- Assess the client's status according to the assessment parameters.
- Record vital signs and ask the client to assess pain, anxiety, tension, or other target symptoms on a numerical scale (1 = comfortable, 10 = extremely uncomfortable).
- Describe to the client the benefits that humor, laughter, and play have on the body (physiologic), mind (psychological), and spirit (emotional and energy level).
- Provide the client with appropriate materials to match his or her preference and some instructions for use.

During the session:
- Use all interventions with sensitivity to the client's needs, responses, and difficulties.
- Provide support for the client through your physical presence, encouragement, or time alone if the client wants to read or watch a videotape.
- Remember that humor is contagious and social. Interventions may be most effective if used within a group (e.g., family and friends) rather than individually.
- Remember that humor and play are spontaneous and therefore are most successful when not precisely planned.

- Continue to evaluate the mood and response of the client and adapt the humor and play intervention to meet the client's perceived needs.

At the end of the session:
- Record vital signs and ask the client to reevaluate the pain, tension, or target symptom on a scale of 1 to 10.
- Discuss the intervention with the client and obtain feedback for future sessions.
- Answer any questions the client may have.
- Encourage the client to continue using the intervention at home and to explore other possible variations.
- Use client outcomes (Exhibit 15-2) and the client's subjective experiences (**Exhibit 15-3**) to evaluate the session.
- Schedule a follow-up session.

Specific Interventions: Humor, Laughter, and Play

Humor interventions can be packaged in many different ways—as humor rooms, comedy carts, humor baskets, laughter libraries, or caring clown programs. The individual caregiver can adapt these programs to meet the specific needs of clients. Several suggestions for starting a humor program follow.

- Create a scrapbook of cartoons. Place the cartoons in a photo album with peel-back pages to protect them and keep them clean. Consider the audience that will read this scrapbook. Try to find humor about situations or problems your clients will be facing. Be careful not to add any potentially offensive or shocking items to the scrapbook. Include a variety of cartoon artists.
- Develop a file of funny jokes, stories, cards, bumper stickers, poems, and songs. When you hear something funny, write it down immediately, before you forget! Many humorous resources are available on the Internet. Books of jokes are available in stores and libraries, but these are rather unreliable resources for usable material. The jokes are often offensive, outdated, or just not funny. A better method of building a collection is to write down jokes you hear from friends, see on television, or read in magazines.
- Collect or borrow funny books, DVDs, videos, and audiocassettes of comedy routines. These can be found in libraries, humor sections of bookstores, mail-order catalogs, or at humor conferences. Create a lending library.
- Keep a file of local clowns, magicians, storytellers, and puppeteers. Invite them to entertain at your facility, at the patient's home, or at a group function.
- Collect toys, interactive games, noisemakers, and costume items. Keep them available for play. Small wind-up toys can be enjoyable. The author has a pair of little shoes that walk around when wound up and a large nose that does the same—it is called the "runny nose." If you will be sharing such

EXHIBIT 15-3   Evaluation of the Client's Subjective Experience with Humor, Laughter, and Play

1. Was this a new experience for you? Can you describe it?
2. Can you describe any physical or emotional shift that occurred during the exercise?
3. Were there any distractions or uncomfortable moments during the exercise?
4. How long has it been since you had this kind of experience?
5. How was this exercise different for you from the last time you took part in a similar one?
6. Would you like to try this again?
7. How could the experience be made more meaningful for you?
8. What are your plans to integrate this exercise into your daily life?

toys with a client, keep in mind safety and infection precautions. (See **Exhibit 15-4.**)

- Create a humor journal or log to record funny encounters or humorous discoveries. On days when you really need a laugh but cannot seem to find anything funny, you will have a collection of amusing stories at your fingertips. A nurse in one of the author's workshops recounted that she had created a journal for the operating room where she worked. She called the book *The Days of Our Knives*.
- Establish a bulletin board in your facility or on your refrigerator at home. Post cartoons, bumper stickers, and funny signs. If the display is public, you must consider the sensitivities of the audience and be careful to exclude potentially offensive (e.g., ageist, sexist, ethnic) material.
- Subscribe to a humorous newsletter or journal to collect new ideas and inspiration.
- Educate yourself about therapeutic humor. Attend conferences, workshops, and conventions. New techniques are developed daily. New research is published, and better resources become available on a regular basis. Stay up to date in this rapidly growing field.

Communication studies have shown that people take in 7% of other people's words, 38% of their vocal characteristics, and 55% of their nonverbal signals.[69] Applying these concepts in the creation and communication of humor can make your efforts even more effective. Because the client will notice less than 10% of your words, choose them carefully. Develop a collection of zingy one-liners, clever riddles, funny stories, and brilliant jokes for every occasion. Vocal characteristics are five times more important than words alone. Try to change the pace and tone of your voice, or speak with an accent, and your words will have more impact. The most powerful communication tool we have is the ability to communicate nonverbally. Facial expressions, physical gestures, costuming, props, and the way we walk or stand or reach for something are nonverbal communication techniques that provide the greatest impact on our audience. Clowns and other physical-comedy artists have perfected these skills and use their body language to deliver the humorous message. Some suggestions for humor program packages follow.

- Laughter libraries offer a selection of funny and informative books about humor and health. Audiocassettes, DVDs, and videos are usually a part of this collection. These resources can be used either at home or within a facility. There are literally hundreds of books that can be included in a laughter library.
- A humor room is a place where clients, their families, and staff can gather to laugh, play, and relax together. These rooms are decorated with comfortable furniture, plants, and artwork. The furniture is arranged in clusters so that groups of three to five people can gather around a game table, television, or reading area.
- A comedy cart is a mobile unit with many of the same supplies available in a humor room. It can be wheeled into a client's room

EXHIBIT 15-4   Supplies for Humor Programs

Joke books	Kaleidoscopes	Wind-up toys
Large sunglasses	Goofy hats	Rubber noses
Giant pacifier	Clown nose	Magic wand
Puppets	Rubber chicken	Smile on a stick
Funny buttons	Funny pictures	Groucho glasses
Squirt guns	Handheld games	Cartoon books
Bubbles	Funny sticky notes	Stickers

to bring mirth aid alongside the frightening medical equipment and monitoring devices. These carts often have clever names such as Laughmobile, Jokes on Spokes, Humor on a Roll, or Humor à la Cart.

- A humor basket is probably the easiest therapeutic humor program to create and is an appropriate place to start if time and resources are limited. This basket is a smaller collection of comedy toys, gadgets, and props. Hospital staff find that humor baskets provide quick and easy access to items with humor potential, stimulate their own creativity, and enhance their spontaneity. (See Exhibit 15-4.)

- Bedside clowning attempts to distract patients from their problems to help them forget their pain. Patients are given a chance to watch or participate in some fun and silliness. Clowns offer a momentary release from personal burdens, inspire joy, and stimulate the will to live.[70] The *Hospital Clown Newsletter* advises performers on routines and precautions that will enhance their bedside skills.

- Scan your local TV program schedule and create a list of humorous entertainment options. Post this list in a common area.

- When using closed-circuit video, be sure to obtain permission for use if the material is copyrighted. In some situations, a license must be purchased to show these films to large audiences.

Case Study/Implementation

CASE STUDY 1

Setting: Hospital room

Client: R. T., a 52-year-old man awaiting open heart surgery

Patterns/Challenges/Needs:
1. Anxiety
2. Coping, ineffective individual
3. Powerlessness
4. Social isolation

R. T. lay quietly in his hospital bed. The doctors had visited and left, the nurses were finished with their morning care. It was quiet. He was alone and feeling lonely. His wife Sally and the kids would not be able to visit until later that evening. What could he do until then? It was hard not to worry about his surgery scheduled for the next day. The more he worried, the more he felt agitated, depressed, and simply scared to death. The next moment, he was given the perfect solution. Evelyn, a smiling hospital volunteer, entered his room pushing a decorated cart. She wore a colorful smock and a funny hat labeled, "Humor Patrol—Department of Energy." R. T. smiled for the first time that day. "Looks like you could use some mirth aid, and we've got a wonderful selection today." R. T. was skeptical but curious. He asked for an explanation. "Well," she replied, "it's difficult for patients to lie around all day waiting for the next medical procedure. They worry and get depressed. These emotions have been proven to inhibit healing, so to prevent them, we provide a therapeutic humor program for our patients. It's part of the hospital's mission statement, to offer care and attention to the whole patient—body, mind, and spirit."

R. T. agreed that his spirits needed a lift and his mind could use some distraction. He asked to see more. First, Evelyn opened the "Yuk-a-Day Vitamin" jar and read a few jokes, riddles, and funny one-liners. Then she opened a drawer and pulled out a few wind-up toys and started them running on his over-bed table. She continued to pull out toys, games, props, puppets, cartoon books, puzzles, and costume items. Soon both of them were laughing, joking, and playing around like small children. After performing a few magic tricks, Evelyn gave R. T. a list of the humorous audiocassettes, videotaped programs, and books that were available from the hospital's laughter library. R. T. chose an audiocassette of Bob Newhart, his favorite comedian, and arranged for a comedy video to be delivered when his family arrived that evening. He selected a few toys to borrow, as well as some rubber vomit to tease the nurses and a squirt gun to defend himself against unwanted interruptions.

R. T. felt like a kid again, filled with enthusiasm and ready to have fun. He looked forward to the fun and laughter he would experience and share with his family. As Evelyn left, she offered one more answer to a problem he had not yet solved: "If you like, we can schedule a clown to visit with you while you're in the hospital." "Great idea," he thought. His son's birthday was on Saturday, and instead of missing his party, now they could share a special celebration right there in the hospital. He scheduled the clown visit. Because of the therapeutic humor program, R. T. was now feeling energized, optimistic, and relaxed. Laughter is the best medicine!

CASE STUDY 2

Setting: Outpatient clinic

Client: J. B., a 45-year-old woman

Patterns/Challenges/Needs: All related to adult-onset intrinsic asthma:

1. Activity intolerance
2. Anxiety
3. Breathing pattern, ineffective
4. Fear
5. Powerlessness

J. B. had visited the clinic for treatment of her asthma over a period of several months. Her bronchodilator medications had been adjusted, she was using a cool mist to thin secretions, her activity level had increased, and she had returned to full-time employment. In the process of teaching breathing techniques to J. B., the nurse noted that she had difficulty in maintaining prolonged exhalation. She was able to lengthen her expiratory time between attacks but would forget the intervention when under the stress of wheezing and shortness of breath.

J. B. arrived at the clinic in mild distress after using an inhaler to open her airways with only partial success. After sitting J. B. in a straight chair, the nurse began coaching her in her breathing pattern while applying gentle pressure on her shoulders with each exhalation. As her breathing became easier, the nurse opened a bottle of bubble solution and invited J. B. to blow bubbles. Although J. B. felt that this was a rather nontraditional approach to her condition, she agreed to participate.

To blow bubbles successfully, one must exhale slowly and for a long period of time. J. B. remembered this from her own childhood and from playing with her children. She was soon blowing long streams of fragile bubbles, and her wheezing disappeared as she did so.

As the attack eased, the nurse coached J. B. to visualize the bubbles as carrying away her tension triggers. J. B. expressed her delight with her new application of an old skill. Her tension decreased, and she returned to work confident in her ability to apply her skill during stressful situations. Linking the skill with an unusual and playful activity made the breathing strategy stand out in her memory and made it easier to recall under stress.

Evaluation

With the client, the nurse determines whether the client outcomes for humor, laughter, and play (see Exhibit 15-2) were successfully achieved. To evaluate the session further, the nurse may again explore the subjective effects of the experience with the client using the evaluation questions in Exhibit 15-3.

Directions for
FUTURE RESEARCH

1. Determine the impact of humor and laughter programs on quality of life, pain control, and symptom management.
2. Examine the cost-effectiveness of humor programs in increasing patient satisfaction, decreasing length of stay, and achieving compliance with the treatment plan.
3. Analyze the impact of laughter and play programs on the immune-compromised patient and the patient at risk for developing infection.

Nurse Healer
REFLECTIONS

After reading this chapter, the nurse healer will be able to answer or to begin the process of answering the following questions:

- What is my inner sense of joy when I hear myself or another laugh?
- Do I nurture my ability, and the ability of my patients, to be playful?
- Can I laugh and play with a sense of freedom and without guilt, even when my work is not yet finished?
- Can I experience playful activities without competing or feeling that I must accomplish a particular goal?

For a full suite of assignments and additional learning activities, use the access code located in the front of your book to visit this exclusive website: http://go.jblearning.com/dossey. If you do not have an access code, you can obtain one at the site.

NOTES

1. A. Klein, *Quotations to Cheer You Up When the World Is Getting You Down* (New York: Sterling Publishing, 1991).
2. V. Robinson, *Humor and the Health Professions* (Thorofare, NJ: Slack, 1991).
3. L. Kronenberger, *The Thread of Laughter* (New York: Knopf, 1952).
4. S. Freud, "Jokes and Their Relation to the Unconscious," in *The Complete Psychological Works of Sigmund Freud*, vol. 8 (London: Hogarth Press, 1905/1961).
5. H. Mindess, *Laughter and Liberation* (Los Angeles, CA: Mansh Publishing, 1971).
6. M. Balick and R. Lee, "The Role of Laughter in Traditional Medicine and Its Relevance to the Clinical Setting: Healing with Ha!," *Alternative Therapies in Health and Medicine* 9 (2003): 88–91.
7. M. L. Apte, *Humor and Laughter: An Anthropological Approach* (Ithaca, NY: Cornell University Press, 1985).
8. R. Dean, A. Kinsman, and D. Gregory, "More Than Trivial: Strategies for Using Humor in Palliative Care," *Cancer Nursing* 28, no. 4 (2005): 292–300.
9. M. Borod, "SMILES: Toward a Better Laughter Life: A Model for Introducing Humor in the Palliative Care Setting," *Journal of Cancer Education* 2, no. 1 (2006): 30–34.
10. M. Walter et al., "Humour Therapy in Patients with Late-Life Depression or Alzheimer's Disease: A Pilot Study," *International Journal of Geriatric Psychiatry* 22, no. 1 (2007): 77–83.
11. C. Hyers, *The Spirituality of Comedy* (New Brunswick, NJ: Transaction Press, 1996), 24.
12. P. Wooten, *Compassionate Laughter*, 2nd ed. (Santa Cruz, CA: Jest Press, 2000), 15, 21.
13. H. Olsson et al., "The Essence of Humour and Its Effects and Functions: A Qualitative Study," *Journal of Nursing Management* 10, no. 1 (2002): 21–26.
14. Personal communication.
15. C. MacDonald, "A Chuckle a Day Keeps the Doctor Away: Therapeutic Humor and Laughter," *Journal of Psychosocial Nursing and Mental Health Services* 42 (2002): 18–25.
16. R. Penson et al., "Laughter: The Best Medicine?" *Oncologist* 10, no. 8 (2005): 651–660.
17. B. Kruse and M. Prazak, "Humor and Older Adults: What Makes Them Laugh?" *Journal of Holistic Nursing* 24, no. 3 (2006): 188–193.
18. M. Wanzer, M. Booth-Butterfield, and S. Booth-Butterfield, "If We Didn't Use Humor, We'd Cry: Humorous Coping Communication in Health Care Settings," *Journal of Health Communication* 10, no. 2 (2005): 105–125.
19. C. Edson, "You Know It's a Long Shift When . . . ," in *Whinorrhea and Other Nursing Diagnoses*, ed. F. London (Mesa, AZ: JNJ Publishing, 1995), 56–57.
20. P. Johnson, "The Use of Humor and Its Influences on Spirituality and Coping in Breast Cancer Survivors," *Oncology Nursing Forum* 29, no. 4 (2002): 691–695.
21. W. Christie and C. Moore, "The Impact of Humor on Patients with Cancer," *Clinical Journal of Oncological Nursing* 9, no. 2 (2005): 211–218.
22. A. Joshua, A. Cotroneo, and S. Clarke, "Humor and Oncology," *Journal of Clinical Oncology* 23, no. 3 (2005): 645–648.
23. J. S. Dowling, "Humor: A Coping Strategy for Pediatric Patients," *Pediatric Nursing* 28, no. 2 (2002):123–131.
24. K. Hammer, *And How Are We Feeling Today* (Chicago, IL: Contemporary Books, 1993).
25. L. Rosenberg, "A Qualitative Investigation of the Use of Humor by Emergency Personnel as a Strategy for Coping with Stress," *Journal of Emergency Nursing* 17, no. 4 (1991): 197–203.
26. J. C. Scholl and S. L. Ragan, "The Use of Humor in Promoting Positive Provider–Patient Interactions in a Hospital Rehabilitation Unit," *Health Communication* 15, no. 3 (2003): 321–330.
27. J. Scholl, "The Use of Humor to Promote Patient-Centered Care," *Journal of Applied Communication Research* 35, no. 2 (2007): 156.
28. A. Klein, *Courage to Laugh* (Los Angeles, CA: Tarcher, 1998).
29. J. Garrick, "The Humor of Trauma Survivors: Its Application in a Therapeutic Milieu," *Journal of Aggression, Maltreatment, and Trauma* 12, no. 1 (2006): 169–182.
30. L. Rosenberg, "A Qualitative Investigation of the Use of Humor by Emergency Personnel as a Strategy for Coping with Stress," *Journal of Emergency Nursing* 17, no. 4 (1991): 197–203.
31. P. Wooten, *Compassionate Laughter* (Santa Cruz, CA: Jest Press, 2000).
32. Personal communication. Barry Sultanoff, MD, December 1988.
33. N. Cousins, *Anatomy of an Illness* (New York: W. W. Norton, 1979).
34. N. Cousins, *Head First—the Biology of Hope* (New York: E. P. Dutton, 1989).

35. L. S. Berk et al., "Modulation of Neuroimmune Parameters During the Eustress of Humor-Associated Mirthful Laughter," *Alternative Therapies Health Medicine* 7, no. 2 (2001): 62–72, 74–76.

36. M. Bennett et al., "The Effect of Mirthful Laughter on Stress and Natural Killer Cell Activity," *Alternative Therapy Health Medicine* 9, no. 2 (2003): 38–45.

37. K. Takahashi et al., "The Elevation of Natural Killer Cell Activity Induced by Laughter in a Crossover Designed Study," *International Journal of Molecular Medicine* 8, no. 6 (2001): 645–650.

38. R. Martin, "Humor, Laughter, and Physical Health: Methodological Issues and Research Findings," *Psychological Bulletin* 127 (2001): 504–519.

39. H. Lefcourt and R. Martin, *Humor and Life Stress* (New York: Springer-Verlag, 1986).

40. P. Wooten, "Humor: An Antidote for Stress," *Holistic Nursing Practice* 10, no. 2 (1996): 49–55.

41. M. Bennett and C. Lengacher, "Humor and Laughter May Influence Health: I. History and Background," *Evidence-Based Complementary and Alternative Medicine* (March 2006): 61–63.

42. M. Bennett and C. Lengacher, "Humor and Laughter May Influence Health: II. Complementary Therapies and Humor in a Clinical Population," *Evidence-Based Complementary and Alternative Medicine* (June 2006): 187–190.

43. M. Bennett and C. Lengacher, "Humor and Laughter May Influence Health: III. Laughter and Health Outcomes," *Evidence-Based Complementary and Alternative Medicine* (May 17, 2007).

44. W. Fry, "The Physiological Effects of Humor, Mirth, and Laughter," *Journal of the American Medical Association* 267 (1992): 1857–1858.

45. Biing-Jiun, S. et. al. 2008.

46. Keicolt 2002.

47. Keicolt 2003.

48. Graham 2006.

49. Kendall-Tackett 2009.

50. McGhee 2010.

51. C. Pert, *Molecules of Emotion* (New York: Charles Scribner's Sons, 1997).

52. Glaser R-Keicolt 2005.

53. L. Kubzansky and R. Thurston, "Emotional Vitality and Incident Coronary Heart Disease," *Archives of General Psychiatry* 64 (2007): 1393–1401.

54. M. Miller et al., "Impact of Cinematic Viewing on Endothelial Function," *Heart* 92 (2006): 261–262.

55. S. Tan et al., "Humor as Adjunct Therapy in Cardiac Rehabilitation," *Advances in Mind Body Medicine* 22, no. 3–4 (Winter 2007/2008): 8–12.

56. J. S. Dowling, "Humor: A Coping Strategy for Pediatric Patients," *Pediatric Nursing* 28, no. 2 (2002). 123–131.

57. M. Stuber et al., "Laughter, Humor and Pain Perception in Children: A Pilot Study," *Evidence-Based Complementary and Alternative Medicine* 6, no. 2 (2009): 271–276. doi:10.1093/ecam/nem097

58. S. Svebak et al., "Sense of Humor and Mortality: A 7-Year Prospective Study of an Unselected County Population and a Sub-population Diagnosed with Cancer," *Psychosomatic Medicine* 69 (2007): A-64.

59. M. H. Brutsche et al., "Impact of Laughter on Air Trapping in Severe Chronic Obstructive Lung Disease," *International Journal of Chronic Obstructive Pulmonary Disease* 3, no. 1 (2008): 185–192.

60. L. Richman et al., "Positive Emotion and Health: Going Beyond the Negative," *Health Psychology* 24 (2007): 422–429.

61. T. Hayashi et al., "Laughter Modulates Prorenin Receptor Gene Expression in Patients with Type 2 Diabetes," *Journal of Psychosomatic Research* 62 (2007): 703–706.

62. T. Hayashi et al., "Laughter Up-regulates the Genes Related to NK Cell Activity in Diabetes," *Biomedical Research* 28, no. 6 (2007): 281–285.

63. T. Matsuzaki et al., "Mirthful Laughter Differentially Affects Serum Pro and Anti-inflammatory Cytokine Levels Depending on the Level of Disease Activity in Patients with Rheumatoid Arthritis," *Rheumatology* 45 (2006): 182–186.

64. L. Berk, "Neuroendocrine and Stress Hormone Changes During Mirthful Laughter," *American Journal of Medical Sciences* 298 (1989): 390–396.

65. E. Erickson, *Toys and Reasons* (New York: W. W. Norton, 1977), 17.

66. A. M. Okimoto, A. Bundy, and J. Hanzlik, "Playfulness in Children with and Without Disability: Measurement and Intervention," *American Journal of Occupational Therapy* 54, no. 1 (2000): 73–82.

67. H. Selye, *The Stress of Life* (New York: McGraw-Hill, 1956).

68. C. Maslach, "Job Burnout: New Directions in Research and Intervention," *Current Directions in Psychological Science* 12 (2001): 189–192.

69. H. Beckman, N. Regier, and J. Young, "Effect of Workplace Laughter Groups on Personal Efficacy Beliefs," *Journal of Primary Prevention* 28 (2007): 167–182.

70. P. Wooten, "Does a Humor Workshop Affect Nurse Burnout?" *Journal of Nursing Jocularity* 2, no. 2 (1992): 42–43.

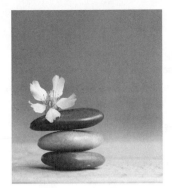

Chapter 16

Relaxation

Jeanne Anselmo

Nurse Healer
OBJECTIVES

Theoretical

- Learn the definitions of relaxation and self-regulation.
- Compare and contrast different relaxation exercises.
- List the body-mind-spirit changes that accompany profound relaxation.

Clinical

- Describe three different types of relaxation exercises and their appropriate clinical application.
- Describe the indications and contraindications for two forms of relaxation practice.
- Identify commonly used technology or equipment from your nursing practice, and describe how it can be used as a biofeedback device.
- Use breathing strategies with a client, and record the subjective and clinical changes that occur with relaxed breathing.

Personal

- Pick one or a combination of relaxation and/or meditation practices and apply them to a stressful moment. Explore the ways they support your well-being and how they affect your ability to transform stress.

- Identify through focused awareness areas in your body where you most often accumulate tension.
- Identify three personally meaningful therapeutic suggestions, and use them as reminders to support your self-care relaxation practice and well-being.

DEFINITIONS

Autogenic training: Developed by Drs. Johannes Schultz and Wolfgang Luthe, this practice teaches relaxation through the repetition of phrases that influence muscle relaxation by bringing an awareness of sensations and feelings of warmth, heaviness, and relaxation to one's body.

Biofeedback: The use of technology or monitors that augment and feed back usually imperceptible signals from the person's psychophysiologic processes for the purpose of cultivating the ability to influence or change stress-related patterns or symptoms. This self-regulation process, which is usually paired with a relaxation practice, offers the person an opportunity to be an active participant in his or her own healing and health maintenance.

Hypnosis: A process for focused awareness and expanded consciousness with diminishing perception of peripheral sensations, thoughts, and feelings.

Mantra: A word, short phrase, or prayer that is repeated either silently or aloud as a focus of concentration during the practice of meditation.

Meditation: Originally based in spiritual traditions, the practice of awareness, focus, and concentration while maintaining a passive yet awake attitude; evolves with discipline and practice and is known to provide health benefits as well as being a road to personal and spiritual transformation.

Pain (medical definition): Localized sensation of hurt, or an unpleasant sensory and emotional experience associated with actual or potential tissue damage, or described in terms of such damage.

Pain (nursing definition): A subjective experience including both verbal and nonverbal behavior.

Power: Barrett's theory of power as knowing participation in change is being aware of what one is choosing to do, feeling free to do it, and doing it intentionally.

Progressive muscle relaxation: The process of alternately tensing and relaxing muscle groups to become aware of subtle degrees of tension and relaxation; originally developed by Edmund Jacobson.

Relaxation (psychophysiologic definition): A psychophysiologic experience characterized by parasympathetic dominance involving multiple visceral and somatic systems; the absence of physical, mental, and emotional tension; the opposite of Canon's fight-or-flight response and Selye's general adaptation syndrome.

Relaxation response: An alert, hypokinetic process of decreased sympathetic nervous system arousal that may be achieved in a number of ways, including through breathing exercises, relaxation and imagery exercises, biofeedback, and prayer. A degree of discipline is required to evoke this response, which increases mental and physical well-being.

Self-hypnosis: An approach for voluntarily fostering a consciousness process for the purpose of influencing one's thoughts, perceptions, behaviors, or sensations.

Stress (psychophysiologic definition): The felt experience of overactivity of the sympathetic nervous system.

■ THEORY AND RESEARCH

People are frequently told to "just relax" or "take it easy" as part of their recovery from illness, as if everyone knew how to practice this skill. Yet the ancients knew that relaxation is a paradox; it is and is not simple. Throughout the ages, in cultures around the world, practitioners of the sacred healing arts and sciences developed and practiced stopping, quieting, and calming on a disciplined and regular basis, offering themselves deep rest to still the bodymindspirit and emotions. They did this not only to access their natural ability to heal, restore, and renew their bodymindspirit, but also to open themselves to the divine, the oneness of being, the numinous. As the waves of the mind stilled and the activity of the body quieted into the deep rest and relaxation found within their meditative refuge and relaxation practice, this oneness of being offered itself to these ancient spiritual voyagers.

Today we continue this voyage to touch shores beyond our unhealthy habit patterns and belief systems through the practice of the ancient arts of relaxation, meditation, yoga, qi gong, and breathing, and their modern counterparts: autogenic training, progressive muscle relaxation, hypnosis, biofeedback, self-regulation, relaxation response, and body scanning.

We now understand relaxation to be an ancient art with many modern interpretations, which have been anchored throughout nursing practice from childbirth education to pre- and postoperative teaching. Relaxation has been defined in medical and scientific terms as a psychophysiologic state characterized by parasympathetic dominance involving multiple visceral and somatic systems. It is also defined as the absence of physical, mental, and emotional tension, and the opposite of Canon's fight-or-flight response.

Relaxation can also be described as an experience or process of calm, comfort, deep rest, natural nurturing, inner connectedness, renewal, and openness that every living creature instinctively and intuitively knows how to access.

Unfortunately, the conditioning in place makes this activity more the exceptional experience than the norm, thereby leading to the development of stress-related illnesses (which account for 75–80% of illness in modern life).

Therefore, the benefits of relaxation practice are great, especially for our hectic, modern, over-scheduled, multitasking, technology-driven lives. Relaxation interventions are useful for people in all stages of health and illness: the critically ill, expectant parents attending childbirth preparation classes, taxi drivers learning to regulate blood pressure while weaving through city traffic, and nursing students dealing with test anxiety.[1] Even in the acute phase of recovery from a myocardial infarction, or during an examination in an emergency room after an accident, clients can derive the clinical benefits of relaxation by learning basic breathing and muscle relaxation exercises (see **Exhibit 16-1**).

Over the past four decades, nurses in all areas of practice can be found who offer relaxation and breathing techniques and some form of meditation to their clients. Yet this is not new to nursing. Florence Nightingale counseled her nurses to support patients' rest and well-being by reducing unnecessary noise, not awakening patients out of their first sleep, and protecting patients from unnecessary disturbances such as conversations of doctors or friends within earshot and the disturbing rustling of crinolines. She advised that "all hurry or bustle is peculiarly painful to the sick."[2] One wonders what Nightingale would say if she were to visit hospitals and healthcare settings today and witness our efforts to follow her legacy in the chaos of our times.

These days, nurses offer relaxation practices in self-care circles for themselves and their colleagues, as well as for clients in hospitals, community and adult education programs, outpatient clinics, and homeless shelters, to promote a variety of personal benefits (see **Exhibit 16-2**). Nurses also offer these practices to individuals, families, groups, children in classrooms, clients and families in home care and hospice, and workers and executives in workplaces and corporations.

Cross-Cultural Context

Relaxation practices are found throughout time in all cultures around the world. Whether these practices are mediated through the use of herbs, acupuncture, movement, or prayer, evidence of the power, impact, and importance of relaxation and the use of breath can be seen in shamanic healing, yoga, meditation, Chinese medicine, and other traditions around the globe. Modern research exploring the area of psychoneuroimmunology demonstrates the vital importance of relaxation in improving immune system function. Thus, psychoneuroimmunologic research suggests the importance of this ancient practice for our modern scientific world. (See Chapter 31 for further information.) Modern psychology uses relaxation as a dimension of systematic desensitization, in which clients learn to relax in the face of mild, then moderate, and then intense stressors. Neuroplasticity research investigates how neuroscience is influenced by practices of mindfulness showing how the structure and function of the brain are much more changeable than originally believed. This new field demonstrates that cultivating the mind also changes

EXHIBIT 16-1   Clinical Benefits of Relaxation

Relaxation training has the following clinical benefits:

- Decreases the anxiety accompanying painful situations, such as debridement or dressing changes
- Eases the muscle tension pain of skeletal muscle contractions
- Decreases fatigue by interrupting the fight-or-flight response
- Provides a period of rest as beneficial as a nap
- Helps the client fall asleep quickly
- Increases the effect of pain medications
- Increases ability to tolerate pain

EXHIBIT 16-2   Whole Self Benefits of Relaxation

Relaxation has the following benefits to self:

- Decreases pain
- Decreases anxiety
- Improves immune system function
- Quiets the fight-or-flight sympathetic response
- Facilitates sleep
- Provides rest
- Increases efficacy of pain medications
- Reduces muscle tension and increases blood flow
- Improves sense of well-being
- Offers insight and creativity

or grows the brain.[3] Practitioners of biofeedback include relaxation practice with their therapy to help clients learn to self-regulate their peripheral temperature, heart rate velocity, muscle activity, and brain wave frequencies.

Jon Kabat-Zinn in his original research at the University of Massachusetts found relaxation breathing and body scanning to be a vital dimension of a mindfulness-based stress reduction practice used for dealing with pain and depression.[4] Dean Ornish includes relaxation, meditation, breathing, and yoga in his pioneering cardiac rehab program to reverse heart disease.[5] Dolores Krieger and Dora Kunz guided nurses to perform sustained centering and presencing, a practice of meditative inner connection and relaxed awareness, before entering into therapeutic touch practice with their clients.[6,7] These modern pioneers all continue to validate the importance of the ancient practice of relaxation through the use of its modern counterparts.

Caring for Ourselves, Caring for Others: A Spiritual Journey

These days the practice of relaxation in its many forms is more important for nurses than it ever was. These challenging times of constant change and global uncertainty require nurses to walk a wellness path of self-care, self-healing, and spiritual awareness. Finding and then cultivating a personal relaxation practice can help nurses restore, renew, deepen professional self-development avoid burnout, as well as model a personal wellness path for their clients. Living this path and sharing by example gives nurses an inner understanding and appreciation of the benefits and challenges their clients face as they start to integrate complementary practice into their everyday lives.

Relaxation practice offers nurses an important refuge, a self-awareness foundation for deepening their spiritual journey as holistic caregivers. Whether individuals are being with themselves and with "all that is" in meditation; exploring their own past issues, traumas, or painful life experiences in counseling and psychotherapy; or expanding their awareness in intuitive practices and energy healing, a foundation of deep relaxation of the bodymindspirit is a fundamental step on the path. Long-time practitioners of healing arts continue to loop back, reconnect, and deepen their abilities to relax and renew with each step of their path (see **Exhibit 16-3**).

The American psyche, poised to do everything with intensity and competitiveness, also enters with us into self-healing and spiritual practices. This intensity and competitiveness can be our undoing, especially if we forget the importance to our bodymindspirit of nondoing, which is different from "doing nothing." Holistic practice, whether offered within the biomedical healthcare system or explored in a retreat setting, offers health and healing benefits with clinical implications but remains in its essence an avenue for spiritual renewal. Achaan Chah offers us guidance in his wise insight on letting go, peace, and nondoing.

EXHIBIT 16-3   Benefits of Relaxation for the Nurse and Holistic Nursing Practice

Relaxation:

- Is an essential element of self-care
- Cultivates a centered, calm presence
- As a self-care practice offers insights into challenges and benefits clients will experience
- Offers a vehicle to modulate and self-regulate the nurse's own stress response in stress-filled work settings
- Supports a therapeutic energetic bond and connectedness when practicing along with clients or colleagues
- Creates opportunity for intuitive exploration, insight, and understanding of self and others, issues, and problems
- Is an excellent vehicle for beginning professional gatherings and staff meetings; offers opportunity to be present, creative, open, and connected
- Can be done anywhere, without any cost or equipment, is easily teachable, and easily practiced
- Can be a spiritual practice for opening ourselves to deeper ways of being

Do everything with a mind that lets go,
Do not expect any praise or reward.
If you let go a little, you will have a
little peace.
If you let go a lot, you will have a lot
of peace.
If you let go completely, you will know
complete peace and freedom.
Your struggles with the world will have
come to an end.[8]

Nurses must reclaim their legacy of caring by cultivating their compassion, wisdom, spirit of service, and heart-centered health care in their culture. Relaxation is a first step along this path. It is easy to learn and practice; its benefits are demonstrated quite readily; and it offers nurses an easy entree to a self-care plan for themselves, their colleagues, and their clients.

The Stress Response

The last decade has brought new awareness to what constitutes an emergency response, both for individuals and for society. Whether we are dealing with a national or international tragedy or disaster or the everyday intense internal reactions we experience when faced with a truck cutting in front of us on the highway, a "code blue" coming over the loudspeaker, or a child darting into the street, we experience what some researchers refer to as an "adrenaline rush," the familiar fight-or-flight response. This response

is actually a complex series of psychophysiologic processes that prepare us to deal with the real or perceived emergency. It is important to note that people respond to an imagined threat in the same way that they respond to an actual threat to their well-being. That is why in times of personal threat, such as facing a possible health crisis or the fear of potential terrorism, these practices help us keep balanced or self-regulated.

The following are the generalized stress responses of the body, mind, and energy field:

- Constriction of blood flow to the hands and feet (cool extremities)
- Tightening of the muscles
- Constriction of one's energy field (closing down or blocking flow)
- Increased heart rate
- Increased oxygen consumption
- Increased brain wave activity
- Increased sweat gland activity
- Increased blood pressure
- Increased anxiety

This stress response readies the bodymindspirit through this instinctive response pattern to prepare for a stress, shock, or trauma. In modern life, the body physically alerts or readies itself far beyond what is needed to deal with a fast-paced stressful life. Most people know how to turn on this stress response but have little familiarity with how to relax or turn it off. Not only do people not know how to relax, but our society typically has a negative view of relaxed people.

The paradox is that masters of ancient practices have learned that, although instinctive responses such as the fight-or-flight response can put one on alert to help protect one in an emergency or a crisis, a more conscious relaxation discipline, practice, and philosophy offer deeper possibilities.

An example for understanding this philosophy is the ancient Chinese hexagram for crisis. The two Chinese characters that make up the word *crisis* are danger and opportunity. Hidden within each crisis is an opportunity, not just a danger. People must learn to face the danger and seize the opportunity. In practice, relaxation offers people that possibility of turning a difficult situation around for the better.

EXERCISE

Imagine a relaxed person. Write as many words as you can to describe that image. After making your list, note how many of those words you consider to represent a positive quality in a person, how many of those words society considers as representing a positive quality, and how many of those words are considered as representing a positive quality of a person in the workplace. Log any awareness or insights you gain from this exercise in a journal. See if these insights help you when you are discussing relaxation practice with clients, colleagues, family members, and others. Look into the real and perceived costs and benefits of multitasking. This exercise may help you to become aware of conscious or unconscious positive and negative attitudes that can affect clients' interest and motivation to learn to relax.

■ MEDITATION

Relaxation Response Meditation

Though many people call the body-mind-spirit effects of relaxation the "relaxation response," this phrase is attributed to Herbert Benson and his colleagues at Harvard University, who used a nonreligious form of meditation that is similar to transcendental meditation to produce the opposite of the fight-or-flight response. Their relaxation response meditation has been introduced into many healthcare settings and has been applied in a variety of studies that demonstrate its efficacy in treating hypertension and anxiety.[9] Both transcendental meditation and relaxation response meditation offer a practice consisting of 20 minutes of daily passive concentration focused on a neutral word, such as the Sanskrit word *Om* in transcendental meditation or *one* in relaxation response meditation. In relaxation response meditation, slow repetition of the word with each exhalation has been shown to bring about the same psychophysiologic responses as other deep relaxation processes (described later). Further studies have documented a deep relaxation response when the client focuses on a short, personally meaningful religious statement or quotation, as was found in what Benson termed the "faith factor."

The changes that occur when an individual reaches a deep level of relaxation are exactly the opposite of those that occur in the fight-or-flight response. Alterations take place in the automatic, endocrine, immune, and neuropeptide systems as follows:

- Deep relaxation increases
  - Peripheral blood flow (warm extremities)
  - Electrical resistance of skin (dry palms)
  - Production of slow alpha waves
  - Activity of natural killer cells (improved immune function)
- Deep relaxation decreases the following functions in the body:
  - Oxygen consumption
  - Carbon dioxide elimination
  - Blood lactate levels
  - Respiratory rate and volume
  - Heart rate
  - Skeletal muscle tension
  - Epinephrine level
  - Gastric acidity and motility
  - Sweat gland activity
  - Blood pressure, especially in hypertensive individuals[10]

Benson calls relaxation response meditation "a very simple technique." For centuries, many elements of the relaxation response have been elicited within a religious context in cultures around the world.

Benson cites four basic elements that are common to all relaxation response practices: a quiet environment, a mental device, a passive attitude, and a comfortable position. To incorporate these four factors, Benson recommends that the practitioner first create a quiet environment devoid of all noises and distractions. Next, the meditator is asked to choose a mental device, that is, the "constant stimulus of a single-syllable sound or word." This word is repeated silently or in a low, gentle tone. To allow rest and relaxation, the person is invited to adopt a passive attitude, not forcing the relaxation response. The meditator also is counseled to simply disregard any distracting thoughts that enter the mind.[11] To reduce any stress or muscular effort, the meditator should assume a comfortable position on the floor or use a chair. Incorporating these elements and focusing on the mental device of the word *one* for 20 minutes each day facilitates the relaxation response.

The holistic nurse may wish to explore and experience each of the relaxation practices presented in this chapter and write her or his insights and experiences in a journal.

Breathing In and Breathing Out

One of the simplest and deepest relaxation practices is right under our noses every moment of every day: breathing. We have special breathing practices to assist childbirth, and we recognize special breathing patterns when we are dying. In between, we breathe each moment, and our breathing patterns reflect our lives' peaks and valleys, our stresses, and our relaxing moments.

Beyond the unconscious breathing pattern that most people are involuntarily practicing is a conscious breathing practice described long ago in the ancient sacred texts of yoga, the Buddha's Four Foundations of Mindfulness, Taoist qi gong practice, native shamanic practices, and spiritual teachings and practices from around the world.

Conscious awareness of breathing—whether the slow, deep, diaphragmatic breaths of hatha yoga or the mindful awareness of breathing in and out in mindfulness meditation—can be practiced in formal sessions of 20 to 45 minutes once or twice a day. Conscious awareness of breathing also can be practiced informally by breathing with mindfulness during everyday activities.

Jon Kabat-Zinn developed a mindfulness-based stress-reduction program that demonstrates how conscious awareness of breathing can help to relieve chronic pain, depression, and anxiety. Participants in the 8-week program practice mindfulness meditation every day; they also practice body scanning (systematically bringing attention to each part of the body, letting the attention rest there, letting go of any judgment about how it is "supposed to feel," being with this part of the body, and then moving on to the next place in the body), and yoga (performance of meditative asanas or postures combined with breathing to create a union of body, mind, and spirit). Several studies in clinics, communities, and prisons have demonstrated that Kabat-Zinn's program, as well as other modern forms of meditation, can improve quality of life and reduce symptoms (see **Table 16-1**).

Breathing and Energy Healing Practice

Breathing practice is also an integral dimension of yoga and qi gong. The breath or life force, called *prana* in yoga and *qi* (or *chi* or *ki*) in Chinese energy practice, is the vital force or energy that animates life. Nurses practicing therapeutic touch center themselves through conscious meditation on their intention to help or to heal, by letting go of outside distractions, and by opening themselves to allow the universal life force to flow through them to their clients. They can use their breathing practice to help enhance this sustained centeredness and their openness to this healing life force.

The ancient yogis knew that by learning to consciously control their breathing and their bodies through practicing a series of yoga postures (asanas), they could open and ready themselves for transcendent awareness. As mentioned previously, yoga practices also have been demonstrated in the work of Kabat-Zinn and Ornish to have great health benefits.

Qi gong practices date back to about 5000 bce. Taoist and Buddhist qi gong masters channeled the flow of qi from nature and the universe through their bodies by practicing simple movements, combined with an awareness of breathing and meditation.

TABLE 16-1   Research-Based Outcomes of Meditation

Practice	Modern Forms	Adapted By	Clinical Benefits	Researcher
Meditation	Mindfulness, insight meditation, vispassana		See list of deep relaxation changes in Relaxation Responses section	
	Transcendental meditation (TM)	Maharashi Mahesh Yogi	TM reduces the affective/motivational dimension of the brain's response to pain.	Orme-Johnson et al. (2006)[12]
	Relaxation response meditation	Herbert Benson (1975)	Decreased hypertension	Benson et al. (1974)[13]
	Mindfulness-based stress reduction	Jon Kabat-Zinn (1977)	Decreased chronic pain	Kabat-Zinn et al. (1987)[14]
			Significant pain reduction for chronic arthritis, back, neck pain. Less pain reduction for headache, migraine	Rosenzweig S, Gresson JM, Reibel DK, et al. (2010)[15]
			Enhanced immune function, QoL and coping in women newly diagnosed with early stage breast cancer	Witek-Janusek L. et al. (2008)[16]
Prayer	Loving Kindness Meditation		Lovingkindness offers improvements in low back pain & psychological distress	Carson JW, et al. (2005)[17]
			Lovingkindness meditation over time "increases mindfulness, purpose in life, social support, decreased illness symptoms"	Fredrickson, B. et al. (2008)[18]
Moving Meditation	Yoga, meditation, stress reduction, nutrition, lifestyle	Dean Ornish	Reversal of heart disease	Ornish (1990)[19]
	Yoga/Meditation		Reduced performance anxiety, improved mood	Khalsa, Shorter, S. et al. (2009)[20]
	Qi Gong, Chi Kung		Decrease in physical pain and emotional distress. Improved sleep, concentration, decision making.	Coleman, J. (2010)[21]
			Qi gong in the treatment of mild essential hypertension	Cheung, et al. (2005)[22]
	Therapeutic Touch	Delores Krieger/Dora Kunz		See Ch 19

These ancient Chinese practices, which are one of the dimensions of traditional Chinese medicine, have long been renowned for producing health benefits and slowing the aging process. These effects are now being researched and documented in scientific literature (see Table 16-1).

Yoga and qi gong practitioners consider these disciplines essential self-care practices for the unitary body-mind-spirit. These practitioners demonstrate a living legacy of self-care that not only offers healing to their patients, but is the fundamental requirement for development of a healer or teacher. In contrast, the Western scientific course of study does not emphasize the cultivation of one's own personal wellness and spiritual development as a prerequisite for becoming a licensed healthcare professional.

Other Forms of Meditation

As illustrated by transcendental meditation and the works of Benson and Kabat-Zinn, there are many forms of meditation. Some say that hundreds of practices can be listed under the heading of meditation. Each practice cultivates a qualitative state of mind that can induce a deep experience of relaxation and calm. In some meditative practices, such as transcendental meditation and relaxation response meditation, the individual focuses on an object of meditation to move away from and minimize thoughts. Other traditions, such as mindfulness meditation, insight meditation, and vispassana meditation, invite practitioners to cultivate greater focus by returning to the breath as sensations, thoughts, and feelings are present.

Centering prayer, a Christian meditation practice developed by Father Thomas Keating, focuses on words or sounds in somewhat the same way that transcendental meditation uses mantras (sacred Sanskrit syllables and words such as *Om*). Other meditation practices invite meditators to gaze at the flame of a candle, a sacred image, or a mandala; to chant aloud; or to concentrate on a nondualist or unanswerable question (or koan), as in Zen practice.

Janet Macrae calls therapeutic touch a moving meditation.[23] Sufi dancing is another form of moving meditation, as are Native American and shamanic ritual dances, which may continue for many hours or many days. The purpose of spiritually focused meditation is to awaken to a higher consciousness, to be at one with the sacredness of "All," and to become one with the Divine. Individuals practice such meditation to open the bodymindspirit to the qualities of compassion, wisdom, forgiveness, skillfulness, no fear, stillness, openness, and interconnectedness.

The healing arts are the underpinning of many cultures' healing traditions. For example, Tibetan healers begin their education at an early age, studying sacred texts on healing and herbs as well as meditating and praying each day to cultivate a heart of compassion and loving kindness and to become one with the compassionate healing energy and wisdom of the limitless realms. After years of study and apprenticeship (some healers apprentice from childhood), they practice their healing art, the science of the bodymindspirit.

What would health care be like if nurses, physicians, and other healthcare practitioners began by cultivating a heart of compassion and service? What would the healthcare system be like? Would burnout exist? (See the section titled "Loving Kindness Meditation" later in this chapter.)

Meditation Practices

This era will give birth to many distillations of ancient meditative practices, including intricate Tibetan meditative practices, because of their health benefits. Finding a meditation practice and learning to explore it deeply offer healing and insight, a gift only gained from committed practice.

Mindful Breathing During Nursing Practice

Nurses who wish to be more present with their clients, to practice self-care, and to awaken to the simple sacredness of everyday nursing practice (e.g., hanging an intravenous bag, writing nursing notes, eating, walking down a hall, feeding a patient) may want to practice mindful breathing each moment, as in the following exercises.

EXERCISE: BREATHING I

Script: Breathing in, I am aware of breathing in.

Breathing out, I am aware of breathing out.

Breathing in, I am aware of introducing this healing medication through this intravenous line.

Breathing out, I send my healing intentions along with the medication to help support this patient's healing.

EXERCISE: BREATHING II

Script: Breathing in, I am walking down this hall.

Breathing out, I smile, enjoying my steps.

Breathing in, I am fresh.

Breathing out, I celebrate my aliveness.

Begin with the breath, reminding oneself to offer self-care in each moment by consciously breathing with each activity, is a gift of self-renewal, freshness, and aliveness that deepens with practice. It is a gift nurses can give to themselves every moment.

Mindful Breathing Meditations

Exploring and practicing relaxation and meditation help the nurse gain insight into specific methods and issues that clients may face as they work to integrate these techniques into their daily lives. It also offers the nurse an opportunity for personal wellness, self-care, and spiritual development. When choosing a meditation practice to explore, the nurse should commit to that practice for at least 4–6 weeks before trying another, while keeping a journal of his or her reflections along the way.

EXERCISE

Mindfulness of the Breath Exercise I (Lying Down)

Mindfulness of breathing is made up of two forms of energy: the energy cultivated by bringing attention to the breath called awareness and the energy of bringing attention back lovingly over and over to the breath called concentration. Our minds naturally wander, so the practice of bringing the attention back to the breath is itself an integral practice of mindfulness meditation. To begin, lie on the floor with your hands on your abdomen. Close your eyes and feel the movement of your body with every rise and fall of the breath. Follow both the inhalation and exhalation fully.

With each inhale, repeat, in your mind, "Breathing in, I am aware of breathing in," and on each exhale, "Breathing out, I am aware of breathing out." As you continue, you may shorten the phrase by repeating gently in your mind "In" on the in breath and "Out" on the out breath. As you are breathing and lying comfortably with your hands on your abdomen, allow a gentle smile to bloom on your lips and at the corners of your eyes. (After all, this is supposed to be an enjoyable practice.) Try this practice for 15 to 20 minutes. Observe and note any awareness, reflections, and insights in your personal journal. To extend this practice during the next week, you may wish to continue lying down in a comfortable position, or you may choose a sitting meditation practice, as described next.

EXERCISE

Mindfulness of the Breath Exercise II (Sitting)

In a quiet place, find a comfortable seated position. Either sit on a chair with your feet on the floor and your back supported and straight, or sit on the floor using a meditation cushion (zafu) or a regular pillow folded in half to create a supportive lift under your buttocks. If you are sitting on the floor, find a comfortable way to place your legs, either (1) crossed in lotus or half-lotus position with or without pillows under your knees, (2) Indian style, or (3) straight out in front of you, with a pillow under your knees and your back supported against a reclining support or against the wall. Focus on a point on the floor in front of you and gently lower your lids until they are almost closed. Gently bring your attention to your breath.

Script: Breathing in, I am aware of breathing in.
Breathing out, I am aware of breathing out.
In.
Out.
Breathing in, I am calm.
Breathing out, I smile.[24]
—*Thich Nhat Hanh*

Continue to bring your attention to your breath, allowing any thoughts, feelings, or sensations to be gently held by your mindful awareness, as you gently bring your attention back to the breath and the repeated phrase. Practice for approximately 15 to 20 minutes. After your practice, note your experience in your journal.

This practice is an example of using meditation to become aware of our minds and to practice just being, being present in this moment, and nondoing rather than "doing nothing." We get so caught up in believing that we always have to be doing or multitasking that we lose the essence of what is of true value. Mindfulness helps us to get back in touch with what is truly healing within and around us.

As you continue, you may want to note Kabat-Zinn's attitudinal foundations of mindfulness practice, which include nonjudging, patience, trust, nonstriving, the cultivated freshness of seeing everything as new (called beginner's mind), acceptance, and letting go.[25]

Walking Meditation

Walking as if one were planting peace with each step—this is the essence of walking meditation.[4pp33-39] This practice can be especially helpful during times of trauma and crisis and can be done to center oneself in the most challenging and traumatic of circumstances.

To practice, start with the left foot and begin walking slowly by synchronizing the in and out of the breathing meditation practice with each step. Sometimes you may take three steps to the inhale and three steps to the exhale. Play with your practice, exploring how carefully you can become aware of the subtle sensations of slowly lifting, moving, and placing each step as you continue your awareness of breathing.

This practice can be interspersed between sitting practice sessions: 20 minutes of sitting, 10 minutes of walking, 20 minutes of sitting, 10 minutes of walking. This also is a wonderful meditation to practice at a more normal pace of walking at work, as well as going to and from work. "Walking down the hall, I am aware of my footsteps and my breathing. Being in this present moment, I know this is the only moment." Practicing walking meditation often allows the practice to be in our bones so that it is there for us when we need it most.

Cultivating the Heart of Compassion Meditation

Loving Kindness Meditation

This meditation for helping professionals is adapted from Thich Nhat Hanh's loving kindness meditation in *Teachings on Love*.[26]

Sitting peacefully, begin as in sitting meditation practice, and then plant each phrase like a healing seed within your heart, following your breath and focusing on your intention to cultivate compassion. Say each line to yourself in your mind, or ask a friend to read this meditation aloud to you, pausing after each line so that you can slowly repeat it silently to yourself.

Part I: May I be peaceful.
May I be happy.
May I look to myself with the eyes of compassion and love.
May I be safe.
May I be free from accidents.

May I be compassionate with my anger and gentle with my fear.

May I be spacious and compassionate to the depths of my true heart.

May I be whole.

May I be well.

May I be free.

May I be peaceful.

May I be happy.

In Part II of this meditation, repeat the same meditation while imagining that someone you care about or are having difficulty with is sitting in front of you, and center your attention on cultivating and offering compassion while repeating silently in your mind:

Part II: May you be peaceful.

May you be happy.

May you look to yourself with the eyes of compassion and love.

May you be safe.

May you be free from accidents.

May you be compassionate with your anger and gentle with your fear.

May you be spacious and compassionate to the depth of your true heart.

May you be whole.

May you be well.

May you be free.

May you be peaceful.

May you be happy.

Then, in Part III, imagine offering compassion to all beings on Earth, to the Earth, to all the planets, and to all beings throughout the universe and beyond time and space:

Part III: May all beings be peaceful.

May all beings be happy.

May all beings look to themselves with the eyes of compassion and love.

May all beings be safe.

May all beings be free from accidents.

May all beings be compassionate with their anger and gentle with their fear.

May all beings be spacious and compassionate to the depths of their true heart.

May all beings be whole.

May all beings be well.

May all beings be free.

May all beings be peaceful.

May all beings be happy.

For other heart-opening meditations, see the St. Francis prayer and www.Beliefnet.com.

Quiet Heart Prayer

One of the most frequently used traditional nursing spiritual therapies is prayer.[27] Prayer is a way of eliciting the relaxation response in the context of one's deeply held personal, religious, or philosophic beliefs. Benson refers to this as incorporating the "faith factor" into relaxation. Many people are comfortable with prayer as meditation, and it requires only seconds to minutes. In healthcare settings, nurses need to accommodate the client's spiritual needs, either by calling on his or her personal spiritual and religious background and resources or by enlisting the help of appropriate family of the client, clergy, or chaplaincy staff.

■ MODERN RELAXATION METHODS

Progressive Muscle Relaxation

In 1935, Edmund Jacobson detailed a strategy leading to deep muscle relaxation. The body responds to anxious thoughts and stressful events with increased muscle tension. This body-mind-spirit tension further provokes subjective sensations of anxiety. In progressive muscle relaxation, the practitioner deliberately tenses muscle groups, focusing on the tightening sensations, and then slowly releases that tension. In this way, the individual learns to manage levels of muscle tension. Progressive muscle relaxation allows the client to deepen the experience of comfort.

Several studies have demonstrated that progressive muscle relaxation reduces subjective feelings of anxiety and increases peak expiratory flow rates in asthmatic clients; it also helps clients with insomnia, headaches, ulcers, hypertension, and colitis (see **Table 16-2**).

TABLE 16-2   Research-Based Outcomes of Relaxation

Modern Form of Relaxation Practice	Developed By	Clinical Benefits	Researcher
Progressive muscle relaxation (PMR)	Jacobson	Immunocompetence in geriatric population: those practicing PMR demonstrated better immunocompetence (increased natural killer cell count and herpes antibodies) and decreased stress	Keicolt-Glaser et al. (1985)[28]
		Immunoenhancement demonstrated through PMR induced relaxation	Pawlow, L. and Jones, G. (2005)[29]
PMR and voice characteristics of therapist		Study supports speaking in a "smooth and quiet, perhaps even monotonous, but not purposely hypnotic" tone while pacing the therapist's voice rhythm with the breathing of patient positively impacts therapeutic PMR training	Knowlton, G. and Larkin, K. (2006)[30]
Autogenic training	Schultz and Luthe	Reduced muscle tone, blood pressure, and skin resistance	Schultz and Luthe (1959)[31]
		Generalized improvement in IBS	Shinozaki, M. et al. (2010)[32]
AT/biofeedback therapy		Reduced idiopathic essential hypertension	Fahrion (1991)[33]
Biofeedback		Heart Rate Velocity Biofeedback plus treatment as usual improved combat-related PTSD symptoms in veterans	Tan, G. et al. (2011)[34]
Biofeedback-assisted relaxation		HRV enhances vagal heart rate control	Nolan et al. (2005)[35]
		Reduced BP in adults with stage 1 or 2 hypertension (78% taking BP medications)	Yucha, CB. (2005)[36]
		Biofeedback and relaxation with Type 2 diabetes demonstrate lower blood glucose for up to 3 months after treatment	McGinnis et al. (2005)[37]

In the original form of progressive muscle relaxation, clients learn to relax 16 of the body's muscle groups. They inhale while tensing their muscles, and then exhale and relax their muscles very slowly. Variations on progressive muscle relaxation, or modified progressive muscle relaxation, are integrated into many relaxation practices.

EXERCISE

Progressive Muscle Relaxation Tension Awareness

The purpose of a tension awareness exercise is to help the client identify subtle levels of mental tension and anxiety and the physical tension that accompanies these mental and emotional states. The client who is aware of the internal differences induced by this exercise can move to threshold levels of tension, holding just enough tightness in the muscle group to be aware of beginning tension and then relaxing the group. By moving from strong contractions to very subtle ones, the client becomes aware of the ability to fine-tune the relaxation process. Read through this script first because you are invited to insert the names of other areas of the body into the text as you go. This exercise requires 10 to 30 minutes depending on how many areas of the body you include.

Script: First take a few moments to focus on your breathing. This will help you to focus better on internal cues of muscle tension and then relaxation. I will guide you as we begin to move through the muscles of your body. Become aware of how you can gain control over the tension found in those muscles. This process involves alternately tightening and relaxing muscle groups. Let yourself tighten each muscle group, hold the tension for 5 to 10 seconds or until mild fatigue is felt in the area, and then release the tension. . . . Begin with the muscles in your feet and calves; tighten that area as much as you can. Pull your toes up toward your head, and become aware that, as the muscles tighten and as you continue to hold that tightness, your legs will perhaps tremble or shake a bit as they fatigue. . . . Now, let the tension slowly dissolve and feel the difference in your lower legs and feet. . . . Let your attention move up to your knees and thighs; tense those muscles by pressing your legs into the surface of the bed (couch, floor, chair).

. . . When you are aware of how they feel, then allow the tension to drift away as you exhale.

The exercise then proceeds to the following areas: hips and buttocks, abdomen and lower back, chest and upper back, shoulders and biceps, forearms and hands, neck and shoulders, jaw and tongue, and finally facial muscles. Insert these areas into the script to continue the exercise.

If the client is experiencing pain or difficulty with a particular part of the body, the exercise should begin as far away from the involved area as possible and conclude with the primary area of difficulty.

Clients should be coached to breathe throughout the session, thereby avoiding the temptation to hold their breath as they tighten their muscles. Clients may learn to exhale as they tighten muscle groups. Tension in muscles should be held short of true discomfort.

Progressive muscle relaxation is particularly effective for clients who are feeling physically tense, anxious, and perhaps agitated. Because it is an active intervention, it may be preferable to other passive exercises, especially early in client training. It should be used with caution for clients with ischemic myocardial disease, hypertension, and back pain, however.

Autogenic Training

In 1932, Johannes Schultz and his student, Wolfgang Luthe, developed a series of brief phrases designed to focus attention on various parts of the body and induce a body–mind shift in those parts. The phrases that were developed are called autogenic because of their ability to assist a person in inducing self- (auto) change from within. This approach to health care was rather new in the 1930s.

Although similar to self-hypnosis, autogenic strategies are a specific present-time-oriented means of gaining access to the natural restorative mechanisms of the mind. Autogenic training has been found to be effective in managing disorders in which cognitive involvement is prominent (see

Table 16-2). These self-healing phrases can be combined with progressive muscle relaxation as an integrative approach to relaxation to help a broader spectrum of clients. Autogenic training is one of the most widely used approaches in teaching clients to warm their hands during biofeedback temperature training.

EXERCISE

Autogenic Training

Clients may find autogenic training helpful to consciously rebalance the internal homeokinetic mechanisms of the cardiovascular and respiratory systems, which simultaneously affect the autonomic, endocrine, immune, and neuropeptide systems. The exercise generally lasts 10 to 20 minutes.

Script: Slowly and silently repeat the following phrases to yourself as I say them out loud to you (repeat each phrase two to four times, pausing a few seconds between each repetition): "I am beginning to feel quiet. . . . I am beginning to feel relaxed. . . . My feet, knees, and hips feel heavy. . . . Heaviness and warmth are flowing through my feet and legs. . . . My hands, arms, and shoulders feel heavy. . . . Warmth and heaviness are flowing through my hands and arms. . . . My neck, jaw, and forehead feel relaxed and smooth. . . . My whole body feels quiet, heavy, and comfortable. . . . I am comfortably relaxed. . . . Warmth and heaviness flow into my arms, hands, and fingertips. . . . My breathing is slow and regular. . . . I am aware of my calm, regular heartbeat. . . . My mind is becoming quieter as I focus inward. . . . I feel still. . . . Deep in my mind I experience myself as relaxed, comfortable, and still. . . . I am alert in a quiet, inward way. As I finish my relaxation, I take in several deep, reenergizing breaths, bringing light and energy into every cell of my body."

Autogenic training should begin in a warm (75°F to 80°F) room to facilitate sensations of warmth. Clients can progress to cooler environments to generalize their training (to simulate being outside). Using the phrases while the mind is relaxed and receptive allows the peripheral circulation to increase and cardiac and respiratory rates and rhythms to slow and stabilize. Several weeks may be required for the client to feel sensations of heaviness and warmth, although the client usually achieves restful heart rate and respiratory patterning much sooner.

Effects of Relaxation Therapies

Over the past four decades, practitioners involved in stress reduction, relaxation training, and biofeedback have questioned whether all the various techniques elicit a single relaxation response, as hypothesized by Herbert Benson in 1975, or whether specific practices render specific effects. The latter view proposes that specific cognitive effects are produced by the use of cognitively oriented methods (see the section on "Autogenic Training" earlier in this chapter), autonomic effects are produced by autonomically oriented methods, and muscular effects are produced by muscularly oriented methods (see the section titled "Progressive Muscle Relaxation" earlier in this chapter). See **Table 16-3**.

Holistic Nurse Learning Experiment I

One of the most effective tools for understanding relaxation is self-exploration and self-experimentation. Within her- or himself, the nurse is a minilaboratory able to explore these various methods and do her or his own inner research. All that is needed is a journal and the commitment to inner exploration and personal and professional self-development.

A commitment must be made to practice the method for at least 4 to 8 weeks to explore beyond initial positive or negative reactions. Practice each day, following your script or recording of the practice, and keep a journal of your awareness observations: how you felt in your body before and after the session, any areas of comfort or discomfort you noted before or after the session, and so on (see **Exhibit 16-4**).

TABLE 16-3   Hypothesized Effects of Relaxation Techniques

Relaxation Technique	Hypothesized Effect	Researcher
Progressive muscle relaxation (PMR)	Modified PMR might be expected to develop muscular skill	Davidson and Schwartz (1976)[38]
Autogenic training (AT)	AT might generate both cognitive and somatic effects because it emphasizes body awareness through repeated self-suggestion.	Linden (1993)[39]
AT vs. PMR	AT is particularly effective in cultivating specific sensations suggested in the self-suggestion statements and has much greater effects in that realm than does PMR.	Lehrer et al. (1980)[40] Shapiro and Lehrer (1980)[41]
Relaxation response meditation	Relaxation response elicited is hypothesized to be universal (i.e., all relaxation techniques are considered equivalent).	Benson (1975)[42]

After practicing, exploring, and writing a journal about your selected practice, you may want to explore another practice in a similar fashion and compare and contrast their effects.

Another method of exploration is to invite others to join you in experimenting with the same practice or different ones. Holding periodic group meetings to review your observations and your inner laboratory journals can help you to explore variations in experiences with the same practice and compare and contrast differences in and preferences for various practices.

Selecting Relaxation Interventions for Clients

No formula exists for determining which relaxation intervention is best for which client. The approach must be tailored to the individual based on his or her condition, personal preferences, and available time. A few clients may initially resist the idea of relaxation practice in spite of the nurse's best efforts to present it in a positive manner. In this situation, the issue need not be forced, for the client may accept the intervention at a later time. Taking some time to explore the client's experience and the source of the resistance may reveal misconceptions or myths that further dialogue can dispel. Recall your list of descriptors of a relaxed person from the beginning of this chapter and its implications for motivation and client participation.

Audio and video relaxation CDs, DVDs, or online versions of relaxation videos or audio instructions present relaxation in a nonthreatening, gentle manner. Often accompanied by soothing music (and images) this format can be offered over hospital closed-circuit television, downloaded onto clients' electronic devices, iPods, or MP3 players, from the Internet, or become part of a nursing comfort cart on each floor. The use of such media may hasten acceptance of this intervention. Relaxation CDs/downloads can also be played on the home or business audio system as a gentle background for daily activities. The following are guidelines for the client in the use of relaxation audio or videos:

1. Listen to an exercise at least once a day, preferably twice a day.
2. Never listen to a relaxation exercise when you are driving or operating a vehicle.
3. Arrange to have uninterrupted privacy while you listen to the practice.
4. Listen with headphones or ear buds to help block out distracting noises from the environment.
5. Listen or watch in a relaxing position in which your body is supported.

EXHIBIT 16-4   Inner Laboratory Journal

Name _____

Date _____   Practice method _____

Session no. _____   _____

Place of practice _____

Method of practice: iPod/MP3/CD/DVD download   ❏ _____
                       Script   ❏ _____
                       Read aloud   ❏ _____
                       Memorized   ❏ _____
                       Other   ❏ _____

Presession Awareness

High comfort,   Low comfort,
high well-being   low well-being

├──┼──┼──┼──┼──┼──┼──┼──┼──┼──┤
10   9   8   7   6   5   4   3   2   1   0

Describe areas of comfort:

_____

_____

_____

No pain   High pain

├──┼──┼──┼──┼──┼──┼──┼──┼──┼──┤
0   1   2   3   4   5   6   7   8   9   10

Where? (Describe) _____

Postsession Awareness

Note areas of: ❏ Tingling   ❏ Heaviness
                  ❏ Pulsing   ❏ Lightness
                  ❏ Throbbing   ❏ Calm
                  ❏ Warmth   ❏ Inner Peace
                  ❏ Numbness   ❏ Energy Flow
❏ Arms   ❏ Head   ❏ Abdomen
❏ Hands   ❏ Neck   ❏ Back
❏ Legs   ❏ Face   ❏ Chest
❏ Feet   ❏ Jaw   ❏ Shoulders
❏ Hips   ❏ Eyes   ❏ Pelvis

Describe any images, thoughts, feelings:

_____

_____

_____

(continues)

EXHIBIT 16-4   Inner Laboratory Journal

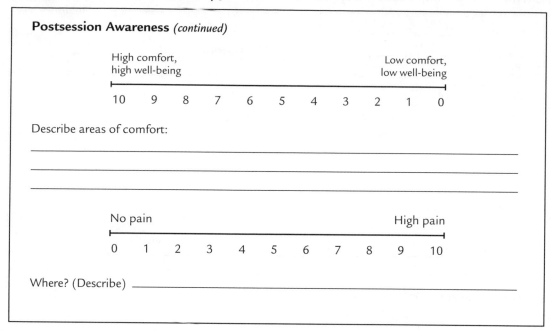

Hypnosis and Self-Hypnosis

Most people misunderstand the use of trance and hypnosis and associate it with stage professionals and entertainment. However, hypnosis and trance have been used for healing and therapeutic purposes from the times of ancient Egypt and Greece. In these ancient societies, priest–healers in healing temples helped their patients evoke a healing process of awareness or trance. Native shamans evoke a trance to seek healing guidance and wisdom for themselves and members of their tribes. In the late 1700s, Viennese physician Franz Mesmer offered "magnetic" treatments to his patients that included hypnosis. The word *mesmerized* is now part of our language—an indication of the impact of Mesmer's work.

Hypnosis has been defined in many ways. Nursing expert Dorothy Larkin, PhD, describes hypnosis as "a process of therapeutic communication, awareness, and behavior within the context of a therapeutic relationship."[43] In hypnosis, attention can be more focused or more mobile, and there is a tendency for greater responsiveness to suggestion. Once the visual, behavioral, and thinking processes and cues associated with hypnosis are understood, they may be seen to occur spontaneously under a variety of circumstances. According to David Cheeks, an expert in the study of trance and hypnosis, "Hypnotic states may occur when people are frightened, disoriented in space, unconscious, very ill, or stammering."[44] These experiences are experiences that nurses' patients and clients experience every day, and thus most nurses first encounter their clients and patients in an already altered process of hypersuggestibility. This naturally occurring trance opens up the client to the influence of nurses' therapeutic presence and therapeutic suggestions.

Recall Cheeks's description of the hypnotic trance of frightened and ill patients, and consider how clients and patients are given the news of their diagnosis and prognosis by their physicians while they are in that state of fear and hypersuggestibility. Many patients today still are told that they have only a few months to live or that nothing can be done for them. This nontherapeutic suggestion is being instilled in a patient's consciousness in a suggestible moment by one of his or her most trusted authorities, the physician. What outcome could be expected? How might the process differ if the client were offered more positive therapeutic suggestions? Nursing experts have been interested in exploring and integrating hypnosis, trance, and therapeutic suggestions because of the history of hypnosis in healing throughout the cultures of the world, because of its natural availability through client hypersuggestibility during healthcare crises, and because of its ease of use and practicality.[45] Larkin and many other nurse experts in hypnosis have explored ways in which therapeutic suggestion can enhance patient cooperation and comfort.[46p88,47]

Nurses can recognize a hypnotic experience in clients who have a faraway stare, glazed eyes, or fixed attention. Larkin notes that nurses

> can utilize this receptive state by offering therapeutic suggestion, reassurance, and health-promoting education. Continual assessment will need to be observed so if the subject's attention suddenly shifts, the nurse can concurrently change the offered therapeutic strategy to meet the patient's needs and altered perceptions.[46]

Learning how to use therapeutic suggestion is not foreign to nurses who have used health education to focus clients on healing and health-promoting phrases to help them reframe their experiences. Norman Cousins, a pioneer in Integrative Health, described an example of reframing an experience and conversational induction in which he supported a man on the street who was having a myocardial infarction. Holding the man's hand, Cousins whispered in his ear that the paramedics were on the way and that the man's body was already beginning to heal itself. He helped the patient begin relaxation breathing and continued to reframe the situation through the use of therapeutic suggestion by introducing simple information about the body's ability to restore, rebalance, and heal during a crisis.[48] Imagine how Cousins's approach contrasts with what usually happens with clients who have heart attacks and do not get any information about their condition, have people speak in terms they can't understand, or have others speak in the room as if they were not present. This form of conversational induction can be most helpful in situations of great crisis or trauma when the patient's capacity for other forms of relaxation may be impeded. "In

daily conversations with patients and families . . . these strategies can help . . . maintain their protective defenses while introducing comfort producing approaches."[47] Learning how to use this skill during usual nursing care embeds this skill deeply into our awareness so that it can be easily accessed in times of crisis or trauma.

Therapeutic suggestion is also a vital accompaniment in disbursing medication. For example, the nurse might say, "This medication will help to quiet your nervous system so that you can relax more comfortably into sleep" rather than, "This pill is for your insomnia." The former emphasizes the possible comfort response, and the latter focuses on the problem. Suggestion and hypnosis have been used in a wide variety of clinical settings. Hypnosis has been used by nurses in hospice care, palliative care, home care, and critical care, as well as in burn units and oncology, obstetrics, medicine, and surgery units, to name only a few areas.

All nurses can learn to use reframing, conversational inductions, and positive therapeutic suggestion, and to recognize an everyday hypnotic trance process of clients in crisis (also see the section titled "Cryptotrauma" later in this chapter). Some nurses may want to pursue hypnosis as an area of expertise by receiving reputable training and may find certification programs through the American Holistic Nurses Association (www.ahna.org) or the American Society for Clinical Hypnosis (www.asch.net). Nurses can also practice self-hypnosis and therapeutic suggestion as part of their personal self-care, in addition to teaching clients this practice so that they can continue self-care at home.

Biofeedback

Another modern form of the ancient healing art of relaxation uses modern technological equipment that most nurses employ daily to monitor body-mind-spirit changes. This combination of ancient awareness practice and technology is called biofeedback. Biofeedback was termed the "yoga of the West" by Elmer and Alyce Green, researchers and early biofeedback pioneers at the Menninger Institute in Topeka, Kansas. When the devices monitoring the unitary bodymind-spirit are turned so that clients can see their displays, clients learn how to read their bodies' signals more accurately and are empowered to make therapeutic changes. Educating clients about how their bodies respond to stress and teaching them how to react more healthfully is the work of biofeedback.

Recall what has just been explored with regard to therapeutic hypnotic suggestion and reframing, and imagine how this new knowledge and awareness might be used to empower clients as they encounter the monitors and other technical equipment in the healthcare setting. If you can imagine turning your monitors around and teaching clients the positive meaning of the monitor's signals so that they can understand how their bodies respond to thoughts and feelings, then you have already begun to understand the impact and usefulness of biofeedback. Biofeedback machines can measure many functions of the unitary bodymindspirit. Whether the biofeedback comes from a temperature monitor measuring hand temperature or from Kirlian photography showing the energy field as displayed on a computer, clients are learning something that, prior to the use of this technology, may have been hidden from their perception. With practice, clients can tune their inner awareness to become like the yogis and learn to influence and control these previously imperceptible and seemingly uncontrollable signals.

The most widely used biofeedback monitors include temperature-sensing units for measuring vasodilatation of extremities, electromyographs for monitoring motor neuron activity of the muscles, electroencephalographs for measuring brain wave frequencies and patterns, and electrodermal response units for measuring electrical activation of the sweat glands. Heart rate variability monitors and blood pressure monitors also are widely used in biofeedback (see **Exhibit 16-5**).

Biofeedback has been practiced since the 1960s. Its focus is to teach clients to create "psychosomatic health," as Elmer Green would put it, instead of psychosomatic illness.[49] This goal is accomplished with the assistance of the biofeedback equipment and the nurse therapist. Specialized training and certification in biofeedback are available through the Association for Applied Psychophysiology and Biofeedback and the Biofeedback Certification Institute of America. Both organizations are established multidisciplinary

groups that integrate the sciences and arts of engineering, psychology, neuroscience, research, education, healing, meditation, and yoga.

Holistic Nurse Learning Experiment II

Biofeedback can offer nurses the opportunity for independent professional practice, whether in private practice or in an institutional setting. Many nurses integrate biofeedback into relaxation therapy, stress management, health counseling, and teaching. Other nurses specialize in neuro-feedback for the care of insomnia, depression, addictions, and attention-deficit hyperactivity disorder. Another area of particular interest to nurses is heart rate variability, as well as the use of electromyography to help

EXHIBIT 16-5   Clinical Indicators for Biofeedback

- Neuromuscular disorders
  - Chronic muscle contraction
  - Movement disorders
  - Spasticity

- Central nervous system disorders
  - Stroke
  - Some epilepsies

- Vascular disorders
  - Raynaud's disease
  - Migraine

- Pain
  - Headache
  - Back pain

- Gastrointestinal and genitourinary disorders
  - Urinary and fecal incontinence
  - Urinary and fecal retention

- Stress reduction
  - Insomnia
  - Anxiety
  - Phobias
  - Alcoholism and addiction
  - Attention-deficit hyperactivity disorder
  - Procedure-related anxiety

clients manage urinary and fecal incontinence (see Table 16-2). All these areas of specialization require extensive study, practice, and mentoring. However, every nurse can benefit from using simple biofeedback principles and techniques in everyday nursing practice. Learning to understand these biofeedback principles from the inside out is the purpose of the following series of experiments. One or two psychophysiologic monitors, paper, and a pen are required. Any monitors available—pulse oximetry, blood pressure, heart rate, incentive spirometer—can be used, or an inexpensive temperature-sensing unit can be purchased through resources found at the Association for Applied Psychophysiology and Biofeedback (www.aapb.org).

Allow 30 minutes for the exercise. Make yourself comfortable. Make sure the environment is relaxing and is as quiet as possible and that there will be no interruptions. Set up the biofeedback equipment, and attach the leads to yourself so that you can easily monitor your responses. Pick only one or two types of equipment, such as an extremity temperature monitor and an automatic blood pressure and/or oxygen saturation rate monitor. If you are setting up a temperature unit, begin by attaching the ceramic end of the wire (called the thermister) to the fleshy, palmar surface of your fingertip (see **Figure 16-1**).

Run the wire down along the length of a finger of your nondominant hand so that the movement of writing your results will not interfere with the temperature and attach the thermister with paper tape so that the tape covers the end of the ceramic tip. You should begin to see changes in the temperature as the heat of your finger warms the thermister. Do not use plastic tape when attaching a thermister because it creates a greenhouse effect and can alter the accuracy of the readings.

The warmer the hands, the greater the blood flow and circulation to the extremities, indicating quieting of the sympathetic nervous system and quieting of the fight-or-flight response. Cooling extremities demonstrate the opposite: decrease in blood flow and circulation in the extremities and an increase in the fight-or-flight response. Normal hand temperature readings can range from 65°F to 99°F.

Sit quietly for 3 to 5 minutes, and then notice your readings on the temperature unit and any other unit you have chosen to monitor. Try to check your readings with as little disturbance to the quiet of the experience as possible. These primary or initial readings are called your baseline readings. Write down these baseline readings. If you are comfortable, remain attached to the biofeedback monitors. Make sure that your

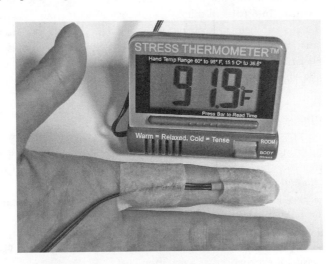

FIGURE 16-1 Biofeedback Temperature Unit. Finger with thermister attached. Ceramic tip of biofeedback thermal probe (thermister) is attached to palmar tip of finger. Tip of thermister is covered with paper tape, and wire is attached to finger as demonstrated in the photograph.

body is supported and that you can easily see the monitors with as little movement as possible. Next, perform one of your favorite relaxation or meditation practices for 10 to 20 minutes.

Take readings immediately at the end of the session in a quiet, unhurried way so as not to disturb your relaxation. Notice any difference in your readings before and after the practice. What did the readings demonstrate about your practice experience? What change did you experience inside? Were these changes reflected in your biofeedback readings?

If you notice a drop in the temperature of your hands during or after a relaxation practice, check the following:

1. Did you feel hurried?
2. Were you trying too hard to relax?
3. Were you thinking about something other than the relaxation practice or wondering what the monitors would show?
4. Was the room warm enough?
5. Were there any interruptions, expected or unexpected, such as people entering the room or phones ringing?

Whatever the results are, they can only help to deepen your understanding of the internal awareness and responses involved in these special practices. Remember to adopt the attitude of the nonjudgmental observer and explore your inner awareness. Examine **Exhibit 16-6** to determine whether any of these factors can help to explain your response. With practice, you may notice an increase in your postrelaxation temperature reading compared to your prerelaxation temperature.

Variation A: Client Practice

Try the biofeedback experiment described earlier on a client. Use an abbreviated form of the experiment (5 to 10 minutes), taking readings before and after relaxation practice. Explore and explain the meanings of the readings, and invite the client to describe what he or she felt inside and what he or she feels the readings mean.

This technique provides an opportunity for healthcare teaching and counseling to move from client compliance into client empowerment. Teaching clients how anxiety, worry, and stress can produce higher blood pressure, cooler hands, and tenser muscles, and how relaxation can produce the opposite responses is an easy way to begin a dialogue providing clients with insight into the stressors of their lives and how they respond to them.

Variation B: Group Self-Care Experiment

Try relaxation or biofeedback in a group. Start with a group of colleagues rather than a group of clients. (You can begin to introduce this technique to a group of clients later as you gain experience and knowledge with the practice.) Schedule a relaxation break for your unit. Take 15 minutes at the beginning of a staff meeting, or schedule the relaxation practice during a lunch break every week or month. A relatively quiet room with chairs arranged in a circle, flowers for the center of the circle, and some music will be helpful. Invite each person to bring a small journal and pen, and obtain a biofeedback temperature monitor for each person. Small

EXHIBIT 16-6   Important Factors in Relaxation Practice

- **Passive volition:** Letting go, being without doing or striving, allowing, being with the process as it unfolds rather than making it happen; planting a seed in the mind of wanting to relax, and then letting go and watching the process.

- **Attention to the here-and-now:** Being oriented toward the present, not caught up in what happened or what might happen.

- **Altered perception of time:** Experiencing time as expanded or contracted. Relaxation practice can change the perception of time so that a very short practice session feels like a long time or a long practice session is experienced as a few moments.

- **Enjoyment of practice:** Committing to practice and, even more important, enjoying practice. Most traditional healers and teachers of the restorative arts ask their students if they are enjoying their practice. Finding a practice that helps one weather the storms of life and enhances one's inner connection is a joy.

alcohol thermometers are the least expensive temperature monitors; liquid crystal cards, dots, or bands also work. If electronic temperature units or finger alcohol thermometers are used, attach the unit to the palmar surface of the finger with paper tape (see Figure 16-1). Agree as a group to meet on a regular basis, keep a journal of individual progress, and begin and end on time so that people can easily return to work or finish lunch.

Set up the room in advance so that the flowers are in the center of the circle of chairs. Have members of the group attach their temperature monitors. Allow 1 to 2 minutes before taking the first baseline reading. Next, introduce a relaxation exercise. You can continue to play music or turn the music down or off, while one of the group members offers a relaxation practice. The role of relaxation leader can be rotated. Depending on the interests of the group, the same practice can be carried out at each meeting, or different practices can be offered each week.

After the relaxation practice, group members take another monitor reading and write journal entries on their experiences and responses. A few minutes should be left for group members to explore and share their experiences with one another. Observe what happens over time. Invite group members to track their medication use and observe overall changes in well-being, blood pressure, headaches, pain, anxiety, and so on.

Special issues for groups. "I don't have time. I'm too busy. I could be/should be catching up on my work, not relaxing." Sandy O'Brien and Jeanne Anselmo developed a staff wellness project using the practices described previously.[50] The answer they found to the challenge of "I don't have time to practice" is that we cannot afford not to take time to center ourselves and care for ourselves to do the best for our own health while offering the best of care to our clients and families.

Although relaxation practice does take time and commitment, most groups learn to avoid giving in to the work-and-hurry sickness and begin to enjoy the benefits of stopping, calming, and letting go.

In fact, according to the Nurses' Health Study from Harvard, the more friends and social ties nurses had the less likely they were to develop physical ailments and the more joyous their life would be. Researchers from UCLA demonstrated that women's social ties reduce the risk of heart disease by lowering blood pressure, cholesterol, and heart rate.[51]

Cautions and Contraindications for Relaxation, Meditation, and Biofeedback

Medications

Clients who take insulin, thyroid replacement medication, antihypertensives, cardiac medications, antianxiety agents, and sleep medications must be monitored for a change in their symptoms and medication needs as they learn to deepen their relaxation response. As clients learn to regulate their stress response, their medication requirements may change. Work closely with clients' prescribing providers to ensure that their medications are titrated properly.

Education and Information

Discussing issues and experiences associated with relaxation before and after each session helps to involve clients, positively empower them, and reframe any of the anticipatory anxiety or questions they may have.

Mental Health History

Clients with a history of dissociative experiences, acute psychosis, borderline personality, and posttraumatic stress disorder are best cared for by nurses and professionals skilled in treating such clients. Check your client's mental health history before beginning relaxation practice.[52]

Cryptotrauma

Many patients have experienced undiagnosed physical or psychological trauma. Many times patients are reluctant to disclose these problems, and many times health professionals are unskilled in or uncomfortable with exploring these issues. Domino and Haber report that 66% of women at a multidisciplinary pain center with chronic headaches had a prior history of physical or sexual abuse (61% had experienced physical abuse; 11%, sexual abuse; and 28%, both physical and sexual abuse). The average duration of abuse was 8 years.

The term *cryptotrauma* indicates that the trauma that is the cause of the patient's pain is hidden or has not been revealed. Signals to watch for in clients with posttraumatic stress disorder (PTSD) and/or cryptotrauma include the following:

- Hypervigilance
- Difficulty falling or staying asleep
- Irritability or outbursts of rage
- Difficulty concentrating
- Exaggerated startle response
- Dissociation
- Addiction
- Flashbacks
- Numbing
- Panic attacks
- Disturbed self-perception, denigration
- Isolation
- Inability to be comfortable with touch
- Nightmares[53]

Even with the most sensitive and careful history taking and preparations, clients with such disorders can have flashbacks related to the underlying trauma. If this occurs, first, do not panic. Remember your intention to help and support, and trust your therapeutic bond with the client. Second, center and ground yourself. Clients in a panic state related to anxiety or flashback are supersensitive to people around them; centering, calming, and grounding yourself will deeply help them. Third, reassure the client, speak to the client in a calm, soothing voice, and use therapeutic suggestions. Have the client open his or her eyes, feel his or her feet on the floor, or touch the furniture; if possible, have the client tighten and release the hands and feet and be aware of the body and of being with you in the present. If appropriate, hold the client's hand; use your judgment. Fourth, remember that the information with which the client is getting in touch is important for the client's wholeness and healing. A simple, short statement explaining this to the client helps to reframe the situation and plant therapeutic suggestions during these most open and suggestible moments. Seek appropriate referrals for the client as needed.

PTSD, Cryptotrauma, and Working in Times of Trauma, Natural Disaster, or Major Crisis

Clients who suffer from cryptotrauma or who have sustained one or more major losses around the time of a disaster are at the greatest risk for developing PTSD. Nurses and other helping professionals who are aware of the previously mentioned symptoms for cryptotrauma could be the first line of help for assessing, recognizing, and helping a client, colleague, child, or even a neighbor or family member suffering from traumatic grief or PTSD after any major community trauma or crisis. In a time of tragedies, such as school shootings; soldiers and military families coping with their uncertainty or the return of traumatized or wounded soldiers from war; or environmental disasters such as hurricanes, earthquakes, floods, tornados, and tsunamis, understanding lessons learned from the lived experience of our colleagues in communities that have been affected can be a great service to all.

Richard Schaedle, director of Crisis Resource Center at LifeNet at the Mental Health Association of New York City, described dealing with trauma in communities after September 11. Though everyone grieves differently, and most people recover without much intervention, "We needed to alert people about a normal reaction to an abnormal event. For the more pathological symptoms, like traumatic grief and PTSD, there were psychotherapy and medication." In a time of crisis or disaster, all members of the community are needed. Schaedle describes how "there were no boundaries" between the spiritual and religious helpers and professionals and paraprofessionals; all were needed to help and all needed to be trained to deal with the enormous needs of the community after the disaster. Volunteers offered massage therapy, yoga, and spiritual counseling along with community counseling and support groups, all of which helped to destress and reduce trauma in the wake of the events of September 11.[54]

Evolution of PTSD After a Community Crisis or Disaster

Immediately after September 11, New York City's mental health/alcoholism/drug addiction 24-hour helpline was transformed into 1-800-LifeNet, a hotline designed to deal with the emotional and mental health issues of the NYC community. In 2002, the number of calls to the LifeNet hotline doubled from the previous year, and almost 2 years after the attack, the number of calls to the hotline continued to grow another 25% by the summer of 2003. Having a helpline already in place prior to 9/11 was a great resource for the community, and the training of 5,000 to 7,000 helping professionals offered a future resource to draw on in case of emergency to address the unprecedented levels of need.

What professionals learned was that even while the rest of the city and country began to move on and feel better, calls related to September 11 continued to come in to LifeNet regarding symptoms, reactions, and PTSD long after the event. This was because as others move on, those with PTSD actually get worse and feel even more isolated and out of synch with the rest of the community and country.

According to John Draper, director of Public Education and the LifeNet Hotline Network, prior to September 11, 1 out of 200 people in the New York metropolitan area would be diagnosed with PTSD. After September 11, 1 out of 3 were diagnosed with PTSD, and during the summer of 2003 that percentage was still high, with 1 out of 10 being diagnosed with PTSD. The antithetical dimension of PTSD is that, left untreated, with time the symptoms do not get better but actually get worse.

Those people who suffered an additional loss around the time of the disaster (e.g., job loss, financial crisis, illness or death in the family) had a four to five times higher possibility of developing PTSD than those who did not have any additional loss or trauma. Those who sustained multiple additional losses around the time of the disaster were 47 to 50 times more likely to develop PTSD.[55]

According to a new study published in 2007 by Canadian researchers, those with PTSD are significantly more apt to have numerous health conditions including cardiovascular diseases, respiratory diseases, chronic pain, gastrointestinal illnesses, and cancer. Those with PTSD were also more prone to "short- and long-term disability, poor quality of life, and suicide attempts."[56] Understanding the significance of these data alerts us to the importance of recognizing PTSD in those we serve and getting those suffering from PTSD the appropriate mental, emotional, and physical help and support.

We as a human community are learning that we live in a time in which major disaster can strike anywhere, whether rural or urban, and no place or group, even those groups such as the Amish, are immune from such tragedy. Those in other parts of the world have had to live with trauma and tragedy as part of their reality every day, but we have found that even the extraordinary preparedness of the Japanese people has been challenged in these times of multiple and concurrent disasters. We in this country are now experiencing natural disasters of floods, hurricanes, and tornados on a unprecedented scale and yet this is still a small percentage of what others in the world have been challenged by for decades. If we allow it, these experiences can help us to enliven and enlarge our hearts as a human family, helping us grow our understanding, compassion, wisdom, and interconnectedness so that we can skillfully develop our ability to help and to heal both locally and globally. As holistic nursing leaders, we know that we can learn from this lived experience and can build the awareness, personal and professional resources, education, and skills needed to help ourselves and our communities in case of a disaster (see Barrett's theory of power below).

We also can recognize that by living in a very mobile society, nurses and helping professionals can be confronted with a client or patient who has moved away from a disaster area or who has friends or family in the disaster and thereby is also at risk for PTSD, which may not be recognized, understood, or supported outside of the area where the original crisis or disaster occurred. Many people have delayed responses and are not immediately diagnosed, as demonstrated by the reports of a 25% increase in calls to the NYC hotline 2 years after September 11. The main statement that trauma therapists treating those with PTSD continue to hear is, "I thought I'd be over this by now." The more time that elapses from the time of the event, the more distressing the symptoms and reactions become for persons with PTSD.[55]

Caring for Those with PTSD

PTSD is characterized by avoidance, numbness, and feelings of helplessness and hopelessness. For those suffering from PTSD, conversational induction and therapeutic suggestion may be even more helpful and appropriate than any form of deep relaxation.[57] As stated earlier, conversational induction helps to support a person's defenses while promoting comfort, important qualities to be cultivated for PTSD sufferers, especially in the immediate time during or after a major trauma. As in any clinical situation, professional experience, clinical judgment, and the client's comfort level with the intervention all help to determine what is the best approach for that client.

Because rescue or relief workers and professionals involved with trauma work of disaster victims may have to continuously return to the disaster site and reexperience the crisis, they, too, may experience vicarious traumatization and feel stuck and isolated while other colleagues move on. They need personal, workplace, and community healing support as well.

■ HOLISTIC NURSING PERSPECTIVES FOR LIVING IN A TIME OF UNCERTAINTY

According to Dr. Elizabeth Barrett:

> Power, from a Rogerian perspective, is the capacity to participate knowingly in the nature of change characterizing the continuous patterning of the human and environmental field. The observable, measurable pattern manifestations of power are awareness, choices, freedom to act intentionally, and involvement in creating change.[58]

So, what awareness, choices, intentions, and involvement do we want to offer, as holistic nurses, to foster community unitary well-being in times of uncertainty? How do we help to support empowered awareness and choices in times of helplessness or uncertainty?

Our own practices of self-healing, meditation, and relaxation support us during times of illness and stress by helping us to build inner skills, awareness, and resiliency. Similarly, communities also can cultivate their inner resiliency by building their own inner capacities and building a more connected interdisciplinary team. Increased training of clergy, child care workers, mental health professionals, teachers, and funeral directors, as well as nurses, social workers, physicians, chiropractors, and nutritionists, to recognize and deal with various forms of trauma and teach self-care practices and group support is one example of developing inner resources of a resilient community. This model of a resilient community fosters a true interdisciplinary team of healers building a lived community of well-being.

Sandra Bloom, president of CommunityWorks (www.sanctuaryweb.com) and an expert in dealing with trauma, makes recommendations for organizations as communities. Bloom recommends that organizations can facilitate healing after trauma by

> viewing the problem as a problem for the entire group and not limited to the individual. A trauma-sensitive workplace culture reverses the effects of trauma emphasizing safety, emotional management, grief resolution, and a vision of recovery, change, growth, and life after trauma.[59]

She also states that a "workplace culture that can respond to the need of trauma survivors will end up being a healthier and more productive environment for everyone."[59]

Cultivating Wellness Preparedness for Professionals, Communities, and Organizations

As holistic nursing leaders, we can build in preparedness within a wellness and healing framework in which communities focus on self-care and community care as shared values. In this way, when times of crisis or disaster arise, community self-care is already in place. One suggestion is to invite your healthcare community to create self-care practice buddies. Make a pact with colleagues to look out for each other's physical, emotional, and mental health by supporting healing breaks and encouraging each other's self-care practice to help maintain our best ability to be present. Though these breaks may take a different form in a time of great challenge, having positive healing patterns in place can help build needed resiliency to cope with uncertainty and trauma or disaster.

Times of crisis offer us choice. The acronym CHOICE is offered by holistic nurse Jeanne Campion as a mnemonic device for remembering the phrase "Consciously Helping One Intentionally Change Energy." She continues in a talk inspired by the first anniversary of September 11: "We always have choices related to our energy/vibration/level of consciousness. One can choose to respond from a place of centered calm (mindful) or one can choose to react from a place of confusion and chaos."[60]

Restorative Practices

Relaxation practice also brings the gifts of restoring, opening, and renewing.

Yoga

In restorative yoga, practitioners open themselves more deeply to the healing energies that flow through them in each posture (asana). They accomplish this by supporting their bodies in yoga poses using bolsters, pillows, and blankets.[61]

Yoga is a philosophy of living that unites physical, mental, and spiritual health. When practiced for the purpose of relaxation, it involves breathing and stretching exercises and postures. The exercises vary greatly in difficulty. Because yoga starts with very gentle stretches and breathing techniques, it is ideally suited for clients with stiff muscles and decreased activity levels who are attempting to begin an active relaxation and exercise program. Clients need not embrace the philosophy to benefit from the activity.

Daily practice of restorative yoga—even 10 to 15 minutes a day—creates energy, restorative rest, spiritual renewal, and calm. Restorative yoga is a wonderful practice to perform during a break at work, and restorative yoga and yoga therapy are evolving as areas of therapeutic practice.[62]

Qi Gong

Seasonal qi gong practices restore, renew, center, and open meridians as the energy field and body changes with the seasons. Some techniques of Chinese qi gong have been practiced for at least 5,000 years. Simple movements are combined with breath and meditation in a flow with nature's healing qi. Restoration and healing come from daily practice. Qi gong practices are a part of Chinese medicine, which includes acupuncture, external qi gong (receiving healing energy from a healer or master), herbal medicine, diet, massage, and self-care.

Restorative Gardens

"Nature alone heals"[2] is one of Nightingale's most famous quotes. What Nightingale knew, and what gardeners and nature lovers also know, is that nature can heal and cure. Many hospitals and healthcare centers are creating healing gardens, restorative gardens, greenhouses, medi-

tative gardens, and labyrinths in their plazas, lobbies, rooftops, and other inner and outer spaces to help cultivate relaxation, renewal, and peace. Bringing nature inside the healing environment is not at all new; it dates back to medieval monastic healing sanctuaries. The medieval architectural designs included low windows so that patients could look out at nature's beauty.

Simply helping clients to be with nature amid the high-tech healthcare system can improve their well-being, reduce their anxiety, and calm their fears. Nurses themselves can benefit from resting in a garden or creating natural spaces within the healthcare setting.[63]

■ HOLISTIC CARING PROCESS

Holistic Assessment

In preparing to use relaxation interventions, the nurse assesses the following parameters and lived experiences:

- The client's perception of personal tension levels and need to relax
- The client's readiness and motivation to learn relaxation strategies, because relaxation is a very subjective and personal endeavor
- The client's past experience with the process of relaxation, hypnosis, or meditation
- The client's personal definition and lived experience of what it means to be relaxed
- The client's ability to remain comfortable in one position for 15 to 30 minutes
- The client's hearing acuity, so that the nurse can speak at an appropriate level while guiding the client in relaxation exercises
- The client's spiritual and religious beliefs, so that the nurse can present the relaxation process in a way that will meld comfortably with the client's belief system
- The client's level of pain or discomfort, anxiety, fear, or boredom
- The client's perception of reality, history of depersonalization states, and locus of control, because deep relaxation may exacerbate the symptoms of psychotic and prepsychotic individuals
- The client's medication intake, particularly of medications that may alter response to relaxation or that may need to be titrated as relaxation progresses

A questionnaire can be used to complete the assessment. The information gathered in the questionnaire provides starting points for discussion and further exploration.

Identification of Patterns/Challenges/Needs

The patterns/challenges/needs (see Chapter 7) compatible with relaxation interventions are as follows:

- Social isolation
- Altered coping; ineffective individual and family
- Activity intolerance, actual or potential
- Deficit in diversional activity
- Powerlessness
- Altered self-concept; disturbance in self-esteem, role performance, personal identity
- Altered sensation and perception: visual, auditory, kinesthetic, gustatory, tactile, olfactory
- Altered thought processes
- Anxiety
- Altered comfort: pain
- Fear
- Potential for violence: self-directed or directed at others

Outcome Identification

Exhibit 16-7 guides the nurse in client outcomes, nursing prescriptions, and evaluations for the use of relaxation as a nursing intervention.

EXHIBIT 16-7   Nursing Interventions: Relaxation

Client Outcomes	Nursing Prescriptions	Evaluation
The client will demonstrate decreased anxiety, tension, and other manifestations of the stress response as a result of the relaxation intervention.	Guide the client in the relaxation exercise. Evaluate for decrease in anxiety, tension, and other manifestations of the stress response as evidenced by heart rate within normal limits, decreased respiratory rates, return of blood pressure toward normal, resolution of anxious facial expressions and mannerisms, decrease in repetitious talking or behavior, and inability to sleep or restlessness.	The client exhibited decreased anxiety, tension, and other manifestations of the stress response as evidenced by normal vital signs; a slow, deep breathing pattern; and decreased anxious behaviors.
The client will demonstrate a stabilization or decrease in pain as a result of the relaxation intervention.	Evaluate for decrease in pain as evidenced by reduction or elimination of pain control medication and increased activities or mobility.	The client's intake of pain medication stabilized and then decreased with relaxation skills practice. The client began to participate in activities previously limited by pain.
The client will link breathing awareness to a commonly occurring cue and use this combination to reduce tension.	Teach awareness of breathing patterns and habitual linking of relaxing breathing to a cue in the environment.	The client used turning in bed as a cue to take a slow, deep breath and relax jaw muscles.

Therapeutic Care Plan and Interventions

Before the session:
- Become personally familiar with the experience of the relaxation intervention before approaching the client.
- If the client has previous positive experience with a particular relaxation intervention, encourage further practice and use of that intervention.
- Review with the client his or her lived experience and gather information from the chart, diaries, and/or verbal self-report concerning pain, anxiety, and activity levels since the last session.

Preparation of the environment (ideal):
- Arrange medical and nursing care to allow for 15 to 45 minutes of uninterrupted time.
- Keep the room warm and ventilated, not cold.
- Shut the door or otherwise decrease extraneous noise and distraction. Place a note on the door indicating a need for privacy until a designated time.
- Turn off the telephone and cell phones or ask a family member or friend to answer the telephone should it ring during the relaxation training session.
- Reduce lighting to a low level.
- Use natural or incandescent lighting if possible; fluorescent lighting can cause headaches in some patients.

Client comfort measures:
- Have the client empty his or her bladder before starting the intervention.
- Help the client find a comfortable sitting or reclining position, with hands resting by the sides or on the thighs.
- Ensure the client's comfort by providing a blanket or by adjusting the thermostat to a comfortably warm setting; have small, soft pillows available for positioning.

Timing of the session (ideal):
- Hold the training session before meals or more than 2 hours after the last meal. A full stomach coupled with relaxation may lead to sleep.

Support tools:
- Have recorded music available.
- If the session is to be followed by drawing, have paper, crayons, or colored markers available.

- Tell the client that you may ask simple yes or no questions during the session to check the comfort level of the music or to confirm the client's understanding of verbal instructions. The client may answer these questions by raising a preestablished "yes" finger or "no" finger or nodding the head.

At the beginning of the session:
- Review briefly the potential benefits of relaxation intervention, and enlist the client's cooperation. Explore the client's lived experience of relaxation and stress.
- Explain to the client that relaxation may be easier if practiced with the eyes closed. The client may drift off to sleep, but this position allows the client to focus attention inward while remaining awake. This may take practice to accomplish, and many times clients fall asleep as a result of exhaustion or lack of sleep. In such a case, the restorative dimension of relaxation is at work, and the nurse has still introduced therapeutic suggestions.
- Explain that one purpose of breathing and relaxation exercises is to experience inward relaxation and become aware of the body-mind-spirit connections associated with relaxation.
- Emphasize that you are merely a guide, and that any therapeutic results obtained from the session are from the client's natural healing ability, involvement, interest, and practice.
- Let go of outcomes. There is an ebb and flow to the learning experience. Encourage the client to practice for comfort and awareness, noting shifts in breathing, anxiety, and sensations.
- Arrive at mutually agreeable goals for the session, such as reduction of pain, decreased time to sleep onset, reduction of anxiety, or enhanced well-being.
- Have the client quantify the level of the parameter to be changed; for example, "My pain or anxiety level right now is 7 on a scale of 0 (none) to 10 (extreme pain)." Record the level before and after the session.
- Record baseline vital signs. If biofeedback equipment is used, record baseline readings.
- Assure the client that sensations of heaviness, warmth, floating, or lightness are

naturally occurring indications of deep relaxation; explain that the client can end the experience at any moment she or he desires by opening the eyes, tightening the fists, or stretching; this will orient the client and enable the exercise to continue.

- Begin soft background music. (See Chapter 18 for suggestions regarding music selection.)
- Guide the client through a basic breathing relaxation exercise. Breathing exercises may be repeated slowly for several minutes as an introduction to deeper relaxation.
- Start the session with short breathing or relaxation exercises (5 minutes); lengthen the exercises to 10 to 20 minutes as the client becomes better able to relax and attend to inner thoughts and feelings.

During the session:

- Phrase all therapeutic suggestions and self-statements in a positive form. For example, say, "I am aware of comfort moving down my arm and into my hand," rather than, "I am not in pain." These therapeutic suggestions enhance the process and reframe the experience.
- Speak in a relaxed manner. Ask the client for feedback concerning the appropriateness of the practice and his or her ability to hear the background music and instructions. Have the client respond with a finger movement (using signals established before the session) or nod of the head, and make adjustments as necessary.
- Pace your instructions according to the following visual cues from the client. Each indicates a deepening of relaxation.
  - Change in breathing pattern: slower, deeper breaths progressing to slow, somewhat shallower breathing as relaxation deepens
  - More audible breathing
  - Fluttering of eyelids
  - Blanching of the skin around the nose and mouth
  - Easing of jaw tightness, sometimes to the extent that the lips part and the jaw drops slightly
  - If client is supine, pointing of toes outward rather than straight up
  - Complete lack of muscle holding (ask client's permission to lift arm gently by the wrist; no resistance should be felt and the arm should move as easily as any other object of similar weight)
- Modify your instructions and strategies to fit the situation. Encourage an intubated and ventilated patient who cannot control respiratory rate or volume to drop the jaw and allow the rhythm of the ventilator to soothe tight muscles, for example. Gently placing your hand over the clavicle or holding the person's hand as you speak enhances the therapeutic relationship and supports relaxation.
- Intersperse your instructions with therapeutic suggestions of encouragement that the client can use after the session as cues to recapture aspects of the relaxation experience. Examples of such phrases are:
  - Perhaps you are noticing a softening of your muscles.
  - As you take your next breath, become aware of how the warmth is flowing down your arm.
  - Deep breathing helps to replenish the oxygen and energy of the body and helps the body heal, relax, restore, and renew.
- As the client relaxes, she or he may experience a release of emotional life issues, which can surface in the conscious mind. Be alert for signs of emotional discomfort or letting go, such as tears or a change in breathing to deeper, faster breaths. If such a sign occurs, ask gentle questions (e.g., "Can you put those feelings into words and express them safely?"), and allow time for the client to express and deal with the material before continuing with or concluding the session. (See the earlier section on cryptotrauma and trauma for more information on helping clients stay grounded if they tap into emotion-laden material.) Often, clients in a deeply relaxed state gain insight into how to resolve problems or which directions to take in their lives.

At the end of the session:

- Bring the client gradually into a wakeful state by suggesting that she or he take deep, energizing breaths, begin to move hands and feet, and stretch; orient the client to the room, talking with the client about the comfort she or he created.

- Have the client reevaluate, on the scale of 0 to 10 used earlier, the level of comfort or severity of the parameter previously selected to be changed. Record the level.
- Allow time for discussion of the experience, including discussion of the techniques that seemed especially effective and the client's physical, emotional, and energy awareness. Invite the client to express his or her experience by writing, making a journal entry, or drawing. Different clients will prefer different methods, such as creating an abstract drawing, offering a story, or writing poetry, to express their experience.
- Ensure that medication changes, if indicated, are appropriately monitored.
- Engage the client in continuing practice on an individually assigned basis until the next session.
- Help the client choose supportive measures for practicing his or her relaxation skill.
- Review a log or journal in which the client records relaxation practice, symptoms, medications, time, and results.

Case Studies (Implementation)

CASE STUDY 1

Setting: Outpatient; multidisciplinary holistic healthcare center

Client: S. D., a 47-year-old African American man with family history of stroke

Medical Diagnosis: Progressive essential hypertension, unresponsive to any antihypertensive therapy

Current Medications: Catapres (clonidine), Lasix (furosemide), Valium (diazepam), Minipress (prazosin), potassium chloride

Patterns/Challenges/Needs:
1. Altered physical regulation (essential hypertension)
2. Anxiety
3. Fear
4. Powerlessness
5. Ineffective coping related to anxiety, stress of job, and parenting of five children
6. Self-esteem disturbance, situational

S. D. had been diagnosed with severe uncontrollable essential hypertension. He scrupulously took his antihypertensive medications and had an extensive clinical workup to rule out any secondary causes. S. D. was very frustrated because his father had died of a stroke, and S. D. did not want to have a stroke or "die young." He and his wife cared for their five children. He worked at a job that required him to perform physical labor and walk up and down three flights of stairs.

His physician sent him to learn biofeedback-assisted relaxation as an adjunctive therapy. His blood pressure at rest while on medication ranged from 160/100 to 200/120 mm Hg. To reduce S. D.'s fear and feeling of powerlessness, the nurse explored his lived experience of his condition and used healthcare teaching and stress management counseling to reframe his understanding of what was happening in his body.

The nurse explained to S. D. that his body knew very well how to respond to stress, but that he needed the opportunity and the time to recover from stress and learn less physically distressing ways to respond. S. D. was shown how to use the temperature trainer and a small galvanic skin response unit that indicated sympathetic outflow by measuring sweat gland response. He was taught simple breathing exercises and autogenic phrases while he learned to monitor his body-mind-spirit response on the biofeedback displays.

Because of the urgency and critical nature of his situation, he was invited to participate in three practice sessions a week for 1 month instead of the usual one session per week. He was asked to practice the relaxation two times a day. Within the first 2 weeks, he had brought his blood pressure down to 140/100 mm Hg. He continued sessions each week during the second month, and then continued practice on his own. After 3 months, his blood pressure was 140/80 mm Hg while he continued on the same level of medication.

After 1 year, his medication level was reduced, and blood pressure was maintained at 140/80 mm Hg. The nurse scheduled a meeting with S. D., his wife, and all their children to explore their needs, fears, and concerns about S. D.'s health. The family agreed to help support S. D. in his healthcare practice by making sure he was not disturbed during his practice time. The opportunity to share their love and support, and to understand how their loved one was working to help himself, offered them a new understanding of their father and husband, his healthcare issues, and how they could be active in his wellness plan.

CASE STUDY 2

Setting: Home care and hospital preoperative and postoperative care

Client: M.C.D., a 76-year-old European American woman undergoing surgery for renal tumor

Patterns/Challenges/Needs:
1. Altered physical regulation (renal tumor)
2. Anxiety
3. Fear
4. Ineffective coping related to renal tumor, possible cancer
5. Powerlessness

M.C.D. complained of back pain. A sonogram revealed a large renal tumor. The surgeon told M.C.D. and her husband the results of the sonogram and recommended surgery within the next 5 days. M.C.D. and her husband were very upset after their visit to the surgeon and consulted with a nurse in private practice about methods of readying for surgery.

Because of M.C.D.'s shock and anxiety, and her fear about the possible outcome of the surgery, the nurse discussed with the client, her family, and the surgeon whether or not the surgery had to be performed immediately. The surgeon had determined that the tumor was a slow-growing mass that had been present for at least 2 years. The surgeon agreed that the surgery could be scheduled 2 weeks later to give M.C.D. time to prepare her bodymindspirit for the experience.

M.C.D. was taught breathing and meditation exercises, began receiving Reiki energy sessions, and, with preoperative teaching, began to create visualizations of surgery as a healing experience. The 2-week delay gave her a chance to reduce the shock and include her family and her parish in her preparation. Members of her women's group at the church prayed for her and were "breathing toward her," sending spiritual energy, love, and support. Her family from out of town had an opportunity to come and escort her to the hospital. Most important, she was able to prepare and practice her relaxation healing surgery experience so that, in the preoperative room, she was so relaxed that she told the nurse she was resting on the "breath of God."

Her relaxation practice included quiet meditation, prayer, deep breathing, and visualization of each of the steps that would occur, from the night before the surgery through the ride to the hospital, the preoperative preparation, surgery, and recovery.

Interspersed throughout her educational preparation were the therapeutic suggestions that there would be very little pain or bleeding and no infection from the surgery, and that everyone who was in contact with her could be a vehicle for sending healing light and energy. Every intravenous line, medication, procedure, and caretaker became a part of her visualization.

M.C.D.'s holistic nurse went with her into the preoperative area and helped her practice her relaxation strategies; the nurse also informed the rest of the surgical team of M.C.D.'s plan to practice during the surgery. The staff wanted to know if their other patients could learn these practices because M.C.D.'s response was so positive.

M.C.D.'s surgery went well. She did have cancer, but she continued to use the practices she had learned and extended them into an ongoing wellness plan. These practices improved her well-being, energy, and spirit; enhanced her immune function; and slowed the progression of the disease. She died 4 years later, practicing relaxation through to the moment of her death. These practices wove together her spiritual life, her desire to be an active participant in her care, and her understanding of her health, wellness, and well-being.

Evaluation

With the client, the nurse determines whether the client outcomes for relaxation interventions (see Exhibit 16-7) were successfully achieved. To evaluate the session further, the nurse may again explore the subjective effects of the experience with the client (see **Exhibit 16-8**). Because the accomplishment of these interventions may take place over a period of days or weeks, they must be reviewed and reevaluated periodically. Continuing support and encouragement are necessary.

Relaxation exercises can be taught to clients under almost any circumstances. They not only reduce the fear and anxiety associated with many medical and nursing interventions but, once learned, may be used in all aspects of a client's life. They increase the overall movement

EXHIBIT 16-8   Evaluation of the Client's Subjective Experience of Relaxation

1. Was this a new experience for you? Can you describe it?

2. Did you have any physical or emotional responses to the relaxation exercises? If so, can you describe them?

3. Do you feel different after this experience? How?

4. How does your body–mind communicate with you when your stress level is at an uncomfortable point?

5. Would you like to do this again?

6. Were there any distractions to your relaxation?

7. What would make this a more pleasant experience for you?

8. How do you see yourself integrating relaxation skills into your daily life?

toward wholeness and balance for both client and nurse, and they facilitate other interventions by allowing the client to move toward learning and participating more fully in his or her own health promotion.

Directions for
FUTURE RESEARCH

1. Correlate the changes in psychophysiology with the specific relaxation interventions used to determine the most effective interventions and their presentation.

2. Conduct tightly structured studies to evaluate specific relaxation techniques, using control groups to validate changes brought about by specific forms of relaxation exercises.

3. Monitor and validate the effect of the "compassionate guide" in the relaxation process.

4. Conduct tightly structured studies to evaluate effects of live guided relaxation and audio- or video-guided relaxation on specific client populations, conditions, and healthcare environments, using control groups to validate changes brought about by live or recorded forms of relaxation exercises.

5. Conduct qualitative studies to explore the meaning of the client's lived experience of phenomena relevant to nursing.

6. Monitor and validate the effect of conversational suggestion and sustained centering for enhancing comfort and calm in crisis situations.

Nurse Healer
REFLECTIONS

After reading this chapter, the nurse healer will be able to answer or to begin the process of answering the following questions:

- How does my inner experience of tension or anxiety shift when I release my muscle tightness?
- How do I model relaxation to my family, friends, colleagues, and clients?
- What is my kinesthetic experience of letting go of tension, concerns, and physical and emotional stresses?
- What cues about my inner experience of tension or relaxation do I receive from my breathing pattern?
- How do I cultivate peace of mind as I move through my potentially stressful job activities?
- Am I aware that my attitudes toward my tasks are contagious to my clients?
- What dimensions of resiliency are found or needed in my workplace and community?

 For a full suite of assignments and additional learning activities, use the access code located in the front of your book to visit this exclusive website: http://go.jblearning. com/dossey. If you do not have an access code, you can obtain one at the site.

NOTES

1. C. Moriconi and S. Stabler-Haas, "Mindfulness-Based Stress Reduction and Its Effect on Test Anxiety and Focused Attention with Baccalaureate Nursing Students: A Pilot Study" (presentation at Mindfulness in Education Conference, American University, Washington, DC, March 19, 2011) .

2. F. Nightingale, *Notes on Nursing, Commemorative ed.* (Philadelphia, PA: Lippincott, 1992): 28.

3. P. de Llosa, "The Neurobiology of 'We,'" *Parabola* (May 15, 2011). http://www.parabola.org/the-neurobiology-of-we.

4. J. Kabat-Zinn, *Full Catastrophe Living: Using the Wisdom of Your Body and Mind to Face Stress, Pain, and Illness* (New York: Bantam Doubleday Dell, 1990).

5. D. Ornish, *Dr. Dean Ornish's Program for Reversing Heart Disease* (New York: Random House, 1990).

6. D. Krieger, *Accepting Your Power to Heal: The Personal Practice of Therapeutic Touch* (Santa Fe, NM: Bear and Co., 1993): 17–20.

7. D. Krieger, "Characteristics of Integration During the Healing Moment" (keynote address at the 5th Annual Holism and Nursing Conference, Zeta Omega Chapter-at-Large of Sigma Theta Tau International, Rye, NY, May 16, 2003).

8. J. Levey and M. Levey, *The Fine Arts of Relaxation, Concentration, and Meditation: Ancient Skills for Modern Minds* (Somerville, MA: Wisdom Publications, 2003).

9. H. Benson et al., "Decreased Premature Ventricular Contraction Through the Use of the Relaxation Response in Patients with Stable Ischemic Heart Disease," *Lancet* 2, no. 7931 (1975): 380.

10. H. Benson, *Beyond the Relaxation Response* (New York: Times Books, 1984).

11. H. Benson, "Your Innate Asset for Combating Stress" in *Relax: How You Can Feel Better, Reduce Stress, and Overcome Tension*, ed. J. White and J. Fodeman (New York: Confucian Press, 1976): 53–54.

12. D. W. Orme-Johnson et al., "Neuroimaging of Meditation's Effect on Brain Reactivity to Pain," *Neuro-report* 17, no. 12 (2006): 1359–1363.

13. H. Benson et al., "Decreased Blood Pressure in Pharmacologically Treated Hypertensive Patients Who Regularly Elicited the Relaxation Response," *Lancet* 1 (1974): 289–291.

14. J. Kabat-Zinn et al., "Four-Year Follow-up of a Meditation-Based Program for the Self-Regulation of Chronic Pain: Treatment Outcomes and Compliance," *Clinical Journal of Pain* 2 (1987): 154–173.

15. S. Rosenzweig, J. M. Gresson, D. K. Reibel et al., "Mindfulness-Based Stress Reduction for Chronic Pain Conditions: Variation in Treatment Outcomes and Role of Home Meditation Practice," *Journal of Psychosomatic Research* 68, no. 1 (2010): 29–36.

16. L. Witek-Janusek, K. Albuquerque, K. R. Chroniak, et al., "Effect of Mindfulness Based Stress Reduction on Immune Function, Quality of Life and Coping in Women Newly Diagnosed with Early Stage Breast Cancer," *Brain, Behavior and Immunity* 22, no. 6 (2008): 969–981.

17. J. W. Carson et al., "Loving-Kindness Meditation for Chronic Low Back Pain: Results from a Pilot Trial," *Journal of Holistic Nursing* 23, no. 3 (2005): 287–309.

18. B. Fredrickson et al., "Open Hearts Build Lives: Positive Emotions, Induced Through Loving-kindness Meditation, Build Consequential Personal Resources," *Journal of Personality and Social Psychology* 95 no. 5 (November 2008): 1045–1062. doi:10.1037/a0013262

19. D. Ornish et al., "Can Lifestyle Changes Reverse Coronary Artery Disease?" *Lancet* 336 (1990): 129.

20. S. Khalsa, E. Shorter, et al. "Yoga Ameliorates Performance Anxiety and Mood Disturbance in Young Professional Musicians," *Applied Psychophysiology and Biofeedback* 34, no. 4 (2009): 279–289.

21. J. Coleman, "Spring Forest Qigong and Chronic Pain: Making a Difference," *Journal of Holistic Nursing* 9 (November 2010). doi:10.1177/0898010110385939

22. B. M. Cheung et al., "Randomized Controlled Trial of Qigong in the Treatment of Mild Essential Hypertension," *Journal of Human Hypertension* 19, no. 9 (2005): 697–704.

23. J. Macrae, *Therapeutic Touch: A Practical Guide* (New York: Knopf, 1987).

24. T. Nhat Hanh, *The Blooming of a Lotus: Guided Meditation Exercises for Healing and Transformation* (Boston, MA: Beacon Press, 1993): 17.

25. T. Nhat Hanh, *The Long Road Turns to Joy: A Guide to Walking Meditation* (Berkeley, CA: Parallax Press, 1996): 8.

26. T. Nhat Hanh, *Teachings on Love* (Berkeley, CA: Parallax Press, 1997): 21.

27. B. Barnum, *Spirituality in Nursing: From Traditional to New Age*, 2nd ed. (New York: Springer, 2003): 165.

28. J. Keicolt-Glaser et al., "Psychosocial Enhancement of Immunocompetence in a Geriatric Population," *Health Psychology* 4 (1985): 25–41.

29. L. Pawlow and G. Jones, "The Impact of Abbreviated Progressive Muscle Relaxation on Salivary Cortisol and Salivary Immunoglobulin A (sIgA)," *Applied Psychophysiology and Biofeedback* 30, no. 4 (December 2005): 375–387.

30. G. Knowlton and K. Larkin, "The Influence of Voice Volume, Pitch, and Speech Rate on Progressive Relaxation Training: Application of Methods from Speech Pathology and Audiology," *Applied Psychophysiology and Biofeedback* 31, no. 2 (June 2006): 173–185.

31. J. Schultz and W. Luthe, *Autogenic Training: A Psychophysiologic Approach in Psychotherapy* (New York: Grune & Stratton, 1959).

32. M. Shinozaki and M. Kanazawa, "Effect of Auto-genic Training on General Improvement in Patients with Irritable Bowel Syndrome: A Randomized Controlled Trial," *Applied Psychophysiology Biofeedback* 35 (2010): 189–198.

33. S. Fahrion, "Hypertension and Biofeedback," *Primary Care* 18 (1991): 663–682.

34. G. Tan, T. Dao, et al., "Heart Rate Variability (HRV) and Posttraumatic Stress Disorder (PTSD): A Pilot Study," *Applied Psychophysiology Biofeedback* 36 (2011): 27–35.

35. R. P. Nolan et al., "Heart Rate Variability Biofeedback as a Behavioral Neurocardiac Intervention to Enhance Vagal Heart Rate Control," *American Heart Journal* 149, no. 6 (2005): 1137.

36. C. B. Yucha et al., "Biofeedback-Assisted Relaxation Training for Essential Hypertension: Who Is Most Likely to Benefit?" *Journal of Cardiovascular Nursing* 20, no. 3 (2005): 198–205.

37. R. A. McGinnis et al., "Biofeedback-Assisted Relaxation in Type 2 Diabetes," *Diabetes Care* 28, no. 9 (2005): 2145–2149.

38. R. Davidson et al., "The Psychobiology of Relaxation and Related States: Multiprocess Theory," in *Behavioral Control and the Modification of Physiological Processes*, ed. D. J. Mostofsky (Englewood Cliffs, NJ: Prentice Hall, 1976).

39. W. Linden, "The Autogenic Training Method of J. H. Schultz," in *Principles and Practice of Stress Management*, 2nd ed., ed. P. M. Lehrer et al. (New York: Guilford Press, 1993).

40. P. Lehrer et al., "Effects of Progressive Relaxation and Autogenic Training on Anxiety and Physiological Measures with Some Data on Hypnotizability," in *Stress and Tension Control*, ed. F. J. McGuigan et al. (New York: Plenum Publishing, 1980).

41. S. Shapiro et al., "Psychophysiological Effects of Autogenic Training and Progressive Relaxation," *Biofeedback and Self-Regulation* 5 (1980): 249–255.

42. H. Benson, *The Relaxation Response* (New York: William Morrow, 1975).

43. D. Larkin, Interview, College of New Rochelle, June 16, 2003.

44. D. Cheeks, "Hypnosis," in *The Complete Guide to Holistic Medicine Health for the Whole Person*, ed. A. Hastings et al. (New York: Bantam Books, 1981): 141–156.

45. B. Rogers, "Therapeutic Conversation and Post-hypnotic Suggestion," *American Journal of Nursing* 72 (1972): 714–717.

46. D. Larkin, "Therapeutic Suggestion," in *Relaxation and Imagery: Tools for Therapeutic Communication and Intervention*, ed. R. Zahorek (Philadelphia, PA: W. B. Saunders, 1988).

47. E. Jacobs et al., "Ericksonian Hypnosis and Approaches with Pediatric Hematology Oncology Patients," *American Journal Clinical Hypnosis* 41, no. 2 (1998): 139–153.

48. N. Cousins, Healers in Healthcare Speakers Series (Advances and Institute of Noetic Sciences, New York chapter, NYU Medical Center Dental School, NY, Fall 1988).

49. E. Green and A. Green, *Biofeedback: The Yoga of the West* (Cos Cob, CT: Hartley Film Foundation, 1970).

50. S. O'Brien, "Staff Wellness Program Promotes Quality Care," *American Journal of Nursing* 98, no. 6 (1998): 16B.

51. S. E. Taylor et al., "Female Responses to Stress: Tend and Befriend, Not Fight or Flight," *Psychological Review* 107, no. 3 (2000): 41.

52. M. Schwartz, "Selected Problems Associated with Relaxation Therapies and Guidelines for Coping with the Problems," in *Biofeedback*, 3rd ed., ed. M. Schwartz et al. (New York: Guilford Press, 2003).

53. J. Domino et al., "Prior Physical and Sexual Abuse in Women with Chronic Headaches: Clinical Correlates," *Headache* 27 (1987): 310–314.

54. R. Schaedle, director of Crisis Resource Center at LifeNet at the Mental Health Association of NYC, unpublished personal interview, June 25, 2003.

55. J. Draper, director of Public Education and the LifeNet Hotline Network, unpublished personal interview, July 9, 2003.

56. J. Sareen et al., "Physical and Mental Comorbidity, Disability, and Suicidal Behavior Associated with Posttraumatic Stress Disorder in a Large Community Sample," *Psychosomatic Medicine* 69, no. 3 (2007): 242–248.

57. D. Larkin, assistant professor, College of New Rochelle School of Nursing, unpublished personal interview, June 16, 2003.

58. E. Barrett, "The Theoretical Matrix for a Rogerian Nursing Practice," *Theoria: Journal of Nursing Theory*, no. 9 (2000): 4.

59. S. Bloom, "After 9/11: Living with Grief: Workplace Strategies for Support and Response" (presentation given at NYU Medical Center, NY, September 24, 2002).

60. J. Campion, "Spirituality and Holism in Nursing Self-Care Practice" (presentation at 5th Annual Holism and Nursing Conference, Zeta Omega Chapter-at-Large of Sigma Theta Tau International, Rye, NY, May 16, 2003).

61. J. Laster, *Relax, Renew: Restful Yoga for Stressful Living* (Berkeley, CA: Rodwell Press, 1995).

62. S. C. F. Tolse, "A Case Report of the Design and Implementation of a Hospital Based Therapeutic Yoga Rehabilitation Program" (abstract presentation at International Association of Yoga Therapists, Los Angeles, CA, January 2007).

63. N. Gerlach-Spriggs et al., *Restorative Gardens: The Healing Landscape* (New Haven, CT: Yale University Press, 1998).

Chapter 17

Imagery

Bonney Gulino Schaub and
Megan McInnis Burt

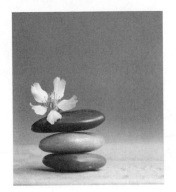

Nurse Healer
OBJECTIVES

Theoretical

- Define and contrast the different types of imagery.
- Discuss the imagery process and different theories of imagery.
- Explain different imagery interventions.

Clinical

- Incorporate imagery interventions into your clinical practice.
- Appreciate the spectrum and variety of clinical responses to imagery.
- Learn techniques to empower your spoken words.
- Train your voice so that your tone of voice and the pacing of selected words and phrases convey the qualities of calmness, reassurance, openness, and trust.

Personal

- Bring awareness of your own imagery process into your daily life.
- Choose a special healing image to focus on throughout the day.
- Learn to trust and be curious about the meaning of your images.

DEFINITIONS

Body–mind imagery: The conscious formation of an image that is directed to a body area or activity that requires attention or increased energy.

Clinical imagery: The conscious use of the power of the imagination with the intention of activating physiologic, psychological, or spiritual healing.

Correct biologic imagery: Biologically accurate images that are visualized to send messages to physiologic processes.

End-state imagery: Images that contain specified imagined hopes and goals (e.g., a healed wound).

Guided imagery: A highly structured imagery technique.

Imagery process: Internal experiences of memories, dreams, fantasies, inner perceptions, and visions, sometimes involving one, several, or all of the senses, serving as the bridge for connecting body, mind, and spirit.

Imagery rehearsal: An imagery technique designed to rehearse behaviors or prepare for activities or procedures.

Impromptu imagery: The nurse's introduction of his or her spontaneous, intuitive images or perceptions into the therapeutic intervention.

Packaged imagery: Commercial tapes that have general images.

Relationship imagery: Imagery designed to explore relationships with other people or with a part of oneself (e.g., the part that is always judgmental) or with a symptom or part of one's body (e.g., connecting with the heart).

Spontaneous imagery: The unexpected reception of an image, as if it "bubbled up," entering the stream of consciousness.

Symbolic imagery: Inner images that represent a person's deeper knowledge, occurring in the form of metaphors or symbols, that may be immediately translatable to rational verbal thought, or their meaning may emerge slowly over time.

Transpersonal imagery: Images that connect one to expanded (i.e., beyond personality) levels of consciousness, such as imagining one's body as a mountain and beginning to feel an inner quality of immovable strength and solidity.

Visualization: The use of external images (e.g., religious paintings, written words, nature photography) to evoke internal imagery experiences that energize desired emotions, qualities, outcomes, or goals.

■ THEORY AND RESEARCH

Imagery is an essential aspect of holistic nursing practice because it brings the natural powers of the mind into the process of health and healing. Distinct from thinking, imagery as a technique interacts with the image-making function of the brain, which, in turn, acts on the entire physiology. Imagery can be used on its own or in conjunction with therapeutic touch, meditation, biofeedback, Reiki, reflexology, massage, and other holistic practices.

The clinical value of imagery has been well documented in the treatment of a wide variety of conditions such as cancer,[1] migraine headaches, irritable bowel syndrome,[2,3] hypertension, anxiety and depression,[4] fibromyalgia,[5,6] post-traumatic stress disorder,[7-9] immune system disorders,[10,11] and asthma.[12]

The Institute of Heartmath (www.heartmath .org), a research center dedicated to the study of the heart and the physiology of emotions, has done extensive research into the resulting physiologic outcomes that arise from the practice of imagining appreciation, gratitude, and compassion. When subjects engaged the imagination in the heartfelt experience of appreciation, studies reflect the outcome of physiologic coherence. The emotional experience of appreciation was found to create a more coherent heart rhythm. This coherent state has been correlated with feelings of emotional well-being and improvements in cognitive, emotional, and physiologic performance.[13,14]

The research definition of imagery is a perception of a stimulus in the absence of that stimulus. For example, if a person imagines a lemon and begins to taste lemon juice, he or she is having a perception (tasting the juice) of a stimulus (lemon) that is not present. Commonly, in addition to tasting the lemon, the person begins to salivate as well, demonstrating a rapid physiologic alteration in response to the imagery suggestion. Research has shown that our physiology reacts to imagined stimuli. For example, research has shown that imagining an odor results in physical changes as if an actual odor has been experienced.[15] Magnetic resonance imaging (MRI) investigations of the brain's recording of tactile information shows that imaged tactile stimulation and actual tactile stimulation are registered in partially overlapping areas of the brain.[16] Researchers also used functional magnetic resonance imaging (fMRI) to examine brain activity in healthy volunteers who mentally imagined walking along a curved path. The outcomes suggest there is a very close neurophysiologic relationship between locomotion and its mental imagery.[17] In other words, the brain processes our images as if they were real.

This "absence of stimuli" definition is relevant to the crucial issue of the placebo effect, a phenomenon in which the patient thinks (imagines) he or she is receiving a potent medication and experiences the anticipated effects, both positive (placebo) and negative (nocebo), of that medication, when in fact a neutral substance was administered.

A practitioner's suggestions regarding expected outcome influences the effect of a placebo. In a study where subjects were instructed to place their hands in ice water, one group was informed of the beneficial effect of this practice, one group was told of the possible hazards, and the control group was given a neutral suggestion. The pain threshold, tolerance, and endurance of the three groups were compared. The tolerance of participants given the positive suggestion was significantly greater than that of the other two groups. In contrast, the group given the negative suggestion had significantly decreased tolerance and endurance of the test condition.[18]

A study compared the impact of language considered compassionate or instructive with words that offered the imagination something it could directly work with, such as imagining being in a safe and comfortable place or imagining coolness or warmth. Words that may have been thought of as instructive or even compassionate, for example, "it's only going to be a small sting," or "don't worry," registered more distress than when the practitioner offered the patient's mind something positive and therapeutic to work with. Soothing, positive imagery suggestions provided more anxiety reduction and decreased distress.[19,20]

This information challenges the holistic nurse to understand and work with the power of a patient's imagination when providing care. Clinical imagery is the conscious use of the power of the imagination with the intention of activating physiologic, psychological, or spiritual healing. The key word in this definition is *conscious*. The power of the imagination, for good or bad, is always affecting people. People imagine negative futures and employ their intelligence to worry about that negative future. Their life becomes focused around a negative future that they imagine to be true. Imagery's clinical focus is to use the imagination to promote life-affirming behaviors and goals. In addition to its contribution in promoting physical healing, imagery has great value in wellness education. It has shown value in improving quality of life through decreasing stress, increasing positive mood, and improving general health status.[21]

The effectiveness of imagery in healing has been recognized and used cross-culturally for thousands of years.[22,23] Imagery, in addition to improving physical symptoms, can be used for promoting psychological and spiritual development. It has the potential for promoting per-sonal transformation through an enhanced sense of the interconnectedness of body, mind, and soul.[24] When bringing imagery into clinical practice, nurses are introducing proven ancient methods of healing into modern health care.

Research on States of Consciousness and Mental Imagery

Several important psychology research findings about the ongoing imagery process, or "stream of consciousness," have implications for the nursing care of patients and clients. Sensory deprivation research in the early 1960s spurred the study of the ongoing imagery process. Initially, the purpose of this research was to examine the functioning of the brain in the absence of sensory input. Much of this research resulted from the space program's need to understand the impact on astronauts of the sensory deprivation, isolation, and confinement of space travel.[25] These studies indicated that an ongoing imagery process is a vital element in human mental experience, particularly when perceptual stimulation is reduced as it is in those who have a sensory impairment, those who are dealing with the monotony of hospitalization—particularly those in intensive care units—and those who work in monotonous environments.

Working with imagery has the potential to tap into memory at extremely deep levels. Wilder Penfield, a Canadian neurosurgeon working in the middle of the twentieth century, did extensive experimentation with direct electrical stimulation and mapping of the brain during surgery. In his research on locally anesthetized, conscious subjects, he identified an area of the brain he labeled the "interpretive cortex." Upon electrostimulation of this region, he discovered that there is a brain mechanism "capable of bringing back a strip of past experience in complete detail without any of the fanciful elaborations that occur in a man's dreaming . . . a record that has not faded but seems to remain as vivid as when the record was made."[26] Penfield went on to indicate that, although the memories recalled in this manner were predominantly visual or auditory, the memory record included all the sensory information that had entered consciousness (e.g., smells, tastes, sounds, tactile sensations). In addition, there was a sense of familiarity about the event. Simultaneous with the experience of these memory records, Penfield's subjects retained an awareness of their present situation, namely, that they were on an operating table having their brain probed by a surgeon.

Penfield's studies illustrate the capacity of consciousness to be absorbed in multiple activities at the same time. Penfield's patients were conscious of complete sensory recall of memories, were conscious of being on an operating room table, and were able to verbalize their experiences to Penfield and his staff. Appreciating the potentials of human consciousness is a key element in imagery work.

Clinical Effectiveness of Imagery

A comprehensive survey of the research on the physiologic effects of imagery cites the following effects on a wide range of systems and symptoms.[27]

- Increased internal blood flow, demonstrated by increased temperature in specific skin areas
- Increased heart rate resulting from imaging sexually or emotionally arousing situations
- Alterations in body chemistry, such as gastric secretions and salivary pH
- Muscle stimulation as shown in electromyography
- Immune system responses
- Wound healing
- Heart rate control in response to either relaxing or anxiety-producing images
- Systolic and diastolic blood pressure changes in response to images of fear and anger

Jacobson demonstrated imagery's effect on motor responses in 1929, when he showed that subtle tensions of small muscles or sense organs result from imagining movement.[28] (See Chapter 15.) This aspect of imagery was applied in working with patients affected with parkinsonism. Mental images of movement were used to help in freeing movement in unmoving body parts.[29]

Imagery has also been applied in poststroke rehabilitation.[30] Patients with chronic hemiparesis worked with imagined wrist movements and imagined movements of reaching and manipulating objects, resulting in significant improvement that remained stable for 3 months.

Simonton and associates explored the effect of imagery on immune function and the application of this information in the treatment of cancer,[31] as did Achterberg and Lawlis.[22,32] Hall studied the effect of hypnosis and imagery on immune modulation, noting increases in the number of lymphocytes and general increased immune system responsiveness.[1,33] Schneider and associates demonstrated enhanced immune responsiveness in subjects working with imagery of white blood cells attacking germs. Schneider and associates also successfully used imagery to increase adherence, or "stickiness," of neutrophils.[34] Two factors affected the successful use of imagery in these studies. First, the biologic accuracy of the imagery appeared to be significant. Second, the ability to work with the imagery without straining at it played a part in significant outcomes.

One of the clearest reflections of the complex body-mind-spirit-environment interaction is in the chronic pain syndromes.[35] A study compared the effectiveness of two different types of imagery in the reduction of daily fibromyalgia pain. In the study, women were assigned to one of three groups: Group 1 received relaxation training and guided instruction in "pleasant imagery" to distract from the pain experience; group 2 received relaxation training and "attention imagery" instruction, encouraging the "active workings of the internal pain control systems"; group 3, the control group, received treatment as usual without any imagery. All the patients in the study were also randomly assigned to treatment with either 50 mg per day of amitriptyline or a placebo pill. The results showed a significant difference in the reduction of pain in the group receiving the pleasant imagery, but not in the attention imagery group when compared with the control group. In addition, it was found that amitriptyline had no significant advantage over the placebo in reducing fibromyalgia pain during the course of the study.[36]

This information also reflects the fact that if an imagery intervention does not prove to be helpful for a particular patient, the practitioner should not be discouraged, but instead should use creativity and try other imagery approaches. The attention imagery may have worked for some, just as the pleasant imagery was not effective with everyone. Statistical significance is helpful and points to a general understanding of effects, but does not give us the final word on what works for an individual. This information may even suggest what works for an individual under one set of conditions, but it may not apply in other circumstances.

Guided imagery with progressive muscle relaxation (PMR) (see Chapter 16) was demonstrated to be effective in the alleviation of pain and mobility difficulties in osteoarthritis (OA). Twenty-eight older women with OA took part in the study. The 14 participants in the treatment group listened to an audiotape of guided imagery and PMR twice a day for 12 weeks. The 14 women in the control group did not do any imagery or PMR. The treatment group reported a significant reduction in pain and increased mobility. This result confirms that this treatment is an effective, cost-effective self-management intervention.[37] Positive outcomes were also found in the introduction of imagery interventions to manage pain in an elderly orthopedic population.[38]

Imagery has the ability to help alter the meaning that patients assign to their pain. This was observed in a study where pain patients learned and used a guided imagery audiotape over 4 consecutive days and the control group received their usual treatment for a 4-day period. At the end of the treatment those patients who used the imagery were able to perceive their pain as changeable as opposed to never ending. They also increased their sense of control, their ability to distract themselves from the pain, and other benefits.[39]

The richness of imagery as an intervention in working with children has been described in many clinical settings. Children's receptivity to imaginative play and interactions is an opening for the nurse's creative use of imagery.[40] The effectiveness of imagery in the reduction of recurrent abdominal pain,[41] in the reduction of postoperative pain,[42] and in pediatric hospice pain management[43] are all areas for additional nursing research.

Our access to our imagination, our inner wisdom, and our inner healing resources are all elements of imagery work. Because anyone's experience of imagery is deeply subjective, imagery is a challenge to quantify and objectify through a process of quantitative research. Although research is a vital element in gaining recognition of the clinical value of this exciting and effective tool, research necessitates, by its nature, reducing the questions asked into dichotomous frame-

works. Do we even know if it is the image, per se, that is effecting the change? Or is it the focus, intentionality, and empowerment that we elicit in our patients when we provide them with education about inner skills and potentials that are ultimately creating the therapeutic effect? Imagery researcher Braud states: "Perhaps images are simply clothed intentions—specific intentions or focused intentions that have been dramatized or personified in imagery forms?"[44]

Clinical Imagery and States of Consciousness

One of the pioneers and influential innovators in the clinical application of imagery into body-mind-spirit medicine was Dr. Roberto Assagioli. He was an Italian psychiatrist who introduced these techniques beginning in 1909.[45,46] His concept of the wholeness of human consciousness, called psychosynthesis, has been extensively applied in the helping professions since 1965. He was personally most interested in developing a science of the higher self, a term that he used to describe the aspect of each person that holds inner wisdom and connection with life purpose. He saw the higher self as a developmental step latent inside each person.

Assagioli used imagery in three forms:

1. Inner images, to explore the various levels of human experience, including biologic, social, and transpersonal experience.
2. Inner images, to represent the intentions and goals of the patient.
3. External images—the actual paintings and statues of his city, Florence, Italy—to help encourage transpersonal feelings in his patients. He often suggested that his patients go to a particular museum or church to meditate on a particular work of art because of the spiritual insights and feelings that the artist expressed in the work.[47]

Within his body-mind-spirit context, Assagioli developed a set of principles he referred to as "psychological laws," which describe the interactive effects among images, ideas, emotions, physical responses, behaviors, attitudes, and impulses. According to one such law, "images or mental pictures tend to produce the physical conditions and the external acts that correspond to them." According to a second law, "attitudes, movements, and actions tend to evoke corresponding images and ideas; these, in turn, evoke or intensify corresponding emotions."[46pp51-52] In these and other laws, Assagioli was seeking to outline the ability of the mind through imagery and intention to interact with, and positively affect, the body–mind for healing and psychospiritual growth.

In a recent study that follows the spirit of Assagioli's work, researchers began with the observation that directing attention to the body is part of the effectiveness of techniques such as imagery and meditation in producing psychophysiologic harmonious states.[48] They wondered what the measurable effect would be of directing attention to particular body organs. Their studies focused specifically on the heart. When simultaneously measuring heart rhythm by electrocardiogram (ECG) and brain wave rhythm by EEG, they instructed subjects to focus attention on their heartbeat. In doing this, they discovered a state of heart–brain electrical wave synchronization. They then postulated that a linear process emerges as a result of the synchronization occurring from this focused direction of consciousness: self-attention to connection to self-regulation to order to ease. They proposed that this existed in contrast to a process of disattention to disconnection to disregulation to disorder to disease. It was also observed that the synchronization was more effective when participants practiced with eyes closed.

CLINICAL TECHNIQUES IN IMAGERY

It is clear that imagery affects our general physical state and our sense of emotional well-being. Patients with negative imagery will go into physical states of fear and nervous vigilance. If, instead, they choose to focus their minds on specific positive imagery, all of their physical systems will move toward states of ease and harmony. Imagery interacts with physiologic processes, sending messages and information from the right brain to the central nervous system.

Nurses may use specific, highly structured, guided body–mind, correct biological, and end-state imagery techniques. The use of symbolic drawing can also be introduced in the explora-

tion process. Perhaps the most available use of imagery is the nurse's own impromptu imagery. Impromptu imagery is the nurse's unplanned use of an image that arises in her own imagery process during a clinical interaction. For example, an emergency room nurse, caring for a woman who had badly injured arms as a result of a car accident, was unable to establish an intravenous (IV) line because the woman's veins were collapsing. The situation was urgent, and there was discussion about the possible need to amputate an arm. The nurse, who had recently started studying clinical imagery, suddenly had an image of this woman holding a baby. She immediately suggested that the woman take a few moments and embrace her injured arm as if it were a tiny baby. She said, "Hold your arm, and send it loving energy." Within moments, the woman was calm, and the nurse was able to start the IV infusion.

Another nurse became aware of a patient's anxiety as she was preparing to administer a transfusion of packed cells. The woman had recently experienced a number of transfusion reactions and was fearful about the procedure. The nurse, who was meeting the patient for the first time, noticed that the cells had come from a source in Florida. She had an image of the blood donor basking on a warm Florida beach. The nurse told the woman where the blood supply had originated and suggested that she imagine these cells bringing the healing energy of the Florida sun and the gentle breeze of the beach to soothe and calm her. The patient immediately responded favorably to this suggestion, happy to have a calming image with which to engage her mind. The transfusion was a success.

Imagery in Holistic Health Coaching

Imagery clearly taps a deep level of self-knowledge in the patient. One example of this occurs in relationship imagery. In one instance, when a patient was asked to describe his relationship with his father, he offered a few familiar comments. But when he was asked to get an image of his father, the patient suddenly got in touch with the feelings of sadness and hopelessness that his father stimulated in him. This deeper level of self-knowledge allowed the patient to appreciate why he struggled with hopelessness in himself.

Nurses are often working with patients and family members who are grieving past or immanent losses. (See Chapter 21.) Imagery is a valuable resource at this time because the connection with the loved one is alive in the imagination. People often feel strongly that they have communicated at an extremely deep, meaningful, and comforting way with internal imagery processes.[49,50] These experiences may be helpful in making decisions, in rehearsing new behaviors, in understanding relationships, in making life choices, and in experiencing equanimity in the face of painful challenges.

Values and Spirituality

Nurses often are caring for patients at a stage in their lives when values and spirituality have become a central concern. Illness, divorce, ethical dilemmas, deaths, or other life crises often cause people to slow down and ask basic questions about how they are going to conduct their lives. Changes in physical capacities, the need to find different employment, decisions about education and lifestyle, and retirement all call upon people to reassess their deepest values and their sense of spiritual purpose in life.

At these times, rational thought processes are not enough because they do not reveal the big picture. Imagery allows someone to imagine the actual results of a decision. For example, a nurse counseling a 59-year-old elementary school teacher struggling with a decision about retirement suggested that she close her eyes, focus on her breath, and imagine herself retired. After a few moments, the woman experienced an image of herself at home, looking bored and unhappy. She was frustrated with this image. She then tried to imagine her retirement as a time of new growth. She went back into the imagery, trying to imagine herself retiring and going back to school to study something new—she was unable to do so. Her imagination literally refused to see it. She then imagined herself doing service work in the community. Suddenly, during this imagery, she felt a peace and an ease settle into her experience.

Imagining pictures of the future helps a person to make specific behavioral and emotional changes. This information is invaluable for decision making because it provides a holistic level of information that is not available at the purely verbal level.

Transpersonal Use of Imagery

The transpersonal (beyond personality) level of human nature is a fact. Cultures throughout the world have used prayer, meditation, imagery, diet, physical training, contemplation and study, ritual, art, and many other methods to experience transpersonal states of consciousness. People seek these states because they tend to provide a subtler understanding of the universal patterns of reality and a more peaceful perspective on the "little self" living in the immensity of creation. Holistic nurses frequently cite their own transpersonal experiences as one of the reasons they became interested in introducing holistic methods into their work. Motivated by their own development through such experiences, they desire to pass the potential of transpersonal experiences on to others.

The role of imagery in transpersonal experience is a crucial one. Holistic nurses can use transpersonal imagery to introduce patients safely to the transpersonal level of consciousness.[51-53] This imagery is referred to as transpersonal because it links and identifies the individual experience with universal processes. Transpersonal imagery taps into an expanded experience of the self, an experience that draws on human beings' capacity to connect deeply with the flow of life energy and creation. This connection, and the imagery that emerges from it, can be interpreted as a connection with God, with all of humanity, with a higher power, with the wonder of the universe and nature, or a connection with the mysterious, nonverbal communication that occurs between people at the level of intuitive knowing and caring. (See Chapters 4 and 32.)

Visualization practice can be helpful for energizing and eliciting transpersonal experiences. Art images, photographs, and picture postcards are all sources for images that can be used in work with transpersonal symbols. The nurse can begin to collect art cards and other images that can be used to help patients. For example, one elderly woman hospitalized with advanced heart disease was feeling lonely, depressed, and fearful. She expressed fear that she was going to die. In sharing this with the nurse, she said she was confused by spirituality and did not know what she believed. The nurse asked if she would like to explore these feelings with imagery, and the woman agreed. The nurse led her in a brief relaxation and then suggested that she experience herself in a place that she felt was sacred. The woman was silent for a long time. The nurse sat silently with her. After a while, the woman opened her eyes. She was surprised by her imagery. She felt herself in Florence, Italy, a place she had never visited. She imagined walking the streets, looking at the beauty of the churches, and feeling deeply connected to the sacredness of the art. She said she always imagined Florence as a sacred place. She deeply loved Renaissance art and imagined the magic of a place where so much beauty had been created. She realized that her love of art was the closest thing she could identify as a spiritual feeling. Recognizing the importance of this imagery for the patient, the nurse said she would bring her a postcard of Florence. This pleased the woman, and the nurse told her that it would be important to honor this inner experience by keeping a reminder of it where she could connect with it over the course of the day.

Working with metaphors and symbols of transcendent experiences is an effective way to help a patient who is experiencing spiritual distress, hopelessness, and helplessness. Bringing a client into deep relaxation and then introducing one of these metaphors in an open-ended, exploratory way can be deeply meaningful. The patient can choose the symbol that he or she wants to explore, or the nurse can create the journey based on information from the patient. In times of illness and crisis, people may have spontaneous spiritual experiences and images. It is advisable to learn about these images so that patients can be supported and derive benefit from their experience (see **Table 17-1**).

TABLE 17-1   Symbols and Metaphors of Transformation

Symbol or Metaphor	Transformative Experience
Introversion	Exploration of the true self; self-knowledge; inner journey to the soul, to beingness
Deepening/descent	Journey to the underworld of the psyche; confronting the difficult aspects of the self, the shadow; entering a cave; the heroic journey of facing fears
Ascent/elevation	Climbing a mountain to reach a higher plane of awareness
Expansion/broadening	Enlarging perspective; taking in the wholeness and seeing beyond one's small, individual perspective
Awakening	Awakening from the dream or from illusions; opening to the truth or reality of what really matters
Illumination	Bringing in the light of the human soul; spiritual light to transform or "enlighten" a situation; moving from darkness to light; bringing in life energy
Fire	Purification; spiritual alchemy; candles, lanterns, and bonfires; ceremonies of transformation
Development	Growth, blossoming; potentials waiting to become real
Love	Opening the heart; compassion and generosity; forgiveness
Path/pilgrimage	"Mystic way"; the journey of outward exploration; seeking to be changed by new experience or knowledge
Rebirth/regeneration	Birth of the new being; resurrection
Freedom/liberation	Liberation of psychic, physical, and spiritual energy to align with creation and creativity

Source: Adapted by permission of Sterling Lord Literistic, Inc. Copyright © 1965 by Robert Assagioli.

Imagery with Disease and Illness

Much emphasis is placed on treating disease, the pathologic changes in organic form either observed or validated by laboratory tests. There is also a great need to address the individual's personal experience of his or her illness, general state of being, anxiety level, state of hopefulness or despair, and the meaning attributed to the situation. The nurse, using imagery, can promote a sense of well-being in clients and help them change their perceptions about their disease, treatment, and their inner resources and innate healing ability. The use of an interactive approach to guided imagery with medical patients, which was designed to promote relaxation and cultivate healing intentions, has been significantly helpful in increasing patients' insights into their health problems.[54]

Fear and negative imagery are not unusual in an individual with an undiagnosed or even a known illness. For example, a woman who discovers a palpable breast lump may conjure up frightening images before any tests or diagnoses. These images may include cancer, mastectomy, chemotherapy, radiation, hair loss, nausea and vomiting, severe pain, metastatic disease, the dying process, funeral, and the actual moment of dying. This process may be conscious or preverbal. It may be noticed in dreams, daydreams, spontaneous images, and kinesthetic sensings.

Concrete Objective Information

Over the last 25 years, nursing research has been conducted on the use of imagery in preparing patients for difficult procedures. Using concrete objective information and descriptions of a procedure is a form of imagery rehearsal. Its effectiveness lies in the importance of the prepared mind. People are fearful of the unknown and of feeling out of control. This technique addresses both these fears.

Clients who receive information about both subjective and objective components of tests, procedures, and surgery recover more quickly. They are able to plan and use more effective coping strategies than clients who receive only one of the components. To prepare a patient for surgery, the nurse would describe what the person will experience at each stage of the procedure, including what will be felt, heard, seen, smelled, or tasted before, during, and after the operation. In addition, the imagery includes the sensory experiences of the postsurgical healing incision (e.g., pressure, smarting, tingling), as well as sensations over time (e.g., fleeting sharp sensations from the incision area when turning in bed or when coughing). **Table 17-2** lists sensations evoked by selected procedures.

Objective experiences are observable and verifiable by someone other than the person going through the procedure. Thus, for the surgical patient, an objective experience may include the time and place of the presurgery nurse's visit, the matters to be discussed in the visit, the preoperative preparation of the skin, placement on the stretcher to go to surgery, awakening in the recovery room, and expected sensations. This process reduces the likelihood that the patient will interpret normal sensations or events as signs that "something's wrong." It also allows the nurse and patient to plan specific strategies for the patient to handle difficult parts of the event.

The following procedural points related to the use of concrete, objective information originate in science-based nursing practice:

- Identify the sensory features of the procedure to be used.
- Determine the individual's perception of the procedure, treatment, or test to be experienced.
- Choose words that have meaning for the person.
- Use synonyms that have less emotional weight, such as *discomfort* instead of *pain*.
- Select specific experiences when giving examples, rather than abstract experiences (see Table 17-2).
- Help individuals reframe any negative imagery. For example, patients often fear chemotherapy and think of it as a poison because of all the precautions and side effects associated with it. It is important to have a way of framing the experience that is positive and focuses on healing. For example, the nurse may say, "Chemotherapy is powerful and effective in fighting the most vulnerable cells, the confused and incomplete cancer cells. The healthy cells—most of the cells in your body—are strong and protected."

TABLE 17-2   Documented Subjective Experience Descriptors by Stressful Healthcare Event

Stressful Event	Descriptors
Gastroendoscopic examination	Intravenous medication; feel needlestick, drowsiness
	As air is pumped into stomach, feeling of fullness like after eating a large meal
	Feel physician's finger in mouth to guide tube insertion
Nasogastric tube insertion	Feeling passage of tube
	Tearing
	Gagging
	Discomfort in nose, throat, mouth
	Limited mobility
Cast removal	Hear buzz of saw
	Feel vibrations or tingling
	See chalky dust
	Feel warmth on arm or leg as saw cuts cast; will not hurt or burn
	Skin under padding looks and feels scaly and dirty
	Arm or leg may feel a little stiff when first trying to move it
	Arm or leg may feel light because cast was heavy
Barium enema	Lying on hard table
	Table feels hard
	Feel fullness
	Feel pressure
	Feel bloating
	Feel uncomfortable
	Feel as if might have a bowel movement
Abdominal surgery	Preoperative medications: feel sleepy, light-headed, relaxed, free from worry, not bothered by most things, dryness of mouth
	Feel incision: tenderness, sensitivity, pressure, smarting, burning, aching, sore
	Sensations might become sharp and feel like they are traveling along incision when moving
	Arm with intravenous tube feels awkward and restricted but not painful
	Feel tired after physical effort
	Feel bloating in abdomen
	Cramping due to gas pains
	Pulling and pinching when stitches are removed
Tracheostomy	When moving about, swallowing, or during suctioning: feel hurting, pressure, choking
Mastectomy—mean of 5.5 years postoperative	Arm or chest wall pain, "pins and needles," numbness, weakness, increased skin sensitivity, heaviness
	Phantom breast sensations, such as twinges, itching
4-vessel arteriography	Before contrast medium: table is hard, head taping is uncomfortable, cleansing solution is cold
	After contrast medium: hot, burning sensation in face, neck, chest, or shoulders

Source: Adapted from *Nursing Interventions: Essential Nursing Treatments*, 2nd ed., by G. Bulechek and J. McCloskey, p. 145, with permission of W. B. Saunders Company, © 1992.

- Plan specific strategies to be used at different stages of the procedure, such as using a breathing technique while waiting for the procedure to begin, and using imagery of a safe place during the procedure as a distraction from uncomfortable sensations.

Fears in Imagery Work

There are three predictable and understandable fears encountered in imagery work:

1. *Nothing will happen.* Patients fear that they will not be able to imagine anything in response to the nurse's imagery suggestion. Coincidentally, the nurse may share the same fear. The nurse may be afraid that the imagery method will produce nothing of worth for the patient.

   The answer to this fear is to be curious about any experience that occurs during the course of the imagery. If, for example, the patient reports that her breathing became faster as soon as she heard the nurse's suggestion to relax, the nurse should be curious about why the patient believes her breathing became faster. The patient may respond that she was afraid of relaxing. On the surface, this may seem a strange statement. How can anyone be afraid of relaxing? In fact, relaxation can be frightening. For example, it can be frightening for someone who has experienced trauma in childhood and feels the importance of maintaining vigilance. Such information can be invaluable in actually helping the patient to enter states of relaxation safely and to engage in imagery work.

2. *Too much will happen.* Patients fear that the imagery will evoke difficult or even overwhelming thoughts and feelings. Coincidentally, the nurse may share the same fear. The nurse may fear the imagery method will be too evocative and will have negative consequences for the patient.

   The answer to this concern is that imagery does not take away a person's defenses. If the imagery suggestion is too evocative, the patient will simply fail to hear it, ignore it, change it into a suggestion that is easier to work with, or open his or her eyes and stop the process. If a patient does have difficult thoughts and feelings in response to the imagery suggestion, these thoughts and feelings will develop because the patient is ready to receive them.

   These statements presuppose that the nurse is skilled in imagery and is not imposing a manipulative imagery practice. Each patient has the potential for important new knowledge and new feeling. The nurse is not using imagery to make something happen. Rather, the nurse is using imagery to evoke what is already present in the patient. Carried out in this spirit, the nurse will not evoke any experiences for which the patient is not ready. The imagery suggestion will instead open the patient to the interior world of latent intuition, knowledge, and creative problem solving already present in the patient's imagination.

3. *It will be done wrong.* Anxious to please the nurse, patients fear they cannot do imagery the "right way." Coincidentally, the nurse may also harbor the fear that there is a "right way" to do imagery, and that his or her personal skills are inadequate for the "right way."

   The answer to this fear is to realize that there is no right way. The processes of the imagination are unique to each person; thus, each imagery experience is unique. Furthermore, a nurse may use the same imagery suggestion twice, and the same patient may experience two totally different responses to the imagery. It is important to realize that the patient's experience is the center of all imagery work. The nurse may suggest imaging a walk in an open field, and the patient may respond by imaging the atmosphere in a dark room. The dark room becomes of importance. The original suggestion of an open field is no longer significant. The meaning of the dark room for the patient becomes the source of interest and new learning. The nurse's imagery suggestion is simply that—a suggestion—to evoke the latent powers and intelligence of the imagination into the service of the patient. Imagery techniques can be studied for many years, imagery skills can be honed, and yet it remains the unique response of the patient that is central to the work.

■ HOLISTIC CARING PROCESS

Holistic Assessment

In preparing to use imagery as a nursing intervention, the nurse assesses the following parameters:

- The client's potential for organic brain syndrome or psychosis to determine if general relaxation techniques should be used instead of imagery techniques.
- The client's anxiety/tension levels to determine which types of relaxation inductions will be most effective.
- The client's hopes in regard to the session and reason for seeking help.
- The client's wants, needs, desires, or recurrent and dominant themes.
- The client's understanding that it is not necessary to literally hear, see, feel, touch, or taste when working with imagery; that it is best to trust the inner experience in whatever form the information comes.
- The client's primary sensory modalities when he or she experiences the imagination—visual, auditory, kinesthetic, and so forth.
- The client's understanding that imagery is basically a way in which we communicate with ourselves at a deep level.
- The client's understanding that imagery can bring us into contact with our body and find out what it needs.
- The client's previous experiences with the imagery process.
- The client's emotional comfort level with closing eyes, bringing attention inside, and opening to states of internal awareness; if the client is not comfortable with closing the eyes, the nurse can suggest just lowering the eyes and gazing at a point on the floor approximately 1 or 2 feet in front of him or her. This will cause the client's peripheral vision to blur, eyelids will usually get heavy, and then the eyes will close effortlessly. Some clients need to learn to

trust that it is safe to relax, that they are experiencing a natural phenomenon.
- The client's knowledge of relaxation skills; if not skilled in relaxation, the client may need an explanation of what the normal sensations will be and time to shift to the "letting go" state. Once the client becomes skilled at entering a relaxed state, a selected word, phrase, or hand posture can become a signal to relax.
- The client's ability to maintain attention and not drowse off in the session.

Identification of Patterns/ Challenges/Needs

The following are the patterns/challenges/ needs (see Chapter 7) compatible with imagery interventions:

- Social isolation
- Role performance
- Caregiver role strain
- Parental role strain
- Spiritual well-being
- Spiritual distress
- Altered effective coping
- Impaired adjustment
- Ineffective denial
- Potential for growth
- Decision conflict
- Health-seeking behaviors
- Sleep pattern disturbance
- Relocation stress syndrome
- Altered self-concept
- Disturbance in body image
- Disturbance in self-image
- Potential hopelessness
- Potential powerlessness
- Pain
- Anxiety
- Fear
- Posttrauma response
- Grief

Outcome Identification

Exhibit 17-1 guides the nurse in client outcomes, nursing prescriptions, and evaluations for the use of imagery as a nursing intervention.

Therapeutic Care Plan and Interventions

Facilitation and Interpretation of the Imagery Process

It is essential for nurses to become aware of their own imagery process and familiarize themselves with the rich variety and individuality of imagery experiences. When nurses come together in a group to listen and share personal and professional stories, they hear many perspectives. They can train themselves to listen to the use of meta-phors and images and learn from the different types of experiences.

To facilitate the imagery process, the nurse serves as a guide. There is absolutely no way to predict what will surface in a client's imagination. Every experience is different, even when the same script is used.

Nurses who are unfamiliar with imagery and guiding should learn a few basic relaxation and imagery scripts and practice on themselves by making tapes of their own voice and following

EXHIBIT 17-1   Nursing Interventions: Imagery

Nursing Prescriptions	Evaluation	Client Outcomes
Following an assessment, guide the client in an imagery exercise.	The client participated in imagery exercise by choice.	The client will demonstrate skills in imagery.
Assess the client's levels of anxiety with this new process.	The client demonstrated no signs of anxiety with imagery process.	
After the imagery process experience, assess effectiveness through client dialogue.	The client stated that the imagery experience was helpful.	
Encourage the client to recognize daily self-talk and the images that lead to balance and inner peace.	The client reported using self-dialogue with imagery.	
Help the client to create images of desired health habits, feelings, desires for daily living.	The client reported creating images of desired health habits, feelings, and desires for daily living.	
Teach the client coping, power over daily events, ability to move toward healthy lifestyle.	The client reported increased coping with daily stressors.	
Teach the client to recognize images leading to self-defeating lifestyle habits.	The client reported recognition of negative images leading to self-defeating behavior; the client created positive images.	
Encourage the client to draw images and symbols as a communication process with self.	The client used drawing as a communication process with self.	

their own guiding. This will help build confidence with the intervention. It is helpful to learn a variety of scripts pertaining to common problems in clinical practice, such as preoperative anxiety, recovery from surgery, postoperative coughing, effective wound healing, fear, anxiety, pain, and relationship problems. For scripts not frequently used, some nurses keep a notebook or reference book handy. In studying clinical imagery, the nurse needs to be willing to open up and learn it from the inside out, using imagery for personal change and development.

Each individual is the best interpreter of his or her own imagery process. Symbolic information that surfaces in the imagination is rich with personal meaning. Many people have been closed off from or afraid of their imagination. Nurses should encourage clients to record their images in a diary or journal for further exploration. It is easy to lose symbolic imagery in the conscious thoughts that dominate one's attention during a busy day.

When teaching imagery, the nurse listens to the way that a client tells his or her story to get a sense of the client's outlook and orientation to the world. Does the client have a materialistic, concrete outlook on problem solving and life in general, or a more intuitive, spontaneous perspective? For the logical, concrete thinker, written information is useful. For example, if using imagery for hand warming, the nurse may prepare an imagery teaching sheet that includes specific physiologic information and instructions such as the following:

- An explanation of normal blood flow physiology
- A drawing of blood flow to the hands via radial and ulnar arteries that branch into intricate blood vessel networks of the hands and the fingers
- Examples of images that warm the hands

Less structure is necessary for the more intuitive patient. The nurse can go directly to working with imagery and use the teaching sheets to support what the vivid imager has learned.

There is no need to follow teaching sheets explicitly. Suggested images are adapted to fit what feels right to the client. Teaching sheets refresh and reinforce the teaching–learning session and provide additional information to be mastered. Clients can add their own notes about specific images and personalize their practice. The nurse can help clients rework weak or erroneous imagery so that it more accurately reflects healthy outcomes (e.g., images focusing on weak, confused, cancer cells and a strong immune system instead of vice versa).

Guided Imagery Scripts

The guidelines that follow help the nurse in the effective implementation of imagery scripts as nursing interventions:

- Start the session with an induction, a general relaxation—focusing on breath, shortened passive progressive relaxation, or body awareness, for example. (Also see Chapter 16.)
- Reaffirm that there is no right or wrong way for the client to do imagery, that whatever occurs is useful information, and that the client has complete control over the process (e.g., deciding whether to go further or to stop).
- Follow the induction instructions for yourself so that you communicate a calming presence.
- Personalize the imagery by using the client's name or other specific references several times during the process.
- Speak slowly and smoothly, allowing for pauses and silence after each suggestion.
- Observe the client's body language and breathing rhythm to assess responses to suggestions.
- If there are signs of tension such as shallow breathing, tightness of muscles, or tense facial muscles in response to an imagery suggestion, ask, "What are you experiencing now?"
- If the client appears to be struggling to get into the imagery, pause in the script and suggest that the client reconnect with the breath and go more deeply into relaxation.
- Avoid saying "yes" or "right" or other words that communicate evaluative reactions to the client's experience. A more supportive comment such as "stay with your experience" can be made.

- Provide encouragement and guidance for those with less vivid imagery. Vivid imagers, on the other hand, prefer more silence: words may be distracting or intrusive to them. Extremely vivid imagers may prefer to keep their eyes partially open to prevent feeling overwhelmed.
- End the session by bringing the person's awareness back to the room. You can do this by encouraging the person to begin to transition back to the room by becoming aware of his or her body in the chair or the bed, by bringing awareness to his or her breath, and then slowly opening his or her eyes. An example of another classic reintegration method is: "At the count of 5, you will be fully awake and alert . . . 1 . . . 2 . . . 3 . . . 4 . . . 5."

Induction for Imagery

A simple breathing technique or other relaxation technique may be useful to focus the client's mind inward and induce imagery. This allows awareness of subtler aspects of experience to become available to the person. This inward focus can be thought of as reducing external stimuli so that the inner awareness is enhanced.

The following induction script can be used as a preparation for most imagery interventions. It is especially appropriate for a person who needs assistance quieting the body. Resting the hands on the lower abdomen and breathing into the belly (diaphragmatic breathing) is an effective calming posture. In this position, the palms of the hands are resting on the body's energy center. By noting the slowing of breathing, relaxation of facial muscles, and changes in skin color, the nurse can assess the effectiveness of the relaxation technique. The induction for imagery can take 5 to 10 minutes. The most common mistake that new imagery practitioners make is to move too quickly through the suggestions. Go slowly. Allow your client time to connect with a subtler awareness. Learn to become comfortable with silent pauses.

> **Script:** Make yourself comfortable and close your eyes. . . . Put your hands gently on your lower abdomen, just below your navel. . . . Bring all your attention to the sensations in your hands. . . . Notice the slight rise and fall of your hands as they move with your breathing. . . . Notice the tactile sensations of the surfaces of your hands and fingers. . . . Bring all your awareness into these sensations. . . . [pause] Now notice the temperature of your hands. . . . [pause] Notice their weight. . . . [pause] Now notice any sensations inside the skin, perhaps tingling or pulsing. . . . [pause] Now bring your attention to the center of your chest and be aware of the sensations . . . notice the movement of your chest with each breath . . . the passage of breath into your lungs . . . the tactile sensations of your skin . . . perhaps an awareness of your heartbeat. . . . [Pause.] Now bring your awareness to your nose and be aware of breath passing through your nostrils. . . . Notice the slight cool sensations of the air touching the inside of your nose.

Connecting with Life Energy Imagery

This imagery, which draws on a person's sense of his or her inner energy, focuses on the fact that the body is not just sick. The life force is operating without any conscious effort. This awareness can reframe a person's attitude, bringing a connection with inner healing mechanisms and with what is functioning healthfully, as opposed to focusing on the disease process.

> **Script:** Bring your awareness to your imagination and take a moment to reflect on all the systems that are functioning in your body–mind at this moment . . . your heart and your circulatory system . . . [pause] your immune system . . . [pause]

your respiratory system . . . [pause] your senses. . . . [pause] Be aware of all of these. . . . [pause] Realize that you don't need to do anything to make these systems function. . . . They are part of your body's wisdom. . . . [pause] And now be aware that deep within you is a source of life energy . . . a vital spark that has been a part of you since the moment of your conception. . . . It has always been a part of you . . . guiding and energizing your body and mind. . . . Use your imagination to get in touch with this source of life energy. . . . Trust whatever information your imagination gives you. . . . Locate this source in your body. . . . Feel its strength and energy. . . . [pause] Allow your intuition to give you an image or symbol for this source and when you have the image, spend some time with it. . . . [pause] If it feels right, communicate with it. . . . What does it need from you? . . . [pause] If there is anything else that needs to happen in relation to this image, let it happen. . . . Take your time. . . . When you feel ready, bring your awareness back to the room.[55]

Special or Safe Place Imagery

Clients need to identify a special place that is a safe retreat. This is an easy place for novices to start. It takes 10 to 20 minutes. Several different approaches can be useful. The first script is more open ended and less specific. The ones that follow are more descriptive. People have different preferences as to what is most helpful.

Script: Let your imagination choose a place that is safe and comfortable . . . a place where you can retreat at any time. This is a healthy technique for you to learn. . . . This place will help you with your daily stressors. [If the client is in the hospital] This safe and special place is very important, particularly while you are in the hospital. . . . Any time that there are interruptions, just let yourself go to this place in your mind.

Form a clear image of a pleasant outdoor scene, using all of your senses. . . . Breathe . . . smell the fragrances around you. Feel . . . feel the texture of the surface under your feet. Hear . . . hear all the sounds in nature, birds singing, wind blowing. See . . . see all the different sights around as you let yourself turn in a slow circle to get a full view of this special space. [Include taste, if appropriate.]

Let a beam of light, such as the rays of the sun, shine on you for comfort and healing. Allow yourself to experience the warmth and relaxation. Form an image of a meadow. Imagine that you are in the meadow. . . . The meadow is full of beautiful grass and flowers. In the meadow, see yourself sitting by a stream . . . watching the water . . . flowing by . . . slowly and gently.

Imagine a mountain scene. See yourself walking on a path toward the mountain. You hear the sound of your shoes on the path . . . smell the pine trees and feel the cool breeze as you approach your campsite. You have now reached the foothills of the mountain. You are now higher up the mountain . . . resting in your campsite. Look around at the beauty of this place.

Imagine yourself in a bamboo forest. . . . You are walking in a large bamboo forest. The bamboo is very tall. . . . You lean against a strong cluster of bamboo . . . hear the swaying . . . and hear the rustling of the bamboo leaves, gently moving in the wind. . . . Look into the sky of your mind. . . . See the fluffy clouds. A cloud gently comes your way . . . the cloud surrounds your body. You climb up on the cloud and lie down. Feel yourself begin to float off gently in a gentle breeze.

Worry and Fear Imagery

Some images can help clients change the internal experience of worry and fear. Clients should set aside 10 to 20 minutes a day to worry, preferably in the morning before they start their daily routines. This approach reassures the subconscious that it has worried, and the person has greater success at stopping the habitual worry during the rest of the day.

Script: Let worries come one by one . . . just watch as one replaces the other. As you do this for a short period of time, feel the experience that occurs with each of those worries and fears. Notice how just having a worry or fear changes your state right now.

Stop the images. Focus on your breathing . . . in . . . and out. . . . Allow yourself to have three complete cycles of breathing before continuing. . . . In your relaxed state, become aware of these feelings of relaxed body–mind. This time, take your relaxed state with you into your imagination. Let one worry come to your mind right now. See and feel it. . . . See yourself in that situation relaxed and at ease.

Right now, just say to yourself, "I can stop this worry." Imagine yourself functioning without that worry or fear. See yourself waving good-bye to that worry and fear. See yourself completely free of that worry and fear. Look at the decisions that you can make for your life that will lead you in new directions. Feel your energy as you breathe in. As you exhale, let go of all of the worry, fear, tension, and tightness.

Experience your comfortable body–mind. Know that you can work with many of your worries and fears that surface daily. Whenever they come, let the dominant worry surface. . . . Then feel what it is like as you gradually give up portions of the worry . . . until it is completely gone. If that seems impossible right now, decide which part of that worry and fear you need to keep and which part you can let go. And now, see yourself waving good-bye to the part that you can let go.

Now, feel what it is like in your mind with part of that worry or fear gone. Experience that and feel the changes within the body. Assess the part of the worry or fear that remains. Again, allow a portion of that worry or fear to move away. See yourself waving good-bye. Feel the change inside as more is released.

Let yourself now be in a place where the worry and fear are diminished. Assess what part remains and see if you can now begin to give up that part. Pay attention to the experiences inside your body as you do this.

This script has many variations: writing worries and fears on a seashell and watching a seagull pick up the shell and drop it into the sea; running along a road, dropping the worries and fears by the road, and watching the wind blow them away; letting a picture of worries and fears flow forward in a moving stream. This basic script can also be individualized by putting into words what the client revealed before the session.

Inner Guide Imagery

The nurse can assist the client in creating purposeful self-dialogue that gains access to inner wisdom and personal truth that naturally reside within each of us. It is advisable to allow 10 to 20 minutes for this exercise.

Script: As you begin to feel even more relaxed now . . . going to a deeper place within . . . feeling deeply relaxed . . . peaceful and safe . . . let yourself become aware of a sense of not being alone. With you right now is a guide . . . who is wise and concerned with your well-being. Let yourself begin to see this wise being with whom you can share your fears or your joys. You have a trust in this wise being.

If you do not see anyone, let yourself be aware of hearing or feeling this wise being, noticing the presence of care and concern. In whatever way seems best for you, proceed to make contact with this wise inner guide. Let yourself establish contact with your guide now . . . in any way that comes. Your guide may appear to you in any form, such as a person, an animal, an inner presence or peace . . . or as an image of the very wisest part of you.

Notice the love and wisdom with which you are surrounded. This wisdom and love are present for you now. . . . Let yourself ask for advice . . . about anything that is important for you just now. Be receptive to what emerges. . . . Let yourself receive some new information. This inner guide may have a special message to share with you.

. . . Listen with openness and pure intention to receive.

Allow yourself to look at any issue in your life. It may be a symptom, a choice, or a decision. . . . Tell your wise guide anything that you wish. . . . Listen to the answers that emerge. Imagine yourself acting on the answers and directions that you received. . . . Imagine yourself calling upon the wisdom and love of this wise guide to help you in the days to come. Now in whatever way is best for you . . . bring closure to the visit with this inner guide. You can come back here any time that you wish. All you have to do is take the time.

This script helps clients gain an awareness of their own inner wisdom. It is best to introduce this exercise after a client has done several imagery sessions. Word choices should take into account the client's dominant sense. If a client prefers the visual, for example, the nurse uses the word *see*; if the client prefers the auditory, the word *hear*; if the client prefers the kinesthetic, the word *feel*.

Seeking an inner guide can be done over many sessions. The client should be aware that many different guides or advisors will surface over time. The guide may also appear as a traditional religious figure such as a shaman, the Virgin Mary, a saint, Moses, or Buddha. It can be interesting and surprising when someone meets a spiritual figure not from his or her own religious tradition. The guide may also emerge as an admired historical or living person such as a favorite author or artist, a philosopher, or a heroic leader such as Martin Luther King, Jr.

There are many versions of this script, so the nurse can add, invent, and explore. Much detail can be added to this imagery script to lengthen the session. When time is extended, a wealth of insight can emerge for the client. The nurse should pause frequently and let a few moments pass in silence during the guiding, as indicated by his or her intuition.

Pain Reduction Imagery

The red ball of pain. To decrease psychophysiologic pain, clients can learn to use distraction. This kind of imagery is good for both acute and chronic pain, as well as for the discomfort or pain of procedures. It takes 10 to 20 minutes.

> **Script:** Scan your body. . . . Gather any pains, aches, or other symptoms up into a ball. Begin to change its size. . . . Allow it to get bigger. . . . Just imagine how big you can make it. Now make it smaller. . . . See how small you can make it. . . . Is it possible to make it the size of a grain of sand? Now allow it to move slowly out of your body, moving further away each time you exhale. . . . Notice the experience with each exhale . . . as the pain moves away.

Give suggestions to the client to change the size of the ball several times in both directions. This serves as a distraction and an exercise in manipulating the pain experience rather than being trapped or overwhelmed by it. This imagery provides a tremendous sense of control as well as pain relief for the client. The person's body cues indicate how many times to go in each of the opposite directions.

Pain Assessment Imagery

Imagery helps access and control both acute and chronic psychophysiologic pain. The following exercise can be done in 10 to 20 minutes.

> **Script:** Close your eyes and let yourself relax. . . . Begin to describe the pain in silence to yourself. Be present with the pain. . . . Know that the pain may be either physical sensations . . . or worries and fears. Let the pain take on a shape . . . any shape that comes to your mind. Become aware of the dimensions of the pain. . . . What is the height of the pain? . . . The width of the pain? . . . And the depth of the pain? Where in the body is it located? . . . Give it color . . . a shape. . . . Feel the texture. Does it make any sound?
>
> And now with your eyes still closed, let your hands come together with palms turned upward as if forming a cup. Put your pain object in your hands. [Once again, the nurse asks these questions about the pain, preceding each question with this phrase, "How would you change the size, etc.?"]
>
> Let yourself decide what you would like to do with the pain. There is no right way to finish the experience. . . . Just accept what feels right to you. You can throw the pain away . . . or place it back where you found it . . . or move it somewhere else. Let yourself become aware . . . of how pain can be changed. . . . By your focusing with intention, the pain changes.

It is not unusual for the pain to go completely away, or at least lessen after this exercise. The client also learns to manipulate the pain so that it is not the controlling factor of his or her life. The exercise is also effective with severe pain. After giving pain medication, the nurse can have the client relax during the imagery process.

Correct Biologic Imagery Teaching Sheets and Scripts

The nurse elicits from a client or patient images and symbols that have special healing meaning and value, and then makes an audiocassette for the client or patient that includes correct biologic images, specific concrete objective information, specific symbols, and specific types of imagery. (See Chapter 18 for guidelines on making an audiocassette tape and establishing an audio library.)

It may seem that the following scripts are suitable only for well-educated, sophisticated individuals, but this is not the case. However, it is necessary for the nurse to assess the individual's education level and adapt these scripts to fit the person's needs and cultural beliefs. Imagery is an important tool, particularly for those clients who do not read.

Bone Healing Imagery

An imagery exercise for bone healing may be done in 20 to 30 minutes.[56] Prior to imagery, to teach basic biologic imagery of bone healing, the nurse should explain the following concepts:

- *Reaction (cellular proliferation):* Within the hematoma surrounding the fracture, cells and tissues proliferate and develop into a random structure (**Figure 17-1a**).

- *Regeneration (callus formation):* At 10 to 14 days after the fracture, the cells within the hematoma become organized in a fibrous lattice. With sufficient organization, the callus becomes clinically stable. The callus obliterates the medullary canal and surrounds the two ends of bone by irregularly surrounding the fracture defect (**Figure 17-1b**).

- *Remodeling (new bone formation):* Approximately 25 to 40 days after the fracture, calcium is laid down within the bone that has spicules perpendicular to the cortical surface (**Figure 17-1c**). Osteonal bone gradually replaces and remodels fiber bone. The fracture has been bridged over by new bone (**Figure 17-1d**). Conversion and remodeling continue up to 3 years following an acute fracture.

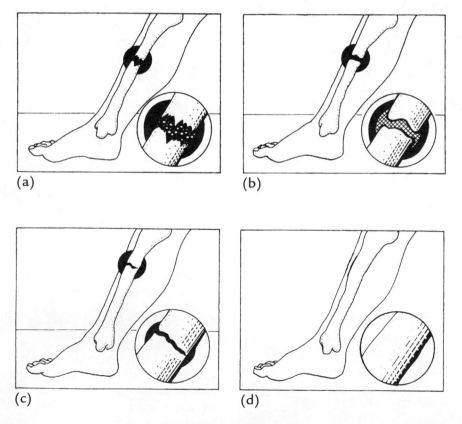

(a)   (b)

(c)   (d)

FIGURE 17-1   Bone Healing Concepts. (a) Reaction: Hematoma and cellular proliferation. (b) Regeneration. (c) Remodeling: Calcium ossification. (d) Healed bone.

Source: Reprinted with permission from J. Achterberg, B. Dossey, and L. Kolkmeier, *Rituals of Healing,* © 1994, Bantam Books.

Script: In your relaxed state, [name], allow yourself to imagine a natural process that is occurring within your body. . . . New cells are gathering very fast at the site of your fracture [cellular proliferation]. This is an important process as it lays the foundation for your bone healing. With your next breath in . . . become aware of the fact . . . that right now your body is allowing those new cells to multiply rapidly [positive suggestion]. Your blood cells . . . at the site of your fracture are arranging themselves in a special healing pattern. You can relax . . . even more . . . if you want to . . . as you continue with this very natural healing process.

In a few days, . . . your wise body will begin to create a strong lattice network of new bone [regeneration]. This will allow your bone to become stable, bridging the new bone that is forming. As you focus in a relaxed way, you help in your healing, for relaxation increases this natural process. Imagine your relaxation to be like a gentle breeze of wind that flows over and throughout your body.

In a few more weeks, your new bone will be formed. . . . Natural deposits of calcium from your body will be taken into the place of healing [remodeling]. Allow an image to come to your mind now of beautiful, healed bone. In about 6 weeks, you will have a beautiful bridge where the calcium has formed new bone. . . . Can you imagine a healing light within you right now? Allow this healing light to radiate throughout your body, bringing its loving energy to every cell in your body. . . . Stay with this experience for as long as you want, and then whenever you feel ready, slowly bring your awareness back to the room.[56pp131-132]

Immune System Odyssey Imagery

Patients can be taught correct biologic images of the normal process of the immune system.[56pp317-328] (See **Figure 17-2**.) The nurse should explain the following concepts previous to the imagery exercise:

- *Neutrophils:* The most numerous cells, billions of neutrophils swim in the bloodstream; when they sense unhealthy tissue, they pass through the blood vessel, move to the unhealthy tissue or cells, surround it, shoot caustic chemicals, and destroy the unhealthy tissue or cells (see Figure 17-2).
- *Macrophages:* Moving throughout the body, always ready to eat, macrophages travel in hordes; each one swells up, consuming the enemy (e.g., bacteria, viruses, yeast, cancer cells).
- *T cells:* Born in the bone marrow, millions of T cells go from infancy to adolescence each minute. They go to the thymus gland, where they get a special imprint; some are designated killer cells, while others become helpers or suppressors. All these specialized cells keep a watchful vigil in the lymph nodes and tissue until needed.
- *B cells:* For years, B cells wait and mature in the bone marrow until needed. They can change like caterpillars to butterflies, becoming plasma cells that manufacture magic bullets—the protein called antibodies. Operating like a guided missile, they can shoot the target, paralyze the enemy, shoot caustic chemicals, and explode the bad cells and tissue. B cells can clone themselves and create whatever number it takes to win the battle.

In 20 to 30 minutes, the nurse can guide the client through an intervention, modifying the script as needed.

Script: You are about to embark on the most incredible journey imaginable, a journey through your own immune system, touching your body's healing forces with your

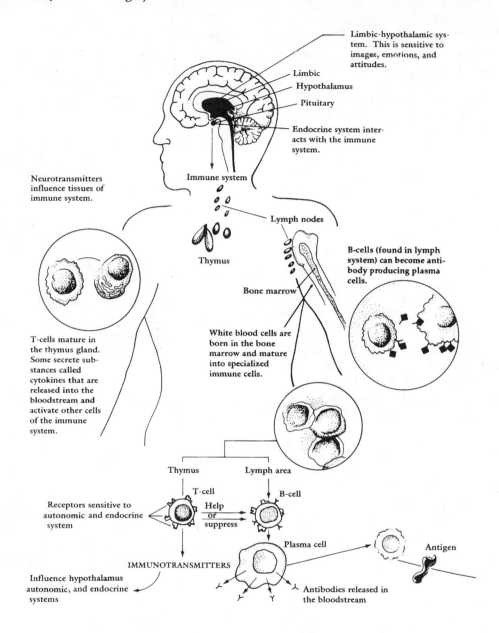

Limbic-hypothalamic system. This is sensitive to images, emotions, and attitudes.

Limbic

Hypothalamus

Pituitary

Endocrine system interacts with the immune system.

Immune system

Neurotransmitters influence tissues of immune system.

Lymph nodes

Thymus

B-cells (found in lymph system) can become antibody producing plasma cells.

Bone marrow

T-cells mature in the thymus gland. Some secrete substances called cytokines that are released into the bloodstream and activate other cells of the immune system.

White blood cells are born in the bone marrow and mature into specialized immune cells.

Thymus   Lymph area

Receptors sensitive to autonomic and endocrine system

T-cell   Help or suppress   B-cell

IMMUNOTRANSMITTERS

Plasma cell

Antigen

Influence hypothalamus autonomic, and endocrine systems

Antibodies released in the bloodstream

FIGURE 17-2   Immune System Components.

Source: Reprinted with permission from J. Achterberg, B. Dossey, and L. Kolkmeier, *Rituals of Healing,* © 1994, Bantam Books.

mind; you will sense, feel, and envision a miracle. A miracle of defense and protection, a miracle of the billions of honorable, persistent warriors within you that have

but one mission: to guard you from disease, injury, and invasion.

To fully appreciate this odyssey, which is as complex as it is magnificent, it is important to clear

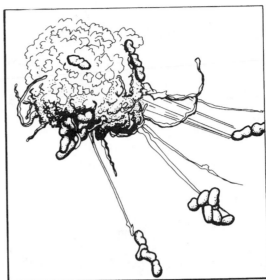

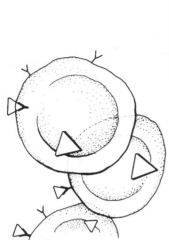

Neuropeptides produced in the brain lock onto specific receptors of immune cells.

Phagocytes, such as neutrophils and the macrophage pictured here literally eat bacteria, viruses, cancer cells, and other foreign particles or destroyed tissue and contain chemicals that break down and destroy the invaders.

The immune system produces memory cells when exposed to an antigen, and the immune system then remembers that encounter and becomes more efficient against it the next time it gets invaded by microorganisms that produce antigens.

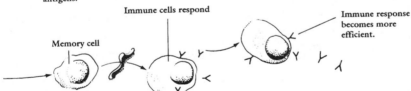

Immune cells respond

Immune response becomes more efficient.

Memory cell

FIGURE 17-2 Immune System Components *(continued)*

and focus your mind, which will help you relax your body. The bridge between your mind and body is easily crossed when your mental distractions are released, when a sense of peace and calm spreads warmly from the top of your head to your toes. As you let go of stress, your immune system is activated. Relax,

now, as you participate in and observe your own healing process.

As your mind becomes clearer and clearer, feel it becoming more and more alert. Somewhere deep inside of you, a brilliant light begins to glow. Sense this happening. . . . The light grows brighter and brighter and more intense. . . . This is your body–mind communication center. Breathe into it. . . . Energize it with your breath. The light is powerful and penetrating, and a beam begins to grow from it. The beam shines through your body into any area you wish. It is your searchlight, your bridge into the glorious mysteries about to unfold. Practice shining it into your body. Sometimes this is easier to do than other times. Just allow it to happen.

The immune journey begins inside your bones. So, take this most intelligent beam of light and shine it into a long bone . . . a leg bone perhaps. Penetrate deeply into the marrow. This is the birthing center for all your blood cells. Just imagine if you can, . . . feel if you can, . . . billions . . . of young cells being born . . . many kinds, each with a task to nurture and protect you. As we go through this exercise, we will focus on a few types of cells that are vital to defending you. They have names: neutrophils, macrophages, T cells, B cells, natural killer cells. One by one, we'll shine the light on them, watching them work to guard, protect, and remove cells that no longer serve you.

The most numerous cells are called neutrophils. They eat and engulf the invaders in a most ingenious way. Imagine them maturing, moving into your bloodstream, floating, ever alert for a call to work in your defense. As a call warns them of an invader, they become exceedingly alert. No longer swimming freely, millions, billions of them sense the danger and move methodically and directly, preparing for attack. The blood vessels become sticky, attracting the neutrophils to their surface. The small opening in the blood vessel walls dilates in the vicinity of the attack. Imagine the neutrophils being attracted to the walls. They move quickly along the vessel walls until they know with absolute certainty that the invader is near. Now, they extend a small foot, a pseudopod, into the walls, and changing shape, they slither through, entering your tissues. Moving forward now, as they approach the invader, they send another small foot out, surrounding the enemy, shooting caustic chemicals into it, wearing it thin. The enemy is halted, destroyed, may even explode into harmless bits. Imagine this happening, constantly, protecting you from the dangers of living in a hostile world. Billions and billions of neutrophils are born every day.

Now, shining the beam of light back into the bone marrow, imagine the macrophages, or the giant eaters . . . fewer of them, but with long lives and many talents. As they mature, watch them move into tissues and organs and blood. They line the walls of the lungs and liver . . . waiting, surveying, watching, constantly ready to move. Bacteria, viruses, yeast cells, even cancer cells trigger the alarm. As the warning of an invader sounds, the macrophages swell up, becoming large and powerful. They may even mesh together with the other macrophages, moving rapidly in a powerful, connecting flank. They reach out for the enemy, lasso it with their armlike extensions, and bring the invader into their bodies, injecting it with potent enzymes. With lightning speed, they consume an enemy. What they can't destroy, they encircle and preserve, protecting you from its dangerous acts. The macrophages are also your scavengers. They can and will digest anything and everything in your body that you no longer have use for. Imagine this happening for a moment.

The macrophages and neutrophils are nonspecific, nondiscriminating in their attack and cleanup activities. Other cells, the lymphocytes, or the T cells and the B cells, have an assigned function, a target that they spend their entire lives stalking. It might be a special virus, or bacteria, or cancer cell, or other foreign tissue. Let's look at these cells in action.

Shining the beam, again, into the bone marrow, observe the T cells being born. Millions . . . more than you could possibly count . . move from infancy to adolescence each minute. The T cells will each be given a special task as they are processed in the thymus gland. Shine your imagery light into the middle of your chest; here is the thymus gland. Feel it pulsating with energy. Watch, now, as the adolescent T cells flow in rapidly, each touched with a spark of wisdom, each challenged with a mission. Some will be killers, assassins with a single target. Others will be helpers for your B cells. Still others will be suppressors, signaling that the battle is over, protecting your body from excessive immune activity. Imagine these—the killers, the helpers, and the suppressors—maturing quickly and with glorious specificity in your thymus. When each has been imprinted, they leave the thymus to go about their tasks. The T cells keep a wakeful vigil in your lymph nodes, your spleen, and other lymph tissue. Think of this for a time. . . .

Back in the bone marrow once again, the B cells are highlighted by the beam. They mature and move into the lymph tissues and blood, waiting for the encounter. Each has a specific enemy to protect you from, and they can wait patiently for years, patrolling, waiting, and watching. When the encounter finally takes place, the B cells change, like cocoons into butterflies, becoming a plasma cell. The plasma cells manufacture magic bullets, which are proteins called antibodies. Each antibody is like a guided missile. . . . It moves directly for its target and hooks on to it, like a key in a lock. The enemy is paralyzed and its surface damaged. Other chemicals are liberated in the blood by this action, and they burn holes in the wall of the enemy, causing an explosion. The B cells also clone themselves, creating whatever number is needed to do pure and perfect battle in your defense.

One last time, peering into the birthing center of the immune system, the light shines onto natural killer cells. The natural killers are wondrous defenses against cancer. Like viruses and bacteria, cancer cells are not especially unusual in the human body. The body simply recognizes them as invaders and sends out the forces of defense. Only in the most unusual circumstances (e.g., when cancer cells wear a disguise) does the immune system fail to find them. Watch now, as the natural killer cells are born and move into the bloodstream. Take the light and shine it on one cell, and watch its action. Ever alert, it senses a cancer cell in the vicinity. Moving at lightning speed, it collides with the cancer cell. Its mere touch paralyzes the cell. Fingers of the natural killer cell reach into the cancer cell, oozing in its power and might. Then, a small cannon-like structure within the natural killer cell tilts, aims, and fires deadly chemicals into the cancer cell. Already paralyzed, the cancer cell develops blisters, peels like an orange. Its cellular matter dissolves, leaving only harmless skeletal remains. The natural killer cell, alive and well, continues its alert patrol of your body.

Before you end this exercise, go over the immune process once more, sensing all the immune cells working in a superbly coordinated team of defense. In the bone marrow, billions of cells are being born each minute, in exactly the number and combinations that you need to stay healthy. As the white blood cells mature, each develops a remarkable intelligence. Each has a dedicated task. Witness these cells moving out of the bone marrow, into blood tissue, watching and waiting for the opportunity to protect and cleanse you. Feel the presence of these magnificent guardians, and sense their power. These dedicated warriors, this system of defense has a universe of its own. That universe is you. By relaxing, as you have just done, and concentrating on this process, you have actively participated in keeping yourself healthy.[32]

Imagery and Drawing

In the imagery process, drawing is an effective way to open up communication with the self and others. It externalizes previously internal mental images and emotions. The emphasis in this intervention is not on how well the client can draw, but on the client's ability to get in touch with feelings and healing potential through drawing. Drawing, as a way of externalizing inner images and deepening understanding of inner processes, may be a safer way to talk about difficult feelings. When clients are overwhelmed with emotions, drawing images of the feelings can be therapeutic. Drawing is especially helpful with children who are not verbally sophisticated.

Drawing after being guided through an imagery exercise can bring further insights. The creativity that is evoked is different from the logical mode of explaining the experiences in words. This creative process can also evoke transcendent experiences and healing energy. Drawing works well when a client is crying and is unable to talk easily but wants to express what he or she is experiencing. When introducing drawing, the nurse can make some of the following suggestions:

- Express yourself with a few images. There is no one correct way to draw. Drawings can be either realistic or symbolic. The most important thing is that you express yourself in a nonlogical way. This can bring new awareness and understanding into your life.

- If you find that you are too focused on the result of the drawing exercise, use your nondominant hand. With your eyes closed, allow yourself to get into the expressive quality of drawing.

- Do not judge your drawing. Allow your body, mind, and spirit to connect as you begin simply to be with the paper and crayons in the present moment.

- Notice the energy flow from you. Let your body energy resonate with your imagery and spirit energy. Let the energies slowly begin to resonate together. Do not try to control the process because this inner quality comes from being immersed in the imagery and drawing experience.

- On the blank piece of paper, allow an image to begin to form that represents your feelings and thoughts in this moment. Choose colors that speak to you. If you wish to change the color that you started working with, feel free to do so.

- After you have drawn, you might want to write some details of your images. Often, what you felt or heard during the imagery drawing may surface into conscious awareness and provide new insights about your important images.

When working with drawing for a client's specific disease or symptoms, it is helpful for the nurse to educate the client about the body processes that are being affected. It is therapeutic for the client to have an understanding of, and an image for, the healthful state; the disease or symptoms and the medication, treatments, and associated procedures; and his or her personal belief systems. Asking the client to draw the disease or symptoms in the way that has self-meaning often reveals a client's constricted view of healing possibilities or misunderstanding of the disease or symptoms, either of which may impair recovery. The drawing process helps the client recognize that the disease need not control his or her life. Insight from drawing helps the client reframe experiences of illness, let go of the inner judgments and struggles, and mobilize his or her creativity for achieving desired outcomes.

Some of the challenges for nurses are to develop innovative teaching worksheets, booklets, and verbal descriptions of body–mind healing; to integrate imagery as part of each nursing interaction and intervention; and to develop assessment tools.[56] The nurse and client should identify the following elements for the best outcome:

- *Disease or disability:* The vividness of the client's view of the disease, illness, or disability and, if the process is ongoing, the strength of the disease or illness to decrease health or the client's focus on the reverse—the vividness and the strength of the client's ability to stabilize the disease or illness or stop the process.
- *Internal healing resources:* The vividness of the client's perception of his or her healing ability and the effectiveness of this ability to combat the disease.
- *External healing resources:* The vividness of the treatment description and the effectiveness of the positive mechanism of action.

CASE STUDY (IMPLEMENTATION)

Setting: Coronary care unit (CCU), followed by outpatient cardiac rehabilitation program

Patient: J. D., a 48-year-old man with acute myocardial infarction complicated by congestive heart failure and pericarditis secondary to the infarction

Patterns/Challenges/Needs:

1. Decreased cardiac output related to mechanical factors (congestive heart failure)
2. Altered comfort related to inflammation (pericarditis)
3. Anxiety related to acute illness and fear of death

The nurse asked J. D. several questions to explore with him his psychospiritual state. Following the interaction, the nurse felt that further exploration of the negative images that he conveyed and the meaning behind them was essential to his recovery. She asked him if he wanted to pursue some new ideas that might help him access his inner healing resources and strengths. He said that he would.

> *Nurse:* In your recovery now with your heart healing, how do you experience your healing?
>
> *J. D.:* There is this sac around my heart, and every time I take a deep breath, my breath is cut off by the pain [pericarditis]. My heart is like a broken vase. I don't think it is healing.
>
> *Nurse:* I can understand why you are discouraged. However, some important things that are present right now show that you are better than when you first came to the CCU. Your persistent chest pain is gone, and your heartbeats are now regular. If you focus on what is going right, you can help your heart and lift your spirits. Let me help you learn how to think of some positive things.
>
> *J. D.:* I don't know if I can.
>
> *Nurse:* I would like to show you how to breathe more comfortably. Place your right hand on your upper chest and your left hand on your belly. I want to show you how to do relaxed abdominal breathing. With your next breath in, through your nose, let the breath fill your belly with air. And as you exhale through

your mouth, let your stomach fall back to your spine. As you focus on this way of breathing, notice how still your chest is.

J. D.: (After three complete breaths) This is the easiest breathing I've done today.

Nurse: As you focused on breathing with your belly, you let go of fearing the discomfort with your breathing. Can you tell me more about the image you have of your heart as a broken vase?

J. D.: I saw this crack down the front of my heart right after the doctor told me about my big artery that is blocked, that runs down the front of my heart, which caused my heart attack.

Nurse: (Taking a small plastic bag full of crayons out of her pocket and picking up a piece of paper) Is it possible for you to choose a few crayons and draw your broken heart using those images you just talked about?

J. D.: I can't draw.

Nurse: This exercise has nothing to do with drawing, but something usually happens when you draw an image of your words.

J. D.: Do you mean the image of a broken vase? (When halfway through with the drawing) I know this sounds crazy, but my father had a heart attack when he was 55. I was visiting my parents. Dad hadn't been feeling well, even complained of his stomach hurting that morning. He was in the living room, and as he fell, he knocked over a large Chinese porcelain vase that broke in two pieces. I can remember so clearly running to his side. I can see that vase now, cracked in a jagged edge down the front. He made it to the hospital, but died 2 days later. You know, I think that might be where that image of a broken heart came from. (See **Figure 17-3a**.)

Nurse: Your story contains a lot of meaning. Remembering this event can be very helpful to you in your healing. What are some of the things that you are most worried about just now?

J. D.: (Tears in his eyes) Dying young. I have this funny feeling in my stomach just now. I don't want to die. I'm too young. I have so much to contribute to life. I've been driving myself to excess as far as work. I need to learn to relax and manage my stress, even drop some weight, start exercising, and change my life.

Nurse: J., each day you are getting stronger. You might even consider that this time of rest after your heart attack can be a time for you to reflect on what are the most important things in life for you. Whenever you feel discouraged, let images come to you of a beautiful vase that has a healed crack in it. This is exactly what your heart is doing right now. Even as we are talking, the area that has been damaged is healing. As it heals, there will be a solid scar that will be very strong, just in the same way that a vase can be mended and become strong again. New blood supplies also come into the surrounding area of your heart to help it heal. Positive images can help you heal because you send a different message from your mind to your body when you are relaxed and thinking about becoming strong and well. You help your body, mind, and spirit function at their highest level. Let yourself once again draw an image of your heart as a healed vase, and notice any difference in your feelings when you do this.

With a smile, he picked up several crayons and began to draw a healing image to encourage hope and healing (**Figure 17-3b**).

When J. D. entered the outpatient cardiac rehabilitation program following his acute myocardial infarction, he was motivated to lower his cholesterol, lose weight, learn stress management skills, and express his emotions. Two weeks into the program, J. D. did not appear to be his usual extroverted self. The cardiac rehabilitation nurse engaged him in conversation, and before long, he had tears in his eyes. He stated that he was very discouraged about having heart disease. He said, "It just has a grip on me." The nurse took him into her office, and they continued the dialogue. After listening to his story, she asked J. D. if he would like to explore his feelings further. He shyly nodded yes.

To facilitate the healing process, she thought it might be helpful to have J. D. get in touch with his images and their locations in his body. She began by saying, "If it seems right to you, close your eyes and begin to focus on your breathing just now." She guided him in a general exercise of head-to-toe relaxation, accompanied by an audio-cassette music selection of sounds in nature. As his breathing patterns became more relaxed and deeper, indicating relaxation, she began to guide him in exploring "the grip" in his imagination.

Nurse: Focus on where you experience the grip. Give it a size, . . . a shape, . . . a sound, . . . a texture, . . . a width, . . . and a depth.

J. D.: It's in my chest, but not like chest pain. It's dull, deep, and blocks my knowing what I need to think or feel about living. I can't believe that I'm using these words. Well, it's bigger than I thought. It's very rough, like heavy jute rope tied in a knot across my chest. It has a sound like a rope that keeps a sailboat tied to a boat dock. I'm now rocking back and forth. I don't know why this is happening.

Nurse: Stay with the feeling, and let it fill you as much as it can. If you need to change the experience, all you have to do is take several deep breaths.

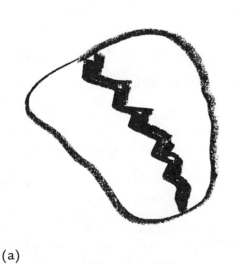

(a)

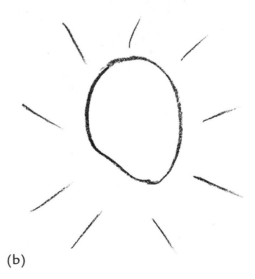

(b)

FIGURE 17-3   Patient Drawings. (a) J. D.'s drawing of his broken heart. (b) J. D.'s drawing of his healed heart.

J. D.: It's filling me up. Where are these sounds, feelings, and sensations coming from?

Nurse: From your wise, inner self, your inner healing resources. Just let yourself stay with the experience. Continue to use as many of your senses as you can to describe and feel these experiences.

J. D.: Nothing is happening. I've gone blank.

Nurse: Focus again on your breath in . . . and feel the breath as you let it go. . . . Can you allow an image of your heart to come to you under that tight grip?

J. D.: It is so small I can hardly see it. It's all wrapped up.

Nurse: In your imagination, can you introduce yourself to your heart as if you were introducing yourself to a person for the first time? Ask your heart if it has a name?

J. D.: It said hello, but it was with a gesture of hello, no words.

Nurse: That is fine. Just say, "Nice to meet you," and see what the response might be.

J. D.: My heart seems like an old soul, very wise. This feels very comfortable.

Nurse: Ask your heart a question for which you would like an answer. Stay with this and listen for what comes.

J. D.: (After long pause) It said practice patience, that I was on the right track, that my heart disease has a message, don't know what it is.

Nurse: Just stay with your calmness and inner quiet. Notice how the grip changed for you. There are many more answers to come for you. This is your wise self who has much to offer you. Whenever you want, you can get back to this special

kind of knowing. All you have to do is take the time. When you set aside time to be quiet with your rich images, you will get more information. You might also find special music to assist you in this process. . . . Your skills with this way of knowing will increase each time you use this process . . . now that whatever is right for you in this moment is unfolding, just as it should. In a few moments, I will invite you back into a wakeful state. On five, be ready to come back into the room, wide awake and relaxed. One . . . two . . . three . . . four . . . eyelids lighter, taking a deep breath . . . and five, back into the room, awake and alert, ready to go about your day.

J. D.: Where did all that come from? I've never done that before.

Nurse: These are your inner healing resources that you possess to help you recognize quality and purpose in living each day. In our future sessions, we will teach and share more of these skills.

Evaluation

With the client, the nurse determines whether the client outcomes for imagery were successful (**Exhibit 17-2**). To evaluate the session further, the nurse may again explore the subjective effects of the experience with the client (see Exhibit 17-1).

Imagery is a tool for connecting with the unlimited capabilities of the body–mind. The client can experience more self-awareness, self-acceptance, self-love, and self-worth. Clients learn a skill for self-care and self-knowledge that will be useful throughout their life. The best way for nurses to develop confidence and skill in using clinical imagery is for them to use it in their own life as a part of self-care and enrichment.

EXHIBIT 17-2   Evaluating the Client's Subjective Experience with Imagery

1. Was this a new kind of imagery experience for you? Can you describe it?
2. Did you have a visual experience? Of people, places, or objects? Can you describe them?
3. Did you see colors while being guided? Did the colors change as the guided imagery continued?
4. Were you aware of your surroundings? Were you able to let the imagery flow?
5. Did you like the imagery?
6. Did the imagery produce any feelings or emotions?
7. Did you notice any textures, smells, movements, or tastes while experiencing the imagery?
8. Was the experience pleasant?
9. Did you feel relaxed and refreshed after the experience?
10. Would you like to try this again?
11. What would make this a better experience for you?
12. What is your next step (or your plan) to integrate this on a daily basis?

Directions for
FUTURE RESEARCH

1. Determine whether a client's specific images increase the client's psychophysiologic healing.
2. Develop valid and reliable tools that measure imagery.
3. Compare the stress level, attitudes, and work spirit of nurses who routinely use imagery as a nursing intervention to those of nurses who do not use imagery.
4. Evaluate the relationship between imagery scripts, physiologic responses, and healing in different clinical settings.
5. Determine whether subjects can learn through manipulation of both imagery scripts and their verbal reports to eliminate or modify negative psychophysiologic responses.
6. Examine cultural diversity through specific types of imagery and symbols.

Nurse Healer
REFLECTIONS

After reading this chapter, the nurse healer will be able to answer or to begin a process of answering the following questions:

- How do I feel about my imagination?
- When I work with imagery, what inner resources can assist me in my life processes?

- How am I able to remove the barriers to my imagery process?
- In what way do I recognize the nonrational part of myself?
- Can I allow my clients to interpret their own imagery to facilitate their own healing?

> **www** *For a full suite of assignments and additional learning activities, use the access code located in the front of your book to visit this exclusive website: http://go.jblearning.com /dossey. If you do not have an access code, you can obtain one at the site.*

NOTES

1. H. Hall, "Imagery and Cancer," in *Healing Images: The Role of Imagination in Health*, ed. A. A. Sheikh, 408–426 (Amityville, NY: Baywood, 2003).
2. V. Miller and P. J. Whorwell, "Hypnotherapy for Functional Gastrointestinal Disorders: A Review," *International Journal of Clinical and Experimental Hypnosis* 57, no. 3 (July 2009): 279–292.
3. M. Shinozaki et al., "Effect of Autogenic Training on General Improvement in Patients with Irritable Bowel Syndrome: A Randomized Controlled Trial," *Applied Psychophysiology and Biofeedback* 35, no. 3 (September 2010): 189–198.

4   J. L. Apóstolo and K. Kolcaba, "The Effects of Guided Imagery on Comfort, Depression, Anxiety, and Stress of Psychiatric Inpatients with Depressive Disorders," *Archives of Psychiatric Nursing* 23, no. 6 (December 2009): 403–411.

5.   V. Menzies et al., "Effects of Guided Imagery on Outcomes of Pain, Functional Status, and Self-Efficacy in Persons Diagnosed with Fibromyalgia," *Journal of Complementary Medicine* 12, no. 1 (2006): 23–30.

6.   V. Menzies and S. Kim, "Relaxation and Guided Imagery in Hispanic Persons Diagnosed with Fibromyalgia: A Pilot Study," *Family and Community Health* 31, no. 3 (2008): 204–212.

7.   J. S. Gordon, J. K. Staples, A. Blyta, M. Bytyqi, and A. T. Wilson, "Treatment of Posttraumatic Stress Disorder in Postwar Kosovar Adolescents Using Mind–Body Skills Groups: A Randomized Controlled Trial," *Journal of Clinical Psychiatry* 69, no. 9 (September 2008): 1469–1476.

8.   J. M. Weis, M. R. Smucker, and J. G. Dresser, "Imagery: Its History and Use in the Treatment of Posttraumatic Stress Disorder," in *Healing Images: The Role of Imagination in Health*, ed. A. A. Sheikh (Amityville, NY: Baywood, 2003): 381–395.

9.   C. M. Nappi, S. P. Drummond, S. R. Thorp, and J. R. McQuaid, "Effectiveness of Imagery Rehearsal Therapy for the Treatment of Combat-Related Nightmares In Veterans." *Behavioral Therapy* 41, no. 2 (June 2010): 237–244.

10.   E. C. Trakhtenberg, "The Effects of Guided Imagery on the Immune System: A Critical Review," *International Journal of Neuroscience* 118, no. 6 (June 2008): 839–855.

11.   O. Eremin et al., "Immuno-modulatory Effects of Relaxation Training and Guided Imagery in Women with Locally Advanced Breast Cancer Undergoing Multimodality Therapy: A Randomised Controlled Trial," *Breast* (November 11, 2008).

12.   C. Lahmann et al., "Effects of Functional Relaxation and Guided Imagery on IgE in Dust-Mite Allergic Adult Asthmatics: A Randomized, Controlled Clinical Trial," *Journal of Nervous and Mental Disorders* 198, no. 2 (February 2010): 125–130.

13.   R. McCraty and D. Tomasino, "Emotional Stress, Positive Emotions, and Psychophysiological Coherence," in *Stress in Health and Disease*, ed. B. B. Arnetz and R. Ekman (Weinheim, Germany: Wiley-VCH, 2006): 342–365. http://www.heartmath.org/research/research-publications/emotional-stress-positive-emotions-and-psychophysiological-coherence.html.

14.   G. Rein, M. Atkinson, and R. McCraty, "The Physiological and Psychological Effects of Compassion and Anger," *Journal of Advancement in Medicine* 8, no. 2 (1995): 87–105. http://www.heartmath.org/research/research-publications/physiological-and-psychological-effects-of-compassion-and-anger.html.

15.   M. Bensafi et al., "Olfactormotor Activity During Imagery Mimics That During Perception," *Nature Neuroscience* 6, no. 11 (2003): 1142–1144.

16.   S. S. Yoo et al., "Neural Substrates of Tactile Imagery: A Functional MRI Study," *Neuroreport* 24, no. 4 (2003): 581–585.

17.   J. Wagner et al., "Mind the Bend: Cerebral Activations Associated with Mental Imagery of Walking Along a Curved Path," *Experimental Brain Research* (August 12, 2008).

18.   P. Staats et al., "Suggestion/Placebo Effects on Pain: Negative as Well as Positive," *Journal of Pain Symptom Management* 15, no. 4 (1998): 235–243.

19.   E. V. Lang et al., "Adjunctive Self-Hypnotic Relaxation for Outpatient Medical Procedures: A Prospective Randomized Trial with Women Undergoing Large Core Biopsy," *Pain* 126 (2006): 155–164.

20.   E. V. Lang et al., "Can Words Hurt? Patient–Provider Interactions During Invasive Procedures," *Pain* 114 (2005): 303–309.

21.   E. Watanabe et al., "Effects Among Healthy Subjects of the Duration of Regularly Practicing a Guided Imagery Program," *BMC Complementary and Alternative Medicine* 5, no. 21 (2005): 1–13.

22.   J. Achterberg, *Imagery in Healing: Shamanism and Modern Medicine* (Boston, MA: Shambhala, 1985).

23.   A. A. Sheikh et al., "Healing Images: Historical Perspective," in *Healing Images: The Role of Imagination in Health*, ed. A. A. Sheikh, 3–26 (Amityville, NY: Baywood, 2003).

24.   H. Elliott, "Imagework as a Means for Healing and Personal Transformation," *Complementary Therapies in Nurse Midwifery* 9, no. 3 (2003): 118–124.

25.   J. Singer, *Imagery and Daydream Methods in Psychotherapy and Behavior Modification* (New York: Academic Press, 1972).

26.   W. Penfield, *The Mystery of the Mind* (Princeton, NJ: Princeton University Press, 1975).

27.   A. A. Sheikh et al., "Physiological Consequences of Imagery and Related Approaches," in *Healing Images: The Role of Imagination in Health*, ed. A. A. Sheikh, 27–52 (Amityville, NY: Baywood, 2003).

28.   E. Jacobson, "Electrical Measurements of Neuromuscular States During Mental Activities: Imagination of Movement Involving Skeletal Muscle," *American Journal of Physiology* 91 (2004): 597–608.

29.   M. Quintyn and E. Cross, "Factors Affecting the Ability to Initiate Movement in Parkinson's Disease," *Physical and Occupational Therapy in Geriatrics* 4 (1986): 51–60.

30. J. A. Stevens and M. E. Stoykov, "Using Motor Imagery in the Rehabilitation of Hemiparesis," *Archives of Physical Medicine Rehabilitation* 84, no. 7 (2003): 1090–1102.

31. C. Simonton et al., "Psychological Intervention in the Treatment of Cancer," *Psychosomatics* 21 (1980): 226–227.

32. J. Achterberg and G. F. Lawlis, *Imagery and Disease* (Champaign, IL: Institute for Personality and Ability Testing, 1978).

33. H. Hall, "Imagery, PNI and the Psychology of Healing," in *The Psychobiology of Mental Imagery*, eds. R. Kunzendorf and A. Sheikh (Amityville, NY: Baywood, 1990).

34. Schneider et al., "Guided Imagery and Immune System Function in Normal Subjects: A Summary of Research Findings," in *Mental Imagery*, ed. R. Kunzendorf, 179–191 (New York: Plenum Press, 1991).

35. W. Lewandowski, "Psychological Factors in Chronic Pain: A Worthwhile Undertaking for Nursing?" *Archives of Psychiatric Nursing* 18, no. 3 (2004): 97–105.

36. E. A. Fors et al., "The Effect of Guided Imagery and Amitriptyline on Daily Fibromyalgia Pain: A Prospective, Randomized, Controlled Trial," *Journal of Psychiatric Research* 36, no. 3 (2002): 179–187.

37. C. L. Baird and L. Sands, "A Pilot Study of the Effectiveness of Guided Imagery with Progressive Muscle Relaxation to Reduce Chronic Pain and Mobility Difficulties of Osteoarthritis," *Pain Management Nursing* 5, no. 3 (2004): 97–104.

38. G. F. Antall and D. Kresevic, "The Use of Guided Imagery to Manage Pain in an Elderly Orthopaedic Population," *Orthopaedic Nursing* 23, no. 5 (September–October): 335–340.

39. W. Lewandowski et al., "Changes in the Meaning of Pain with the Use of Guided Imagery," *Pain Management Nursing* 6, no. 2 (2005): 58–67.

40. M. M. Huth et al., "Playing in the Park: What School-Age Children Tell Us About Imagery," *Journal of Pediatric Nursing* 21, no. 2 (2006): 115–125.

41. J. A. Weydert et al., "Evaluation of Guided Imagery as a Treatment for Recurrent Abdominal Pain in Children: A Randomized Controlled Trial," *BMC Pediatrics* 6 (2006): 29. http://www.ncbi.nlm .nih.gov/pmc/articles/PMC1660537/.

42. M. M. Huth et al., "Imagery Reduces Children's Post-Operative Pain," *Pain* 110, nos. 1–2 (2004): 439–448.

43. C. Russell and S. Smart, "Guided Imagery and Distraction Therapy in Paediatric Hospice Care," *Paediatric Nursing* 19, no. 2 (2007): 24–25.

44. W. Braud, "Transpersonal Images: Implications for Health," in *Healing Images: The Role of Imagination in Health*, ed. A. A. Sheikh, 448–470 (Amityville, NY: Baywood, 2003).

45. R. Assagioli, *Psychosynthesis: A Manual of Principles and Techniques* (New York: Hobbs, Dorman, 1965).

46. R. Assagioli, *Act of Will* (New York: Viking, 1973).

47. B. G. Schaub and R. Schaub, *Dante's Path: A Practical Approach to Achieving Inner Wisdom* (New York: Gotham Books, 2003).

48. L. Song et al., "Heart-Focused Attention and Heart–Brain Synchronization: Energetic and Physiological Mechanisms," *Alternative Therapies in Health and Medicine* 4, no. 5 (1998): 44–62.

49. J. K. Morrison, "The Dynamic, Clinical Use of Imagery to Promote Psychotherapeutic Grieving," in *Healing with Death Imagery*, ed. A. A. Sheikh and K. S. Sheikh, 139–164 (Amityville, NY: Baywood, 2007): 139–164.

50. R. G. Kunzendorf, "Confronting Death Through Mental and Artistic Imagery," in *Healing with Death Imagery*, ed. A. A. Sheikh and K. S. Sheikh, 47–65 (Amityville, NY: Baywood, 2007).

51. M. R. Lane, "Spirit Body Healing—A Hermeneutic, Phenomenological Study Examining the Lived Experience of Art and Healing," *Cancer Nursing* 28, no. 4 (2005): 285–291.

52. B. G. Schaub and R. Schaub, "Imagery and Spiritual Development," in *Healing Images: The Role of Imagination in Health*, ed. A. A. Sheikh, 489–498 (Amityville, NY: Baywood, 2003).

53. B. G. Schaub and R. Schaub, "Spirituality and Clinical Practice," *Alternative Health Practitioner* 5, no. 2 (1999): 145–150.

54. L. W. Scherwitz et al., "Interactive Guided Imagery Therapy with Medical Patients: Predictors of Health Outcomes," *Journal of Alternative and Complementary Medicine* 11, no. 1 (February 2005): 69–83.

55. B. G. Schaub, "Imagery in Health Care: Connecting with Life Energy," *Alternative Health Practitioner* 1, no. 2 (1995): 113–115.

56. J. Achterberg et al., *Rituals of Healing* (New York: Bantam Books, 1994).

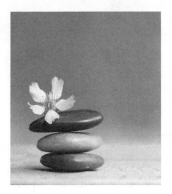

Chapter 18

Music: A Caring, Healing Modality

Shannon S. Spies Ingersoll
and Ana Schaper

Nurse Healer
OBJECTIVES

Theoretical

- Discuss the current state of research evidence on music in developing best nursing practice.
- Review new research on the effectiveness of music in clinical practice with an open mind to the strengths and limitations of the research being reported.
- Be proactive in supporting new research using strong qualitative and quantitative research methodology.

Clinical

- List factors to consider when using music as a caring, healing modality.
- Practice caring moments with patients using music as a caring, healing modality.
- Explore using music listening in providing spiritual-based holistic care to individuals.
- Partner with a music therapist to support the use of music as a caring, healing modality in health systems.

Personal

- Set aside time in your life to feel and reflect on your body's response to different music

genres, different music tempos, and your favorite songs.

DEFINITIONS

Caring consciousness: A "deeper" level where the nurse is mindful, intentional, and present and chooses how he or she portrays "being" in the interaction (achieved through centering).

Caring, healing modality: Auditory, visual, olfactory, tactile, gustatory, cognitive, and kinesthetic in nature and essential for holistic caring, healing practices and health in the twenty-first century.

Caring moment(s): Influencing both individuals through a relationship and by being together in that given moment in time.

Centering: A mind-body-spirit activity (breathing exercises, meditation) to prepare the body to enter into, prepare for, and begin caring consciousness in a relationship.

Entrainment: Synchronization where the vibrations of one object cause the vibrations of another object (usually the less powerful one) to oscillate at the same rate.

Genre: Category of artistic works of all kinds can be divided by form, style, or subject matter.

Intentionality: Deliberately focusing consciousness on something, for example, a belief, will, expectation, attention, or action.

Transpersonal nursing: Human-to-human interaction that entails wholeness, caring consciousness, and intentionality.[1]

Wholeness: The inner sense of unity with all life on Earth (universal oneness and connectedness of all).[2]

■ THEORY AND RESEARCH

One may ask, "Why is music so much a part of our everyday lives?" Music is with us whenever we want to listen, at the touch of a button on a phone or an iPod tucked in a pocket. Every moment of the day, most Americans can listen to an unlimited selection of music. Music has been a part of human history since the first records created. Today, people can download self-selected music to provide individualized music listening sessions that can be endlessly re-created. With such instant availability, how can nurse healers explore the conscious and intentional use of music as a modality for care and healing of their patients and themselves? What do nurse healers need to know to use music as a caring, healing modality?

As healers in the nurse–patient interaction, nurses employed in health systems are challenged to defend their use of music as a caring, healing modality. When nurses express the desire to include music (or another complementary care modality) as a standard of care for patients, they are told to provide outcome-based research demonstrating strong evidence (see Chapters 34 and 35) that music makes a difference in patient outcomes. Nurses are not only challenged in having to show "strong" evidence for their use of music listening when caring for individuals but are confronted with having limited time to carry out these caring, healing modalities in the busy healthcare industry.

In the effort to build a strong evidence base for music and its inclusion as a standard of care, the vast majority of new research addresses the functionality of music. Research questions most frequently asked include: What is music's capacity to produce a clinical change in the patient's condition? How does music produce this change?

In this chapter, the nurse healer is asked to carefully reread these questions in light of the research being published. The nurse healer is asked to reflect on the power of music as a therapeutic modality in holistic nursing care. Therefore, the nurse healer must consider: What research questions are not being asked? To begin exploring this journey in understanding music as a caring, healing modality, consider a quote from the book *Musicophilia* by Oliver Sacks:

> Music is part of being human, and there is no human culture in which it is not highly developed and esteemed. Its very ubiquity may cause it to be trivialized in old songs going through our minds for hours on end, and think nothing of it. But to those who are lost in [some neurologic condition or some other condition such as] dementia, the situation is different. Music is no luxury to them, but a necessity, and can have a power beyond anything else to restore them to themselves . . . at least for a while.[3]

Music has a long, rich history in the care of patients. The Greek philosopher Pythagoras, considered the founder of music therapy, promoted music for health in the sixth century.[4] Pythagoras prescribed a specific diet and music to restore harmony of the body and soul. During the Crimean War, Florence Nightingale advocated the use of music in hospitals to aid in the healing of soldiers. As a critical observer of environmental effects on the human body, Nightingale noted that wind instruments producing a continuous sound had a beneficial effect and instruments that did not produce continuous sounds were detrimental. In *Notes on Nursing*, Nightingale wrote: "The effect of music upon the sick has been scarcely at all noticed. . . . wind instruments, including the human voice, and stringed instruments, capable of continuous sound, have generally a beneficent effect."[5p33]

The invention of the phonograph in the late 1800s made recorded music available for use in hospital settings. In 1926, another nurse led the world in utilizing music to create a healing environment. Isa Maud Ilsen founded the National Association for Music in Hospitals. Ilsen believed that music should be used for physical ailments and pain. She proposed rhythm to be the basic therapeutic component in music.[4]

Music use in the care of hospitalized patients continued to gain popularity through the World Wars. However, with the advent of new medications for pain and anxiety, the popularity of music declined. With the recognition of the side effects associated with pharmaceutical management, there was a resurgence of interest in music in the 1990s. Research is supported by technical advancements in neuroimaging, and clinical application of music has increased as a result of technological advancements in music moving away from records, radio, and compact disc players to smart phones, iPods, and the iTouch.

■ THE CAPACITY OF MUSIC TO PRODUCE A CLINICAL CHANGE

Does the research currently reported support the historical role of music in care and healing? With the thrust for evidence-based practice, a multitude of studies on the effectiveness of music has been produced in the last decade. On a very happy note, research interest in music and health care has expanded into the natural setting. On a more dissonant note, the overall quality of the majority of clinical research studies has been poor as a result of heterogeneity of samples, small sample size, lack of randomization, and inconsistencies in the delivery of music interventions. Cochrane Reviews are one of the most highly regarded sources of evidence on a given topic, even if the results of the review indicate that not enough evidence is available for making a recommendation, results are conflicting, or results do not support a practice.[6] Several recent Cochrane Reviews have been published and report very limited support for the use of music in clinical practice. Notably, these reviews consistently report that there was no difference in outcomes between interventions when music was selected by the researchers compared with self-selected music. Reviewers also consistently suggest the need for better study design and larger sample sizes in research evaluating the effects of music.

What is important for the nurse healer to know about Cochrane Reviews? First, Cochrane Reviews synthesize the results of clinical intervention research trials. Second, very stringent quality criteria must be met. At the present time, very few large clinical trials on the efficacy of music have been conducted. As a result, the Cochrane Reviews for music have been based on a very few ($N = 4$) to a moderate number of studies ($N = 31$). In addition, Cochrane Reviews as well as many other systematic review papers make a clear distinction between research in which the interventions are delivered by a certified music therapist (music therapy) and music interventions delivered by a health provider (also referred to as music medicine).[7] According to the American Music Therapy Association, music therapy "is the clinical and evidence-based use of music interventions to accomplish individualized goals within a therapeutic relationship by a credentialed professional who has completed an approved music therapy program."[8] Certified music therapists individualize their interventions to meet patients' specific needs through a clinical assessment, the delivery of a tailored music experience, and evaluation. Music therapy as delivered by a music therapist includes: (1) listening to live, improvised, or prerecorded music; (2) performing music on an instrument; (3) improvising music spontaneously using voice or instruments or both; (4) composing music; and (5) music combined with other modalities. Overall, music therapy interventions demonstrate more effectiveness than music delivered by a health provider. Strengths of music therapy interventions are the use of multiple modalities including active music participation, an individualized music therapy regime adapted over time, and direct interaction with a music therapist. When reading research on the effectiveness of music, it is important to note whether the intervention was delivered as a structure therapy approach by a music therapist or a music listening session delivered by a health provider. When considering using music as a caring, healing modality, nurses' collaboration with a music therapist may enhance patients' music experience, particularly for the use of music in the management of chronic illnesses.

Effectiveness of Music Therapy Delivered by a Music Therapist

Music therapy plays a unique role in holistic care for people striving for recovery and/or maintenance of wellness when coping with chronic illness. The majority of music therapy research involves people with cognitive deficits and mental illness.[9] Although too few studies of music therapy for people with dementia were available for a Cochrane Review,[10] Witzke, Rhone, Backhause, and Shaver report that music therapy may decrease the need for physical and chemical restraints in older adults with dementia or Alzheimer's disease living in assisted care or nursing homes.[11] In a qualitative synthesis of research on home-based music therapy in a predominantly elderly population in cancer care or the hospital, the reviewers conclude that music was effective in decreasing pain and symptoms of depression.[12] Not only were patients responsive to the music, their families similarly appreciated the music therapy interventions.

In patients with acquired brain injury, music therapy may be beneficial for improving measures of walking.[13] For adults recovering from stroke or in therapy for Parkinson's disease, a systematic review reports consistent positive and significant improvement in gait parameters, along with fine and gross motor functioning.[14] Music therapy has been shown to be effective for people with schizophrenia or schizophrenia-like illness, who demonstrate improvement in global state, mental state, and functioning.[15] These gains can support the person in developing relationships or address issues for which the person does not have words. For adults with depression, short-term music therapy programs, delivered over the course of 6 to 10 weeks, resulted in greater reduction of symptoms, including improved mood.[16] Improvements in general functioning were significant for therapy delivered in 20 or more sessions.

Effectiveness of Music Delivered by a Health Provider

Research utilizing music delivered by a healthcare provider focuses primarily on the short-term management of pain, anxiety, and distress while patients undergo invasive procedures or hospitalization for surgery. A recent Cochrane Review of 23 research studies (21 studies without a music therapist) involving cardiac patients assesses the effectiveness of a music intervention.[7] Outcomes were measured immediately following the listening session. The data indicate that music listening has a moderate effect on anxiety and may have a beneficial effect on systolic blood pressure and heart rate. Anxiety reduction from music listening was highest in patients experiencing a myocardial infarction. This review reports no evidence for the anxiety-reducing effects of music for patients undergoing a cardiac procedure (intracardiac catheterization, coronary angiography, coronary artery bypass grafting). However, in a recent study of patients undergoing coronary angiographic procedures, Weeks and Nilsson report that anxiety was reduced in patients listening by headphones or by loudspeakers compared with controls.[17] Patients preferred listening to music via audio or music pillow. Staff reported that loudspeaker music was distracting. A Cochrane Review of music interventions for mechanically ventilated patients supports the small but consistent effect of music in reducing patient anxiety.[18]

Music listening is effective as an adjunct therapy in pain relief. A Cochrane Review published on the effectiveness of music in pain relief concludes that the use of music reduced postoperative pain, increased the number of patients who reported at least 50% pain relief, and lowered morphine-like analgesic use.[19] However, the magnitude of the music effect was very small. On a 0 to 10 pain rating scale, there was only a 0.5 difference in these pain outcomes compared with the control groups. The Cochrane Review on the effectiveness of music on anxiety in patients with coronary disease adds evidence on pain reduction.[7] When two or more music listening sessions were used for anxiety reduction, patients reported less pain.

Nilsson conducted a systematic review of 42 randomized clinical trials involving 3,936 patients who underwent surgery to evaluate the anxiety- and pain-reducing effects of music.[4] In 59% of the trials, patients listening to music rated the pain significantly lower. Among studies measuring analgesic use ($n = 15$), 47% of trials reported a decrease in the use of analgesics. Similarly, 57% of the trials demonstrated an effect on vital signs, with 27% demonstrating a lower heart rate, 27% demonstrating a decrease in blood pressure, and 38% reporting a significant decrease in respiratory rate. In 50% of studies measuring anxiety ($n = 22$), the music significantly reduced anxiety. Nilsson's report supports the Cochrane reviewers' summary finding that there were no differences in the effectiveness of music when the music was selected by the researchers compared with self-selected music. Nilsson excludes seven clinical trials, all of which were conducted before 2006, from this review because of poor quality scores. These data suggest that the quality of research evaluating music is improving. Although nurse healers need to critique all research carefully before using a specific research study to demonstrate support for a music intervention, nurses should use greater caution when reviewing research conducted before 2006.

Newman, Boyd, Meyers, and Bonanno reviewed studies evaluating the effectiveness of music listening in the operating room during monitored anesthesia care (MAC).[20] The Bispectral Index (BIS) monitor was used to assess the effect of music on the level of sedation or anesthesia. Procedures consisted of total abdominal hysterectomies, colonoscopies, and extracorporeal shock wave lithotripsies. They also cite a study by Maeyama et al. that evaluated music for patients undergoing spinal anesthesia. Overall, the reviewers report a reduction in sedation requirements during anesthesia, faster recovery, and decreased likelihood for converting to a general anesthetic. No qualitative data were collected, and establishing a nurse-to-patient relationship during music listening was lacking. Newman and colleagues share a sample protocol for music listening during MAC cases for clinical practice.

Research on music listening in the postanesthesia area has also been conducted. Fredriksson, Hellström, and Nilsson studied patients' well-being in regard to listening to music during their early postoperative care.[21] This study demonstrates that patients experiencing two music listening sessions were more aware of their environment, indicating they had a positive response to the music and an awareness that music helped them refocus attention on a more pleasing, soothing stimulus. Good et al. found that a combination of jaw relaxation techniques while listening to relaxing music resulted in less immediate pain relief for patients on day 1 and day 2 after surgery compared with controls.[22] Lin et al. tested listening to 30 minutes of preselected music the night before spinal surgery, 1 hour before surgery, and

on day 1 and day 2 after surgery.[23] Compared with controls, mean anxiety and pain scores were lower along with lower mean systolic blood pressure levels. In contrast, there were no differences in urine lab measurements of cortisol, norepinephrine, or epinephrine. A Cochrane Review on the effectiveness of music on preoperative anxiety is in progress.[24]

The effectiveness of music in the care of cancer patients is a recent focus of research. Huang, Good, and Zauszniewski demonstrated that cancer patients with pain greater than a rating of 3 on a 0 to 10 scale who received 30 minutes of relaxing music reported significantly less pain compared with patients provided with a 30-minute rest period.[25] In this study, 42% of the music listening group experienced a 50% reduction in pain compared with only 8% of the resting group. Lin et al. report that music had a greater effect on postchemotherapy anxiety compared to verbal relaxation and usual care.[26] Patients with the high-state anxiety experienced the most benefit from music listening. A Cochrane Review of music for improving psychological and physical outcome in care of cancer patients is under way.[27]

Another area of research focuses on the effect of music in older adults. Witzke et al. conducted a qualitative review of studies using music in Alzheimer's dementia.[11] Music listening reduced the need for chemical and/or physical restraints, with 9 of 11 studies reporting reductions in agitation after music intervention. In a study assessing acute confusion following hip or knee surgery in older adults, McCaffrey reports lower levels of confusion in the music group, which received music listening sessions for 3 days following surgery, compared with controls.[28] Participants chose music from 20 offered selections and could listen to music selections at any time, in addition to scheduled sessions.

In contrast to positive outcomes of the preceding studies, other research in older adults demonstrates no differences between music listening groups and controls. Nilsson reports no difference in subjective response to pain or anxiety in a music group compared to a rest-only control group of patients undergoing cardiac surgery.[29] Chan evaluates the effect of music on sleep quality of older adults but reports there was no statistical difference between the music listening group and the control group over a 4-week period.[30]

Music listening has also been evaluated in infants and children. Hodges and Wilson report an integrative review of preterm infants' response to music.[31] Despite limitations in study methodologies, the reviewers conclude that music appears to have positive effects, including increased oxygen saturation levels, lower heart rates, reduced behavioral stress responses, improved weight gain, and shorter length of hospitalization. Preterm infants receiving music experienced increased levels of quiet awake and quiet sleep states with improved parent–infant interactions. A recent study evaluated the effectiveness of music listening in children aged 7 to 12 years undergoing a lumbar puncture.[32] Compared with controls, the music group reported lower anxiety before and after the procedure, consistent with lower pain scores, heart rate, and respiration rates. In short interviews following the procedure, there was a notable difference between groups. Children enjoyed listening to music and reported feeling more calm/relaxed. Children in the control group wore headphones for noise reduction. Children with headphones but no music talked about their fears and anxiety related to the procedure and their disease and death. Among adolescents receiving immunizations, music listening groups reported less pain compared to the control group.[33] In this study, there were two music listening groups, with and without headphones. Whereas both groups reported less pain than the control group, adolescents with headphones were frequently observed removing their headphones to reengage with the nurse.

Overall, review papers and research reports that incorporate a large variety of study designs consistently suggest that music may be a helpful adjunct to usual practice. Findings from the preceding studies support using music listening as part of a healing environment for patients. The most frequently reported arguments in support of music are the following: music appears to have a positive effect in a majority of studies, music can be easily administered, music is low cost, and there is a very low probability of harm.[17] Other researchers suggest caution in using music, suggesting that music can elicit strong negative emotions, which may be unexpected.[34-36] In a qualitative review of music experiences of terminally ill patients, the reviewers indicate that the use of music needs to be a personal decision.[36] The researchers provide examples of patients rejecting the use of music and suggest that music listening may not be a positive experience when the music is unfamiliar, is experienced as unpleasant, or is associated with loss. Thus, the nurse healer's initial assessment of a person's interest in music, the decision on the genre of music and tempo to use, and ongoing evaluation of the person's response to music are important in using music as a caring, healing modality. The same process is important when nurse healers choose to use music as a caring, healing modality for themselves.

Several individual research studies include a qualitative component in which patients are asked about the use of music. Patients consistently report high satisfaction and well-being.[17,21,32] Few recent qualitative studies have been reported. Using a qualitative approach, Daykin et al. report key themes reflecting the experiences of participants in a 3-month group music therapy program: choice and enrichment, power, freedom and release, music and healing, balance, individuation, and creativity and loss.[37] The importance of identity and the role of creativity in the processes of individuation of cancer patients using music therapy were evident in the study. McCaffrey and Good, as reported in McCaffrey (2008), identified three themes capturing the effectiveness of listening to music postoperatively: feeling comfort in a discomforting and frightening situation, distraction from pain, and a feeling of being at home.[38] The last theme reflects patients' statements indicating that music transported them out of the hospital to their own homes, a familiar, comforting environment.

Little attention, outside of structured music therapy interventions, has been given to gaining insight on music as a means for people to relate and share a health-related experience. Few research studies explore how music contributes to a person's development of the capacity to strive, endure, recover, heal, live, or die. A small and older body of qualitative work shows that listening to music can foster a sense of identity, expressions of joy, a release from negative emotions, experiences of creativity, and feelings of freedom and release "to let go."[37,39] O'Callaghan et al., in summarizing their qualitative study in children with cancer, states that music facilitated communication, self-reflection, self-expression, and creativity.[39]

Summary of Research Evidence

The research on music continues to grow rapidly, providing more and perhaps stronger evidence in support of music for therapeutic purposes. Nonetheless, current research evidence, with its many limitations, must be considered in clinical decision making today. At this point in time, there are a great number of unknowns in the effectiveness of music.

Currently, what does research on music listening tell nurse healers?

- The vast majority of research has been conducted using Caucasian and Asian population samples. Identifying culturally appropriate music for patients is a key element.
- Music is effective in reducing anxiety for patients, in particular, for patients with a high level of anxiety.
- Music is effective in reducing pain, but only to a limited extent. Only 50% of the trials demonstrate a significant effect of music on pain and anxiety in patients undergoing an elective surgical procedure.
- A highly variable response to music is likely among patients. Different effects of music may result from a combination of internal and external factors.
- Delivery of two or more music listening sessions increases the likelihood of a positive outcome. Listening to music before and after an invasive procedure may enhance effectiveness.
- Music in combination with other healing modalities may enhance effectiveness.
- Time duration for a listening session does not make a difference, although the majority of sessions were approximately 30 minutes in length.
- Music genre does not make a difference, although the majority of studies used classical music.
- Music tempo does make a difference such that a slower tempo along with calming, soothing music appears to be the most important music element in enhancing music effectiveness in reducing pain and anxiety. In several studies by Nilsson, a selection of "genreless" music was used for music listening groups, available from MusiCure (www.musicure.com).[40]
- Decision making on the choice of music selection is important. A key component to positive outcomes may be the determination of an intended goal with specific music chosen to meet that goal.
- Music has meaning beyond its function in producing outcomes.

Given the state of research today, what questions still need to be asked? What approach to music has not been evaluated? Can the limited effectiveness of music be enhanced?

Outcome indicators for the majority of studies are defined by the researchers as traditional physiologic markers (heart rate, respiratory rate, cortisol levels) or as traditional standardized psychological measures of anxiety (predominantly used is the State-Trait Anxiety Index). Although these indicators help to provide a consistency of measurements across studies, perhaps they are not the best markers to capture the effectiveness of music. Do we need more qualitative research conducted to capture the wider aspects of meaning and possibilities in musical relating? This is to say that more research using larger sample sizes and stronger designs is needed, and qualitative research should be conducted independently or within a triangulated approach to evaluating music in health care.

To date, the vast majority of research studies evaluate the effects of music either delivered as a structured music therapy intervention through interaction with a music therapist or as just listening to music. No research tests a holistic nursing approach in which the nurse creates a therapeutic relationship with the patient using the modality of music. The emphasis has been placed on providing music as a "to-do" element of care, as an adjunct to usual best care. However, this recommendation does not capture the value of nurse–patient interaction and neither does it identify the nurse as an integral person who can influence the effectiveness of music. The nurse interacting with the patient while using music as a caring, healing modality may enhance the patient's psychophysiologic outcomes and heighten the patient's experience of feeling cared for. The nurse values this reciprocal relationship as well.[41] Quinn, Smith, Ritenbaugh, Swanson, and Watson state that research on healing modalities delivered by nurses must take into account the nurse–patient relationship because the healing relationship involves "(at least) two individuals engaged in a mutual, simultaneous process."[42] The health and well-being of the nurse affects his or her self-care as well as the care of others. Whereas all studies recruit volunteer participants, not all people are sensitive to the nuances of music. It is notable that 4% of the general population suffers from "amusia," or tone-deafness. This is usually inherited but may be a consequence of brain damage, often coupled with aphasia.[43] Assessing the role that music plays in a person's daily life can give the nurse healer insights for developing a "deeper" relationship that may enhance the use of music as caring, healing modality.

The effectiveness of music in the delivery of this relationship-based care has not yet been evaluated. Here lies the future of nursing research on use of personal healing modalities. Perhaps the new phase in music research studies should be based on an increased understanding of the human body's response to music, the nurse–patient relationship, and human caring theory. The next section describes new laboratory research followed by thoughts on application of this knowledge within nurse–patient interactions.

■ THEORETICAL BASIS FOR THE CAPACITY OF MUSIC TO PRODUCE A CLINICAL CHANGE

The goal of laboratory research addressing the functionality of music is to understand the mechanisms of action on a cellular or molecular level. These mechanisms remain unclear. Research in the last decade shows that music can reduce the stress hormone cortisol.[29,35,44] Music, which elicits a strong pleasurable response, may lead to a release of endogenous dopamine.[45] The newest proposed marker for hormonal changes is oxytocin, which is synthesized in the hypothalamus and released in response to stress. Oxytocin has been shown to create a sense of calmness and diminish the sensation of pain.[46,47] Mrázová and Celec propose that molecular science intersecting with new understandings of the endocrine mechanisms and neurophysiology will lead to better understanding of the effects of music.[35]

In the last decade, advancements of neuroimagery have provided for rapid developments of theory on the functional neuroanatomy of music. A traditional model of music response suggests that music listening is predominantly a right brain activity and music composition is a left brain activity. With the utilization of positron emission tomography (PET), functional magnetic resonance imagery (fMRI), and magnet encephalography (MED), researchers have identified distinct neural circuits that are stimulated in response to music.[48] Ongoing research suggests that music listening, composing, and performing engage regions throughout the brain through an integrative system of music processes. In Western tonal music (almost exclusively used in neuroimagery research), which is based on groups of two, three, or four primary beats, major and minor tonal notes are the principal distinctions. Neuroimagery studies show that major and minor tones generate a response in the bilateral inferior frontal gyri, medial thalamus, and dorsal cingulate cortex. However, minor cords also activate the amygdala, retrosplenial cortex, cerebellum, and brain stem. Whereas all music is processed through the auditory association areas, emotionally neutral music is also processed in the insula. Happy music, which elicits strong feelings of pleasure, is associated with activity in the bilateral ventral and left dorsal striations, left anterior cingulated, and left parahippocampus gyrus. Sad music activates the hippocampus, amygdala, and auditory association areas. Dissonant music (not harmonic; sounds that clash) evokes unpleasant sensations by both altering neuroactivity and blood flow. Insights on the complexity of brain responses to music demonstrate the degree to which the right and left hemispheres work in harmony. For an in-depth discussion of the neurological mechanisms induced by music, refer to Levitin and Tirovolas.[48]

While several researchers are mapping the complex nature of neurophysiologic responses of the human body to happy and sad music tones, other researchers are working to gain new insights into psychological values of varying emotions generated by music.[44,49] According to this line of research, more attention and sensitivity needs to be paid to the specific effects of music tone and tempo on varying emotions people experience while listening to music. Music elicits not only feelings of happiness or sadness, but also feelings of joy, sorrow, fear, peacefulness, anxiety, or excitement. Researchers assessing the psychological influence of music report that music often elicits mixed feelings and perceptions.[49] Typically, a nurse healer can expect that music perceived as happy or sad or relaxing will create a parallel emotional response. However, this emotional response may be subtle. In the study by Hunter, Schellenberg and Schimmack, emotional responses could be enhanced with the consistent delivery of happy (major key) or sad (minor key) music and by varying the tempo. Faster tempo of major key music resulted in higher happy ratings. Slower tempo of minor key music was associated with higher sad ratings. Mixed music cues (fast-pace minor key) resulted in feelings of ambivalence. Researchers suggest that when music is used for therapeutic purposes, it may elicit mixed feelings and perceptions in contrast to the intended purpose of the music selection, such as mood regulation or relaxation. Nilsson, in her systematic review of music, cautions against the use of music that evokes strong emotions resulting from music memories associated with various life events.[4] Jeong and colleagues demonstrate that environment affects the emotions elicited by music.[50] In a new study to test the effects of congruence and incongruence between visual imagery and music, the research suggests an additive effect can occur in a person's emotional response, such that when happy music is combined with a happy visual, subjects rated their happiness higher. The congruence between music stimuli and visual stimuli across modalities appears to enhance an intended emotional effect. Music combined with another congruence stimulus, such as art or external imagery, may strengthen more subtle effects of music and reduce the possibility of mixed effects resulting in feelings of ambivalence.

In most studies reporting researcher-selected music, participants were offered a choice of selections, all of which provide continuous, soothing sounds at a slower tempo. In studies reporting the use of self-selected music, frequently there was no description of a discussion that took place regarding the choice of music. Little attention has been paid to the importance of guiding a person in choosing music selections for optimal, desired effects. In past research, self-selected music may have included songs with a variety of tempos, with mixed major, minor, and dissonant tones stimulating more complex networks in the brain and mixed feelings and perceptions of the music itself. The result may have been a personal experience of ambivalent feelings compared to feelings of relaxation that appear to accompany consistently soothing, slow-tempo music. The nurse healer can interact with each person to help him or her become conscious of the psychological and physical effects of the music the person enjoys. As people identify their unique responses to various music selections, they can become conscious and intentional in the selection of the music that will meet their goals, whether the goal is to motivate, distract, relax, manage pain, or to decrease anxiety.

Entrainment theory is frequently provided as the theoretical framework in music research and may help to illustrate the importance of making a best choice in the self-selection of music for a specific goal. Entrainment theory is a physics theory used to understand the body's response to music. Entrainment is the synchronization process whereby the vibrations of one object cause the vibrations of another object (usually the less powerful) to oscillate at the same tempo or rate.[51] Entrainment theory suggests that music is a natural pacemaker, influencing the rate or tempo of heartbeat and brain waves. The human body, including individual cells, has a number of rhythms and vibrations. According to entrainment theory, sound vibrations from musical instruments can influence the body's rhythms (such as brain rhythms and vital signs) to match or be in harmony with the rhythm of the music. For this to occur, the music stimulus should have a consistent rhythm and amplitude.[52] According to entrainment theory, music used for relaxation should have a tempo of 60 to 80 beats per minute with a slow, repetitive nature. The human body will synchronize the heart beat to the slow tempo with a reduction in sympathetic nervous control and lowered metabolism, muscle tension, and gastric activity. Another example of entrainment theory is the human body's response to sound created by Tibetan singing bowls.[53] Buddhist teachings state that nothing exists independently of itself, which is reflective of sound made by the Tibetan singing bowls. These calming, high-resonance bowls represent holism because one note is dependent on another to produce this mystical, healing, tranquil sound. **See Figure 18-1.**

Entrainment theory may also account for the effectiveness of music in regaining walking and gait functions following stroke. The tempo of music acts as a cue or rhythmic auditory stimulation (RAS) for each step and can serve as an anticipated and continuous time reference for movements. Similar to the relaxation response, the body is responsive to different repetitive tempos.[11] Neuroimaging studies by Thaut suggest that music stimulates the spatiotemporal functioning of the motor cortex networks of the brain.[54] Finger tapping, toe tapping, swaying to the music, and even head nodding reflect

the human body's response to the rhythm and tempo of music.

Movement to music is the basis for a novel midrange nursing theory of music, mood, and movement (MMM Theory), systematically developed with the purpose of guiding research on music to improve health outcomes.[55] Murrock and Higgins propose that a person's psychological, physiologic, and social responses to music influence health outcomes. The first theoretical statement of the MMM Theory is "Music produces the psychological response of altered mood leading to improved health outcomes." Music affects moods both through neurophysiologic responses (as noted previously) and through social interaction. Music is perceived as playing an important role in communication of feelings and identity, which is integrated into selections of music for enjoyment. The second theoretical statement of MMM Theory is "Physiologic responses to music are a cue for movement leading to initiation of and maintenance of physical activity." The third theoretical statement is "Both the psychological response of altered music and physiologic response of movement to music promotes the initiation and maintenance of physical activity leading to improved health outcomes." **See Figure 18-2.**

Although the MMM Theory is designed to guide research and be tested, the authors suggest that the framework can also guide the nurse–patient interaction in the selection of music for enjoyment. The person can select music that will purposefully cue movement for activity during an exercise period and sustain the physical activity through the discomfort of exercise. Research has consistently shown that regular sustained exercise results in positive health outcomes. The major challenge has been to initiate and sustain physical activity. Murrock and Higgins actively invite the nurse to engage patients in the development of exercise goals for good outcomes using music.

■ MUSIC: A CARING, HEALING MODALITY

This chapter repeatedly identifies the value of conscious and purposeful decision making in the selection and evaluation of music listening. It suggests that the nurse–patient interaction may

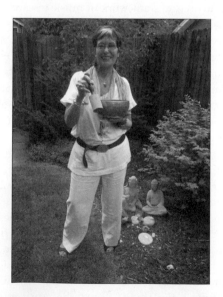

FIGURE 18-1   Jean Watson and the Tibetan Singing Bowl
Source: Courtesy of Jean Watson.

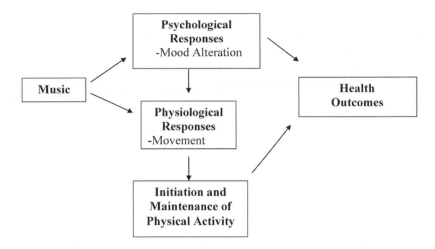

FIGURE 18-2   The Theory of Music, Mood, and Movement to Improve Health Outcomes.
Source: Courtesy of Carolyn J. Murrock, PhD.

be key to enhancing the effectiveness in music. The MMM Theory is presented as a new mid-range theory designed to promote the nurse–patient interaction. However, there is still a major missing component that helps frame the larger picture of holistic care nursing.

From the time of Nightingale, the caring, healing arts were a part of the nurse–patient relationship.[1] According to Watson, Nightingale viewed the nurse–patient and nurse–God relationships as sacred pledges. Through these sacred relationships, the patient and nurse are one, in body and soul, a conceptualization that is similar to transpersonal nursing in the twenty-first century. Watson explains how Nightingale used the basic care essentials (light, clean air, nutrition) and the environment (outdoors, flowers, paintings, and music) to promote this body-to-soul connection for healing. On the one hand, modern medicine consists of "doing" tasks such as administering drugs, carrying out procedures, and using technology and does not attend to "deeper" human-to-human interactions using caring, healing modalities to promote health and intentional caring. On the other hand, transpersonal nursing brings to light explicit caring consciousness and intentionality through caring, healing modalities in the nurse–patient interaction. Within this interaction, Watson espouses that the nurse develops a connection with the

person and utilizes caring, healing modalities to change individual moments of a difficult experience into caring moments. One modality that nurses can use in the context of this nurse–patient interaction is music.

Watson states that the caring, healing modalities "potentiate wholeness, harmony, integrity and beauty, and preserve dignity and humanity with every act."[1] Watson bases transpersonal caring, healing modalities such as music listening on caring consciousness and intentionality. Caring consciousness involves a deeper spiritual awareness between the nurse and patient through the interaction. The nurse is mindful, present, and chooses how he or she portrays "being" in the interaction. This deeper level of caring consciousness is not a primary nursing characteristic but is reciprocal (transpersonal) between the nurse and the patient through the interaction. When nurses and patients can consciously connect spiritually in these relationships, both individuals are changed positively or negatively by the interaction and the nature of the experience itself.[56] Caring consciousness is present in caring moments when nurses intentionally interact with a patient for the purpose of a deeper human-to-human connection.

The concept of intentionality, according to Watson, involves direct purpose and effectiveness toward action. Intentionality is consciously placing focus on something, for example, a belief, will, expectation, attention, or action. Setting intention serves to remind nurses of what is important, what the focus should be, and provides the opportunity to be present. In transpersonal nursing, nurse healers become holistic spirits of caring for patients and themselves by the interactions (caring moments) they engage in. A strong human-to-human connection between the nurse and patient can be established using complementary modalities such as music listening. Music listening in the context of a caring moment applying caring consciousness and intentionality exemplifies a value for human life and promotes quality caring, healing experiences for patients and nurses.[41]

How can nurse healers apply the research evidence guided by the Theory of Human Caring in practice? Music therapy is more effective than music listening in part because of the therapist–patient interaction and goal-setting components. Through interactions with patients, nurse healers can use caring consciousness and intentionality to enhance patients' experiences with music. Using the Theory of Human Caring, the nurse healer consciously engages the patient in a caring moment with the intention of using music as a healing modality. Consider the following example of a caring moment: music is playing on a TV station (dedicated to music) in the background. The nurse healer consciously brings the patient's attention to the music and begins an intentional dialogue. The dialogue can focus on music's relaxing or distracting effects, on music as a cue for deep breathing or range of motion exercises, on sharing a memory of music and a better time, or exploring how music can be added to the patient's day. By exploring music's healing effects together, the nurse and patient can create significant life-changing recollections through their relationship, which influences their very being.

In a caring moment that may take only a few minutes, nurse healers can apply caring consciousness and intentionality that exemplify value for human life and promote high-quality caring, healing experiences for both patients and nurses.[57] Consider the use of other artistic expressions in a caring moment. External imagery (visual imagery) such as paintings, sculptures, pottery, and other forms of artwork synergistically work with music listening. Just as music can transform moods, so can external imagery.[58] The combination of visualizing a painting (external imagery) and listening to music can have an intense impact on well-being. A greater sense of healing can evolve that cannot be achieved by each caring, healing modality alone. The music and imagery can promote escape of the bodymindspirit to "a place" viewed in the imagery or in the imagination. See **Figure 18-3a and 18-3b.**

Individual Musical Preferences

Music, like art, is a subjectively perceived phenomenon. Music encompasses many types of genres that individuals may or may not connect with on a personal level. Music listening can affect individuals' current state of mind, mood, feelings, and eventually actions. Morris explains the International Organization for Standardization (ISO) principle that focuses on matching types of music (genres) to individuals' moods.[51] The ISO principle is two sided and works on altering individuals' moods. Altering moods can accomplish a "state of consciousness." The mind and feelings vibrate at a certain frequency and the music listening is in resonance with that same frequency. This state of consciousness resembles caring consciousness in the nurse–patient relationship. There is a deeper level achieved, and the individual is mindful, intentional, and present in that given moment. The individual chooses how to act through the interaction with music compared to expressing one's self in the nurse–patient relationship.

Individuals must be aware of what, how, and why music affects their mood, feelings, and/or attitudes. As Morris points out, keeping track of experiences with music can lead to establishing an appreciation for sound and music's healing potential.[51] Journaling on specific types of genres and how and why they have affected emotions, actions, and life overall is an excellent way for nurses to start using music personally as a caring, healing modality.

Future research and evidence-based practice centering on music as a caring, healing modality will pave the way for modifications in individual musical preferences.

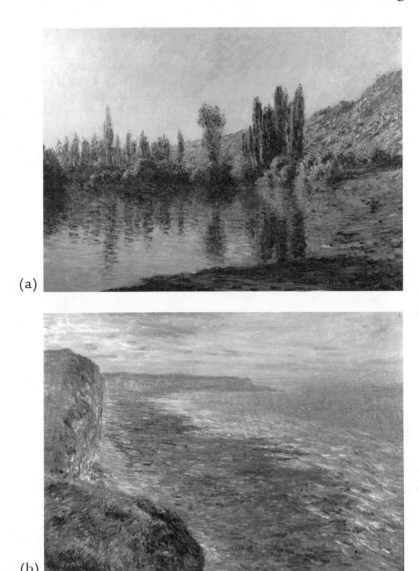

(a)

(b)

FIGURE 18-3   a. Painting with trees and water. b. Painting with cliff and water.
Source: Courtesy of Minnesota Marine Art Museum, Winona, Minnesota.

■ HOLISTIC CARING PROCESS

In the use of music as a caring, healing modality, the nurse healer utilizes the nursing process to integrate music into a patient's plan of care during a procedure, treatment, or hospitalization.

Holistic Assessment

Using the nursing process, nurse healers assess individuals' interest in the use of music, the genre they enjoy, their history of using music in their daily lives, and hearing ability. In a teaching moment, nurses can share that music can be effective in itself and as an adjunct to other pharmacologic and nonpharmacologic therapies. Together the nurse, the patient, and the family can then explore the various types of music that may fit the context of the situation (consciousness) and the purpose for using music (intentionality). Frequently, the intention or goal for listening to music is to relax, reduce anxiety, or mediate a pain response. However, music can be used for goals of supporting deep breathing, promoting both active and passive exercises, and establishing a caring, healing relationship with each other.

Identification of Patterns/Challenges/Needs

- Hard of Hearing
- Deaf
- Confusion
- Anxiety
- Pain
- Relaxation
- Depression
- Loss of Memory
- Loneliness
- Spiritual Distress
- Stress
- Motivational
- Fear
- Fatigue
- Hopelessness
- Outcomes

In planning for the use of music for the reduction of anxiety and/or pain, music selections should be flowing, nonlyrical, with 60–80 beats per minute, with low tones and minimal brass percussion.[59] A volume of 60 dB is recommended. Patients should be asked to select music they would describe as quiet, soft, peaceful, dreamy, soothing, serene, undramatic, slow-speed, regular rhythm, or a pleasant combination of instruments. Music selections should be played for approximately 30 minutes. Self-selected music can be brought from home as either downloads for an MP3 player/iPod or chosen from a music library developed for a floor or institution.[51] Nurse healers are conscientious in the prevention of infection when using headphones. Using individual ear buds or music pillows and changing pillow cases are options.

Holistic Care Plan and Interventions

At the beginning of the session:
- If in a clinical or hospital setting, inform others of the need for minimal noise and disruptions (you can post a sign on the patient door requesting no interruptions for 30 minutes).
- If the patient has a hearing loss, consider a variety of methods for delivering music.

Headphones provide for individual control of sound level. Music pillows are available or the nurse may simply find the most effective placement of the music player.

- Discuss how listening to music can help the patient reach intended goals (relaxation, anxiety reduction, mediating pain).
- Discuss the length of the session, usually 20 to 30 minutes.
- Ask the person to empty his or her bladder, if needed.
- Ask the person to remove eyeglasses.
- Minimize environmental stimuli from the environment, such as lowering the light level, closing a curtain or door.
- Assist the patient in finding a comfortable position, and offer an extra pillow or blanket if needed.
- Have the patient begin playing the music to make sure the equipment is functioning properly.

Evaluation

At the end of the session:
- Assess the patient's response and tolerance to the session.
- Create a caring moment by connecting with the person during a 5–10 minute interaction.
- Use the following script to begin this caring moment:[41]
  1. What did you listen to today?
  2. Tell me what you thought of when you listened to this music (memories)?
  3. How does listening to (specific music selection) music make you feel?
  4. Share a personal experience of how listening to music makes you feel.
  5. In what ways did listening to the music help you? Did the music help you reach your goal?
  6. What are your thoughts about having music listening available during your time here?
  7. What would be helpful to make this a better experience for you?
- If appropriate, schedule a follow-up session.

Documentation of Session and Plan of Care

Record the following information:
- Person's goal or intention for listening to music
- Song or genre the person selects

- Time and tolerance of the listening session
- Outcome of the music listening experience
- Update of the plan to use music listening session in the future

Today, nurse healers are challenged to define best practice for documentation of music as a caring, healing modality in their current and future record systems. With a move to electronic medical records, nurses have the opportunity to document how music listening is used and the patient's responses to inform not only the next nurse caring for the patient, but also future nursing care, when another procedure, treatment, or hospitalization takes place. The nurse healer's message to others can define the nature of patient-centered care in a future care context.

CASE STUDY

Setting: Adult hematology/oncology outpatient center

Clients: Male and female patients (20 to 50 years and older) and female nurses (20 to 50 years and older)

Patterns/Challenges/Needs:

1. Limited choices for distraction and relaxation during chemotherapy treatments
2. Providing spiritual-based care

A therapeutic music pilot program was instituted in an adult chemotherapy unit at a midwestern medical center. Many of the patients who participated in the therapeutic music pilot (self-selected music listening with CD players or MP3 players) were fond of music and had a musical history (choir, singing, playing). Selected patient and nurse experiences from this pilot exemplify the use of music as a caring, healing modality. A music therapist was also present on the unit at the time of the trial pilot.

When the pilot began, D. S. was asked if she was interested in listening to music during her treatments. D. S. stated that treatments were long and boring. "There is nothing to do except sleep during this time because the chemo makes me so tired." Following the music session, D. S. went on to say that "music" took her to another place and she was no longer in the four-walled treatment room. Another patient, S. I., expressed

feeling a sense of autonomy with selecting her music for listening. She stated, "It's nice to have a choice; I had no choice in getting cancer." Experiencing a sense of relaxation and calmness each time S. I. listened to music in the treatment room was important to her. F. G., an older gentleman, verbalized his enjoyment of the "healing effects of listening to music." F. G. shared that in his past he played the banjo in bands and for his church on occasion. Listening to music took his mind off his cancer and the chemotherapy he was getting. "I have always enjoyed music and playing my banjo, it brings me joy!"

Music as a caring, healing modality moved beyond listening to flowing with the music in a married couple, A. K. and B. K., who came to the clinic together while the wife was receiving chemotherapy for breast cancer. Each time music was offered to the couple, they would share their memories of ballroom dancing together. They had met years ago on a dance floor. Dancing was one thing they both loved and shared during their 58 years together. The couple told the nurses that they should not be surprised to find them dancing during treatment one day. "The music takes me back to our dancing days and how much fun we had doing it," A. K. stated. Her husband had a twinkle in his eye as he looked at her. He was reliving the lovely memories of their time together dancing. B. K. went on to say, "Everything was so peaceful and carefree on the dance floor, I miss that." A few weeks later, as the nurses looked through the window leading to the treatment room, they saw this lovely couple finally dance.

As part of the therapeutic music pilot project nurses were asked to interact with their patients by focusing on the patients' music listening experiences. Focus groups with the nurses were conducted following the pilot.[41] The nurses taking part in this music listening pilot also enjoyed personal benefits from music and shared the healing, caring benefits their patients' experienced in their care. One nurse who frequently floated to the chemotherapy center gave this patient insight: "Music brings a 'new' side to my patients; calmness and healing are what I am seeing." She also commented on how the nurse–patient relationship seemed "closer." She sensed cohesiveness in the relationship and felt herself regrouping and centering during her encounters with her patients. "I feel this music project has brought passion back into the profession and my practice." She continued to share that she saw the chemotherapy nurses using music to care for themselves. "We are seeing our own values and purposes for listening to music. . . . We are seeing how our patients are relating music listening to healing and caring." Another nurse commented on how "music touches the soul." "Music almost always comes with a 'story,' so this is an ideal tool for patients and us to tell 'our' stories." Overall, nurses thought this was fantastic and viewed music as an "open door" to the soul and heart. At the end of the workday, nurses began to tune in music while they prepared the unit for the next workday. Other healing activities involving music soon followed with the establishment of a choir, care clowning, and get-togethers involving music and food.

As a result of the music pilot, the chemotherapy nurses openly addressed the challenge of providing spiritual care for their patients. During the focus groups, spiritual-based care was identified as the most challenging to provide. Nurses stated their feelings of "uncomfortableness" with assessing spirituality in their patients. One nurse expressed that nurses in general put up a "boundary" between spirituality/religion and work. Many felt time constraints had a negative impact in establishing these time-sensitive patient conversations. Through this pilot project, nurses began to view music as a pathway to "open doors" to spiritual-based care with caring moment discussions of spiritual music and hymns. The chemotherapy nurses created new venues for integrating music, such as inclusion of music offering in the sanctuary and a commitment to devoting more "quality" time to listening to patients and getting to know them on a "deeper" level (caring moments). Nurses felt the need to be "aware" of clues patients leave that "open doors" for telling their stories. Stories that may lead to clues in assessing music listening for future research and guided pathways to uncovering "why is music so much a part of our everyday lives."

Spirituality

Music can be a spiritual practice and have a calming effect, enabling people to get in touch with a higher being (God). In Samuel 1 16:23, when David would play the harp King Saul would feel a sense of relief, feel better, and the evil spirit would disappear from his body.[60] The different tones and rhythms can resemble the beauty, creativity, and wonder of the Maker if the listener surrenders and becomes one with the notes.[57] When one listens to music with an open heart and mind, the sense of calmness present can resemble prayer and listening to a higher being.

Music can be an avenue that goes beyond everyday existence. It can speak to the soul and move a person from despair to hope and from sadness to joyfulness. Music can encourage action, taking someone to the next destination in life's journey.[60]

Nature sounds encompass many wonders of the world. Birds singing, trees blowing, rain falling, waves crashing, and fire crackling can represent creations by the Maker. These sounds of music can symbolize spirituality and can be another path in providing spiritual-based holistic care. Nursing's spiritual practice is caring moments that are time-sensitive periods that lead to critical turning points for self and others.[56] According to Avery Brook, "Particularly when the turmoil in our mind is great, the simple tune and words of a spiritual song may lift our hearts and minds to a quieter plane."[60]

As nurses develop and sustain deeper human-to-human connections with their patients using music listening as a caring, healing modality, they practice the core philosophy of holistic care. Nurses can incorporate caring, healing values and beliefs into their practice and promote health and well-being for their patients and themselves. Nurses can be more in touch with who they are and what they contribute to their practice. By separating the heavily emphasized "doing" tasks from a nursing model centering on roles of "being" in the context of Watson's Human Caring Theory, nurses can rejuvenate their work and experience satisfaction, pride, and passion for holistic care nursing.

Directions for
FUTURE RESEARCH

1. Investigate long-term effects of music as a caring, healing modality with a patient's plan of care in chronic disease management.
2. Contrast outcomes based on dosage of music received (once a day, twice a day).

3. Evaluate the influence of a diversity of music genres on the stress response.

4. Research the use of music listening in a culturally diverse group.

5. Increase understanding of different outcomes on subsets of populations, for example, patients who have a strong history of including music in their lives and patients who enjoy music but who have not engaged in music listening on a regular basis.

6. Increase understanding of health conditions for which music may not be helpful, including varying outcomes.

7. Assess the relationship between coping styles and the effect of music. For example, a person whose preferred coping style is distraction may be very responsive to the anxiolytic effect of music in contrast to a person who copes with a more active style.

8. Conduct qualitative studies to explore the meaning of the patient's music experience relevant to healing, recovery, and lifestyle changes.

9. Develop valid and reliable evaluation tools that assess a client's subjective response to music based on qualitative studies.

10. Conduct quantitative studies with strong methodology with sample size based on power analysis.

11. When developing research, follow recommendations for music-based interventions that support the Consolidated Standards for Reporting Trials (CONSORT) and the Transparent Reporting of Evaluations with Non-randomized Designs (TREND) statements for transparent reporting.[61]

Nurse Healer
REFLECTIONS

After reading this chapter, the nurse healer will be able to answer or to begin the process of answering the following questions:

- How do I feel about using music as a caring, healing modality within the nurse–patient relationship?

- How can I promote and use music as a caring, healing modality for individuals I care for and myself?

- Next time I turn on the iTouch, iPod, radio, or any other music listening device, I will be aware of why I did this action and how the music makes me feel. (You can journal your insights, which may "open doors" to the answers in using music beyond its ordinary function as a caring, healing holistic practice.)

---

www. *For a full suite of assignments and additional learning activities, use the access code located in the front of your book to visit this exclusive website: http://go.jblearning.com /dossey. If you do not have an access code, you can obtain one at the site.*

NOTES

1. J. Watson, *Postmodern Nursing and Beyond* (Philadelphia, PA: Churchill Livingstone, 1999).

2. W. R. Cowling 3rd, M. C. Smith, and J. Watson, "The Power of Wholeness, Consciousness, and Caring: A Dialogue on Nursing Science, Art, and Healing," *Advances in Nursing Science* 31, no. 1 (January 2008): E41–E51.

3. O. Sacks, *Musicophilia: Tales of Music and the Brain*, rev. and expanded ed. (New York: Vintage Books, 2008).

4. U. Nilsson, "The Anxiety- and Pain-Reducing Effects of Music Interventions: A Systematic Review." *AORN Journal* 87, no. 4 (April 2008): 780.

5. F. Nightingale, *Notes on Nursing: What It Is and What It Is Not* (New York: Cambridge University Press, 2010).

6. Cochrane Collaboration, homepage. http://www.cochrane.org/.

7. J. Bradt and C. Dileo, "Music for Stress and Anxiety Reduction in Coronary Heart Disease Patients," *Cochrane Database of Systematic Reviews* no. 2 (June 2009).

8. American Music Therapy Association, "What Is Music Therapy?" http://www.musictherapy.org /faq/#38.

9. H. Tang and T. Vezeau, "The Use of Music Intervention in Healthcare Research: A Narrative Review of the Literature," *Journal of Nursing Research* 18, no. 3 (September 2010): 174–190.

10. A. C. Vink et al., "Music Therapy for People with Dementia," *Cochrane Database of Systematic Reviews* 1 (2009).

11. J. Witzke et al., "How Sweet the Sound: Research Evidence for the Use of Music in Alzheimer's

Dementia," *Journal of Gerontological Nursing* 34, no. 10 (October 2008): 45–52.

12. W. Schmid and T. Ostermann, "Home-Based Music Therapy—A Systematic Overview of Settings and Conditions for an Innovative Service in Healthcare," *BMC Health Services Research* 10 (2010): 291.

13. J. Bradt et al., "Music Therapy for Acquired Brain Injury," *Cochrane Database of Systematic Reviews* 10 (2010).

14. C. M. Weller and F. A. Baker, "The Role of Music Therapy in Physical Rehabilitation: A Systematic Literature Review," *Nordic Journal of Music Therapy* 20, no. 1 (February 2011): 43–61.

15. C. Gold et al., "Music Therapy for Schizophrenia or Schizophrenia-Like Illnesses," *Cochrane Database of Systematic Reviews* 1 (2009).

16. A. Maratos et al., "Music Therapy for Depression," *Cochrane Database of Systematic Reviews* 1 (March 2008).

17. P. B. Weeks and U. Nilsson, "Music Interventions in Patients During Coronary Angiographic Procedures: A Randomized Controlled Study of the Effect on Patients' Anxiety and Well-being," *European Journal of Cardiovascular Nursing* 10, no. 2 (June 2011): 88–93.

18. J. Bradt, C. Dileo, and D. Grocke, "Music Interventions for Mechanically Ventilated Patients," *Cochrane Database of Systematic Reviews* 12 (2010).

19. S. M. Cepeda et al., "Music for Pain Relief," *Cochrane Database of Systematic Reviews* 8 (2010).

20. A. Newman et al., "Implementation of Music as an Anesthetic Adjunct During Monitored Anesthesia Care," *Journal of PeriAnesthesia Nursing* 25, no. 6 (December 2010): 387–391.

21. A. Fredriksson, L. Hellström, and U. Nilsson, "Patients' Perception of Music Versus Ordinary Sound in a Postanaesthesia Care Unit: A Randomised Crossover Trial," *Intensive and Critical Care Nursing* 25, no. 4 (August 2009): 208–213.

22. M. Good et al., "Supplementing Relaxation and Music for Pain After Surgery," *Nursing Research* 59, no. 4 (2010): 259–269.

23. P. Lin et al., "Music Therapy for Patients Receiving Spine Surgery," *Journal of Clinical Nursing* 20, no. 7 (April 2011): 960–968.

24. C. Dileo, J. Bradt, and K. Murphy, "Music for Preoperative Anxiety," *Cochrane Database of Systematic Reviews* 4 (2010).

25. S. Huang, M. Good, and J. A. Zauszniewski, "The Effectiveness of Music in Relieving Pain in Cancer Patients: A Randomized Controlled Trial," *International Journal of Nursing Studies* 47, no. 11 (November 2010): 1354–1362.

26. M. Lin et al., "A Randomised Controlled Trial of the Effect of Music Therapy and Verbal Relaxation on Chemotherapy-Induced Anxiety,"

27. C. Dileo et al., "Music Interventions for Improving Psychological and Physical Outcomes in Cancer Patients," *Cochrane Database of Systematic Reviews* 10 (2010).

28. R. McCaffrey, "The Effect of Music on Acute Confusion in Older Adults After Hip or Knee Surgery," *Applied Nursing Research* 22, no. 2 (May 2009): 107–112.

29. U. Nilsson, "The Effect of Music Intervention in Stress Response to Cardiac Surgery in a Randomized Clinical Trial," *Heart & Lung* 38, no. 3 (2009): 201–207.

30. M. F. Chan, "A Randomised Controlled Study of the Effects of Music on Sleep Quality in Older People," *Journal of Clinical Nursing* 20, no. 7 (April 2011): 979–987.

31. A. L. Hodges and L. L. Wilson, "Preterm Infants' Responses to Music: An Integrative Literature Review," *Southern Online Journal of Nursing Research* 10, no. 3 (May 2010).

32. T. N. Nguyen et al., "Music Therapy to Reduce Pain and Anxiety in Children with Cancer Undergoing Lumbar Puncture: A Randomized Clinical Trial," *Journal of Pediatric Oncology Nursing* 27, no. 3 (2010): 146–155.

33. O. Kristjánsdóttir and G. Kristjánsdóttir, "Randomized Clinical Trial of Musical Distraction with and Without Headphones for Adolescents' Immunization Pain," *Scandinavian Journal of Caring Sciences* 25, no. 1 (March 2011): 19–26.

34. D. Austin, "The Psycholophysiological Effects of Music Therapy in Intensive Care Units," *Pediatric Nursing* 22, no. 3 (April 2010).

35. M. Mrázová and P. Celec, "A Systematic Review of Randomized Controlled Trials Using Music Therapy for Children," *Journal of Alternative and Complementary Medicine* 16, no. 10 (October 2010): 1089–1095.

36. Q. M. Leow, V. B. Drury, and W. Poon, "Experience of Terminally Ill Patients with Music Therapy: A Literature Review," *Singapore Nursing Journal* 37, no. 3 (July 2010): 48–52.

37. N. Daykin, S. McClean, and L. Bunt, "Creativity, Identity and Healing: Participants' Accounts of Music Therapy in Cancer Care," *Health: An Interdisciplinary Journal for the Social Study of Health, Illness & Medicine* 11, no. 3 (July 2007): 349–370.

38. R. McCaffrey, "Music Listening: Its Effects in Creating a Healing Environment," *Journal of Psychosocial Nursing and Mental Health Services* 46, no. 10 (December 2008): 39–44.

39. C. O'Callaghan, M. Sexton, and G. Wheeler, "Music Therapy as a Non-pharmacological Anxiolytic for Paediatric Radiotherapy Patients," *Australasian Radiology* 51, no. 2 (April 2007): 159–162.

Journal of Clinical Nursing 20, no. 7 (April 2011): 988 999.

40. MusiCure Music as Medicine, homepage. http ://www.musicure.com/.

41. S. Spies Ingersoll and A. Schaper, "Therapeutic Music Pilot in the Context of Human Caring Theory," in *Measuring Caring: International Research on Caritas as Healing,* ed. J. Nelson and J. Watson (New York: Spring Publishing, 2011).

42. J. F. Quinn et al., "Research Guidelines for Assessing the Impact of the Healing Relationship in Clinical Nursing," *Alternative Therapies in Health and Medicine* 9, no. 3 (May 2, 2003): A65–79.

43. G. Cervellin and G. Lippi, "From Music-Beat to Heart-Beat: A Journey in the Complex Interactions Between Music, Brain and Heart," *European Journal of Internal Medicine* 22, no. 4 (2011):371–374.

44. M. Suda et al., "Emotional Responses to Music: Toward Scientific Perspectives on Music Therapy," *Brain Imaging* 19, no. 1 (2008): 75–78.

45. V. N. Salimpoor et al., "Anatomically Distinct Dopamine Release During Anticipation and Experience of Peak Emotion to Music," *Nature Neuroscience* 14, no. 2 (February 2011): 257–262.

46. U. Nilsson, "Soothing Music Can Increase Oxytocin Levels During Bed Rest After Open-Heart Surgery: A Randomised Control Trial," *Journal of Clinical Nursing* 18, no. 15 (2009): 2153–2161.

47. M. H. Whitaker, "Controlling Pain. Sounds Soothing: Music Therapy for Postoperative Pain," *Nursing* 40, no. 12 (December 2010): 53–54.

48. D. J. Levitin and A. K. Tirovolas, "Current Advances in the Cognitive Neuroscience of Music," *Annals of the New York Academy of Sciences* 1156 (March 2009): 211–231.

49. P. G. Hunter, E. G. Schellenberg, and U. Schimmack, "Feelings and Perceptions of Happiness and Sadness Induced by Music: Similarities, Differences, and Mixed Emotions," *Psychology of Aesthetics, Creativity, and the Arts* 4, no. 1 (2010): 47–56.

50. J. W. Jeong et al., "Congruence of Happy and Sad Emotion in Music and Faces Modifies Cortical Audiovisual Activation," *NeuroImage* 54, no. 4 (February 14, 2011): 2973–2982.

51. D. L. Morris, "Music Therapy," in *Holistic Nursing: A Handbook for Practice,* 5th ed., ed. D. M. Dossey and L. Keegan (Sudbury, MA: Jones & Bartlett, 2009).

52. K. Sand-Jecklin and H. Emerson, "The Impact of a Live Therapeutic Music Intervention on Patients' Experience of Pain, Anxiety, and Muscle Tension," *Holistic Nursing Practice* 24, no. 1 (2010): 7–15.

53. Bodhisattva, "Tibetan Singing Bowl History." http://www.bodhisattva.com/singing_bowl_history.htm.

54. M. H. Thaut, "Neurologic Music Therapy in Cognitive Rehabilitation," *Music Perception: An Interdisciplinary Journal* 27, no. 4 (2010): 281–285.

55. C. J. Murrock and P. A. Higgins, "The Theory of Music, Mood and Movement to Improve Health Outcomes," *Journal of Advanced Nursing* 65, no. 10 (December 2009): 2249–2257.

56. J. Watson, *Nursing: The Philosophy and Science of Caring,* rev. ed. (Boulder, CO: University Press of Colorado, 2008).

57. J. Watson, "Caring Theory as an Ethical Guide to Administrative and Clinical Practices," *Nursing Administration Quarterly* 30, no. 1 (January 2006): 48–55.

58. T. R. Stein et al., "A Pilot Study to Assess the Effects of a Guided Imagery Audiotape Intervention on Psychological Outcomes in Patients Undergoing Coronary Artery Bypass Graft Surgery," *Holistic Nursing Practice* 24, no. 4 (2010): 213–222.

59. "The Joanna Briggs Institute Best Practice Information Sheet: Music as an Intervention in Hospitals," *Nursing and Health Sciences* 13, no. 1 (March 2011): 99–102.

60. J. E. Vennard, *The Way of Prayer: Companions in Christ* (Nashville, TN: Upper Room Books, 2007).

61. S. L. Robb, J. S. Carpenter, and D. S. Burns, "Reporting Guidelines for Music-Based Interventions," *Journal of Health Psychology* 16, no. 2 (March 2011): 342–352.

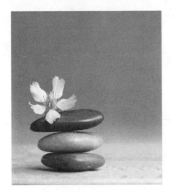

Chapter 19

Touch and Hand-Mediated Therapies

Christina Jackson and Corinne Latini

Nurse Healer
OBJECTIVES

Theoretical

- Describe various types of touch therapies.
- Compare and contrast the various touch therapies.
- Articulate physiologic changes that can result from touch therapies.
- Describe psychoemotional changes that can result from touch therapies.

Clinical

- Develop your abilities to become calm and focused before you use touch therapies in your practice.
- Experiment with soothing music, guided imagery, and aromatherapy as adjuncts to the touch session.
- Observe subjective and objective changes in the client experiencing a touch therapy session.

Personal

- Examine the significance of touch in your personal and professional relationships.
- Notice whether there are any changes in your emotions and sense of well-being during or after you use touch therapy.
- Create opportunities to practice touch therapies in your clinical practice.

DEFINITIONS

Acupressure (Shiatsu): The application of finger and/or thumb pressure to specific sites along the body's energy meridians for the purpose of relieving tension, reestablishing the flow of energy along the meridian lines, and restoring balance to the human energy system.

Body therapy and/or touch therapy: The broad range of techniques that a practitioner uses in which the hands are on or near the body to assist the recipient toward optimal function.

Centering: A calm and focused sense of self-relatedness that can be thought of as a place of inner being, a place of quietude within oneself where one feels integrated and focused.

Chakra or energy center: Specific center of consciousness in the human energy system that allows for the inflow and directing of energy from outside, as well as for outflow from the individual's energy field. There are seven major energy centers in relation to the spine and many minor centers at bone articulations in the palms of the hands and the soles of the feet.

Energy meridian: An energy circuit or line of force. Eastern theories describe meridian lines flowing vertically through the body, culminating at points on the feet, hands, and ears.

Foot reflexology: The application of pressure to points on the feet thought to correspond to other structures and organs throughout the body. Access to the entire nervous system is accomplished through the proprioceptive network of the feet.

Grounding: The process of connecting to the Earth and the Earth's energy field, to calm the mind and focus one's inner flow of energy as a means to enhance healing endeavors.

Healing Touch: A specific system of techniques that make use of the human energy system for healing.

Human energy system: The entire interactive, dynamic system of human subtle energies, consisting of the energy centers, the multidimensional field, the meridians, and acupuncture points.

Intention: The motivation or reason for touching; the direction of one's inner awareness and focus for healing.

M Technique: A registered method of gentle, structured touch suitable for the very fragile or actively dying, or when the giver is not trained in massage. Simple to learn, the M Technique is profoundly relaxing to both the giver and receiver. Essential oils are used in specific ways with this technique.

Procedural touch: Touch performed to diagnose, monitor, or treat an illness; touch that focuses on the end result of curing the illness or preventing further complications.

Reiki: A form of energy healing in which the practitioner uses light touch through a series of hand positions over chakras to channel energy. *Reiki* means "universal life force energy" and is composed of two Japanese words, *rei* meaning universal and *ki* meaning life force.

Therapeutic massage: The use of the hands to apply pressure and motion to the recipient's skin and underlying muscle to promote physical and psychological relaxation, improve circulation, relieve sore muscles, and accomplish other therapeutic effects.

Therapeutic touch: A specific technique of centering intention while the practitioner moves the hands through a recipient's energy field for the purpose of assessing and treating energy field imbalance.

■ THEORY AND RESEARCH

Touch is unique among all the senses in that although we can see or hear without being seen or heard ourselves, we cannot touch another without being touched ourselves. A profound exchange occurs whenever we touch, and the power of this exchange cannot be underestimated. By respecting this potential, we can better learn to use touch to promote healing in others and ourselves.

Touch in Ancient Times

Healing through touch is as old as civilization itself. Practiced extensively in all cultures, this ancient treatment is instinctive—it feels natural to rub or hold any part of one's body that hurts and to do so for others. The ancient Egyptians used bandages, poultices, touch, and manipulation. Inside the Pyramids, illustrations thousands of years old show representations of one person holding hands near another, with waves of energy depicted moving from the hands of the healer to the body nearby. The oldest written documentation of the use of body touch to enhance healing comes from Asia. The *Huang Ti Nei Ching* is a classic work of internal medicine that was written 5,000 years ago. The *Nei Ching*, a 3,000- to 4,000-year-old Chinese book of health and medicine, records a system of touch based on acupuncture points and energy circuits. The ancient Indian Vedas also described healing massage, as did the Polynesian Lomi practice and the traditions of Native Americans.

During the height of classical Greek civilization, Hippocrates wrote of the therapeutic effects of massage and manipulation; he also gave instructions for carrying out these practices. He wrote during the time of the great Aesculapian healing centers, at which many whole-body therapies included touch. Touch therapies were also employed at the healing centers to assist individuals who wished to make the transition to a higher level of functioning. Massage was used as a mode of preparation for dream work, which was a significant part of therapy in the healing rites. The Roman historian Plutarch wrote that Julius Caesar was treated for epilepsy by being pinched over his entire body every day.

Biblical accounts of the healings performed by Jesus of Nazareth frequently include the use of touch in the form of laying hands on the body. In two New Testament passages (using the new revised standard version [NRSV]), the human energy field is described. In Mark 5:25–34, a woman who had been bleeding for 12 years touched the back hem of Jesus' garment with an inner sense of knowing that this would heal her. Jesus felt that "power had gone forth from him" and turned around quickly, asking who had touched his clothing. Luke 6:18–19 tells of a crowd that had come to be healed of their diseases and demons through Jesus' touch, for "power came out from him and healed all of them."

Both shamans and traditional practitioners used touch widely until the rise of the Puritan culture during the 1600s, including the shift from primitive healing practices to modern scientific medicine. Puritan culture equated touch with sex, which was associated with original sin. During the late nineteenth and early twentieth centuries, health care moved away from anything associated with superstition and primitive healing and was directed toward scientific medicine. All unnecessary touch was discouraged because of the association of touch with primitive healing, and because of the prevailing Puritan ethic. Consequently, touch as a therapeutic intervention remained undeveloped in U.S. health care until research into its benefits began in the 1950s.

Cultural Variations

The fact that many cultures, both ancient and modern, have developed some form of touch therapy indicates that rubbing, pressing, massaging, and holding are natural manifestations of the desire to heal and care for one another. However, attitudes toward touch vary among cultures. One society may view touch as necessary, whereas another may view it as forbidden. The nurse must be aware of personal and cultural views and reactions to touch in addition to particular gender prohibitions within cultures.

Philosophic and cultural differences have influenced the development of touch in various areas of the world. The Eastern worldview is founded on energy, whereas the Western worldview is based on reductionism of matter. This basic cultural difference has led to the evolution of widely differing approaches to touch. The Eastern worldview holds that qi (or chi), also described as energy or vital force, is the center of body function. A meridian is an energy circuit or line of force that runs vertically through the body. Magnetic or bioelectrical patterns flow through the microcosm of the body in the same way that magnetic patterns flow through the planet and the universe. Meridian lines and zones are influenced by pressure placed on points along those lines.

Expert practitioners in acupuncture and acupressure purport to send healing energy to the recipient via an energy flow that moves through the body and out through their hands. In contrast, the Western worldview holds that it is the physical effect of cellular changes occurring during touch that influences healing. For example, massage stimulates the cells and aids in waste discharge, promotes the dilation of the vascular system, and encourages lymphatic drainage.[1] Swedish and therapeutic massage techniques were developed to produce these physical changes.

A blending of Eastern and Western techniques has resulted in an explosion of new and widely practiced modalities. The modern-day renaissance in body therapies is probably a healthy response to the fast-paced technologic revolution that has swept Western culture, bringing back a sense of balance and caring.

Modern Concepts of Touch

Evidence is mounting that supports what healers have intuitively known—touch is a vital aspect of human health and well-being. Some of the first studies documenting the significance of touch involved infant monkeys and surrogate mothers.[2] In the 1950s, Harlow caged one group of infant monkeys with a monkey-shaped wire form that served as a surrogate mother, and a second group with a soft cloth mother surrogate. When frightened, the monkeys housed with the wire form reacted by running and cowering in a corner. The other group reacted to the same stimuli by running and clinging to the soft cloth surrogate for protection. These infant monkeys even preferred clinging to an unheated cloth surrogate mother to sitting on a warm heating pad. Although the cloth surrogate was unresponsive, the offspring raised with it developed basically normal behavior. This and other classic studies conclusively documented the significance of touch in normal animal growth and development.

Studies of human development soon followed. A study examining abandoned infants and infants whose mothers were in prison found that infants whom the nurses held and cuddled thrived, whereas those who were left alone became ill and died.[3] These studies led to the development of the concept of touch deprivation.

These early studies in the 1950s and 1960s awakened scientific interest in the phenomenon of healing touch. Bernard Grad, a biochemist at McGill University, was one of the first to investigate healing by the laying on of hands. He conducted a series of double-blind experiments with the renowned healer Oskar Estebany.[4] In these studies, wounded mice and damaged barley seeds were separated into control and experimental groups. After Estebany used therapeutic touch to manipulate the energy fields of the mice and seeds in the experimental groups, these groups demonstrated a significantly accelerated healing rate in comparison to the control groups. In a subsequent study, an enzymologist worked with Grad using the enzyme trypsin in double-blind studies.[5] After the trypsin was exposed to Estebany's treatments, its activity was significantly increased.

Within the past two decades there has been a renaissance in the use of touch as a therapeutic practice. A proliferation of research publications, books, continuing education offerings, and web resources document the effectiveness of these practices. Both the American Nurses Association and the National League for Nursing endorse the use of biofield and touch therapies. The North American Nursing Diagnosis Association includes the diagnosis *Disturbed Energy Field*, defined as a disruption of energy flow surrounding a person that disrupts harmony of body, mind, and/or spirit. Many healers who use biofield therapies claim that they either direct or channel energy to the recipient. Others say that energy will go where it is needed. Nurses are using hand-mediated therapies with increasing frequency as they seek ways to help or heal those for whom they care.

Touching Styles

Data collected through in-depth interviews with eight experienced intensive care nurses reveal two substantive processes—the touching process itself and the acquisition of a touching style—neither of which had been previously reported in the literature. The touching process is more than skin-to-skin contact; it involves entering the patient's space, connecting, talking, following nonverbal cues, and eventually touching. Nurses learn about touch from their culture, family, street knowledge, personal experience, and nursing school. The phenomenon of the healer's touch has been researched and there are distinct characteristics that emerged. Touch is gestural, impactful, and reciprocal. This is inclusive of the fact that the practitioner will also experience these three responses. Emotions, past experiences, and receptivity to healing can emerge from the touch experience. As the practitioner touches the client, relaxation of the muscles may be felt and a change in the breathing pattern may be observed. An openness for the healing power of touch is necessary between the patient and the client, which constitutes the "I–Thou relationship."[6]

There is power demonstrated through the use of touch and it is important for nurses to be mindful of this when using touch techniques. In Gueguen and Vion's study, touch was used to emphasize and anchor a particular message regarding the taking of antibiotics. Those clients who were touched by the general practitioners while instructions were given had significantly higher compliance rates. This underscores the risk for touch to become coercive or to facilitate hierarchical relationships. Our intention as practitioners should always be examined and touch should be offered with the best of intention for our patients/clients.[7]

Body–Mind Communication

Touch is perhaps one of the most frequently used and yet least acknowledged of the five recognized senses. It is the first sense to develop in the human embryo and the one most vital to survival. Touch can vary from subtle fleeting brush strokes to violent physical attacks. Touch evokes the full range of emotions from hatred to the most intimate love. Figurative references to touch in our daily language such as "That speech really touched me," or "This conversation helped me get in touch with my feelings" attest to its deep importance and value to us. As the largest and most ancient sense organ of the body, the skin enables us to experience and learn about the environment. We use touch to help us perceive the external world.

A piece of skin the size of a quarter contains more than 3 million cells, 12 feet of nerves, 100 sweat glands, 50 nerve endings, and 3 feet of blood vessels. There are estimated to be approximately 50 receptors per 100 square centimeters—a total of 900,000 sensory receptors over the human body.[8] Viewed from this perspective, the skin is a giant communication system that, through the sense of touch, brings messages from the external environment to the attention of the internal bodymindspirit.

Because health care is increasingly delivered in complicated technologic settings, nurses are concerned with ensuring that the human, spiritual, and social needs of patients are not overlooked. This is particularly valuable when working with the geriatric population, an often touch-deprived group. Yet nurses must take into account social contexts and cultural differences before engaging in efforts to provide touch therapy. In addition, it is important to remember that for many an experience of unwanted touch in the form of physical and/or sexual abuse may have occurred, leaving lasting fears related to receiving and giving touch. Nurses must respect and be vigilant about their own boundaries as well as their clients' as related to touch. A nurse should never assume that a client will find touch comforting and should always ask before touching. If the suggestion evokes no response or a wary expression, the nurse may try a tentative touch and observe the client's response carefully. To be truly effective, touch must be given authentically by a warm, genuine, caring individual to another who is willing to receive it. Unwelcome, uncaring, or boundary-violating touch is likely more upsetting than none at all.

Like any other nursing intervention, hugging and touching demand careful assessment. Nurses need to recognize their own feelings, as well as consider the client's age, sex, and ethnic background. A few key questions (e.g., "Would a back massage help you relax?" or "Would it help if I held your hand?") can help the client clarify his or her own beliefs, values, and desires regarding different types, locations, and intensities of touch.

There are many variations in and names for the touch therapies available for use as nursing interventions. Some are basic human contacts, such as hand holding and hugging. Holding hands with patients who have dementia has been noted as a form of communication by volunteers in a nursing home. This form of touch can be more profound than words for clients with moderate to advanced stages of Alzheimer's disease.[9] However, some clients react strongly to touch, especially if they have been exposed to inappropriate or uncomfortable touch at other times. The touch therapies described here are used by holistic practitioners who often advocate and teach healthy lifestyle behavior patterns to their clients to augment well-being during the course of the touch therapy treatments. The addition of guided imagery and/or music before and during treatment may heighten the relaxation response elicited during touch therapies. The type of setting—acute care, long-term care, home care, rehabilitation center, or wellness center—also affects the focus and length of the treatment.

■ OVERVIEW OF SELECTED TOUCH INTERVENTIONS AND TECHNIQUES

Although touch therapy is as old as civilization, documentation of how and why it works is relatively new in the nursing, medical, and allied health literature. In addition, many special approaches to working with the body and energy field are emerging. The following overview addresses the techniques most frequently encountered and practiced by nurses, including current research findings when available. Touch therapies can be classified into several categories: somatic and musculoskeletal therapies; Eastern, meridian-based, and point therapies; energy-based therapies; emotional bodywork; manipulative therapies; and other holistic touch therapies.

Except for therapeutic touch, Healing Touch, and Reiki, most body therapies involve actual physical contact. The contact usually consists of the practitioner's touching, pushing, kneading, or rubbing the recipient's skin and the underlying fascia. Each of the therapies has an explanatory theory, body of knowledge, history, and techniques. Some techniques are derived from other methods and represent a synthesis of these approaches. Some methods require special licensure or certification, and others can be incorporated into a nurse's practice after minimal instruction via audiovisual media, conference, or classroom presentation.

Somatic and Musculoskeletal Therapies

The category of somatic and musculoskeletal therapies encompasses the generic work known as therapeutic massage. As a nursing intervention, therapeutic massage is effective in stimulating circulation of blood and lymph, dispersing nutrients, removing metabolic wastes, and enhancing relaxation. Several basic strokes are involved, including long smooth strokes (i.e., effleurage), kneading motions (i.e., petrissage), vibration, compression, and tapping (i.e., tapotement). Although they may be called by different names (e.g., Swedish massage, medical massage), many of the techniques of therapeutic massage are similar. Varying degrees of pressure and various types of oils or creams can be used, depending on client preference and the intention for the treatment. Therapeutic massage has also been referred to as "soft massage" and has been associated with helping the recipient reestablish balance and as a means to draw attention away from suffering. [10]

Nurses have routinely performed therapeutic massage primarily on the backs and sometimes on the hands and feet of their clients. Back care is not new; for decades, it has been incorporated into the standard bathing and evening care routine of most hospitals. Because of time constraints and traditional neglect of the body therapies in institutions, these patients receive only a portion of the complete range of touch therapies.

Learning full-body massage greatly augments and expands the nurse's basic knowledge of massage techniques. Most practitioners learn these techniques in continuing education classes, but books on massage that illustrate the techniques are also available. Myriad styles of bodywork literally offer something for everyone. To use these specific techniques, the nurse must take special courses, which often grant a certificate of completion. Massage licensure laws vary from state to state; some states require that even registered nurses take an additional course to become certified prior to practicing massage therapy.

Because no two clients, either within or outside the institutional setting, have the same needs, the nurse must become skilled at adapting the therapy to the setting and the time available. Massage techniques that can be performed quickly—massage for the hands, feet, or neck and shoulders—may have beneficial results in short time periods. In randomized, controlled trials, acute care hospital nurses were assigned to either a group that received a weekly 15-minute back massage, or to a no-intervention control group. Data collected throughout the 5-week protocol included physiologic as well as psychological measures of stress. Urinary cortisol and blood pressure were measured at weeks 1, 3, and 5, and the State-Trait Anxiety Inventory (STAI) was administered at weeks 1 and 5. Although differences in the physiologic measures between groups did not reach statistical significance, the STAI scores of the experimental group decreased significantly, while the control group's STAI scores increased. It was concluded that massage therapy can be a beneficial tool for reducing psychological stress levels in nurses. [11]

Evidence supports the use of somatic and musculoskeletal therapies to enhance mood, cardiac health, immune function, pain relief, and treatment of clients with cancer. Over the last 20 years, evidence supports the use of massage therapies to relieve chronic lower back pain, cancer pain, and migraine headache; enhance natural killer cell function; and help relieve depression and anxiety. [12]

In a study involving 150 massage clients, it was found that the type of massage technique, length of session, and degree of pressure affected blood pressure (BP). In particular, Swedish massage was correlated with the greatest reduction in BP, while potentially painful styles of massage such as trigger point therapy and sport massage were associated with elevations in BP. [13] Another study involving 151 clients with advanced cancer emphasized the effectiveness of massage therapy in palliative care. Outcomes included improved lymph drainage, increased relaxation, and improved attitude by the recipients toward touch. Many of the clients had previously associated touch with negative experiences such as needle sticks and invasive exams. [14]

Thirty-nine women with breast cancer undergoing chemotherapy, recruited from an oncology clinic in Sweden, were randomly assigned to either a massage group or a no-massage control group.

Both groups were seen for 20 minutes on five different occasions, and measures of nausea and anxiety were recorded on a visual analogue scale before and after each visit. They also completed the hospital anxiety and depression scale with each visit. Although the differences in anxiety and depression between the groups did not reach statistical significance in this study, the experimental group reported significant reductions in nausea when compared to the control group.[15]

Sixty-eight adults with osteoarthritis of the knee were assigned to either a treatment group (Swedish massage twice weekly for 4 weeks followed by 4 weeks of one session a week) or to a control group (no massage). The results showed significant improvement in the massaged group in the areas of pain, stiffness, range of motion, and physical function domains when compared with the control group.[16]

Massage is frequently combined with other therapies to amplify therapeutic benefit. Aromatherapy is frequently used in conjunction with massage through the use of essential oils, scented creams, and fragrant candles. The M Technique is an example of this. (See Chapter 25.) In a multicenter, randomized, controlled trial involving four cancer centers and a hospice, 288 cancer patients were randomly assigned to either a course of aromatherapy massage or to standard care. Patients who received aromatherapy massage reported significant improvement in clinical depression and/or anxiety 6 weeks into the trial when compared with control group participants. However, this effect was not as significant at 10 weeks into the trial. Interestingly, the patients receiving aromatherapy massage described greater improvements in anxiety at both the 6- and 10-week markers.[17]

Infants and children can benefit from massage therapy, and researchers are examining its use for this population. In a meta-analysis of literature examining potential benefits of massage for children with cystic fibrosis (CF), researchers hypothesized that this modality could provide relaxation, pain relief, decreased anxiety, improved mood and sleep, and enhanced pulmonary function. This information was based on known physiologic effects of massage, related research, and subjective reports of many youth with CF who were known to the researchers. These hospitalized youth received massage

from an RN who was also licensed as a massage therapist. The youth routinely reported that massage made them feel more comfortable, more relaxed, and able to move more freely.[18] The meta-analysis reveals that more research is needed to support the use of massage therapy from an evidence standpoint. In other words, these researchers conclude that the risks of negative side effects are small, and based on the subjective reports of the children with CF, the massage therapy will continue, but the research evidence is not yet in place. This illustrates the conundrum that pervades many complementary nursing modalities—their effects cannot always be measured in the same ways as, for example, pharmacologic agents. (See Chapter 34.)

So, although participants may not demonstrate pain reduction or other specific symptom reduction after receiving massage, they may actually have a greater sense of well-being. However, if well-being is not measured, a modality can be dismissed as having no significant, measurable, therapeutic benefit. Whenever pain reduction is desired, all of the factors that influence resistance to pain are important in the overall subjective experience for the client. Thus, improvement in well-being is a significant part of pain reduction because the overall degree of suffering is lessened.

The immune status of young, HIV-positive Dominican children improved as a result of massage therapy twice a week. Eligible children who had no access to antiviral drugs were assigned to the massage treatment group or to a "friendly-visit" control group. Blood was drawn at the beginning of the study and at the end of the 3-month intervention. Despite similar baseline immune parameters, the children receiving massage therapy had significant improvements in CD4 and CD8 cell counts as well as CD41CD251 cells, and an increase in natural killer cells, particularly in the younger children.[19]

Infants in Ecuador, recruited from two orphanages, received massage therapy and demonstrated statistically significant differences in incidence of diarrhea. The massaged infants had 50% less risk of diarrhea than their nonmassaged control group counterparts.[20] In another study, 50 low-birth-weight (LBW) babies were cross-matched, controlled, and assigned to a massage group or a nonmassaged group. The massage consisted of gentle rubbing, stroking, and passive movements of the limbs. The intervention lasted for 6 months. The findings suggest that infants receiving massage had better quality of sleep with greater daytime alertness than control group infants did.[21]

In another study involving infants, 68 preterm babies were randomly assigned to either moderate or light pressure massage therapy, and each received 15-minute massages three times per day for 5 days. The moderate versus light pressure massage group gained significantly more weight per day. In addition, they demonstrated greater relaxation and reduced arousability, both of which may have contributed to the significant increase in weight gain.[22]

Infants in neonatal intensive care units are subject to a highly stressful environment with continuous, high-intensity noise and bright light, as well as to a lack of the tactile stimulation that they would otherwise experience in the womb or in general mothering care. As massage seems to both decrease stress and provide tactile stimulation, it has been recommended as an intervention to promote growth and development of preterm and low-birth-weight infants. However, concerns about the method quality of many studies, particularly with respect to selective reporting of outcomes, weaken credibility of findings pertaining to developmental outcomes.

Mary Ann Finch, a one-time seminary professor, is dedicated to "touching the untouchable." The Care Through Touch Institute, which she founded 25 years ago, offers homeless clients massage therapy. In the dangerous neighborhoods of San Francisco she and her team of massage therapy interns, staffers, and volunteers provide foot, neck, and shoulder massages to those who would otherwise not receive any type of touch. Her work has provided the homeless with a sense of being cared for that has had a profound effect on many of their lives.[23]

In general, massage has been shown to be a safe and comforting way for parents and grandparents to connect with their infant or child. The parents of children with chronic pain or other conditions may feel helpless watching their child wander through myriad interventions. Massage can benefit the parents by giving them a therapeutic role and reducing their anxiety. While offering the reciprocal act of touch to their child, they too feel the effects of being touched. This facilitates a shift in the direction of healing for all concerned.

Eastern, Meridian-Based, and Point Therapies

The category of Eastern, meridian-based, and point therapies include modalities that are derived from an Eastern medical approach that is very different from that in our Western training and education. Interested nurses must study these methods in a program that teaches about fields that emanate from our bodies, meridians, pressure points, reflex points, imbalances in the energy system, and Eastern healing philosophy. New programs and modalities are being created regularly in this rapidly growing field of energy-based interventions. Several instruments have been used to measure the human energy field, including Kirlian photography and the superconducting quantum interference device. Some of the better-known and well-studied healing methods used by nurses include therapeutic touch, Healing Touch, Reiki, acupressure, and reflexology. These modalities are described in more detail.

Energetic touch therapies typically involve four phases:

1. Centering oneself physically and psychologically; that is, finding within oneself an inner reference of calm focus
2. Exercising the natural sensitivity of the hand to assess the energy field and/or chakras of the client for clues to understand the quality and balance of energy flow
3. Use the hands and intention to mobilize areas in the client's energy field that appear to be nonflowing (e.g., sluggish, congested, or static), smooth and harmonize areas that seem perturbed, or work with balance and flow within chakras and along meridians
4. Allowing energy flow and exchange to assist the client to repattern and balance his or her energies; some modalities emphasize directing energy, others view the practitioner as a conduit to channel energy, and many practitioners state that energy will move and go where it is needed

The energetic healing process should be halted when there are no longer any differences in body symmetry relative to density or temperature variation, or when balance is perceived. Four commonly observed responses are (1) flushed skin, (2) deep sighs, (3) physical relaxation, and (4) verbalized relaxation. A caution when using these therapies is to limit the amount of time spent and/or energy spent in working with the very young, the old, and the infirm. When the client's energy field is full, the energy pushes the nurse away. Nurses can monitor clients for physical and emotional responses throughout the session and be supportive of the client.

Healing modalities that involve touching with the conscious intent to help or heal, therapeutic touch (TT), Healing Touch (HT), and Reiki, decrease anxiety, relieve pain, and facilitate the healing process. Most of the energy-based touch therapies have certain common tenets, although the methods for applying them can vary. Nurses are becoming increasingly involved in the use of energy-based modalities for reducing anxiety and pain, inspiring balance, and bringing the body–mind connection into focus. They can be used in any type of environment, and interest in using these low-tech interventions in high-tech environments such as critical care is growing.[24] Over the past three decades, Krieger, Hover-Kramer, Quinn, and others have documented the importance of therapeutic touch.[25-28]

Therapeutic Touch

Therapeutic touch can be learned by anyone, and there are no certifications offered as the founders hoped that everyone would learn and practice this modality. It is taught at beginning, intermediate, and advanced levels in continuing education programs (visit www.therapeutic-touch.org and www.therapeutictouch.com for more information). A recent study examining the effects of TT on hemoglobin (Hgb) and hematocrit (Hct) levels in basically healthy but anemic women (test groups of 92 women) found that both TT and sham (mimic of the action but without the intention) TT groups exhibited significant increases in Hgb and Hct, whereas the control group receiving no treatment had no changes in Hgb or Hct.[29] This highlights another difficulty in researching these modalities—it is often difficult to construct control conditions that will not, in themselves, produce a therapeutic effect.

In a descriptive study examining the effects of TT on adult tension headache pain, 10 sufferers were randomly assigned to control and experimental groups. Data were collected through interviews, and results suggest that one session of TT was useful in reducing headache pain in all subjects receiving TT.[30]

Healing Touch

Healing Touch involves working with the energy fields (auras) as well as with energy centers (chakras). Janet Mentgen, founder of Healing Touch, believed that anyone can learn to facilitate healing if they have a compassionate heart and a desire to help others. During an HT session, the practitioner moves his or her hands over the client to assess for disturbances in the energy field. Treatment can be done by holding the hands just above the body or by applying gentle touch to parts of the body to clear and balance the energy. The premise is that by restoring balance, the human energy system will promote healing for the mind, body, and spirit.[31]

Healing Touch is also taught in levels and offers a certificate of completion at each stage with eventual certification upon completing level 5. Level 6 is the instructor level for those who would like to teach HT. Formal training and certification are available through the Healing Touch Program. (Visit www.healingtouch program.com for curriculum and class information, www.healingtouch.net for more information, and www.healingtouchinternational.org for research findings. The Healing Touch Program curriculum is endorsed by the American Nurses Credentialing Center [ANCC] and American Holistic Nurses Association [AHNA] for continuing education credits.)

A mixed method study (test groups of 12 people) assessed the role of HT in modulating chronic neuropathic pain and associated psychological stress after a spinal cord injury. The participants were assigned to either HT or guided progressive relaxation (control group) for six weekly home visits. The HT group showed a reduction in pain, fatigue, and confusion and increased well-being when compared to the control group.[32] In a response to this study published in the same journal, the lack of concrete measures for many of the phenomena (such as the "quality of participants' energy fields") and the use of scientific terminology to mask "pseudoscience" were cited as serious concerns and cause for interpreting results with great caution.[33] An editorial written in this same issue illuminates the conundrum researchers face when designing methods for investigating these modalities and is important reading for all who are interested in complementary and integrative therapies.[34]

A pilot study investigating the effects of HT on patients with dementia used the Cohen-Mansfield Agitation Inventory to measure agitation before and after HT. Those who received HT were significantly less agitated, and the researchers recommend further investigation with larger groups.[35]

Promising results of a pilot study of children (*n* = 9) who were diagnosed with acute lymphoblastic leukemia and were pediatric clinic oncology outpatients showed a significant decrease in stress and heart rate variability (HRV) when HT was compared with rest. Patients completed visual analogue scales (VAS) for relaxation, vitality, overall well-being, anxiety, and depression before and after a 20-minute rest period and an HT treatment. The HT treatment was significantly more effective than the rest period at decreasing stress, with lowered stress and changes in HRV demonstrated. The researchers note that although the sample size was small, it is possible to complete a HT study in the pediatric population. More research is needed as to how HT can be added to outpatient pediatric oncology clinic care as a supportive therapy.[36]

Healing Touch has also been implemented as a complementary modality for pediatric patients and their families at Nemours/AI duPont Hospital for Children in Wilmington, Delaware. The facility supports and encourages the use of some complementary therapies and has a special room where Healing Touch practitioners can offer patients HT therapy. Families are also taught how to perform Healing Touch on their loved ones (www.nemours.org/service/medical/cancer/nchaidhc.html). Nemours/AI duPont Hospital for Children also is sensitive to the needs of its staff and offers a Day of Caring during Nurses Week to minister to the mind, body, and spirit. Healing Touch sessions, chair massages, healthy snacks, and peaceful music give attendees an opportunity for self-care during breaktimes. Recognizing the need for self-care is an important part of practice.

Reiki

Reiki, another energy/biofield modality, also involves training and levels of certification (visit www.reiki.org and www.reikialliance.com for more information). The term *Reiki* (universal life force energy) is derived from the Japanese words *rei* meaning universal and *ki* meaning life force. Originating more than 3,000 years ago and practiced in Tibet, it was rediscovered in the late 1900s in Japan by Dr. Mikao Usui. The practitioner uses various hand positions to facilitate the flow of life force energy.

Healing can be at any level and the premise is for the practitioner to come into intention with the client and have the energy flow to the client's greatest area of need. Reiki may be used alone or in conjunction with nursing and medical interventions. Research has been done on the results of using Reiki and it has been reported to produce a decrease in pain, alleviation of anxiety, and a reduction in depression. Improved well-being in the mind, body, and spirit has been reported by many who have experienced Reiki therapy.[37] Reiki gives power and control for healing to the receiver. The intention for healing is set by the practitioner and the client, and through the relaxation response, healing is encouraged at all levels within the body.[38]

In a study of 25 community-dwelling older adults, using an experimental design, Reiki was found to provide relaxation with the effects lasting longer after the second session. Sessions were 45 minutes, which included 30-minute Reiki treatments, 1 day a week for 8 weeks. Participants also reported decreased back spasms, decreased shoulder and neck pain, and improved sleep patterns. The authors of the study also found that there was potential for Reiki to be used as a coping resource for older adults.[39]

A pilot study was conducted using a triangulated methodology aimed to determine if level 1 Reiki training would affect the caring perceptions of healthcare providers. The data demonstrate positive changes in participants' caring behaviors. Twelve nurses were interviewed and asked to complete caring efficacy scales (CES) pre- and post-Reiki training. The nurses described heightened levels of spirituality and greater attention to self-care, healing presence with clients, and increased personal awareness.

Neither the actual CES nor reliability and validity data were included for evaluation.[40] In a related study, TT and HT were taught to medical students to see if such content would cultivate compassion in these students. Students reported significant improvements in confidence, practice, feelings and practice of compassion, and sense of personal achievement after taking the course. In addition, they felt more optimistic about future practice. One medical student stated, "I am confident in being calm, peaceful, and focused (centered) before and during patient encounters."[41]

A quasi-experimental pilot study compared reports of pain and anxiety in two groups of women after abdominal hysterectomy. The experimental group (test group of 10 women) received three 30-minute sessions of Reiki and the control group (test group of 12) received traditional nursing care. Pain at 24 hours postsurgery was significantly less for the Reiki group, yet was not significantly less at 48 and 72 hours postsurgery. Use of medication and anxiety levels were significantly less in the Reiki group.[42]

Continued research and studies carefully documenting the therapeutic effects of Reiki are important to validate its usefulness. In 2009, vanderVaart, Gijsen, de Wildt, and Koren completed a systematic review of the literature on studies that had been published up to December 2008. Their review resulted in the conclusion that although many Reiki studies have been done, there are "serious methodological and reporting limitations which preclude a definitive conclusion on its effectiveness."[43]

Energy Field Disturbance

In the 1995–1996 *Nursing Diagnoses: Definitions and Classification*, by the North American Nursing Diagnosis Association, the definition of energy field disturbance made its entry into the world of professional nursing. Energy field disturbance is defined as

> a disruption of the flow of energy surrounding a person's being which results in a dis-harmony of the body, mind, and/or spirit. Defining characteristics include temperature changes (warmth/coolness); visual changes (image/color); disruption of the field (vacant/hold/

spike/bulge); movement (wave/spike/tingling/dense/flowing); and sounds (tonewords).[44]

Nursing Intervention Classifications

In addition to including a new nursing diagnosis related to energy healing, the nursing interventions classification, which lists therapeutic touch, also specifies simple massage and touch as a means to enhance the effects of these modalities.[45]

Acupressure and Shiatzu (Shiatsu)

The Eastern energy system of meridian lines and points is the foundation of acupressure and Shiatzu. The word *shiatzu* comes from the Japanese words *shi* (finger) and *atzu* (pressure). The technique is a product of 4,000 years of Eastern medicine and philosophy. Although widely known and practiced in Japan, Shiatzu was virtually unknown in Western culture until acupuncture began receiving widespread public attention. Shiatzu is based on the same 657 energy points running along 12 pathways or meridians that are used in acupuncture. Instead of inserting needles, however, the practitioner applies pressure on these points with the thumbs, fingers, and heel of the hand. According to the theory underlying these practices, the application of pressure releases congestion and allows energy to flow. Another difference between acupuncture and Shiatzu is that the main function of Shiatzu is to maintain health and well-being (prevention), rather than to treat imbalance, as often occurs in acupuncture.[46]

Reflexology

In the early 1900s, William FitzGerald noted that application of pressure to certain points on the hands caused anesthesia in other parts of the body. Another physician, Edwin Bowers, learned of FitzGerald's work and joined him in the exploration and development of this zone therapy. The technique became more specific as it evolved into reflexology, which encompasses many more pressure points.

Reflexology is based on the theory that 10 equal longitudinal zones run the length of the body from the top of the head to the tips of the toes. This number corresponds to the number of fingers and toes. Each big toe matches to a line that runs up the medial aspect of the body, through the center of the face, and culminates at the top of the head. The reflex points pass all the way through the body within the same zones. Congestion or tension in any part of a zone affects the entire zone running laterally throughout the body. More than 72,000 nerves in the body terminate in the feet. A problem or disease in the body often manifests itself through formation of deposits of calcium and acids on the corresponding part of the foot. It is thought that hand and ear reflexology work in the same way, with points corresponding to distant structures.[12]

The purpose of reflexology is twofold. First, relaxation itself is an important goal. Good health is dependent on one's ability to return to homeostasis after injury, disease, or stress. From this perspective, reflexology is effective in helping the body–mind restore and maintain its natural state of health because foot manipulation triggers deep relaxation. The second goal

of this therapy is to stimulate the proprioceptive reflexes in the feet, thereby triggering a corresponding release that affects the endocrine, immune, and neuropeptide systems. Manuals with specific diagrams are used to instruct the therapist. An example of a foot reflexology chart is shown in **Figure 19-1**. (Visit www.reflexology .org for more information.)

In a quasi-experimental study comparing anxiety levels of 30 oncology patients undergoing chemotherapy, the experimental group received reflexology foot massage, while the control group did not. The reflexology recipients reported significantly less anxiety on the STAI both immediately and 24 hours post intervention. The researchers conclude that foot reflexology can be an important support treatment to help cancer patients feel and cope better with their disease.[47]

For menopausal women experiencing sleep disturbances, reflexology can provide needed relief. Eight women experiencing moderately

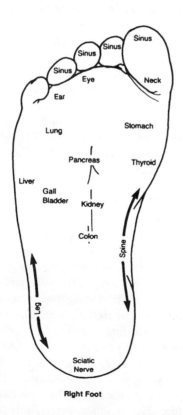
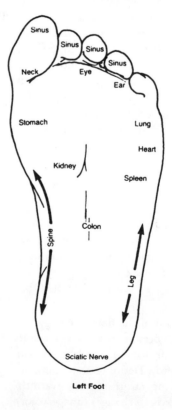

FIGURE 19-1   Foot Reflexology Chart

severe to severe menopausal symptoms received a 6-week trial of hand, ear, and foot reflexology. Preliminary results indicate that the women experienced relaxation and enhanced sleep, with a cumulative benefit after the third or fourth session, which lasted 3 to 4 days. A larger replication study is being planned.[48]

In an interesting case study, HT and foot reflexology were used together for a 40-year-old woman who had been unable to conceive after 18 months of trying. The intent was to facilitate conception and a normal pregnancy, and to avoid pharmacologic and invasive procedures. She did conceive and had a healthy pregnancy, delivery, and baby without pain or other medications. This use of modalities in conjunction with each other is typical of how complementary therapies are often used.[49]

Deep Tissue Techniques

This approach to bodywork aims to affect structure by releasing chronic patterns of muscle tension and held trauma or restriction in connective tissue. This work is done with great intention, and deep finger pressure is used to penetrate through layers of muscle, fascia, and tendons. This work can involve crossing or following the direction of muscle fibers. Sports massage, myofascial release, somatic neuromuscular integration (i.e., soma), Aston-Patterning, Zentherapy, Rolfing, and Hellerwork are examples of this type of massage.[50] (Visit www.rolf.org and www.zentherapy.org for more information.)

Emotional Bodywork

The category of emotional bodywork includes numerous techniques developed by individuals operating in the various fields that combine psychotherapy and bodywork. Some of the specific techniques include Lomi, Rosen Method, somatic experiencing, Trager, and psychoenergetic balancing. Some of these methods derive from ancient traditions, others from established health fields, such as chiropractic care. In general, it is important to remember that all touch therapies can trigger memories, physical and emotional release, and catharsis. This can be unexpected and frightening to clients, and they should be reassured that this is a common occurrence. This release can be related to

the assumption of a body position that triggers state-dependent memory or to cellular memory stimulation.[1]

Occasionally, individuals who have experienced abuse or trauma will release long-held emotional or physical tension during a touch session. This can manifest as laughter, tears, uncontrollable twitching, shaking, deep sighs, anger, or a variety of other expressions. Displaying calm acceptance, touching a neutral area of the body (determine this ahead of time with the client), and allowing the client time to release emotion are all therapeutic responses to this type of occurrence.[51] Appropriate referral for counseling is important.

Manipulative Therapies

Manipulative therapies often involve more invasive bodywork and demand a complete program of education often considered separate from nursing. Some nurses study these techniques to augment their nursing endeavors. Manipulative therapies include chiropractic and osteopathy (which involve manipulation of bones, ligaments, and soft tissue areas, including work on the head and dura). A similar, related field of practice is physical therapy.

Other Holistic Therapies and Programs Related to Touch

The number of bodywork, somatic therapies, and touch-related programs is too extensive to cover completely in this chapter. A sampling is included here to awaken nurses to the magnitude and scope of what is available. Additional touch therapies not discussed in this chapter are noted in **Table 19-1**.

Various types of massage and therapies have been developed for those with specific needs. Chair massage, geriatric massage, prenatal and perinatal massage, and infant massage are but a few examples. Healing Touch International has a program called "Bosom Buddies" for those with breast cancer. Manual lymphatic drainage is available for postmastectomy patients who have lost lymph nodes. Craniosacral therapy is available for infants who have experienced birth trauma. With the proliferation of approaches, a style of touch is available for anyone who may benefit.

TABLE 19-1   Additional Touch Therapies

Therapy	Originator	Primary Purpose and Function
Applied kinesiology	George Goodheart	Focuses on the relationship of muscle strength and energy flow. The theory is that, if muscles are strong, then circulation and other vital functions are also strong.
Chiropractic	D. D. Palmer	Based on alignment of spinal vertebrae. This therapy involves manipulations to restore natural alignment.
Feldenkrais method	Moshe Feldenkrais	Gives the client gentle manipulations to heighten awareness of the body. As awareness increases, clients can make more informed choices about how to move the body in daily situations.
Jin shin Jyutsu	Master Jiro Murai of Japan in early 1900s	A milder form of acupressure that involves pressure along eight extra energy meridians.
Kofutu touch healing	Frank Homan	Developed in the early 1970s when a series of symbols for use in touch came to the originator during meditation. It is called "Kofutu" for the symbols and "touch" healing because the auras of the healer and recipient must touch. This therapy uses higher consciousness energy symbols to promote self-development and spiritual healing.
Lomi	R. K. Hall, R. K. Heckler	Directs attention to current muscle tension to aid learning of postural alignment to enhance free flow of the body's physical and emotional energies.
Polarity therapy	Randolph Stone	Repatterns energy flow in the individual by rebalancing positive and negative charges. The practitioner places finger or whole hand on parts of the client's body of opposite charge to facilitate energy balancing where it is needed. Through these contacts, with the help of pressure and rocking movements, energy can reorganize and reorder itself.
MaríEL	Ethel Lombardi	A 1980s variation of Reiki.
Neuromuscular release		Involves movement of the limbs toward and away from the body by the practitioner to assist the client in learning to let go for the purpose of enhanced circulation and emotional release.
Rolfing	Ida P. Rolf	A form of bodywork that reorganizes the fascia (connective tissues) that permeate the entire body, thus enabling the body to regain the natural integrity of its form. Rolfing enhances structural alignment, postural efficiency, comfort and freedom of movement.
Trager work	Milton Trager	Involves rhythmically rocking the limbs and often the whole body to aid relaxation of the muscles and promote optimal flow of blood, lymph, nerve impulses, and energy.

HOLISTIC CARING PROCESS

Holistic Assessment

In preparing to use touch interventions, the nurse assesses the following parameters:

- The client's perception of his or her body–mind situation
- The client's potential physical problems that may require referral to a physician for evaluation
- The client's history of emotional and psychiatric disorders (The nurse must modify the approach with clients who have present or past psychiatric disorders. Touch itself may present a problem, and the deeply relaxed, semihypnotic state that a balanced person finds enjoyable may actually frighten or alarm an unbalanced individual.)
- The client's values and cultural beliefs about touch and energy therapies
- The client's past experience with body therapies

The knowledge levels of clients vary widely. The approach will differ markedly depending on the client's previous experience. Assisting a client in transferring prior learning such as from childbirth preparation classes to a new situation is helpful.

Identification of Patterns/ Challenges/Needs

The following patterns/challenges/needs (see Chapter 7) are compatible with the interventions for touch:

- Altered circulation
- Impairment in skin integrity
- Social isolation
- Altered spiritual state
- Impaired physical mobility
- Altered meaningfulness
- Altered comfort
- Anxiety
- Grieving
- Fear

Outcome Identification

Exhibit 19-1 guides the nurse in client outcomes, nursing prescriptions, and evaluation for the use of touch as a nursing intervention.

Therapeutic Care Plan and Interventions

Before the session:

- Wash your hands.
- Have the client empty his or her bladder to reduce muscle tension.
- Prepare the hospital bed, therapy table, or surface on which you will be working. If you will be using a therapy table, drape it with a cotton blanket and place a sheet over the top. Lay out a blanket or sheet for the client to use as a cover when he or she lies on the table. Adjust the height of the table or bed to protect your back.
- Have small pillows, bolsters, or towel rolls available for supporting the head, back, or lower legs.
- Control the environment so that the room is warm, dimly lit, and quiet. If you are in a client's hospital room, draw the curtain and turn off the television set.
- Use relaxation and breathing techniques, imagery, or music to elicit the relaxation response.
- After you have talked with the client, spend a few moments to quiet and center yourself, focus on your healing intention, and then begin.

At the beginning of the session:

- Explain to the client the steps in the touch process to be used. Ask permission to proceed.
- As you progress through the intervention, explain what you are about to do before you actually begin. Encourage the client to address concerns or discomfort at any time.
- Position the head comfortably. If the client has long hair, pull it up and away from the neckline.
- If you are using massage techniques, have the client disrobe to his or her level of comfort. The client lies on a padded therapy table or hospital bed that is covered with a cotton blanket and sheet. The sides of the sheet and blanket are then wrapped over the client so that he or she feels protected and warm. (This procedure is used for physical touch therapies and is not needed for TT, HT, Reiki, or other energy-based interventions, which may be done with the client fully clothed. However, remember

EXHIBIT 19-1   Nursing Interventions: Touch

Client Outcomes	Nursing Prescriptions	Evaluation
The client is relaxed following a touch therapy session.	Encourage the client to receive touch therapy to evoke the relaxation response.	The client willingly accepted touch therapy.
	During the touch therapy session, help the client ■ Decrease anxiety and fear ■ Decrease pulse and respiratory rate ■ Recognize a feeling of body–mind relaxation ■ Develop a sense of general well-being ■ Increase effectiveness in individual coping skills ■ Increase a sense of belonging and lessened loneliness ■ Feel less alone and express that feeling	The client ■ Exhibited decreased anxiety and fear ■ Demonstrated a decrease in pulse and respiratory rate ■ Reported muscle relaxation ■ Exhibited satisfied facial expression and expressed inner calmness ■ Reported greater satisfaction in individual coping patterns
The client has improved circulation.	Provide the client with information about how touch therapies improve circulation and tissue perfusion.	Clients with white skin had a reddened color in the area where the nurse had used effleurage and pétrissage massage strokes. Skin in the massaged area is warmer than before the therapy.
The client receives touch therapy to maintain and enhance health.	Encourage the client to ask for touch therapy. Suggest that the client seek out the nurse. Recommend that the client accept touch when offered by the nurse.	The client asked for touch therapy.

that when the client experiences the relaxation response, the body may undergo cooling, so a blanket may be necessary.)

■ Uncover only the body area that is being massaged or pressed as the therapy proceeds. You may leave the client covered during energetic treatments.

■ In most cases, begin with the client lying on his or her back.

■ Encourage the client to take slow, deep, releasing breaths.

■ During the turning process, slide the sheet or towel around the client's body to ensure that the client will not be exposed.

During the session:

■ Be attuned to the client's responses to therapy. This will help the client build trust and achieve optimal relaxation. Be prepared for an emotional or physical release, and calmly remain with the client should this happen.

■ In initial sessions, continue to explain what the client can expect to happen so that he or she feels comfortable with the continued direction of the touch sessions. After trust has been established and the relaxation response is learned, the client will relax more quickly and move to deeper levels in subsequent sessions.

At the end of the session:

- When you have finished the touch therapy session, verbally let the client know that it is time to return gradually to the here-and-now, to begin to move around slowly, and to awaken fully.
- Anticipate that the client will take a few minutes to reorient to time and place after being in a deep state of relaxation.
- Allow a period of silence for the client to appreciate fully the experience and benefits of his or her relaxed body–mind.
- Stay in the room while the client rouses and sits up. Give necessary assistance to ensure a safe transfer to an ambulatory position.
- Allow time to receive the client's verbal feedback about the meaning of the session if the client feels the need to talk. If this does not occur spontaneously, ask for feedback. The insight gained provides guidelines for further sessions or specific ideas that the client can follow up in daily life.
- When the touch therapy is used for relaxation or sleep induction for hospitalized patients, close the session by softly pulling the bedcovers up over the patient's back and quietly turning off the light as the patient moves into sleep. Let the client know in advance that you will leave quietly at the end.

- Use the client outcomes that were established before the session (see Exhibit 19-1) and the client's subjective experience (**Exhibit 19-2**) to evaluate the session.

Case Study (Implementation)

CASE STUDY 1

Setting: Medical/surgical unit of a general hospital

Patient: E. S., a 68-year-old single man with COPD

Patterns/Challenges/Needs:

1. Anxiety
2. Altered comfort
3. Social isolation (related to chronic obstructive pulmonary disease [COPD] and pneumonia)

E. S. was oxygen dependent and no longer ambulatory. After a history of heavy smoking for 40 years, his lungs continued to deteriorate in spite of quitting smoking at age 60. His stomach frequently felt upset, and it was difficult for him to eat much. He could not tolerate liquid nutritional supplements, he worked very hard to breathe, and his weight had dropped from 160 to 100 pounds over a 2-year period. He had become very weak. Because E. S. had become sedentary and very bony, he was uncomfortable most of the time, with stiffness and body aches.

EXHIBIT 19-2   Evaluation of the Client's Subjective Experience of Touch Therapies

1. Was this a new kind of experience for you? Can you describe it?
2. Did this feel like a comforting or stimulating tactile sensation or both?
3. Was it pleasurable on all planes—physical, mental, emotional, and spiritual—or more focused in one area than another?
4. Were you aware of your surroundings during the experience, or did you sink into a sense of timelessness?
5. Did emotions surface during the experience? If so, what were they? Can you focus on them now?
6. Did you experience any imagery during the touch session?
7. Did you feel comfortable with the therapist? Is there anything that you want to do to increase your comfort level with the touch therapist?
8. Did you feel relaxed and refreshed after the experience?
9. Would you like to try this again?
10. What would be helpful to make this a better experience for you?
11. Can you develop a plan or strategy to integrate more of the touch therapies into your life on a regular basis?

E. S. had grown up in the city in which he now found himself hospitalized. He had never married and had no remaining living family.

E. S. declined massage because he was afraid it would hurt him. He felt very fragile and very much alone. He became especially anxious and fearful at nighttime. One of the nurses caring for him had attended a local course and learned the basics of therapeutic touch. She knew that TT would not cause any physical pain for E. S. because it did not involve actually touching him. She also knew that it might be very relaxing for him, perhaps even easing his respiratory effort. She offered E. S. a "trial" session for 10 minutes to see if this might be a helpful modality for him. Pulling the curtain around his bed, she encouraged him to relax and breathe slowly and fully. She calmed herself and took a few deep slow breaths to increase her sense of focus. Working about 7–10 inches away from his body, she began to move her hands through his field from head to toes with the intention of moving energy and balancing his field. After only 5 minutes, she saw E. S. relax as his shoulders released and his facial expression softened.

E. S. reported that he slept better that night than he had for a long while. It was decided that he would receive a TT session each evening for the remainder of his hospitalization. The nurse who had performed the first session taught several of the other nurses how to do the basic techniques she had used. As they saw the positive effects of their interventions with E. S., they became interested in learning more and sought their own formal training in energetic healing.

CASE STUDY 2

Setting: Long-term care facility

Client: J. S., a 76-year-old widow

Patterns/Challenges/Needs:

1. Anxiety related to painful arthritis in hands
2. Altered self-image related to deformity of hands

J. S. is a delightful woman who has lived in the long-term care facility for 2 years. She is generally healthy and has loving family who visits her regularly. The pain in her hands from arthritis has increased, and she has become increasingly

intolerant of the medications used to ease her pain and inflammation. Nurses who care for J. S. have decided to incorporate hand massage twice daily into her routine care. Although they are very busy, they plan to spend at least 5 minutes per hand, using gentle stroking and kneading motions along with lotion. J. S. likes the smell of lavender, and essential oil of lavender is mixed into the lotion that is kept in her room because it is thought to enhance relaxation and pain relief.

Sometimes, when the nurses are very busy, they massage one of her hands, and then come back later to do the other hand. J. S. loves this time and says that it is giving her noticeable pain relief and a feeling of greater relaxation. The nurses enjoy this time as well and report that it gives them a chance to get more information from J. S. as to how she is doing in general. Over time, J. S.'s daughter and granddaughter start to massage her hands when they come to visit. Other residents request hand massage, and those clients who are able begin to offer this to each other as well.

CASE STUDY 3

Setting: Patient's home

Client: J. H., a 45-year-old single female minister

Patterns/Challenges/Needs:

1. Anxiety related to pain
2. Ineffective breathing pattern
3. Altered spiritual state

J. H., who was suffering from end-stage pancreatic cancer, gently closed her eyes. The practitioner explained the Reiki treatment that the patient was about to experience. J. H.'s breathing began to slow and her body relaxed. She had been short of breath and unable to get comfortable for most of the morning. The music played softly, the lavender candle flickered gently, and the light touch of the Reiki practitioner began to have an immediate effect on the client. As the hour-long treatment ended, the client opened her eyes and said she had been able to breathe more deeply and to experience a sense of well-being and comfort that had not been present for several months. The calmness in her expression and the deep, rhythmic breathing pattern lasted for several hours after the session. J. H. died a few weeks later. Her experience and testimony demonstrate how comfort can be brought into the lives of others through the use of energetic touch therapies and the practitioner's healing presence.

Evaluation

With the client, the nurse determines whether the client outcomes for touch therapies were successfully achieved (see Exhibit 19-1). To evaluate the session further, the nurse may again explore the subjective effects of the experience with the client using the evaluation questions in Exhibit 19-2.

Directions for
FUTURE RESEARCH

1. Develop valid and reliable tools to measure the effects of touch and hand-mediated therapies.
2. Investigate hand-mediated techniques practiced in conjunction with other modalities to mirror real-world usage of these modalities.
3. Continue to strengthen the evidence base for practicing touch and hand-mediated therapies.
4. Discern which therapies are best suited for various health concerns and populations.
5. Examine the use of touch and hand-mediated therapies in ambulatory and community settings.
6. Examine long-term cost-effectiveness of touch and hand-mediated techniques.
7. Investigate whether periodic hand-mediated therapy sessions can increase work performance or productivity.
8. Evaluate length of stay, complications, and well-being as related to the use of touch techniques.
9. Examine the responses to touch and hand-mediated therapies related to developmental stage.
10. Investigate how touch can be taught effectively in nursing schools and what methods are best suited to accomplish this.
11. Explore ways in which nursing students' cultural learning pertaining to touch affects performance of clinical care.
12. Measure parental and caregiver satisfaction when taught to offer touch and hand-mediated therapies to loved ones.

Nurse Healer
REFLECTIONS

After reading this chapter, the nurse healer will be able to answer or to begin the process of answering the following questions:

- How do I feel about using touch and hand-mediated therapies as healing interventions?
- What does the process of centering myself feel like?
- How does the use of my intention alter my experience of offering touch?
- How astute am I at observing my client's response to touch interventions?
- How can I increase my skill pertaining to the use of touch and hand-mediated therapies?
- Who might be a good mentor for me as I increase my repertoire of healing modalities?
- What other modalities can I learn and include to enhance the effectiveness of touch?

 For a full suite of assignments and additional learning activities, use the access code located in the front of your book to visit this exclusive website: http://go.jblearning.com /dossey. If you do not have an access code, you can obtain one at the site.

NOTES

1. K. Fontaine, *Complementary and Alternative Therapies for Nursing Practice*, 3rd ed. (Upper Saddle River, NJ: Prentice Hall, 2010).
2. H. Harlow, "Love in Infant Monkeys," *Scientific American* 200 (1958): 68–74.
3. R. Spitz, *The First Year of Life* (New York: International Universities Press, 1965).
4. B. Grad, "Some Biological Effects of the Laying on of Hands: A Review of Experiments with Animals and Plants," *Journal of the American Society for Psychical Research* 59 (1965): 95–127.
5. M. J. Smith, "Enzymes Are Activated by the Laying on of Hands," *Human Dimensions* (1973): 46–48.
6. D. Leder and M. W. Krucoff, "The Touch That Heals: The Uses and Meanings of Touch in the Clinical Encounter," *Journal of Alternative and Complementary Medicine* 14, no. 3 (2008): 321–327.

7. N. Gueguen and M. Vion, "The Effect of a Practitioner's Touch on a Patient's Medication Compliance," *Psychology, Health, & Medicine* 14, no. 6 (2009): 689–694.

8. A. Montagu and F. Matson, *The Human Connection* (New York: McGraw-Hill, 1979): 89.

9. J. Ellis, "The Touch That Means So Much," *Nursing Older People* 22, no. 8 (2010): 10.

10. I. Beck, I. Runeson, and K. Blomqvist, "To Find Inner Peace: Soft Massage as an Established and Integrated Part of Palliative Care," *International Journal of Palliative Care* 15, no. 11 (2009): 541–545.

11. N. Bost, "The Effectiveness of a 15-Minute Weekly Massage in Reducing Physical and Psychologic Stress in Nurses," *Australian Journal of Advanced Nursing* 23, no. 4 (2006): 28–33.

12. N. Cuellar, *Conversations in Complementary and Alternative Medicine: Insights and Perspectives from Leading Practitioners* (Sudbury, MA: Jones & Bartlett, 2006).

13. J. A. Cambron, "Changes in Blood Pressure After Various Forms of Therapeutic Massage: A Preliminary Study," *Journal of Alternative and Complementary Medicine* 12, no. 1 (2006): 65–70.

14. M. C. Smith, T. E. Yamashita, L. L. Bryant, L. Hemphill, and J. S. Kutner, "Providing Massage Therapy for People with Advanced Cancer: What to Expect," *Journal of Alternative and Complementary Medicine* 14, no. 4 (2009): 367–371.

15. A. Billhult, I. Bergbom, and E. Stener-Victorin, "Massage Relieves Nausea in Women with Breast Cancer Who Are Undergoing Chemotherapy," *Journal of Alternative and Complementary Medicine* 13, no. 1 (2007): 53–58.

16. S. Ayas et al., "Massage Therapy for Osteoarthritis of the Knee: A Randomized Controlled Trial," *American Journal of Physical Medicine and Rehabilitation* 166, no. 22 (2006): 2533–2538.

17. S. M. Wilkinson et al., "Effectiveness of Aromatherapy Massage in the Management of Anxiety and Depression in Patients with Cancer: A Multicenter Randomized Controlled Trial," *Journal of Clinical Oncology* 25, no. 5 (2007): 532–539.

18. M. Huth, K. Zink, and N. Van Horn, "The Effects of Massage Therapy in Improving Outcomes for Youth with Cystic Fibrosis: An Evidence Review," *Pediatric Nursing* 31, no. 4 (2005): 44–52.

19. G. Shor-Posner et al., "Impact of a Massage Therapy Clinical Trial on Immune Status in Young Dominican Children Infected with HIV-1," *Journal of Alternative and Complementary Medicine* 12, no. 6 (2006): 511–516.

20. V. Jump, J. Fargo, and J. Akers, "Impact of Massage Therapy on Health Outcomes Among Orphaned Infants in Ecuador," *Family and Community Health* 29, no. 4 (2006): 314–319.

21. A. Kelmanson and E. Adulas, "Massage Therapy and Sleep Behavior in Infants Born with Low Birth Weight," *Complementary Therapies in Clinical Practice* 12, no. 3 (2005): 200–205.

22. T. Field et al., "Moderate Versus Light Pressure Massage Therapy Leads to Greater Weight Gain in Preterm Infants," *Infant Behavior Development* 29, no. 4 (2006): 574–578.

23. R. Jones, "Touch for Homeless Clients: San Francisco's Care Through Touch Institute," *Massage & Bodywork* (September/October 2008): 71–79.

24. V. S. Eschiti, "Healing Touch: A Low-Tech Intervention in High-Tech Settings," *Dimensions of Critical Care Nursing* 26, no. 1 (2007): 9–14.

25. D. Hover-Kramer, *Healing Touch: A Guidebook for Practitioners*, 2nd ed. (Albany, NY: Thomson Delmar Learning, 2001).

26. D. F. Bruce and D. Krieger, *Miracle Touch: A Complete Guide to Hands-on Therapies That Have the Amazing Ability to Heal* (New York: Three Rivers Press, 2003).

27. D. Krieger, *Accepting Your Power to Heal: The Personal Practice of Therapeutic Touch* (Santa Fe, NM: Bear and Co., 1993).

28. J. F. Quinn and A. J. Strelkauskas, "Psychoimmunologic Effects of Therapeutic Touch on Practitioners and Recently Bereaved Recipients: A Pilot Study," *Advances in Nursing Science* 15, no. 4 (1993): 13–26.

29. Z. Movaffaghi et al., "Effects of Therapeutic Touch on Blood Hemoglobin and Hematocrit Level," *Journal of Holistic Nursing* 24, no. 1 (2006): 41–48.

30. M. MacNeil, "Therapeutic Touch, Pain, and Caring: Implications for Nursing Practice," *International Journal for Human Caring* 10, no. 1 (2006): 40–48.

31. C. Hutchison, C. Komitor, and K. M. Layte, eds., *Healing Touch Level 1 Notebook*, 6th ed. (San Antonio, TX: Healing Touch Program, 2009).

32. D. Wardell et al., "A Pilot Study of Healing Touch and Progressive Relaxation for Chronic Neuropathic Pain in Persons with Spinal Cord Injury," *Journal of Holistic Nursing* 24, no. 4 (2006): 231–240.

33. K. Bowman, commentary on "A Pilot Study of Healing Touch and Progressive Relaxation for Chronic Neuropathic Pain in Persons with Spinal Cord Injury," *Journal of Holistic Nursing* 24, no. 4 (2006): 241–242.

34. T. Cox, "Caught on the Horns of a Conundrum," *Journal of Holistic Nursing* 24, no. 4 (2006): 228–230.

35. K. Wang, "Pilot Study to Test the Effectiveness of Healing Touch on Agitation in People with Dementia," *Geriatric Nursing* 27, no. 1 (2006): 34–40.

36. K. J. Kemper, N. B. Fletcher, C. A. Hamilton, and T. W. McLean, "Impact of Healing Touch on Pediatric Oncology Outpatients: Pilot Study,"

Journal of the Society for Integrative Oncology 7, no. 1 (2009): 12–18.

37. L. Bourne, "The Art of Reiki and Its Uses in General," *Practicing Nursing* 20, no. 2 (2009): 11–14.

38. L. Barnett and M. Chambers, *Reiki Energy Medicine* (Rochester, NY: Healing Arts Press, 1998).

39. N. E. Richeson, J. A. Spross, K. Lutz, and C. Peng, "Effects of Reiki on Anxiety, Depression, Pain, and Physiological Factors in Community-Dwelling Older Adults," *Research in Gerontological Nursing* 3, no. 3 (2010): 187–199.

40. A. Brathovda, "Reiki for Self-Care of Nurses and Healthcare Providers," *Holistic Nursing Practice* 20, no. 2 (2006): 95–101.

41. K. Kemper, D. Larrimore, and C. Woods, "Impact of a Medical School Elective in Cultivating Compassion Through Touch Therapies," *Complementary Health Practice Review* 11, no. 1 (2006): 54.

42. A. Vitale and P. O'Connor, "The Effect of Reiki on Pain and Anxiety in Women with Abdominal Hysterectomies: A Quasi-Experimental Pilot Study," *Holistic Nursing Practice* 20, no. 6 (2006): 263–272.

43. S. vanderVaart, V. M. Gijsen, S. N. de Wildt, and G. Koren, "A Systematic Review of the Therapeutic Effects of Reiki," *Journal of Alternative and Complementary Medicine* 15, no. 11 (2009): 1157–1169.

44. North American Nursing Diagnosis Association, *Nursing Diagnoses: Definitions and Classification 1995–1996* (Philadelphia, PA: NANDA, 1994): 37.

45. M. E. Doenges, M. F. Moorhouse, and A. C. Murr, *Nursing Diagnosis Manual: Planning, Individualizing, and Documenting Client Care*, 6th ed. (Philadelphia, PA: F. A. Davis, 2008).

46. M. Micozzi, *Fundamentals of Complementary and Integrative Medicine*, 3rd ed. (St. Louis, MO: Saunders Elsevier, 2006).

47. R. Quattrin et al., "Use of Reflexology Foot Massage to Reduce Anxiety in Hospitalized Cancer Patients in Chemotherapy Treatment: Methodology and Outcomes," *Journal of Nursing Management* 14 (2006): 96–105.

48. D. Morris, "Pilot Study Using Reflexology," *Beginnings* 26, no. 5 (2006): 28–29.

49. J. Kissinger and L. Kaczmarek, "Healing Touch and Fertility: A Case Report," *Journal of Perinatal Education* 15, no. 2 (2006): 13–20.

50. D. Rakel and N. Faass, *Complementary Medicine in Clinical Practice* (Sudbury, MA: Jones & Bartlett, 2006).

51. D. Hover-Kramer and K. H. Shames, *Energetic Approaches to Emotional Healing* (Albany, NY: Delmar Publishers, 1997).

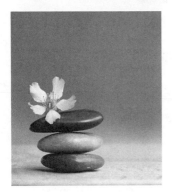

Chapter 20

Relationships

Mary Blaszko Helming

Nurse Healer
OBJECTIVES

Theoretical

- Define three areas in which nurses are required to develop effective relationships.
- List seven issues that either strengthen or interfere with relationships.
- Identify ways in which selected nursing theorists inform therapeutic relationships.
- Identify ways that the humanistic psychologies of Rogers and Maslow, as well as the positive psychology of Seligman, expand holistic thinking.
- Identify four archetypes of human relationships that address physical, emotional, mental, and spiritual domains, using Jung and Arrien.

Clinical

- Identify core elements that lead to establishing and maintaining effective relationships.
- Implement and evaluate effective negotiating styles that address issues while maintaining a sense of relatedness.
- Gain insight into problematic aspects of relationships and how to manage them more effectively.

Personal

- Increase your use of key effective personal relationship characteristics.
- Develop strategies to incorporate effective boundaries in relationships.
- Strengthen your concepts of spiritual relationship.

DEFINITIONS

Archetype: Name given by Jung and Arrien to specific patterns of human collective awareness that symbolically represent human potentials, such as the Healer, the Warrior, the Mother, or the Wise Person.

Boundaries: Artificial separations between people that define the perimeters of the relationship.

Complementary transaction: An interaction in which the ego states match (e.g., adult-to-adult communication). Complementary transactions support and strengthen relationships.

Defense patterns: Protective mechanisms that justify individual action while detracting from relationship building.

Emotional intelligence: Awareness and attention to personal emotional needs that allow individuals to be in a position of equality with others, rather than seeking power and control or becoming overly passive.

Forgiveness: A willingness to acknowledge one's own mistakes and shortcomings and to allow others room to acknowledge their shortcomings as well.

■ THEORY AND RESEARCH

Relationship refers to kinship, passionate attachment, or a connection between those having relations or dealings. A relationship refers to two or more persons or things working together, belonging together, or being part of a whole, as in relatives within a family. John Donne wrote these famous words, "No man is an island, entire of itself."[1] Throughout history, relationships have existed between human beings, between the divine and human beings, and between the earthly environment and human beings. It is evident that no human being was intended to live alone. This concept is repeated in many world religions. Throughout the ages, the great religions have spoken of the necessity of loving, caring human relationships. Keegan and Drick explain the term *interconnectedness* as implying that people may share the "universal reciprocity of love and responsibility" without regard to their culture, politics, or religion.[2]

■ RELATIONSHIP THEORIES

The Theory of Human Relatedness, according to Hagerty and Patusky, suggests that people are "relational beings who experience some degree of involvement with external referents, including people, objects, groups, and natural environments."[3] The theory emphasizes that some human relationships serve to lessen anxiety and improve wellness, and others promote distress and anxiety. The following are the four stages of human relatedness:

1. Connection means there is active involvement with another, associated with enhanced comfort and wellness.
2. Disconnection involves lack of involvement and is associated with lack of wellness and distress.
3. Parallelism implies disengagement, or the lack of involvement with others. This can

have a positive effect of creating solitude with associated physical and psychological replenishment.
4. Enmeshment often describes negative, overinvolved relationships, fraught with anxiety, distress, and functional disability.

It is also possible for people to be in relationships in all these quadrants simultaneously. Hagerty and Patusky further suggest that there are four social competencies vital for relationships:

1. Sense of belonging means there is an appropriate "fit" with the environment, group, or individual. There is a sense of being valued and needed in the relationship.
2. Reciprocity is a positive aspect of relationship in which there is a perceived equal exchange between parties.
3. Mutuality represents how people tend to join with those they believe share similarities to them, or with whom they share an acceptance of differences.
4. Synchrony is a person's perception of congruent feelings or behaviors with another with whom the individual shares a relationship.

The term *interrelationship* implies the existence of a subtle web of life that connects all human beings, their environment, and spirituality. Each person's actions can directly and indirectly affect others and can create a healing or toxic response or energy. Holistic nurses have identified interrelationship as a key element of their practice. For holistic nurses, relationship transcends patient care and includes patient families and significant others, interactions with coworkers, interdisciplinary associates, and authority figures. Jackson cites 12 essential values to guide relationship-based care, evolving from care theory, holistic concepts, and loving care, as referenced in Koloroutis's (2004) classic work, *Relationship-Based Care: A Model for Transforming Practice*.[4] Seven of the 12 values include relationship, and they are as follows:

1. The meaning and essence of care are experienced in the moment when one human being connects with another.
2. Feeling connected to one another creates harmony and healing; feeling isolated destroys spirit.

3. The relationship between patients and their families and members of the clinical team belongs at the heart of care delivery.

4. Care providers' knowledge of self and self-care are fundamental requirements for high-quality care and healthy interpersonal relationships.

5. Healthy relationships among members of the healthcare team lead to the delivery of high-quality care and result in high patient, physician, and staff satisfaction.

6. The value of relationship in patient care must be understood, valued, and agreed to by all members of the healthcare organization.

7. A therapeutic relationship between a patient/family and a professional nurse is essential to high-quality patient care.

■ THERAPEUTIC RELATIONSHIPS IN HOLISTIC NURSING

The *therapeutic relationship* has more traditionally been associated with psychological counseling processes, but it is highly adaptable to holistic nursing. A therapeutic relationship is a professional alliance between the nurse and the client or patient, working together for a defined period of time to accomplish specific health-related goals.[5] Further, a therapeutic relationship can occur even if a patient is in the end stages of life or is generally uncooperative on health and wellness initiatives.

The patient must feel supported as well as listened to, and the nurse should feel valued in his or her role. A significant point is that patients may not listen well to their healthcare providers unless they themselves feel listened to. Discontent with healthcare providers can cause patients to avoid treatment, take longer to recover, have more complications, and misunderstand vital information.

The therapeutic relationship is considered to be essential to psychiatric nursing, yet Dziopa and Ahern note that it is not instinctive, but requires high-level skills, including advanced practice skills.[6] Nine primary concepts explain the therapeutic relationship, according to their review of the literature: (1) demonstrating respect; (2) being genuine; (3) being there/being available; (4) accepting individuality; (5) hav-ing self-awareness; (6) maintaining boundaries; (7) demonstrating understanding and empathy; (8) providing support; and (9) promoting equality. However, therapeutic relationship in the past has not been well defined, and those who practice it have some difficulty describing it. Scanlon also studied psychiatric nurses' perceptions of what constitutes a therapeutic relationship and determined there is difficulty measuring the amount of positive change associated with the therapeutic relationship, plus the ability to provide a therapeutic relationship is dependent on the interpersonal skills of the provider and the life experience of the recipient.[7]

Other areas of nursing find the therapeutic relationship essential. In palliative care, the therapeutic relationship is considered the most important aspect of nursing care.[8] In critical care, the therapeutic relationship often extends to family members and requires the nurse to use sound emotional intelligence. Porr describes the importance of therapeutic relationship for public health nurses working with vulnerable and disadvantaged populations.[9]

Likewise, many psychotherapists consider the therapeutic relationship vital to therapy. Zuroff and Blatt studied patients with depression and determined that a positive therapeutic relationship between client and therapist played a vital role in the therapeutic outcome.[10] The authors prove that the positive therapeutic relationship is much more than merely an outcome of clinical improvement, having developed as the client became less depressed and saw the therapist in a positive light. They also determine that the particular therapy technique used (cognitive behavioral therapy, for example) had no relationship to positive therapeutic presence. If a high-quality therapeutic relationship existed early in treatment, this predicted improved treatment response, reduction in symptoms, and overall better functioning.

In this light, it is important to discuss selected psychological theorists whose work encourages the use of the therapeutic relationship. Many other healthcare workers, such as licensed clinical social workers, marriage and family counselors, psychologists, psychiatrists, peer counselors, occupational therapists, physical therapists, and psychotherapists, utilize the concept of the therapeutic relationship, which promotes a healing relationship. *Being therapeutic* implies using oneself as an agent of healing in the dynamic relationship between provider and patient or client. Although holistic nurses may not have expertise in a variety of psychological approaches, it is meaningful for them to have a basic understanding of selected psychological modalities that have influenced models of therapeutic relationship, counseling, and therapy. For human beings to relate well to one another, it is vital to comprehend some of the primary psychological theories that influence understanding of human behaviors and relationships. To understand others, it is first necessary to understand ourselves and why we do the things we do. Because human lives are built on interrelationships, it is understandable that the sources of our conflicts and troubles are associated with unhealthy relationships to a Higher Power, to other human beings, to the environment, and to one's self.

Therefore, **Table 20-1** highlights selected influential psychologists and their theories, ranging from traditional theories to humanistic psychology to the new positive psychology. First, Pavlov described *behavioral psychology*, with the belief that most human actions are conditioned behaviors. This concept was followed by traditional *psychoanalytical psychology*, which looks at the subconscious as the key motivator for human behavior, as exemplified by Freudian psychology. Then, in the 1960s, the *humanistic psychology* movement brought with it the concept that caring, trust, and understanding of human complexity are key. The person is viewed holistically, and human creativity and transcendence are valued.[11] The distinction with humanistic psychologists is their belief that human beings are not just controlled by subconscious forces or their environments, but are people of free will who maintain the ability to reach for their highest potential. Key concepts of humanistic psychology include self-actualization, creativity, intrinsic nature, individuality, becoming, and meaningfulness. *Positive psychology* developed on the heels of human psychology.

Holistic nurses may select which theories they find most reasonable to use in their practice settings and in their own sphere of personal relationships.[12] (See also **Table 20-2**.)

The Healing Relationship

In addition to pursuing a therapeutic relationship with their patients or clients, holistic nurses have identified that the act of relating to another human being can be accomplished in a healing environment, and this is termed the *healing relationship*. Nightingale characterized the healing relationship as that which puts the patient in the best position for Nature to act on him or her. She spoke of the healing nurse–patient relationship.[13] Dossey describes Nightingale as a mystic, visionary, and healer.[14] Nightingale, as a visionary, described many aspects of healing with which nurses can empower patients. Promoting a healing relationship is both an art and a relational skill.

Patients and clients are very often in crisis states, compromised health, or in states of varying degrees of vulnerability. It is most often at these times that patients and clients realize they must rely on others for assistance. The greatest healing can occur when patients and clients can place their trust in the abilities of other healthcare professionals. In crisis and emergent situations, it is highly evident that one's well-being is in the hands of others.

Healthcare providers, including holistic nurses, can create healing relationships by becoming more *patient centered*. Too often, the fast pace of care causes providers only to nod to patients' stories and move on to complete the exam or tasks at hand. Providers, especially nurses and physicians, are so busy and short on time in this era of managed care that it is difficult to find the time to really listen to patients. Healthcare reform is a powerful concept in the United States at this time. A return to the ideals of patient-centered care includes the following concepts for all healthcare providers:[15]

- Provide dignity and respect; honor patient and family choices. Incorporate the cultural background, values, and beliefs of the patient/family into health care.
- Encourage patients and families to participate in decision making about their healthcare needs.

TABLE 20-1　Relationship Theorists

Psychologists	Theory and Applications
Eric Berne	Transactional Analysis (TA).
	Concept: Three ego states, people move among states; unconscious games played between people may be a substitute for true intimacy. Three ego states are Adult (rational, objective), Parent (authoritative figure), and Child (playful, curious, stubborn). All human beings need social interaction, even if it is negative interaction.
	Book: *Games People Play: The Psychology of Human Relationships* (1964)
Erik Erikson	Eight psychosocial stages of life; psychoanalytic approach:
	1. Trust vs. mistrust (infancy)
	2. Autonomy vs. shame (early childhood)
	3. Initiative vs. doubt (preschool)
	4. Competence vs. incompetence (elementary school)
	5. Identity vs. role confusion (middle/high school)
	6. Intimacy vs. isolation (college)
	7. Generativity vs. stagnation (adult)
	8. Ego integrity vs. ego despair (older age)
	Concept: Tasks of each age group must be completed; youth often develop identity crisis in their 20s after completing higher education.
	Book: *Identity, Youth, and Crisis* (1968)
Carl Jung	Freudian psychoanalytic psychology.
	Concepts: Collective unconscious as the inherited human unconscious composed of universal mental images and thoughts, which are archetypes.
	Archetypes: Concepts of personality expressed in myths and fairy tales; people fit into these roles interchangeably.
	Mother archetype: Most important, role of nurse, Mother of God, grandmothers, church, Earth, and Nature.
	Crone archetype: The wise old woman who is a visionary, who at the crossroads of life chooses the path of the soul rather than the ego, and she speaks the truth always.
	Book: *Development of Personality* (1981)
Angeles Arrien	Transpersonal psychology; views life holistically.
	Concepts: Evolved Jungian archetypes, four primary archetypes identified.
	Healer archetype: Holistic nursing professionals manifest this archetype by relating to others compassionately and with love. Other essential characteristics of the Healer include bringing caring to human relationships, viewing others in a positive light, and bringing emotional comfort.
	Teacher archetype: The Teacher represents the mental quality in relationships, helping learners to achieve new knowledge, wisdom, and insight. Teachers are also very open to learning. Holistic nurses often exhibit the teacher quality as well.
	Warrior archetype: The Warrior symbolizes physical qualities of relationship building. This archetype uses courage to help improve behaviors of self and others, is firm, and uses knowledge, especially facts, effectively. Holistic nurses are very interested in helping patients improve their health and wellness behaviors and can use facts and their knowledge very effectively in this endeavor.

(continues)

TABLE 20-1 Relationship Theorists *(continued)*	
Psychologists	**Theory and Applications**
Angeles Arrien *(continued)*	Visionary archetype: The Visionary archetype symbolizes the spiritual aspect of relationship. The Visionary is nonjudgmental and assists in conflict resolution. This personality model exemplifies sound intuitive knowing to assist others in achieving their highest good. Holistic nurses need to focus on the spiritual aspect of relationship, which, in itself, tends to move others toward their highest potential.[15]
	Book: *The Four-Fold Way* (1993)
Isabel Briggs Myers	Concept: Jungian based. Myers-Briggs Type Indicator (MBTI) test widely used to identify personality types. Basis of much psychometric testing; often used to gauge appropriate career choices for individuals, to describe marriage compatibility, and for personal development
	The MBTI results are expressed in four-letter codes representing how personalities fall into four different domains. Possible to have total of 16 combinations of domains. Manner in which a person perceives reality is described as either "sensing" type (relies on the five senses) or "intuiting" type (relies on the unconscious to confirm what is real and what is not). Second area of personality involves the way a person judges, either through "thinking" (using logic in interpersonal relationships) or "feeling" (interpreting what something means to themselves as individuals). The third domain involves being an "extravert" (outgoing, makes quick decisions, attempts to influence situations) or an "introvert" (more interested in the inner world of ideas, needs time to develop ideas and insights, quieter). The final domain involves deciding between dominant and auxiliary processes. Sensing (S), intuition (N), thinking (T), and feeling (F) are placed together in pairs. Of these pairs, one function is "dominant" and the other is "auxiliary" (additional), which helps in ordering the letters. Extraverts (E), introverts (I), judgment (J), and perception (P) round out the personality symbols.
Abraham Maslow	Father of human psychology.
	Concept: Hierarchy of needs. People move from lowest physiologic needs (food, water, oxygen) to safety and security, to love and belonging, to esteem and respect, to the highest level, self-actualization (need to do and be the person one is meant to be).
	Other significant concepts of humanistic psychology:
	▪ Identifying one's own voice as the self, rather than listening to society or the parental figure
	▪ Realization that life is a series of choices, one leading to personal growth and the other to regression
	▪ Being honest and taking responsibility for one's feelings, even if not popular
	▪ Being the best one can be in one's work; think outside box, creative
	▪ Seeing others at their best, finding the good in others
	▪ Abandoning psychological defense mechanisms
	Book: *Toward a Psychology of Being* (1968)
Carl Rogers	Humanistic psychologist.
	Concept: Patient-centered or client-centered therapy; some people have experienced being in open, trusting dialogue with another, without being judged, and having felt a sense of healing from this relationship. Based on Buber's I-Thou philosophy of treating the other as person, not object.

TABLE 20-1   Relationship Theorists *(continued)*

Psychologists	Theory and Applications
Carl Rogers *(continued)*	Preferable to listen to what clients were saying, rather than trying to "fix" them. Therapist did not need to remain detached and objective; could respond emotionally to the client. Book: *On Becoming a Person: A Therapist's View of Psychotherapy* (1995)
Daniel Goleman	Concept: Began new movement looking at significance of emotional vs. intellectual intelligence. Qualities such as optimism, empathy toward others, resilience (the ability to recover from adversity), and ability to adapt to change are considered part of emotional intelligence. Also conscientiousness, goal orientation with delayed gratification to achieve goals, awareness of one's own shortcomings, confidence in being able to handle most problems, having ability to interact well with others, be cooperative, and manage close personal relationships. Book: *Emotional Intelligence* (1995)
Martin Seligman	Father of Positive Psychology. ■ The study of emotions that are positive ■ The study of traits that are positive, including virtues, intelligence, strength, and athleticism ■ The study of social institutions or concepts that possess positive qualities (e.g., functional family units, freedom of inquiry, and democracy) and support a virtuous life. Virtues include integrity, loyalty, valor, and equity. Concepts: Positive emotions such as trust, hope, and confidence help us most in times of distress. Optimistic people interpret problems as controllable, transient, and limited to one situation. Pessimistic people believe troubles last forever, are uncontrollable, and undermine them. Learned helplessness: Concept that studied human and animal responses to uncontrollable events. Linked to passivity in emotionally stressed and traumatized human beings. Linked to depression and victim abuse because of learned helplessness. Book: *Authentic Happiness: Using the New Positive Psychology to Realize Your Potential for Lasting Fulfillment* (2002)

Source: Adapted from T. Butler-Bowden, *50 Psychology Classics: Who We Are, How We Think, What We Do* (Boston, MA: Nicholas Brealey, 2007).

TABLE 20-2   Case Studies Using Theoretical Models

Using the Rogerian model	The nurse provides client-centered care in her psychiatric setting. She listens to Shelly, a 16-year-old female who has just lost her mother, and she allows her to tell stories of how her mother was her best friend. The nurse nonjudgmentally allows Shelly to describe her guilt over having an argument with her mother the day before she died.
Using the Myers-Briggs Type Indicator	The nurse is providing care to 43-year-old JoEllen who talks excessively about her past. The nurse recognizes that JoEllen may have the Feeler personality type, and talking is her way of expression. Another patient, Ryan, is a 35-year-old executive who has a Thinker personality, consistent with his job as a manager. The nurse recognizes that Thinkers prefer direct information rather than excessive conversation.
Using Seligman's Positive Psychology	The nurse assists 28-year-old Amy, a victim of physical abuse, to avoid the passivity and pessimism that often comes with being abused. The nurse points Amy in the direction of hope, positive change, lack of acceptance of this "learned helplessness," and optimism about a new future.

- Share complete and unbiased information with patients/families, and make certain the information in accurate, timely, and complete.
- Healthcare leadership should collaborate with patients/families to develop and implement patient-centered policies, programs, education, and care delivery.

The Nurse–Patient Relationship

By walking alongside patients who are on healing journeys, nurses can foster truly mutual healing relationships using patient-centered care. Beyond establishing rapport, holistic nurses utilize authentic relationships, which represent true sharing of self and a willingness to be open and genuine within certain limits that protect patient well-being. Patient-centered care has been represented as a key means to achieve a healing relationship. Analogous to patient-centered care is the concept of the nurse–patient relationship or the nurse–client relationship.

Hagerty and Patusky assert that the nurse–patient relationship (NPR) is foundational to good nursing care. The interpersonal process that grows over a period of time defines the NPR.[2] This relationship is traditionally defined as having three distinct phases: a beginning phase involving the development of trust; a middle phase, which is the active working phase; and the ending phase, in which the relationship may be terminated. However, Hagerty and Patusky disagree with this traditional approach because even single encounters or short-term relationships with patients/clients can possess as much value as this three-step NPR. Shorter hospital stays and quick primary care or urgent care visits exemplify this shortened relationship; some nurses believe these short stays and the nursing shortage disallow building patient relationships. It has been observed that some NPRs are superficial and task oriented, which is infinitely less satisfying to most nurses. Interestingly, research has shown that nurses believe patients should desire relationships with them to work on identifying and improving healthcare needs. If patients reject the offered relationship and assistance, they may be seen as noncompliant and uncooperative. Evidence demonstrates that nurses obtain greater relationship satisfaction with patients who respond to their offered care.

Jackson[3] describes Halldorsdottir's classic qualitative research on nurse–patient relationships, which are categorized as uncaring and destructive to caring and healing using four terms: the biocidic relationship is considered toxic, the biostatic relationship in considered cold, the biopassive relationship is considered detached and apathetic, while the ideal relationship is bioactive. The bioactive relationship is described as concerned, kind, and life sustaining, as well as being the classic ideal nurse–patient relationship.

Biogenic relationships are described as loving, full of compassion, fostering of spiritual growth and freedom, and restoring of dignity and well-being. These are high-level interactions and are likely the most supportive of healing. Perhaps truly optimal, biogenic, healing relationships place people in the best settings for Nature to act on them, as Nightingale theorized.

Theories About Relationships

Barbara Dossey's Theory of Integral Nursing, a grand theory, transcends holistic nursing theory and includes multiple dimensions of interrelationships. Within the theory are four quadrants demonstrating how human beings experience their world through relationships. The "I" quadrant represents the individual; the "We" quadrant demonstrates relationship to others within the context of culture, values, and vision, for example; the "It" quadrant represents the physical body; and the "Its" quadrant represents relationships to environment and social systems. Further, integral nursing values the patient–practitioner relationship, the community–practitioner relationship, and the practitioner–practitioner relationship. The patient–practitioner relationship is an ideal combination of psychosocial spiritual care along with biotechnological care that favors holistic ideals. The community–practitioner relationship involves working with families, coworkers, companions, community, hospital, and religious organizations within the sphere of the practitioner. The practitioner–practitioner relationship involves collaborative and interdisciplinary work with the goal of improving patient care. See Chapter 1 for more detail.

Nurse theorists Paterson and Zderad describe the importance of person-to-person relationships in their humanistic nursing theory. Relationship occurs through presence, inferring, being with, and doing with another. These theorists believe "through relating with other persons as presences, individuals become more and realize their uniqueness" and so that presence is a gift of self.[16] This concept implies that people grow and improve through relationship. Learning to understand others gives each person the opportunity to appreciate the uniqueness of his or her self. Presence is characterized by spontaneity, availability, and reciprocity in a mutual nurse–patient relationship. Reciprocity is considered a flow between two people in a shared situation. The nurse's goal is to nurture well-being. The nurse–patient relationship is a type of community, implying two or more people moving toward a common goal. Paterson and Zderad utilize Martin Buber's concept of "I-Thou" as the ideal relationship, as compared with "I-It." "I-Thou" refers to viewing the other as a valued, integral whole, while "I-It" refers to viewing others without relationship and caring. The theorists mold Buber's work into a nursing framework emphasizing that a person comes to know himself or herself as a unique person primarily through relationship to others.

Nurse theorist Jean Watson has developed a Science of Caring over the past 3 decades, drawing from the work of Florence Nightingale and Martha Rogers, and this science is said to be the hallmark of nursing practice. One of the major concepts of *Caring Science* is that it is *transpersonal*, defined as a subjective human-to-human relationship in which the nurse affects and is affected by the person of the other. Both are fully present in the moment and feel a union with the other, and thus share a phenomenal field that becomes part of the life history of both. Transpersonal Caring affirms both the unity of life and the fact that relationship connections are made with individuals, groups, communities, the planet, and the universe (spiritually speaking).[17] Nightingale actually described the concept of transpersonal caring long ago by advocating that nurses maintain full use of self, connect with humanity, the environment, Nature, the cosmos, and the divine within and without.[18]

Relationships, according to Watson, may develop a spiritual dimension as in the transpersonal human relationship that transcends person-to-person relationship and evolves into spirit-to-spirit relationship within what Watson terms a "caring moment." This segment in time is capable of connecting the spirits of two or more people on a spiritual level. According to Watson, a transpersonal caring relationship, such as that typifying the nurse–patient relationship, involves an energetic communication of intentionality (i.e., desiring the highest good of the other), consciousness, and full presence. Outcomes of transpersonal healing include improved self-knowledge, self-healing, and self-control. The Ten Caritas Processes affiliated with Caring Science, as shown in **Exhibit 20-1**, describe values in the ideal nurse–patient relationship and transcend to describe other life relationship ideals.[19]

Erickson, Swain, and Tomlin use the work of Maslow, Erikson, Piaget, Selye (Adaptation Response), Seligman (Positive Psychology), and Bowlby (Attachment Theory) to develop their theory titled *Modeling and Role-Modeling*. This theory posits that the nurse–client relationship is the essence of nursing and that it should be interactive and interpersonal. Concepts integral to modeling and role modeling include assisting patients to adapt to adversity and maintain their biopsychosocial functioning, as well as promoting self-care among nurses. Five significant goals of nursing interventions include creating trust, assisting the client to maintain control, encouraging a positive orientation, promoting client strength, and assisting the client to set goals as well as promoting needs such as love, belonging, self-esteem, safety, and biophysical wellness. It is evident that Modeling and Role-Modeling is a theoretical framework that promotes a therapeutic healing relationship as well as a patient-centered nurse–client relationship.[20] Key concepts for nurses to consider in using this holistic nursing theory include the following: unconditional acceptance of the patient, no matter what his or her background is; facilitating the identification of personal strengths; and nurturing the client to utilize his or her affective and cognitive abilities, as well as physical abilities, toward improved health.[21]

A nurse who matches her breathing pattern to that of her patient or who paces with a patient who is manic to engage him is using

EXHIBIT 20-1   Ten Caritas Processes

1. Embrace altruistic values and practice loving kindness with self and others.
2. Instill faith and hope and honor others.
3. Be sensitive to self and others by nurturing individual beliefs and practices.
4. Develop helping–trusting–caring relationships.
5. Promote and accept positive and negative feelings as you authentically listen to another's story.
6. Use creative scientific problem-solving methods for caring decision making.
7. Share teaching and learning that addresses the individual needs and comprehension styles.
8. Create a healing environment for the physical and spiritual self that respects human dignity.
9. Assist with basic physical, emotional, and spiritual human needs.
10. Open to mystery and allow miracles to enter.

Source: Watson Caring Science Institute, "Dr. Jean Watson's Human Caring Theory: Ten Caritas Processes." http://www.watsoncaringscience.org/caring_science/10caritas.html.

synchrony to facilitate the NPR and maximize the potential for healing. By matching and modeling the patient's pattern, the nurse can then role-model a different way of being, should the patient desire that. This modeling behavior is an example of Erickson, Tomlin, and Swain's theory of care. Progressive relaxation, imagery, guided imagery, breathing, and hypnosis are techniques that can be used to carry out the concepts of this nursing theory. These modalities are all within the scope of nursing practice. A nurse who has learned how to use his or her whole self as an instrument of healing will be more sensitive to cues from others and can make a profound healing difference in someone's life in a very short time using his or her expanded repertoire of healing interventions.

■ RELATIONSHIP TO OTHER LIVING BEINGS

For many people, relationships with animals are as important as relationships with other people. Pets, in particular, dogs and cats, are capable of providing love, affection, companionship, and fidelity in an unconditional manner. Animal-assisted therapy has become very popular, and studies have shown remarkable health benefits. Animals can be taught to enhance their human bonding and provide remarkable services to those with hearing and vision impairments. Matuszek performed an extensive literature review on the use of various animals for animal-assisted therapies.[22] In addition to the services just mentioned, animals, especially dogs, have been used to provide an incredible number of services in such areas as palliative care, geriatrics, Alzheimer's units, pediatrics, physical therapy and correctional facilities. Animal-assisted therapy can help patients with psychological disorders, multiple sclerosis, spinal cord injuries, developmental disabilities, post-myocardial infarction, and veterans with posttraumatic stress disorder. The relationship between human beings and animals is considered mutually beneficial, and studies reveal such benefits as reduction in lipid levels, heart rate, blood pressure, depression, and loneliness. More than 60% of U.S. households include pets, and people bond so greatly with their pets that these relationships may supersede human–human relationships for some. Holistic nurses need to be aware of the myriad of benefits of animal-assisted therapies, or just of owning or being with a pet.

Relationship to Nature is yet another means to interact with living things. Many people feel at peace being in Nature, hiking on a tree-shaded forest path, sitting by the ocean in the salt air and feeling the sea breezes, or lovingly tending a home garden. All of these, and other activities involving Nature, demonstrate relationship to living plants, living waters, and living ecosystems. Kline describes four studies that used visual and auditory nature scenes and sounds to promote improved pain relief.[23] McCaffrey studied the benefit of garden walking on older adults with depression and found it efficacious.[24] She notes that gardens have been shown to be a distraction from negative stimuli, relaxation enhancers, and also a means to promote positive attitude. Anecdotally, it is said that plants often thrive by being "talked to"!

■ SPIRITUALITY AND RELATIONSHIP TO A HIGHER POWER

Physician Herbert Benson, cardiologist and a legendary mind–body researcher, stated years ago that human beings are "wired" for God,[25] and others have agreed. This implies that no human being can achieve true happiness without a relationship with a Higher Power, also variably called the Source, the Divine, God, Christ, Buddha, Yahweh, Spirit, Universal Energy, and so forth. Maslow's hierarchy of needs suggests that those moving closer to self-actualization also move closer in their search for the Source. Nurses need to acknowledge that people of different religions may view relationship with a Higher Power in myriad ways, and some religions do not worship one God or they may worship many gods.

How does a human being develop a relationship with the Divine? According to Burkhardt and Nagai-Jacobson, prayer is considered the most fundamental and primordial language human beings use.[26] Through prayer, which can be accomplished at any moment of the day or at a set time, in such modalities as silence, contemplative prayer, meditation, chanting, music, reading of scripture, or simple conversation with God, human beings can form increasingly intimate relationships with the Divine. Helming describes the lived experience of being healed through prayer.[27,28] Sixteen of 20 participants who attributed most of their healing to prayer, even if they utilized allopathic and integrative modalities, described the essence of this healing as *spiritually transformative*.

In monotheistic religions, such as Christianity, Judaism, and Islam, many feel that God reaches out to people through the Old or New Testament or the Koran. Some religions assist people to find spirituality in themselves; through other inspirational readings; through Nature, art, and music; and through silent times spent in meditation or contemplative prayer. Other religions, such as Buddhism and Hinduism (God is Brahma, but there are other gods as well), emphasize doing good in life. Buddhists do not believe in one God but still place much importance on spirituality and peace.

Some feel that people never reach their potential without having a right relationship with the Divine. Communicating with and about a Higher Power may take many forms, such as prayer, journaling, inspirational writing about spirituality, sermons, prayer groups, meditation, and contemplation. For some, it is necessary to have periods of solitude away from the noise and chaos of daily life, to "hear" the still, small voice of God within. Some people believe that "Higher Power" does not need to be God but may be Nature or a sense of spirituality outside of oneself, a power larger than oneself. This is the concept expressed in Alcoholics Anonymous, to allow nonbelievers to receive hope and help from their Higher Power, however they conceive it.

It is indeed possible to develop an enhanced relationship with the Divine, just as one gets to know a friend better by spending time with him or her. Shirer says, "Our desire shouldn't be to impress God, but to have a relationship with Him. That's how we get close to Him and learn to recognize His voice."[29] This requires daily thought and constant communication, not only once a week or in crisis communication. As with any other healing relationship, this requires complete honesty with the Supreme Being and complete trust in Him. It requires time to build and work to maintain this relationship. This may be the most significant relationship that any human being needs to develop, and it is a two-way relationship. In the famous novel *The Shack*, the main character meets God and is told by Him: "The friendship is real, not merely imagined. We're meant to experience this life, your life, together, in a dialogue, sharing the journey. You get to share in our wisdom and learn to love with our love."[30]

Qualities That Enhance Relationships

Three of the most vital concepts in healthy relationships are trust, forgiveness, and appropriate boundary setting.

Trust

It has been traditionally felt that an ideal nurse–patient relationship requires the development of trust before patients can open up and engage in active problem resolution. Trust is an essential element of the therapeutic and healing relationship as well.

Messina and Messina term trust "the glue or cement of relationships" and further describe trust as having several beliefs and attitudes implicit in its development.[31] First, people who believe in a Higher Power tend to develop an intrinsic trust that God is ever present and caring. The popular phrase "Let go and let God" implies a willingness to trust the Higher Power's direction, assistance, and concern. Second, a sense of hope in the essential goodness of humankind assists people to trust rather than distrust on most occasions. Third, a healing environment where acrimony, blame, and hurtful actions are nonexistent allows trust to flourish. In this environment, health communication, forgiveness, and openness promote the development of trust.

Another vital step in building trust includes the ability to risk being vulnerable, implying risking hurt from others through self-revelation of one's weaknesses as well as one's strengths. This self-disclosure is usually necessary in the growth of trust. Self-acceptance is a meaningful component of building trust because it implies self-trust and self-love, vital to the development of strong, healthy, trusting relationships. The following statements are some of the roadblocks and false beliefs that impair the building of trust:

- Excessive hurt in the past, creating fear of being hurt again
- Being hurt by loved ones
- A belief that people cannot be trusted
- A belief that people manipulate others and use them
- A history of physical, sexual, or emotional abuse or neglect
- Having been put down repeatedly for one's beliefs or feelings
- Unresolved grief, leading to fear of opening up to others because of the possibility of abandonment
- Being the victim of a hostile or violent relationship, or of an acrimonious divorce
- Being raised in an unpredictable and often volatile environment

- Having such low self-esteem that one believes he or she is not worthy of trust or love
- A fear that being vulnerable (opening up and revealing one's true self) is dangerous and can be used against you[31]

Forgiveness

One of the most significant hallmarks of healing relationship is forgiveness. To be empowered to forgive, it is necessary to release the anger and struggle that is part of resentment. This can alter a relationship immeasurably. There are all levels of forgiveness: of self, of spouse or significant other, of children, of parents, of coworkers, of friends or family, and of God.

Dincalci believes that forgiveness is transformative.[32] He states: "People who have completely forgiven all the people and situations in their lives have a much more joyful existence. They get sick less often. In fact, some say they don't get sick at all as long as they hold no grudges or resentments toward people. Their interactions with others are much more pleasant and productive than they were before their forgiveness transformations." Through his work in Forgiveness Therapy, he has found that some clients who learn to forgive encounter a religious experience, develop a deeper understanding of life, and discover that all of their relationships tend to improve and are less subject to turmoil.

Delaney, Barrere, and Helming completed a research study that included community-dwelling older adults utilizing a Heart Touch meditation technique to help heal and appreciate personal relationships.[33] Forgiveness was a prominent theme as noted by such statements as: "I had not spoken to my sister for several years and I realize now that it is time for us to reconnect. I was able to let go and to focus on bringing in joy to my life and spreading it around. I called her last week for the first time in years." The Heart Touch, used in addition to meditation, encouraged the participants to feel connected to others by imagining a circle of light moving from their heads to their hearts, along with remembering a time of feeling loved or loving. This Heart Touch technique enhanced connection to the Higher Power and the sending of loving energy to the persons being visualized.

Boundaries

Boundaries are artificial separations between people that can be either healthy or unhealthy. They define the perimeter of a relationship. In psychotherapeutic work and in the therapeutic nurse–patient relationship, it is vital to recall that the nurse or therapist should have therapeutic neutrality, that he or she should not give directives about major life decisions to the patient or client. Nurses and others in therapeutic roles are often held in high esteem, and the patient should not assume the "child" role of adhering to major life decisions set forth by the nurse or therapist. The patient–provider relationship assumes that the provider has power because the patient is seeking help from him or her. This is an asymmetrical relationship. The nurse or therapist is not intended to remain totally neutral, and emotion can be expressed, but neither should the nurse or therapist reveal significant personal information to the patient. This is a healthy boundary issue, with attempts to keep the relationship objective and helpful.

Therapeutic relationships between a provider and patient are often considered a dyad of two, but in reality, they are really a triad because the family is always the third aspect of the relationship triangle, even if they are not physically present. This is because most people act within family relationships and are highly influenced by them. Parents may feel they are to blame for their child's emotional disorders, and this is exaggerated by keeping parents out of child counseling. It is suggested that family counseling and individual child counseling go together, for this reason. Family members can be extremely useful in counseling because they give the nurse or therapist another perspective on the patient's life, and they can become engaged in being helpful in recovery. Family therapy allows the nurse or therapist to view family interactions, but this dynamic can be just as visible in a hospital setting or home care visit where the patient is observed interacting with family members in front of the nurse.

Boundaries can be considered rigid, permeable, or semipermeable. A formal relationship may be seen as more rigid and family relationships as more permeable (i.e., diffuse with ease of exchange between parties). An example of a boundary issue occurs when a parent acts as too much of a "friend" or "peer" to his or her adolescent child, and thus the boundary is too permeable to promote executive decisions that the parent must make regarding the adolescent.[34]

Nurses are constantly faced with boundary issues. In hospital and home situations, nurses see very personal sides of their patients and their families. Nurses must maintain professional boundaries, not revealing too much personal information, and keeping safety always in mind. However, the nature of nursing and therapeutic relationship is such that we may transcend ordinary conversation and converse with patients and clients on a much deeper level.

Signs of ignored boundaries include the following:

- *Disassociation:* "Blanking out" during a stressful circumstance keeps a person out of touch with his or her feelings and may impair memories of the circumstance.
- *Excessive detachment:* People in families or groups operate too independently and there are no common goals or identities. The union is not healthy.
- *Chip on the shoulder:* As a result of anger over past emotional or physical violations or one's rights being ignored, the person creates distance.
- *Over enmeshment:* Everyone must follow the same rules and think the same way; uniqueness is not permitted.
- *Martyrdom or victim state:* Victims isolate themselves defensively to avoid further hurt or allow themselves to continue to be victimized by others in the martyr state.
- *Distant and cold:* Barriers are set up to prevent others from entering one's emotional or physical space. These are usually related to avoidance of past hurt or rejection.[33]

Table 20-3 reveals distinctions between healthy and unhealthy boundaries, as described by Messina and Messina.[34]

■ DISORDERS IN RELATIONSHIPS

Selected psychological issues that create unhealthy relationships are discussed in this section. These include an explanation of psychological defense

TABLE 20-3 Distinctions Between Healthy and Unhealthy Boundaries	
Healthy Boundary	**Unhealthy Boundary**
I have a right to say "no" to others if it is an invasion of my space or a violation of my rights.	I can never say "no" to others.
I have a right and a need to explore my own interests, hobbies, and outlets so that I can bring back to this family or group my unique personality to enrich our lives, rather than be lost in a closed and overenmeshed system.	I should do everything I can to spend as much time together with you or else we won't be a healthy family or group.
I have a right to take the risk to grow in my relationships with others. If I find my space or rights are being violated or ignored, I can assertively protect myself to ensure I am not hurt.	I can never trust anyone again.
I have a right to take care of myself. If they want to stay together as a family or group, it is up to each individual to make such a decision.	It is my duty to hold them together.
There is a line I have drawn, which I do not allow others to cross. This line ensures me my uniqueness, autonomy, and privacy. By drawing this line I am able to be me the way I really am rather than the way people want me to be. With this line I let others know that this is who I am, where I begin, and you end.	I can never tell where to draw the line with others.

Source: Adapted from J. J. Messina and C. M. Messina, Building Healthy Boundaries. http://www.coping.org/growth/trust.htm.

mechanisms, anger, power and control issues, and attachment disorders.

Defense Mechanisms

According to Freud, defense mechanisms are thought processes that protect the ego and help us to deal with stress.[35] In their daily interactions, nurses frequently encounter the six most commonly used defense mechanisms. *Denial* is used to distance oneself from a perceived threat. It often appears that the person in denial is ignoring or denying reality. This mechanism can be helpful, as in the case of a family who gives a loved one the gift of a good death by laughing with the dying person and living life as fully as possible despite the knowledge that this loved one will likely not live for much longer. It can be harmful, as in the case of an addicted person who does not address his or her addiction.

Rationalization is a process of filtering or reframing reality to make that reality more acceptable. It can involve not taking full responsibility for one's actions, and it can sometimes lessen the emotional impact of one's circumstances. *Projection* is used when one does not want to take responsibility for one's own thoughts and feelings. With this mechanism one ascribes one's own intentions, feelings, or motives to another person and does not take ownership of the thoughts or feelings. This defense mechanism can be particularly tricky to identify and is very threatening to clear communication.

Displacement involves transferring unpleasant emotional pain from the direct source of the pain to another, less threatening person or thing. For example, someone who is angry with his or her boss but who does not feel comfortable confronting the boss instead may become angry with a colleague or a family pet.

Repression is the unconscious denial of painful thoughts or feelings. For example, by repressing potentially upsetting memories, the conscious mind is not confronted with uncomfortable material. However, this unconscious material may affect a person's behaviors, moods, and health in undesirable ways until the content is brought to conscious awareness and healed.

Humor is frequently used to share otherwise unpleasant, unacceptable, or unwelcome thoughts and feelings. It involves the body and the mind and can release stress associated with negative thoughts and feelings. Although humor is not always perceived in a positive way (for example, gallows humor), laughter can provide physiologic benefit and assist in coping with difficult circumstances.

Defense mechanisms can interfere with healthy relationships. They can create distance from the truth and block honest dialogue. Many of the psychological frameworks discussed in this chapter address why people use defense mechanisms and how to manage them effectively in counseling.

Anger

Anger is a transient but forceful emotion arising out of a threat. It may be expressed openly, or it may be suppressed quietly and persist as chronic resentment. Resentment is the long-term persistence of the pain of anger, long after the initial situation that sparked the anger has subsided. People may suppress their anger because it makes them feel ashamed or is inconsistent with their image of themselves as good people. Anger can serve the following functions:

- It may give a sense of power, strength, and pride.
- It can be a motivator of change, but it generates fear and opposition as well.
- It can control others by manipulating them or making them feel guilty.
- It may keep others away so that the angry person feels less vulnerable and safer.
- It can be used as a defense mechanism to avoid communicating about painful or difficult topics, including the situation that caused the anger.
- It can keep a person in the role of victim, and there is sometimes secondary gain to feeling the victim or the martyr.[36]

Psychologically, some people are passive-aggressive. This implies that they remain passive and quiet externally, but they are repressing anger internally. The anger seeps out in small ways, such as going behind another's back to gossip about him or her in a spiteful way, while remaining superficially pleasant to the other. Defensive mechanisms that are commonly used in anger include a penchant to withdraw and isolate oneself, as well as the impulse to express anger openly in out-of-control rage, verbal abuse, and insults. Anger can become extreme and manifest in explosive anger and rage. Holistic nurses frequently have to handle patients and clients who are angry at life, at others, at themselves, and at their illnesses. Helping patients to comprehend their anger, particularly when it is repressed, and assisting them to move toward forgiveness are essential aspects of the therapeutic nurse–patient relationship.

Power and Control Issues

Dominant personality patterns can cause relationship conflicts. Controlling people tend to assert themselves over others and exert power over them. Although there are people who are willing to be subservient to controlling personalities, others reject this and power battles ensue. People with obsessive-compulsive personality disorder tend to be highly controlling, rigid, and perfectionistic. They often fail to allow others to participate in projects or discussions, feeling that their way is the only right way. These people are capable of being highly devoted to their work, which can be seen in a positive or negative light. There is a preoccupation with inflexible rules, details, and lists. The disorder termed obsessive-compulsive personality disorder is different from obsessive-compulsive disorder, in which the person feels compelled to repeat specific behaviors, such as hand washing and counting.

The nurse seeking to develop and maintain caring relationships understands the inherent inequities of power that exist in most encounters between health providers and patients. Inequities regarding the hierarchical structure of institutions, race, sex, gender, education, occupation, and socioeconomic status must be monitored as the nurse seeks to collaborate with patients and families in promoting health and planning care. The unique language of health care, the schedules and routines within these environments, and the lack of partnership between patients and their care providers all reinforce these power differentials. By offering clients more choices, using language that is free of jargon, and sharing important information relevant to their care, nurses can reduce the power differential between patients and providers. Reducing the power differential between patients and professionals increases the likelihood of a partnership and aids the facilitation of healing. Nurses are in an ideal position to maximize the potential benefits of this healing alliance because they are inherently often more approachable than, for example, physicians. Truly, the core of healing power is in the exchange within the healing relationship itself.

Without establishing relationships, nurses cannot do their often intimate work sensitively and accurately. The quality of nursing care is greatly affected by the quality of relationships between nurses and those they care for, as well as by the relationships among caregivers in the professional setting. This web of relationships creates a community complete with its own cultural norms, and this environmental context has a tremendous effect on the delivery of care.

Attachment Disorders and Inability to Form Relationships

One of the most essential components of being able to relate to others is a sense of trust. This ability to trust is established in the first months of life. If the primary caretaking process of an infant is disrupted in any way by any means, the individuals' ability to trust fully may not develop and all future relationships can be adversely affected. This is termed reactive attachment disorder (RAD) and is essentially a form of early posttraumatic stress disorder. The *Diagnostic and Statistical Manual of Mental Disorders*, 4th edition (*DSM-IV*) acknowledges that severe deprivation or multiple, successive caregivers are etiologic factors in RAD. RAD begins in children younger than 5 years old and, often, in infancy; it is considered a relatively new diagnosis and is seen with greater frequency among adopted or foster care children. The *DSM-IV* essentially defines two subtypes of RAD:

1. *Inhibited RAD*. Children fail to initiate or respond to social relationships as appropriate for their age. Theoretically, the etiology of this abnormal attachment is the loss of the primary attachment figure and the inability of the child (usually the infant) to attach to a new primary caregiver. Also, an infant may never have had the chance to develop a relationship with a sustained caregiver.

2. *Disinhibited RAD*. The child is indiscriminate in relationships, overly familiar with strangers, and has diffuse attachments, rather than a primary attachment figure. The etiology may be the loss of the primary attachment figure(s) or multiple caregivers without consistency. Stranger anxiety is lacking because the child is accepting of any caregiver and acts with strangers in a familiar way.[37]

There are numerous, typical signs and symptoms of inhibited RAD, including failure to thrive; blank expression; lifeless eyes; avoidance of eye contact; avoidance of closeness, hugs, and touch of others; lack of awareness of body language; lack of focus; and lack of ability to note others' facial expressions. This generates a lack of trust in others, such that psychological defense mechanisms, including ambivalence and avoidance, dominate relationships so that the child is not disappointed with the caregivers. This creates a negativity surrounding the child's lifelong relationships, causing deep insecurity. Disinhibited RAD signs and symptoms include overfriendly approaches to strangers without normal stranger anxiety, hugging people who approach them, and asking strangers to give them food, toys, or comfort. This child is typically exposed to multiple caregivers simultaneously, and there is no ability to develop trust in just one person. Therefore, the child often copes using psychological defense mechanisms, including no expectation of being comforted or cared for by adults, suppression of fear, inability to trust, and total self-reliance for survival. There is usually an indiscriminate use of anyone available (e.g., strangers) to provide pseudo comfort. Children with disinhibited RAD may be seen climbing onto the laps of total strangers, seeking comfort and leading to risk of abuse and endangerment.

These children require the care of mental health professionals trained in attachment disorders. Play therapy, family, and skilled parenting are essential. It is interesting to note that RAD is often misdiagnosed as other disorders, such as attention deficit hyperactivity disorder, oppositional defiant disorder, and bipolar illness, and comorbidities with other mental illness are common as well.

Fraley notes that this same system of attachment that serves to bond children and parents is also relevant for adults to develop emotionally intimate relationships.[38] Research of Brennan, Clark, and Shaver suggests that adult attachments have two primary variables:[39]

1. *Attachment-related anxiety.* High scorers worry whether their adult partners are attentive and available, and low scorers are more secure about their partners.
2. *Attachment-related avoidance.* High scorers usually fail to rely on other people or discuss personal issues with them, and low scorers are more at ease with depending on others, having others depend on them, and being intimate and open with others.

Kassel, Wardle, and Roberts studied the association between adult attachment security and the development of substance abuse (cigarettes, alcohol, and marijuana) among college students.[40] Those with insecure attachment, represented by dysfunctional attitudes and self-esteem, as well as fear of abandonment, had a higher incidence of substance abuse, especially alcohol abuse.

■ HOLISTIC CARING PROCESS

Holistic Assessment

In preparing to use relationship interventions, the nurse should assess the following parameters:

- The client's social support system and social network
- The quality of the client's relationships as perceived by the client, including the client's satisfaction with these relationships
- The client's use of clear communication and patterns of relating
- Predominant relational styles (e.g., shy and withdrawn, outgoing and gregarious, controlling, passive, aggressive, mutual)
- Use of defense mechanisms
- Evidence of boundaries
- Boundary issues (e.g., evidence of codependency in relationship)

Identification of Patterns/ Challenges/Needs

The patterns/challenges/needs (see Chapter 7) compatible with relationship interventions are as follows:

- Withdrawal
- Denial
- Repression
- Rationalization
- Regression
- Changes in parenting and family structure
- Human sexual dysfunction
- Lack of social coherence
- Spiritual disconnectedness and distress
- Altered family process
- Ineffective coping
- Self-care deficits
- Self-care dysfunction
- Anxiety
- Grief
- Fear
- Response to trauma

Outcome Identification

Exhibit 20-2 guides the nurse in client outcomes, nursing prescriptions, and evaluations for effective relationship interventions.

In addition to effective outcomes with clients, it is important to examine possible outcomes for nurses and clients as follows:

- The nurse will recognize family and relationship patterns.
- The nurse will identify healthy boundaries in each interaction, assertively confronting any putdowns or defense patterns.
- The nurse will recognize opportunity for effective negotiations and conflict management, using the characteristics of effective communicators.
- The nurse will work from the dimension of mutual respect, valuing both self and others without discounting either.
- The nurse will increasingly see opportunities for new relational patterns in challenging situations.

Therapeutic Care Plan and Interventions

The holistic nurse's careful planning and preparation enhance the effectiveness of relational

EXHIBIT 20-2   Nursing Interventions: Relationships

Client Outcomes	Nursing Prescriptions	Evaluation
The client will recognize personal and relationship patterns and how they support or detract from quality of life.	Assist the client in identifying the following: ▪ The importance of relationships ▪ The patterns that increase comfort and effective communication ▪ Family relationship patterns and areas that could be improved ▪ Sources of emotional stress in his or her relationships ▪ The human needs that are fulfilled by quality relationships ▪ The impact of relationships on health and illness	The client verbalized the dynamics within the family relationship patterns. The client stated the importance of his or her relationships to quality of life. The client identified areas in which relationships could be improved. The client recognized factors that create stressors in relationships. The client stated understanding of the interconnection between relationships and health or illness.
The client will recognize and identify harmful defense mechanisms in relationships.	Demonstrate examples of defense mechanisms and help the client to identify such problems in family and caregiver relationships.	The client identified defense mechanisms in use within the relationship.
The client will increase awareness of parent, adult, and child ego states.	Demonstrate examples of the differences among the three ego states.	The client identified his or her personal use of parent, adult, and child ego states.
The client will identify personal response patterns to others' ego states.	Assist the client in identifying personal response patterns to others' ego states, and help the client to improve the effective expression of inner feelings. Describe the four archetypes and their applications in communicating physical, emotional, mental, and spiritual perspectives.	The client recognized another person's use of an ego state and his or her personal response.
The client will incorporate new strategies to improve the quality of interpersonal relationships.	Provide the client with techniques to improve relationships, such as making "I" statements (e.g., "This is how I feel . . . My feeling is . . ."), noting ego states in a transaction, and activating the four archetypes.	The client showed interest in the four archetype patterns and willingness to try out new communications from each perspective.

EXHIBIT 20-2   Nursing Interventions: Relationships *(continued)*

Client Outcomes	Nursing Prescriptions	Evaluation
The client will increase awareness of the physical, emotional, mental, and spiritual aspects of relationship interactions.	Teach the client to express awareness of physical needs and take responsibility for practical aspects of his or her care, such as need for more information and understanding of optimal outcomes.	The client demonstrated the ability to express personal feelings using "I" statements.
The client will recognize opportunities for effective negotiations with willingness to reconsider ineffective aspects.	Assist client to identify areas where he or she can negotiate, make choices, or reconsider previous decisions; to see the open-ended nature of present relationships, especially with caregivers and family; and to view the present disease as an opportunity for learning and change.	The client negotiated effectively after considering options. The client reconsidered relationship interactions that were ineffective. The client expressed interest in the open-ended nature of learning from his or her illness and treatment.

interactions. The following are guidelines for planning and implementing effective relational patterns.

Before the session:
- Take a moment to set your intent and focus, allowing yourself to breathe fully, to sense your center, and to align with your sense of purpose.
- Take several deep breaths and relax the body.
- Rehearse a new pattern, such as giving accurate facts, in your mind.
- Imagine the successful outcome.
- Acknowledge your positive intent.
- Be willing to learn from each experience.

During the session:
- Notice the ego states that are in evidence, specifically the feelings that are triggered within yourself.
- Be aware of ways that finding common ground enhances rapport.
- Consider options that can achieve the goal of the communication.
- Make "I" statements when speaking about your personal point of view or experience; avoid "you" statements, which can be taken defensively and negatively.

- Set limits by determining time frames, topics to be discussed, the context, and the environment.
- Be willing to change direction or reconsider a point to come to feasible compromises.
- Above all, keep the intent of the communication positive and maintain a relationship of mutual respect, even though specific content areas may be questioned and differing viewpoints may be expressed.

At the end of the session:
- Use the client outcomes (see Exhibit 20-2) to assess the ways in which you assisted the client in moving toward goals of understanding relationship patterns.
- Consider alternatives and make concrete plans for future action.
- Evaluate your own relational skills, your use of different ego states, your use of the archetypes, your own personality style, your Myers-Briggs pattern, and so forth.
- Honor your learning process by accepting mistakes and thinking about what you might have done differently.
- Consider methods that will make trying new behaviors safe and enjoyable, such as sharing your process with a friend or mentor.

Suggestions for Implementation

The following eight major personal characteristics are ones that have been found most helpful in moving toward more effective relationship styles, according to Hover-Kramer:[41]

1. Willingness to look at personal defenses and "blind spots"; identifying and letting go of defense patterns
2. Holding an accurate sense of self-worth, confidence, and self-esteem; neither with an overinflated sense of self nor putting oneself down unnecessarily
3. Flexibility; looking at things from different perspectives, "walking in another's shoes," and thinking "outside the box"
4. Willingness to take personal responsibility for feelings or actions, known as emotional intelligence; using "I" statements rather than blaming and using indirect "you" language
5. Intentionality and boundary setting that allow a clear sense of purpose, goal orientation, and direction
6. Motivation to be understood and perseverance to find common ground; seeking and integrating feedback
7. Empathy and mutual respect for others without appeasing, complying, or attempting to be overly pleasant
8. Willingness to revisit, rethink, and redefine previous decisions; accepting the possibility of being wrong and thereby allowing others the space to acknowledge their mistakes as well

The following topics also demonstrate ways in which holistic nurses can assist in improving relationship issues of their patients and clients.

- *Facing fears:* People may have difficulty altering relationship patterns because of fear. Holistic nurses can help patients and clients become aware of their nonverbalized fears and rationally evaluate them. People tend to expect the worst, when in fact, that is not usually what happens.
- *Improved communication:* Nurses can assist clients to verbalize their emotions and fears by identifying them and labeling them. Nursing knowledge of psychological defense mechanisms, factors that improve or destroy relationships, and psychological theories all play a role in identifying appropriate communication styles that create healthy relationships.
- *Counseling:* Nurses are skilled at interpersonal relationship work and can counsel patients effectively. Nurses are fully capable of counseling patients for wellness interventions, such as smoking cessation, weight control, and proper nutrition. Many nurses without advanced psychiatric skills are still capable of beginning therapeutic counseling, and then referring patients over to higher-level mental health care. Understanding the basic psychological theories and concepts within this chapter can assist holistic nurses in beginning levels of counseling.
- *Storytelling:* It is recognized that telling stories about one's experiences and problems can be highly therapeutic. It is common to feel a sense of relief in sharing personal experiences and thoughts with another. This is a very significant nursing role. Nurses can help clients to acknowledge their strengths, as well as weaknesses, through the power of story. Use of story may enhance relationship building by helping the client empathize or understand the life stories of others. If the nurse repeats the story back to the client, there is the potential for the client to see relationships in a new light.
- *Nurses' relationships with others, including co-workers:* First and foremost, nurses accept responsibility for bringing caring and sensitivity into their relationships with their patients or clients. If effective relating to clients were enough, nursing professionals would have an easy task because most nurses demonstrate deep caring and respect for those for whom they have responsibility. It is also necessary, however, to address intricate interactions with coworkers, who possess a wide variety of backgrounds, skills, and educational levels. Thus, nurses may have ongoing transactions with colleagues ranging from a sophisticated medical specialist who focuses solely on a single domain, to a nursing aide who may have little training

in interpersonal skills or understanding of person-centered values. Bringing these various interactions into harmony with holistic ethics, theory, and philosophy is a challenging task. It also offers a grand opportunity for building teamwork through effective relationship interventions.

Time Urgency in Nursing

Unfortunately, relationships take time. The single most frequent complaint from practicing nurses—whether nurse practitioner, operating room nurse, or nursing faculty—is the lack of time. We are oriented to view the nursing process as a linear one that requires time to first establish rapport and trust. How can healing take place when there is no time to listen to patients?

Jean Watson refers to the importance of "caring moments" between nurses and others. These moments of eye contact or touch can be transforming, even though they take only seconds. Amplified by the intention of the nurse, powerful healing can be facilitated even while doing other, seemingly task-oriented nursing activities. Hagerty and Patusky explicate a different way of viewing the brief but essential relationships nurses often encounter.[2] When viewed as a dynamic interaction, each encounter between a nurse and patient can be a valuable relational moment where mutual goals can be attained, even within a very brief time period. Ideally, nurses should have as much time as possible to be with patients. However, when this is not possible nurses need not feel all is lost.

Often there is no time to establish trust, yet trust on specific levels occurs all of the time—for example, one trusts a nurse one has only just met at a physician's office to give a safe injection of a correct substance at an appropriate dose. Through reciprocity (i.e., the idea that the patient has something to give to the nurse as well), patients can feel empowered. The importance of here-and-now interactions is emphasized. So, rather than being discouraged with time restrictions, nurses should see their interactions as nonetheless effective. Mottram describes how nurses working in day surgery developed therapeutic relationships with their patients; most patients reported they felt the nurses' presence, befriending, and comfort giving.[42]

Healing the Healer

Wise educators and nurse leaders build systems into the routine that decrease the isolation of the healer, enabling nurses to regularly share feelings and responses to the difficult physical, emotional, and intellectual work that is nursing, as in staff debriefings. These gatherings can be interdisciplinary.

Nurses represent the largest professional group within the healthcare field. Nurses, nurse educators, advanced practice registered nurses, and nurse leaders are in need of enhanced training in self-healing and self-care to avoid burnout that is so typical of healers. In 1951, Carl Jung first wrote about the concept of the *wounded healer*.[43] The concept is that all healers (physicians, nurses, etc.) are "wounded" in some ways in their own life histories, and this wounding enables them to care for their patients in a more collegial fashion than with a supervisory style. Wounded healers may also react negatively to patients, without being aware of their subconscious motivations, for example, when a nurse whose father was an alcoholic cannot tolerate alcoholic patients and displays no empathy toward them. Conti describes two types of wounded healers:

- *Walking wounded:* "An individual who remains physically, emotionally and spiritually bound to past trauma. This wounding can be reflected in the nursing practice of the individual in many ways. The walking wounded have limited consciousness related to how their pain is manifested in their lives."
- *Wounded healer:* "Through self reflection and spiritual growth, the individual achieves expanded consciousness, through which the trauma is processed, converted and healed."[44]

The ideal situation is for healers to work through their own traumas and woundings so that they can use themselves therapeutically in healing patients.

■ CONCLUSION

How, then, can holistic nurses apply these skills to therapeutic relationships with patients or clients? First, the holistic nurse brings a sense of

EXHIBIT 20-3 Evaluating the Nurse's Subjective Experience with Relationship Interventions

1. Can you continue to identify and be aware of a relationship that is troublesome to you?
2. Is it possible for you to be clear about your wants and expectations in this relationship?
3. Have you tried out new patterns, such as making a conscious choice of a different ego state? What was the result?
4. Have you considered the transactions in this relationship to make them more complementary? Have you considered how to make the transactions in this relationship more complementary?
5. Is it possible for you to communicate your strengths in this relationship? What are the strengths and intent of the other person that you could also acknowledge?
6. Can you imagine how the Healer in you could approach this relationship? How about the Teacher? The Visionary? The practical, grounded Warrior?
7. What would a healed relationship with this person be? How would you feel?
8. Can you identify the steps you could take to move in this direction?
9. What interventions would be most helpful in moving toward healing this relationship?
10. Do you have any questions about any of the new strategies that you have learned for healing this relationship?
11. What is your next step?

presence to the encounter. He or she becomes more self-aware and pays attention to self-care and personal growth so that he or she can be present with clients. He or she can calmly focus on the here-and-now and be totally present for the "other." Current research supports mindfulness practices and training (such as Kabat-Zinn's Mindfulness-Based Stress Reduction program) that involve breath awareness, body scan, and yoga as increasing self-awareness and compassionate presence in helping professionals.[45] In this way, cues and perceptions are attended to in the dialogue, in the "space between." As explained by the concepts of Watson, the energy fields of the nurse and patient may overlap. In a momentary glimpse of time, the nurse and patient or client may become one in relationship.

Right relationship implies a therapeutic and, therefore, helpful relationship. As explained, there are many ways for relationships to become destructive. However, holistic nurses are focused on helping patients and clients achieve healing of the bodymindspirit. Even without extensive psychiatric training, nurses can incorporate tenets of one or more psychological models in their therapeutic and healing relationship skills. We know it is vital for patients and clients to

tell their stories. People need to be heard, and in this day of abbreviated medical and nursing encounters, it is difficult to have the time simply to listen to detailed patient and client stories. Nonetheless, there is a universal human need to be heard, and if nurses bear that in mind, the accuracy and compassion of the nursing care are amplified, enriching the healing relationship for both the client and the nurse. **Exhibit 20-3** lists several questions that help to evaluate a nurse's subjective response to relationship interventions.

Directions for
FUTURE RESEARCH

1. What tools can be used to measure the quality of the nurse–patient relationship?
2. How does the quality of the nurse–patient relationship influence patient outcomes?
3. How does the quality of the nurse–patient relationship influence nurse satisfaction?
4. Is it feasible to include the quality of a nurse's therapeutic relationships as part of the nurse's performance evaluation?
5. Does a program of "relationship training" for nurses enhance patients' perceptions of quality of care?

Nurse Healer
REFLECTIONS

After reading this chapter, the nurse healer will be able to answer or to begin a process of answering the following questions:

- How do I feel at the end of the workday?
  - Can I acknowledge the child within?
  - What gives me pleasure?
  - What bothers me?
  - Which defenses do I use?
  - What do I wish I had done differently?

- Were there any unpleasant interactions?
  - What other options could have been considered?
  - Do I need to forgive anyone?

- Are there repeated patterns in my relationships?
  - Are there anger or control issues?
  - How can I change the pattern?

- Will I be able to practice new responses with a friend or coworker?
  - What will I do differently?
  - Will I have support from trusted friends?
  - Will I honor and acknowledge myself as a growing, learning being, aligned with inner light and truth?

 For a full suite of assignments and additional learning activities, use the access code located in the front of your book to visit this exclusive website: http://go.jblearning.com/dossey. If you do not have an access code, you can obtain one at the site.

NOTES

1. John Donne, "Devotions upon Emergent Occasions" (circa 1600).
2. L. Keegan and C. Drick, *End of Life: Nursing Solutions for Death with Dignity* (New York: Springer, 2011): 108.
3. B. M. Hagerty and K. L. Patusky, "Reconceptualizing the Nurse–Patient Relationship," *Journal of Nursing Scholarship* 35 (2003): 145–150.
4. C. Jackson, "Using Loving Relationships to Transform Health Care," *Holistic Nursing Practice* (July–August 2010): 181–186.
5. E. C. Arnold and K. U. Boggs, *Interpersonal Relationships* (St. Louis, MO: Elsevier, 2011).
6. F. Dziopa and K. Ahern, "What Makes a Quality Therapeutic Relationship in Psychiatric/Mental Health Nursing: A Review of the Research Literature," *Internet Journal of Advanced Nursing Practice* 10, no. 1 (May 28, 2009): 11–19.
7. A. Scanlon, "Psychiatric Nurses' Perceptions of the Constituents of the Therapeutic Relationship: A Grounded Theory Study," *Journal of Psychiatric Mental Health Nursing* 13 (2006): 319–329.
8. D. Canning, J. P. Rosenberg, and P. Yales. "Therapeutic Relationships in Specialist Palliative Care Nursing Practice," *International Journal of Palliative Nursing* 13, no. 5 (May 2007): 222–229.
9. C. J. Porr, "Establishing Therapeutic Relationships in the Context of Public Health Nursing Practice" (doctoral dissertation, University of Alberta, Canada, 2009).
10. D. C. Zuroff and S. J. Blatt, "The Therapeutic Relationship in the Brief Treatment of Depression: Contributions to Clinical Improvement and Enhanced Adaptive Capacities," *Journal of Consulting and Clinical Psychology* 74 (2006): 130–140.
11. Association for Humanistic Psychology, "Humanistic Psychology Overview." http://www.ahpweb.org/aboutahp/whatis.html.
12. T. Butler-Bowdon, *50 Psychology Classics: Who We Are, How We Think, What We Do* (Boston, MA: Nicholas Brealey, 2007).
13. J. Watson, *The Philosophy and Science of Caring.* (Boulder, CO: The University Press of Colorado, 2008, p. 86). Retrieved June 12, 2011, from http://www.nightingaleexpressed.com/images/FloQuotesWeb.pdf12
14. B. M. Dossey, *Florence Nightingale: Mystic, Visionary, Healer,* Centennial ed. (Springhouse, PA: Springhouse, 2010).
15. Remaking American Medicine: Health Care for the 21st Century, "Receiving Patient-Centered Care." http://www.pbs.org/remakingamericanmedicine/care.html.
16. N. O'Connor, *Paterson and Zderad: Humanistic Nursing Theory* (Newbury Park, CA: Sage, 1993).
17. Watson Caring Science Institute, "Caring Science Ten Caritas Process." http://www.watsoncaringscience.org/index.cfm/category/62/theory.cfm. www.watsoncaringscience.org/index.cfm/category/62/theory.cfm
18. J. Watson, "Florence Nightingale and the Enduring Legacy of Transpersonal Human Caring-Healing," *Journal of Holistic Nursing* 28, no. 1 (2010): 107–108.

19. Watson Caring Science Institute, "Dr. Jean Watson's Human Caring Theory: Ten Caritas Processes." http://www.watsoncaringscience.org/index.cfm/category/61/10-caritas-processes.cfm.

20. H. Erickson, *Modeling and Role-Modeling: A View from the Client's World* (Austin, TX: Unicorns Unlimited, 2006).

21. H. Erickson, Swain, and Tomlin, derived from http://www.mrmnursingtheory.org/

22. S. Matuszak, "Animal-Assisted Therapy in Various Patient Populations," *Holistic Nursing Practice* 24, no. 4 (July–August 2010): 187–203.

23. G. Kline, "Does a View of Nature Promote Relief from Chronic Pain?" *Journal of Holistic Nursing* 27, no. 3 (2009): 159–166.

24. R. McCaffrey, "The Effect of Healing Gardens and Art Therapy on Older Adults with Mild to Moderate Depression," *Holistic Nursing Practice* 21, no. 2 (2007): 79–84.

25. H. Benson, *Timeless Healing: The Power and Biology of Belief* (New York, NY: Simon and Schuster, 1996).

26. M. A. Burkhardt and M. G. Nagai-Jacobson, "Spirituality and Health," in *Holistic Nursing: A Handbook for Practice*, 5th ed., ed. B. M. Dossey and L. Keegan (Sudbury, MA: Jones and Bartlett, 2009): 617–645.

27. M. A. Helming, "The Lived Experience of Being Healed Through Prayer Among Adults Active in a Christian Church" (doctoral dissertation, Union Institute & University, 2007).

28. M. Helming, "The Lived Experience of Healing Through Prayer: A Qualitative Study," *Holistic Nursing Practice* 25, no. 1 (January–February 2011): 33–44.

29. P. Shirer, *He Speaks to Me: Preparing to Hear from God* (Chicago, IL: Moody Publishers, 2006): 162.

30. W. P. Young, *The Shack: Where Tragedy Confronts Eternity* (Newbury Park, CA: Windblown Media, 2007): 189.

31. J. J. Messina and C. M. Messina, "Building Trust," http://www.coping.org/growth/trust.htm.

32. J. Dincalci, "Forgiveness Transforms!" http://howtoforgivewhenyoucant.com/whyforgive.php.

33. C. Delaney, C. Barrere, and M. Helming, "The Influence of a Spirituality-Based Intervention on Quality of Life, Depression, and Anxiety in Community-Dwelling Adults with Cardiovascular Disease: A Pilot Study," *Journal of Holistic Nursing* 29, no. 1 (March 2011): 21–32.

34. J. J. Messina and C. G. Messina, "Establishing Healthy Boundaries." http://jamesjmessina.com/growingdowninnerchild/healthyboundaries.html.

35. B. L. Seaward, *Managing Stress: Principles and Strategies for Health and Well-Being* (Sudbury, MA: Jones and Bartlett, 2006).

36. R. Casarjian, *Forgiveness: A Bold Choice for a Peaceful Heart* (New York: Bantam, 1993).

37. R. Lubit, "Child Abuse and Neglect: Reactive Attachment Disorder." http://www.emedicine.com/ped/topic2646.htm.

38. R. C. Fraley, "A Brief Overview of Adult Attachment Theory and Research." http://internal.psychology.illinois.edu/~rcfraley/attachment.htm.

39. K. A. Brennan, C. L. Clark, and P. R. Shaver, "Self-Report Measurement of Adult Romantic Attachment: An Integrative Overview," in *Attachment Theory and Close Relationships,* ed. J. A. Simpson and W. S. Rholes, 46–76 (New York: Guilford Press, 1998).

40. J. D. Kassel, M. Wardle, and J. E. Roberts, "Adult Attachment Security and College Student Substance Use," *Addictive Behaviors* 32 (2007): 1164–1176.

41. D. Hover-Kramer, "Relationships," in *Holistic Nursing: A Handbook for Practice*, 4th ed., ed. B. M. Dossey, L. Keegan, and C. E. Guzzetta, 672 (Sudbury, MA: Jones and Bartlett, 2005).

42. A. Mottram, "Therapeutic Relationships in Day Surgery: A Grounded Theory Study," *Journal of Clinical Nursing* 20 (2009): 2830–2837.

43. S. Daneault, "The Wounded Healer: Can This Idea Be of Use to Family Physicians?" *Canadian Family Physician* 54, no. 9 (September 2008): 1218–1219.

44. M. Conti, "The Theory of the Nurse as Wounded Healer: Finding the Essence of the Therapeutic Self." http://www.drconti-online.com/theory.html.

45. S. Shapiro, W. Brown, and G. Biegel, "Teaching Self-Care to Caregivers: Effects of Mindfulness-Based Stress Reduction on the Mental Health of Therapists in Training," *Training and Education in Professional Psychology* 1 (2007): 105–115.

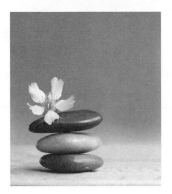

Chapter 21

Dying in Peace

Melodie Olson and
Lynn Keegan

Nurse Healer
OBJECTIVES

Theoretical

- Use theories of grief, self-transcendence, and culture to guide the process of helping the dying to experience their deaths peacefully and meaningfully.
- Discuss with colleagues difficult issues surrounding the care of dying people.
- Interview patients who have experienced nearing death awareness.

Clinical

- Explore personal myths and beliefs about death with colleagues.
- Use comeditation to help a dying patient experience peace.
- Use the life review process to help a person experience a sense of integration.

Personal

- Plan your ideal death.
- Record several imagery scripts and experience "letting go" with these exercises.

DEFINITIONS

Culture: Socially transmitted ways of life including but not limited to language, arts and sciences, thought, spirituality, social activity, and interaction.[1]

Death: A moment in time.

Dying: A stage of life that fits into a broader philosophy, giving both death and life meaning.

Grief: A response to loss, characterized as dynamic, pervasive, individual, yet normative.

Loss: The absence (or anticipated absence) of someone or something of real or symbolic meaning.

Mourning: The expression of a sadness or sorrow resulting from a loss.

Myth: Story lines created by individuals and cultures about meaning and journeying in life.

Nearing death awareness: The dying person's knowledge of death and attempts to describe this experience to healthcare providers, family, and friends.

Perideath: The last hours of life, the actual death, and the care of the body after death.

Self-transcendence: A spiritual concept referring to moving one's self into a wider sense of consciousness and understanding.[2]

Spirituality: "The essence of our being." (See also Chapter 32.)

■ THEORY AND RESEARCH

To die peacefully, to die with the knowledge that life has had meaning and that one is connected through time and space to others, to God, and to the universe, is to die well. Helping people to die well requires knowledge and skill, as well as a willingness to be intensely involved in the most intimate phases of another's life. Physical, spiritual, psychological, and social distress must be addressed with concern and compassion. The nurse, in being present "in the moment" with the patient and family, inevitably confronts her or his own mortality. Care for the caregiver (professional and family) is a requirement, a part of the care of the dying. The patient and the family are the unit of care.

One approach to easing the burden for those who are caring for the terminally ill is based on Watson's Theory of Caring.[3] Her theory of human caring focuses on the relationship between the whole person of the caregiver (nurse) and the whole self of the client/family as it protects and preserves the humanity and dignity of the client. In this partnership or relationship between caregiver and client and family, the burden becomes shared; each can ease the other's burden. Developing theories to guide end-of-life care are based on standards of care, like those identified by professional associations, state laws, and culture. Theories related to grief and loss, self-transcendence, myths and beliefs (two components of culture), and nearing death awareness are particularly useful in formulating effective plans of care for the dying.

Grief and Loss

Grief theory links concepts of loss, bereavement, and mourning into a fabric of ideas that help decide action on the part of caregivers, family members, and patients. Grief is not only normative, but dynamic, pervasive, and individual. Each individual moves through bereavement at a different pace and copes in a different manner, depending on inner resources, support, and relationships. Society may think that the period of mourning has been long enough (a normative statement), but the individual may need more (or less) time before beginning to take charge of a changed life.[4]

Grief is a necessary process for both the dying person and his or her significant others. The more bonded and intimate two people have been, the more intense the grief. Grief is pervasive, affecting every area of life. Therefore, it affects relationships, physical symptoms, feelings, spirituality, and one's sense of meaning in life and schedules of care. The person who is dying integrates care (e.g., regular laboratory tests, visits to the healthcare providers, various therapies) into a full schedule. As death grows closer, visits by family and friends may be welcome. But there comes a time when the one who is dying needs time to become introspective, to consider life's messages and meanings. At any of these stages, caregivers may feel excluded from the dying one's life, wanting to be present yet having difficulty "reaching" the loved one.

Hope increases as death approaches, but the nature of hope changes. Hope for less pain, for example, is common, when hope for a cure has been abandoned. Hope is a basic construct of spirituality and has been recognized as having both physiologic and psychological value. Families and staff caregivers share in hope as it relates to spirituality and the end of life. The whole team grieves, and the whole team helps each other through the process.[5,6]

Spiritual development is related to the phases of grief originally identified by Kübler-Ross.[7] Nursing care during each of the phases takes into account the spiritual maturity of the griever, whether it is the dying person or those who love that person. A person who is in the early stages of spiritual maturity, whether a child or an adult, needs much external help, information, communication, and developing trust. This person may not achieve acceptance (and transcendence) without moving to a higher level of spiritual development. For comfort persons who have a more formal spiritual practice may use rituals, rites, symbols, and activities that incorporate them; thus, they may find comfort in planning their own funeral. Skeptics may build on the comfort found in the formal structures but often add intellectual processes, such as bargaining with medical science (e.g., becoming part of experimental studies), reading books on death and dying, considering their contributions in this life, yet acknowledging a fear of the final moments—fear of pain and loss. Those in the final spiritual stage believe in a common bond uniting humanity, the world, and the universe. They are attracted to the mystery of faith.[8] Therefore, the dying person in this stage may worry more about others, become angry about the effect the disease or the dying has on loved ones, choose humanitarian goals, become introspective and prayerful, and contact family and friends to say goodbye.

Nursing care requires a careful assessment of a dying person's spiritual resources to assist with peaceful death. Dossey's description of the last moments of her mother's life shows a beautiful integration of past ways of her mother's worship practices (Bible verses) and modern, familial ritual created especially for her.[9]

The nurse's own developing spiritual maturity can be a useful support, as when one accompanies an acquaintance for a while along a road. The nurse maintains an attitude of being open, listening, and assessing the client's path even when his or her own journey changes directions. Successfully dealing with grief allows the dying client to achieve peace and allows the family and significant others to move on with a changed life, cherishing memories while creating new ones.

Self-Transcendence

Many people have studied self-transcendence, the sense of a temporal integration of self, the feeling that past and future enhance the present. In studying survivors of concentration camps, Frankl discovered that those who survived seemed to transcend (beyond self) either toward other people or toward meaning.[10] Transcendence may occur through creativity, the family, or works of art; through receptivity toward others; or through acceptance of a situation that cannot be changed. People who can be identified as self-transcendent at the end of life tend to have less depression, less self-neglect, and less hopelessness.[11] They have a greater sense of well-being and a greater ability to cope with grief. The self-transcendent person lives in the present and usually sees death as a normal part of life. Encouraging people to seek meaning and connections, either in the present or through the ages, helps people move toward self-transcendence to achieve peace.

Measures to support one's movement toward self-transcendence build on the need to look inward for connectedness and a sense of timelessness. Life review—the systematic review of one's life to see that it was meaningful, to remember those who are loved, and to know

one's own place in history—is one example of a useful process.[12] Life review is the story of this life, of living in this space on this Earth in this time. Studies show that systematic life review helps reduce depression and anxiety, and it promotes a feeling of "This was my life, no one else would have done it this way, and I have a unique place in this universe."[13]

Myths and Beliefs

Myths are our story lines, values, beliefs, and images; they are our personal manual about the meaning and the journeys of the human spirit.[14] Myths help us seek the unfolding mystery in life. In seeking life's meaning and purpose, personal myths help us manifest hope, learn to accept daily struggles and challenges, and deal with ambiguity and uncertainty. Myths help us recognize strengths, choices, goals, and faith. They also help us to assess our perception of our world, recognize our capacity to pursue personal interests, and demonstrate love of self and self-forgiveness. Myths provide a sense of connection and of oneness with all of life and nature.

Throughout life, we create many myths; some serve us well, while others hinder our healing journey. More than 30 years ago, the Senior Actualization and Growth Exploration (SAGE) study began to question society's beliefs about older people and their potential.[15] The researchers taught seniors deep relaxation, biofeedback, breathing exercises, meditation, yoga, and ways to expand creativity through movement, music, art, education, and group discussion. This project not only helped the participants reshape their declining years to an understanding of healthy aging and lifestyles that promote the goal of healthy aging, but also gave them new, practical ways to cope with personal problems and a more confident self-image. With healthier lifestyles, most people can add a vital 30 or more years to their life span. There is also more time to practice a new way of living so that dying in peace is a clear choice for each person.

Nearing Death Awareness

When people become aware that they are approaching death, they often talk about two things. They may attempt to describe what they are experiencing while dying, and they may request something that they need for a peaceful death. This awareness is not to be confused with near-death experiences that happen as a result of cardiac arrest, drowning, or trauma in which a person feels the self suddenly leave this life, but quickly return. In a state of nearing death awareness, a person's dying is slower, often because of a progressive illness such as acquired immunodeficiency syndrome (AIDS), cancer, or heart or lung disease. The person becomes aware of a dimension that lies beyond, a drifting between this world and another, perhaps a space of transcendence, yet not one that touches "an Ultimate." The slower dying process allows the dying person to have more time to assess his or her life and to determine what remains to be finished before death. Some dying patients try to describe being in two places at once or somewhere in between. It is a time for a caregiver to respond to the dying person's wishes and needs and to listen to what dying is like for that person. It is at this time that discussions about the patient's wishes about cardiopulmonary resuscitation should be heard if this topic has not been discussed prior to this time.[16] This can be a period of challenge for many caregivers, and yet it can help each of us to prepare for what may happen in our dying. Those individuals who are tired of living but who do not believe that it is time to die describe the dying process differently from those who are truly ready to depart. The statements of those who are truly ready are different in the clarity with which the words are spoken, the look in their eyes, or their touch. Their statements, looks, or touches are like no others that have been made before or during the dying process.

■ HOLISTIC CARING PROCESS

Holistic Assessment

In preparing to use interventions for promoting peaceful dying, the nurse assesses both the dying person and the family or significant others in the following areas:

- The different emotions that surface during the process:
  - *Guilt:* Blame of self and others over management of the dying person; distress over inability to decrease pain
  - *Anger:* Toward God, disease, family or significant others, doctors, or survivors, over inability to fix things physically, emotionally, and spiritually
  - *Ability to laugh:* The shortest distance between two people; relationship between comedy and tragedy (joy and sadness pathways cannot operate simultaneously)
  - *Love:* An essential element in living and in dying; a state of self-giving and presence of being a person, where openness and willingness exist for self or another; the network that brings and weaves families and significant others together to work through the dying process and move into total acceptance of death
  - *Fear:* Often evocation of separateness and aloneness, but can become a path leading deeper into the present moment; useful in that it reveals areas of resistance; return to unconditional love and a sense of equanimity after release of fear
  - *Forgiveness:* Essential element for inner peace; an exercise in compassion that is both a process and an attitude; not necessarily reconciliation
  - *Faith:* The larger vision of existence, which is different for each person; helps to harness energy to evoke healing resources and power
  - *Hope:* Support of patient or family and significant others during death's darkness; an inner moment that perceives lightness when in the midst of darkness and has the potential for leading to deeper love; hope for decreased pain and increased physical and spiritual comfort, for a miracle, for peace of mind, for a remission, for peaceful death transition, and for acceptance of a shorter life than expected or the death of a loved one
- The patient's interactions with others and the effect of the patient's emotions on these interactions
- The need for education about what will happen and what can be done to help, for the family and the patient
- Comfort needs, assessed according to the patient's culture and wishes for
  - Pain control and symptom management
  - Hydration

- Nutrition
- Respiratory assistance
- Movement
- Touch
- Signs of psychiatric illness, under- or over-medication that may interfere with a patient's ability to cope with dying
  - Hallucinations
  - Delusions
  - Depression
  - Denial that interferes with the ability to move toward comfort and peace
  - Excessive anxiety
  - Confusion, agitation, or memory loss, especially in older adults
  - Advanced dementia

Identification of Patterns/Challenges/Needs

Following are the patterns/challenges/needs compatible with dying in peace interventions. (Also see Chapter 7.)

- Altered circulation
- Altered oxygenation
- Altered body systems
- Altered communication
- Effective communication (see the section titled "Nearing Death Awareness" earlier in this chapter)
- Spiritual distress
- Spiritual well-being (see the section titled "Nearing Death Awareness" earlier in this chapter)
- Ineffective individual or family coping
- Self-care deficit
- Body image disturbance
- Powerlessness
- Hopelessness
- Pain
- Anxiety
- Death anxiety
- Grieving
- Fear

Outcome Identification

Exhibit 21-1 guides the nurse in identifying patient outcomes, nursing prescriptions, and evaluation for assisting patients and their families and significant others during the dying process.

Therapeutic Care Plan and Interventions

The following guidelines are appropriate both for the dying person and the caregivers, whether family, friends, or nurse. They are helpful in all settings. The guidelines apply from the first awareness of a coming interaction with a patient and family who are moving through the dying process, through dying, and afterward.

Before the interaction:

- Spend a few moments centering yourself to recognize and honor your presence there. Become a healing presence, be in the present moment with the client/family . . . believing in and affirming their dignity and wholeness.
- Begin the session with intention to facilitate healing and peaceful dying. This may be a prayer.

At the beginning of the interaction:

- Encourage the patient and the family and significant others as the caregiver(s) to do the following:
  - Set realistic goals.
  - Identify different behaviors that have surfaced in their interactions with each other during this period.
  - Gather a healing team and honor the patient's personal needs and feelings to avoid more suffering.
  - Accept current circumstances, and release things that are beyond their control. Accept the fact that release may not be possible at this time, but they can work toward it.
  - Take frequent breaks, at least 20 minutes daily, to evoke high-quality quiet time with relaxation, imagery, music, meditation, prayer, journal keeping, or dream work to assist in the process of letting go.
  - Exercise, take long hot baths or showers, eat nutritious foods, eliminate excess caffeine or junk food, and ask other people for relief.
- Encourage the patient and caregivers to tell themselves over and over what a good job they are doing and that it is the best job that they can do. Repeating it helps in releasing guilt, anger, and frustration.

EXHIBIT 21-1   Nursing Interventions: Dying in Peace

Client Outcomes	Nursing Prescriptions	Evaluation
The patient will demonstrate an understanding of reasons for ongoing assessment and management of anxiety, including ■ Quiet environment ■ Explanations of all personnel, procedures, and equipment ■ Touch and reassurance by nurse ■ Relaxation skills	Continue to reassess states of anxiety and provide ways to decrease anxiety. ■ Provide quiet environment. ■ Explain all interventions. ■ Offer reassurance. ■ Teach relaxation and imagery skills.	The patient demonstrated an understanding of the reasons for assessment and management of anxiety.
The patient will verbalize feelings of anxiety and will talk spontaneously about fears. (If the patient is intubated, the patient and the nurse use specific communication codes.)	Provide high-quality time for the patient to share worries and fears. Use common symbols for communication if the patient is intubated.	The patient verbalized anxiety and fears.
The patient will use effective coping mechanisms during course of illness.	Focus on the patient's strengths.	The patient used effective coping mechanisms during the course of illness. (List specific examples.)
The family will communicate stressors associated with the patient's illness to staff.	Allow time for the family to express worries and fears.	The family or significant others communicated stressors to staff.
The patient will verbalize fears of death.	Be present with the patient, and allow time for the patient to talk about fears of dying.	The patient talked of death.
The family and significant others will verbalize fears that the patient may die and what this means to them.	If death seems imminent, be with the patient and family to assist them through the death.	The patient's family or significant others acknowledged the impending death and shared feelings about death.
The family and significant others will receive support from nurses and clergy.	Provide spiritual support for the patient through presence, life review, prayer, talking, and handholding. Allow the family to be with the patient. Call clergy for assistance, if requested.	The family or significant others received spiritual support and talked to nurses and clergy.
The patient, family, and significant others will express fears and other feelings associated with dying and death.	Assist the patient and family to focus on what has been accomplished in life. Provide as much privacy as possible.	The patient and the patient's family focused on life accomplishments.

EXHIBIT 21-1   Nursing Interventions: Dying in Peace *(continued)*

Client Outcomes	Nursing Prescriptions	Evaluation
The patient will experience closure on matters of daily living.	Provide the opportunity to complete "unfinished business." Fulfill the patient's requests to see a member of the family, lawyer, member of the clergy, or a physician.	The patient and the family completed unfinished business.
The patient will be comfortable and participative until death occurs.	Evaluate the procedures and treatments that can be discontinued to make the patient more comfortable. Make provisions for someone to remain with the patient all the time if so desired by the patient.	Procedures and treatments were used for comfort only.

During the dying process:

- Recognize the one who is dying as the person who is usually the best teacher about what is right. The place of death is not as important as the care, trust, compassion, acceptance, and love that was provided and shared in the perideath interactions.
- Determine the care needed. The whole family should consider the following questions and issues:
  - Will the dying person receive better care in a hospital, in a hospice, or at home?
  - What kinds of medical treatment, technology, and equipment are needed?
  - What information is needed to make decisions about care choices (e.g., providing hydration, withholding nutrition)?
  - Can a hospice nurse or healthcare professional assist with treatments and medication?
  - Is a parish nurse or congregational nurse available for liaison with the congregation involved?
  - What expenses will be involved? What expenses will be covered by insurance? Is the patient eligible for state or federal disability payments, veterans or Social Security benefits, or Medicaid or Medicare?
  - Who will assume the care 24 hours a day? Who will provide respite care? Are there children at home who also need continu- ous care? Can the care of the dying person and young children both be managed?
  - Will some or all of the organs be donated?
- Explore the advantages and disadvantages of dying at home (or alternative sites). Advantages for staying in the home include the freedom of the patient and the family to do anything they wish because they can change or alter routines and schedules at will. In addition, staying in the home makes the continuous support of family, friends, and even pets available. It allows meals to be prepared fresh and served with attention to details; it eliminates the stress of traveling to and from the hospital or hospice; it provides the unique beauty of familiar surroundings; it makes high-quality time available to focus on inner work for the moment of death; and permits the patient and family to experience feelings and emotions in a different way because their closeness is subject to fewer interruptions. Finally, the patient and family can make most of the decisions regarding care, medication, and treatments and can ask advice from professionals when needed. Disadvantages to staying at home may include inadequate support for coping with care needs or competing needs for care by small children, older adults, and other sick or disabled family members. When available, inpatient hospice units may help

blend some of the advantages of care in the home with the additional support an individual may need that significant others cannot provide.

- Integrate therapies.
  - Does the dying person believe that medical and nonmedical modalities are complementary?
  - How motivated is he or she to try nonmedical resources (e.g., acupuncture, aromatherapy, touch therapies, music)?
  - What nonmedical resources are available?
  - Does the dying person really want to try different modalities, or is he or she receiving so much advice about therapies that the response is passive rather than active?
  - Is the dying person choosing to try therapies to please caregivers? A patient should feel free to choose not to include complementary therapies if they are not wanted.
- Incorporate the senses in rituals.
  - *Touching:* Lovingly, freely, and joyfully convey through your hands what your heart is feeling. Touching is a powerful way to break the illusion of separateness, loneliness, and fear; it may evoke laughter, calmness, or tears. Create times to give and get hugs. Hold a hand now and then. Avoid touching if it is not welcome.
  - *Smelling:* Use lotions and colognes with mild fragrances, remembering that illness will probably change the types of fragrances that can be tolerated. Use caution because some odors cause nausea and unpleasant feelings. Try light, natural scents such as rosemary or vanilla, perhaps as a plant growing in the room or a candle in the bathroom (remembering safety considerations with an open flame).
  - *Tasting:* Remember that taste varies with degrees of illness but stays with us until the end of life. Tasting and eating have social and symbolic meaning to patients and family. Explain what will happen if the patient stops eating within the progression of terminal illness, that it may be normal and may not cause undue suffering. Provide tastes and foods that are desired.
  - *Seeing:* Arrange in a pleasing manner healing objects and different touchstones that have special meaning and symbolize people, places, and events in the patient's life. A room that receives soft, subdued rays from the sun can bring balance to surroundings. Sitting out on the patio in good weather allows the patient to feel the sun as well as see the sunlight. Light colors are usually more soothing than dark colors.
  - *Hearing:* Remember that the sense of hearing is often sharp to the end of life, so special words at death can be heard. Be present in silence also, sitting or holding one another. Music can be nice, but not all the time.
- Practice sitting quietly with relaxation, meditation, or prayer. Gentle sounds from wind chimes or environmental recordings of ocean waves, wind, rain, birds, and music (e.g., harp, flute, stringed instruments) can offer a sense of peace. Music thanatology, referred to as sung prayer, uses the human voice when chanting or singing to bring balance to the dying, dissolving fears and lessening the burden, sorrows, and wounds.[17] Use words ending in *ing* such as *releasing, letting, floating, softening* or words ending in *ness* such as *openness, beingness, awareness, vastness* to help the patient to relax.
- Recognize the patient's going in and out of awareness. The moment of death itself has no pain but is a reflex last breath. It opens up very special exchanges of intention, intimacy, and bonding where the patient may share the dying spaces. The patient's eyes can take on a staring, a glazing, a spaciness so different that the patient appears to be going to another realm of knowing or to be focusing on something that the caregiver cannot see; the dying person can return with a smile and possibly share that he or she was in a space of peace.
- Learn about changes in the body during dying. Knowing what body changes to expect as death approaches helps the family anticipate personal healing rituals and removes the fear, shock, and mystery from the moment of death.
- Understand and accept the body's shutting down. The conscious dying person knows that it is time to leave the physical body and

can choose to shut physical life down. The caregiver and family journey with the dying person as far as possible, and then tell the person it is all right to leave; this can evoke the purest, most special moments for all involved. For those people who wish to experience every morsel of life, even if that morsel is physical agony, respect the choice. For them, it may be inappropriate to suggest that they leave. Tell them that you love them and will stay with them as long as they need you (or a significant other).

At the moment of death:

- Prepare rituals for the moment of death. The dying person usually has serenity and inner calm, particularly if healing rituals have been carried out prior to death. Before the dying person's eyes close, tight brow muscles may become relaxed; the peace in the face or within the room is often palpable. Trust your inner wisdom for how to touch, hold, talk, and be with the dying one in ways that deepen hope and faith for a peaceful crossing into death and beyond.

- Surround yourself and the dying person with the peace and the light of love, taking the energy of love and light in with each breath; imagine and experience literally going inside the breath, flowing inside the breath with comeditation (see scripts in the section titled "Specific Interventions," which follows) into the death of each moment.

- Continue to communicate with family caregivers and those there to support the dying patient. Talk to the dying loved one as restlessness or agitation moves to unresponsiveness; give gentle love squeezes, touches, and hugs; play favorite music; read poems; or say mantras and prayers. Shut the half-closed eyes, stroke and hug the physical body, and adjust the loved one's head on the pillow for the last time. Give permission for this special person to be free, to soar, to meet God and others who have died before, if this is appropriate. Say all you need to say, and share your own kind of blessings for the smooth transition.

- If appropriate, when the person has taken a last breath, carry out additional rituals that may be helpful to those present. Holding hands around the bed, saying a blessing or prayer, or anointing with healing oil, for example, may be planned ahead of time for this moment.

- Schedule a follow-up session or visit with family and significant others, if appropriate. If grief support groups are available, a referral may be helpful.

- Take care of yourself. Adequate rest, relaxation, exercise, and nutrition are always important; the person who cares for dying people needs to "go apart for a little while." Center, meditate, celebrate, or plan your own self-renewal times. There are retreat centers and sanctuaries for those who wish to use them. Simply sharing your experience with others, either verbally or in writing (e.g., journaling, writing poetry or narratives), is helpful. Be glad for the opportunity to share such a sacred moment with others, and use those special times for your own growth.

Specific Interventions

Planning an Ideal Death

To help patients and families experience peace in the dying process, it is important to engage them in planning. To be of maximum assistance to someone else on the journey toward his or her own death, it is helpful for the nurse to explore this journey as well. The following reflective questions provide enormous insight about death myths, beliefs, problem solving, loving, and forgiving:

- What would an ideal death be like?
- When are you going to die?
- Where are you going to die?
- Who do you want to be with you, or do you want to be alone?
- What legal matters, relationships, or other personal business must be finished?
- What have been and what are the most precious events in your life?
- Who are the important people in your life?
- Have you told them why they are important?
- Are there family or friends who need to be told special things that you have never shared?
- Do you need to forgive or be forgiven?
- Have you written your obituary or your epitaph?

- Have you completed advance directives, in writing, and shared them with those involved?
- Who do you want to care for your pets?
- What are your assets?
- What treasures do you wish to leave to specific family members or friends?
- Who have you appointed to be in charge of your medical decisions? Does this person know what you want done?
- Have you planned rituals for your burial, or a funeral, memorial service, or cremation? Are they recorded and available to those who will perform them, whether family, religious institution, or funeral home?
- If you are to be buried, what do you want to be buried in?
- What kind of a coffin or container do you want for your body?
- Who will perform your burial ceremony?
- What kind of a ceremony do you want?
- Do you prefer a wake or another form of ceremony?
- What prayers, passages, poems, or music do you want to have used?
- Who will direct the ceremony? Or do you want a death day celebration for people to celebrate your life during or in place of a funeral, and to be celebrated in subsequent years?

Part of confronting death is deciding how to use medical care and technology. As part of their right to die, individuals can decide whether they want medical treatment; what kind of treatment; and under what circumstances to start, continue, or stop treatment. A power of attorney for health care records the appointment of someone to make medical decisions for the individual, should that become necessary. An individual can record his or her wishes as a living will for four different life situations: (1) mental incompetence, (2) terminal illness, (3) irreversible coma, or (4) persistent vegetative state. Recording information about the individual's wishes regarding organ donation is also important. Most hospital and hospice organizations have documents called advance directives available. These documents can be changed by the dying person as long as he or she is competent.

States vary in the legislative details of such documents. Specific information about the details to include in such a document can be found in the office of the state attorney general or by consulting an attorney. Furthermore, because these wishes often reflect philosophic, personal, religious, and spiritual desires, individuals should discuss these matters with the family and friends who will function on their behalf should they become incompetent. It is important for those who will be asked to make decisions to understand fully the nature of the request. Withholding of nutrition and fluids is often thought to be a cruel decision and a cause of suffering, yet history suggests that artificially feeding and hydrating a person who is clearly dying is an anomaly and reflects society's denial of death. Some research indicates that patients who stop taking food and fluids slowly sink into unconsciousness and coma over a period of 5 to 8 days and die several days later. Any discomfort that they experience, such as dry mouth, can be addressed with routine care. Those who make these kinds of decisions need to be fully informed, both about the patient's desires and about the effects of their wishes. Those who cannot do what the patient asks of them should have the choice of withdrawing from the decision-making role.

Learning Forgiveness

Forgiveness is important because it helps us get on with life. Many people are "stuck" in feeling guilt or assigning blame. Self-guilt leads to depression, and blaming others leads to anger. Both of these conditions steal energy and focus, reduce coping ability, and rob a person of precious time that could be used in establishing a positive relationship and attending to end-of-life goals. Dunn compares forgiveness to removing a thorn (the hurt that needs forgiveness) so that healing cam commence.[18] Many authors have described steps to forgiving self and others. They include: (1) taking responsibility for what we have done; (2) confessing the nature of the wrongs to ourselves, another human being, or God; (3) atonement, or being willing to make amends where possible, as long as we can do this without harm to ourselves or other people; (4) asking for forgiveness, if that is possible; (5) looking to God for help; and (6) receiving or accepting forgiveness. Steps to forgiving others are (1) acknowledging that a wrong has occurred; (2) recognizing that we are responsible for what we are holding onto; (3) confessing our story to ourselves, another person, and God; (4) receiving atonement, or considering whether any specific action needs to be taken; (5) looking to God for help; and (6) offering forgiveness.[19-20] These steps take time to complete. As the awareness of forgiving self and others is developed, we recognize unconditional love. Because it helps us connect more with our source of joy, not focusing on loss, sadness, or pain, unconditional love helps release us from fear.

Becoming Peaceful

Use relaxation and imagery scripts. To learn how to let go of attachments, what is right and wrong, and what is good and bad, requires commitment and practice. Nurses encourage patients to hear their inner voice of judging and to release the judging. Nurses encourage patients just to listen, be ready for the next moment of listening, and to be in the present moment. Centering, meditation, and contemplative prayer are helpful in learning to listen to the inner self. The skill of opening and releasing ordinary fears allows a person to emerge with awareness in the healing moment and to be fully present when assisting another during death.

Patients who are dying and their caregivers may set aside 20 minutes or more several times a day to practice opening to the moment. It may be helpful to create a special relaxation and imagery tape as part of a personal ritual to practice releasing and letting go. The breathing, relaxation, imagery, and music scripts that follow are important experiential exercises to help you and others learn the letting-go experience of calming the mind and creating a sense of spaciousness within the body. (See Chapters 16, 17, and 18.) Recording one or several of these scripts, after a 5- to 10-minute relaxation exercise, allows the dying patient and caregivers to use them repeatedly, even when professionals are not present. It is important to be sensitive about which scripts are likely to be useful for particular individuals. A person who has suffered from a respiratory disorder such as emphysema for many years may

not do well with a script focused primarily on breathing, for example. The following scripts are adapted from the work of Stephen Levine, and Anees Sheikh and Katrina Sheikh, who developed their work in the 1970s and 1980s.[21-23]

> *Script:* ***Introduction. (Name),*** as your mind becomes clearer and clearer, feel it becoming more and more alert. Somewhere deep inside of you, a brilliant light begins to glow. Sense this happening. The light grows brighter and more intense. Breathe into it. Energize it with your breath. The light is powerful and penetrating, and a beam begins to grow out from it. The beam shines into the core of your spirit.

> *Script:* ***Letting go.*** Notice the rhythm of the breath . . . becoming more aware of all the sensations that arise from the breath. Watching . . . noticing . . . feeling . . . as the breath begins to breathe you. As you become more aware of the breath, let your conscious awareness release the notion of breathing . . . becoming more and more aware as the breath arises in each moment. As interfering thoughts arise, let them float on . . . dissolving into awareness . . . quieting the constant chatter of the ego . . .

> *Script:* ***Opening the heart.*** Relax into the moment of the awareness of the breath . . . Let the rhythm of the breath just breathe you. Allow a fearful image to emerge in thought . . . noticing where it is in the body . . . letting the feelings of fear be in the body. In a way that seems right for you . . . let the fear move

to the center of your chest . . . to the center of your heart. There is space within your heart to let the fear be . . . noticing the sensations of fear as they rest in the spaciousness of your heart center . . . opening and softening . . . opening and releasing denial . . . letting the fears become what they need to be . . . opening and accepting. Within the center of your heart . . . your love and compassion are present to let the fear(s) be present.

Script: **Forgiving self and others.** Relax into the moment of the awareness of the breath . . . Let the breath just begin to breathe you. Allow yourself to let an image emerge of a person . . . alive or dead . . . who brings forth feelings of resentment. As that image is forming, . . . notice the spaciousness of your heart . . . and the openness of your heart center. Send the image of the person who causes you to feel resentment into your heart center. From the spaciousness of the center of your heart . . . hold the image of this person as you repeat, "I forgive you for anything you may have done in the past . . . in thoughts, words, or actions that may have caused you or me pain. I forgive you."

As you do this, . . . notice any change in the feelings of resentment . . . opening and softening to the moment. If any feelings such as pain . . . tightness . . . or any other body sensation arises . . . just let them be . . . watching . . . noticing . . . all changes . . . opening into the moment. Just continue to focus on the image of this person . . . speaking from your heart . . . releasing resentment . . . pain . . . forgiving yourself . . . forgiving others.

Script: **Releasing grief and pain.** With one or both thumbs or the palms of your hands, locate the point just at the base of your sternum, and press into this area; feel the point of maximum pressure for you. Notice any sensations of tension, pain, or aches that result from sadness, grief, and loss. Continue to hold the thoughts, feelings of yourself, the loved one you have lost, or any other person or issues that cause you to feel loss. If it seems right, as often as needed, return yourself to the power of the awareness of your own breath as it breathes you.

Relax into the moment of the awareness of the breath . . . Let the breath just begin to breathe you. Within your heart just now may be grief and pain . . . the feelings of loss . . . the heaviness of sadness. With your thumbs or the palms of your hands, . . . press into the area below your sternum . . . Become aware of any sensations of pressure, pain, or any aches. Continue to hold the pressure. As you notice the pressure in this area, . . . breathe slowly into the sensations as they arise . . . emerging through the many levels of protection. Let yourself open into the pain . . . being with the feelings that come . . . not holding back . . . not pushing away . . . opening . . . softening. Observing and experiencing . . . allowing the pain . . . the fear . . . the sadness . . . the loss . . . just to be . . . not evaluating. Continuing to hold the pressure . . . releasing control . . . become aware of the fear . . . all fears that come as you feel the fear of losing your loved one . . . all loved ones. And become aware of your fear of your own death . . . any pain, fear . . . anger . . . sadness.

Let all your feelings now penetrate to the center of your heart . . . opening to the moment . . . receiving the love . . . the caring . . . the warmth . . . coming from the center of your heart. And now . . . let yourself release the physical pressure . . . continuing to receive the love and caring from your heart center.

While consciously living, it is possible to experience conscious dying. It is helpful to use a relaxation or imagery technique to become grounded before the exercise. After the exercise, this same technique can facilitate the return to full alertness and readiness to proceed with daily activities. These scripts are intended to be a rehearsal, not an actual shutting down and leaving of the physical body.

Learning to confront our own death helps us be more present to assist others in facing their death. It reaffirms that we really need to do nothing but be present with another and speak with our hearts in dying time. The nurse may begin with an extended head-to-toe general relaxation or other breathing exercise (see the previous scripts). Because the experience of dying can be described as melting or dissolving away at the moment of death, the words *dissolving* and *melting* are used in the script. To continue this script, the four elements of the body described by the ancients—earth, water, fire, and air—are used to represent decomposition as the body dissolves.

Script: **Conscious dying.** Relax into the moment of the awareness of the breath. Let the breath just continue to breathe you. As you focus on the breath, . . . begin to notice how the breath lets you move from heavy sensations in the body to the lighter . . . subtle body of awareness . . . all awareness on the breath . . . the breath in . . . and the breath out . . . Let yourself be in the heavy body . . . and now all awareness on being in the light body . . . The breath is all that there is . . . just breathing . . . let each thought dissolve into the breath . . . melting into the breath . . . awareness of the light body . . . and now letting the breath go . . . this is the final breath . . . let the breath in . . . and the breath out . . . dissolving . . . opening to death . . . and let yourself die.

Script: **Earth.** The body . . . solid . . . heavy . . . mass . . . compact . . . all changing as death comes . . . the vital body losing its form . . . weakening and dissolving . . . becoming thinner like the elements of Earth . . . changing . . . dissolving . . . all parts dissolving . . . organs . . . extremities . . . muscles . . . all senses dissolving . . . fading away . . . melting away . . .

Script: **Water.** All feelings becoming one . . . dissolving . . . all sensations dissolving . . . body fluids that flow through you . . . drying up . . . all body organs closing down . . . dissolving. . . .

Script: **Fire.** The fire of life within you . . . going out . . . all body warmth and heat leaving . . . all organs ceasing to function . . . your body becoming cooler and cooler . . . your sense of boundary is dissolving . . . all senses dissolving . . . breath is dissolving . . .

> *Script:*   ***Air.*** Your body is without func-
> tion . . . The air is the element of
> consciousness . . . dissolving . . .
> all sensation . . . all feeling . . . all
> senses have gone . . . body bound-
> aries are no more . . . light . . .
> melting . . . dissolving . . . no sepa-
> rate body . . . no separate mind . . .
> all separateness dissolving . . . all in
> the vastness of oneness . . .
>
> Take a few slow, energizing breaths
> and, as you come back to this
> awareness, know that whatever is
> right for you at this point in time is
> unfolding just as it should and that
> you have done your best, regardless
> of the outcome.

Adapted from Levine's work, the following
script is useful for someone who is preparing
for the death moment or for a family member or
friend whose loved one has just died.[24] It can be
expanded as needed. The four-elements part of
the imagery script may also be used to assist one
whose death is imminent.

> *Script:*   ***Moving into the light.*** Fill yourself
> with an awareness of brilliance of
> clear light . . . a pure light within
> you and surrounding you . . . go
> forward . . . releasing anything that
> keeps you separate . . . pushing
> away nothing . . . spaciousness . . .
> releasing . . . dissolving . . . all body
> . . . dissolving into consciousness
> itself . . . Let go of all distractions
> . . . Listen and be with the transi-
> tion . . . what is called death has
> arrived . . . You are not alone . . .
> many have gone before you . . . let
> yourself go . . . into the clear light.

The dying person may move in and out of sleep
or comatose states after this script or the conscious dying script. The nurse or family member

sits with the person as long as necessary to bring
closure to this time. If the person lingers a while
longer, the nurse or family member may close
with the following phrases.

> *Script:*   ***Closure.*** Take a few slow, energiz-
> ing breaths and, as you come back
> to this awareness, know that what-
> ever is right for you at this point in
> time is unfolding just as it should,
> and that you have done your best,
> regardless of the outcome.

The Pain Process

In 90–99% of cases, pain can be managed. Pain
medication response patterns should be evaluated at least every 72 hours, as well as after each
administration. When giving the medication, the
nurse reminds the patient that the pain medication is in the body and working. Nurses should
understand and use the most current pain
management strategies and treatments. These
include new medications, methods of administration, physical treatments (e.g., massage, ice,
and movement), combinations of treatments,
documentation, and evaluation techniques. The
administration of medication should precede
activity (e.g., positioning).

Although the physical body can experience
pain, the mind's fear of the pain is often more
intense. Acute pain has qualities of suddenness
and surprise that can evoke anxiety and fear.
The best thing to do with this suddenness is to
encourage the dying person to breathe rhythmically and soften into the pain to decrease the
resistance to the experience. Relaxation, imagery,
or acupressure may be combined with pain medication. Even the worst of pain can be shifted in
many ways. For example, shifting the pain experience by calling it sensations rather than pain
often reduces discomfort. It also helps to encourage the person to make decisions over which he
or she has control, such as decisions about medications, treatments, and daily routines.

When guiding the person in pain, the nurse
may suggest allowing pain images and the different felt experiences to emerge. Each person

enters pain in a way that opens in the moment, and each person will know how far to go in exploring the pain. Common expressions an individual may have about the pain (e.g., pain attacks, it has a grip on me and takes my breath away, it has a loud and deafening pulsation, it is violent and unrelenting) create negative images that may interfere with the emergence of healing images. These negative images may become positive if the person focuses on the grip of pain being released, a deep belly breath coming forth evenly and effortlessly, or the pulsating sound becoming like the falling of gentle raindrops or falling snowflakes. Different relaxation and imagery exercises help the person practice letting go of the perception of the physical body. This letting go helps ease both physical pain, such as difficult procedures, and emotional pain, such as conflicts, and allows the person to experience death with peace and dignity.

With continued gentle exploration of opening and releasing into the pain, the person may begin to experience the pain as floating and diminishing. This is also a way of expanding one's sense of time. Another suggestion is to have the patient step aside in the mind and watch the pain to see how it might be changed to release some of the pressure, resistance, and holding on to the pain. Such guidance and presence over time will help the person to stay with a focused attention, opening and softening and expanding into the pain.

Blending Breaths and Comeditation

The simple release of the breath and the *ah-h-h-h* sound is an ancient ritual for dying into peace. Comeditation is based on the principle that respiration evokes a particular state of mind and serves as a direct link to the nervous system. There is a direct correlation between breathing and thinking. At first, the *ah-h-h-h* sound may be like an echoing of words, but staying with the sound allows the release of tension, fears, and pain.

Following are the steps for comeditation:

1. Position yourself comfortably close to the patient. A session may last 20 to 30 minutes or longer. Obtain whatever is necessary to make you and the person comfortable, such as pillows or a light blanket.

2. Suggest to the person that watching the breath is an ancient method of calming the body and the mind. Let the person first begin noticing the rise and fall of his or her abdomen with each breath in and each breath out.

3. Sitting at the person's midsection, focus on the rise and fall of the abdomen with each inhalation and each exhalation. Focus your attention on the person's lower chest area, and observe closely for the natural flow of the exhalation from the person. With this focused attention, you can begin breathing in unison with the person. At the beginning of the exhalation, begin softly and out loud to make the sound *ah-h-h-h*, matching the respiration of the person.

4. Occasionally, say simple, powerful phrases, such as *peaceful heart* or *releasing into the breath*. The fewer words spoken, however, the more powerful the breath work. If the person should fall asleep, you may wish to sit with the person for a while or sit until he or she awakes.

Mantras and Prayers

A mantra is the repetition of a word or sound, either aloud or silently. The word may be given by another or discovered. It has meaning to the individual. Repetition moves one toward peace.

A prayer may be special phrases or repeated words, or it may be a unique and spontaneous communication with God. There is considerable evidence for the effectiveness of at least two forms of prayer, the directed and the nondirected. In direct prayer, the individual has a specific goal or outcome in mind. In the nondirected form, the individual takes an open-ended, nonspecific, non-goal-oriented approach. In one form of contemplative prayer, *Lectio Divina*, one listens for the word of the Divine following a meditative focus on a few words of scripture.[25,26] In centering prayer, individuals seek a place deep inside themselves, where they live in rich harmony and connection with other people and with God and in the place of wisdom. Every faith group has prayers of the faithful that provide comfort and joy in the last moments.

Saying mantras and prayers can decrease the number of lonely hours at home, as well as in the hospital, although this is not the main reason for the practice. They serve as an affirmation of a deeper faith. In asking the dying person about wishes for prayers or repeated phrases, we may encourage him or her to select phrases that are short, easy to remember, and rhythmic. The personal selection of focus words enhances the faith factor. It may be helpful to pray for the highest good for the dying one or ourselves rather than for what we want. If we are praying for another, we need to hold the person for whom we are praying in our conscious thought, not ourselves. If we are totally focused on the patient, we cause ourselves less grief, frustration, and fear, recognizing that we are not responsible for outcomes. The nurse and the patient should agree on what to pray for before the prayer begins, and the nurse must be sensitive to the individual's formal system of belief.

Reminiscing and Life Review

A process basic to human existence is reminiscing and recounting past events, either alone or with friends. We spend much of our time talking, thinking, or writing about plans, goals, resources, successes, disappointments, and failures. This is especially true when facing death. Life review is a more formal process that involves reviewing present and past experiences. A life review experiencing form is useful in ordering questions related to each stage of life from earliest memories to old age.* To conduct a life review, it is best to plan six to eight sessions. Each session requires approximately 45 minutes. During each session, the patient tells the story of that phase of life. Open-ended questions are preferable, and it may be helpful to record the session. The first session is primarily an introduction. The last session is the most important because it is a summing up or discussion of the meanings of the story. The patient may feel emotions of all kinds during any session, reflecting the emotions that he or she felt during the stage of life being discussed. It is the acknowledgment of emotional content, in part, that facilitates

---

* Note: A new version of this tool appears in B. K. Haight and B. S. Haight, *The Handbook for the Structured Life Review* (Baltimore, MD: Health Professions Press, 2007).

integration. In the summary, perhaps earlier, an individual usually begins to feel a sense of integration with the past and present, a kind of wholeness to life. Unfinished business becomes finished. This is helpful in achieving peace.[12]

Where We Die

The environment in which people die, by choice or not, affects the ability of the person to achieve peace. Hospice and palliative care has evolved and helped to change the way and places where people die. Nurses seek to continue to look for ways to help people die with dignity and without needless suffering. As a culture, we are still debating when to stop life-prolonging interventions when one has reached the definitive time to die. However, even as these discussions continue, when it is time to die, where we die becomes a most important consideration.

Many people are alone at their time of death. Countless hundreds come to their end in the nursing homes that permeate every state in the nation. And of these hundreds, many are alone without living or able-bodied family members. Still others face death at home, many hopefully with hospice care nearby. Unfortunately, many more are surrounded by machines and invaded with tubes in the busy ICU.[27] Those interventions to help them last a few more hours or day are still in force, and thus they die wrapped in technology and seldom in the arms of caring people.[28] It is encouraging to know that there are alternatives.

One of the newest options is a place called *the Golden Room*. This concept is a place that offers a new and expanded way to provide care for the terminally ill. A definitive place is particularly important when you realize that about half of all Americans who die in hospitals spend their last 3 days of life in the ICU. In this ICU setting where the dying receive aggressive life-sustaining interventions, suffering is common and death is expected in up to 20% of these patients.[29] The new concept of the Golden Room removes the dying patient from the acute care setting into either a cluster of rooms separated from the regular patients in the general hospital and/or the nursing home. Another place for Golden Rooms is a free-standing building entirely dedicated to caring for the dying. These rooms are similar to contemporary hospice care but offer expanded facilities and personnel.

> The purpose of *The Golden Room* is to facilitate and honor the dying process, both for the patient and their loved ones. To create that place all elements of the design are taken into consideration. The physical room reflects calm and inclusion for all members present in the environment. Certain features designed into the space augment the sense of peace and security. A sense of spirit is reflected from the center-piece ceiling mural. Scenes depicting the cosmos with ethereal themes draw the supine patient below upward into a dimension of cosmic design. Some patients may sense a feeling of being drawn upward into their personal conception of spirit. Others may not consciously relate to a star-studded mural or painting of angels bursting from clouds, but subconsciously they will likely be relating to something much greater than themselves.[28]

These Golden Rooms will be designed with color schemes, furniture, technology, and comfort features to put the dying person and his or her caregivers in the best possible place for a comfortable, dignified, and peaceful death. Caregivers who render care in this setting will have special skills and, for example, be knowledgeable of the scripts and methods detailed in this chapter.

When these places for end of life are developed, we reason that pending death will not seem so formidable and frightening. Compassionately educated caregivers will be able to ease the transition from life into a peaceful death.

Death Bed Ritual (Basic)

Easing the transition from life to a peaceful death can be helped by integration of planned ritual into the process. This may occur at the moment of death or immediately after. If anointing has not already been done, it may be done at this time. Family, special friends, care staff, and clergy may choose to hold hands, surround the bed of the deceased, and share a moment of silence, a prayer, a song, or hugs. They may choose to touch the body, prepare the body according to rituals within the faith community involved, and say goodbye. It is important to allow as much time as needed.

Leave-Taking Rituals (Basic)

A nurse who works with survivors must remember that their grief period is unique for them. Furthermore, grief has no timetable. Healing grief requires a commitment to imagine a fulfilling life without a loved one. Action steps toward continued self-discovery after the death of a loved one may include dream work, meditation, movement, drawing, journal keeping, crying, sighing, drumming, chanting, singing, and music, as well as the following rituals.[24]

- *Celebrating holidays:* Special holidays, birthdays, anniversaries, and other important dates can be a time for creating rituals to ease the pain of loss and acknowledge feelings. For example, a widow fixed a place at the Christmas dinner table for her deceased husband. She and her six children gave him a farewell toast and shared special memories of him before they ate. A young couple who had a stillborn child asked several of the nurses and the attending physician to a memorial service in the hospital chapel before the baby was taken to the funeral home. After her mother died, a woman chose to have her healing team of eight friends with her at a memorial service by the sea. The family of a teenaged girl who died in an automobile accident had a gathering for her class and gave each person an opportunity to say special things about the girl. Her favorite music was played while dancing and singing began in her honor.
- *Rearranging and giving away:* If a loved one has died at home, the family member who shared the bedroom must decide what is best to do. Some wish to rearrange the room and remove hospital beds and other equipment quickly after death. Giving away a loved one's possessions, such as special mementos of jewelry, clothes, shoes, makeup, shaving equipment, and other personal possessions, is healing. Some people

need a shrine or memorial for a period of time, however.

- *Letting grief be present:* There are periods after death when a person appears brave, in control, or strong to others. Grief will come, however. It is important to share with the grieving person that there is no special way to grieve. When pain, fear, and anger can dissipate, the bodymindspirit knows the best way to grieve. Grieving allows love to heal the loss one feels for self and the person who has died.

- *Sustaining faith and hope:* There are many ways to sustain faith and awareness toward life, meaning, and purpose during grieving time. For example, survivors sometimes have a sense of talking to deceased loved ones, being enveloped in their love, and feeling their presence. People have described experiences such as having a faith in oneness, feeling an energy, vaguely sensing the presence of the deceased person, hearing the voice of the deceased giving guidance, or working on the same problem at different energy levels. One woman said, "My [deceased] husband told me how to finish this business deal." Another woman created a healing ritual after the death of her husband. When the weather permitted, she would get in her truck in the evening and drive to her husband's favorite hill on their big Texas ranch. As she looked out over the prairie and gazed into the Milky Way, she would choose a bright star and carry on a dialogue with the star, experiencing a sense of unity with her deceased husband somewhere in infinity. This provided her with calmness, wisdom, and clarity of thought.

- *Releasing anger and tears:* The release of anger, sadness, and tears is a cleansing process of the human spirit that makes a person more open to experience living in the moment. Holding grief in increases the suffering, fear, and separation.

- *Healing memories:* It is not necessary to stop thinking about the person who has died. Often, a grieving person who feels that the grief process is over finds that a memory, a song, or a meal suddenly evokes a sense of loss so deep that it seems as though it

will never heal. The person needs to stay with the pain, sadness, guilt, anger, fear, or loneliness. Love and joy will begin to fill the heart again. The wisdom is to let pain in and to stay open to it, to let the pain penetrate every cell in your body, to trust pain, to know that what emerges from the pain is a new level of healing awareness.

- *Getting unstuck:* Grieving can bring on suffering; therefore, it may be helpful for survivors to ask for assistance from friends, family, or a healthcare professional to help them move past the blocks. Some people think, "It's been 6 months since my mother died [or a year since my husband, son, or wife died], why am I still depressed and cry so frequently?"

Case Study (Implementation)

CASE STUDY 1

Setting: Critical care unit where visiting schedule was one visitor every 2 hours

Patient: S. R., a 30-year-old mother of three children

Patterns/Challenges/Needs:
1. Decreased cardiac output related to end-stage heart failure
2. Grieving related to imminent death
3. Spiritual strength related to dynamic belief systems and family and friend support

S. R. said to the nurse, "I feel death over my right shoulder. Call my husband. I need him to come and bring my children, my parents, and my three friends. Tell them to come as soon as possible." The nurse also had an inner felt sense of the presence of death and began calling S. R.'s family. Four hours before her death, all her family was present. Her friends sang her favorite songs as one played a guitar.

CASE STUDY 2

Setting: Writing thoughts about healthy grief in a letter, 4 years after son's death

Client: V. D. J., a 45-year-old professional and mother

Patterns/Challenges/Needs: Spiritual strength related to ability to deliberate the meaning of life, death, grief, and suffering

There is a holy purpose in grief and nothing should stand in its path. Grief begins with so few words. Sounds take shape traveling from a great distance. Within, a reserve is sensed. Something sacred that holds a luminous darkness that stills the mind even as the heart shudders with waves of deep sorrow. The natural quality of grief is ancient and bone bare. It tolerates nothing false. Grief is unrestrained; conscious effort is not required.

A mother who has lost a child learns what true freedom is. It is being cut free from the knot of habit, customs, rules. It is not being bound by considerations or even fear, for the worst has happened. Your child is dead, and you live. A mother's lament begins.

Your heartbeat creates a tone for your body to hear. It drums and moves you slowly forward with your family even as you weep and prepare to say your last goodbye. Now is not the time to be a bystander. It is crucial that you support and include your other children and family in the vigil, the wake, the funeral, and burial or cremation ceremonies. They, too, are in shock and disbelief. And it doesn't end there.

Let nothing be left undone, unsaid, unwritten, or unsung in this farewell. This is not the place to lose courage or even your humor, for you will need both to sustain the intense suffering you have yet to bear. Nature provides the exact dosage for dealing with the constant strikes of pain experienced. Usually there is no real need for outside medication. Your body in its perfect wisdom gauges your requirements and numbs you accordingly. You will feel cold, but your mind–body will not allow more pain than you can tolerate. To disrupt the natural safeguards may only postpone the initial pain in your mourning process.

During the vigil and the wake your only thought is to do everything you can do to console your children and other family members. You realize they have the same concern for you. Plan the funeral ceremonies together. In the process, some small consolation may be experienced. The path of grief leads inward when you watch and listen. Didn't you bring this spirit child into the world, flesh of your flesh? This last goodbye may enable you to complete the circle; keeping a vigil through the night allows you to be closer to your child.

The vigil with your child provides a place to begin to say goodbye, the goodbye you were both denied, by sudden, unexpected death. You hear yourself talking and reassuring your son. You must now help your child to take the first steps into the great mystery, by talking aloud and guiding, much as you did when he was very young. Empty your mind and your heart, and give him all your love and spiritual strength for his journey.

The week following the funeral I moved everything from my bedroom except basic essentials. I felt driven to sleep on a mat and to make a low altar that I filled with family photographs, mementos, childhood treasures belonging to Sean and my children, family poetry, drawings, vigil candles, prayer fans, fresh flowers, and ceremonial sage.

Prayers became conversations and chants and death songs for the son who had no time to create them for himself. Forty-nine days of talking-prayer asking the angelic beings to guide my son on his journey. Each member of the immediate family scattered Sean's ashes in places special to him. A spirit bundle was placed and kept before the altar for him. Always the moving between worlds; letting go of the loneliness through weeping, sound and moving prayer to returning to repose, listening, and sitting. A year goes by.

You find it difficult to speak. Your breathing habits are changing. You become aware of differences in your breath. You sense your heart breathing, your brain breathing. You notice that when you breathe out, you see thought. Some days you don't remember breathing at all.

You keep a journal as an ongoing discussion with your child, seeking solace. You somehow deal with daily life, guilt, illness, helplessness, and the grief of your other children.

Four more years go by; 4 years of dreams, voices, and mourning. I begin to understand the innate usefulness of creative work and humor as an antidote to loneliness and pain. My children need me and continually pull me onto the more solid ground where they stand. Dream walks, drumming, chanting, and round dancing lead me to my tribal traditions. My children personify the creative weaving of compassion, intelligence, and courage and remind me of how precious each individual life is and the miracle of being together with Sean and with each other in this life and in this time and in this place.

My son Sean has taught me that the true object of death is life. I have learned that a dream can be shaped by the dreamer; that in the act of sacrifice, the sacred is manifested through surrender of all that is.

CASE STUDY 3

Setting: Bedroom at home of daughter (M. L.), who recently brought her ill mother (L. Y.) home to care for her

Patient: L. Y., a 90-year-old mother of two middle-aged adults, grandmother of two, who has been ill for 4 months. She had lived alone for the last 40 years.

Patterns/Challenges/Needs:

1. Moderate pain related to diagnosis of cancer
2. Decreased cardiac output (including altered oxygenation) related to multisystem organ shutdown
3. Family grieving related to imminent death
4. Spiritual well-being and effective individual coping related to patient desire to care for her grieving family

M. L. checked with her mother to see that she was not in pain or distress prior to going out of the house on a short errand. L. Y. told her daughter to go, adding that she was quite comfortable and would be fine. M. L. noticed her mother's skin was mottled and cool, but her breathing was unlabored and she seemed peaceful. Her husband remained in the home. When M. L. returned, she found that her mother had stopped breathing. The bedclothes were unruffled, and her mother's face was peaceful. Her husband had heard nothing to indicate when the passing occurred. M. L. called the hospice nurse, the nun who was her neighbor and belonged to the same church, and other family members, and they carried out the ritual that they had planned for this moment. They held hands around the bed, prayed together in the ways of their tradition, and played a hymn that had been taped. After this, they informed the doctor, called the funeral director, and took care of legal obligations. A woman who had lived alone for 40 years had chosen to die alone, but cared for, to the end. The family grieving needs were also addressed.

Evaluation

With the patient (family and significant others), the nurse evaluates whether the patient outcomes for planning and implementing a peaceful death (see Exhibit 21-1) were successfully achieved. To evaluate the interventions further, the nurse may explore the subjective effects of the experience with the patient (family and significant others), using questions such as those shown in **Exhibit 21-2**.

Like peaceful living and dying, the care of a dying person and the family and significant others is an art. Preparing for death can be a series of

---

EXHIBIT 21-2   Evaluating the Patient's (Family's and Significant Others') Subjective Experience with Perideath Nursing Interventions

1. Can you continue to be aware of ways to recognize your anxiety, fear, and grief at this time?
2. Which of your strengths can best serve you as you move through this difficult time?
3. What are the things that you will do to take care of yourself at this time?
4. Do you have any questions that I can help you with just now?
5. Will you call on others to help you?
6. Whom can you ask for help?
7. Were the imagery exercises helpful for you? Do you pray?
8. Are there images, feelings, or emotions that surfaced during the imagery exercises that I can help you with?
9. Can I help you with anything just now?
10. Are there rituals that you can begin to create to help you deal with your grief?

Note: These subjective experiences may be used in helping a patient, family members, and significant others during the dying process or with the family or significant others during the grieving process.

conscious, spirit-filled, light-filled moments that lead to the ultimate peaceful moment of death. It is different for each person. True healing and dying in peace come from integrating the creative process and the art of healing into our daily lives. The paradox is that, although this healing awareness may appear at first to be rare, it is a very ordinary and natural event that is available to each of us at all times. As each of us seeks to understand and integrate our spirit-filled lives as meaningful and connected with others throughout the ages, we learn about life and death. The more we integrate solitude, inward-focused practice, and conscious awareness into daily life, the more peaceful is dying and the moment of death.

Directions for
FUTURE RESEARCH

1. Evaluate the attitudes and stress levels of nurses who work with death; determine whether rituals for nurses to use following death of patients might be useful in decreasing stress and helping grief.
2. Determine effective responses and nursing interventions for the increasing vulnerability of the dying person.
3. Develop empirically based therapeutic interventions to preserve dignity at the end of life.
4. Evaluate the use of life review in assisting patients with a sense of integration of life at the end of that life.
5. Determine the special needs of nurses who work with dying people who are friends and relatives or who have special experiences while dying (such as negative near-death experiences).

Nurse Healer
REFLECTIONS

After reading this chapter, the nurse healer will be able to answer or to begin a process of answering the following questions:

- Do I feel a greater sense of healing intention when I include relaxation, imagery, or music in my life every day?
- What are the effects on me when I guide others in healing modalities to facilitate peace in dying?

- How do I know that I am actively listening?
- What new death mythologies and skills can assist me in releasing attachment to my physical body, possessions, and people?

> **www** *For a full suite of assignments and additional learning activities, use the access code located in the front of your book to visit this exclusive website: http://go.jblearning.com/dossey. If you do not have an access code, you can obtain one at the site.*

NOTES

1. Roshan Cultural Heritage Institute, "Definition of Culture." http://www.roshan-institute.org/474552.
2. L. Keegan and C. A. Drick, "Theoretical Frameworks," in *End of Life: Nursing Solutions for Death with Dignity*, ed. L. Keegan & C. A. Drick, 118 (New York: Springer Publishing, 2011).
3. J. Watson, *The Philosophy and Science of Caring*, rev. ed. (Boulder: University Press of Colorado, 2011).
4. B. Davies and R. Steele, "Supporting Families in Palliative Care," in *Textbook of Palliative Care Nursing*, ed. B. F. Ferrell and N. Coyle (New York: Oxford University Press, 2011, pp. 613–629).
5. M. Erseck and V. T. Cotter, "The Meaning of Hope in the Dying," in *Textbook of Palliative Care Nursing*, ed. B. F. Ferrell and N. Coyle (New York: Oxford University Press, 2011, pp. 579–597).
6. J. Lynn, J. L. Schuster, A. Wilkinson, and L. N. Simon, "Supporting People in Difficult Times: Relationships, Spirituality, and Bereavement" in *Improving Care for the End of Life: A Sourcebook for Health Care Managers and Clinicians*, 133–162 (New York: Oxford University Press, 2008).
7. E. Kübler-Ross, *On Death and Dying* (New York: Macmillan, 1969).
8. J. W. Fowler, *Stages of Faith: The Psychology of Human Development and the Quest for Meaning* (New York: Harper & Row, 1981).
9. B. Dossey, "She Is Now Wherever We Are," in *Mother Stories: Through Our Mothers Death and Dying*, ed. C. A. Drick, 25–36 (Charleston, SC: BookSurge, 2009).
10. V. Frankl, *Man's Search for Meaning*, 3rd ed. (New York: Simon & Schuster, 1963).
11. P. Reed, "Self-Transcendence Theory," in *Middle Range Theory for Nursing*, ed. M. Smith and P. Liehr, 105 (New York: Springer, 2008).
12. B. K. Haight and B. S. Haight, *The Handbook for the Structured Life Review* (Baltimore, MD: Health Professions Press, 2007).

13. Growth House, *Life Review and Reminiscence Therapy* (San Francisco, CA: Growth House, 2011). http://www.growthhouse.org/lifereview.html.

14. P. Burns, "Myth and Legend from Ancient Times to the Space Age." http://www.pibburns.com/myth.htm.

15. G. Luce, *Your Second Life: The SAGE Experience* (New York: Delacorte Press, 1979).

16. ELNEC (End-of-Life Consortium), *Graduate Curriculum: Faculty Guide* (Washington, DC: City of Hope and American Association of Colleges of Nursing, 2010).

17. J. L. Hollis, *Music at the End of Life: Easing the Pain and Preparing the Passage* (Santa Barbara, CA: Praeger, 2010).

18. L. L. Dunn, "Spiritual Needs: Focus on Forgiveness" [editorial], *Online Journal of Rural Nursing and Health Care* (2009). http://www.rno.org/journal/index.php/online-journal/article/viewFile/188/235.

19. B. M. Reik, "Transgressions, Guilt and Forgiveness: A Model of Seeking Forgiveness," *Journal of Psychology and Theology* 38, no. 4 (Winter 2010): 246–254. http://sccn612final.wikispaces.com/file/view/Transgressions,+Guilt+and+Forgiveness.pdf.

20. I. Rahman, "The Seven Steps to Genuine Forgiveness," *Free Online Library* (September 3, 2009).

21. http://www.thefreelibrary.com/The+Seven+Steps+to+Genuine+Forgiveness-a01073981047.

21. S. Levine, *A Gradual Awakening* (New York: Anchor Press, 1979).

22. S. Levine, *Healing into Life and Death* (New York: Doubleday, 1989).

23. A. Sheikh and K. Sheikh, *Death Imagery* (Milwaukee, WI: American Imagery Institute, 1991).

24. C. Hammerschlag, *Healing Ceremonies*, Kindle ed. (Amazon Digital Services, 2011).

25. T. Gray, *Praying Scripture for a Change: An Introduction to Lectio Divina* (Westchester, PA: Ascension Press, 2009).

26. T. Keating, *Spirituality, Contemplation and Transformation: Writings on Centering Prayer* (Brooklyn, NY: Lantern Books, 2008).

27. S. O'Mahony et al., "Preliminary Report of the Integration of a Palliative Care Team into an Intensive Care Unit," *Palliative Medicine* 24, no. 2 (2010): 154–165.

28. L. Keegan and C. A. Drick, *End of Life: Nursing Solutions for Death with Dignity* (New York: Springer, 2011).

29. R. A. Mularski et al., "Pain Management Within the Palliative and End-of-Life Care Experience in the ICU," *Chest* 135, no. 5 (2009): 1360–1369

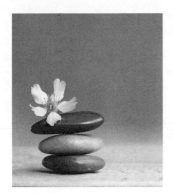

Chapter 22

Weight Management Counseling

Sue Popkess-Vawter

Nurse Healer
OBJECTIVES

Theoretical

- Discuss the strengths and weaknesses of biological, behavioral, psychological, and cognitive theories of weight management.
- Describe and explain the cognitive restructuring Balance from the Inside Out (BIO) strategies for healthy weight management.

Clinical

- Describe three differences between unidimensional and multidimensional interventions for long-term weight management.
- Discuss and adapt the basic principles of the Holistic Self-Care Model for long-term weight management to clients in your nursing practice.
- List one positive self-talk statement to replace the three negative self-talk statements most frequently used by your clients, and identify in which of the eight metamotivational states the negative statements originated.

Personal

- Discuss how you base your eating habits on the food pyramid and the American Diabetic Association diet using the EAT (Eat, Ask, Tell) for Hunger strategy.

- Describe your personal aerobic and strength exercise program using the Exercise for LIFE (Learn the habit, I am important, Friends, Enjoy) strategy.
- Describe how you nourish your self-esteem through spiritual connections each day (Energy, Spirit, Time, Eating, Exercise, Meditation).

DEFINITIONS

Body mass index (BMI): Weight in kilograms divided by height squared (m²), with healthy weight less than or equal to 24.9.

Obesity: Body mass index greater than or equal to 30.

Overeating: Eating when not hungry or eating more than is required to satisfy hunger.

Overfat: Percentage of body fat greater than recommended for a client's gender and age (e.g., 28% for women and 20% for men).

Overweight: Body mass index of 25–29.9.

Self-talk: Mental verbalizations that elicit emotional responses.

Weight cycling/yo-yo dieting: Repeated weight loss greater than 10 pounds followed by weight gain, in a repetitive pattern three or more times over the past 2 years.

Weight management: Holistic, long-term lifestyle adjustments in clients' bio-psycho-sociocultural-spiritual dimensions to promote a high level of individual wellness;

caring for and assisting clients to reach sufficient self-acceptance, self-love, and self-responsibility to adjust their lifestyles to support eating for hunger, exercising regularly, and esteem.

■ THEORY AND RESEARCH

The Weight Gain Epidemic in the United States

Obesity has been a serious healthcare epidemic for more than 3 decades. More than two-thirds of adults in the United States are overweight or obese despite efforts and national initiatives to abate this unchecked problem.[1] Progress in the past 10 years toward *Healthy People 2010* objectives for overweight and obesity was of little consequence, thus requiring retention and revision of objectives for healthy weight and obesity in the new *Healthy People 2020* objectives.[2]

For adults aged 20 years or older, overweight is defined as a body mass index (BMI) of 25–29.9, Class 1 obesity is defined as a BMI of 30–34.9, Class 2 obesity is a BMI of 35–39.9, and Class 3 obesity is a BMI greater than 40.[3] Weight management failures result from lack of practical, long-term interventions to address holistic influences of weight gain (e.g., biological, psychological, sociocultural, and spiritual).[4] Experts agree that environmental influences, rather than biological reasons, explain the obesity epidemic of the past 3 decades. There is general agreement that four key factors can explain the environmental stimulus–response nature of the rise in obesity in the United States: (1) fast-paced eating style of fatty, glycemic "fast foods" and super sizing; (2) excessive calorie intake; (3) reduced physical activity and greater use of high-tech devices; and (4) heightened sensitivity to food as a stimulant from the media.

Only recently has the weight gain epidemic in the United States been recognized as multifactorial, and as such calls for multifactorial and multidimensional approaches to abate the problem. Although classic theories of energy balance remain accurate in describing why body weight is gained, cognitive and behavioral theories may better address the multifactorial overweight situation. Weight management approaches need to account for energy in (food), energy out (exer-

cise), psychological aspects such as self-esteem and stress management, "toxic environments" that do not support healthy eating and exercise, comorbidity and obesogenic medications, and family–job influences. The current trend, in light of consistent failures, is to correct and reprogram thinking of American citizens, healthcare providers, community planners, and policymakers to promote small, consistent lifestyle changes that encompass all multifactorial influences. The Surgeon General and national healthcare professional organizations advise consideration of all influencing factors to promote modest weight loss. Improvements in insulin sensitivity, type 2 diabetes, blood lipids, and blood glucose/A1c, sleep apnea, and blood pressure were demonstrated with 5–10% weight loss (for example, a 10- to 20-pound loss in a 200-pound person or a 15- to 30-pound loss in a 300-pound person).[5]

History may shed light on the context of the recent weight gain epidemic in the United States. During the Great Depression and through World War II, people focused on peace and financial security. Times were literally lean because of financial and nutritional shortages. As the economic struggles began to resolve and people gained greater wealth, they also gained weight. Advances in automation rapidly mechanized a once physically active society, making it faster paced but paradoxically slowing it down physically. People learned to overeat in celebration of their new-found freedom and prosperity, and, at the same time, they learned to use eating as a coping mechanism. From an operant conditioning perspective, food acted as the powerful positive reinforcer that stopped the unpleasant feeling of physical and emotional hunger (i.e., the negative reinforcers). Eating to feel better, in the presence or absence of hunger and a wide variety of pleasant and unpleasant feelings, soon became a habit in U.S. culture as foods (usually those high in fat, sugar, and starch) became more affordable and convenient.

Around 1950, dieting to lose weight came into style to achieve the thinness of fashion models and movie stars, which constantly flashed before Americans' eyes in the burgeoning media. Soon, feelings of deprivation and preoccupation with food and dieting yielded a rise in eating disorders and weight cycling.

Long-term habits of overeating without hunger and little or no physical exercise in a fast-paced society can explain the U.S. weight crisis. To date, most weight loss interventions in the United States have not contributed to long-term weight loss and probably have exacerbated the overweight problem. Comorbid conditions associated with overweight and obesity include heart disease and hypertension, stroke, gallbladder disease, osteoarthritis, sleep apnea, respiratory problems, and cancers (e.g., endometrial, breast, prostate, colon); the most dramatically rising overweight comorbidity is type 2 diabetes.[6]

Approaches to Weight Management

Most weight management approaches are based on at least one of four categories of theories—biological, behavioral, psychological, and cognitive.

Biological Theories

Interventions based on biological theories aim to correct excess weight and fat by reducing the number of available calories so that excessive fat is not deposited and fat stores are used. Traditionally, four biological theories explain excess weight gain from genetic and energy balance perspectives.

According to two genetic theories, individuals have a genetic predisposition to an excessive accumulation of fat, either by hypertrophy (enlarged size) or hyperplasia (excessive numbers) of fat cells. The Hypertrophy Theory focuses on the size of the fat cell as a regulatory mechanism for food consumption; that is, when existing adipocytes have expanded to their size limitation, a signal causes the individual to stop eating. According to the Hyperplasia Theory, individuals are destined to continue their degree of fatness according to the number of fat cells present in childhood and adolescence. The adipocyte Hypertrophy Theory supports adult-onset obesity, while the adipocyte Hyperplasia Theory supports child-onset obesity. Neither genetic theory leaves much room for therapeutic interventions.

Set Point Theory, another popular theory, gained attention in the 1980s and 1990s. Nesbitt, who introduced this theory in 1972, claims that individuals have but one body weight at which their energy expenditure is normal.[7]

Despite changes in the rate of energy expenditure, be it higher or lower, individuals eventually will gain or lose weight to return their weight to its set point.[8]

Energy Balance Theory has been widely used as the basis of weight loss interventions.[9] Simply put, the theory holds that an excessive number of calories ingested, but not required for metabolic needs, results in an excessive body weight. Conversely, fewer calories in the presence of demanding exercise and work create a deficit that allows weight loss to occur. No matter what the source of energy (e.g., carbohydrate, protein, fat), excessive calories are converted to be stored as fat. Excessive body weight, then, usually is from excessive intramuscular and subcutaneous fat stores.

Behavioral Theories

The primary focus of behavioral theories in weight management is that behaviors such as overeating are learned responses. Interventions such as behavior modification techniques (based on Skinner's Stimulus–Response Theory) aim to control stimuli that result in actions that perpetuate overeating.[10] Some believe stimulus control strategies can permanently change external motivations related to eating. Thus, stimulus control strategies are designed to control eating by restricting calories, choices, locations, and timing, while avoiding environmental or external stimuli that may lead to eating outside those limitations.

Many calorie-restricted diets and food supplements are a type of stimulus control strategy that concentrate on controlling antecedent stimuli (i.e., controlling what, when, where, and how much to eat). At one end of the nutritional continuum are extreme and unhealthy diets (e.g., a grapefruit diet or a high-protein diet); at the other end are balanced, healthy diets from the food pyramid. Even healthy diets can be difficult to comply with over the long term when they are aimed at controlling hunger. No matter how healthy they may be, stimulus-controlled diets focus on avoiding or eliminating hunger. When the body's natural, physiologic, internal signals of hunger are erased or minimized, individuals are forced to focus on external cues to tell them when they need to eat.

A behavioral change theory that healthcare providers have found useful is Prochaska and DiClemente's Stages of Change, or Transtheoretical, Model (TTM).[11] The TTM posits that health behavior change involves progress through five stages of change: precontemplation, contemplation, preparation, action, and maintenance. Authors found consistent patterns among individuals' reasons for changing and the stages of change. Improvements have been demonstrated in program recruitment, retention, and progress using stage-matched, proactive recruitment procedures and interventions. Healthcare providers and health promotion program designers are beginning to recognize greater long-term behavioral change using the TTM as a guide.

The Holistic Self-Care Model for long-term weight management is based on the premise that stimulus control addresses only part of the reasons for weight gain—the external reasons. The other reasons for weight gain are internal. For individuals to make long-term lifestyle changes that promote fat loss, it is necessary to emphasize healthy eating for hunger rather than the elimination of hunger.

Clients should be assisted in calculating the number of calories that they require to meet their basic metabolic and exercise metabolic needs, based on American Dietetic Association guidelines (daily calories greater or equal to 1,200). Health-promoting behavioral techniques help clients learn how to distribute calories among the food pyramid groups and record daily intake according to time, place, kinds, amounts, pyramid groups, social situation, and hunger level. Most behavioral programs require individuals to monitor and record their compliance with prescribed dietary restrictions. Often they are assisted with setting up a meaningful reward system, such as money, special gifts, and entertainment. Individuals usually are weighed weekly because weight loss becomes the external indicator of progress. Generally, less emphasis is placed on internal indicators of progress, such as changes in thinking and feelings, than on external indicators, such as weight, body shape, and body size. Although the National Heart, Lung, and Blood Institute (NHLBI) recommends keeping records and weighing regularly, tailoring these techniques to individual clients can

help them transition from external to internal monitoring. Behavioral therapy is effective on a short-term basis but is less effective for helping obese individuals address disturbed thinking, emotions, and body image related to overeating and poor self-esteem.

Psychological Theories

Weight management interventions based on psychological theories usually are directed toward decreasing stress-induced eating and helping to find ways to control eating in the presence of stressful situations. Similarly, negative body image, poor self-esteem, depression, and issues of social discrimination become the focus of psychotherapy, while dietary and exercise prescriptions usually receive less emphasis during therapy. Binge eating disorder, bulimia, and compulsive overeating are treated as relationship disorders that have similar etiologies but that manifest differently. Usually, in psychotherapy individuals with eating disorders are encouraged to focus on related issues of abandonment and verbal, sexual, and physical abuse rather than the eating problem per se, unless physical well-being is threatened. Depression and obesity as related concerns are on the rise in the United States, especially among younger age groups.[12]

Cognitive Theories

Beck explains how unrealistic, negative thinking triggers unpleasant emotional responses, which can lead to overeating and not getting regular exercise.[13] Interventions based on cognitive theory are aimed at providing rapid symptomatic improvement, understanding of mood changes, coping strategies for self-management when upset, and guidance for personal growth. Individuals are assisted in assessing their basic values and attitudes that lead to negative feelings, as well as in reevaluating and challenging basic assumptions about their self-worth. Problem-solving and coping techniques help clients to deal effectively with major, realistic problems (e.g., low self-esteem, guilt) and minor vague irritations (e.g., frustration, apathy) that seem to have no obvious external cause.

Beck offers cognitive restructuring techniques to help identify and eliminate cognitive distortions that elicit irrational emotional responses.

Beck's approach to cognitive restructuring uses three steps:

1. Identify automatic thoughts that are self-critical.
2. Identify any cognitive distortions and unrealistic beliefs underlying the thoughts.
3. Provide rational responses that defend the self.

Cognitive restructuring aims to substitute objective rational thoughts for illogical, harsh self-criticisms that predominate in response to negative events. Overall, clients learn how underlying beliefs relate to thinking, thinking relates to feelings, and feelings relate to actions. As seen in the following cognitive theory progression, actions must be addressed through feelings and thinking to identify underlying beliefs that initiate the chain of events: Beliefs → Thoughts → Feelings → Actions. Focusing only on actions is a behavior modification and stimulus–response approach. A more in-depth and lasting approach is exploration of basic beliefs as a means to change thinking, feelings, and actions.

Failure of Traditional Weight Management Interventions

In 1994, failure rates for most weight reduction programs were estimated to be as high as 90–95%.[14] These high dieting failure rates may be indirectly reflected in the National Health and Nutrition Examination Survey (NHANES) report of the prevalence of overweight and obesity in adults. Overweight adults comprised 47% of the population in 1976, 56% in 1988, and 65% in 1999. The prevalence of obese adults rose from 15% in 1976, to 23% in 1988, and to 31% in 1999.[15] Weight gain trends appeared to reach a relatively steady state from 1999 to 2008; people were not gaining weight at the rapid rates since 1976, but overweight and obesity prevalence remained about the same, especially for women. Men, on the other hand, showed a somewhat upward trend in weight gain. The NHANES report for 2007–2008 showed overall prevalence of overweight and obesity for adults was 68% (approximately 72% among men and 64% among women).[1] Obesity prevalence for women was 35.5% and 32.2% for men. Class 3 obesity was reported to have increased at greater rates than

any other class of obesity in the United States.[16] Over the past 3 decades, childhood obesity has more than doubled among children ages 2–5 years, has tripled among youth ages 6–11 years, and has more than tripled among adolescents ages 12–19 years. About 17% of American children ages 2–19 years were obese—a 1 in 6 incidence rate. Overweight and obesity have a greater effect on minorities; blacks had 51% and Hispanics had 21% higher obesity prevalence compared with whites.

Over these past decades, many interventions that fail to promote long-term weight management have characteristics in common: (1) they are restrictive in calories, choices, and times to eat; (2) they are unidimensional, using only one major means to achieve weight loss, and do not include regular exercise; (3) they do not permit individuals to tailor weight management to their preferences, lifestyles, and humanness; and (4) they do not focus on internal motivations for overeating and not exercising regularly.

Restrictions on Calories, Choices, and Times

Interventions that restrict calories, choices, and times to eat offer a temporary and artificial modification that is unrealistic for the long term. In the 1960s, 7% of men and 14% of women were on reducing diets (21% total). In the 1990s, 24% of men and 40% of women were on diets.[17] Despite dieting attempts, the prevalence of overweight Americans increased from 25% to 33% between 1980 and 1991. Although Americans were trying to eat less fat, they were getting fatter. In a 1994 U.S. Department of Agriculture survey of 5,500 U.S. citizens, one in three adults was overweight.[18] In an effort to follow recommendations to reduce fat intake, they reported eating more grains, but in doing so increased their intake of snacks by 200% and their intake of ready-to-eat cereals by 60%. It seems that their responses to dietary restrictions and deprivation ultimately resulted in overeating, which may have led to weight gain reflected in the current 68% incidence of overweight and obesity. When calories and choices are restricted, human beings often revert to old patterns that led to being overweight in the first place. In response, the national guidelines on weight management have become less restrictive and provide for human fallibility, which is the necessary ingredient for long-term weight management.

Unidimensional Treatment

Many medical interventions that yield weight loss in the short term usually fail in the long term. Such interventions include surgical reduction of the gastrointestinal tract, stomach expansion devices and lap band restriction devices to produce a full feeling, and drugs to suppress the appetite and block fat absorption—all aimed at reducing amounts of ingested and metabolized foods. Sibutramine hydrochloride (satiety-enhancing agent) and orlistat (inhibits intestinal lipase) were approved pharmacologic support for weight management despite distressing physiologic side effects.[19] Often dramatic weight regain occurs when surgical procedures fail and medications are withdrawn because clients lack insight into why they overeat and do not exercise. It is vital that clients learn healthy eating, exercise, and self-esteem before or concurrently with other weight management treatments. Perhaps equally disconcerting about use of surgery and pharmacologic agents are the detrimental side effects. Dietary, pharmacologic, and surgical treatments that reduce intake and restrict calories, choices, and when to eat offer temporary modifications that are unrealistic for the long term and often are accompanied by rebound weight gain and damaging psychological consequences.[20]

Regular exercise as part of weight management is no longer controversial. Researchers have found supportive evidence that exercise plays a vital role in weight loss. Research findings suggest that exercise can prevent a reduction in the resting metabolic rate, either by elevating it following the exercise or by maintaining or increasing fat-free mass (lean body mass). Research supports both aerobic and strength (i.e., resistance) exercises to promote healthy weight. Short 10-minute bouts of exercise throughout the day, three to five times per day, have been shown to be equally beneficial in healthy weight management.[21]

Insulin resistance syndrome, or metabolic syndrome, formerly called syndrome X, is a condition of insulin resistance associated with a cluster of abnormalities typical for type 2 diabetes and its comorbidities.[22] Most individuals who display metabolic syndrome are hypertensive, overweight, glucose intolerant, and have lipid abnormalities, all of which put them at a higher risk for cardiovascular disease. Non-insulin-dependent diabetes mellitus, or adult-onset diabetes, is now called type 2 diabetes and accounts for almost 95% of all diagnosed cases of diabetes.[23] As the degree to which a person is overweight increases, so does the risk for developing type 2 diabetes, especially when visceral adiposity increases, as evidenced by greater waist circumference, or an "apple shape." Waist measurements greater than 35 inches for women and 40 inches for men may indicate a higher disease risk than that of people with smaller waist measurements. Increased central obesity among Americans may be related to greater intake of high glycemic index foods (e.g., high sugar and starch, low fiber, refined and processed foods), in addition to recognized overindulgence of fatty, fast foods. High sugar and starch content in low-fiber, refined foods may be directly related to the growing incidence of insulin resistance. The "good news" about this disheartening evidence is that modest weight loss of 5% to 10% of initial body weight can improve glucose tolerance and reduce blood pressure, lipids, and mortality.[24] Healthcare providers are urged to assess those at risk for insulin resistance and related health risks and offer long-term lifestyle interventions to reverse this growing epidemic.

The U.S. media potentiates magical thinking and encourages individuals to seek "quick-fix, magic bullet" programs. Some individuals hold to the magical thinking that they can rapidly achieve slimmer images and will have lasting results without extended and consistent use of nutritional and exercise strategies. In the author's experience, women who do not think magically about weight loss are usually older (35–45 years old), have tried many weight loss methods, failed frequently, and learned from their experiences that quick-fix weight loss methods only lead to more failures. Realistic thinkers can articulate what they want in life and are more willing to expend effort to achieve "a healthier, more energetic body, mind, and lifestyle."

Inability to Tailor Weight Management Programs to the Individual

Interventions that do not permit individuals to tailor weight management to their preferences, lifestyles, and humanness do not last. Weight loss interventions fail when program directives are too stringent for individuals to gain a sense of ownership and to accept the weight management strategies as a way of life. Instead, individuals view weight management as something that will happen magically if they can endure program directives long enough. Usually, they do not view "the program" as a long-term lifestyle change and, therefore, do not address their individual preferences (e.g., dislike for certain foods and types of exercise), way of life (e.g., working nights, family versus single), and "being human" along the way (e.g., not feeling guilty or dropping out when they deviate from the plan).

The American Dietetic Association states that to achieve long-term weight management adults must make a lifelong commitment to healthy lifestyle changes.[25] Both daily physical activity and eating should be *sustainable* and *enjoyable*—terms that imply personal tailoring of healthy, yet livable lifetime habits. Without individualization, a lifelong program is not possible, because life is always changing and adaptation is the norm.

Inability to Focus on Internal Motivation for Overeating and Lack of Exercise

Interventions that are not focused on internal motivations for overeating and for lack of regular exercise generally do not uncover important underlying reasons for being overweight. This idea is reminiscent of the old saying, "Don't look where you fell, but where you slipped." Weight management programs often do not help overweight individuals uncover motivations for weight regain or reasons for staying overweight. Perhaps the reason that stimulus control techniques have had limited success is because they seek to control the diet and environment but do not take into account that eating may be a coping mechanism to manage unpleasant feelings.[26] Weight management should include biological, psychological, and social interventions to normalize eating and separate physical from emotional hunger.

Toxic stress is the uncontrollable, chronic type of stress that causes sustained high levels of serum cortisol, the powerful stress hormone necessary for fueling stressful events.[27] Sustained high cortisol levels can lead to fatigue, impaired immune response, lower mental sharpness, and stimulated appetite, all of which can contribute to metabolic syndrome. Attempts to lower stress usually include relaxation exercises and physical exercise. Techniques to prevent a toxic stress response involve seeking a different, healthier perception of troublesome stressors through healthy self-esteem. Healthy self-esteem can be cultivated through daily spiritual nurturance and spiritual coping, which conceptually can lower levels of the stress response and, thus, can lower cortisol. Healing from the "inside out" may be the only lasting intervention to address America's overstressed, overweight epidemic. Support books such as *The Language of Letting Go* and *10 Secrets for Success and Inner Peace* can help clients reach the inner healing necessary to make lifelong lifestyle changes.[28,29]

Multidimensional Weight Management Interventions

Successful weight management programs focus on internal motivations for overeating and not exercising regularly and are multidimensional and flexible. According to the 2009 American Dietetic Association position statement, multidimensional long-term weight management comprehensive programs should comprise dietary and physical activity strategies to lose and maintain weight loss as well as multiple cognitive behavioral strategies.[25] Suggested cognitive-behavioral strategies are self-monitoring, stress management, stimulus control, problem solving, contingency management, cognitive restructuring, and social support.

Weight management professionals need to be aware of differences between behavioral strategies and cognitive behavioral strategies in weight management. Behavioral strategies, or behavior modification, focus on changing individuals' behaviors with little or no concern for their underlying reasons for overeating, not exercising, and unhealthy coping behaviors. For example, large multisite clinical trials, such as the Action for Health in Diabetes Look AHEAD studies, incorporate both successful meal replacement and exercise behavioral strategies;[30] nevertheless, little or no attention may be paid to help participants transition to "normal eating," exercise that is realistic for their lifestyles, and related emotional issues. Such programs could be termed "multifaceted unidimensional" programs because they use several behavioral strategies that emphasize stimulus control of intake and output by dieting and weight-related behavior modification. Unidimensional programs focus on overweight behaviors without regard for individuals' beliefs, thinking, feelings, and related behaviors (cognitive behavioral theory). Researchers and professionals may believe that eating and exercise behavioral programs should "cover" the major etiologic factors to promote weight reduction and maintenance. Failure to address the cognitive factors of weight management, however, may sabotage long-term maintenance and could be partly responsible for continued escalation of the overweight and obesity epidemic.

Many multidimensional programs claim to use cognitive restructuring techniques, but only focus on thinking about food, relationships with others around food, and restructured thinking about hunger and satiation. *Cognitive restructuring* is defined as reprogramming of negative, derogatory self-talk to positive, constructive self-talk. *Self-talk* is defined as automatic thoughts in one's mind, often derived from parents, authority figures, and religious teachings. Few programs directly address how negative beliefs and negative self-talk about one's shortcomings and interactions with others can repeatedly increase tension, distort attitudes, and lead to negative behaviors, such as overeating and skipping exercise.

The Centers for Disease Control and Prevention (CDC) lists psychological disorders associated with obesity, including depression, eating disorders, distorted body image, and low self-esteem, which can be associated with suboptimal weight loss.[12] Nondieting weight programs usually focus on emotional overeating, including programs such as 12-step Overeaters Anonymous,[31] religious-oriented Weigh Down Workshops,[32] and the Solution Developmental Method.[33] These programs are multidimensional (psychological, sociocultural, religious, spiritual) and help people maintain healthy weight loss without undue dieting, exercise, and constant monitoring of both.

Cognitive therapy based on Reversal Theory serves as the basis of the holistic self-care approach to healthy weight management. A brief overview of cognitive therapy and Reversal The-ory sets the stage for clear understanding of the Holistic Self-Care Model.

Cognitive Therapy Based on Reversal Theory

Beck describes cognitive therapy as helping clients restructure self-statements to be more realistic and positive, which in turn elicits positive responses.[13] Cognitive theories by themselves cannot explain why people can cope with stressors some of the time (and do not overeat to cope) and not at other times (leading to overeating to cope). Reversal Theory, a relatively new theory, offers an added dimension to cognitive restructuring. It provides the necessary organizing structure to locate tension stress in motivational states where negative self-talk originates and can be targeted for positive self-talk replacements to decrease tension stress.

Reversal Theory

Reversal Theory is explained as the basis of the Holistic Self-Care Model. *Tension stress*, defined as the discrepancy between where individuals are and where they want to be, is reviewed as the foundation for cognitive strategies used in holistic self-care for healthy weight management.

Apter's theory of psychological reversals, commonly referred to as Reversal Theory, provides a framework to explain factors related to overeating and lack of exercise in overweight individuals.[34] According to this phenomenologic theory of arousal, motivation, and action, Apter posits that personality is inherently inconsistent and that individuals reverse between opposing, paired states called metamotivational states because they are not, in themselves, concerned with motivation, but rather with the way in which motivation is experienced. Psychologically healthy individuals experience their motivations and actions in different ways, depending on metamotivational states. Four pairs of opposing states have been identified: telic and paratelic, conformist and negativistic, mastery and sympathy, and, last, alloic and autic (see **Exhibit 22-1**). At a given point in time, individuals are in combinations of the different states, consisting of one state of each of the four pairs, but never in both states of a pair at the same time.

When in the telic state, individuals are serious-minded and goal oriented; when in the paratelic

EXHIBIT 22-1   Apter's Reversal Theory Metamotivational States Pairs and Characteristics

---

Eight Ways of Being Human

Telic
Serious-minded
Goal-oriented
Plan ahead
Try to accomplish something
Future-oriented
*Anxiety   **Calmness

Paratelic
Playful
Spontaneous
Emphasize good feelings
Have fun for fun's sake
Present-oriented
*Boredom   **Excitement

Conformist
Don't make waves or disagree with others
Follow the rules
Feel embarrassed or guilty if I break a rule
Compliant
Agreeable
Stay in line
Do what others do
Worry about what others think
*Unprotected   **Protected

Negativistic
Stick up for what I think when I disagree with others
Bend and break the rules
Feel angry
Stubborn
Rebellious and defiant
Want to be difficult
*Trapped   **Free

Mastery
Do your best
Give it your all
Be strong, don't show feelings of weakness
Be tough, stay strong
Compete
Be in control
*Soft   **Hardy

Sympathy
Let my feelings tell me what to do
Deserve a break
OK to show and tell feelings of weakness
Be tender, OK to not be strong
Don't compete
Be nurturing
*Insensitive   **Sensitive

Alloic
Think of others first
Put self last
Others are most important
*Shame   **Modesty
*Guilt   **Virtue

Autic
Think of self first
Put others after self
I am most important
*Humiliation   **Pride
*Resentment   **Gratitude

* Unpleasant feelings or responses (tension stress) associated with specific metamotivational states.
** Pleasant feelings and responses associated with specific metamotivational states.

Source: S. Popkess-Vawter, "Weight Management," in *American Holistic Nurses' Association Core Curriculum for Holistic Nursing,* ed. B. M. Dossey, 211–219 (Gaithersburg, MD: Aspen, 1997).

---

state, they are playful and spontaneous. When in the conformist state, people prefer to go along with rules and regulations; when in the negativistic state, they prefer to break rules and want to be rebellious or noncompliant. When in the mastery state, individuals feel that being tough and being in control are important; when in the sympathy state, they feel that being tender and noncompetitive are important. In the alloic state, people derive pleasure from thinking of others before themselves in an altruistic way; in the autic state, they derive pleasure from thinking of themselves before others. Healthy individuals reverse between states easily and often throughout the day. The balance that results when individuals reverse easily between the four pairs of motivational states is termed "Eight Ways of Being Human."

Unpleasant Feelings and Tension Stress

Each metamotivational state has pleasant and unpleasant feelings and responses associated with it (indicated by asterisks in Exhibit 22-1). Pleasant responses, depending on the metamotivational state, include feeling calm, excited, free, and proud. Unpleasant responses include feeling anxious, bored, angry, trapped, ashamed, humiliated, guilty, and resentful, all which represent tension stress. According to Reversal Theory, tension stress is the discrepancy between desired and actual feelings. Individuals can take actions to reduce levels of tension stress within the same metamotivational state or may experience a spontaneous reversal to the opposing state within the metamotivational pair when attempting to lower stress levels. The following is an example of tension stress leading to overeating.

EXAMPLE

K. Z., 29 years old, reported how she repeatedly used overeating as an attempt to reduce tension stress within the same reversal theory state. "While I'm eating, I'm oblivious to everything else. I'm not thinking about what is hurting me. . . . It's just like an escape . . . to be able to eat is just an escape from everything. . . . The only time I can turn myself off is when I'm eating." K. Z. spontaneously described a happening referred to in the literature as the escape phenomenon and in clinical practice as "numbing out." She obtained relief from unpleasant feelings (tension stress) by "numbing out" during eating, even though she knew she would not feel good later.

On the particular occasion that K. Z. related her overeating, she had an unpleasant telephone exchange with her mother. She was saying to herself in her mind, "It's always my fault! I'm always the bad guy!" She related that these negative self-talk words represent many old interpersonal conflicts experienced with her mother and family members.

Repeated negative thoughts can evoke negative feelings that, in turn, can evoke negative behavior such as coping by eating favorite foods to feel better. Another client shared about a similar unpleasant incident on the telephone with her sister. "Even though I had eaten breakfast and was not hungry, while still on the phone I knew I was going to go get donuts to feel better."

Self-report questionnaires based on Reversal Theory were developed and tested for use as weight management assessment and progress measures.[35] The original questionnaire assessed stress-related overeating. Later, two additional questionnaires were developed using the same Reversal Theory–based questions, but measured stress-related skipping planned exercise and feeling low or bad.[36] Measures have been converted for computer administration and are being tested for psychometric properties. Preliminary testing shows overweight participants to have higher stress related to overeating and skipping exercise compared to normal-weight participants. Interventions, guided by the Holistic Self-Care Model and designed to address stress-related unhealthy behaviors, are accompanied by pre- and ongoing assessment using the Overeating, Exercise, and Feelings Tension questionnaires.

Holistic Self-Care Model

The Holistic Self-Care Model is designed to assist overweight clients with individualized nutritional, exercise, and psycho-social-spiritual strategies for a long-term pursuit of healthier and happier lifestyles. Healthcare professionals help overweight clients become sensitive to their bodies, motivations, self-talk, feelings, and actions. Holistic self-care emphasizes concurrent work in nutritional, exercise, and psycho-social-spiritual dimensions to reduce the percentage of body fat and increase physical fitness.

Externally focused, "quick-fix" methods have limited effects and may compound the overweight problem through, for example, a reduction in metabolic rate and serious pharmaceutical side effects. In contrast, the Holistic Self-Care Model takes an internal perspective to seek insight about negative self-talk that obstructs long-term guidance from the body's natural hunger and satiety signals, as well as the positive benefits and sensations of regular exercise. The challenge that faces healthcare professionals is to design multidimensional interventions aimed at correcting what researchers know causes individuals to drop out of weight programs—namely, feelings of restriction and deprivation, no time for exercise, and hassles of daily living that habitually send overweight clients to seek relief from stressors by eating.

The Holistic Self-Care Model provides a unique plan of face-to-face counseling appointments to continually support, guide, individualize, and adjust lifelong strategies. The model is based on the following principles for long-term weight management:

- There is continual feedback among the three dimensions of eating, physical exercise, and esteem, as in the integration among mind, body, and spirit.
- Both nurses and clients who gain and lose weight in a cycle must give equal consideration to the mind, body, and spirit trinity as they develop permanent life changes.
- Clients are in charge of redesigning lifestyle patterns in these three areas, consistent with self-care tenets.
- Permanent life changes take a very long time. Old habits can be changed through small, steady efforts that lead to greater success, as opposed to drastic changes that lead to feelings of deprivation, burnout, relapse, and eventual failure.

The Holistic Self-Care Model emphasizes integrated care and empowerment of clients in mind, body, and spirit. Nurses sometimes find performing interventions for the mind and body more familiar and comfortable, but supporting and intervening for spirituality concerns may be the most important contribution that they can make to promote health. Spirituality can reunite parts of individuals so that they become whole. Spirituality includes belief in a power greater than that which humans possess—a higher authority and guiding spirit, and existential beliefs of positive values, meanings, and sense of purpose.

Nurses who address clients' spirituality as part of caregiving can help strengthen clients' sense of meaning, dignity, worth, and identity. Healing becomes possible not only for the body, but for low self-esteem, feelings of isolation, anger, powerlessness, and hopelessness. Human practices of honesty, love, caring, wisdom, imagination, and compassion can create a flowing, dynamic balance that allows and creates healing. Cognitive restructuring called BIO strategies are part of the Holistic Self-Care Model—the glue that can hold together bio-psycho-social-spiritual beings to make long-lasting, healthy lifestyle changes.

BIO Strategies

BIO strategies are defined as spiritually based, cognitive strategies designed to expand and maximize people's ability to manage healthy weight with long-term results. *BIO*, which stands for Balance from the Inside Out, is shown in the model's logo as an upside-down triangle. Upside-down triangles, used to express all BIO strategies, are divided down the middle to represent the two sides of each content area covered in the Holistic Self-Care Model. Each side of the triangle is further divided into four sections, thus representing the Eight Ways of Being Human (i.e., Reversal Theory), as well as representing all strategies as multidimensional. Emphasis is placed on keeping the triangle balanced on its tip by practicing both sides—all eight aspects daily. The theme of balance is carried through all BIO strategies and is represented in handouts. For example, clients can receive handouts with triangles representing eating, exercising, and esteem activities of daily living and positive self-talk (**Exhibit 22-2**). Spiritually based cognitive strategies promote internal self-awareness to guide self-care from moment to moment. Negative self-talk can block the body's natural signals of hunger and satiety, the need for regular exercise, and the inner voice of guidance for healthy self-care. BIO strategies are consistent with characteristics of successful weight management programs that include multiple intervention strategies focusing on lifestyle changes (e.g., self-monitoring, stimulus control, stress management, social support, physical activity, relapse prevention) to help people achieve gradual, consistent weight loss.

The BIO strategies are as follows: EAT for Hunger, Exercise for LIFE, and ESTEEM for Self and Others. Cognitive restructuring is defined for clients as reprogramming of negative, derogatory

EXHIBIT 22-2   BIO-Eating-Exercise-Esteem

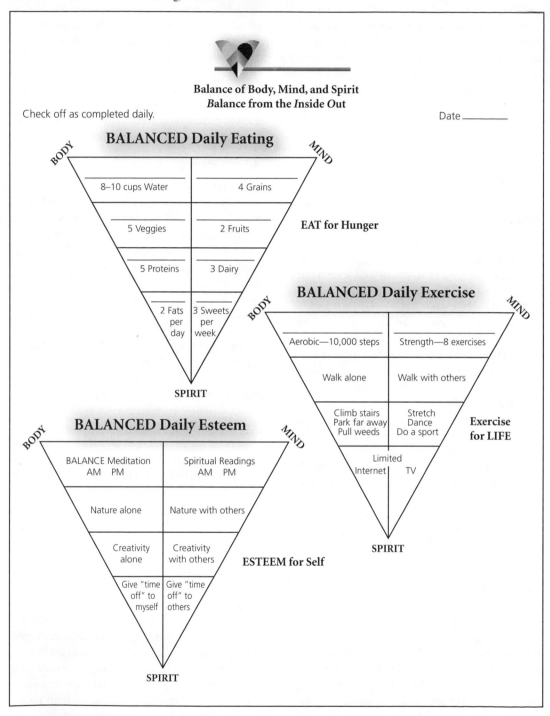

Balance of Body, Mind, and Spirit
Balance from the Inside Out

Check off as completed daily.   Date _____

BALANCED Daily Eating

BODY   MIND

_____   _____
8–10 cups Water   4 Grains

_____   _____   **EAT for Hunger**
5 Veggies   2 Fruits

5 Proteins   3 Dairy

2 Fats | 3 Sweets
per | per
day | week

SPIRIT

BALANCED Daily Exercise

BODY   MIND

_____   _____
Aerobic—10,000 steps   Strength—8 exercises

Walk alone   Walk with others

Climb stairs   Stretch   **Exercise
Park far away   Dance   for LIFE**
Pull weeds   Do a sport

Limited
Internet | TV

SPIRIT

BALANCED Daily Esteem

BODY   MIND

BALANCE Meditation   Spiritual Readings
AM   PM   AM   PM

Nature alone   Nature with others

Creativity   Creativity   **ESTEEM for Self**
alone   with others

Give "time | Give "time
off" to | off" to
myself | others

SPIRIT

Source: Reprinted with permission from Dr. Sue Popkess-Vawter, © 2003.

self-talk to positive, constructive self-talk. Self-talk, as mentioned earlier, is defined as automatic thoughts in one's mind, often derived from parents, authority figures, and religious teachings. EAT for Hunger is used to promote awareness for eating in response to hunger and satiety cues instead of emotional eating. Exercise for LIFE is a cognitive strategy to support daily exercise and physical activity. ESTEEM for Self and Others is a cognitive strategy to support self-esteem and coping through daily meditation, spiritual reading, and personal creativity. All three strategies use a mnemonic device of letters (i.e., EAT, LIFE, ESTEEM) to help clients to commit strategies to memory. Each letter stands for a part of the strategy that replaces unhealthy behaviors, such as overeating, skipping exercise, and negative self-talk. For example, in the EAT for Hunger strategy, EAT stands for Eating only when hunger occurs, Asking the body what it needs, and Telling the self to stop when hunger is satisfied, not full (**Exhibit 22-3**). People are taught to think of their hunger on a 10-point continuum (1 = starving to 10 = stuffed, 5 = feel nothing). This approach is cognitive because it requires individuals to limit portions to what their bodies need at the time, which means slowing eating to at least 20 minutes to recognize the absence of hunger. EAT for Hunger supports spiritual strategies because it emphasizes nourishment for energy needs only, not for emotional needs. EAT for Hunger emphasizes stopping eating when hunger is gone, which is a finer distinction than stopping when full. Thus, EAT promotes ingesting smaller portions using internal limits versus overeating to fullness or to a predetermined amount specified by a diet (i.e., external limits). This strategy was found to reduce overeating significantly.[20,37,38] Clients use this strategy to separate eating from emotional needs by using the STOP Emotional Eating strategy (Exhibit 22-3). They also learn to increase healthy food intake with more fiber and water, eat in five to six smaller portions daily, and decrease fat, sugar, and starches.

BIO self-talk for eating, exercise, and esteem accompanies each BIO strategy to promote reprogramming of negative thinking that can lead to negative feelings and unhealthy behaviors. Clients are assisted to create their own positive statements, as seen in **Exhibit 22-4**. The top line

EXHIBIT 22-3   EAT for Hunger/STOP Emotional Eating

EAT for Hunger

Eat	ONLY when hungry. Am I a "3" or "4"?
	1 2 3 4 5 6 7 8 9 10
	←————————————————→
	Starving Stuffed
Ask	Self, what am I hungry for?
	Eat slowly to enjoy (20 minutes or more) and to satisfy hunger.
Tell	Self, stop when hunger is gone.
	Eat to a "5," similar to drinking until thirst is gone.

STOP Emotional Eating

Stop	Do BALANCE Meditation
Tell	What am I FEELING? What do I NEED right now? Negative self-talk?
Options	For Positive self-talk?
Plans	To deal directly with my feelings and needs?

Source: Reprinted with permission from Dr. Sue Popkess-Vawter, © 2003.

EXHIBIT 22-4   BIO-Self-Talk

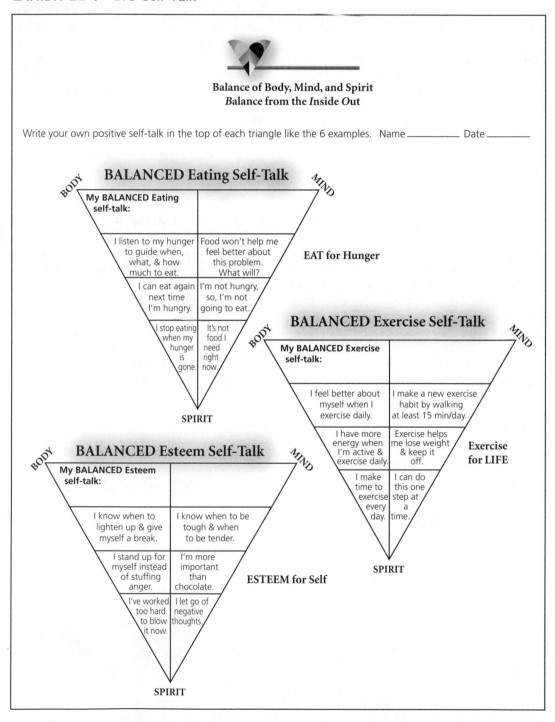

Balance of Body, Mind, and Spirit
Balance from the Inside Out

Write your own positive self-talk in the top of each triangle like the 6 examples.   Name _____   Date _____

BALANCED Eating Self-Talk

BODY   MIND

My BALANCED Eating
self-talk:

I listen to my hunger | Food won't help me
to guide when, | feel better about
what, & how | this problem.   EAT for Hunger
much to eat. | What will?

I can eat again | I'm not hungry,
next time | so, I'm not
I'm hungry. | going to eat.

I stop eating | It's not
when my | food I
hunger | need
is | right
gone. | now.

SPIRIT

BALANCED Exercise Self-Talk

BODY   MIND

My BALANCED Exercise
self-talk:

I feel better about | I make a new exercise
myself when I | habit by walking
exercise daily. | at least 15 min/day.

I have more | Exercise helps
energy when | me lose weight   Exercise
I'm active & | & keep it   for LIFE
exercise daily.| off.

I make | I can do
time to | this one
exercise| step at
every | a
day. | time.

SPIRIT

BALANCED Esteem Self-Talk

BODY   MIND

My BALANCED Esteem
self-talk:

I know when to | I know when to be
lighten up & give | tough & when
myself a break. | to be tender.

I stand up for | I'm more
myself instead | important
of stuffing | than   ESTEEM for Self
anger. | chocolate.

I've worked | I let go of
too hard | negative
to blow | thoughts.
it now. |

SPIRIT

Source: Reprinted with permission from Dr. Sue Popkess-Vawter, © 2003.

of all upside-down pyramids is provided for them to write personal statements that they believe can replace negative, self-sabotaging statements that currently lead to overeating, skipping planned exercise, and feeling bad about one's self.

Exercise for LIFE involves regular daily exercise that includes planned aerobic and strength exercises (e.g., walking, swimming, biking, resistance machines and weights) and simply moving more often through the day. Exercise for LIFE uses the acronym LIFE to represent the following: Learn the habit, I am important, Friends, and Enjoy myself. Although research has shown that 60–90 minutes per day of moderate-intensity physical activity is needed to maintain a significant weight loss,[39] Exercise for LIFE emphasizes beginning with whatever amount of exercising and movement that clients are doing presently and building on that baseline, using small increases of planned exercise and movement (e.g., parking farther away, taking the stairs, pulling weeds). Clients must believe they are important enough to take time each day for exercise to become a habit. Exercising companions, such as friends and family, help clients enjoy a variety of exercises and view their daily exercise as a lifelong habit.

ESTEEM for Self and Others involves a regular personal practice of seeking solitude for a specified time in a private, quiet setting to read, meditate, pray, and journal. ESTEEM stands for Energy, Spirit, Time, Eating, Exercise, Meditation. Esteem for self can emerge from time spent in solitude and meditation to provide spiritual energy that guides healthy eating and exercise. Solitude (i.e., purposeful, quiet time alone) and a connected sense of spirit can provide wholeness and balance in physical, psychological, and sociocultural aspects of life. According to cognitive theory, positive feelings arise from positive beliefs and positive self-talk. On the other hand, negative beliefs of not being a worthy person can elicit worthless self-talk, negative feelings, and behaviors of overeating to comfort the self. To stop this negative chain response, the BIO strategies begin with helping individuals redefine basic values through spirituality. Sustained behavioral change begins at the spiritual level by taking care of the spirit or soul. Spiritual activities may act as nutrition for the spirit as actual food does for the body. Unknowingly, people may try to fulfill spiritual needs with food and other substances, whereas vital nurturance may only be found through inner spiritual connections for internal decision making. Spiritual activities can help clients connect, in solitude, with a power greater than one's self in "internal self-talk" about needs and internal decision making. Without a sense of inward direction from a power greater than the self, people may not feel a genuine sense of energy and balance, and thus not have positive self-esteem. Clients may be given handouts and daily meditation books such as those by Beattie,[28] Dyer,[29] and Easwaran,[40] and a personal journal that has blank pages for participants to write about thoughts and feelings as they experience personal growth throughout the intervention. Journaling serves as an emotional release that can improve depressive symptoms. The BIO balance meditation (**Exhibit 22-5**) can be given to clients as an example of a relaxation, affirmation, and coping strategy to guide development of their own version of the meditation, which facilitates regular, individualized spiritual connections.

■ HOLISTIC CARING PROCESS

Holistic Assessment

In preparing to use weight management interventions, the nurse should assess the following parameters:

- Body composition (baseline and at least every 6 months)
  - Body mass index
- Resting heart rate and blood pressure
- Blood profile (baseline and at least every 6 months)
  - Lipid profile
  - Blood glucose level
  - Thyroid level
  - Hemoglobin and hematocrit
- Physical fitness
  - If possible, exercise testing using submaximal bicycle ergometer or maximal treadmill
  - Strength testing using repetition maximum for chest press and leg press (or comparable exercises)
  - BIO Eating-Exercise-Esteem (Exhibit 22-2)

EXHIBIT 22-5 Balance Meditation

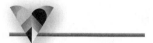

Balance of Body, Mind, and Spirit
Ten-Minute Relaxation-Meditation Exercise*

Relaxation

- I sit, close my eyes, and take three deep breaths.
- I let go of all negative self-talk and feelings.
- I gently tighten and relax muscles head to toe.
- I feel balanced, healthy, and at peace.
- Slowly repeat the BIO Affirmation.

BIO Affirmation

Balance of Body-Mind-Spirit

BIO = **B**alance from the **I**nside **O**ut

Balance means accepting myself totally as I am . . .

- I accept my **body** as I am right now as I take positive actions to be healthier.
- I accept all **feelings** as they come to me. I can choose to quickly let go of negative feelings and negative self-talk so that my **mind** can think **positive self-talk** to be healthier.
- I believe I am a good person. As a human, I make mistakes. My **spirit** can connect with a power greater than myself for healthy guidance.

Balance is accepting my body-mind-spirit and trusting my inner voice's direction to

- Think positive self-talk
- Feel positive feelings
- Act in healthier ways every day, to receive

Balance from the **I**nside **O**ut

BALANCE to Cope

- Relaxed, I repeat over and over the word, *BALANCE*
- To cope with any negative feelings and negative self-talk today, I take a deep breath, close my eyes if possible, and slowly repeat the BALANCE Affirmation to slow down, think positive self-talk, feel peaceful, and make good choices that honor myself and others.

▪ *Note:* Change any part of this meditation to make it meaningful to you.
Source: Reprinted with permission from Dr. Sue Popkess-Vawter, © 2003.

- Psychological profile
    - Life review and dieting history, from clients' stories of their lives and the evolution of their weight problem; identification of lifestyle patterns
    - BULIT (bulimia test) scale to screen for bulimia[38]
    - Body image according to a 10-point visual analog scale (1 being the best)
    - Overeating, Exercise, Feelings, Tension Stress questionnaires[36]

Identification of Patterns/ Challenges/Needs

The patterns/challenges/needs (see Chapter 7) compatible with weight management interventions are as follows:

- Altered nutrition (more than body requires)
- Spiritual distress
- Ineffective individual coping
- Decreased physical mobility
- Disturbance in body image
- Disturbance in self-esteem
- Hopelessness
- Knowledge deficit
- Anxiety

Specific patterns/challenges/needs related to the Holistic Self-Care Model and BIO strategies include the following:

- Overeating related to increased tension stress
- Decreased aerobic and resistance exercise related to a poor body image and a feeling of being unworthy to take time for exercise
- Infrequent episodes of play and creativity related to early modeling and values that consider work to be more important than play
- Lack of skills to express anger and disagreement, related to a belief that it is unacceptable behavior
- Lack of skills to express feelings, related to early suppression of feelings as a self-protective mechanism
- Inability to put the self first, related to early teaching that others have greater value and worth

Outcome Identification

Prochaska and DiClemente developed the Transtheoretical Therapy Model to expand the applicability of change theory.[11] Their stages of change have been applied to a wide variety of healthcare problems, including weight management. They propose that individuals may move through five stages of motivational readiness when confronted with lifestyle changes: (1) precontemplation, (2) contemplation, (3) preparation, (4) action, and (5) maintenance. Nurses can tailor their assessments, interventions, prescriptions, and evaluations to the individual's stage to attain long-term weight management (**Exhibit 22-6**).

Most clients begin sessions at either the precontemplation or the contemplation stage. It is possible for an individual to be in different stages of the nutritional, exercise, and psychosocial-spiritual dimensions of the program. For example, in the case of K. Z., she may be starting to exercise two to three times per week (preparation stage) but refuses to even discuss nutritional interventions (precontemplation stage). She apparently has no insight into her negative self-talk and, therefore, has no intention of changing (also precontemplation state).

Therapeutic Care Plan and Interventions

Before the session:

- Spend a few moments centering yourself to recognize your presence and to begin the session with the intention to facilitate healing.
- Create an environment in which the client is encouraged to share his or her story.

At the beginning of the session:

- Show a listing of the stages of change to the client and have him or her explain any differences between his or her stage at the last session and now. Proceed accordingly with the Holistic Self-Care Model as shown in Exhibit 22-6.

At the end of the session:

- Ask the client to review what he or she gained from the session and answer any questions. Give the client a copy of any

EXHIBIT 22-6   Nursing Interventions: Long-Term Weight Management According to Prochaska and DiClemente's Stages of Change

Client Outcomes According to Stage of Change	Nursing Prescriptions	Evaluation
1. *Precontemplation (no intention of changing in the next 6 months):* The client will verbalize reasons for not wanting to reduce weight and fat, and perform regular exercise.	Measure client's body mass index, body fat, resting heart rate and blood pressure, cholesterol, lipids, and blood glucose. Administer life review and dieting history, BULIT (bulimia test) scale to screen for bulimia, and body image 10-point visual analog scale.	The client received a clinic weight management brochure with a written report of his or her physical and psychological findings. The client verbalized understanding of the report, implied risks, and invitation to learn more about the clinic weight program.
2. *Contemplation (considering changing in the next 6 months, but not active yet):* The client will report fewer overeating episodes and less tension stress during daily eating.	Assist the client to apply the EAT for Hunger cognitive restructuring nutritional strategy based on Reversal Theory. Administer tension stress scale.	The client verbalized the three steps of the EAT for Hunger strategy and shared one difficulty with the strategy to work on in the next 6 months. The client was pleased with freedom of eating for hunger.
3. *Preparation (making some changes, but not at goal):* The client will report exercising more frequently, resulting in greater muscle strength, less fatigue, and more energy.	Assist the client to apply the Exercise for LIFE strategy based on Reversal Theory.	The client described aerobic and strength exercises that he or she is willing to do and shared one difficulty with the strategy to work on in the next 6 months. The client reported lower tension stress.
4. *Action (6 months of active behavior change):* The client will have lower levels of total cholesterol and low-density lipoproteins, a higher level of high-density lipoproteins, and blood glucose levels within normal limits.	Assist the client to apply the STOP Emotional Eating cognitive restructuring psycho-social-spiritual strategy based on Reversal Theory.	The client verbalized the four steps of the STOP Emotional Eating strategy and shared one difficulty with the strategy to work on in the next 6 months. The client is pleased with exercise progress.
5. *Maintenance (sustained change past 6 months):* The client will have a lower percentage of body fat, lower weight, lower resting heart rate, and lower blood pressure.	Assist the client to apply the acceptance of obstacles cognitive restructuring psycho-social-spiritual strategy.	The client verbalized the acceptance strategy and shared one difficulty with the strategy on which to concentrate efforts in the next 6 months. The client is pleased with lipid levels, weight, and blood pressure.

relevant support materials, and ask him or her to explain how to use them. Ask him or her to complete a copy of the BIO Eating-Exercise-Esteem worksheet (Exhibit 22-2) and verbalize what he or she has written and the times allotted for the behaviors.

Specific Interventions

Specific interventions used in the Holistic Self-Care Model are listed and interpreted according to the five stages of change as described in Exhibit 22-6.

Precontemplation

When clients are not ready to make lifestyle changes, a nurse cannot "motivate" or manipulate them to do so. The nurse can inform them about his or her assessment of their situation, risks involved, and options available to them. Raising their consciousness without demands can do more to move them to the next level of readiness than giving them "pep talks" and trying to force them to see other perspectives. Thus, the nurse should teach the client the basic principles of the Holistic Self-Care Model for long-term weight management as follows:

- There is no need to diet, count calories, and weigh one's self daily or weekly. The percentage of body fat is a more accurate way to determine whether clients weigh too much because weight can be normal but consist of a high percentage of body fat.
- Both physical and psychological reasons that clients are not losing excess pounds must be addressed to be successful for the rest of their lives.
- Most people with weight problems have lost weight successfully at some point in their lives, but regained the weight. Often, they are very knowledgeable about food and exercise, and they may even be somewhat in touch with the psychological reasons that they "go off" of their weight reduction programs.
- When young, many people learned to eat to feel better when they experienced unpleasant feelings; their active lifestyles kept them from having an overweight problem until adult years. Greater responsibilities in adult life forced them to be more sedentary, allowing fat to accumulate and reducing lean body mass.
- Increasing pressures, stressors, and short-term bouts of weight gain (e.g., because of pregnancy, loss of a job) put extra pounds on individuals' bodies.
- Eating must be separated and disconnected from emotions and reconnected with naturally occurring hunger. Emotions, then, must be recognized, felt, and acted on in healthy ways.
- The Holistic Self-Care Model for long-term weight management is the combination of stopping overeating, getting challenging exercise four to six times every week, and reprogramming negative, self-destructive self-talk to realistic and personally valued self-talk.

Contemplation

Clients in the contemplation stage still believe that the reasons for not changing their behaviors (e.g., too tired, too hungry, too busy, don't have enough money) overbalance the reasons that they should. When past dieters view a future of dietary restrictions, their negative feelings toward past failures tip the balance of the scales in the negative direction.

EAT for Hunger Strategy

Under the EAT for Hunger strategy, clients learn to eat according to their internal control (hunger) with as many food choices as desired; regulation of eating is according to internal satiation of their hunger.

The purpose of this nutritional strategy is to bring physiologic hunger and the pleasure of eating into balance. Clients should weigh only weekly or monthly, or wait until the nurse weighs them at an appointment to increase the accuracy of true weight fluctuations and avoid unnecessary emotional responses to false readings of temporary water weight loss and gain. Group exercises, such as participating in a taste-testing exercise or eating a meal together, can reinforce new principles. Topics discussed in group or individual sessions can include why people overeat, why they lose weight, how thin people think and eat, why diets do not work, and why people choose fat over thin. Essential content in this nutritional strategy includes learning healthy balance of nutrients; reading food labels for sugar, fiber, fat, and sodium content; and the need for healthy choices (e.g., low sugar, starch, fat, and high fiber).

Before beginning the strategy, the nurse should administer the BULIT and the tension stress scale to determine the client's risk for overeating and tension stress level before overeating, respectively. Scores on these measures serve as evaluation outcomes over time. The nurse should also encourage clients to think about the meaning that hunger has for them. In most cases, feeling hungry is associated with negative feelings of deprivation, past restriction, and physical discomfort. They can learn to manage negative feelings associated with hunger and begin to think of hunger as a positive signal that tells them to eat.

Ways to Stop Overeating

Naturally thin people eat differently compared to overweight people. Naturally thin people do not overeat often, exercise more, and have less negative emotional associations with food. Overweight weight cyclers often have a sense of deprivation that can lead to binge eating of "forbidden foods."

The three steps to stop overeating are written as positive self-talk (i.e., affirmations):

1. I eat only when I'm hungry, after rating my hunger on a scale of 1 to 10.
   a. Ravenously starved = 1
   b. Uncomfortably stuffed = 10
   c. Feeling nothing = 5
   d. Eating to satisfy hunger = between 3 and 5
2. I eat exactly what I want. My body has the natural ability to know what it wants and needs. When I crave "unhealthy, forbidden" foods, I ask myself if it is truly a physical craving; if so and I am hungry, I can eat it. If the food does not taste good, I don't eat it. I eat slowly, enjoying every bite. Eating slowly helps me fully experience the pleasure of eating the food. Eating slowly allows time for my brain to get the messages of satisfaction and feeling nothing.

This usually takes about 20 minutes. Conscious, enjoyable eating satisfies cravings so that they will not return for a while.

3. I stop eating when my hunger is gone and I feel nothing (a rating of 5 on the 1 to 10 hunger scale). When I eat to a rating of 5, it is like drinking water until my thirst is gone. If hunger is still present, I take and enjoy three more bites slowly and then stop.

Minimum daily requirements may be met over 2 or 3 days rather than every day. When clients take in all of their calories to meet minimal daily requirements from foods that they "should" eat, extra calories eaten to satisfy natural cravings will be beyond their needs and result in stored fat. The American Diabetic Association diabetic diet consists of taking in five to six small feedings at regular intervals throughout waking hours. The purpose is to keep blood glucose at a relatively stable level, preventing dramatic peaks and valleys. Similarly, the EAT for Hunger pattern does not allow dramatic swings between hunger and fullness. Current emphasis on portion control can be accomplished using the EAT for Hunger strategy. Increasing water intake to the recommended 8 to 10 cups per day is also essential for effective metabolic processes.

Old overeating habits come from self-talk that clients may need to become aware of and discuss, such as the following examples:

- I always eat a "good breakfast"—even when I'm not hungry.
- I had better eat now because I may not have time later.
- I always finish off my meals with a little something sweet.
- I always clean my plate (for the starving children).
- I cannot stand to throw away perfectly good food.
- I eat it whether it tastes good or not.
- I can't eat the foods I want until I eat the healthy foods I should eat first.

Later, clients can learn new positive self-talk replacements to overcome these overeating habits. The STOP Emotional Eating strategy (Exhibit 22-3) can also be discussed later as clients move into the preparation stage.

Preparation

In the preparation stage, clients begin to make lifestyle changes, but they perform the new behaviors sporadically and have not yet incorporated them as a permanent part of their lifestyles. The nurse can play an important supportive role at this time as the clients gradually override their individual reasons not to incorporate new behaviors into their lifestyles. After each success, they gain confidence in their new behaviors and find ways to adapt daily habits to accommodate them. The nurse should not push clients at this stage, but rather should be available when they have questions and need suggestions. The Exercise for LIFE strategy is introduced at this stage because individuals often need to be at a higher level of change to put forth the effort and time demanded by regular exercise habits.

Exercise for LIFE Strategy

The purpose of the Exercise for LIFE strategy is to introduce regular, challenging exercise as a means to express self-value and love (Exhibit 22-2). When clients learn to accept exercise as part of their life, they learn to truly love themselves and their bodies. Valuing the self enough to schedule and maintain regular exercise is an act of self-love. When they exercise for others (e.g., physician, spouse, friend, child), efforts are usually short lived and can end in resentment. When they hold to a regular and challenging exercise plan, while at the same time allowing themselves to miss a few days without panic or guilt, they have learned to Exercise for LIFE.

Clients can be given the book *Fit to Live*.[27] Sessions may be divided equally to discuss the book's topics: reasons that women are fatter than men, use of aerobic and strength exercises to reduce fat, design of a personal aerobic and strength exercise program, and incorporation of exercise into one's lifestyle. A healthcare professional should assess risks involved in performing aerobic and strength training before the client begins training. Once the client's safety is ensured, it is time to prescribe beginning, intermediate, and advanced levels of combined aerobic and strength training protocols based on physical exercise pretesting results. When possible, the assistance of a colleague educated in exercise physiology or physical therapy is helpful for exercise testing. If colleagues cannot assist clients directly, they can assist the nurse in developing a step test that is easily administered in most settings.

In 2007, the American College of Sports Medicine and American Heart Association recommended that healthy adults ages 18–65 years need moderate-intensity aerobic physical activity for at least 30 minutes on 5 days each week, or vigorous-intensity aerobic physical activity for at least 20 minutes on 3 days each week.[41] Further, they recognized that 10-minute bouts of exercise three or more times per day and routine activities of daily life (walking, cleaning) add to physical fitness. Clients may use any mode of aerobic exercise to sustain heart rate within their working heart range for duration according to their fitness levels. To maintain fat-free mass and increase muscular strength and endurance, the American College of Sports Medicine recommends strength training (i.e., weight lifting) with one to three sets of 8 to 12 repetitions using moderate-intensity resistance at least 2 days per week. Clients should receive instruction about exercising all muscle groups using no equipment, minimal equipment, and strength training gym equipment. Muscle group and related exercises include leg press, bench press, leg curl, lateral pull shoulder press, calf raises, arm curls, triceps press, rowing, back extension, pectorals, and abdominals. Clients usually can begin training for the first month with one set of 12 repetitions at a resistance they can perform with ease (to minimize muscle damage and soreness).

By the second month, clients will perform according to beginning, intermediate, and advanced levels. The usual goal by the end of the first year is to participate in aerobic and strength exercises two to three times per week for each type of exercise, for a total of 4 to 6 exercise days per week (consistent with American College of Sports Medicine recommendations). If clients need regular, anticipated support, they may find it helpful to join a gym.

Ways to Get Regular, Challenging Exercise

To get ready for a regular and challenging exercise program, clients should seek physician approval and should ensure that their risks are minimal. They should wear loose-fitting, environmentally proper clothes and supportive shoes matched for the type of exercise (e.g., walking, jogging, cross-training). Clients should be knowledgeable about and plan for physical and environmental safety. The nurse should educate and help clients design exercise to fit their lifestyles.

Clients can learn that having a healthy percentage of body fat (22–28%) is necessary for metabolic rate to be driven by fat-free or lean body mass. Excess fat is metabolically less active than muscle and results in a slow metabolism, making it more difficult to lose weight.

Clients can learn about differences between aerobic and anaerobic exercise. Aerobic exercises (e.g., walking, slow jogging, swimming, biking) use more oxygen, use large muscle groups, and are at lower intensities and of longer duration. Anaerobic exercises (e.g., running, swimming, stair-climbing, biking, weight lifting at a very fast or vigorous pace) use more glucose stores, usually use isolated muscle groups, and are at higher intensities and of shorter duration.

An exercise schedule should address frequency, duration, and intensity. Frequency of aerobic exercises should be three and four times per week; frequency of strength training or weight lifting exercises should be two and three times per week. Strength training should not be done two consecutive days using the same muscle groups; an every other day schedule allows for maximum muscle repair. Duration of an aerobic workout should be 20 to 60 minutes; duration of a strength workout should be 30 to 60 minutes. Intensity of an aerobic workout is at 70–80% of the maximum heart rate. The following is a quick method to calculate working heart range (the range within which rate should be kept to gain aerobic benefit):

EXAMPLE

Working Heart Range = (220 − Age) × 70% (for lower end) and × 80% (for upper end)

Example: $220 - 40 = 180$

$180 \times 0.80 = 144$

$180 \times 0.70 = 126$

Working Heart Range = 126 to 144 beats per minute

Intensity of a strength workout should be one to two sets of 12 to 15 repetitions of lifting weights. Sample workout plans may be prescribed in the following four levels:

Level 1: Exercise 3 days per week; 1 strength day and 2 aerobic days

Level 2: Exercise 4 days per week; 2 strength days and 2 aerobic days

Level 3: Exercise 5 days per week; 2 strength days and 3 aerobic days

Level 4: Exercise 6 days per week; 3 strength days and 3 aerobic days

---

An exercise workout should start with stretching the arms and legs in a static stretch without bouncing. Next is the warm-up, lasting 3–5 minutes to increase the heart rate slowly. After the exercise is the cool-down phase, which is slow-paced, continuing aerobic exercise, again followed by stretching the arms and legs in a static stretch without bouncing. A slight soreness 12–24 hours after exercise shows that the muscles have been sufficiently challenged to require energy-expending repair to rebuild muscle and indicates an increased excess postexercise oxygen consumption (EPOC). Often called afterburn, EPOC helps clients lose excess fat even at rest, particularly with resistance exercise. For maximum benefit, the client should not do the same workout repeatedly because the body adapts and will not be challenged.

Scheduling exercise ahead of time by week helps develop a new habit. Writing workout days and times in the personal calendar can build the client's commitment to exercise. Great variability in workouts from day to day prevents boredom and maximizes use of different muscle groups. Workouts with friends and family add interest and challenge.

Action

Around 3 to 6 months, clients usually have their eating and exercise habits started well and have experienced pride and satisfaction in their lifestyle changes. They still can resume former habits if boredom, illness or injury, life crises, and burnout occur, however. Thus, it is especially important at this stage to introduce the esteem and spiritual portion of the intervention to help prevent relapse. They can truly understand that their new eating and exercise habits are for a lifetime. By learning to be aware of their self-talk, they can decrease negative self-talk and increase positive self-talk to support long-term, holistic self-care weight management. By using the STOP Emotional Eating strategy (Exhibit 22-3) and BIO self-talk worksheets (Exhibit 22-4), clients can learn to pinpoint and change their most threatening triggers and sabotaging self-talk.

STOP Emotional Eating Strategy

The purpose of the STOP Emotional Eating strategy is to separate emotions from eating responses and to learn actions for managing underlying stress without eating to cope. Clients learn to hear internal self-talk that describes their true underlying needs. Clients can be given copies of books such as *The Language of Letting Go*[28] and *Fit to Live*[27] to support separating emotions from overeating.

Clients can complete homework using self-talk worksheets for identifying and reframing negative self-talk into positive self-talk replacements (Exhibit 22-4). Discussion topics include how beliefs, thoughts, feelings, and actions are related. Individual and group discussions can include real-life examples of each type of irrational thinking:

- All-or-nothing thinking—perceiving absolute, black-and-white categories
- Overgeneralization—seeing negative situation as never ending
- Mental filter—dwelling on negatives and ignoring positives
- Mind reading and fortune telling—interpreting others and events as negative without the facts
- Magnification or minimization of importance—blowing situation out of proportion or shrinking it unrealistically
- "Shoulding" and blaming—saying *should*, *shouldn't*, *have to*, and taking too much or not enough responsibility
- Labeling—naming self instead of behavior (instead of *I made a mistake, I am a mistake*)

To counter each type of irrational thinking, clients can review and practice the challenges to irrational thinking:

- Where is the evidence that this thought is true or not true?
- Would an informal survey of those I trust show that this thought is realistic?
- Would I talk to and treat my best friend the way I talk to and treat myself?
- Can I consider shades of gray instead of black-and-white thinking?
- How can "should thinking" be restated with *preferably* and *sometimes*?

Ways to Change Negative Self-Talk Triggers

Helping clients use BIO strategies and self-talk to balance their Eight Ways of Being Human begins with an examination of the frequent emotions found to trigger overeating, skipping planned exercise, and feeling bad about one's self. At this point, the effort focuses on desensitizing, practicing, and accepting being in the negative state. Clients can use these guidelines for writing positive self-talk:

- Write in a positive tone.
- Write in the present as if you had already done it.
- Write as specifically and succinctly as possible.
- Write about yourself rather than "fixing" others.
- Write in your usual everyday language.
- Write from the heart.

The BIO self-talk worksheet is used to tailor personal positive self-talk statements to replace negative, self-sabotaging statements. Several samples are listed in the BIO triangles, but clients are encouraged to write their own personal statements in the top spaces provided in each triangle for eating, exercise, and esteem.

Maintenance

After 6 months of clients practicing and refining lifestyle changes, the nurse can be very instrumental in helping them maintain their lifestyle changes by continuing supportive actions such as being available to answer questions, providing resources, and assisting with modifications in eating and exercise routines. By allowing clients to stay in touch and approaching them when the nurse has innovative ideas, the nurse may spark their new and continued interest in their programs. The nurse may help clients examine their patterns when they overeat and do not exercise to discover ways to reinforce and strengthen areas of deficit. For example, the nurse may suggest that clients examine the last months of BIO Eating-Exercise-Esteem worksheets for the following:

- What emotional trigger or situation gets me off my healthy eating plan?
- What emotional trigger or situation gets me off my healthy exercise plan?
- What emotional trigger or situation gets me off my healthy esteem plan?

The final key to lasting change is acceptance. When clients fully accept sadness, anger, and the bad, irritating things in life, rather than try to change perfectly, manipulate, succumb to, and overpower these things, a peace can settle into their spirits. Acceptance opens new possibilities that can help move them ahead to grow beyond obstacles that occurred in the past. The nurse may point out that constantly "fighting it" (like trying to break the door down) actually can keep them stuck in the past. As a key in a locked door, acceptance can move them to places they have never been or even fathomed.

The nurse guides clients to write in a journal about problematic obstacles in simple, succinct statements. Obstacles are the triggers that repeatedly set off negative self-talk that keep clients overeating, not exercising, and feeling bad about themselves. Acceptance of the obstacle statements are written as positive self-talk (Exhibit 22-4). Clients can be encouraged to individualize their own personal balance meditation (Exhibit 22-5). Personally meaningful versions of the relaxation, affirmation, and balance meditations can be used as mantras to build new habits to promote lower stress response and preventive actions to meet negative obstacles of everyday life.

CASE STUDY (IMPLEMENTATION)

A. W., a single 34-year-old high school English teacher, experienced all the stages of change over a period of approximately 1 year. At each stage, the A. W. was asked to rate her readiness in response to a listing and descriptions of the stages of change.

A. W. in the Precontemplation Stage

Setting: A. W. is at an afternoon appointment in a health clinic for Pap test and breast examination

Patterns/Challenges/Needs:

1. Altered nutrition, more than body requirements (167 pounds; 5 feet, 2 inches tall; BMI = 31; 35% body fat)
2. Body image disturbance (8 on a 10-point scale, 1 being best)
3. Hopelessness related to 17 years of past failures at weight management

After her regular wellness check, Pap smear, and breast examination, A. W. told her story in a brief life review and weight management history. She had a 17-year history of weight cycling that began when she was in high school. She had always been active in sports and aerobic exercise. In high school, she had a muscular build and average weight. When she entered college, she was less active because she studied more to keep her grades above average. She always felt a lot of pressure from her parents to make all As and become a college professor like her father.

In high school and college, A. W. developed a habit of munching on chips and candy while studying. She continued the habit as she prepared lectures and graded papers as a high school teacher. As she gradually gained weight and became more self-conscious about her physical appearance, she did not pursue relationships with men. She remained healthy except for occasional sinus headaches. Because she dieted and exercised throughout the 17 years of weight cycling, she was very pessimistic about her ability to lose and maintain a healthy weight. She became tearful when she told of her repeated failures and said that she was much too busy to exercise regularly.

A.W. was in relatively good physical health other than being mildly obese and inactive. She was to return to the clinic for blood work to be drawn within the next 2 weeks. She was rated "at risk" for binge eating on the BULIT scale, and she ranked her body image as an 8 on a 10-point scale (1 being best). She rated herself as being in the precontemplation stage; she was given a brochure that contained a section in which the nurse wrote a report of the physical findings to date, the health risks involved, and a summary of the Holistic Self-Care Model weight management program offered at the clinic. The nurse answered questions and encouraged A. W. to call her for more information about the program whenever she was ready.

A. W. in the Contemplation Stage

Setting: A. W. has a return appointment 1 month later in a health clinic for blood work (blood glucose and lipid levels)

Patterns/Challenges/Needs:

1. Altered nutrition, body requirements
2. Body image disturbance
3. Hopelessness

A. W.'s blood glucose level was within normal range, but her total cholesterol level and cholesterol to high-density lipoprotein ratio was slightly elevated. She said that she had been thinking about the program and wondered if individuals could choose to attend individual or group sessions. She asked for clarification about the fact that the brochure specified no type of diet—only eating according to hunger. When the nurse asked if A. W. was considering making some changes in eating and exercise, A. W. said that she was intrigued about a "no-diet" diet. The nurse noted A. W.'s interest in attending a group session and gave her the month's schedule of meetings about the EAT for Hunger strategy in the clinic's weight management program.

A.W. in the Preparation Stage

Setting: A. W. attended the last evening group meeting about the EAT for Hunger strategy in the clinic's weight management program (1 month later, after four group meetings).

Patterns/Challenges/Needs:

1. Altered nutrition, more than body requirements
2. Body image disturbance
3. Hopelessness
4. Decreased mobility related to no regular exercise program
5. Increased tension stress before overeating episodes—"at risk" scores on the tension stress scale

A. W. related that she enjoyed the group meetings about EAT for Hunger and felt great relief not dieting. She said that she realized how much she had been eating when she was not hungry, especially when she felt pressured to complete her teaching responsibilities. She expressed more hope that she could cut down on overeating by using the new EAT for Hunger strategy. Her major difficulty with the strategy was stopping at a "5" when her hunger was gone (preparation stage). A. W. also said that she was planning to attend next month's sessions on the Exercise for LIFE strategy, although she had not changed her activity level to date (contemplation stage for exercise).

A. W. in the Action Stage

Setting: A. W. attended the last evening group meeting about the Exercise for LIFE strategy in the clinic's weight management program (1 month later).

Patterns/Challenges/Needs:

1. Altered nutrition, more than body requirements—loss of 6 pounds
2. Body image disturbance—rated 7 on a 10-point scale (1 is best)
3. Hopelessness—more hopeful to make long-term lifestyle changes in new program with group support
4. Decreased mobility related to no regular exercise program—attending group meetings regularly and beginning a 3- to 4-day per week workout program
5. Increased tension stress before overeating episodes—overeating less often, but tension stress still high with overeating

A. W. began walking with a friend twice every week and came early to walk with two group members before meetings once a week. She bought videotapes of combined aerobics and strength exercises and did a 30-minute workout before leaving for work once a week. She lost 3 more pounds at the end of the third month of participating in the program and lost inches in her body proportions almost equal to one dress size.

A. W. began the third month of the program using the STOP Emotional Eating strategy. She described the pressures in her high school teaching job that kept her eating when anxious. Others in the group explained how troubled relationships with husbands, friends, and family members often precipitated overeating. A. W. could not relate to their stories because she almost never had disagreements with her father, mother, and women friends. Gradually, through the use of the self-talk worksheets, she discovered sources of anxiety, boredom, and anger of which she was unaware. Perhaps her most startling discovery was her new awareness of feeling angry with her father's high expectations and her resultant perfectionism. She did not feel comfortable expressing her feelings in the group; she felt guilty and thought she was being a dishonorable daughter.

A. W. announced to her group 3 weeks later that she was so confident in her progress that she was going to continue working on her own and not return to the group. She said that she needed the extra time for her increasing work demands. She expressed sadness about leaving the group but was excited to live her new lifestyle on her own.

A. W. did not return to the group until 3 months later after she came to the nurse for a bout with the flu and a sinus infection. She said that it was more difficult to continue the EAT, LIFE, and ESTEEM strategies on her own without the group support. She had regained 4 pounds but continued to exercise twice a week most weeks. She thought of returning to the group several times but said that she thought the discussions were too personal at times. When the nurse asked for specifics, she learned about the anger that A. W. felt toward her father and the consequent guilt she experienced.

A. W. and the nurse agreed to have two or three private, individual sessions to learn more about A. W.'s angry feelings and how they relate to overeating and not getting regular exercise. A. W. was able to understand her perfectionist behaviors and need for others' approval. After two weekly individual sessions, she said that she wanted to return to the group to continue work in the program.

A. W. in the Maintenance Stage

Setting: A. W. was in attendance at the last evening group meeting about the acceptance of obstacles in the clinic's weight management program (about 11 months after the first meeting A. W. attended).

Patterns/Challenges/Needs:

1. Altered nutrition, more than body requirements—from 167 to 148 pounds, from 31 to 27 body mass index, from 35% to 32% body fat
2. Body image disturbance—from an 8 to a 6 on a 10-point scale (1 being best)
3. Hopelessness—diagnosis resolved after individual counseling and continued group work
4. Decreased mobility related to no regular exercise program—improving; need more strength exercises added to workout to maximize metabolic rate
5. Increased tension stress before overeating episodes—lowered "at risk" scores (i.e., within normal range on the tension stress scale)

A. W. returned to group meetings at least monthly but found individual help from a psychologist recommended by the nurse to work on issues of self-esteem, perfectionism, and approval needs. A. W.'s EAT for Hunger and Exercise for LIFE habits were becoming integrated into her lifestyle. She found that her own version of the BIO meditation and writing in her journal were helpful ways to work on her own issues when not in the group or in counseling. Her major focus was on acceptance and love of herself. Although the experience was painful at times, A. W. said that she was thankful to have greater insight into her past overeating and no-exercise habits.

Evaluation

With clients, the nurse determines whether their outcomes for weight management were achieved (Exhibit 22-6). To evaluate clients' progress on goals, the nurse examines their BIO worksheets with them. Together, the nurse and clients may explore the subjective effects of their experiences in the program by answering the questions found in **Exhibit 22-7.**

EXHIBIT 22-7   Evaluating the Client's Subjective Experience with Weight
Management Interventions

1. How am I feeling about myself and my progress right now?
2. Do I have any questions about my eating and exercise programs?
3. What new insights have I gained about my self-talk?
4. What is my next step, and do I need help to take that step?
5. Are my goals realistic for me right now?
6. What pain and joy can I expect in reaching my goals?
7. Am I seeking my higher power to accept the things that I cannot change, and am I thinking positively about changing the things I can change?

Directions for
FUTURE RESEARCH

1. Contrast and evaluate discrepancies between nurses' and clients' perceptions of client readiness according to the transtheoretical stages of change for eating, exercise, and psycho-social-spiritual work.
2. Analyze clients' progress toward outcome variables listed in Exhibit 22-6, and describe differences among individuals within and between different stages of change.
3. Analyze clients' progress toward outcome variables listed in Exhibit 22-6 according to whether they received primarily individual, group, or a combination of individual and group counseling sessions.

Nurse Healer
REFLECTIONS

After reading this chapter, the nurse healer will be able to answer or to begin a process of answering the following questions:

■ How did I accommodate my eating within the food pyramid and the American Diabetic Association diet using the EAT for Hunger strategy?
■ How did my personal aerobic and strength exercise program incorporate the Exercise for LIFE strategy?
■ How did I deal directly with unpleasant feelings, instead of eating to cope, using the STOP Emotional Eating strategy?

 For a full suite of assignments and additional learning activities, use the access code located in the front of your book to visit this exclusive website: http://go.jblearning.com/dossey. If you do not have an access code, you can obtain one at the site.

NOTES

1. K. M. Flegal et al., "Prevalence and Trends in Obesity Among U.S. Adults, 1999–2008," *Journal of the American Medical Association* 303 (2010): 235–241.
2. E. J. Sondik et al., "Progress Toward the *Healthy People 2010* Goals and Objectives," *Annual Review of Public Health* 31 (2010): 271–281.
3. WHO Expert Committee on Physical Status, *Physical Status: The Use and Interpretation of Anthropometry* (Geneva, Switzerland: WHO, 1995).
4. U.S. Department of Health and Human Services, *The Surgeon General's Vision for a Healthy and Fit Nation* (Rockville, MD: U.S. DHHS, Office of the Surgeon General, 2010).
5. American Heart Association, *Heart Disease and Stroke Statistics—2005 Update* (Dallas, TX: AHA, 2005).
6. Centers for Disease Control and Prevention, *Obesity: Halting the Epidemic by Making Health Easier: At a Glance 2010* (2010). http://www.cdc.gov/chronicdisease/resources/publications/aag/obesity.htm.
7. D. W. Reiff and K. K. Reiff, *Eating Disorders* (Gaithersburg, MD: Aspen Publishers, 1992).
8. R. Keesey, "A Set-Point Theory of Obesity," in *Handbook of Eating Disorders*, ed. K. Brownell and J. P. Foreyt, 103–123 (New York: Basic Books, 1986).

9. National Heart, Lung, and Blood Institute, "Why Is a Healthy Weight Important?" (2011). http://www.nhlbi.nih.gov/health/public/heart/obesity/lose_wt/index.htm.

10. B. F. Skinner, *About Behaviorism* (New York: Random House, 1974).

11. J. O. Prochaska and C. C. DiClemente, "In Search of How People Change," *American Psychologist* 47 (1992): 1102.

12. Centers for Disease Control and Prevention, "An Estimated 1 in 10 U.S. Adults Report Depression" (2011). http://www.cdc.gov/Features/dsDepression/.

13. A. T. Beck, *Cognitive Therapy and the Emotional Disorders* (New York: International Universities Press, 1976).

14. K. D. Brownell et al., "The Dieting Maelstrom: Is It Possible and Advisable to Lose Weight?" *American Psychologist* 49 (1994): 781–791.

15. Centers for Disease Control and Prevention, "U.S. Obesity Trends: Trends by State 1985–2010" (2011). http://www.cdc.gov/obesity/data/trends.html.

16. G. L. Blackburn, S. Wollner, and S. B. Heymsfield, "Lifestyle Interventions for the Treatment of Class III Obesity: A Primary Target for Nutrition Medicine in the Obesity Epidemic," *American Journal of Clinical Nutrition* 9 (2010): 289S–292S.

17. R. J. Kuczmarski et al., "Increasing Prevalence of Overweight Among U.S. Adults: The National Health and Nutrition Examination Surveys, 1960–1991," *Journal of the American Medical Association* 272 (1994): 205–211.

18. R. Green, "Americans Eat Less Fat but Are Getting Fatter," *Kansas City Star* (January 17, 1996): A1, A6.

19. L. H. Powell, J. E. Calvin III, and J. E. Calvin Jr., "Effective Obesity Treatments," *American Psychologist* 62 (2007): 234–246.

20. S. Popkess-Vawter, E. Yoder, and B. Gajewski, "The Role of Spirituality in Holistic Weight Management," *Clinical Nursing Research* 14 (2005): 158–174.

21. K. Goto et al., "A Single Versus Multiple Bouts of Moderate-Intensity Exercise for Fat Metabolism," *Clinical Physiology and Functional Imaging* 31 (2011): 215–220.

22. National Heart, Lung, and Blood Institute, "What Is Metabolic Syndrome?" (2011). http://www.nhlbi.nih.gov/health/dci/Diseases/ms/ms_diagnosis.html.

23. National Institute of Diabetes and Digestive and Kidney Diseases, "Fast Facts on Diabetes" (2011). http://diabetes.niddk.nih.gov/dm/pubs/statistics/#fast.

24. National Heart, Lung, and Blood Institute, "Facts About Healthy Weight" (2011). http://www.nhlbi.nih.gov/health/prof/heart/obesity/aim_kit/healthy_wt_facts.htm.

25. American Dietetic Association, "Position on Weight Management," *Journal of the American Dietetic Association* 109 (2009): 330–346.

26. S. Popkess-Vawter, C. Brandau, and J. Straub, "Triggers of Overeating and Related Intervention Strategies for Women Who Weight Cycle," *Applied Nursing Research* 11 (1998): 69–76.

27. P. Peeke, *Fit to Live* (London: Pan Macmillan, 2007).

28. M. Beattie, *The Language of Letting Go: Daily Meditations for Codependents* (New York: Harper Collins, 1990).

29. W. Dyer, *10 Secrets for Success and Inner Peace* (Carlsbad, CA: Hay House, 2001).

30. T. A. Wadden et al., "One-Year Weight Losses in the Look AHEAD Study: Factors Associated with Success," *Obesity* 17 (2009): 713–722.

31. Overeaters Anonymous, "Welcome to Overeaters Anonymous" (2011). http://www.oa.org/.

32. G. Shamblin, "The Weigh Down Approach" (2011). http://www.weighdown.com/AboutUs/TheWeighDownApproach.aspx.

33. L. Mellin, M. Croughan-Minihane, and L. Dickey, "The Solution Method: 2-Year Trends in Weight, Blood Pressure, Exercise, Depression, and Functioning of Adults Trained in Developmental Skills," *Journal of the American Dietetic Association* 97 (1997): 1133–1138.

34. M. Apter, *Reversal Theory: Motivation, Emotion, and Personality* (London: Routledge, 1989).

35. S. Popkess-Vawter, M. M. Gerkovich, and S. Wendel, "Reliability and Validity of the Overeating Tension Scale," *Journal of Nursing Measurement* 8 (2000): 145–160.

36. K. Kramer-Jackman and S. Popkess-Vawter, "Method for Technology-Delivered Healthcare Measures," *Computers, Informatics, Nursing* (in press).

37. K. Kramer et al., "Nursing Practice Mailed Client Surveys as a Source of Evidence-Based Data," *Nurse Practitioner World News* 9 (2004): 9–11.

38. S. Popkess-Vawter and V. Owens, "Use of the BULIT Bulimia Screening Questionnaire to Assess Risk and Progress in Weight Management for Overweight Women Who Weight Cycle," *Addictive Behaviors* 24 (1999): 497–507.

39. J. O. Hill and H. R. Wyatt, "Role of Physical Activity in Preventing and Treating Obesity," *Journal of Applied Physiology* 99 (2005): 765–770.

40. E. Easwaran, *Take Your Time: Finding Balance in a Hurried World* (New York: Hyperion, 1994).

41. American College of Sports Medicine, "Updated Physical Activity Guidelines Released Today" (2007). http://www.acsm.org/AM/PrinterTemplate.cfm?Section=Home_Page&template=/CM/ContentDisplay.cfm&ContentID=7769.

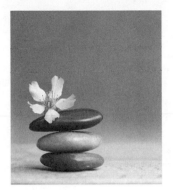

Chapter 23

Smoking Cessation

Christina Jackson

Nurse Healer
OBJECTIVES

Theoretical

- Explore antecedents to smoking behavior.
- Analyze the mind–body responses to nicotine.
- Examine theoretical strategies for successful smoking cessation.

Clinical

- Interview a client who smokes and listen to the client's story, including reasons the client gives for starting and continuing smoking. Ask if the client has ever tried to quit smoking or will attempt smoking cessation again.
- Through the interview, try to gain insight into what the meaning of smoking is to the client, and explore ways to teach smoking cessation that may be most effective for this individual.
- Design interventions that correspond to the stages and processes of change as appropriate to the client.

Personal

- If applicable, examine the effect of passive smoking on you and what changes you can facilitate in your environment.
- Consider your own coping mechanisms, and how you can make changes for greater health.

- If you are a smoker, explore your need for healthier coping mechanisms, and identify habit breakers (behaviors) to become a successful nonsmoker.

DEFINITIONS

Habit breakers: New action behaviors that replace old "smoke signals" or triggers.

Quit Line: A telephone smoking cessation resource available 7 days a week to support tobacco cessation efforts.

Smoke signals/triggers: Phenomena in the internal and external environment that create a desire to smoke.

■ THEORY AND RESEARCH

Many smokers who have achieved sobriety from drugs or alcohol might say that quitting smoking is an even more formidable challenge than quitting those other substances! In fact, nicotine is highly addictive for several reasons. It has powerful effects on brain function and the feel-good neurotransmitters dopamine, endorphins, and norepinephrine. Second, it can both calm the user who is feeling anxious or stimulate the user who is feeling sluggish. What an ideal drug—and it is legal and does not alter level of consciousness or ability to function; in fact, many believe it enhances thinking and performance. An older nurse who sought smoking cessation treatment said, "I've always had 20 friends in this pack who have helped me any time I needed them. I will miss them dearly." Indeed, smokers have an emotional attachment to their drug of choice and have often bypassed the development of other (healthier) coping mechanisms because smoking became the default mode of adaptation.

It is probably most helpful to view tobacco use as a coping mechanism indicative of underlying issues in need of healing, rather than viewing smoking as the chief problem in and of itself. Smokers often report starting the habit at a young age—even 10 or 11 years—not only to impress peers, but to cope with "stress." This is an indication of the plethora of adverse childhood events and traumas from which children must recover and heal. By viewing smoking as an attempt (albeit unhealthy) to handle the stresses and traumas of life, we can get a more complete picture of a holistic plan to support the cessation of tobacco use.

The Prevalence of Smoking and Its Health Consequences

Whereas rates of smoking in the United States declined by 3.5% between 2001 and 2008, rates have remained unchanged in recent years, and smoking continues to be a major health hazard as well as the chief cause of preventable morbidity and mortality today.[1] With an estimated 44.5 million smokers in the United States, it is thought that 430,000 premature deaths are caused annually because of smoking.[2] One out of every five adults is a smoker, and there is a disproportionately higher prevalence of smoking among adults with lower educational attainment.[1] Less than half of smokers ever achieve long-term abstinence even though approximately 75% want to quit, and at least a third have made serious attempts to quit.[3] These statistics are sobering and underscore the need to focus on smoking *prevention*.

Currently, there are about 1.3 billion smokers in the world, 84% of whom live in developing countries.[4] Tobacco use is responsible for an estimated 5 million deaths worldwide each year and is projected to cause 10 million deaths per year by 2030.[5] Between direct healthcare costs and loss of productivity from smoking-related illness around the world, tobacco use is projected to cost governments more than $200 billion per year.[4]

Cigarette smoking (and secondhand smoke) contributes to four of the five leading causes of death per year in the United States, including lung cancer, coronary heart disease, chronic lung disease, and stroke. In May 2007, the state of Arizona put into effect a comprehensive statewide smoking ban. Research into the impact of this ban reveals significant reductions in hospital admissions for smoking-linked diagnoses including acute myocardial infarction, angina, stroke, and asthma.[6] The American Heart Association–American Stroke Association (AHA-ASA) strongly recommends smoking cessation because of the direct correlation between smoking and both coronary artery disease and ischemic stroke.[7] It is estimated that tobacco is responsible for 85% of deaths caused by lung cancer.

Smokers constitute 20.9% of the U.S. population. Twenty-three percent of men and 18.3% of women smoke cigarettes, and 22% of white adults and 21.3% of black adults use tobacco.[1] Rates of smoking prevalence continue to be high among certain population groups, especially American Indians and Alaska Natives (32.4%) and are highest among those with low educational attainment (grades 9–11) and those with a General Educational Development certificate (GED) (41.3%). Conversely, rates of smoking are lowest among adults with graduate degrees. Adults who live below poverty levels also experience a high prevalence of tobacco use (31.5%).[1]

Women and Smoking

Though the use of tobacco by women in the United States was 6% in 1924, peaked at 33% in 1965, and is now at 18.5% (including 18% of pregnant women), it is estimated that 250 million women throughout the world smoke, and most of these are in developed countries. In Europe, South Africa, and Australia, 20-45% of pregnant women smoke.[8] Smoking during pregnancy harms both mother and baby and is a leading cause of morbidity and mortality during the intrauterine and early childhood stages of life. These preventable problems include premature birth and miscarriages; implantation, placental, and membrane issues; and infant respiratory, cognitive, and behavioral issues.[8]

Marketing campaigns over the years have used glamorous imagery to promote cigarettes and offer "light" or low-tar alternatives that falsely claim safety advantages. Chronic obstructive pulmonary disease (COPD), once thought of as a predominately male disease, now kills more women than breast cancer, and the number of new cases of COPD in women is increasing three times faster than in men.[9] Growth and development of lung and airway tissue are different in males and females, and the airways of females are vulnerable to hormonal effects. Estrogen affects the metabolism of nicotine, and this also affects addiction and cessation in women smokers. Healthcare providers tend to diagnose COPD more readily in men than in women, offering spirometry evaluation more often to men than to women, even in women with more severe dyspnea and cough.[9]

Smoking is a problem among nurses. The prevalence of smoking is higher in licensed practical nurses (LPNs; 28%) than in registered nurses (RNs; 15%). The rate among RNs is lower than the 18% average for females in general, and LPNs have higher smoking rates than women in general and other health professionals. These findings are significant because those who smoke are less likely to encourage cessation in others.[10]

Smoking cessation should be a priority in women's health, and it should be geared toward the unique needs of females. For example, one study reported increased smoking relapse rates among women during the premenstrual (luteal, progesterone predominant) phase of the cycle. Another found no difference in relapse rates according to stage of menstrual cycle, but did find the withdrawal symptoms of craving and anger to be the most frequently associated with relapse, but only in women who quit during the follicular phase of the cycle.[9]

Although some research shows increased difficulty for women to quit, other studies show women to have greater receptivity to smoking cessation. Women tend to be more afraid of weight gain as a result of cessation than male smokers do. Smoking cessation has been associated with increased body fat in several studies; however, one study also found an increase in functional muscle mass.[11] This potential for increased functional capacity in women who quit could be used as a motivator, especially when designing holistic approaches to cessation

that include exercise and other lifestyle changes. In a study of female prisoners who participated in a group smoking cessation intervention with nicotine replacement, significant weight gain (net difference of 10 pounds) was experienced by abstainers when compared to continuing smokers. This effect did slow down at 1 year post intervention, however.[12] The fear of weight gain should be taken into account when designing cessation programs for women.

Various mood states such as depression and anxiety have been correlated with higher rates of exacerbation and hospitalization in patients with COPD and are more frequently seen in women. Among COPD patients with psychiatric comorbidity, 60% of women had psychiatric disorders as compared to 38% of men.[9] So, though research on women and smoking is often contradictory, there is evidence that hormone fluctuation, physiology, mood, and differences in motivation play roles in smoking and cessation that make women different from men.

Environmental Tobacco Smoke

In addition to smoking cigarettes and inhaling smoke directly, there is also the problem of passive smoking (sometimes referred to as "secondhand smoke"), better known as environmental tobacco smoke (ETS). ETS is a combination of smoke from the burning end of a cigarette, cigar, or pipe and the smoke exhaled from a smoker's lungs. This environmental perspective on exposure has now been expanded to include "thirdhand smoke," or the residual chemical contamination that remains in an environment (clinging to furniture, carpets, walls, and the like) even 24 hours after a cigarette has been extinguished.[13] ETS contains more than 4,000 highly toxic chemicals, such as formaldehyde, nitrogen oxide, acrolein, Group A carcinogens (asbestos), cadmium, nickel, and carbon monoxide. In addition, ETS contains a radioactive substance from tobacco leaves that have been subjected to high-phosphate fertilizers.[14]

Children and adults exposed to ETS have a greater risk for respiratory illness, including lung cancer; higher rates of respiratory tract infections; exacerbation of asthma; otitis media; and sudden infant death syndrome (SIDS).[14-16] One study found higher rates of mental health disorders among adolescents and children exposed to ETS.[17] Increased exposure to ETS nearly doubles a woman's risk of heart attack.[15] Measures of cotinine, a metabolite of nicotine in the bloodstream, demonstrate that 37% of adult nonsmokers and 43% of U.S. children, aged 2 months through 11 years, are exposed to ETS in their homes or workplaces.[16]

A study of nonsmoking bar workers in Scotland revealed a remarkable (89%) and lasting reduction in salivary cotinine levels after smoke-free legislation (public smoking ban) was put into place.[17]

In the United States, approximately 59% of children aged 4–11 years are exposed to second-hand smoke in their homes. Young children are especially vulnerable to the damaging effects of ETS, including risk for asthma, bronchitis, pneumonia, and SIDS. Because mothers usually spend more time in the home and more time with their children than do fathers, maternal smoking has been linked with childhood respiratory problems and some facial deformities.[18] Children of mothers who smoke more than 10 cigarettes per day are twice as likely to develop asthma as are children of nonsmokers. These same youngsters are 2.5 times more likely to develop asthma in their first year of life and 4.5 times more likely to need medicine to control asthma attacks.[19] Maternal smoking remains an indicator of childhood asthma even after variables such as gender, race, presence of both biologic parents in the household, and number of rooms in the house are taken into account.

Physiologic Responses to Smoking

Smoking and tobacco contribute directly to death. Yet, deaths from smoking do not receive the same amount of attention from the news media as do airplane crashes, violence, and disease epidemics, situations resulting in far fewer deaths. Smoking causes more deaths, but these deaths take a very long time to develop; therefore, the significance of the problem is often minimized.

Over time, smoking strips the lungs of their normal defenses and completely paralyzes the natural cleansing processes. The early morning cough associated with smoking results from attempts by the bronchial cilia to clear the thick, yellow or yellow-green mucus that accumulates in the air passage to an abnormal amount because toxic cigarette smoke interferes with the cilia's normal function. This cleansing action triggers the cough reflex. As exposure continues, the bronchi begin to thicken, which predisposes the person to bacterial and viral infections, asthma, emphysema, and cancer.[20]

The smoker's heart rate speeds up an extra 10 to 25 beats per minute, with a predisposition to dysrhythmias. The blood pressure increases by 10–15%, thus exposing the person to risks of myocardial infarction, stroke, and vascular disease.[19]

Within seconds after the smoke is inhaled, irritating gases (e.g., formaldehyde, hydrogen sulfide, ammonia) begin to affect the eyes, nose, and throat. With each inhaled breath of smoke, carbon monoxide enters the bloodstream, and its concentration eventually rises to a level 4 to 15 times as high as that of a nonsmoker. The carbon monoxide passes immediately to the bloodstream, binding to the oxygen receptor sites and, thus, depleting the cells of oxygen. Hemoglobin, which normally carries oxygen throughout the body, becomes bound to the carbon monoxide and is converted to carboxyhemoglobin, which is unable to deliver oxygen to the cells. In addition, smoking increases platelet aggregation, allowing the blood to clot more easily.[9,19]

The constriction of tiny blood vessels decreases the delivery of oxygen to the skin and contributes to "smoker's face," where deep lines appear around the mouth, eyes, and center of the brow. The muscular puffing action also contributes to lines around the mouth. There is an established link between nicotine and erection problems in male smokers, and smoking is believed to be the leading cause of impotence in the United States today. Smoking also adversely affects fertility by decreasing sperm count and sperm motility. Female smokers are significantly more likely than nonsmoking females to be infertile, and heavy smoking amplifies this decline in fertility.

Recent research demonstrates a clear correlation between smoking and gene expression (individual genes as well as entire networks of gene interaction) that corresponds to smoking-related pathologies including cancer, cell death, and immune response.[21]

Nicotine is the drug inhaled from cigarettes that quickly reaches the smoker's brain. As the average smoker takes an estimated 10 puffs per cigarette, a pack-a-day smoker gets about 200 puffs per day. Each nicotine "hit" goes directly to the lungs, and the nicotine-rich blood travels to the brain in approximately 7 seconds. This time is twice as fast as that of an intravenous injection of heroin, which must pass through the body's systemic circulatory system before reaching the brain.[19,22]

As nicotine enters the brain, it acts as a "mood thermostat" and can help users to maintain a steady and pleasant sensation of psychological neutrality. Nicotine stimulates people when they are drowsy and calms them when they are tense; it affects cognitive processes of concentration and emotional states. Unlike other powerful street drugs, nicotine does not interfere with the capacity to work and create, and it may actually enhance individuals' capabilities.

The action of nicotine causes the brain to release norepinephrine, endorphins, corticosteroids, and dopamine.[4] The brain then adapts to accept these chemicals by increasing the number of nicotine receptors and becomes physically dependent on nicotine. Thus, the general level of arousal is adjusted up or down by introducing nicotine levels that allow the smoker to feel stimulated or relaxed. The effects of nicotine are reached in a matter of seconds; the smoker experiences drug-induced contentedness, all in a legally sanctioned manner.

Norepinephrine controls arousal and alertness. Beta-endorphin, referred to as the brain's natural analgesic, can decrease pain and anxiety. Dopamine is part of the brain's pleasure center and also can decrease pain and anxiety. Smoking's "attention thermostat" effect is mediated through the brain's limbic system, where the major neurotransmitters are adrenaline and dopamine, both of which are influenced by nicotine. It appears that nicotine helps the smoker concentrate by promoting selective attention to important tasks, which increases learning and memory. So, nicotine can enhance cognitive processes and reduce fatigue. In addition, nicotine can exert a sedating effect, reducing anxiety and inducing euphoria.[4] Continued smoking also prevents the unpleasant side effects of nicotine withdrawal, such as irritability, irrational mood changes, low energy levels, inability to feel stimulated, and increased sensitivity to light, touch, and sound.

The overall effect of smoking is a shift in brain chemistry that creates the mood needed for the situation at hand, that is, increased relaxation, alertness, or pleasure and decreased pain or anxiety. But, even though nicotine is a powerful and effective drug, concerned smokers can create and sustain new behaviors to achieve the same positive effects without the health risk to themselves or those around them. The physiologic dependency declines sharply in the first week of cessation; however, the behavioral or habitual pattern triggering the desire to smoke is more difficult to modify. Success in smoking cessation requires a plan of action and a great deal of body-mind-spirit self-care. A growing body of research underscores the fact that successful cessation plans must address any issues pertaining to mood disorders and focus on underlying or withdrawal-related depression. Although some smokers go it alone and quit "cold turkey," for many, smoking cessation is a process that can take time and a great deal of emotional and physical support. The hopeful reality is that cessation can be achieved by anyone who is motivated, open to addressing concomitant depression, and willing to try a variety of strategies to find what works.

Cultural Considerations and Special Populations

Research supports the effectiveness of smoking cessation counseling and programming for people from all cultural backgrounds.[23,24] Resources must be linguistically appropriate, and accessible, including for those with sensory impairments such as deafness or blindness. The Internet is a valuable resource for those with special needs of any kind and can link almost anyone to resources tailored to help with cessation. Those with mental illness (including psychosis) can benefit from cessation counseling and resources, but again, the mode of delivery must be accessible and tailored to accommodate special needs.[25] Smoking cessation in those with mental illness is also more complex because smoking is a pervasive behavior in most mental health environments, so triggers are difficult, if not impossible, to avoid. In addition, nicotine often calms and enhances well-being in a way that the other drugs persons with mental illness take do not. So, motivation to quit among this population of clients is often a problem.

Native American tobacco users often have difficulty with smoking cessation because for them tobacco use is part of sacred ceremony. The deep cultural, spiritual, and social ties to smoking and tobacco can make addressing the addiction component more complex. Careful exploration of perceived benefits, motivation, and supportive resources is necessary to assist in quitting.

■ SMOKING CESSATION

Measuring Successful Cessation

Because smoking cessation is not an easy task, success is often measured in small increments. Smoking quit rates vary with the different approaches to cessation. Over the years, research has evaluated a variety of public and private multicomponent cessation programs, healthcare provider–directed counseling, and community-based programs. Researchers have compared types of programs, for example, one such study looked at group interventions compared to individual interventions offered in pharmacies in Scotland. It was found that the group interventions were significantly more successful.[26] Measures of success also vary, and smoking cessation may be defined as point prevalence (a measure taken at one point in time) at the end of a cessation program or long-term abstinence lasting for 1 year or more.[27] Fourteen meta-analyses of 17 different treatments for cessation demonstrated efficacy with 100% agreement, and the researchers conclude that clinicians should offer a variety of treatments and be reimbursed on par with other medical and behavioral disorders.[28] Smoking cessation treatments can be extremely powerful in aiding those who want to quit.

Self-Quitters, Healthcare Provider Counseling, and Nurse Follow-up Advice

There are conflicting data as to the best way to quit smoking. Research reports estimate 90% of successful quitters kick the habit on their own each year , and quit rates are twice as high for those who quit on their own as for those who participated in a cessation program.[22] Other studies demonstrate that smokers who quit cold turkey were more likely to remain abstinent than were those who gradually decreased their daily consumption of cigarettes, switched to cigarettes

with lower tar or nicotine, or used special filters or holders. Yet other researchers claim that those who use medications to support cessation efforts are more likely to be successful. All agree that the quitter must be motivated and must be ready to quit. Careful exploration of these factors with the client, and strategic support to bolster strengths and minimize challenges, can amplify chances of quitting.

Smokers who received nonsmoking advice from their healthcare providers were nearly twice as likely to quit smoking. Heavy smokers (25 cigarettes a day) and more addicted smokers were much more likely to participate in an organized cessation program than were people who smoked less. A recent Cochrane review looked at 14 studies involving more than 10,000 smokers that used motivational interviewing as an intervention. (See Chapter 10.) This focused, goal-directed interview lasts between 20 and 45 minutes and explores the smoking behavior from the client's perspective in a nonjudgmental manner, aiming to help them gain insight and formulate a quit plan. Most of the studies also involved provision of self-help materials and telephone follow-up. Participants receiving motivational interviewing had 23% improved success rates for quitting, with better results if they were offered by primary care providers or counselors and the interviews lasted longer than 20 minutes. In fact, for those who were offered motivational interviewing by their primary care providers, the success rate was three times higher than in those who received "usual care."[29] Details regarding specific content of the counseling were lacking in the study reports, making application difficult. One could extrapolate these findings to suggest that nurses could have a significant impact on smoking cessation using motivational interviewing and could hone the skills needed to amplify this effect. (Chapter 10 can assist in developing skills for motivational interviewing.)

Healthcare providers and nurses have considerable opportunity to reach all demographic subgroups of the population.[27] Seventy percent of smokers see a healthcare provider at least once per year. Nurses working in hospitals regularly encounter patients who are smokers. These represent ideal opportunities for motivational interviewing whereby the smoker is asked about the behavior, encouraged to quit, and given the opportunity to explore cessation strategies.

The Tobacco Free Nurses (TFN) initiative was launched in 2003 as an effort to reduce smoking among nurses as well as to encourage nurses to become more involved in tobacco control efforts. The "5 As" behavioral approach has been adopted by TFN and can be readily used by nurses and other healthcare providers during encounters with patients in any setting.[30] Key elements of this approach include the following:

Ask: Always ask about tobacco use during every patient encounter.

Advise: Provide any and all tobacco users with strong verbal encouragement to quit.

Assess: Determine motivation to quit and stage of readiness.

Assist: Provide counseling, refer to cessation resources, and arrange support.

Arrange: Plan follow-up visits to encourage ongoing abstinence or new attempts to quit.

A survey of 3,482 nurses working in Magnet-designated hospitals in the United States were found to be deficient in addressing smoking cessation among their patients. Although 73% of nurses asked and assisted with cessation, only 24% recommended pharmacotherapy, 22% referred to community resources, and only 10% recommended use of the Quit Line. Nurses who were familiar with the TFN were significantly more likely to deliver all aspects of the 5 As, including assisting with cessation and recommending medications.[31]

Although the impact of healthcare provider advice varies, many smokers say that they would quit if urged to do so by a healthcare provider. For smoking interventions to become a routine part of healthcare practice, however, medical and nursing education must integrate smoking cessation strategies into the curriculum. Research findings support the value and effectiveness of treatment and follow-up by nurses and other healthcare providers.

Quit Lines

Initially developed with input from psychologists and available 7 days a week and (most often) 24 hours a day, telephone quit lines offer personal, convenient, accessible, and comprehensive support for those endeavoring to quit tobacco use.[32] Trained counselors are available to talk with callers about their readiness and motivation to quit, their smoking triggers, their support system, local referral resources, and more. These counselors can customize a quit plan with the client and are also available during a craving or to answer questions like "I have redness under my nicotine patch, is that normal?" Most states have quit lines, and most state departments of health can connect callers with a quit line. Most services are free of charge, including free medications such as nicotine replacement patches. When medication support is determined to be appropriate, a brief medical interview is conducted, and medications are sent through the mail. In some cases, a caller's healthcare provider must sign for the medications, as in the case of someone with a cardiac history or a pregnant caller. The quit line counselors also link individuals with local resources (such as smoking cessation support groups or local chapters of the 12-step program Nicotine Anonymous) and assist them in maximizing relevant benefits available through their health insurance. The American Cancer Society (1-866-784-8454) and American Lung Association (1-800-586-4872) have quit lines, and Great Start has a quit line for pregnant women (1-866-667-8278). All of these resources are easily explored on the Internet.

Pharmacologic Therapies in Support of Cessation

Seven medications have been shown to support long-term smoking cessation, including five forms of nicotine replacement therapy (NRT). NRT decreases intensity of withdrawal symptoms and the urge to smoke. Nicotine gum, lozenges, and the transdermal patch are available over the counter, and nicotine cartridge inhalers, nasal spray, and higher-dose patches are available by prescription.[33] By using NRT, maintaining nicotine levels is divorced from cigarettes, helping the smoker to break the emotional ties with smoking. Nicotine replacement therapy does not release the client from the bad effects of nicotine including nausea, dyspepsia, altered cardiac rhythms, dizziness, headache, and local irritations of the nose, mouth, and skin that vary with mode of delivery.[34] Approximately 25% of those using NRT experience adverse effects in the first 2 weeks of use, and 40% experience adverse effects within 2 to 3 months of use; however, these effects are usually described as mild. Still, NRT should be discontinued as soon as possible.

There are four major controversies regarding the use of NRT: (1) the use of NRT while a person continues to smoke; (2) how long to use NRT before weaning from the drug; (3) the recommended dose of the NRT product; and (4) misusing and abusing NRT, especially becoming addicted to over-the-counter gum.

Because of nicotine's potentially dangerous side effects, NRT must be used with caution in cardiac patients and should not be used within 4 weeks of myocardial infarction.[33] Although NRT is a means for achieving short-term smoking cessation for nicotine-addicted individuals, it does not seem to reduce relapse rates and is not a substitute for learning new and healthier coping behaviors. NRT should always be used in tandem with a smoking cessation program that addresses behavior and lifestyle changes.

Many tobacco cessation experts believe that sufficient doses of NRT are needed for sufficient lengths of time to support cessation, and that the risks of smoking far outweigh the risks of NRT. And, although NRT is expensive and carries with it the potential for adverse effects, many believe the benefit is estimated to outweigh the risks. A simulation model using a large body of survey data estimated the number of premature deaths (caused by smoking) avoided because of NRT use to be 40,000 over a 20-year period. After factoring out the potential risks from long-term NRT use, a net projection of 32,000 premature deaths because of smoking would still be avoided.[35] Although significant, this is a small portion of smoking-related deaths over a 20-year period of time.

The other two drugs that are currently identified as first-line cessation therapies are bupropion SR (Zyban) and varenicline (Chantix). Bupropion, an atypical antidepressant, is used to improve abstinence in smokers independent of a history of depression.[33] Cigarette smoking is closely associated with a history of depression that often predicts failure with cessation efforts.[36] Smoking cessation may also trigger the onset of depression as a serious nicotine withdrawal

symptom in otherwise healthy individuals. This may be the result of removing a primary coping mechanism—the cigarettes—thus leaving the person vulnerable and without a way to cope with the many feelings that are likely to arise. Again, this reinforces the need for therapeutic support and behavioral and lifestyle modifications to be used along with any plan of pharmacotherapy. Clients who need psychotherapy should be referred to an appropriate professional.

Bupropion is contraindicated in those with seizure disorders, eating disorders, and those who take monoamine oxidase inhibitors (MAOIs). It is recommended to be taken for 12 months and may be taken concurrently with NRT. It often causes constipation. Varenicline is classified as a smoking deterrent that reduces cravings and withdrawal symptoms, prevents nicotine from binding to receptors, and lessens the satisfaction derived from smoking. Varenicline should not be used for clients with a prior diagnosis of depression. Both bupropion and varenicline carry boxed warnings about increased risk for suicide, and frequent assessment for suicidal ideation is necessary. Both drugs interfere with normal sleep patterns and can induce bizarre dreams. Both drugs have been associated with lessening weight gain in abstainers, though this effect is limited.[33]

Nortriptyline, a tricyclic antidepressant, is identified as a second-line drug when first-line therapy is not tolerated or effective. The mechanisms behind these antidepressants (bupropion and nortriptyline) are observed through their direct interactions with nicotine in the brain. When nicotine is inhaled through smoking or ingested through chewing tobacco it binds to receptors in the brain and causes release of the neurotransmitters dopamine and norepinephrine. These drugs mimic the neurochemical effects of nicotine on noradrenergic and dopaminergic systems in the brain, thus relieving withdrawal symptoms and alleviating negative affect and depression. Interestingly, a randomized clinical trial using St. John's wort (SJW) showed that SJW did not attenuate withdrawal symptoms, nor did it increase smoking abstinence rates.[37]

Life Span Considerations

A large body of research suggests that children with attention deficit hyperactivity disorder

(ADHD) are more likely to start smoking in their teens when compared with non-ADHD peers.[38] It makes sense that they may seek tobacco as a way to self-medicate, given the positive physiologic effects of nicotine on focus and attention.

It is critical to identify teens in need of cessation counseling because this is when so many smokers become addicted. Providing smoking cessation counseling to adolescents may be different from working with adults. Facilitators of smoking programs aimed at youth must be able to connect in nonjudgmental ways with teens. Research suggests that personality characteristics such as trustworthiness, caring, and the ability to hold confidence matter a great deal to teens.[39]

The concept of self-efficacy is very important because teens who perceive that they are capable of executing a cessation plan are more likely to make the attempt. Antecedents to self-efficacy include developmental stage, emotional support and past experiences with support, available resources, and preferred (healthy) coping strategies. In the absence of any of these conditions that would promote self-efficacy and therefore successful smoking cessation, nurses can facilitate strategic support and growth.[40,41]

In a meta-analysis of randomized controlled trials measuring effectiveness of pharmacologic therapies in adolescent smokers, results show no significant effects on abstinence rates. This study also reveals few adverse events resulting from the medications used.[42]

When reviewing research on cessation in older smokers, it is clear that they derive significant health and financial benefits, and that it is never too late to offer support and strategies to assist quit efforts. Doing so may also protect others from ETS.[43] Many older smokers (and their healthcare providers) may shy away from cessation because they think that the damage is already done, they do not know of appropriate resources, or that it is not worth giving up one of few remaining life pleasures. In reality, research on older smokers hospitalized with cardiovascular disease shows they can quit at high rates with proper support. In addition, the use of NRT may be safe and effective in this population.[44] With increased likelihood of hospitalizations in this age group, these times can provide opportunities for nurses to offer cessation encouragement using the 5 As.[30] As with any habit, the person who smokes must want to quit and must be ready to do so before he or she will be successful.

Online and Social Network Resources as Cessation Support Mechanisms

Online resources to support cessation have burgeoned. A systematic review and meta-analysis of the literature from 1990 to 2008 reveals that interactive, web-based interventions were acceptable to users and effective, especially when used by those motivated to quit.[3]

A study of 1,790 nurses using an online quit resource called "Nurses QuitNet" shows that most participants most often used the "read-only social support" feature of the site. Data from the site registration intake questionnaire reveal that 92.5% were female, 34% were between 45 and 54 years old, 84.5% were Caucasian, and 57.5% were college graduates. More than 68% smoked 10–20 cigarettes/day, and 66.4% smoked within 30 minutes of waking.[10] This online quit modality was deemed acceptable to nurses and convenient no matter their work schedules.

A recent Cochrane review of 20 studies describing short- and long-term effectiveness of a variety of Internet-based interventions found that appropriately tailored content including frequent automated contact with users was most effective.[45] Interactive sites seemed the most effective, and one trial demonstrated cessation success was boosted if NRT was used along with the Internet resource.

Risks Associated with Quitting

Smoking cessation alters the physiology of the abstainer in powerful ways and may affect the metabolism of certain drugs that are being taken. Be aware that the client who is taking theophylline, clozapine, warfarin, insulin, or olanzapine while smoking may need to have dosage adjustments (most likely reductions) once he or she abstains from tobacco.[46]

Psychoemotional risks of cessation include a tendency toward depression, especially if other coping mechanisms and outlets for emotional issues are not facilitated and developed. Certainly, the risk for suicide should be taken into account when assessing individuals who are abstaining, particularly if they are taking bupropion or varenicline.

Smokers may experience flu-like symptoms and/or cough as they withdraw from smoking and the body detoxifies itself. They also may experience feelings of loss. These are natural processes and are often dose related (varying with the amount smoked and duration of the habit), yet may be frightening to the smoker who does not know what to expect. Nutritious foods and appropriate supplements, fluids, and exercise can support healing and feelings of well-being as the former smoker goes through a process of detoxification.

The Transtheoretical Model of Change

There is often no truly effective means for measuring individual readiness to change smoking behavior. Within the dynamics of smoking cessation, there are many issues of resistance to change and recidivism. Smoking cessation is not a dichotomous product of smoking but often a long and laborious process of progress and regression, ups and downs, successes and failures. The Transtheoretical Model of Change provides a theoretical basis for explaining when and how people change behaviors.[47] The model is useful for comprehending self-initiated, as well as professionally facilitated, change. The model supports the notion that change occurs in a cyclic rather than linear fashion, often causing certain sequences and phases to be repeated before a change goal is reached. There are also varying rates of change. Some individuals move through the change sequence rapidly, while others never move beyond a particular stage.[48]

Prochaska and colleagues began investigating and developing the Transtheoretical Model of Change by integrating diverse theories of change from the psychotherapy literature. They examined the cognitive, affective, and behavioral processes as individuals moved through different levels of change. Specifically, the researchers studied attrition and relapse, which were more the rule than the exception.[48]

Two major constructs organize the framework of the Transtheoretical Model—the stages and the processes of change. Other important concepts are self-efficacy, pros and cons of decisional balance, and temptations for relapse.[47]

Five stages of change that provide a temporal structure for monitoring the change process include the following:

1. *Precontemplation:* No intention of quitting within the next 6 months
2. *Contemplation:* Seriously considering quitting within the next 6 months
3. *Preparation:* Seriously planning to quit within the next 30 days and has made at least one quit attempt in past year
4. *Action:* Former smoker continuously quit for less than 6 months
5. *Maintenance:* Former smoker continuously quit for greater than 6 months

The stages are important for measuring progress toward quitting and help to predict relapse.

Precontemplators have no intention of changing their behaviors in the near future. They cannot really see that they have a problem. Contemplators are aware that a problem exists and are thinking seriously about changing their behaviors, but they have not yet made a commitment to take action.[49] Individuals in the preparation stage combine intention with preliminary actions to change behaviors in the near future. They may have made a past attempt to change that was unsuccessful. Smokers in the preparation stage may begin with small changes, such as smoking fewer cigarettes in a day, delaying the first cigarette of the morning, and changing some of their smoking habits (e.g., forgoing the "pleasant" cigarette with coffee after a meal). People who move into the action stage actually shift from thinking about the problem to doing something about the problem. They dedicate a considerable amount of commitment, time, and energy to the change. Finally, individuals who make a change and stick with it move into the maintenance stage and work to prevent relapse. They begin to stabilize the behavior change and make it a way of life.[49]

Behavioral and Lifestyle Approaches to Smoking Cessation

Smoking cessation is stressful to the body, and careful planning and scrupulous self-care on the part of the quitter can help a great deal. The smoker may like the image of being "in training," as an athlete would be. Using a variety of preferred strategies in combination can bolster the client's ability to be successful.

Smoking Diary

Recording habits in a smoking diary increases self-awareness. Smoking is such a pervasive, automatic habit that it is helpful for clients to keep a smoking diary of when, where, how often, and what moods are associated with smoking. The client records the feelings associated with smoking and begins to think about new habits to replace these urges. Keeping such a record for several weeks before the quit date allows the client to identify patterns, and knowing the smoking triggers leads to permanent changes. To strengthen the new awareness, the client may record thoughts, feelings, urges, and observations about smoking. With each cigarette that is smoked, for example, the client should consider the following questions:

1. What internal cues made me think that I needed a cigarette (e.g., breathing patterns, mouth watering, tense muscles, fidgety hands)?
2. What external cues made me think that I needed a cigarette (e.g., talking on the phone, watching television, finishing eating, drinking alcohol, sitting down with friends)?
3. Now that I've smoked that cigarette, did I enjoy it?

Preparing for the Quit Date

Preparation for quit date makes the process a reality. The desire to be a nonsmoker should build. Becoming smoke free requires preparation. The client should take the time to identify personal reasons for quitting, such as to reduce the risk of heart, lung, or circulatory disease; to increase endurance and productivity; to improve sense of smell and taste; to increase self-esteem; to be in control; or to decrease the risk to family health from ETS. Once certain that it is time to quit, the client's goal is to be a nonsmoker in 5 days. The nurse may encourage the client to identify family members, friends, or a specific person who may want to join the effort as a quit-smoking partner. The client should tell significant people the quit date and solicit their support.

Preparing for Nicotine Withdrawal

Preparation for nicotine withdrawal facilitates the process of being a nonsmoker. There is no one best way to quit smoking. Some people are successful at just quitting cold turkey and going through the nicotine withdrawal, with the worst part usually lasting 5 days or less. Others require a gradual decrease of nicotine with the use of nicotine replacement therapy (NRT). The client must decide which approach to try.

Preparing a Smoke-Free Environment

Creating a smoke-free body and environment can be a creative process for the client. During the first few nonsmoking days, the client rids the body of toxic waste left from the cigarettes by bathing, brushing teeth, drinking water, exercising, relaxing, imaging, resting, and ingesting good nutrition. A fresh nonsmoking living environment can be accomplished by placing clean filters in heating and cooling units and cleaning carpets, drapes, clothes, office, and car. Signs may be placed on the office door: "Thank you for not smoking." The more energy that the client puts into these activities, the more likely the client will quit and become a permanent nonsmoker. The client should become aware of how quickly the senses of smell and taste increase and how disgusting the smell and taste of cigarettes become.

Identifying Smoking Triggers and Creating Habit Breakers

Identification of personal smoking triggers (smoke signals) and creating habit breakers can also be a creative process for the client. Becoming smoke free is directly related to minor changes in daily routines, referred to as habit breakers. Many ex-smokers report that the first 5 days of being smoke free are the hardest. Minor or major changes in daily activities can be less stressful if accompanied by a healing state of awareness. If the client should slip and fall back into old routines, these relapses can become learning situations. The client can identify negative self-talk or a stressful situation in which a new habit breaker may not have been used soon enough. The following events are the times when smoking is most likely:

Before starting the day:

- Getting out of bed
- Taking a bath or shower
- Eating breakfast
- Reading the newspaper
- Starting work or driving to work

Mornings:

- During telephone calls
- During coffee
- While driving
- During office work or housework
- In meetings
- In morning breaks
- Before, during, and after lunch

Afternoons:

- During telephone calls
- During office work or housework
- In meetings
- With coffee
- During afternoon breaks
- While completing and organizing your work for the next day
- While driving home or resting in late afternoon
- With alcohol

Evenings:

- Before, during, and after dinner
- If stressed or lonely
- With alcohol
- While relaxing, watching television, or out with family or friends
- While preparing for bed

It is helpful to create habit breakers for each of these events. Success with habit breakers requires commitment to identifying them, writing them down, creativity, and finding ways to personalize this list. For example, the client can take this list, divide a piece of paper into two columns, and write down new habit breakers:

Nutritional Counseling

Nutritional counseling should encourage the client to choose nutrient-dense foods. (See Chapter 13.) In general, vegetables, fruits, whole grains, and high-quality protein are essential. Nuts, seeds, vegetable juices, lots of good water to maintain generous hydration and flush out toxins, a high-potency multivitamin/mineral supplement with omega-3 fish oils, B supplement, vitamin C, and vitamin D are indicated. Avoidance of highly processed foods, sweets, and alcohol is helpful because these foods may dysregulate blood glucose and increase inflammation in the body, negatively affecting mood and increasing withdrawal symptoms and cravings. Miso soup is thought to cleanse the body of nicotine, and leafy greens, lemon juice, carrots, and celery promote alkalinity and decrease cravings. Green tea, white tea, and red (rooibos) tea contain valuable antioxidants and less caffeine and are also recommended. Chewing natural licorice sticks found in health food stores helps manage cravings as well as tactile and oral urges. Using licorice root chew sticks (not candy) is sometimes recommended and can be helpful, but must be used in moderation since too much can lower potassium and raise blood pressure. Sugarless gum may help for the same reason.

Exercise

Exercise is a powerful ally in the effort to quit smoking. Regular exercise has been shown to reduce stress in the body and improve mood. Because these are key aspects of the motivation to smoke, as well as problematic issues during withdrawal, it is beneficial for the client to engage in a regular program of enjoyable movement at the highest level of vigor possible. This reduces cravings and mood disturbance, improves self-esteem, promotes self-concept as a person who engages in healthy behaviors

Routine	Habit Breaker
Smoke cigarette upon awakening	Play relaxing music or shower on awakening
Two cups of coffee at breakfast	Hot tea instead of coffee at breakfast
Frequent lighting of cigarettes	Keep sugarless gum or natural licorice sticks nearby
Midmorning smoke break for energy	Eat an apple, drink water, take a walk
Smoking while driving in the car	Listen to music or educational CD, think, breathe

(reinforcing identity as a nonsmoker), and reduces weight gain, a significant deterrent to smoking cessation. (See Chapter 14.)

A recent Cochrane review identified three large studies demonstrating that those who engaged in regular, vigorous exercise were more likely to abstain from smoking, even at 12 months post quit date.[50] Several smaller studies did not show significant improvement in abstinence in those who exercised; however, the frequency and intensity of exercise programs were not clearly described, or adherence was poor. Many studies that did not meet Cochrane criteria have demonstrated short-term benefits of exercise on cravings and withdrawal symptoms, including a yoga intervention.[51] One study looked at the effects of body scanning and isometric exercise on cigarette cravings and withdrawal symptoms and found both to be helpful but only for 5 minutes after the intervention.[52] Still, these may be helpful strategies for the mindful quitter getting from moment to moment without tobacco.

Yoga postures that are particularly helpful for smoking cessation include spinal twists (seated and standing), back bends (seated and standing), Camel, Bridge, Bow, and Corpse pose. In general, the breathing, stretching, strengthening, and meditative aspects of yoga practice are of benefit to those seeking a release from addictive behaviors.

To the person becoming smoke free, an exercise program serves as a stress manager (as an alternative to smoking), helps with weight management, and increases energy levels. If the client does not have an exercise program, the nurse offers assistance and helps the client decide what lifestyle patterns to approach first. It usually takes about 3 months for an exercise program to become a regular part of life, so the client may look for an exercise partner who is serious about exercising or being a nonsmoker.

Weight gain can be avoided. It occurs because the nonsmoker eats too much, lacks aerobic exercise, or consumes too much alcohol. If weight management is a challenge, it is helpful to set a target date for establishing and following an exercise program 2 to 3 months before the quit date. (Refer to Chapter 22 for specific strategies to maintain healthy weight.) Then, as the client commits to quitting smoking, one component of an effective stress management program has already begun.

Client Bill of Rights

Clients engaged in smoking cessation should recite their bill of rights. They can be creative and add to this list:

I have a right to

- Be smoke free in any situation
- Review my list of reasons to stop smoking frequently, particularly before any social gathering
- Ask others not to smoke in my home, office, or car
- Choose a network of people who will support me in my efforts to quit
- Avoid those who rob me of energy or motivation to stay smoke free
- Avoid environments and situations where people smoke
- Remind myself that cigarettes leave toxic substances in my body and in my environments, sometimes harming others
- Throw away all objects associated with smoking
- Keep sugarless gum and natural licorice sticks close at hand
- Practice my relaxation, imagery, and coping skills anywhere and at any time
- Seek healing for underlying emotional wounds revealed through my quit process
- Seek therapy to support new coping behaviors and address any underlying trauma
- Keep healthy beverages close by at work and at home
- Support legislation to protect nonsmokers from the dangers of passive smoking in public places

Integration of Rewards

The client should plan a reward at least every 5 to 7 days for having a smoke-free lifestyle. These rewards should continue as long as the client needs to be aware of new lifestyle habits. The client is considered smoke free when his or her habits are indeed nonsmoking behaviors. Continued use of the listed habit breakers always helps a client anticipate when smoke signals can surface and, thus, quickly take actions to prevent relapse.

Reinforcement of Positive Self-Talk

Feelings, moods, behaviors, and motivation affect physiologic changes. As the client learns to recognize the self-talk that sabotages his or her positive outlook, it is possible for the client to remain in control and not give in to the urge to smoke. Positive affirmations such as "I am feeling more free," "I am feeling in control," "every day I am getting healthier" can help the client be successful. The nurse can also assist with cognitive restructuring of automatic negative thoughts (ANTs) of those who are quitting. (See Chapter 11.) Negative rationalization must be recognized because it can gradually lead to doubt about the ability to change. The client may reframe negative statements, for example, changing "I've become more nervous since I quit smoking" to "I am noticing a change in my moods since quitting and I am adding a relaxation and imagery practice. This makes me feel much better than the short burst of nicotine energy." Similarly, negative thoughts must be identified and replaced with positive thoughts. For example, "I'll never get over this urge to smoke; I'll never be successful at breaking the habit" may be reframed as "Of course, I can get over this urge. I am learning new coping strategies, and I can really imagine myself smoke free."

Journaling and Self-Reflection

Journal writing and self-reflection (see Chapter 12) may help to get feelings up and out through the quit process, rather than the client holding them in. Self-reflection can lead to self-awareness, and by journaling clients may identify changes they can make. For example, setting good boundaries in relationships can help to keep out "energy-draining people" and naysayers (those who may not support quit efforts), thus helping the former smoker stay on course with the quit plan. Staying away from other smokers, even loved ones, may be well worth the effort.

Breathing Techniques

Breathing is a powerful strategy to aid in smoking cessation. There are as many ways to breathe as there are smokers, but it is helpful to teach deep breathing exercises to soothe, energize, and calm the client. Breathing, like nicotine, can serve many purposes! The *4-2-8 count breath* can be very

helpful, and the counts can be varied to meet the needs of the individual client because breathing rhythm mimics smoking behavior. In this technique, the client breathes in slowly and fully to the count of 4, holds it for 2 counts, and then exhales slowly and fully to the count of 8. By repeating this pattern, the parasympathetic nervous system (the "rest and digest" response) is triggered.

Another breathing technique that may be helpful is the "Butt Kicking Breath" demonstrated online at www.sadienardini.com. To practice this technique, place hands on sides of ribcage, drop shoulders down away from ears, inhale to the count of 4 through the nose, hold to the count of 2, exhale through pursed lips to the count of 8. Repeat, keeping shoulders down and adding abdominal contractions with the belly tucked in toward the spine.

Alternate nostril breathing can soothe and shift mood in a positive direction, therefore enhancing quit efforts. Clients can use the thumb and forefinger of one hand to alternately occlude one nostril and breathe fully in and out of the open nostril each time. Repeating for at least 12 cycles/switches elicits an effect. Online videos clearly demonstrate this technique.

Guided Imagery and Hypnosis

Hypnosis, a process that includes relaxation techniques, guided imagery, and suggestion, is often used in behavioral approaches to smoking cessation. A dearth of research evidence documents effectiveness of this strategy, yet anecdotal evidence abounds that hypnosis is effective, and it makes intuitive sense to harness the power of the mind–body connection to promote cessation. The imagery scripts that follow enable the nurse to begin working with a client using this process.

Guided imagery with suggestions (hypnosis) enhances the client's success at becoming smoke free. The nurse can use the following scripts to create a live session with the client or create a relaxation and imagery recording, or the nurse can provide the scripts to the client to make his or her own recording. The scripts help the client form correct biological images of being smoke free. They can be modified or expanded, depending on present habits and which new skills the client wishes to develop to break the nicotine habit. A relaxation exercise from Chapter 16 may be used/recorded for 5 to 10 minutes to induce a relaxed and receptive state; then, the script for smoking cessation is used/recorded for 15 minutes. The nurse should encourage the client to listen to the tape daily or several times a day throughout the first week of cessation when physiologic withdrawal is occurring. Then, the client can listen every other day for a week, and then as often as needed thereafter.

Excellent smoking cessation guided imagery CDs and MP3 downloads created by therapist Belleruth Naparstek and marketed by Health Journeys are available at www.healthjourneys.com. Physiologically correct, specific, and well constructed, these resources are readily available and reasonably priced.

Script: **Introduction. (Name)**, as your mind becomes clearer and clearer, feel it becoming more and more alert. Somewhere deep inside of you, a brilliant light begins to glow. Sense this happening. . . . The light grows brighter and more intense. . . . This is your mind–body communication center. Breathe into it. . . . Energize it with your breath. The light is powerful and penetrating, and a beam begins to grow from it. The beam shines into your body now as you prepare to focus on being smoke free. . . .

In your relaxed state, affirm to yourself at your deep level of inner strength and knowing . . . that you are already becoming a nonsmoker. Say it over and over as you begin to see the words and feelings in every cell in your body. Feel your relaxed state deepen. You can get to this space anytime you wish. . . . All you have to do is give yourself the suggestion and stay with the suggestion as you move into your relaxed state. This is a skill that you will use repeatedly as you move into being smoke free.

Script: **Quit date.** You are at a place in time where smoking no longer suits you. It is no longer a comfortable behavior for you. Congratulate yourself on reaching this point in your life journey and for setting your quit date. You are aware of all the resources available to help you quit. With your mind's eye now . . . see your calendar and experience yourself reading your quit date. With full intention to quit, mark your quit date on the calendar. Enlist the help of your family or a friend as you set your quit date. The process has begun.

Script: **Cleansing your body and environment.** It is now time to rid your body of toxins left from the cigarettes. Begin to cleanse your body. . . . Feel the toxins flowing out of your body as you increase the liquids you drink. Practice your deep breathing exercises, remembering to exhale completely . . . enjoying this new awareness of how healthy your lungs will become with the cleansing and clearing of toxins. Experience your breath, skin, hair . . . fresh as a spring breeze. See yourself making your surroundings smoke free day by day. Notice the pleasant changes in your new, nonsmoking environment. . . . First, begin to notice how you are becoming more sensitive to smells. . . . Enjoy the freshness of your clothes, home, office, and car being free of smoke.

As you keep your records, become aware of your progress. Reward yourself regularly. Imagine you have had 5 smoke-free days. The worst of any withdrawal is over. What is your first reward going to be? Give yourself that reward!

As you continue to deepen your relaxation, inhale to the count of 4, hold to the count of 2, then exhale to the count of 8. Repeat to yourself the words "I am calm" as you exhale. Let your body experience these words in your own unique way.

Register this feeling throughout your body. Begin to increase your awareness of feeling good about being alive, to be conscious of beginning new habits . . . free of smoking.

Script: ***Triggers/smoke signals.*** Starting now, as a nonsmoker, reflect on your wonderful decision to release the habit of smoking . . . a habit that could cause illness and take away your energy and vitality. Get in touch with your smoke signals/ smoking triggers. Is it a certain time of day, a person, a place, or social gathering? As you bring them into awareness. . . rehearse in your mind the healthy behaviors you will use to replace the urges. . . . Is it drinking a glass of water . . . chewing sugar-free gum, going for a walk, listening to music, chewing on a toothpick, or taking a hot shower or bath? And as you think about smoking urges . . . those unconscious habits . . . you realize that from now on, you will never unconsciously reach for a tobacco product again. . . . As a nonsmoker, you have simply lost the desire and urge to smoke. . . . You are very aware of your body, mind, and spirit. . . . You can hear your powerful inner voice repeating clear affirmations, . . . "I have stopped smoking . . . I am free of smoking . . . I feel strong and healthy . . .

I can taste, and smell fragrances. My cough has gone."

Hear your own voice saying, "I no longer crave a habit negatively affecting my health. I no longer unconsciously reach for a cigarette or smoke. This habit is diminishing steadily, and I can envision being completely free of this addiction. My mind–body is functioning in such a manner that I no longer crave tobacco. . . . I value my lungs and heart and care for them. I no longer place unnecessary strain on these organs so vital to life."

When you feel the urge to smoke, hear yourself saying, "Stop!" followed by inhaling to the count of 4, holding to the count of 2, and exhaling to the count of 8. Then, tell yourself, "Smoking no longer suits me. It is no longer a part of who I am. I am free." These words will become more powerful the more you say them. Feel a warm inner glow of healthy pride that grows every day. It fills you with warmth and a sense of freedom and control on deep levels of your being. Remember this message of freedom and pride is always with you . . . and you are no longer a smoker. That is behind you. Any feelings of loss have already been replaced by the stronger feelings of freedom, control, vitality, and hope.

Script: ***Nutritious eating and exercise.*** "As I stop smoking, I will not be excessively hungry or eat excessively. Because of my body-mind-spirit connection, I am free of my addiction. Because of increasing feelings of energy, I take any and all opportunities to move my body. I increase my exercise to three or four times a week for 20 minutes or longer. I am conscious of using deep breathing exercises regularly, and certainly any time I feel stressed or have a craving. I increase my fluid intake and chew sugar-free gum. I sleep soundly at night. My environment is fresh. Food tastes and smells wonderful. I have more money to use as I choose. I am in control at deeper levels of my being. I am free of smoking. I am free." You can access this inner wisdom any time that you wish. . . . All you have to do is get calm and easy, breathe deeply, and focus inward.

Script: ***Closure.*** Take a few slow, energizing breaths and, as you come back to full awareness of the room, know that you are on a body-mind-spirit journey, and whatever is right for you at this point in time is unfolding just as it should and that you have done your best, regardless of the outcome.

Prevention as the Best Protection from Smoking

Because smoking is highly addictive, it is best not to start in the first place. The average age of first use is 14.5 years, and approximately 40% of teens who smoke become addicted to nicotine.[4] With that knowledge, prevention efforts must start when children are young, with school-based programs beginning in later elementary and middle school years. An interesting study revealed that parents who quit smoking enhanced their children's negative attitudes toward smoking, especially if the parent quit before the child was in third grade. These parents are often actively engaged in relapse-prevention behaviors, and this has a protective and deterring effect on children.[53]

Evidence shows that tobacco control programs reduce smoking behavior, and that

tobacco advertising and public health counter-advertising measures vie for the attention of youth. In the last two decades, improvements have been documented in terms of the prevalence of high school students who smoke. In 1991, the prevalence of current high school student smoking was 27.5%, and by 1997 it had grown to 36.4%; however, the rate for teen smoking in the United States dropped to 19.5% in 2009.[54] These data support the findings of other studies that indicate youth smoking has reached its peak and is now in decline, though the rate of decline has slowed in recent years.

Factors that discourage smoking in youth include more aggressive school health policies and school-based prevention and cessation programs, strict restrictions on selling to minors, harnessing the power of media images and messages by having effective role models on television and in magazines, and strong counteradvertising campaigns that depict smoking and tobacco use in a negative light. In addition, measures that discourage smoking across the life span include high cigarette prices through taxation, smoking bans in public places, restricted access to tobacco products, and ongoing public education campaigns depicting the harmful health effects of tobacco.[4]

Unfortunately, the *Healthy People 2010* goal to reduce the high school smoking rate to 16% or less was not met. However, the Family Smoking Prevention and Tobacco Control Act (TCA) enacted in 2009 offers new opportunities for comprehensive reductions in tobacco use. By giving the Food and Drug Administration (FDA) additional authority to regulate the tobacco industry, the TCA imposes specific marketing, labeling, and advertising requirements and establishes restrictions on youth access and promotional practices that are targeted toward youth. Evidence of this act may be seen in the new, gruesome pictures that are now included on cigarette packaging depicting harmful consequences of smoking.

Research demonstrates that living farther away from stores that sell tobacco products enhances abstinence after a quit attempt.[55] Therefore, zoning restrictions in residential areas could be an effective means to bolster existing strategies aimed at reducing tobacco use. As described in the 2007 Institute of Medicine report titled *Ending the*

Tobacco Problem: A Blueprint for the Nation, the regulation of tobacco products is an essential aspect of a comprehensive national tobacco prevention and control strategy that will strengthen the impact of the growing body of evidence-based interventions already in use.

Educating our youth and offering healthy strategies to cope with the stresses of life is probably the best way to keep them away from cigarettes. Mindful exercise such as yoga classes that include breathing and meditation should be a part of this approach. Developing healthy behaviors begins early and sets the pattern for life.

■ HOLISTIC CARING PROCESS

Holistic Assessment

In preparing to use smoking cessation interventions, the nurse assesses the following parameters:

- The client's level of addiction to cigarettes
- The meaning of smoking to the client
- The client's attitudes and beliefs about successful and sustained smoking cessation
- The client's motivation to learn interventions to become a permanent nonsmoker
- The client's stage of change in terms of smoking cessation
- The client's eating patterns and exercise program
- The client's existing stress management strategies
- The client's support and encouragement from family and friends

Identification of Patterns/ Challenges/Needs

The following patterns, challenges, and needs (see Chapter 7) compatible with smoking cessation interventions are as follows:

- Exchanging:
  - Altered circulation
  - Altered oxygenation
- Valuing:
  - Spiritual distress
  - Spiritual well-being
- Choosing:
  - Ineffective individual coping
  - Effective individual coping
- Moving: Self-care deficit
- Perceiving:
  - Disturbance in body image
  - Disturbance in self-esteem
  - Hopelessness
- Knowing: Knowledge deficit
- Feeling:
  - Anxiety
  - Fear

Outcome Identification

Exhibit 23-1 guides the nurse in client outcomes, nursing prescriptions, and evaluation for successful smoking cessation.

Therapeutic Care Plan and Interventions

Before the session:

- Spend a few moments centering yourself to become mindfully present and to begin the session with the intention to facilitate healing.
- Gather any materials you will use during the session.
- Create a quiet place to begin guiding the client in smoking cessation strategies.

At the beginning of the session:

- Review the smoking diary, if client has been keeping one. Explore the meaning of smoking patterns with the client. Elicit insight into changing behaviors.
- Establish prequitting strategies. Suggest that the client identify and combine the methods that can work best.
- Encourage the client to take a few days before the quit date to rid the body of toxins and to clean the house, office, and car of any evidence of cigarettes or odors.
- Advise attention to exercise and nutrition ahead of quit date.
- Have the client establish the quit date and sign a contract that specifies the quit date.
- Encourage the client to call on family and friends on the first smoke-free days, particularly when confidence is low. Remind them that their support is very important.
- Encourage the client to practice small acts of control (such as delaying gratification). This enhances feelings of self-control and has been shown to enhance quit efforts.

EXHIBIT 23-1   Nursing Interventions: Smoking Cessation

Client Outcomes	Nursing Prescriptions	Evaluation
The client will demonstrate attitudes, beliefs, and behaviors that indicate the desire to be a nonsmoker.	Determine the client's desire to be a nonsmoker.	The client demonstrated attitudes, beliefs, behaviors, and the desire to be a nonsmoker.
	Assist the client in setting realistic plans for being a nonsmoker by ■ Establishing quit date ■ Self-assessing bodymind-spirit health to see which areas need bolstering ■ Drawing up a nicotine withdrawal schedule ■ Cleansing self and environment of nicotine ■ Developing habit-breaker strategies ■ Keeping a smoking diary ■ Practicing relaxation and imagery ■ Assessing support network ■ Integrating behavior changes ■ Deciding on rewards for attaining goals	The client set a realistic plan and became a nonsmoker over 1 week as follows: ■ Focused on quit date goal and stopped use of cigarettes ■ Cleansed body and environment of nicotine ■ Adhered to habit-breaker strategies ■ Kept a smoking, exercise, food diary ■ Practiced relaxation and imagery daily ■ Integrated behavior changes daily ■ Rewarded self for attaining goals

During the session:

■ Reinforce the quit date, and have the client imagine being smoke free in 5 days.

■ Teach basic relaxation and imagery skills to shape mind–body changes for internal and external smoke-free images. These images create a new self-perception and will enhance the client's success. Rhythmic breathing and progressive muscle relaxation are most helpful in teaching body-centered awareness and effective coping. Relaxation and imagery help the client to recognize and block triggers/smoke signals. Combine this practice with a stop smoking CD once or twice a day.

■ Teach the client to create specific imagery patterns (see Chapter 17):
   ■ *Active images:* Cleansing the body of nicotine and other toxins; finding a safe place

that establishes a feeling of security and comfort; envisioning a protective bubble that receives what is needed from others and blocks out negative images, such as smoke signals.

   ■ *Process images:* People, events, and situations that trigger the desire to smoke. Have the client rehearse being in a situation where smoking normally occurs, but now using a new behavior, such as breathing deeply and saying, "I am calm" on exhalation or reaching for a glass of water.

   ■ *End-state images:* Being smoke free; accessing feelings of control and freedom.

■ Have the client create strategies to break smoke signals and become smoke free—waking up and having a glass of water, reading the morning paper in a different room, taking a break and drinking water or juice, brushing teeth, talking on the telephone, and practicing relaxation and rhythmic breathing.

- Encourage the client to be patient in making this major lifestyle change and to remember that smoking is about self-protective control. The old, superficial (and unhealthy) sense of control must be replaced with a new, deeper (healthy) sense of control. Identify internal and external experiences as new health behaviors are being shaped. Some are easy to change; others take longer.

- Ask the client to become aware of new opportunities for being with family, friends, and self while being smoke free. Discuss options for new patterns of socializing.

- Discuss the people who form the client's support network. Who is supportive and energy giving? Who is energy draining? In what ways can social patterns change to support being smoke free? It can be helpful to identify who to reduce time with until new patterns of nonsmoking become stronger.

At the end of the session:

- Suggest that the client create a series of personal rewards—establishing a schedule that will be motivating. Perhaps having a reward after 5 smoke-free days, or having a small reward each day, with a larger reward after 5 days.

- Evaluate with the client the goals of behavior changes—reduction of smoking urges and development of new habit patterns.

- Encourage the client to make a list of anticipated high-risk situations and decide (in advance) ways to prevent a relapse. The most frequent high-risk situations are social situations, emotional upsets, home or work frustration, interpersonal conflict, driving, and relaxing after a meal. In general, when a person is hungry, angry or anxious, lonely or tired (HALT), vulnerability to addictive behaviors is heightened. Using the breathing techniques described in this chapter can help the client get through a craving or relapse-prone situation.

- Reinforce the fact that the client can avoid relapse. Having learned to recognize high-risk situations for relapse, the client can be ready quickly to use strategies to resist smoking temptations. Successful coping strategies must honor internal responses (mind–body feelings and thoughts) and action-oriented responses (action steps).

- Suggest that the client become a support person for someone else who is trying to become smoke free to decrease chances of relapse.

- Use the client outcomes (see Exhibit 23-1) that were established before the session to evaluate the session.

- Schedule a follow-up session.

CASE STUDY (IMPLEMENTATION)

Setting: Nurse-based wellness clinic smoking cessation program

Client: J. N., a 48-year-old interior designer, telling her story to the new clients after she has been smoke free for 5 years

Patterns/Challenges/Needs: Health maintenance related to engagement in strategies to remain smoke free

"You can call it midlife crisis or whatever; I just happened to wake up and tell myself that I'm worth a better state of health and mind. How did I do it? Lots of determination and reprogramming my mind with successful images. I never dreamed that I could be so successful at quitting smoking. I'd tried to quit on many occasions, but the reason I never was able to sustain change is that I had tried to quit before I really was ready to do so.

"I'd been smoking for 27 years, and I just got tired of my chronic cough and feeling tired. Other things began to happen also. My family and friends began to ask for nonsmoking sections in restaurants and gave me 3 months before they declared the house a nonsmoking house. They also placed a disgusting, ugly series of pictures of me smoking with a title on it saying, 'We Love You—Quit Smoking!' The first time I looked at the pictures, I burst into tears and heard their message loud and clear. I got in touch with why I began smoking in the first place as a teenager—I thought I looked important and glamorous. Those pictures certainly didn't convey that image.

"The last straw that really got my attention was when a friend and I were driving along with our windows down on a nice spring day. My friend said to me, 'Who do you think is smoking?' We could see no person smoking, but my friend could smell it. Sure enough, there was a smoker three cars in front of us in the left lane to us. I was driving, and, as we passed the car, smoke came in our window. I couldn't smell it even though I could see the smoke coming in the window.

"I really planned a ritual for my quit date for ending smoking—which has changed my life in many ways. I have now been smoke free for 5 years. Let me begin by saying that, in the previous 15 years, I had tried to quit smoking seven times; each time I was successful for 1 month at the longest, so I knew that it was possible. As I look back on it now, the reason that I didn't have any sustained change was that I didn't shape any new behaviors or thoughts.

"Let me share with you my rituals. I planned a 5-day period to be by myself to focus on shaping new behaviors. The reason I chose to stay at home was the importance of preparation and concentration of new thoughts and behaviors prior to my quit date.

"Prior to that special week, I began my 'detox' process. I decided to buy a new bright blue toothbrush, which I placed in a beautiful small wicker basket. I also placed this on the opposite side of where I usually kept my toothbrush. When brushing my teeth gently, frequently followed by a mouthwash, I was aware of repeating words to myself about cleansing and purifying. I used these same thoughts when I bathed. I would stand in the shower and concentrate on the water washing the toxins from my skin. For the internal removal of toxins, I increased my fluid intake of water and herb teas to 6 to 8 glasses a day. Exercise also became part of my ritual. I would get up each day and start my morning with a 30-minute walk. On the walk, I used the time to see myself smoke free.

"Well, my home environment reeked of smoke and staleness. My drapes and fabric chairs and couches had not been cleaned in 16 years; my carpets, in 8. I allowed myself the luxury of having them professionally cleaned. Not only did the house smell fresh, but all the colors were very fresh and seemed new. Air-conditioning filters were changed. I cleaned clothes that were well overdue. I aired the house.

"The biggest task was to gather all the cigarette packages throughout the house. They were in every room, and I had about three full cartons when I finally gathered them all up. This was really scary for me, because when I saw them all together, the thought that came to me was, 'I'm really addicted. There is no way I can break this habit.' Out of nowhere, this very loud, powerful voice blurted out, 'Yes, you can, and you have already begun.' I have never heard such volume from my own voice. It was as if it was a voice other than my own. Prior to that, I also removed all of the ashtrays and bought a beautiful door sign which read "Thank You For Not Smoking." When I placed it above the door bell, I felt this inner sensation of glee and energy. It was very affirming to me, and, from that moment on, there was no stopping my success. I really believed for the first time that I was going to be successful, and I felt an inner strength that I had never experienced before. I also received so much encouragement from my husband and two children when they came home that evening. I cleaned my car as well as I had the house.

"During this period of 1 week of cleaning my body, house, and car, I recorded my internal and external cues of why I smoked. It was when I was hungry, talking on the phone, when I was putting on my makeup in the morning, and after meals. During this time, I let myself smoke no more than three cigarettes a day—outside standing up. I concentrated on what a disgusting habit smoking was. As I focused on these messages to myself, I not only slowed down the smoking, I also didn't enjoy the cigarettes and found that it was really not as pleasant as in the past. I had tried this before, but my thoughts were also on how much I was going to miss the smoking and pleasure of the buzz from smoking. I was so aware of not really enjoying it as much as I used to.

"I well remember my quit date 5 years ago. It is so clear; it is as if I planned it just yesterday. The reason it seems so recent is that my preparation and commitment to stopping smoking spilled over into other areas in my life. Do I miss smoking? Frankly, I'll say yes. I have those urges on

EXHIBIT 23-2   Evaluating the Client's Subjective Experience with Smoking Cessation Interventions

1. Did you gain any new insight today about your smoking patterns?
2. Do you have any questions about preparing for a quit date?
3. Do you have any questions about recording your habits?
4. Can you identify two new habit breakers right now to be smoke free?
5. Are you aware of your mind–body signals that trigger your desire to smoke?
6. What relaxation exercises are most helpful to you in replacing smoking habits? What breathing exercises are most helpful?
7. What coping behaviors may help you heal in bodymindspirit as you become a nonsmoker?
8. What will be your exercise program?
9. Do you have any questions about the active imagery, process imagery, and the end-state imagery exercises that you experienced today?
10. Do you find the imagery exercises to be effective? What might make them more effective for you?
11. Have you gained any new insights from monitoring your self-talk?
12. What are three affirmations to help you create an image change of being smoke free?
13. Who are the people in your life who can provide support as you make changes for health? Who are the people in your life who are not likely to provide support? What do you want to do with this awareness?
14. What aspects of your life are in need of further healing? What is your next step?

occasions. However, as I've integrated relaxation, imagery, and positive affirmations in my life, my commitment to being smoke free is stronger. I honor that inner voice that says, 'Light Up.' For me, what works best is to hear the message, honor that I heard it, but to replace smoking with something that is always with me—the power of relaxed breathing. I also use a saying a friend taught me, which is Avoid H.A.L.T.—Avoid becoming too Hungry, too Angry, too Lonely, or too Tired. Time, commitment, and believing in my success are part of every day for me. Quitting smoking is one of the hardest things I've ever done. I can't remember planning so well for any event in my life. I believed I could do it, and that is exactly what continued to happen."

Evaluation

With the client, the nurse determines whether the client outcomes for smoking cessation (see Exhibit 23-1) were achieved. To evaluate the session further, the nurse may again explore the subjective effects of the experience with the client (**Exhibit 23-2**).

In becoming an ex-smoker, a client must understand that it is a gradual step-by-step process that requires learning new skills. Smoking cessation involves (1) recognizing smoking habits and triggers, (2) establishing habit breakers, (3) preparing for detoxification of the body and environment, (4) establishing a support network, (5) modifying behavior including using habit breakers, and following good nutrition and exercise programs, (6) using medications and community resources as needed, and (7) addressing underlying emotional issues and mood disturbances to enhance healing and prevent relapse. The integration of these seven areas helps clients achieve new levels of self-awareness and increase the chance of being smoke free.

Directions for
FUTURE RESEARCH

1. Determine the nursing interventions that most effectively minimize stress and enhance emotional healing as clients begin a smoking cessation program.
2. Evaluate combinations of smoking cessation content and teaching methods to determine which are most effective in assisting a client in sustained smoking cessation.
3. Determine the nursing interventions that are most effective in helping a client explore underlying emotional issues to enhance cessation and prevent relapse.

Nurse Healer
REFLECTIONS

After reading this chapter, the nurse healer will be able to answer or to begin a process of answering the following questions:

- What rituals can I create or assist others in creating to detoxify and cleanse the body and environment of all traces of nicotine?
- What underlying emotional issues need healing so that the client can let go of unhealthy behaviors?
- What coping mechanisms and resources can be used to facilitate healing?
- What are specific process, end-state, and general healing images for teaching myself or others about releasing attachments to smoking and moving forward in being smoke free?

 For a full suite of assignments and additional learning activities, use the access code located in the front of your book to visit this exclusive website: http://go.jblearning.com/dossey. If you do not have an access code, you can obtain one at the site.

NOTES

1. Centers for Disease Control and Prevention, "Cigarette Smoking Among Adults and Trends in Smoking Cessation—United States, 2008," *Morbidity and Mortality Weekly Report* 58, no. 44 (2009): 1227–1233.
2. National Institutes of Health State-of-the-Science Panel, "National Institutes of Health State-of-the-Science Conference Statement: Tobacco Use: Prevention, Cessation, and Control," *Annals of Internal Medicine* 145, no. 11 (2006): 839–844.
3. L. Shahab and A. McEwen, "Online Support for Smoking Cessation: A Systematic Review of the Literature," *Addiction* 104 (2009): 1792–1804.
4. R. G. Lande et al., "Nicotine Addiction: Overview, Clinical Presentation, Treatment, and Follow Up" (2011). http://emedicine.medscape.com/article/287555.
5. N. Cobb, A. Graham, and D. Abrams, "Social Network Structure of a Large Online Community for Smoking Cessation," *American Journal of Public Health* 100, no. 7 (2010): 1282–1289.
6. M. Herman and M. Walsh, "Hospital Admissions for Acute Myocardial Infarction, Angina, Stroke, and Asthma After Implementation of Arizona's Comprehensive Statewide Smoking Ban," *American Journal of Public Health* 101, no. 3 (2011): 491–498.
7. L. B. Goldstein et al., "Guidelines for the Primary Prevention of Stroke. A Guideline for Healthcare Professionals from the American Heart Association/American Stroke Association," *Stroke* 42 (December 6, 2010): 517–584.
8. G. Karatay, K. Gulumser, and O. Emiroglu, "The Effect of Motivational Interviewing on Smoking Cessation in Pregnant Women," *Journal of Advanced Nursing* 66, no. 6 (2010): 1328–1337.
9. S. Rahmanian et al., "Tobacco Use and Cessation Among Women: Research and Treatment-Related Issues," *Journal of Women's Health* 20, no. 3 (2011): 349–357.
10. S. Bialous et al., "Characteristics of Nurses Who Used the Internet-Based Nurses QuitNet for Smoking Cessation," *Public Health Nursing* 26, no. 4 (2009): 329–338.
11. A. Kleppinger et al., "Effects of Smoking Cessation on Body Composition in Postmenopausal Women," *Journal of Women's Health* 19, no. 9 (2010): 1651–1660.
12. K. Cropsey et al., "The Impact of Quitting Smoking on Weight Among Women Prisoners Participating in a Smoking Cessation Intervention," *American Journal of Public Health* 100, no. 8 (2010): 1442–1448.

13. J. P. Winickoff et al., "Beliefs About the Health Effects of 'Thirdhand' Smoke and Home Smoking Bans," *Pediatrics* 123, no. 1 (2009): 74–79.

14. T. D. Skorge et al., "Exposure to Environmental Tobacco Smoke in a General Population," *Respiratory Medicine* 101 (2007): 277–285.

15. M. A. Honein et al., "Maternal Smoking and Environmental Tobacco Smoke Exposure and the Risk of Orofacial Clefts," *Epidemiology* 18 (2007): 226–233.

16. O. K. Magas, J. T. Gunter, and J. L. Regens, "Ambient Air Pollution and Daily Pediatric Hospitalizations for Asthma," *Environmental Science and Pollution Research International* 14 (2007): 19–23.

17. F. C. Bandiera et al., "Secondhand Smoke Exposure and Mental Health Among Children and Adolescents," *Archives of Pediatric and Adolescent Medicine* 165, no. 4 (2011): 332–338.

18. S. Semple, "Bar Workers' Exposure to Second-Hand Smoke: The Effect of Scottish Smoke-Free Legislation on Occupational Exposure," *Annals of Occupational Hygiene* 51, no. 7 (2010): 571–580.

19. K. Fagerstrom, "The Epidemiology of Smoking: Health Consequences and Benefits of Cessation," *Drugs* 62 (2002): 1–9.

20. J. Grossman et al., "5 A's Smoking Cessation with Recovering Women in Treatment," *Journal of Addictions Nursing* 19 (2008): 1–8.

21. J. Charlesworth et al., "Transcriptomic Epidemiology of Smoking: The Effect of Smoking on Gene Expression in Lymphocytes," *BMC Medical Genomics* 3, no. 29 (2010). http://www.biomedcentral.com/1755-8794/3/29.

22. R. West, "Tobacco Control: Present and Future," *British Medical Bulletin* 77–78 (2006): 132–136.

23. B. Borelli et al., "Motivating Latino Caregivers of Children with Asthma to Quit Smoking: A Randomized Trial," *Journal of Consulting and Clinical Psychology* 78, no. 1 (2010): 34–43.

24. M. Webb et al., "Cognitive-Behavioral Therapy to Promote Smoking Cessation Among African American Smokers: A Randomized Clinical Trial," *Journal of Consulting and Clinical Psychology* 78, no. 1 (2010): 24–33.

25. K. Morrison and M. Naegle, "An Evidence-Based Protocol for Smoking Cessation for Persons with Psychotic Disorders," *Journal of Addictions Nursing* 21 (2010): 79–86.

26. L. Bauld, J. Chesterman, J. Ferguson, and K. Judge, "A Comparison of the Effectiveness of Group-Based and Pharmacy-Led Smoking Cessation Treatment in Glasgow," *Addiction* 104 (2009): 308–316.

27. R. West, "The Clinical Significance of 'Small' Effects of Smoking Cessation Treatments," *Addiction* 102 (2007): 506–509.

28. J. Hughes, "How Confident Should We Be That Smoking Cessation Treatments Work?" *Addiction* 104 (2009): 1637–1640.

29. D. T. Lai et al., "Motivational Interviewing for Smoking Cessation," *Cochrane Database Systematic Review* 1 (2010): CD006936.

30. U.S. Preventive Services Task Force, *Counseling to Prevent Tobacco Use and Tobacco-Related Diseases: Recommendation Statement* (Rockville, MD: Agency for Healthcare Research and Quality, November 2003).

31. L. Sarna et al., "Frequency of Nurses' Smoking Cessation Interventions: Report from a National Survey," *Journal of Clinical Nursing* 18 (2009): 2066–2077.

32. E. Lichtenstein, S. Zhu, and G. Tedeschi, "Smoking Cessation Quitlines: An Underrecognized Intervention Success Story," *American Psychologist* 65, no. 4 (2010): 252–261.

33. J. Feigenbaum, "Pharmacological Aids to Promote Smoking Cessation," *Journal of Addictions Nursing* 21 (2010): 87–97.

34. G. Huber and V. Mahajan, "Successful Smoking Cessation," *Disease Management and Health Outcomes* 16, no. 5 (2008): 335–343.

35. B. Apelberg et al., "Estimating the Risks and Benefits of Nicotine Replacement Therapy for Smoking Cessation in the United States," *American Journal of Public Health* 100, no. 2 (2010): 341–348.

36. R. Branstrom et al., "Positive Affect and Mood Management in Successful Smoking Cessation," *American Journal of Health Behaviors* 34, no. 5 (2010): 553–562.

37. A. Sood et al., "A Randomized Clinical Trial of St. John's Wort for Smoking Cessation," *Journal of Alternative and Complementary Medicine* 16, no. 7 (2010): 761–767.

38. K. Flory, P. Malone, and D. Lamis, "Childhood ADHD Symptoms and Risk for Cigarette Smoking During Adolescence: School Adjustment as a Potential Mediator," *Psychology of Addictive Behaviors* 25, no. 2 (2011): 320–329.

39. T. Jarrett, K. Horn, and J. Zhang, "Teen Perceptions of Facilitator Characteristics in a School-Based Smoking Cessation Program," *Journal of School Health* 79, no. 7 (2009): 297–303.

40. R. Heale and M. Griffin, "Self-Efficacy with Application to Adolescent Smoking Cessation: A Concept Analysis," *Journal of Advanced Nursing* 65, no. 4 (2009): 912–918.

41. J. Bricker et al., "Social Cognitive Mediators of Adolescent Smoking Cessation: Results from a Large Randomized Intervention Trial," *Psychology of Addictive Behaviors* 24, no. 3 (2010): 436–445.

42. Y. Kim et al., "Effectiveness of Pharmacologic Therapy for Smoking Cessation in Adolescent Smokers: Meta-Analysis of Randomized Controlled Trials,"

American Journal of Health-System Pharmacists 68 (2011): 219–226.

43. N. Rowa-Dewan and D. Ritchie, "Smoking Cessation for Older People: Neither Too Little nor Too Late," *British Journal of Community Nursing* 15, no. 12 (2010): 578–582.

44. D. Doolan and E. Froelicher, "Smoking Cessation Interventions and Older Adults," *Progress in Cardiovascular Nursing* 23 (2008): 119–127.

45. M. Civljak et al., "Internet-Based Interventions for Smoking Cessation," *Cochrane Database Systematic Review* 9 (2010): CD007078.

46. S. Schaffer, S. Yoon, and I. Zadezensky, "A Review of Smoking Cessation: Potentially Risky Effects on Prescribed Medications," *Journal of Clinical Nursing* 18 (2009): 1533–1540.

47. J. O. Prochaska et al., "Multiple Risk Expert Systems Interventions: Impact of Simultaneous Stage-Matched Expert Systems for Smoking, High-Fat Diet, and Sun Exposure in a Population of Parents," *Health Psychology* 23 (2004): 503–516.

48. J. O. Prochaska et al., "Stage-Based Expert Systems to Guide a Population of Primary Care Patients to Quit Smoking, Eat Healthier, Prevent Skin Cancer, and Receive Regular Mammograms," *Preventive Medicine* 41 (2005): 406–416.

49. E. D. Boudreaux et al., "Predicting Smoking Stage of Change Among Emergency Department Patients and Visitors," *Academic Emergency Medicine* 13 (2006): 39–47.

50. M. Ussher, A. Taylor, and G. Faulkner, "Exercise Interventions for Smoking Cessation," *Cochrane Database of Systematic Reviews* 4 (2008): CD002295.

51. B. C. Bock et al., "Yoga as a Complementary Treatment for Smoking Cessation: Rationale, Study Design and Participant Characteristics of the Quitting-in-Balance Study," *Complementary and Alternative Medicine* 10, no. 14 (2010). Retrieved from http://www.biomedcentral.com/1472-6882/10/14

52. M. Ussher et al., "Effect of Isometric Exercise and Body Scanning on Cigarette Cravings and Withdrawal Symptoms," *Addiction* 104 (2009): 1251–1257.

53. C. Wyszynski, J. Bricker, and B. Comstock, "Parental Smoking Cessation and Child Daily Smoking: A 9-Year Longitudinal Study of Mediation by Child Cognitions About Smoking," *Health Psychology* 30, no. 2 (2011): 171–176.

54. Centers for Disease Control and Prevention, "Cigarette Use Among High School Students—United States, 1991–2009," *Morbidity and Mortality Weekly Report* 59, no. 26 (2010): 797–801.

55. L. Reitzel et al., "The Effect of Tobacco Outlet Density and Proximity on Smoking Cessation," *American Journal of Public Health* 101, no. 2 (2011): 315–320.

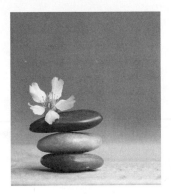

Chapter 24

Addiction and Recovery Counseling

Bonney Gulino Schaub
and Megan McInnis Burt

Nurse Healer
OBJECTIVES

Theoretical

- Discuss factors leading to addiction.
- Identify patterns of thinking and behavior associated with addictions.
- Identify the reasons that spiritual development is important in long-term recovery.

Clinical

- Develop skills in assessing clients' relationships to drugs, alcohol, and addictive patterns of behavior.
- Learn to recognize the patterns of denial that perpetuate and protect addictive behaviors.
- Become knowledgeable about the long-term issues in recovery and in relapse prevention.
- Identify support systems within the community for the person in recovery, such as support groups, psychotherapists knowledgeable about issues in recovery, meditation or prayer groups, and other resources for spiritual development.

Personal

- Take the self-assessment about problem drinking (Exhibit 24-4) and determine if drinking is a problem in your life.
- Assess your responses to stress from the perspective of addictive patterns of behavior (e.g., alcohol or drug use, smoking, excessive

sugar consumption), and learn more effective stress management strategies.
- Recognize your own feelings of vulnerability and your characteristic responses to these feelings.
- Assess your environment, and determine whether there are any people with addictions in your personal or work life; notice whether you have any patterns of denial and enabling in relating to them.

DEFINITIONS

Addiction: A physiologic or psychological dependence on a substance (e.g., alcohol, cocaine) or behavior (e.g., gambling, sex, eating).

Denial: A major dynamic in the process of addiction in which the person willfully refuses to accept the reality of his or her behavior and its effect on self and others.

Detoxification: The physical process of withdrawing from using drugs or alcohol.

Dry drunk: Referring to alcoholism (*dry* refers to not drinking) where a person has stopped drinking but has not extended this change to developing mentally, emotionally, and spiritually.

New consciousness: A concept used in Alcoholics Anonymous (AA) that refers to a movement away from addictive thinking and toward an understanding of one's life purpose or spiritual purpose.

Recovery: The mental, emotional, physical, and spiritual actions that support conscious living and freedom from addictive behaviors.

Relapse: A return to addictive behavior.

Spiritual awakening: An expansion of awareness that results in a realization that the isolated individual is, in fact, participating in a universe of divine intention and order.

■ THEORY AND RESEARCH

Drug abuse and addiction have negative consequences for individuals and for society. Estimates of the total overall costs of substance abuse in the United States, including health, productivity, and crime-related costs, exceed $600 billion annually. This includes approximately $181 billion for illicit drugs, $193 billion for tobacco, and $235 billion for alcohol. As staggering as these numbers are, they do not fully describe the breadth of destructive public health and safety implications of drug abuse and addiction, such as family disintegration, loss of employment, failure in school, domestic violence, and child abuse. It is generally accepted that chemical dependency, along with associated mental health disorders, has become one of the most severe health and social problems facing the United States.[1]

Addiction is a chronic, often relapsing brain disease that causes compulsive drug seeking and use, despite harmful consequences to the addicted individual and to those around him or her. Although the initial decision to take drugs is voluntary for most people, the brain changes that occur over time challenge a person's self-control and ability to resist intense impulses urging him or her to take drugs. Similar to other chronic, relapsing diseases, such as diabetes, asthma, or heart disease, drug addiction can be managed successfully. And as with other chronic diseases, it is not uncommon for a person to relapse and begin abusing drugs again. Relapse, however, does not signal treatment failure—rather, it indicates that treatment should be reinstated, adjusted, or that an alternative treatment is needed to help the individual. Treatment of chronic diseases involves changing deeply embedded behaviors.[2-4]

It can be wrongfully assumed that drug abusers lack moral principles or willpower and that they could stop using drugs simply by choosing to change their behavior. In reality, drug addiction is a complex disease, and quitting takes more than good intentions. In fact, because drugs change the brain in ways that foster compulsive drug abuse, quitting is difficult, even for those who are ready to do so.

Drugs of abuse such as cocaine trigger epigenetic changes in certain brain regions, affecting hundreds of genes at a time. Some of these changes remain long after the drug has been cleared from the system. Research in this area suggests that some of the long-term effects of drug abuse and addiction (including high rates of relapse) may be written in epigenetic code.[5-7]

It is estimated that more than 28 million children are living in homes with adults who have alcohol use disorders.[8] Children raised in homes with substance-abusing parents are at increased risk for chronic anxiety disorders and social phobias as well as at increased risk for their own substance abuse.[9] In the United States in 2008, almost one-third of adolescents aged 12 to 17 years drank alcohol in the past year, around one-fifth used an illicit drug, and almost one-sixth smoked cigarettes. Caffeine is a widely used psychoactive substance that is legal, easy to obtain, and socially acceptable to consume. Although once relatively restricted to use among adults, caffeine-containing drinks are now consumed regularly by children. Children and adolescents are the fastest growing population of caffeine users with an increase of 70% in the past 30 years. Energy drinks sales have grown by more than 50% since 2005 and represent the fastest growing segment of the beverage industry.[10]

Because of the prevalence of alcoholism and other addictions, nurses in every practice setting inevitably will work with individuals who are addicted, who are in recovery, or whose lives are affected by the addiction of a friend or family member.

Addiction Defined

Alcoholics Anonymous (AA), in its basic book (referred to by people in AA as the "Big Book"), describes alcoholism as a "mental obsession and a physical compulsion."[11] This description of a pattern of thinking and behaving applies to many things besides alcohol, most obviously the use of other substances such as cocaine, heroin, methamphetamine, and marijuana. The elements of obsession and compulsion are evident in the actions of people with unhealthy relationships to food, exercise, work, gambling, Internet use, television viewing, shopping, sexual behaviors (including compulsive use of pornography), and other activities. A recent study suggests that the use of tanning beds can be addictive. The study proposes that tanning beds that emit ultraviolet (UV) rays caused a release of cutaneous endorphins that created a sense of well-being in the tanner. When opioid antagonists were administered this feeling was blocked.[12] Indoor tanning was seen as a common adolescent risk behavior, and the mood-altering effect of the UV rays was a factor that motivated maintenance of the behavior.[13]

Certain elements distinguish the process of addiction from the healthy or recreational use of any of these substances or behaviors. The key difference is in the individual's relationship to the substance or behavior. In the addictive process, the element of choice is absent. A woman no longer chooses to relax with a glass of wine at a dinner party—she goes to the party because it is an opportunity to drink a great deal. A man no longer enjoys watching a sporting event—he watches it only because he has a bet on it. A young college student takes up running to lose weight and feels compelled to go for a run despite her knee injury because she will be depressed and obsessing about her weight without a run of at least 5 miles a day. In other words, the mental obsession has overruled the ability to reflect on behavior and has bypassed any self-awareness that could lead to alternative behaviors. These addictive behaviors often coexist with various forms of substance abuse. The addictive use of any of these activities serves the same purpose as alcohol or drugs: the person is seeking relief and distraction from painful, unsafe, and vulnerable feelings.

The Cycle of Addiction

All addictions have a basic cycle. Understanding this cycle makes it possible to understand the specific kinds of help that a person with an addiction needs to facilitate the healing process. In the early stage of addiction, people use a substance or substances as a means of changing unsafe or vulnerable feelings. Some commonly heard descriptions of these feelings are phrases like, "I feel like I don't have any skin," "Everything gets to me," and "Everything is just too much." Typically, there are physical signs of anxiety such as light-headedness, palpitations, painful levels of self-consciousness and social discomfort, and generally heightened degrees of agitation or irritability.

Vulnerability is a normal human emotion that everyone has experienced, but the person vulnerable to addiction feels it more intensely and more frequently. Characteristics such as a low frustration tolerance, a low pain threshold, and a need for instant gratification go along with this vulnerability. These characteristics present challenges for nurses when caring for addicted clients.

Most people who have become addicted to a substance have a vivid memory of their first experience of relief from the feelings of discomfort as a result of using the substance. This first encounter typically occurs in early adolescence, a time of normal emotional turmoil and struggle for social identity and acceptance. Getting high may have alleviated social anxiety or the pain of family conflicts. The incidence of substance abuse is high among young people in conflict about their sexual identity because they often lack support and positive role models in their life. For some young people, sharing drugs or alcohol becomes a way of being accepted into a peer group and changing the feeling that do not feel they "fit in." Thus, the stage is set for dependence and progression to addiction. The process of building emotional and social skills, which is a major developmental task of adolescence, stops because an instant solution has been found. Picking up where they have left off in this process of emotional and social skill building is one of the major challenges for people in recovery.

The Early Stage of the Addictive Cycle

In the early stage of addiction, a person has some awareness of seeking relief from discomfort. It may simply be an awareness of feeling stressed, anxious, or self-conscious. The following is a typical progression of feelings and responses in the early stage of addiction:

1. Unsafe feelings
2. Mental focus on the feelings
3. A desire to get rid of the feelings
4. The use of chemicals to get rid of the feelings
5. Nervous system disturbance caused by the chemicals
6. The return of unsafe feelings[14p5]

The Middle Stage of the Addictive Cycle

In the middle stage of addiction, the unsafe feeling is not experienced as a thought. It is experienced only as danger or discomfort. The person knows that immediate relief comes with use of the substance. The following is the typical progression and recurring pattern in the middle stage of addiction:

1. Unsafe feelings
2. The use of chemicals to get rid of the feelings
3. Nervous system disturbance caused by the chemicals
4. Unsafe feelings[14p8,15]

The Late Stage of the Addictive Cycle

People in the depths of addiction rarely talk about feeling high. The need is more frequently described as a desire to feel "normal." The impulse is to escape a feeling that is intolerable. At the late stage of addiction, physical instability replaces the emotional vulnerability. The addiction has come full circle. What was initially used as an answer to unsafe feelings has become the source of unsafe feelings. Mental instability and confusion, mental terrors and paranoia, and hallucinations or feelings of unreality are all possible results of the neurological damage from the substances. The following is the recurring pattern of the late stage of addiction:

1. Nervous system disturbance
2. The use of chemicals
3. The return of nervous system disturbance[14p11,16]

Models of Addiction

Many models have been put forth to explain why a person develops an addiction. Any nurse who has worked with addicted patients can recognize recurring themes such as familial and environmental patterns of addiction or early childhood trauma and loss. Clearly, addiction defies simple explanation. Each of these models offers a piece of a complex puzzle.

Medical Model

In the medical model, the emphasis is on the physiologic effect of the substance itself. The body's tolerance for the drug leads to the need for greater and greater amounts to achieve the desired effect, which results in addiction. The absence of the drug leads to cravings, and then to a withdrawal or abstinence syndrome characterized by symptoms such as fever, nausea, seizures, chills, hallucinations, and delirium tremens. In this model, the progression toward addiction is a property of the drug's effect. Those in the media often demonstrate this attitude toward addiction when they describe a celebrity who has attended a 30-day alcohol or drug rehabilitation program as "free" of drugs. In fact, 30 days is just the beginning of treatment. Most drugs of abuse directly or indirectly target the brain's reward system by flooding the circuit with dopamine. Dopamine is a neurotransmitter present in regions of the brain that regulate movement, emotion, cognition, motivation, and feelings of pleasure. The overstimulation of this system, which rewards our natural behaviors, produces the euphoric effects sought by people who abuse drugs and teaches them to repeat the behavior.

Genetic Disease Model

Research in the area of genetics has focused primarily on alcoholism. Much research points to strong patterns of alcoholism within families. People with close relatives who are alcoholic are at a greater risk for alcoholism by three to four times. The closer the genetic tie and the higher the number of affected relatives, the greater the risk. Adoption studies show a three times greater incidence of alcoholism in children of alcoholics, even if they have been raised in a nonalcoholic family.[15] There is evidence that alcohol and tobacco both act on a part of the brain that is involved in rewards, emotions, memory, and thinking. Both alcohol and tobacco have an impact on the neurons that release dopamine binding at the receptor sites. The presence of a common mechanism of action may shed light on the interplay of alcohol and tobacco addiction.[16] The possibility that genetics play a role in a greater vulnerability to these addictions in some individuals fits in with the idea that genetically based differences in biochemistry are a factor in being susceptible to addiction.

The emerging field of epigenetics is advancing our understanding of the role of genetics in addictions. Epigenetics is the study of changes in the regulation of gene expression and gene activity that are not dependent on DNA sequence. The field of epigenetics refers to the science that studies how the development, functioning, and evolution of biological systems are influenced by forces operating outside the DNA sequence, such as environmental and energetic influences. Studies indicate that there is an alteration in gene expression by repeated substance abuse that can produce lasting changes in gene expression within the reward pathways of the brain. Epigenetic mechanisms are providing insight into how drugs alter genetic expression. Insights into the long-lasting adaptations that underlie the chronic relapsing nature of addiction are on the edge of research and have implications for new treatments.[17]

Dysfunctional Family System Model

The frequent appearance of addictions within the families of addicts may indicate that substance abuse can be a learned behavior. In effect, children learn by daily close observation of the adults in their environment that conflicts and stressors are to be dealt with using drugs and alcohol. Children usually do not have a conscious awareness of this message. They may not have a full understanding of the role that addiction played in their home life until they reach adulthood and begin their own recovery. It is important to acknowledge that many other people who have grown up in such an environment are aware of the damage done and make a conscious choice to abstain from alcohol or other substances.

Self-Medication Model

According to the self-medication model, the addict has an underlying psychiatric disorder and is, in effect, self-prescribing to alleviate symptoms. For example, in a Canadian survey of more than 14,000 residents ages 18 to 76 years, there was a significantly greater use of alcohol among those who were suffering from depression.[18] Addicts characteristically have tried a variety of substances and have found that they have a strong preference for a particular category of drug and drug effect. It is not unusual for addicts to say that their preferred substance makes them feel "normal."

Psychosexual, Psychoanalytic Model

Emerging from Freud's conceptualization of psychosexual stages of development, addiction appears to be a fixation at the oral stage of development. In the psychosexual, psychoanalytic model, an infant or child whose basic needs are unmet becomes focused on seeking gratification of those unmet needs. Emotional development becomes fixated at the age of this early trauma.[14p23]

Oral gratification is the most basic need of the infant, as seen in the way an infant receives nourishment and pleasure through sucking. In adulthood, people continue to seek comfort and pleasure from gratification of oral needs through behaviors such as eating, smoking, talking, touching their mouth, and various chewing behaviors. Whereas healthy human activity includes some limited seeking of oral gratification, the addict is fixated at this developmental phase. The compelling need for comfort derived from oral gratification then becomes focused on the consuming of substances.

Ego Psychology Model

Also emerging from Freudian theory, ego psychology suggests that when an infant's or child's environment does not provide an adequate degree of nurturance and acknowledgment, the child grows into adulthood with an impaired sense of self. This results in feelings of emptiness and hypersensitivity that lead to a self-absorbed and narcissistic relationship with the world. The addict's behaviors are then seen as self-soothing attempts to relieve the basic feelings of emptiness.[14p24]

Cultural Model

Our culture may be a contributing factor in addiction because it teaches us to seek materialistic answers outside ourselves to experience well-being. People in the United States are confronted with a relentless message of consumerism and quick fixes. This then leads to a society of consumers with impulse disorders who seek instant gratification and believe that there is a pill for every ill.

In recent years, media advertising has bombarded people with messages about both over-the-counter (OTC) and prescription medications. In light of this, it is interesting to note the following information. The total number of drug-related emergency department (ED) visits increased 81% from 2004 (2.5 million) to 2009 (4.6 million). ED visits involving nonmedical use of pharmaceuticals increased 98.4% over the same period, from 627,291 visits to 1,244,679. The largest pharmaceutical increases were observed for oxycodone products (242.2% increase), alprazolam (148.3% increase), and hydrocodone products (124.5% increase). Among ED visits involving illicit drugs, only those involving Ecstasy increased more than 100% from 2004 to 2009 (123.2% increase). For patients aged 20 years or younger, ED visits resulting from nonmedical use of pharmaceuticals increased 45.4% between 2004 and 2009 (116,644 and 169,589 visits, respectively). Among patients aged 21 years or older, there was an increase of 111.0%.[19,20]

There is also an increased awareness of the abuse of substances among athletes. The primary abuse is of "recreational" drugs such as cocaine and alcohol. There is a significant increase in the use of performance-enhancing (i.e., ergogenic) drugs such as amphetamines, as well as "designer" stimulants such as Ecstasy (i.e., methylenedioxymethamphetamine, or MDMA). Two readily available drugs that are amphetamine mimicking when taken in high doses are pseudoephedrine, available in cold medications, and ephedrine marketed as a dietary supplement. Anabolic steroids and other drugs are taken in an attempt to enhance performance and build muscle mass. Additionally, human growth hormone (HGH) precursors are marketed in various forms, promising increased muscle mass, increased energy, and performance enhancement.[21] This is another situation in which to consider the role of media and other cultural influences in the patterns of abuse and choice of substances.

Character Defect Model of AA

Alcoholics and other addicts are seen having different characters and morals from nonaddicts in the character defect model of AA. Although the idea of a "moral" defect is not used extensively in addiction treatment settings, it is a concept that pervades the AA literature. A person in recovery may explain his or her "character defect" as the reason for his or her difficulty in making behavioral and attitudinal changes.

Trance Model

Derived from learning theory and the principles of hypnosis, the trance model proposes that the memory of the intense pleasure experienced in response to a substance is never forgotten. The experience is recorded by the pleasure-seeking, pain-avoiding part of the brain and remains, in effect, a deeply planted, posthypnotic suggestion that repeatedly seeks expression. The addict essentially falls in love with the feelings that the addictive behaviors produce. The AA literature speaks to this idea in stating, "The urge to repeat the experience of becoming 'high' is so strong that we will forsake . . . our responsibilities and values, . . . our families, our jobs, our personal welfare, our respect, and our integrity . . . to satisfy the urge."[22]

Transpersonal Intoxication Model

According to the transpersonal intoxication model, the desire to break free of a limited, time-bound, socially defined sense of self as well as the desire to expand consciousness are the driving forces in addiction. Many people have experimented with lysergic acid diethylamide (LSD), marijuana, psilocybin mushrooms, peyote cactus, and other psychedelic substances and have experienced expanded states of awareness that have resulted in spiritual and creative breakthroughs. The challenge then is to integrate these insights into daily life.

There is a significant degree of substance abuse and addiction among artists, writers, performers, and musicians. This model suggests that their desire to break free of mental and emotional limitations is at the heart of their substance use. One part of the artistic process is about finding a way to express the most intimate, subtle, and spiritual aspects of human experience. Artists often mention a fear of losing this creative capacity—of becoming "ordinary"—as they enter recovery. They have given the creative power to the substance rather than trusting that it resides within themselves. The ability to practice their creative endeavor while sober then becomes a major milestone in the recovery process.

Transpersonal–Existential Model

In the transpersonal–existential model, the human condition is such that humans are inherently anxious because they have knowledge of their mortality. Everyone finds ways to bypass or deny this awareness of reality. Becker, in a book authored when he was dying of cancer, wrote that a person

> has to protect himself against the world, and he can do this only as any other animal would—by . . . shutting off experience and developing an obliviousness both to the terrors of the world and to his own anxieties. Otherwise he would be crippled for action . . . some people have more trouble with their lies than others. The world is too much with them.[23]

This heightened awareness and sensitivity to the human condition can lead to addiction as a solution to the existential pain.

■ VULNERABILITY MODEL OF RECOVERY FROM ADDICTION

A holistic nursing model of the recovery process, the Vulnerability Model of Recovery honors the biological, emotional, social, familial, neurochemical, and spiritual aspects of addiction. It focuses on the lived experience of the addict, which is that of essential vulnerability. The model points to specific ways that the holistic nurse can facilitate the healing journey of full bio-psycho-social-spiritual recovery. The basic points are presented in **Exhibit 24-1**.

Recognition of Addiction

Given the prevalence of alcoholism and other addictions, it can be assumed that nurses in every clinical area are working with people whose lives are affected by this problem—even when the issue is never directly addressed. Therefore, it is essential that all nurses become skilled in assessing the possibility of addiction, as well as recognizing risk factors and behaviors suggestive of

substance abuse. Nurses must first examine any preconceived notions that they may have about what an addict or alcoholic looks like. Addiction is a problem that occurs in every profession, in every educational and socioeconomic group, in every ethnic group, and in every age group from early adolescence through senescence.

Fifty percent of patients admitted to trauma centers are intoxicated with alcohol. Studies have shown that alcohol interventions initiated in these settings result in a 50% reduction in reinjury rates and a 66% reduction of drunk driving arrests. In addition, introducing alcohol intervention is extremely cost effective, saving $4 for every dollar spent.[24]

The most challenging, and potentially frustrating, aspect of working with people at the stage of active addiction is their pervasive denial of the problem, even when confronted with blatant evidence of their addiction. Alcoholics Anonymous uses the phrase "self-will run riot" in describing this behavior. It is the key obstacle to entering into the healing process of recovery. (See **Exhibit 24-2** for definitions of denial.)

The addict's loyalty to the substance is profound. It surpasses loyalty to family and friends and is the cause of the addict's manipulations. The nurse should not personalize these manipulations. Attempts to be of help often meet outright rejection or failure. The root of the addict's behaviors is an intense fear of living without the mood-altering effects of the alcohol or drugs. The behaviors are attempts to control the world and avoid painful feelings. The first step of recovery is relinquishing this control effort and admitting to oneself and others that the addictive process is not working, that it is actually making everything worse, that he or she does not know what to do, and that he or she must learn a new way to be in the world. This new way means a change in attitude to recognize that people who want to help stop the addictive behaviors are acting from a place of caring.

Detoxification

The simplest, most straightforward aspect of the recovery process is detoxification. When medical management of detoxification is necessary, brief inpatient or outpatient treatment is available in many hospitals and addiction treatment centers. Acupuncture has been successfully used in

EXHIBIT 24-1   The Vulnerability Model of Recovery

- Addiction is a repetitive, maladaptive, avoidant, substitutive process of getting rid of vulnerability.
- This addictive process is triggered by an experience of vulnerability that is believed to be intolerable.
- Vulnerability is anxiety ultimately rooted in the human condition of being conscious, separate, and mortal. As such, this vulnerability is a normal emotion and an elemental aspect of our actual human situation.
- People who have a greater degree of vulnerability (explanations for which include genetic, biochemical, characterological, familial, cultural, and spiritual) have a greater degree of need to get rid of it.
- Getting rid of vulnerability is accomplished by trying to feel powerful or by trying to feel numb. Trying to feel powerful is an act of willfulness. Trying to feel numb is an act of will-lessness. Drugs are selected to help produce these results. Trying to feel powerful and trying to feel numb are both choices. Made repeatedly, they become addictive, producing predictable but brief episodes of relief from vulnerability.
- People in recovery from addiction begin to heal their feelings by recognizing and respecting their vulnerability.
- Continued recovery is based on developing new, nonavoidant responses to vulnerability.

- However, this vulnerability cannot be effectively responded to on a long-term basis by the separate, ego-level, temporary sense of self because it is that sense of self that is at the very root of the vulnerability.
- Advanced recovery therefore requires the development of an expanded sense of self that is communal and spiritual in awareness. Such spiritual development is a normal aspect of adult development, despite the fact that it is ignored by most Western psychology.
- Communal awareness is provided by Alcoholics Anonymous and other 12-step programs through fellowship and service to others in recovery. Spiritual awareness requires development, which has been studied by the world's wisdom traditions and, more recently, by transpersonal psychology.
- Many people in recovery do not experience spiritual awareness because this aspect of human nature has been neglected and poorly understood in modern culture. Pioneering transpersonal psychiatrist Roberto Assagioli referred to this issue as "repression of the sublime."
- Transpersonal approaches offer insights and practices that can lift repression of the sublime, energize spiritual awareness and increase inner peace, and work at the deepest root of the addictive process.

Source: Reproduced by permission. *Healing Addictions* by Schaub and Schaub. Delmar Publishers, Albany, NY. 1997.

detoxifying many people from alcohol, heroin, nicotine, and other drugs. Its use was pioneered in New York City in the 1970s by Dr. Michael O. Smith. In recent years, it has gained wider acceptance and has been found to be a powerfully effective, natural treatment that is simple, safe, and inexpensive by improving patient outcomes in terms of program retention, reductions in cravings, anxiety, sleep disturbance, and need for pharmaceuticals.[25,26]

Alcoholics Anonymous

With its 12-step, self-help treatment approach, AA offers one of the most important, effective,

and widely accepted interventions in addiction treatment. The 12 steps of Alcoholics Anonymous put forth a systematic progression of actions to take that, when followed, will assist the person in recovery to find a new way to be in the world (**Exhibit 24-3**). Ongoing peer support as well as support for spiritual development were cited as significant factors in the effectiveness of this program.[27-29]

An important element in AA is the practice of providing service to other members of the program by becoming a sponsor. Members who have achieved a strong recovery are encouraged to be available to newer participants to help them in

EXHIBIT 24-2   Definitions of Denial

- Continuous negative behavior in the face of obvious negative physical, emotional, and social consequences, as in, "My girlfriend is constantly bugging me and threatening to break up with me because of my drinking. She's really got hang-ups about drinking because her father is an alcoholic."

- Prideful insistence that he or she has control of behaviors that are out of control, as in, "I didn't get into that car accident because of the coke. I actually am a better driver when I've done a few lines. It keeps me alert and my reflexes are better."

- A maladaptive strategy for achieving security, as in, "I don't really have a problem with alcohol, I just need a few drinks when I get home from work because I work the evening shift. My job is very stressful and it's hard to relax enough to fall asleep."

- The energy used to maintain a destructive lie, as in, "I only use drugs because my girlfriend does. I can stop whenever I want."

- A narrowing of awareness to shut out anything that makes the person vulnerable, as in, "When I get high I just don't give a damn. All this crap just fades away."

- An unwillingness to experience the feelings the truth provokes, as in, "My boss was a total hypocrite. He was always on my case. All the guys have a few beers at lunch time. He fired me because he never liked me."

Source: Reproduced by permission. *Healing Addictions* by Schaub and Schaub. Delmar Publishers, Albany, NY. 1997.

EXHIBIT 24-3   The 12 Steps of Alcoholics Anonymous

1. We admitted we were powerless over alcohol—that our lives had become unmanageable.

2. Came to believe that a power greater than ourselves could restore us to sanity.

3. Made a decision to turn our will and our lives over to the care of God as we understood Him.

4. Made a searching and fearless moral inventory of ourselves.

5. Admitted to God, to ourselves, and to another human being the exact nature of our wrongs.

6. Were entirely ready to have God remove all these defects of character.

7. Humbly asked Him to remove our shortcomings.

8. Made a list of all persons we had harmed, and became willing to make amends to them all.

9. Made direct amends to such people whenever possible, except when to do so would injure them or others.

10. Continued to take personal inventory, and when we were wrong promptly admitted it.

11. Sought through prayer and meditation to improve our conscious contact with God as we understood Him, praying only for knowledge of His will for us and the power to carry that out.

12. Having had a spiritual awakening as the result of these steps, we tried to carry this message to others, and to practice these principles in all our affairs.

Source: The Twelve Steps of Alcoholics Anonymous have been reprinted with permission of Alcoholic Anonymous World Services, Inc. (A.A.W.S.). Permission to reprint the Twelve Steps does not mean that AA is in any way affiliated with this publication, or that it has read and/or endorses the contents thereof. AA is a program of recovery from alcoholism only—inclusion of the steps in this publication, or use in any other non-AA context, does not imply otherwise.

their sobriety. They may attend meetings with the new participant, be available by phone on a regular basis, and generally serve as a role model and guide toward effective use of the program.

Family Awareness

A person in the addictive process has fears about change, and the people closest to him or her usually have fears as well. It is in the nature of the addictive process that the people living and working closest to the person with the addiction have made accommodations to compensate for and cover up the addicted person's behaviors. The nurse who takes on the role of working with a person in recovery will find it necessary to help the people closest to the person change their behavior as well. The individuals in this close circle need to look at their own patterns of enabling the addicted person's behavior and be willing to keep the focus on their own process of growth and change.

Al-Anon is a self-help program for the friends and family members of alcoholics and other substance abusers. Family members, particularly spouses and partners, who have undoubtedly expended much energy in trying to help the addicted person, learn in Al-Anon how to accept their powerlessness to control others. The emphasis of Al-Anon is on reorienting priorities and supporting the group members to focus energy on making positive life changes for themselves.

Early Recovery

Detoxification is the initial step in early recovery, and it is just the beginning of the addicted person's process of making new choices, moment by moment, hour by hour, and day by day. The nurse can help the person in recovery to make healthy choices by intensive questioning about old patterns of substance abuse and other behaviors. This information can then be used to develop new ways of responding. Because behaviors associated with addiction are totally integrated into the person's life, he or she needs help in recognizing them and accepting the fact that they are no longer possible. The following are some important questions for the nurse to ask:

- Where did the addictive behavior take place? Some people stay isolated in their home or car when using drugs, while others prefer social settings such as bars, clubs, or the work environment.

- What special rituals were a part of the addictive behavior? People typically have a routine associated with their substance use. For example, a marijuana abuser may purchase her favorite foods before using the drug.

- What locations served as cues for the addictive behavior? For the alcoholic, particular liquor stores or bars may have strong memories and pulls. A particular street sign or exit on the expressway may trigger the desire to go to the neighborhood where drugs were bought and shared.

- What people in the environment were associated with the addictive behavior? The person in recovery may come to realize that everyone he or she knows is associated with the drug use. People in recovery often cannot name a single person they can count on to be drug free. The feeling of loss of family and friends associated with this realization can be profound.

Nutritional Factors

Alcohol has high caloric content, but it is useless as a source of nutrients. Malnutrition is common in alcoholics because they often fail to consume adequate amounts of food. In addition, alcohol interferes with the absorption of vitamins and minerals. Alcoholics typically are deficient in B vitamins, especially thiamine, pyridoxine, and vitamins B_{12} and folate. There is also some evidence that the B vitamin deficiency itself may increase alcohol cravings.

Some studies indicate that alcoholics who followed healthy dietary plans that included both nutritional and vitamin supplementation, along with nutrition education, were more successful at maintaining sobriety.[30] The effectiveness of this approach may be attributed not only to the actual physiologic impact of improved nutrition, but also to the individual's commitment to making significant lifestyle changes. As stated earlier, recovery is a process of repeatedly choosing healthy, life-affirming actions.

For the recovering alcoholic or other addict, working with a holistic nurse to develop a nutritious eating plan may be an important first step on the path to health. As with any treatment plan, the key to its success depends on compliance. Having a variety of approaches helps to develop personalized care and increase the likelihood of acceptance.

Body Work and Energy Work

In the early phase of recovery, shortly after cessation of use and resolution of any primary withdrawal symptoms, the person in recovery may experience difficulty sleeping, general agitation, and irritability. Acupuncture has been found to be very effective in the reduction of withdrawal symptoms and in the overall rebalancing of the physical system. Other types of body work such as Reiki, therapeutic touch, massage, and reflexology can be of help in calming the body. Modalities offering direct physical touch or energy work are of value in the very early stages of recovery.

The energy-based approach of Healing Touch (HT) has been effectively used with patients in recovery from alcoholism.[31] The person in recovery from an addiction typically experiences irritability, anxiety, tremors, and weakness among other symptoms. In addition, there is the stigma associated with addiction that is usually internalized by the person in recovery. Healing Touch is seen as promoting self-healing and integration of mind, body, and spirit. Another innovative practitioner has introduced the use of drumming circles into recovery work. One aspect of this treatment's effectiveness is in creating a sense of connectedness with self and others.[32]

Techniques requiring concentration, such as meditation and imagery for self-care, may be too difficult in the early phase of recovery; relaxation exercises that focus on very simple breath awareness and counting may be all the person can handle. Avoiding caffeine, drinking plenty of water and soothing herbal teas, exercising, and taking warm baths or showers are all helpful during this period when the body is literally releasing and cleansing itself of a buildup of toxins.

Relapse

A person can achieve abstinence and still not make life changes at the level of emotions and spirit. A person can, in fact, stop drinking and continue to be hostile, rageful, blaming, and irresponsible. These people are controlling their behavior through force of will. Alcoholics Anonymous calls these individuals "dry drunks." The person functioning in recovery in this way is at greater risk for relapse.

Relapse is an ongoing issue in every stage of recovery. Many people stop completely without treatment, or with very brief intervention, but others relapse repeatedly. In AA, there is a saying, "The further you are from your last drink, the closer you are to your next." It is helpful to differentiate between someone who very briefly returns to drinking and then returns to abstinence versus someone who resumes heavy drinking. The brief episode is referred to as a lapse rather than a full relapse. This distinction is important to avoid the "all-or-nothing," black-and-white thinking that can sabotage the process of recovery.

It is estimated that up to 75% of people in recovery relapse within the first year. It is significant to note that the figure is estimated to be even higher, up to 90%, for women with a history of sexual abuse and trauma. This information points back to the Vulnerability Model. If sexual abuse and trauma caused the unbearable feelings of vulnerability that led to the person's addiction, then abstaining from the substances that served as the emotional anesthesia results in a return of these feelings. It becomes important to connect the painful feelings to the trauma rather than to attribute them all to the absence of the substance. This opens the door to the need for a second recovery process—the treatment and recovery from trauma.[14p75]

Alcoholics Anonymous has a helpful acronym that identifies the times that a person in recovery may be most vulnerable to drinking: HALT. This is shorthand for hungry, angry, lonely, tired. If the person in recovery notices the impulse to drink, it is advised that he or she stop and take time to determine whether any of these factors are creating this feeling. It is also advised to avoid, whenever possible, letting these situations develop. This simple advice is a very helpful tool for a person in recovery.

Gorski and Miller outline the signs that lead back toward addiction.[33] Nurses can use this list to evaluate a relapse trend in the person's recovery process. Paraphrased from Gorski and Miller, the signs leading to relapse include the following:

- Active denial in many areas of life
- Efforts to convince others of their need for sobriety, referred to in AA as taking someone else's inventory
- Compulsive behaviors
- Impulsive behaviors
- Tendencies toward isolation and bitterness
- Failure to see the big picture
- Idle daydreaming with wishful and magical answers to complex problems
- Helplessness and hopelessness
- An immature wish to be happy always
- Frequent episodes of confusion
- Tendency to judge other people
- Quick anger
- Irregular eating habits
- Listlessness
- Irregular sleeping habits
- Progressive loss of daily structure
- Irregular attendance at treatment meetings
- Development of an "I don't care" attitude
- Open rejection of help
- Self-pity
- Opinion that social drinking is manageable
- Conscious lying
- Complete loss of self-confidence

These are simply warning signs, not inevitable signs of relapse, and constructive responses are possible. The person in recovery will have these thoughts and feelings, to one degree or another, on a recurring basis throughout his or her life. Each time the person lives through the experience and finds that it passes, and each time the person tolerates the feeling effectively and responds to it in a healthy manner, recovery and satisfaction in living deepen.

Deepening of the Recovery Process

Choosing to take new actions in response to vulnerability is the key to recovery. If the element of choice is absent in the obsession and compulsion of addiction, then reclaiming the ability to make life-affirming choices—reclaiming free will—is the essence of recovery. The use of will can be considered the use of one's life energy. If someone is "willing" to do something, he or she is choosing to give energy to the task at hand. If he or she is "unwilling" to do something, he or she is withholding life energy. There are three different ways to use energy: willfully, will-lessly, and willingly. "Willingness and willfulness become possibilities every time we truly engage life. There is only one other option—to avoid engagement entirely [will-lessness]."[34]

The energy of willfulness is reflected in behaviors of force, exertion, strain, contraction, constriction, violence, manipulation, controlling actions, and drive. It is the fight aspect of the fight-or-flight response to perceived danger. Will-lessness—the withdrawal of energy—is seen in behaviors reflecting withdrawal, escape, giving up, immobilization, collapse, and numbness. Will-lessness is the flight response to fear and vulnerability.

Every person tends to favor one of these patterns of behavior. Typically, a person who is predominantly willful eventually becomes exhausted and collapses into will-less behaviors. A person following a very restrictive and rigid weight loss diet, for example, ultimately binges. In contrast, a person who has fallen into a pattern of total will-lessness (e.g., has gone on an extended alcohol binge) suddenly becomes scared, vows to stop drinking, and goes on a "health kick." This grasp of control cannot be sustained because it is not grounded in any deeper changes. Consequently, the person swings back to the will-less behavior.

The array of behaviors that can be identified as willful and will-less is shown in **Figures 24-1** and **24-2**. These models are useful in teaching a person in recovery about patterns of behavior. People readily recognize and identify with these descriptions, and they generally appreciate the nonjudgmental presentation. As can be seen in these charts, these behaviors can be observed in every aspect of a person's life—in the physical, mental, emotional, and spiritual realms.

Willfulness and will-lessness are extreme uses of energy. They each represent an energetic state of imbalance. The goal in recovery from addictions is to lead a life of balance, harmony, and increasing serenity. Willingness is the active state of living life from the place of dynamic balance, as opposed to the extremes. It can be likened to the ideal of many of the world's wisdom traditions. It is spoken of in the Buddhist path of the

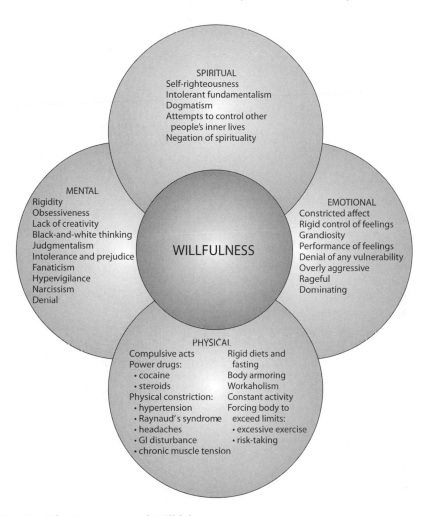

FIGURE 24-1   The Spectrum of Willfulness
Source: Reproduced by permission. *Healing Addictions* by Schaub and Schaub. Delmar Publishers, Albany, NY. Copyright 1997.

middle way, in the Taoist concept of the balance of yin and yang energies, in the Greek ideal of the golden mean, and in the common sense of moderation in all things. The qualities of life lived from this ideal are depicted in **Figure 24-3**.

Spiritual Development and Transformation

Spiritual development is an innate evolutionary capacity within all people. Spirituality is not a concept, but a process of learning about love, caring, empathy, and meaning in life. (See Chapter 31.) This process leads a person to connect with his or her psyche, soul, or spirit and to have

a lived experience of inner peace and harmony that allows access to inner wisdom.

Participants in AA and other 12-step programs are encouraged to seek spiritual growth and connection with their own higher power. There are studies that find people in recovery who score higher in standardized spirituality measures are more successful in maintaining abstinence than those with lower scores. Spirituality in these studies was not equated with participation in religion. Rather, individuals in treatment spoke of experiencing a turning point in their life, feeling "protection and support from a higher power, guidance of an inner voice, life meaning, gratitude,

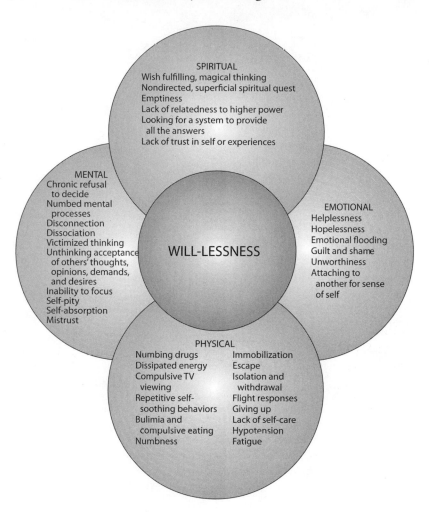

FIGURE 24-2   The Spectrum of Will-lessness
Source: Reproduced by permission. *Healing Addictions* by Schaub and Schaub. Delmar Publishers, Albany, NY. Copyright 1997.

and an appreciation of service work."[35] These experiences point to the fact that long-term recovery is a process that goes beyond abstinence and can lead to deep healing and an enriched sense of meaning and purpose.[36,37]

In a qualitative phenomenological study conducted by Bowden, eight recovering alcoholics described the importance of integrating spiritual practices into their daily lives.[38] In addition to developing self-acceptance, those who were doing well in recovery were also participating in an ongoing search for connections with the transpersonal realm. This information confirms that it is important to encourage the person in recovery to explore his or her spiritual nature (see Exhibit 24-1).

There is much cynicism and discouragement in addiction treatment because professionals in rehabilitation and treatment centers often witness the "revolving door syndrome." Yet, unlike so many other conditions that nurses work with, an addiction is completely reversible. There is a real possibility for a person to transform his or her life dramatically and to begin living a healthy and sane life.

Because of their compatibility with 12-step programs and the AA philosophy, spiritually oriented therapies and psychotherapy are important components of care. Addiction treatment is one of the few areas in health care where spiritual development and exploration are not only openly addressed, but are recognized as

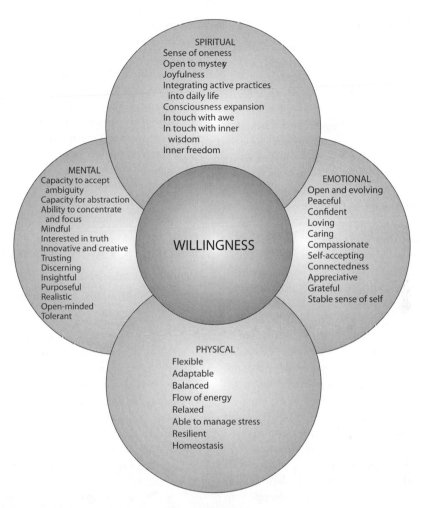

FIGURE 24-3 The Spectrum of Willingness
Source: Reproduced by permission. *Healing Addictions* by Schaub and Schaub. Delmar Publishers, Albany, NY. Copyright 1997.

an integral aspect of care. As nurses and other healthcare professionals interested in addictions counseling explore their own spirituality, they can serve as role models for grounding spirituality in real, human terms. Furthermore, it is genuinely difficult for spiritually repressed nurses or psychotherapists to assist clients who are working through AA's 12-step program.

No single nurse or therapist can provide enough support and reinforcement for the recovery process. Thus, the nurse must be aware of a client's degree of participation in AA and any resistance to the spiritual aspect of the AA meetings. A person who feels alienated by the spiritual components of AA is unlikely to participate

in meetings. Some individuals hear the word *God* or *Higher Power* in meetings and begin to reject AA's "God talk." If this is the case, the nurse can find out if there is a way the person can translate the concepts into personally acceptable ideas to facilitate a broader approach to spirituality. For some people, the idea of a higher power can be translated into Mother Nature, or the healing energy and intention of the people in their AA group. Clients may benefit from developing a more open view of spirituality by seeking out books on different spiritual philosophies or exploring spiritual practices such as yoga, tai chi, or meditation that offer people ways to experience expanded awareness. (See Chapter 31.)

Body-Mind Responses

Benson and Wallace conducted a classic early study on the application of meditation to the treatment of substance abuse. Their study had 1,862 participants, and they found that those who used prescription and illicit drugs began reducing their intake of drugs as they learned to enter a deep state of relaxation. After 21 months of regular meditation, most had stopped using drugs completely. The investigators looked closely at alcohol use in these same subjects. They classified drinkers as light users (three times a month or less), medium users (once to six times a week), and heavy users (once a day or more). After 21 months of meditation, heavy use of alcohol had dropped from 2.7% to 0.6%, medium use dropped from 15.8% to 3.7%, and light use dropped from 41.4% to 25.8%. The percentage of nonusers of alcohol rose from 40.1% to 69.9%. More than half of the participants in this study, 61.1%, reported that meditation was "extremely important" in helping to reduce their alcohol consumption. The more the participants meditated, the less they drank.[39]

A study at the Addictive Behaviors Research Center at the University of Washington in Seattle explored whether Vipassana meditation (VM), a Buddhist mindfulness-based practice, can provide an alternative for individuals who find traditional addiction treatments incompatible or unattractive. The investigators evaluated the effectiveness of a VM course on substance use and psychosocial outcomes in an incarcerated population. Results indicated that after release from jail, participants in the VM course, as compared with those in a treatment-as-usual control condition, showed significant reductions in alcohol, marijuana, and crack cocaine use.[40]

Researchers at the University of Maryland School of Medicine in Baltimore investigated the efficacy of adding qi gong to a residential treatment program for substance abuse. Qi gong, which blends relaxation, breathing, guided imagery, inward attention, and mindfulness to elicit a tranquil, healing state, was introduced into a short-term residential treatment program. Participants whose qi gong meditation was of acceptable quality reported greater reductions in craving, anxiety, and withdrawal symptoms.

The investigators conclude that qi gong meditation appears to contribute positively to addiction treatment outcomes, with results at least as good as those of an established stress management program.[41]

Brain wave biofeedback also has been used successfully with people in recovery. It is a process in which electroencephalographic feedback helps participants go into deep states of relaxation. This heightened awareness also assists clients in recognizing their feelings of tension and then learning that deep relaxation can replace the chemically induced relief gained from addictive substances.[42]

■ HOLISTIC CARING PROCESS

Holistic Assessment

In preparing to use strategies to assist clients in overcoming alcoholism, the nurse should assess the following:

- The client's characteristics that may suggest alcoholism:
  - Restlessness, impulsiveness, anxiety
  - Selfishness, self-centeredness, lack of consideration
  - Stubbornness, irritability, anger, rage, ill humor
  - Physical cruelty, brawling, child and spouse abuse
  - Depression, isolation, self-destructiveness
  - Aggressive sexuality, often accompanied by infidelity, which may give way to sexual disinterest or impotence
  - Arrogance that may lead to aggression, coldness, or withdrawal
  - Low self-esteem, shame, guilt, remorse, loneliness
  - Reduced mental and physical function leading to eventual blackouts
  - Susceptibility to other disease
  - Lying, deceit, broken promises
  - Denial that there is a drinking problem
  - Projection of blame onto people, places, and things
- The client's current drinking patterns (**Exhibit 24-4** provides a self-scoring test that can be taken by a client or by a family member or friend concerned about the client's drinking.)

EXHIBIT 24-4   Are You a Problem Drinker?

1. Have you ever tried to stop drinking for a week (or longer), only to fall short of your goal?
2. Do you resent the advice of others who try to get you to stop drinking?
3. Have you ever tried to control your drinking by switching from one alcoholic beverage to another?
4. Have you taken a morning drink during the past year?
5. Do you envy people who can drink without getting into trouble?
6. Has your drinking problem become progressively more serious during the past year?
7. Has your drinking created problems at home?
8. At social affairs where drinking is limited, do you try to obtain "extra" drinks?
9. Despite evidence to the contrary, have you continued to assert that you can stop drinking "on your own" whenever you wish?
10. During the past year, have you missed time from work as a result of your drinking?
11. Have you ever "blacked out" (had a loss of memory) during your drinking?
12. Have you ever felt you could do more with your life if you did not drink?

Did you answer YES four or more times? If so, chances are you have a serious drinking problem or may have one in the future.

Source: The preceding 12 questions have been adapted from questions appearing in the pamphlet *Is A.A. for You?*, with permission of Alcoholics Anonymous World Services, Inc. Permission to use this material does not mean that Alcoholics Anonymous has reviewed and/or endorses this publication. AA is a program of recovery from alcoholism only—use of AA material in any non-AA context does not imply otherwise.

- The client's attitudes, beliefs, and motivation to learn interventions to become non-addicted
- The client's available family and friends
- The client's eating and exercise patterns
- The client's existing stress management strategies
- The client's willingness to join a support group

Identification of Patterns/Challenges/Needs

The patterns/challenges/needs (see Chapter 7) compatible with addiction interventions are as follows:

- Altered nutrition (more or less than body requirements)
- High risk for trauma
- Impaired verbal communication
- Altered social interaction
- Altered family processes
- Altered sexuality patterns
- Spiritual distress
- Ineffective individual and family coping
- Noncompliance
- Health-seeking behaviors
- Decreased physical mobility
- Sleep pattern disturbance
- Disturbance in self-esteem
- Disturbance in personal identity
- Hopelessness
- Powerlessness
- Knowledge deficit
- Altered thought processes
- Anxiety
- Potential for violence
- Fear

Outcome Identification

Exhibit 24-5 guides the nurse in client outcomes, nursing prescriptions, and evaluation for overcoming addictions.

EXHIBIT 24-5 Nursing Interventions: Overcoming Addictions

Client Outcomes	Nursing Prescriptions	Evaluation
The client demonstrated attitudes, beliefs, and actions that reflect an intention to overcome addiction.	The client set realistic plans for overcoming addiction as evidenced by the following actions: ■ Accepted support of healthy family or friends ■ Attended AA daily ■ Contacted AA sponsor regularly ■ Detoxified self and environment of drugs and alcohol ■ Practiced relaxation and imagery daily ■ Integrated behavioral changes on a daily basis ■ Rewarded self for attaining set goals	The client will demonstrate attitudes, beliefs, and behaviors that result in overcoming addictions. Determine the client's intention to overcome addiction by assessing follow-through on the following actions: ■ Seeking support from healthy family and friends ■ Attending AA meetings ■ Seeking support of a sponsor ■ Detoxifying self and environment of alcohol and drugs ■ Practicing relaxation and imagery ■ Integrating behavioral changes ■ Selecting ways to reward self for attaining goals

Therapeutic Care Plan and Interventions

Before the session:
- Spend a few moments centering yourself, connecting with your inner wisdom and intention to facilitate healing.
- Create a quiet place to begin guiding the client in strategies to overcome addiction(s).

At the beginning of the session:
- Review the results of the self-assessment.
- Reinforce the concept that overcoming addictions is a process requiring commitment, new behavioral skills, and support from family and friends.
- Ask the client to tell his or her personal story.
- Assist the client in identifying the steps necessary for overcoming addictions. If necessary, assist the client in going through detoxification.

During the session:
- Teach the client general relaxation and imagery exercises with a focus on awareness of body sensations and their connection to feelings.

- Teach the client how to create specific imagery patterns (see Chapter 17) and to practice and integrate the following:
  1. *Active images:* Images such as cleansing the body of impurities, possibly by a gentle waterfall; creating a safe place where the client can feel secure and comfortable; and using a protective shield to let the client receive what is needed from others and to block out negative images, such as alcohol or drug signals, places, or events.
  2. *End-state images:* Images of feeling healthy, of living with a sense of accomplishment and satisfaction, and of having healthy, supportive relationships.
  3. *Healing images:* Images such as connecting with the inner healer, inner wisdom, and with spiritual resources.
  4. *Process images:* Imagining successfully overcoming drink or drug signals and making healthy, alternative choices.
- Teach the client to reframe current situations and problems. For example, instead

of the client saying, "I can't admit publicly that I'm an alcoholic," help the client rehearse being at a 12-step meeting and saying, "Thank you for letting me share my story with you. I have been an alcoholic for 10 years, and I am ready to quit."

- Teach the client to use HALT, checking to notice if being hungry, angry, lonely, or tired is a contributing factor when experiencing alcohol or drug signals. Encourage the client to avoid these conditions whenever possible.
- Encourage the development of creative skills as a means of working with strong emotions and experiences. This may include actively working with dreams; journal keeping; letter writing (see Chapter 12); using artistic expressions by drawing, painting, or sculpting with clay; playing evocative music to enhance images or dance with the emotions (see Chapters 14 and 18).
- Have the client identify his or her habit breakers (see Chapter 23).
- Have the client learn forgiveness (see Chapter 32).

At the end of the session:

- Encourage the client to explore the value of a 12-step program as an adjunct to treatment.
- Emphasize the value of selecting someone in the program as a sponsor so that a support person is available to be contacted on a daily basis.
- Reinforce the idea that the client can outwit relapse by learning how to recognize high-risk situations. Reinforce the value of using HALT when experiencing signals for substance use. Is hunger, anger, loneliness, or tiredness contributing to these feelings? Encourage the client to make a list of particular high-risk situations and decide in advance quick action steps to prevent relapse.
- Reinforce the importance of integrating healthful habits into daily life. Encourage the client to select one or two practices to which he or she is willing to make a commitment to include in daily life. Imagery, breathing exercises, meditation, yoga, jogging or other physical activities, and dietary changes are all of value.
- Use the client outcomes (see Exhibit 24-5) that were established before the session to evaluate the session.
- Schedule a follow-up session.

Holistic Interventions

Imagery

As previously noted, addicted individuals are not in touch with their bodies or feelings. Basic relaxation and imagery training can help them to experience themselves with new awareness. The daily practice of relaxation and imagery exercises not only reverses stress and depression, but also increases clients' recognition of inner knowledge. People who have been addicted have lost trust in themselves because of all the poor choices they have made while in their addiction. In addition, they experience a deep shame when thinking of all the people they have hurt or disappointed. There is a harsh, condemning, inner voice with which these clients must contend.

Clients must become aware of their physical responses to stress (e.g., heart palpitations, muscle tightness, headaches, stomachaches). The abuse of alcohol, drugs, food, or other substances or behaviors numbs awareness of body responses, short-circuiting mind–body communication. Clients must learn to practice stress management skills daily rather than waiting until a vulnerable moment occurs. For example, the nurse can teach diaphragmatic breathing as a very basic skill. Shallow chest and shoulder breathing is a common stress response, one that often becomes chronic. Simply breathing diaphragmatically can bring about significant physiologic and psychological responses. Changing to this breath pattern efficiently slows the heart rate, increases oxygenation of the blood, strengthens weak intestinal and abdominal muscles, and can bring about a sense of well-being and inner calm.

Teaching a client the concept of "constant instant practice" is a way of linking a new behavior to an activity that is done repeatedly during the course of the day. For example, if the person spends a great deal of time on the telephone, he or she can let the telephone be the reminder to take a few deep, cleansing breaths. If the telephone is ringing, the person can let it ring a few extra times and take a deep breath before answering. This practice can be linked with any activity that occurs frequently during the client's day.

The mind responds best when it is given positive images about new ideas and new behavior patterns. A nurse may start by guiding clients in rhythmic breathing exercises. When the clients are in a quieted state, they can be guided to imagine being clean and sober and walking down a street where they went to use drugs or alcohol with friends, now experiencing this place from a sober perspective. The image of experiencing their world from a new perspective can then be practiced and reinforced, resulting in the breakdown of addictive responses and the strengthening of positive coping strategies.

Imagery Scripts

To assist in the client's recovery process, the nurse can take time to create special relaxation and imagery tapes that the client can listen to several times a day. The following three imagery scripts focus on substance abuse, but they can be modified for other addictions. A relaxation exercise from Chapter 15 may be recorded for 5 to 10 minutes, followed by one or several of the scripts for overcoming addictions for 15 minutes or longer.

It is best to use these scripts as suggestions. The most effective imagery tapes take advantage of the nurse's creativity, intuitions, and clinical insights—in combination with words and images the client has used—to create an imagery script that is designed for a particular person. (See Chapter 16.)

Script: **Introduction. (Name)**, as your mind becomes clearer and clearer, feel it becoming more and more alert. Somewhere deep inside of you, a brilliant light begins to glow. Sense this happening. The light grows brighter and more intense. This is the body–mind communication center. Breathe into it. Energize it with your breath. The light is powerful and penetrating, and a beam begins to grow out of it. The beam shines from the core of your spirit.

Script: **Affirming strengths.** In your relaxed state, affirm to yourself at your deep level of inner strength and knowing that you can stop drinking [or taking drugs]. Say it over and over as you begin to imagine the words and feelings in every cell in your body. Feel your relaxed state deepen. You can get to this space anytime that you wish. All you have to do is give yourself the suggestion and stay with the suggestion as you move into your relaxed state. This is a skill that you will use repeatedly as you move into your new healthy life patterns.

You have gone through detox . . . you are sober. Notice what you are feeling. Increase your awareness of deepening your relaxation. You have come a long way and are on your path toward healing.

The client provides affirmations and repeats them several times. For example, "I am at peace," "I am totally relaxed," "I feel safe and calm," "I can drink water or other kinds of liquids that will satisfy my oral needs," and "I am secure in my inner knowledge that I have the strength for recovering."

Script: **AA meeting rehearsal.** Imagine yourself attending an AA meeting. You have opened your body and mind to receive many positive messages and support from others about being sober. Imagine now that you have entered the meeting room and are pleased with yourself for being there. Look around the room. Is there any one person that you might like to meet? If yes, see yourself going over to meet this person, and hear your voice as you introduce yourself. If there is no one you wish to meet, that is

OK. See yourself finding a place to sit, and continue to focus on your relaxed breathing. With your relaxation you are able to be more present during the meeting . . . to be open to hear other people share their stories.

Imagine that you are ready to share part of your story. Remember, there are many ways to share your story . . . sharing with a friend . . . a counselor . . . or your AA sponsor. Listen to your inner wisdom . . . you will know what is right for you. Can you imagine sharing something special about your journey? What would it be? How would you like to feel? The meeting is now over. Is there anyone that you wish to greet? If so, see yourself doing so.

Script: ***Closure.*** Take a few slow, energizing breaths and, as you come back to full awareness of the room, know that whatever is right for you at this point in time is unfolding just as it should . . . that you are willing to enter on this healing journey . . . and that you have done your best.

CASE STUDY (IMPLEMENTATION)

Setting: AA meeting

Client: S. W., a successful, married professional with two children. At the time he told us his story, he had been free of alcohol and amphetamines for 3 months and had begun his path toward recovery.

Patterns/Challenges/Needs: Health maintenance related to engaging in actions supportive of remaining free of addiction

"My healing began when I finally admitted to myself, my family, and my friends that I was addicted to alcohol and drugs. I began to explore and own my dark side. I've created some wonderful healing rituals, which include getting the nerve up to attend my first AA meeting—which gave me the opportunity to hear other people tell their story. I've been regularly attending AA meetings and have a sponsor who I've called several times when I felt myself slipping. I realized I didn't know how to do anything to relax except drink. If I needed energy, I didn't know any way to get it but to take speed. So, I've learned relaxation and imagery skills, started an exercise program, and am taking time for myself.

"Here I was at 45 feeling lost and wondering if this was all life had to offer. How could I feel lost? I had so much. My career was going well. I had good kids, a loving and supportive wife, good looks, and I was involved in several civic projects. Everyone was always telling me how wonderful I was and stressing my contributions to the community. But I was searching for more to fulfill my life. I had been a secret drinker and had taken speed off and on since college in order to do all that I needed to accomplish. Everybody saw me as perfect, but I could feel my world falling apart. I got scared.

"For the past 5 years or so my wife had said that she thought I was drinking too much, which had recently become a source of tension between us. I told my wife to take the kids and go on a holiday while I worked at home alone. As soon as they left, I got drunk. When I fractured my ankle from a fall in my own house the first day they were gone, I really began to look at my life. I had a month of deep depression. During that time, my inner voice was screaming at me about all the abuse I was into. It was as if I was having a conversation with a part of myself that I had never heard. The message was so clear I could not turn it off.

"I'm not like many addicts who lose family, money, jobs, and friends. During a month of struggling to perform and continuing to hear my inner dialogue, one day my depression lifted enough for me to find a local AA meeting and hear myself say, 'I've had it; I need help.' I finally admitted in public that I was addicted to alcohol and drugs and used them to be successful. I began educating myself about addictions. I asked for help. What I recognized was that previously I sought ways to connect with sources outside of myself to make me feel good. The real

EXHIBIT 24-6   Evaluating the Client's Subjective Experience with Overcoming Addictions

1. What new awarenesses have you had today?
2. Do you understand how to keep a journal of your habits?
3. Can you identify two habit-breaker strategies that you are planning to utilize?
4. Are you aware of your body–mind's signals of wanting a drink?
5. Which relaxation exercises are you finding most beneficial?
6. Do you have any questions on how best to practice your imagery and meditation?
7. What physical activities are you including in your daily routine?
8. Have you been monitoring the pattern of your craving by using HALT?
9. What affirmations are you working with to reinforce your intentions to be conscious and sober?
10. What have you observed about your patterns of response to vulnerability? Do you tend toward willfulness or will-lessness?
11. What have you discovered is your preferred way of connecting with your spiritual nature?
12. What is your next step?

healing came when I learned to connect with the core of my spirit, which awakened my inner resources for feelings of wholeness."

Evaluation

With the client, the nurse determines whether the client outcomes for overcoming addictions (see Exhibit 24-5) were achieved. To evaluate the session further, the nurse may explore the subjective effects of the experience with the client (**Exhibit 24-6**).

Directions for
FUTURE RESEARCH

1. Determine the effectiveness of imagery and breathing techniques in assisting clients to manage cravings.
2. Determine the effectiveness of cognitive strategies (e.g., teaching about willfulness and will-lessness, using HALT) in helping clients to manage feelings of vulnerability.
3. Study the role of spiritual perspective and practice in long-term recovery.

Nurse Healer
REFLECTIONS

After reading this chapter, the nurse healer will be able to answer or to begin a process of answering the following questions:

- What addictive patterns do I recognize in my own life?
- What patterns of response to vulnerability do I observe in myself?
- What practices and changes am I willing to bring into my life to encourage my own healing?
- Who are the people in my life who would support me in making healthy changes?
- Can I allow an image to emerge that represents my inner wisdom?
- Can I identify what interferes with my connection to my inner wisdom?
- How do I connect with my spiritual nature and how do I support this in my daily life?

> *For a full suite of assignments and additional learning activities, use the access code located in the front of your book to visit this exclusive website: http://go.jblearning.com/dossey. If you do not have an access code, you can obtain one at the site.*

NOTES

1. SAMHSA (U.S. Substance Abuse and Mental Health Services Administration)
2. Office of National Drug Control Policy, *The Economic Costs of Drug Abuse in the United States, 1992–*

2002, Publication No. 207303 (Washington, DC: Executive Office of the President, 2004). http ://www.ncjrs.gov/ondcppubs/publications/pdf /economic_costs.pdf.

3. Centers for Disease Control and Prevention, *Best Practices for Comprehensive Tobacco Control Programs* (Atlanta, GA: U.S. Department of Health and Human Services, Centers for Disease Control and Prevention, National Center for Chronic Disease Prevention and Health Promotion, Office on Smoking and Health, October 2007). http ://www.cdc.gov/tobacco/stateandcommunity/best _practices/pdfs/2007/bestpractices_complete.pdf.

4. J. Rehm et al., "Global Burden of Disease and Injury and Economic Cost Attributable to Alcohol Use and Alcohol-Use Disorders," *Lancet* 373, no. 9682 (2009): 2223–2233.

5. A. Kumar et al., "Chromatin Remodeling Is a Key Mechanism Underlying Cocaine-Induced Plasticity in Striatum," *Neuron* 48, no. 2 (2008): 303–314.

6. I. Maze and E. J. Nestler, "Epigenetic Landscape of Addiction," *Annals of the New York Academy of Sciences* 1216 (January 2011): 99–113. doi: 10.1111/j.1749-6632.2010.05893.x

7. S. C. McQuown and M. A. Wood, "Epigenetic Regulation in Substance Use Disorders, " *Current Psychiatry Report* 12, no. 2 (April 2010): 145–153.

8. C. E. Rice, D. Dandreaux, E. D. Handley, and L. Chassin, "Children of Alcoholics: Risk and Resilience," *Prevention Researcher* 13, no. 4 (2006): 3–6.

9. M. Pagano et al., "Impact of Parental History of Substance Use Disorders on the Clinical Course of Anxiety Disorders," *Substance Abuse Treatment, Prevention, and Policy* 2, no. 13 (2007): 2–13.

10. Office of Applied Studies, *Results from the 2008 National Survey on Drug Use and Health: National Findings*, HHS Publication No. SMA 09-4434, NSDUH Series H-36. (Rockville, MD: Substance Abuse and Mental Health Services Administration, 2009). http://oas.samhsa.gov/nsduh/2k8nsduh /2k8Results.cfm.

11. Alcoholics Anonymous, *Alcoholics Anonymous* (New York: AA World Services, 1976).

12. M. Kaur et al., "Induction of Withdrawal-Like Symptoms in a Small Randomized, Controlled Trial of Opioid Blockade in Frequent Tanners," *Journal of the American Academy of Dermatology* 54, no. 4 (2006): 709–711.

13. S. Zeller et al., "Do Adolescent Tanners Exhibit Dependency?" *Journal of the American Academy of Dermatology* 54, no. 4 (2006): 589–596.

14. B. Schaub and R. Schaub, *Healing Addictions* (Albany, NY: Delmar Publishers, 1997).

15. American Psychiatric Association, *Diagnostic and Statistical Manual of Mental Disorders-TR* (Washington, DC: APA, 2000).

16. National Institute of Alcohol Abuse and Alcoholism, *Alcohol Alert* (January 2007). http://www .niaaa.nih.gov/Publications/AlcoholAlerts/Pages /default.aspx.

17. S. C. McQuown and M. A. Wood, "Epigenetic Regulation in Substance Use Disorders," *Current Psychiatry Report* 12, no. 2 (April 2010): 145–153. doi:10.1007/s11920-010-0099-5

18. K. Graham and A. Massak, "Alcohol Consumption and the Use of Antidepressants," *Canadian Medical Association Journal* 176, no. 5 (2007): 633–637.

19. Substance Abuse and Mental Health Services Administration, Center for Behavioral Health Statistics and Quality (formerly the Office of Applied Studies), *The DAWN Report: Highlights of the 2009 Drug Abuse Warning Network (DAWN) Findings on Drug-Related Emergency Department Visits* (Rockville, MD: SAMHSA, December 28, 2010). http://www.oas.samhsa.gov/2k10/DAWN034 /EDHighlights.htm.

20. Substance Abuse and Mental Health Services Administration, Center for Behavioral Health Statistics and Quality, Drug Abuse Warning Network, "DAWN Emergency Department Publications." http://dawninfo.samhsa.gov/pubs/edpubs/.

21. P. Agostino, "Unsportsmanlike Conduct," *Nurse Week*. http://www.nurseweek.com/news/Features /05-04/Abuse.asp.

22. Hazelden Foundation, *The Twelve Steps of Alcoholics Anonymous* (New York: Harper/Hazelden, 1987): 2.

23. E. Becker, *The Denial of Death* (New York: Free Press, 1973): 178.

24. L. M. Gentilello, "Let's Diagnose Alcohol Problems in the ER and Successfully Intervene," *Medscape General Medicine* (2006). http://www .medscape.com/viewarticle/518824_print.

25. NIH Consensus Conference, "Acupuncture," *Journal of the American Medical Association* 280, no. 17 (1998): 1518–1524.

26. T.-T. Liu, J. Shi, D. H. Epstein, Y.-P. Bao, and L. Lu, "A Meta-Analysis of Acupuncture Combined with Opioid Receptor Agonists for Treatment of Opiate-Withdrawal Symptoms," *Cellular Molecular Neurobiology* 29 (2009): 449–454.

27. E. A. Robinson, A. R. Krentzman, J. R. Webb, and K. J. Brower, "Six-Month Changes in Spirituality and Religiousness in Alcoholics Predict Drinking Outcomes at Nine Months," *Journal of Studies on Alcohol and Drugs* 72, no. 4 (July 2011): 660–668.

28. C. A. Bradley, "Women in AA: 'Sharing Experience, Strength and Hope' the Relational Nature of Spirituality," *Journal of Religion and Spirituality in Social Work*, 30, no. 2 (April–June 2011): 89–112.

29. S. A. Straussner and H. Byrne, "Alcoholics Anonymous: Key Research Findings from 2002–2007," *Alcoholism Treatment Quarterly* 27, no. 4 (2009): 349–367.

30. M. R. Werbach, *Nutritional Influences on Mental Illness* (Tarzana, CA: Third Line Press, 1991): 15.

31. R. J. Brey, "The Role of Healing Touch in the Treatment of Persons in Recovery from Alcoholism," *Counselor: The Magazine for Addiction Professionals* (November 30, 2006). http://www.counselormagazine.com/feature-articles-main menu-63/29-alternative/550-the-role-of-healing-touch-in-the-treatment-of-persons-in-recovery-from-alcoholism.

32. M. Winkelman, "Complementary Therapy for Addiction: Drumming Out Drugs," *American Journal of Public Health* 93, no. 4 (2003): 647–651.

33. T. Gorski and M. Miller, *Counseling for Relapse Prevention* (Independence, MO: Independence Press, 1982).

34. G. May, *Addiction and Grace* (San Francisco, CA: Harper, 1991): 104.

35. W. White and A. Laudet, "Spirituality, Science and Addiction," *Counselor: The Magazine for Addiction Professionals* 7, no. 1 (2006): 56–59.

36. A. B. Laudet, K. Morgan, and W. White, "The Role of Social Supports, Spirituality, Religiousness, Life Meaning and Affiliation with 12-Step Fellowships in Quality-of-Life Satisfaction Among Individuals in Recovery from Alcohol and Drug Problems," *Alcohol Treatment Quarterly* 24, nos. 1–2 (2006): 33–73.

37. E. A. R. Robinson et al., "Six-Month Changes in Spirituality, Religiousness, and Heavy Drinking in a Treatment Seeking Sample," *Journal of Studies on Alcohol and Drugs* 68, no. 2 (2007): 282–290.

38. J. W. Bowden, "Recovery from Alcoholism: A Spiritual Journey," *Issues in Mental Health Nursing* 19, no. 4 (1998): 337–352.

39. H. Benson and R. K. Wallace, "Decreased Drug Abuse with Transcendental Meditation," *Drug Abuse—Proceedings of the International Conference* (Philadelphia, PA: Lea & Febiger, 1972): 369–376.

40. S. Bowen et al., "Mindfulness Meditation and Substance Use in an Incarcerated Population," *Psychology of Addictive Behavior* 20, no. 3 (September 2006): 343–347.

41. K. W. Chen, A. Comerford, P. Shinnick, and D. M. Ziedonis, "Introducing Qigong Meditation into Residential Addiction Treatment: A Pilot Study Where Gender Makes a Difference," *Journal of Alternative and Complementary Medicine* 16, no. 8 (August 2010): 875–82.

42. T. M. Sokhadze, R. L. Cannon, and D. L. Trudeau, "EEG Biofeedback as a Treatment for Substance Use Disorders: Review, Rating of Efficacy, and Recommendations for Further Research," *Applied Psychophysiology and Biofeedback* 33, no. 1 (March 2008): 1–28.

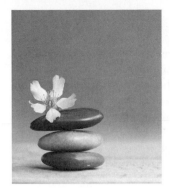

Chapter 25

Aromatherapy

Jane Buckle

Nurse Healer
OBJECTIVES

Theoretical

- Describe the historical path of aromatherapy, from ancient times to the present renaissance.
- Describe the relevance of learned memory in the choice of essential oil.
- Compare the different methods of using essential oils.
- Discuss the safety issues of using essential oils.

Clinical

- Describe the use of aromatherapy for insomnia.
- Describe the use of aromatherapy for chronic pain.
- Describe the use of aromatherapy for infection.
- List three uses for essential oil of *Lavandula angustifolia*.
- List three uses for essential oil of *Eucalyptus globulus*.
- List three uses for essential oil of *Mentha piperita*.
- List three uses for essential oil of *Melaleuca alternifolia*.
- List three uses for essential oil of *Boswellia carteri*.

Personal

- Integrate aromatherapy into your daily life to enhance your well-being.
- Experience each of the five essential oils mentioned previously, both inhaled and topically.

DEFINITIONS

Aromatherapy: The use of essential oils for therapeutic purposes.

Chemotype: A cloned variety of a plant that always has the same chemistry.

Clinical aromatherapy: The use of essential oils for specific, measurable outcomes.

Essential oil: The distillate from an aromatic plant, or the oil expressed from the peel of a citrus fruit.

Learned memory: The ability of the mind to condition the response to an aroma based on previous experience.

Limbic system: The oldest part of the brain; it contains the amygdala, hippocampus, thalamus, and hypothalamus.

'M' Technique: A registered form of very gentle, structured touch suitable when the receiver is very fragile, actively dying, or the giver is not trained in massage. Recognized as part of holistic nursing care.

■ HISTORY

Aromatherapy is often misunderstood and maligned because many people think aromatherapy is just about inhaling aromas. Aromatherapy is part of herbal medicine that dates back 6,000 years and has been used in many parts of the world. According to the World Health Organization, more than 85% of the world population still relies on herbal medicine, and many of the herbs are aromatic.

The renaissance of modern aromatherapy began in France just prior to World War II, at about the same time the first antibiotics were being introduced. A medical doctor, Jean Valnet, a chemist, Maurice Gattefosse, and a surgical assistant, Marguerite Maury, were key figures in the rediscovery of this ancient art of healing. They did not use aromatherapy for nice aromas or for stress reduction, two of the most popular ways aromatherapy is used today; they used aromatherapy clinically to help wounds heal, to fight infections, and to reduce skin problems, and they used essential oils topically.

This more clinical approach to aromatherapy has survived in France and Germany, where aromatherapy is seen as an extension of orthodox medicine. German doctors and nurses are tested in the use of essential oils to become licensed. The clinical use of aromatherapy is easy to understand, as many of today's drugs originally came from plants: for example, aspirin from willow bark and digoxin from foxglove. Even the contraceptive pill originally came from a plant— the humble yam—and the yew tree produces a cytotoxic drug to fight cancer.

■ THEORY AND RESEARCH

Aromatherapy uses essential oils obtained from aromatic plants for the physical, psychological, and spiritual benefit of the patient. Essential oils are powerful; they can be up to 100 times more concentrated than the herb itself. Many essential oils have familiar smells, such as lavender, rose, and rosemary. Essential oils are highly volatile droplets created by the plant to prevent (or treat) infection, regulate growth, and mend damaged tissue. These tiny droplets are stored in veins, glands, or sacs by the plant, and when they are crushed or rubbed, the essential oil and its aroma are released. Some plants store large amounts of essential oil, some store very little. This, along with the difficulty of harvesting the essential oil, dictates the price of each type of oil. More than 220 pounds (100 kilograms) of fresh rose petals are needed to produce a little more than 2 ounces (60 grams) of essential oil, making rose one of the most expensive essential oils, and therefore one of the most frequently adulterated.

There are a few important things to know about essential oils before they can be used safely: extraction, the botanical name (for clear identification), method of application, safety, storage, and contraindications. These topics are discussed in the following subsections as well as in Exhibit 25-2, later in this chapter.

Extraction

Only steam-distilled or expressed extracts produce essential oils. These two methods give a product with no additional solvent or impurity. However, many "essential oils" on the market are actually extracted with solvent, which can produce allergic or sensitive reactions in the user. A bottle of essential oil should state that the contents are pure essential oils: steam distilled or expressed. (Only the peel from citrus plants such as mandarin, lime, or lemon produces an *expressed* oil.)

Identification by Botanical Name

It is very important to know the botanical name of a plant because there can be many different species of the same plant, and using just the common name can lead to confusion. For example, there are three species of lavender and many hybrids, each with different chemistry and, therefore, very different therapeutic effects. There are 400 different species of eucalyptus. Identification is simple if the full botanical name is given. This should include the genus, species, and where relevant, the chemotype. The genus of lavender is *Lavandula*, and so all lavender plant names begin with *Lavandula*. The species is the second part of the name. The chemotype, if there is one, comes last. See **Table 25-1** for a list of the botanical and the common names for the essential oils mentioned in this chapter.

Do not buy just anything that is labeled "lavender oil" because there is no way of knowing

TABLE 25-1   Essential Oils Mentioned in This Chapter

Common Name	Botanical Name
Aniseed	*Pimpinella anisum*
Basil	*Ocimum basilicum*
Chamomile, German	*Matricaria recutita*
Chamomile, Roman	*Chamaemelum nobile*
Clary sage	*Salvia sclarea*
Coriander seed	*Coriandrum sativum*
Eucalyptus	*Eucalyptus globulus*
Fennel	*Foeniculum vulgare var. dulce*
Geranium	*Pelargonium graveolens*
Ginger	*Zingiber officinale*
Hyssop	*Hyssopus officinalis*
Lavender, true	*Lavandula angustifolia*
Lemongrass	*Cymbopogon citratus*
Neroli	*Citrus aurantium var. amara*
Palmarosa	*Cymbopogon martinii*
Parsley	*Petroselinum sativum*
Pennyroyal	*Mentha pulegium*
Peppermint	*Mentha piperita*
Rose	*Rosa damascena*
Rosewood	*Aniba rosaeodora*
Sage	*Salvia officinalis*
Sandalwood	*Santalum album*
Tarragon	*Artemisia dracunculus*
Wintergreen	*Gaultheria procumbens*

which lavender is in the bottle. One lavender is soothing, calming, and exceptional for burns, but another lavender is a stimulant and expectorant (helps someone to cough up mucus). This second lavender will not promote sleep or soothe burns.

Methods of Application

Essential oils can be absorbed by the body in three ways: through ingestion, through olfaction, and through topical application. For methods of using essential oils that are congruent with holistic nursing practice, see **Exhibit 25-1**.

Touch in Aromatherapy

Aromatherapy often is used with massage or the 'M' Technique.[1] This registered method of touch is suitable when massage is inappropriate, either because the receiver is too fragile or the giver is not trained in massage.[2] The 'M' Technique is used in hospitals, hospices, and long-term care facilities in the United States, the United Kingdom, the Netherlands, and South Africa. It is simple to learn and produces a profound relaxation response in just a few minutes, reducing perceptions of chronic pain, agitation in dementia,[3] and at the end of life.[4] The 'M' Technique appears to be more relaxing than conventional massage and to have an accumulative effect.[5] Gentle stroking enhances absorption of essential oils through the skin into the bloodstream. (For more details on this method of very gentle, structured touch, the how-to DVDs, the 2-day practitioner, and 4-hour

EXHIBIT 25-1   Methods of Application

1. Inhalation: 1–5 drops undiluted
2. Topical
    - In baths: 1–8 drops
    - Compresses: 1–8%
    - 'M' Technique or massage: 1–10%
    - Wounds: 12–40% (depending on chemistry of essential oil)
    - Burns, bites, and stings (first aid): 100%
    - Radiation burns: 3–10%
3. Vaginal: Useful for yeast infection or cystitis. Use 1–5% diluted on tampon.
4. Ingestion: This is not accepted as part of holistic nursing care.

hand and foot 'M' Technique training programs, please see www.rjbuckle.com.)

Olfaction

The fastest effect from aromatherapy is through olfaction.[6] Essential oils are composed of many different chemical components that travel via the nose to the olfactory bulb. There is debate as to whether the components are recognized by shape or vibration;[7] either way, they trigger responses in the limbic system of the brain—the oldest part of the brain—where the aroma is processed. The limbic part of the brain contains the amygdala, where fear and anger are analyzed; the thalamus, where pain is analyzed; and the hippocampus, which is involved in the formation and retrieval of explicit memories. This is why an aroma can trigger memories that have lain dormant for years. Smell is very important, beginning with the newborn baby's identification of its mother and continuing into old age, where studies show that the depression of residential older adults can be reduced with the aromas of familiar fruits and flowers.

The effect of odors on the brain was "mapped" using computer-generated graphics.[8] Brain Electrical Activity Mapping (BEAM) indicates how a subject, linked to an electroencephalogram (EEG), rates different odors even when the subject is asleep.[9] These maps indicate that aromas can have a psychological effect even when the aroma is subliminal (i.e., below the level of human awareness), and that, provided the olfactory nerve is intact, the aroma still has a measurable effect on the brain.

Topical Applications

Components within essential oils are absorbed into, and through, the skin via diffusion. The two layers of the skin, the dermis and fat layer, together act as a reservoir before the components within the essential oils reach the bloodstream. There is some evidence that massage or hot water enhances absorption. Essential oils, because they are lipophyllic (dissolve in fat), can be stored in the fatty areas of the body and can pass through the blood–brain barrier and into the brain itself.

Negative Reactions

Essential oils are commonly used in the pharmaceutical, perfume, and food industries.[10] Pure essential oils rarely produce an allergic effect, unlike synthetics. Today, increasingly more essential oils are being replaced with synthetic copies.

Nursing Theory

Aromatherapy links into many of the most recognized nursing theories. Certainly, it resonates with Watson's Theory of Caring because aromatherapy allows nurses a method of showing their care at a deep level.[11] It resonates with Barrett's Theory of Power because it allows the patient to participate knowingly in change and offers a model for change through empowerment.[12] Nightingale put forward the first theory of nursing—putting the patient in the best condition for Nature to act—and thus aromatherapy clearly fits here because it allows the patient to relax sufficiently for the healing process to occur from within.[13] Nightingale also suggested creating an environmental space conducive to healing—aromatherapy fits very well here as well, because essential oils create a safe environment at many levels. Erickson's work led to the Modeling Theory,[14] which requires building trust, promoting positive orientation, promoting strength, and setting mutual health-directed goals—these requirements also fit exceptionally well with aromatherapy. Rogers's theory suggests that human beings are more than just physical entities and have specific energy fields. Aromas clearly affect both the psyche and the human energy field.

How Aromatherapy Works

The term *aromatherapy* refers to the therapeutic use of essential oils—the volatile organic constituents of plants. Essential oils are thought to work at psychological, physiologic, and cellular levels. This means that they can affect our body, our mind, and all the delicate links in between. The effects of aroma can be rapid, and sometimes just thinking about a smell can be as powerful as the actual smell itself. Take a moment to think of your favorite flower. Then, think about a smell that makes you feel nauseated. The effects of an aroma can be relaxing or stimulating depending on the previous experience of the individual (called the *learned memory*), as well as the actual chemical makeup of the essential oil used.

Who Uses Aromatherapy?

Aromatherapy is used by nurses in the United Kingdom, France, Germany, Switzerland, Sweden, Australia, New Zealand, Korea, and Japan. In France and Germany, medical doctors and pharmacists also use aromatherapy as part of conventional medicine, often for the control of infection. Aromatherapy is the fastest growing therapy among nurses in the United States.[6]

Although essential oils are very safe to use, there are some guidelines that need to be followed. Reference-backed, patient-centered clinical training is strongly recommended (see www.rjbuckle.com for classroom or home study courses). See **Exhibit 25-2** for relevant warnings, contraindications, and precautions. Possible drug interactions are listed in **Exhibit 25-3**.

Adverse Reactions

There is some evidence of adverse skin reactions caused by sensitivity in rare instances. The majority of cases were from extracts rather than pure essential oils. Bergamot used in conjunction with sunshine or tanning beds can result in skin damage ranging from redness to full-thickness burns.[15] It is recommended that essential oils should be used with caution during pregnancy, although the risk is extremely small when the essential oils are used only topically or inhaled; however, sage, pennyroyal, camphor, parsley, tarragon, wintergreen, juniper, hyssop, and basil should be avoided.[16] Tisserand and Balacs state that there is "no evidence that essential oils are abortificient in the amounts used in aromatherapy."[17]

Administration

Essential oils can be used topically or inhaled. A typical topical application uses a 1–5% mixture: 1–5 drops of essential oils diluted in 5 cc (a teaspoon) of cold-pressed vegetable oil such as sweet almond oil. Some wound infections may require higher concentrations—up to 20%. Certain essential oils, such as lavender and tea tree, can be topically applied undiluted for stings or bites. Others, like clove and thyme, should never be used undiluted on the skin because their high phenol content would cause burning. For insomnia, nausea, or depression, the client should inhale the correct oil for 5–10 minutes as necessary. The nurse can use touch methods such as massage or the 'M' Technique where appropriate. Simple stress management can be incorporated into an everyday regime with the use of baths and foot soaks, vaporizers, and sprays. Oral intake of essential oils, while extremely effective for acute infection or gastrointestinal problems, is not recognized as part of holistic nursing care at this time.

Self-Help

Aromatherapy can be very useful when self-applied for stress management, insomnia, or depression because the oils are portable and can be used anywhere at any time. A drop of peppermint can help clear your mind at the end of

EXHIBIT 25-2   Warnings, Contraindications, and Precautions When Using Essential Oils

1. Avoid with patients with severe asthma or multiple allergies.
2. Do not take by mouth (unless guided by a person trained in aromatic medicine).
3. Do not use essential oils near the eyes. If essential oils get into eyes, rinse out with milk or carrier oil (essential oils do not dissolve in water), and then water.
4. Store away from fire or naked flame. Essential oils are volatile and flammable.
5. Store in cool place out of sunlight, in colored glass—amber or blue. Store expensive essential oils in a refrigerator.
6. Ensure you have accountability by being properly trained. For a clinical home study course see www.rjbuckle.com.
7. Don't use phenol-rich essential oils undiluted on the skin (for example, red thyme).
8. Keep away from children and pets.
9. Only use essential oils from a reputable supplier who can supply the correct botanical name, place of origin, part of plant used, method of extraction, and batch number when possible. See **Table 25-2** for suggested suppliers.
10. Always close the container immediately.
11. Use carefully during pregnancy.
12. Be aware of which essential oils are photosensitive, such as bergamot.

TABLE 25-2   Essential Oils Distributors Used by the Author

Elizabeth Van Buren Inc.
P.O. Box 7542
Santa Cruz, CA 95061
Phone: 1-800-710-7759
www.elizabethvanburen.com

Floriahana France
Les Grands Pres
06460 Caussols, France
Phone: 1-513-576-9944
https://www.florihana.com

Nature's Gift Ltd.
316 Old Hickory Boulevard
East Madison, TN 37115
Phone: 1-615-612-4270
www.naturesgift.com

SunRose Aromatics
P.O. Box 98
Bronx, NY 10465
Phone: 1-718-794-0391
www.sunrosearomatics.com

Recommended Diffusers
Plants Extracts International
10921 Excelsior Boulevard, Suite 111
Hopkins, MN 55343
1-877-999-4236
www.plantextractsinc.com

EXHIBIT 25-3   Drug Interaction When Using Essential Oils

1. Avoid strong aromas such as peppermint and eucalyptus with patients receiving homeopathy.
2. People who are allergic to ragweed may be allergic to chamomile.
3. The effect of tranquilizers, anticonvulsants, and antihistamines may be slightly enhanced by sedative essential oils.

a busy day, or a drop of ylang ylang can help soothe nerves. It is simple to choose an essential oil that is pleasing as well as efficacious.

Credentialing

At the moment there is no recognized national certification for aromatherapy. The closest thing is the Aromatherapy Registration Council (ARC) exam set by the Aromatherapy Registration Board (ARB), a nonprofit entity that provides a national exam for lay people (www .aromatherapycouncil.org). Details of the exams are available from the website. The exam is open to anyone who has studied aromatherapy for 200 hours and meets the criteria. There is little, if any, clinical content in the exam. There are two professional bodies: the National Association of Holistic Aromatherapy (NAHA) and Alliance of International Aromatherapists (AIA). At present, there are no requirements to become certified or accredited, and aromatherapy training can range from 1 day to several years. However, because nurses are accountable, if a nurse wants to use aromatherapy in his or her nursing care, it is strongly recommended that he or she be able to show documented evidence of clinical training, preferably one that is nurse taught and patient centered. Please see the AHNA website for endorsed and approved aromatherapy courses for nurses (www.ahna.org).

Aromatherapy for Dementia

Lin et al. conducted a cross-over randomized trial on 70 Chinese older adults with dementia.[18] Half the subjects were randomly assigned to the active group (lavender inhalation) for 3 weeks and then switched to the control group (sunflower inhalation) for another 3 weeks; the other half did the opposite. Clinical outcomes were evaluated using the Chinese versions of Cohen-Mansfield Agitation Inventory (CCMAI) and Neuropsychiatric Inventory (CNPI). The mean CCMAI total scores decreased from 24.68 to 17.77 ($t = 10.79$, df = 69, $p < .001$). The CNPI scores changed from 63.17 (SD = 17.81) to 58.77 (SD = 16.74) ($t = 14.59$, df = 69, $p < .001$) after receiving Treatment A (*Lavandula angustifolia*). Also, Fowler shows aromatherapy could help crisis management during the night shift for adolescents in a residential treatment center.[19]

An in vitro study by Huang et al. in 2008 demonstrates that lavender essential oil reversibly inhibited GABA-induced currents in a concentration-dependent manner whereas no inhibition of NMDA- or AMPA-induced currents was noted.[20] Lavender essential oil elicited a significant dose-dependent reduction in both inhibitory and excitatory transmission, with a net depressant effect on neurotransmission (in contrast to the classic GABA[A] antagonist picrotoxin, which evoked profound epileptiform burst firing in these cells). Lavender is commonly used to relax and soothe patients with dementia.

Five R. J. Buckle students chose to do their research projects on dementia between 1999 and 2003. The most common essential oil chosen was lavender, but there were also good results from mandarin and frankincense. Sadly, none of the studies has been published.

Aromatherapy for Pain

Previous studies using aromatherapy for pain suggest that both inhaled and topically applied essential oils may affect the perception of pain. More recent research indicates that some essential oils might have analgesic properties. Also, aromatherapy uses touch, particularly the 'M' Technique, and this technique has profound effects on chronic pain on its own, which are enhanced with essential oils. Please see Case Study 2 on chronic pain later in this chapter.

In 2006, Han et al. found a mixture of essential oils topically applied to the abdomen of 67 nurses had a statistically significant effect on reducing menstrual pain.[21] This randomized, placebo-controlled study is one of several exciting studies carried out by nurses to come out of Korea. The essential oils used were *Lavandula angustifolia*, *Salvia sclarea*, and *Rosa centifolia*. Subjects were nurses who rated their pain less than 6 on a 10-point visual analog scale and who did not use contraceptive drugs. Kim et al. explored the use of 2% lavender oil inhaled immediately postoperatively in a randomized, controlled study of 50 patients undergoing breast biopsy surgery.[22] A visual analog score (0–10) was used at 5, 30, and 60 minutes postoperatively, as well as patient pain satisfaction scores and time required to discharge from the postanesthesia care unit. It is strange that such a low percentage was used for inhalation

(2%)—normally full-strength essential oil is used—and hardly surprising that pain scores were not affected. However, subjects did report a higher satisfaction pain control rate in the lavender group. Perhaps it might have been simpler to have evaluated the difference in "comfort." This was the outcome measure in a study by Nord looking at promoting comfort in pediatric perianesthesia.[23] She used lavender and ginger on 91 patients: the control group received a nonactive vegetable oil with a slight aroma (jojoba). The mean distress was lower for the experimental group.

Aromatherapy for Infection

There is considerable published research available on the in vitro antibacterial, antifungal, and antiviral effects of a great number of essential oils. A search on Medline using the botanical name of the individual aromatic plant coupled with the term *essential oil* produces between 20 and 100 papers per essential oil.

The world is experiencing a soaring increase in resistant infections. Methicillin-resistant *Staphylococcus aureus* (MRSA) has become endemic.[24] Even vancomycin, often used to treat MRSA, has shown disappointing cure rates: 44% failure in treating bacteria and 40% failure in treating lower respiratory tract infections.[25] Some antifungal drugs are no longer working,[26] and some antivirals are no longer effective.[27]

Warnke et al. tested tea tree against several *Staphylococcus* strains including MRSA, four *Streptococcus* strains, and three *Candida* strains including *Candida krusei*.[28] Tea tree showed considerable efficacy. Bowler et al. used tea tree in conjunction with conventional antibiotics to control MRSA spread in residents of five nursing homes in Wisconsin.[29] After intervention and follow-up for 12 months or more, the prevalence of MRSA carriage at the nursing homes decreased by 67% ($p < .001$), and 120 of 147 (82%) nursing home residents and 111 of 125 (89%) clinic patients remained culture negative for MRSA. Tea tree was one of the essential oils originally tested by Edwards-Jones et al. in a wound dressing pack.[30] They looked at both the vapor and topical effect of essential oils and found geranium and tea tree were the most effective against MRSA in a dressing. In another study, Thomson et al. presented a research protocol for a randomized controlled

trial of tea tree oil (5%) body wash versus standard body wash to prevent colonization with MRSA in critically ill adults.[31] The actual study ($n = 1,080$) has just been completed in Northern Ireland in two intensive care units, so watch for the research results.

Sherry and Warnke broke new ground when they applied essential oils directly into the bones of patients suffering from osteomyelitis (MRSA) and presented their findings at the American Academy of Orthopedic Surgeons.[32] Twenty-five patients with MRSA infections were treated: 16 involved bone, 6 a joint, and 3 soft tissue. Ten patients were diabetic. Following debridement, diluted essential oils were applied to the infected sites. In the case of bone, calcium (Osteoset) beads soaked in essential oils were used. In 22 cases, the infection was completely resolved either without antibiotics (19) or with antibiotics (3). In Australia, 90% of hospital-acquired infections are MRSA. In vitro studies on tea tree and eucalyptus show that both were effective within 1 minute against 90% of the five multiple-resistant tuberculosis (TB) organisms tested. The paper concludes that essential oils could be a possible mass treatment for TB.

Finally, three other studies that might be useful in nursing care include the following. An essential oil mixture of diluted tea tree, peppermint, and lemon reduced malodor and volatile sulfur compounds (VSC) in intensive care unit patients.[33] Black pepper stimulated swallowing reflex in people with swallowing dysfunction following stroke. This Japanese study found inhalation of black pepper essential oil for 1 minute reduced the delay in swallowing, compared with lavender oil or distilled water ($p < .03$) ($n = 105$).[34] A paper by Lesho suggests that essential oils would be useful to reduce the incidence of hospital-acquired and ventilator-associated pneumonia.[35]

Several exhibits follow that contain descriptions of the therapeutic value of five of the most useful and commonly available essential oils suitable for holistic nursing care. See **Exhibit 25-4** for applications for lavender. Applications for peppermint can be found in **Exhibit 25-5**. Applications for tea tree oil can be found in **Exhibit 25-6**. Applications for eucalyptus can be found in **Exhibit 25-7**. Applications for frankincense

EXHIBIT 25-4   Properties of Lavender *(Lavandula angustifolia)*

1. Skin regenerative: For burns, wound healing, insect bites, mild eczema[36]
2. Calming,[21,37] good for insomnia and depression,[38] good for stress[39,40]
3. Reduces agitation in dementia[19]
4. Enhances sense of well-being[41]
5. Effective against ticks[42]
6. Fungistatic, not fungicidal[43]

EXHIBIT 25-5   Properties of Peppermint *(Mentha piperita)*

1. Analgesic,[44] migraine,[45] postherpetic neuralgia[46]
2. Antinausea,[47-49] opiate detoxification[50]
3. Useful in treatment of irritable bowel syndrome (antispasmodic)[51]
4. Antibacterial;[52-54] useful in sinusitis[55]
5. Effective against MRSA and TB;[33] viriducidal[56]

EXHIBIT 25-6   Properties of Tea Tree *(Melaleuca alternifolia)*

1. Bacterial infections,[57] acne.[58]
2. Fungal infections including athlete's foot, tinea.
3. Most skin infections, including impetigo, cold sores, herpes,[59] and warts.[60]
4. Mouth infections.[61]
5. Effective against MRSA.[29-31,62]
6. Antiviral, including influenza.[63,64]
7. Antitumoral.[65,66]
8. Vaginal infections, especially *Candida albicans*.[67] Tea tree can be diluted and used as a vaginal douche for infections, or it can be diluted in carrier oil and used on tampon: put 2 drops of tea tree oil in 1 teaspoonful of carrier oil, roll tampon in mixture, and insert into vagina. Repeat with fresh tampon every 4 hours and leave in overnight. Relief should occur within 48 hours. Vaginal thrush should not reoccur.

EXHIBIT 25-7   Properties of Blue Gum *(Eucalyptus globulus)*

1. Respiratory complaints, including TB[55,68-70]
2. Effective against pneumonia in ventilated patients[36,71]
3. Antibacterial;[72] effective against MRSA[73]
4. Effective against head lice[74]

can be found in **Exhibit 25-8**. The kind of application depends on whether a psychological or physiologic response is required. Nurses should remember to ask their patients if they like the aroma before beginning their aromatherapy treatment and make sure to have some clinical training. Essential oil companies used by the author are listed in Table 25-2.

■ CONCLUSION

There is tremendous emphasis on "doing" in the Western world, where we are judged (and tend to judge others) on what we "do" rather than our ability "to be." But illness takes away a patient's ability "to do" and forces him or her to address his or her "being" on a much broader scale. This can be quite frightening. However, it allows the nurse an opportunity to share with the patient a glimpse of a multidimensional world, which until then has remained hidden. Aromatherapy gives caring to the soul, the mind, and the body—a true holistic therapy. And it smells good!

■ HOLISTIC CARING PROCESS

Holistic Assessment

In preparing to use essential oils clinically, the nurse assesses the following parameters:

- The client's like or dislike of particular aromas because this affects the choice of essential oils
- The client's like or dislike of touch because this affects what method is chosen
- The client's perception of the problem because this indicates the targeted outcome
- The client's level of stress because this directly affects the oils chosen

- The client's understanding of aromatherapy—this indicates whether the client is expecting cure or care
- The client's skin integrity because certain essential oils are inappropriate with poor skin integrity
- The client's age—very young or elderly clients need low percentages of essential oils
- The client's medical history because previous illness could be related to the current problem
- The client's current medical status because this indicates which essential oils are safest to use
- The client's sleep pattern because this indicates if this is one of the main areas for improvement
- The client's weight and height because these indicate the amount of essential oil required
- The client's blood pressure because this indicates hypotensive or hypertensive essential oils
- The client's medication because certain medications could be affected by essential oils
- The client's respiratory pattern because this indicates whether there is chronic obstructive pulmonary disease or asthma
- The client's reproductive status because this indicates whether the patient is pregnant, reducing the choice of essential oils
- The client's allergy status, particularly to ragweed, because some essential oils would then be inappropriate
- The client's close proximity to others who may be affected by the aromas because this will affect which essential oils are chosen

EXHIBIT 25-8   Properties of Frankincense *(Boswellia carteri)*

1. Good for relaxation, meditation, and spiritual renewal
2. Very useful in terminal agitation[75]
3. Good for scars[76]
4. Anti-inflammatory[77,78]
5. Useful in asthma[79]
6. Antiparasitic[80]
7. Anticancer[81,82]

Identification of Patterns/ Challenges/Needs

The following patterns/challenges/needs (see Chapter 7) compatible with aromatherapy are as follows:

- Altered circulation
- Risk of infection
- Constipation
- Perceived constipation
- Risk for constipation
- Altered tissue perfusion (peripheral)
- Ineffective breathing pattern
- Dysfunctional ventilatory weaning response
- Impaired tissue integrity
- Risk for impaired skin integrity
- Energy field disturbance
- Impaired verbal communication
- Social isolation
- Risk for loneliness
- Sexual dysfunction
- Caregiver role strain
- Ineffectual individual coping
- Defensive coping
- Ineffective family coping
- Family coping with potential for growth
- Decisional conflict
- Impaired physical mobility
- Impaired bed mobility
- Activity intolerance
- Fatigue
- Sleep pattern disturbance
- Delayed surgical recovery
- Adult failure to thrive
- Ineffective breastfeeding
- Bathing or hygiene self-care deficit
- Relocation stress syndrome
- Body image disturbance
- Chronic low self-esteem
- Sensory or perception alterations, such as olfactory or tactile
- Hopelessness
- Powerlessness
- Chronic confusion
- Impaired memory
- Chronic pain
- Nausea
- Dysfunctional grieving
- Chronic sorrow
- Post trauma response
- Anxiety
- Fear

Outcome Identification

Exhibit 25-9 guides the nurse in client outcomes, nursing prescriptions, and evaluations for the use of aromatherapy as a nursing intervention.

Setting Goals

It is important to establish mutually acceptable goals prior to beginning an aromatherapy and 'M' Technique session. These outcomes may be immediate or long term, but should be relevant to aromatherapy and the role of holistic nursing care. Clients are more likely to be content with the outcomes if they are perceived to be achievable within a specified time frame and are deemed successful with recognizable tools such as a visual analog. It is recommended that such goals are judged by using a visual analog scale (0–10), where 0 is lack of the symptom (such as pain) and 10 is the worst imaginable symptom (such as pain). Informed consent (with written consent where possible) is required before using essential oils.

Therapeutic Care Plan and Interventions

Before the session:

- If in a clinical area, inform other people that aromatherapy will be used and assess if they are comfortable with the aromas that will be used.
- Request no interruptions for the period required. This could be 5 minutes for a hand 'M' Technique using essential oils, or 15 minutes for hand, face, and feet. Allow 5–15 minutes for inhalation, 5 minutes for wound application, 5–10 minutes for sitz or hand bath, and 10–15 minutes for compress.
- Discuss the length of the session, the required outcome, and the method to be used.
- Ask the client to empty the bladder for comfort.
- Prepare the hospital bed or surface on which you will be working. Adjust the bed height for your convenience.
- Ensure that the temperature of the room is appropriate.
- Ask the client to remove eyeglasses if using direct inhalation as a method.

EXHIBIT 25-9   Nursing Interventions: Aromatherapy

Client Outcomes	Nursing Prescriptions	Evaluations
The client will choose aromas from a selection offered by the nurse.	Provide the client with various aromas to choose from that are suitable for client's condition.	The client chose aromas from a selection offered by the nurse.
The client will demonstrate positive physiologic outcomes in response to the aromatherapy and the 'M' Technique sessions, such as the following:	Assess the client's physiologic outcomes in response to aromatherapy and the 'M' Technique before and immediately after each session. Evaluate the client for the following:	The client demonstrated the following:
■ Decreased respiratory rate	■ Decreased respiratory rate	■ Decreased respiratory rate
■ Decreased heart rate	■ Decreased heart rate	■ Decreased heart rate
■ Decreased blood pressure	■ Decreased blood pressure	■ Decreased blood pressure
■ Decreased muscle tension	■ Decreased muscle tension	■ Decreased muscle tension
■ Decreased fatigue	■ Decreased fatigue	■ Decreased fatigue
■ Decreased pain	■ Decreased pain	■ Decreased pain
■ Improved physical mobility	■ Improved physical mobility	■ Improved physical mobility
■ Improved bed mobility	■ Improved bed mobility	■ Improved bed mobility
■ Improved activity tolerance	■ Improved activity tolerance	■ Improved activity tolerance
■ Improved sleep pattern	■ Improved sleep pattern	■ Improved sleep pattern
■ Improved surgical recovery	■ Improved surgical recovery	■ Improved surgical recovery
■ Improved ability to thrive	■ Improved ability to thrive	■ Improved ability to thrive
■ Improved breast-feeding	■ Improved breast-feeding	■ Improved breast-feeding
■ Improved self-care	■ Improved self-care	■ Improved self-care
■ Reduced nausea	■ Reduced nausea	■ Reduced nausea
■ Reduced constipation	■ Reduced constipation	■ Reduced constipation
■ Reduced risk of infection	■ Reduced risk of infection	■ Reduced risk of infection
The client will demonstrate positive psychological outcomes in response to the aromatherapy and the 'M' Technique sessions, such as the following:	Assess client's psychological outcomes in response to aromatherapy and the 'M' Technique before and immediately after each session. Evaluate the client for the following:	The client demonstrated the following:
■ Improved body image	■ Improved body image	■ Improved body image
■ Improved self-esteem	■ Improved self-esteem	■ Improved self-esteem
■ Improved olfactory ability	■ Improved olfactory ability	■ Improved olfactory ability
■ Improved tactile ability	■ Improved tactile ability	■ Improved tactile ability
■ Reduced hopelessness	■ Reduced hopelessness	■ Reduced hopelessness
■ Reduced powerlessness	■ Reduced powerlessness	■ Reduced powerlessness
■ Reduced confusion	■ Reduced confusion	■ Reduced confusion
■ Improved memory	■ Improved memory	■ Improved memory
■ More functional grieving	■ More functional grieving	■ More functional grieving
■ Reduced sorrow	■ Reduced sorrow	■ Reduced sorrow
■ Improved trauma response	■ Improved trauma response	■ Improved trauma response
■ Reduced anxiety	■ Reduced anxiety	■ Reduced anxiety
■ Reduced fear	■ Reduced fear	■ Reduced fear
■ More effective coping	■ More effective coping	■ More effective coping
■ Less decisional conflict	■ Less decisional conflict	■ Less decisional conflict
■ Better family coping	■ Better family coping	■ Better family coping

- Prepare the environment for optimal relaxation if this is the purpose of the session.
- Place a clean towel under the hand or foot for 'M' Technique.
- Wash hands.
- Prepare mixture of essential oils in carrier oil if being applied topically to the skin.
- Prepare diffuser with mixture of undiluted essential oils if inhalation is being used.
- Prepare compress with either water or carrier oil for wound care.
- Prepare bath for immersion of limb or body.
- Prepare basin with very hot water for steam inhalation.
- Prepare basin with warm water and essential oils for body wash.
- Focus on your healing intention, and then begin.

At the beginning of the session:
- Tell the client what you are going to do before you do it.
- Tell the client which part of the body you are going to touch before you touch it.
- Make sure that the limb is supported.
- Ask the client to tell you what the pressure feels like to him or her (on a level of 0–10) if you are using the 'M' Technique. It should be a level 3.
- Warm your hands by rubbing them together.
- Apply a small amount of dilute essential oil into one hand if using the 'M' Technique.
- Put required drops of essential oil in basin for steam inhalation.
- Put required number of drops of essential oil in diffuser.
- Begin slowly and rhythmically if using the 'M' Technique.
- Help position the client above steaming bowl for inhalation, and place towel over head and shoulders.
- Begin applying dilute essential oils to wound or burn.

During the session:
- Maintain constant pressure, rhythm, and speed if using the 'M' Technique.
- Discourage conversation.
- Encourage client to focus on the treatment.
- If client is using inhalation method, encourage him or her to breathe deeply.

- Have tissues available for expectoration if steam inhalation is used.
- Have empty basin available if essential oil is being used for nausea.
- Stay with a confused, elderly, infirm, or very young patient if inhalation or bath is being used.
- Reassess the client as you move through the session.

At the end of the session:
- Remove any apparatus used for aromatherapy (basin, bath, diffuser).
- If the client has gone to sleep, gently wake him or her after a few moments.
- Tell the client that you have finished the session.
- Dry skin if bath has been used.
- Wash your hands.

Specific Interventions
- Have the client discuss any changes or experiences that occurred during the session.
- The nurse may reassess physical parameters such as blood pressure, pulse, and respiration.
- The nurse may suggest that the treatment be self-applied at regular intervals.
- The nurse may make up a series of treatments in a bottle for such self-application.
- The nurse may schedule a follow-up treatment.

Case Study (Implementation)
CASE STUDY 1

Setting: Outpatient unit

Client: G. D., a 54-year-old Caucasian woman with mild asthma

Patterns/Challenges/Needs:
1. Altered physical regulation
2. Anxiety
3. Fear
4. Powerlessness
5. Ineffective coping related to anxiety around asthma attacks

G. D. is a 54-year-old woman who has had asthma with frequent wheezing and coughing problems for the last 10 years and fears each attack when she feels she "just cannot get enough air." The attacks are triggered by very cold weather, exercise, and stress. She has tried relaxation techniques, but none has really worked. G. D. developed asthma as a child, but during her teenage years her symptoms resolved and only reappeared about 10 years ago. She has been wheezing on a daily basis for the last 9 months, and currently the wheezing is controlled with fluticasone propionate (Advair).

Prior to commencing Advair, G. D. required emergency department treatment as a result of an asthma flare-up. At the time, she was prescribed a course of oral corticosteroids and antibiotics, albuterol and amoxicillin. This resolved the asthma completely, and she was much better for a month. But after a month, she felt the albuterol did not really help, so her physician switched her to Advair. This seems to be controlling the asthma; however, when she exercises, her chest tightens and she coughs. She particularly resents that the asthma prevents her from exercising because she is trying to lose weight. She has allergies to mold and some animals, she does not smoke, and there are no pets in the house. Her father has eczema.

The nurse outlined the use of inhaling essential oils and their effect on opening up the respiratory tract. She invited G. D. to smell the aromas of *E. globulus*, *E. smithii*, *E. citriadora*, *Ravansara aromatica*, *L. latifolia*, and *Boswellia carteri*. The client liked *E. globulus* and *B. carteri* best. The nurse prepared a bowl of steaming hot water and added two drops of *E. globulus* and two drops of *B. carteri* and asked the client to close her eyes, lean forward, and inhale the aroma. The client did so. The nurse reassured her that she (the nurse) would stay with her, and asked if it would be acceptable to place a towel over her head and shoulders to make a steam tent. This steam tent could be removed at any time. The client agreed. The client was encouraged to breathe slowly in and out through her mouth as the water cooled, and then in and out through her nose. The client was asked if she could feel the essential oils deep within her chest, and the client said yes. The session was concluded after 8 minutes when the client felt that she had received enough.

The client stated that the effect of inhaling the essential oils and the steam was quite remarkable and appeared to open up her airway almost immediately. The steam was comforting to her chest, she felt the aromas were familiar and calming—and she felt it was a very reassuring treatment to receive although she had been dubious of whether aromatherapy would have any effect. The nurse offered the client a towel to wipe her face that was very wet from the steam.

The nurse told G. D. where she could obtain essential oils if she wished to continue treatment on her own and to come back in a week to reassess the situation. G. D. continued to use daily inhalations of *E. globulus* and *B. carteri*. She found that the effects of the essential oils and steam on her asthma lasted for about 3 hours, but that the calming effect lasted considerably longer. She felt the aromatherapy session was quite intense initially because of the steam and the heat. However, it was a very simple and inexpensive way to help herself: she felt empowered and no longer helpless. She was particularly pleased that she did not need to go and see her physician, and her supply of Advair lasted a long time, as she needed to use it only once a day and sometimes would go for several days without needing to use it at all.

The nurse showed G. D. how to apply the essential oils topically to her chest if she did not want to use steam. She found the topical method very useful although not as effective on the asthma as the steam inhalation. The nurse also told G. D. that she could purchase a blank personal inhaler—it looks a little like a Vicks inhaler. The essential oils could be added to a small amount of scent-free soap to fix the aroma and placed inside the inhaler tube. The personal inhaler was something small and easy to use that G. D. could have with her at all times that could help her until she was able to get home and use a steam tent.

Evaluation

The nurse determined with G. D. if the desired outcomes had been achieved. Both the nurse and G. D. felt that the inhaled essential oils had proved effective on all five outcomes:

1. Altered physical regulation (asthma) went from a 7 to a 3.
2. Anxiety went from an 8 to a 2.
3. Fear went from a 7 to a 2.

4. Powerlessness went from an 8 to a 2.
5. Ineffective coping related to anxiety around asthma attacks went from a 7 to a 3.

CASE STUDY 2

Setting: Hospital inpatient

Client: B. S., an 82-year-old Caucasian woman with unresolved chronic pain resulting from severe spinal degeneration

Patterns/Challenges/Needs:

1. Chronic pain
2. Anxiety
3. Fear
4. Powerlessness
5. Ineffective coping related to chronic pain

B. S. is an 82-year-old woman who had been experiencing severe back pain. X-rays revealed spondylolisthesis of L4 and L5 secondary to severe degenerative changes, a central spinal stenosis of L1 through L4, and a mild compression fracture of L2. B. S. had a caudal epidural block without relief. For the following 10 days, she had been on bed rest with bathroom privileges only. She was on 6-hour medication for pain control, but the medication (morphine derived) left her nauseated and confused. The pain remained at a 5–6 on a scale of 0–10. Prior to the aromatherapy session, she was lying rigid in bed with her eyes closed, her respirations were shallow, and her skin was very pale. When she was called by name her eyes seemed glazed and her lips stuck to her teeth when she tried to reply. She said that she had been given pain medication about 3 hours previously, but it "hadn't helped much." She had been unable to eat because she felt so nauseated. Her oxygen saturation was 94%, her heart rate was 89 beats per minute, and her breathing was shallow (24 breaths per minute).

The nurse asked B. S. if she had any likes or dislikes when it came to aromas. She said she liked flowery smells and disliked the smell of food at the present time. She was open to being touched and said she would prefer her hands and face to be touched rather than her feet and legs. The nurse chose specific essential oils to alter perception of pain (*Rosa damascena* and *L. angustifolia*), to relieve nausea (*Zingiber officinalis*),

and to give comfort and relaxation (*Salvia sclarea* and *Chamaemelum nobile*). She made a 5% solution of the essential oils in jojoba oil.

The nurse centered herself before making her touch known so that B. S. would know the texture and temperature of her touch. Then, the nurse carried out a 5-minute 'M' Technique with 5% solution of *L. angustifolia, Z. officinalis, C. nobile, S. sclarea,* and *R. damascena* (one drop each essential oil in 5 cc of grapeseed carrier oil) on each of her hands. She worked slowly and rhythmically, keeping her pressure light. She checked with B. S. that the pressure was a 3 (on a scale of 0–10). B. S. nodded but did not say anything. The nurse wrapped each hand in a hand towel at completion. Then, the nurse completed an 'M' Technique of B. S.'s face; this took an additional 5 minutes. B. S.'s face began to soften a little toward the end of the technique and her breathing became less shallow. She sighed several times. At the end of the treatment B. S. was nearly asleep. The nurse checked oxygen saturation (97%) and her heart rate (74 beats per minute). Her respirations were down by 14 breaths a minute.

B. S. slept for 2 hours and later stated it was the first time she had been without pain since the accident. The nurse continued to return to give the aromatherapy treatment using the 'M' Technique each day. Each time, B. S. experienced profound pain relief that was unobtainable through medication. Immediately following the 'M' Technique, her pain was rated as a 1. This effect lasted for 3 hours. The relaxing effect of the 'M' Technique coupled with the analgesic effect of the essential oils seemed to enable B. S. to relax into her pain and thus achieve relief.

Evaluation

The nurse determined with B. S. if the desired outcomes had been achieved. Both the nurse and B. S. felt that the 15 minutes of 'M' Technique with dilute essential oils had proved effective on all five outcomes:

1. Chronic pain went from a 5 to a 1.
2. Anxiety went from a 7 to a 1.
3. Fear went from a 7 to a 2.
4. Powerlessness went from a 9 to a 2.
5. Ineffective coping related to chronic pain went from a 7 to a 2.

Directions for
FUTURE RESEARCH

1. Evaluate the outcome of inhaled essential oils on sinusitis and/or asthma.
2. Evaluate the outcome of inhaled aromas on chemo-induced and/or postoperative nausea.
3. Evaluate the effect of topically applied dilute essential oils on postradiation burns.
4. Evaluate the effect of topically applied essential oils and the 'M' Technique on chronic pain.
5. Evaluate the effect of topically applied dilute essential oils on wound healing, both noninfected and infected.

Nurse Healer
REFLECTIONS

After reading this chapter, the nurse healer will be able to answer or to begin the process of answering the following questions:

- What is important for me to know before I begin using essential oils?
- How do I know whether to apply an essential oil topically or ask the patient to inhale it?
- What is my experience of inhaling the five essential oils discussed in this chapter?
- What do I feel about using aromatherapy with the 'M' Technique for chronic pain?
- What do I feel about using essential oils for infection?
- What do I feel about using aromatherapy as part of holistic nursing care?

For a full suite of assignments and additional learning activities, use the access code located in the front of your book to visit this exclusive website: http://go.jblearning.com/dossey. If you do not have an access code, you can obtain one at the site.

NOTES

1. J. Buckle, *Clinical Aromatherapy: Essential Oils in Practice* (New York: Churchill Livingstone, 2003).
2. J. Buckle, "Take Five and Relax," *Nursing Spectrum* (New York and New Jersey edition) 18A, no. 11 (2006): 23–23.
3. J. Buckle, "The 'M' Technique for dementia," *Working with Older People* 13, no. 3 (2009): 22–24.
4. J. Buckle, "The 'M' Technique: Touch for the Critically Ill or Actively Dying," *Positive Health* 152, no. 1 (2008). http://www.positivehealth.com/article/bodywork/the-m-technique-touch-for-the-critically-ill-or-actively-dying.
5. J. Buckle et al., "Measurement of Regional Cerebral Blood Flow Associated with the 'M' Technique—Light Massage Therapy: A Case Series and Longitudinal Study Using SPECT," *Journal of Alternative and Complementary Medicine* 14, no. 8 (2008): 903–910.
6. J. Buckle, "Should Nursing Take Aromatherapy More Seriously?" *British Journal of Nursing* 16, no. 2 (2006): 116–120.
7. C. Burr, *The Emperor of Scent* (New York: Random House, 2003).
8. C. Brownlee, "Mapping Aroma: Smells Light Up Distinct Brain Parts," *Science News* 167, no. 22 (2005): 340–341.
9. N. Goel, H. Kim, and R. Lao, "The Olfactory Stimulus Modifies Nighttime Sleep in Young Men and Women," *Chronobiology International* 22, no. 5 (2005): 889–904.
10. Y. Fu et al., "Antimicrobial Activity of Clove and Rosemary Essential Oils Alone and in Combination," *Phytotherapy Research* 21, no. 10 (2007): 989–994.
11. J. Watson, *Caring Science as Sacred Science* (Philadelphia, PA: F. A. Davis, 2005).
12. E. Barrett, "The Theoretical Matrix for a Rogerian Nursing Practice," *Theoria: Journal of Nursing Theory* 9, no. 4 (2000): 3–7.
13. B. Dossey, *Florence Nightingale: Mystic, Visionary, Healer* (Philadelphia, PA: F. A. Davis, 2009).
14. H. Erickson, "Philosophy and Theory of Holism," *Nursing Clinics of North America* 42 (2007): 139–163.
15. K. Kejlovia, D. Jirova, H. Bendova, P. Gajdos, and H. Kolarava, "Phototoxicity of Essential Oils Intended for Cosmetic Use," *Toxicology in Vitro* 24, no. 8 (2010): 2084–2089.
16. J. Bastard and D. Tiran, "Aromatherapy and Massage for Antenatal Anxiety: Its Effect on the Fetus," *Complementary Therapies in Clinical Practice* 12, no. 1 (2006): 48–54.
17. R. Tisserand and T. Balacs, *Essential Oil Safety* (London, England: Churchill Livingstone, 1995).
18. P. Lin, W. Chan, B. Ng, and L. Lam, "Efficacy of Aromatherapy (*Lavandula angustifolia*) as an Intervention for Agitated Behaviors in Chinese Older Persons with Dementia: A Cross-Over Randomized Trial," *International Journal of Geriatric Psychiatry* 22, no. 5 (2007): 405–410.
19. N. Fowler, "Aromatherapy Used as an Integrative Tool for Crisis Management by Adolescents in a Residential Treatment Center," *Journal of Child and Adolescent Psychiatric Nursing* 19, no. 2 (2005): 69–76.

20. L. Huang et al., "Both *Melissa officinalis* (Mo) and *Lavandula angustifolia* (La) Essential Oils Have Putative Anti-Agitation Properties in Humans, Indicating Common Components with a Depressant Action in the Central Nervous System," *Journal of Pharmacy and Pharmacology* 60, no. 11 (2008): 1515–1522.

21. S. Han, M. Hur, J. Buckle, J. Choi, and M. Lee, "Effects of Aromatherapy on Symptoms of Dysmenorrhea in College Students: A Randomized, Placebo-Controlled Clinical Trial," *Journal of Complementary and Alternative Medicine* 12, no. 6 (2006): 38–41.

22. J. Kim et al., "Evaluation of Aromatherapy in Treating Postoperative Pain: Pilot Study," *Pain Practice* 6, no. 4 (2006): 273–276.

23. D. Nord. "Effectiveness of the Essential Oils Lavender and Ginger in Promoting Children's Comfort in a Perianesthesia Setting," *Journal of Perianesthesia Nursing* 24, no. 5 (2009): 307–312.

24. C. Arias and B. Murray, "Antibiotic-Resistant Bugs in the 21st Century: A Clinical Super Challenge," *New England Journal of Medicine* 360 (2009): 439–443.

25. D. Wegner, "No Mercy for MRSA: Treatment Alternatives to Vancomycin and Linezolid," *Medical Laboratory Observer* (January 2005). http://findarticles.com/p/articles/mi_m3230/is_1_37/ai_n9770627/.

26. A. Espnel-Ingroff, "Mechanisms of Resistance to Antifungal Agents: Yeasts and Filamentous Fungi," *Revista Iberoamericana de Micologia* 25, no. 2 (2008): 101–106.

27. C. Gilbert and G. Bolvin, "Human Cytomegalovirus Resistance to Antiviral Drugs," *Antimicrobial Agents and Chemotherapy* 49, no. 3 (2005): 873–883.

28. P. Warnke et al., "The Battle Against Multi-Resistant Strains: Renaissance of Antimicrobial Essential Oils as a Promising Force to Fight Hospital-Acquired Infections," *Journal of Craniomaxillofacial Surgery* 37, no. 7 (2009): 392–397.

29. W. Bowler, J. Bresnahan, A. Bradfish, C. Fernandez, "An Integrated Approach to Methicillin-Resistant *Staphylococcus aureus* Control in a Rural, Regional-Referral Healthcare Setting," *Infection Control and Hospital Epidemiology* 31, no. 3 (2010): 269–275.

30. V. Edwards-Jones, R. Buck, S. Shawcross, M. Dawson, and K. Dunn, "The Effect of Essential Oils on Methicillin-Resistant *Staphylococcus aureus* Using a Dressing Model," *Burns* 30, no. 8 (2004): 772–777.

31. G. Thompson et al., "A Randomized Controlled Trial of Tea Tree Oil (5%) Body Wash Versus Standard Body Wash to Prevent Colonization with Methicillin-Resistant *Staphylococcus aureus* (MRSA) in Critically Ill Adults: Research Protocol," *BMC Infectious Disease* 28, no. 8 (2008): 161.

32. E. Sherry and P. Warnke, *Alternative for MRSA and Tuberculosis (TB): Eucalyptus and Tea Tree Oils as New Topical Antibacterials* (paper presented at Orthopedic Surgery Conference, February 13–17, 2002, Dallas, TX).

33. M. Hur, J. Park, W. Maddock-Jennings, D. Kim, and M. Lee, "Reduction of Mouth Malodor and Volatile Sulphur Compounds in Intensive Care Patients Using Essential Oil Mouthwash," *Phytotherapy Research* 21, no. 7 (2007): 641–643.

34. T. Ebihara, S. Ebihara, M. Maruyama, et al., "A Randomized Trial of Olfactory Stimulation Using Black Pepper Oil in Older People with Swallowing Dysfunction," *Journal of the American Geriatric Society* 54, no. 9 (2006): 1410–1416.

35. E. Lesho, "Role of Inhaled Antibacterials in Hospital-Acquired and Ventilator-Associated Pneumonia," *Expert Review of Anti-Infective Therapy* 3, no. 3 (2005): 445–451.

36. J. Valnet, *The Practice of Aromatherapy* (Rochester, VT: Healing Arts, 1990): 146.

37. F. Xu et al., "Pharmaco-physio-psychologic Effect of Ayurvedic Oil-Dripping Treatment Using an Essential Oil from *Lavandula angustifolia*," *Journal of Alternative and Complementary Medicine* 14, no. 8 (2008): 947–956.

38. I. Lee and G. Lee, "Effects of Lavender Aromatherapy on Insomnia and Depression in Women College Students," *Taehan Kanho, Hakhoe Chi* 36, no. 1 (2006): 136–143.

39. E. Pemberton and P. Turpin, "The Effect of Essential Oils on Work-Related Stress in Intensive Care Unit Nurses," *Holistic Nursing Practice* 22, no. 2 (2008): 97–102.

40. B. Bradley, N. Starkey, S. Brown, and R. Lea, "Anxiolytic Effects of *Lavandula angustifolia* Odour on the Mongolian Gerbil Elevated Plus Maze," *Journal of Ethnopharmacology* 111, no. 3. (2007): 517–525.

41. J. Lehrner, G. Marwinski, S. Lehr, P. Johren, and L. Deecke, "Ambient Odors of Orange and Lavender Reduce Anxiety and Improve Mood in a Dental Office," *Physiology and Behavior* 86, nos. 1–2 (2005): 92–95.

42. K. Pirali-Kheirabadi and J. Teixeira da Silva, "*Lavandula angustifolia* Essential Oil as a Novel and Promising Natural Candidate for Tick (*Rhipicephalus (Boophilus) annulatus*) Control," *Experimental Parasitology* 126, no. 2 (2010): 184–186.

43. F. D'Auria et al., "Antifungal Activity of *Lavandula angustifolia* Essential Oil Against *Candida albicans* Yeast and Mycelial Form," *Medical Mycology* 43, no. 5 (2005): 391–396.

44. H. Gobel, "Mint Oil Solution in Tension Headache Is Comparatively as Effective as Paracetamol or Acetylsalicylic Acid," *Notfall Medizin* 27 (2001): 12.

45. A. Borhani et al., "Cutaneous Application of Menthol 10% Solution as an Abortive Treatment of

Migraine Without Aura: A Randomized, Double-Blind, Placebo-Controlled, Cross-Over Study," *International Journal of Clinical Practice* 64, no. 4 (2010): 451–456.

46. S. Davies and L. Harding, "A Novel Treatment for Postherpetic Neuralgia Using Peppermint Oil," *Clinical Journal of Pain* 18, no. 3 (2002): 200–202.

47. A. Piotrowski, "Inhale Peppermint to Relieve Postoperative Nausea" (R. J. Buckle Associates certification no. 293, 2005).

48. S. Irby, "Peppermint for Chemo-Induced Nausea" (R. J. Buckle Associates certification no. 322, 2005).

49. G. Lowdermilk, "Peppermint and Ginger for Chemo-Induced Nausea" (R. J. Buckle Associates certification no. 348, 2007).

50. M. Chalifour, "Peppermint as Anti-Emetic in Opiate Detox" (R. J. Buckle Associates certification no. 270, 2005).

51. R. Kline et al., "Enteric Coated, pH-Dependent Peppermint Oil Capsule for the Treatment of Irritable Bowel Syndrome in Children," *Journal of Pediatrics* 138, no. 1 (2001): 125–128.

52. H. Salari, G. Amine, M. Shirazi, R. Hafezi, and M. Mohammadypour, "Antibacterial Effects of *Eucalyptus globulus* Leaf Extract on Pathogenic Bacteria Isolated from Specimens of Patients," *Clinical Microbiology Infection* 12, no. 2 (2006): 194–196.

53. A. Tyagi and A. Malik, "Antimicrobial Action of Essential Oil Vapours and Negative Air Ions Against *Pseudomonas fluorescens*," *International Journal of Food Microbiology* 143, no. 3 (2010): 205–210.

54. S. Inouye, H. Yamaguchi, and T. Takizawa, "Screening of the Antibacterial Effects of a Variety of Essential Oils on Respiratory Tract Pathogens, Using a Modified Dilution Assay Method," *Journal of Infection and Chemotherapy* 7, no. 4 (2001): 251–254.

55. L. Pitcher, "*Mentha piperita* to Reduce Sinus Pain and Congestion" (R. J. Buckle Associates certification no. 153, 2000).

56. A. Schumacher, J. Reichling, and P. Schnitzler, "Viriducidal Effect of Peppermint Oil on the Enveloped Viruses Herpes Simplex Virus Type 1 and Type 2 in Vitro," *Phytomedicine* 19, no. 607 (2003): 504S–510S.

57. J. Kwiecinski, S. Eick, and K. Wojcik, "Effects of Tea Tree (*Melaleuca alternifolia*) Oil on *Staphylococcus aureus* in Biofilms and Stationary Growth Phase," *International Journal of Antimicrobial Agents* 33, no. 4 (2009): 343–347.

58. S. Enshaieh, A. Jooya, A. Siadat, and F. Iraji, "The Efficacy of 5% Topical Tea Tree Oil Gel in Mild to Moderate Acne Vulgaris: A Randomized, Double-Blind Placebo-Controlled Study," *Indian Journal of Dermatology, Venereology, and Leprology* 73, no. 1 (2007): 22–25.

59. A. Astani, J. Reichling, and P. Schnitzler, "Comparative Study on the Antiviral Activity of Selected Monoterpenes Derived from Essential Oils," *Phytotherapy Research* 24, no. 5 (2010): 673–679.

60. B. Millar and J. Moore, "Successful Topical Treatment of Hand Warts in a Paediatric Patient with Tea Tree Oil (*Melaleuca alternifolia*)," *Complementary Therapies in Clinical Practice* 14, no. 4 (2008): 225–227.

61. J. Bagg et al., "Susceptibility to *Melaleuca alternifolia* (Tea Tree) Oil of Yeasts Isolated from the Mouths of Patients with Advanced Cancer," *Oral Oncology* 42, no. 5 (2006): 487–492.

62. A. Brady, T. Farnan, J. Toner, D. Gilpin, and M. Tunney, "Treatment of a Cochlear Implant Biofilm Infection: A Potential Role for Alternative Antimicrobial Agents," *Journal of Laryngology and Otology* 124, no. 7 (2010): 729–738.

63. A. Garozzo et al., "In Vitro Antiviral Activity of *Melaleuca alternifolia* Essential Oil," *Letters in Applied Microbiology* 49, no. 6 (2009): 806–808.

64. F. Mondello, A. Girolamo, M. Scaturro, and M. L. Ricci, "Determination of *Legionella pneumophila* Susceptibility to *Melaleuca alternifolia* Cheel (Tea Tree) Oil by an Improved Broth Micro-Dilution Method Under Vapor Controlled Conditions," *Journal of Microbiology Methods* 77, no. 2 (2009): 243–248.

65. S. Greay et al., "Inhibition of Established Subcutaneous Murine Tumour Growth with Topical *Melaleuca alternifolia* (Tea Tree) Oil," *Cancer Chemotherapy and Pharmacology* 66, no. 6 (February 21, 2010): 1095–1102. http://www.springerlink.com/content/0wnt5366k2lh1r17/.

66. G. Bozzuto, M. Colone, L. Toccacieli, A. Stringaro, and A. Molinari, "Tea Tree Oil Might Combat Melanoma," *Planta Medica* 77, no. 1 (2011): 54–56.

67. A. Catalán, J. Pacheco, A. Martínez, and M. Mondaca, "In Vitro and In Vivo Activity of *Melaleuca alternifolia* Mixed with Tissue Conditioner on *Candida albicans*," *Oral Surgery, Oral Medicine, Oral Pathology, Oral Radiology, and Endodontology* 105, no. 3 (2008): 327–332.

68. E. Sherry and M. Reynolds, "Inhalational Phytochemicals as Possible Treatment for Pulmonary Tuberculosis: 2 Case Studies," *American Journal of Infection Control* 32, no. 6 (2004): 369–370.

69. A. Sadlon and D. Lamson, "Immune-Modifying and Antimicrobial Effects of Eucalyptus Oil and Simple Inhalation Devices," *Alternative Medicine Review* 15, no. 1 (2010): 33–47.

70. E. Ben-Ayre et al., "Treatments of Upper Respiratory Tract Infections in Primary Care: A Randomized Study Using Aromatic Herbs," *Evidence-Based Complementary and Alternative Medicine* (2011). doi:10.1155/2011/690346

71. C. Cermelli, A. Fabio, G. Fabio, and P. Quaglio, "Effect of Eucalyptus Essential Oil on Respiratory Bacteria and Viruses," *Current Microbiology* 56, no. 1 (2008): 89–92.

72. H. Daroui-Mokaddem et al., "GC/MS Analysis and Antimicrobial Activity of Essential Oil of Fresh Leaves of *Eucalyptus globulus* and Leaves and Stems of *Smyrnium olusatrum* from Constantine (Algeria)," *Natural Products Communication* 5, no. 10 (2010): 1669–1672.

73. A. Todidpur, M. Sattari, R. Omidbaigi, A. Yadegar, and J. Nazemi, "Antibacterial Effect of Essential Oils from Two Medicinal Plants Against Methicillin-Resistant *Staphylococcus aureus* (MRSA)," *Phytomedicine* 17, no. 2 (2010): 142–145.

74. A. Toloza, A. Lucia, E. Zerba, H. Masuh, and M. Picollo, "Eucalyptus Essential Oil Toxicity Against Permethrin-Resistant *Pediculus humanus capitis*," *Parasitology Research* 106, no. 2 (2010): 409–414.

75. K. Eaton-Kelley, "Frankincense and the Terminally Ill Patient" (R. J. Buckle Associates certification no. 303, 2006).

76. P. Calzavara-Pinton, C. Zane, E. Facchinetti, R. Capezzera, and A. Pedretti, "Topical Boswellic Acids for Treatment of Photoaged Skin," *Dermatology Therapy* 23, Suppl. 1 (2010): S28–32.

77. E. Blain, A. Ali, and V. Duance, "*Boswellia frereana* (frankincense) Suppresses Cytokine-Induced Matric Metalloproteinase Expression and Production of Pro-Inflammatory Molecules in Articular Cartilage," *Phytotherapy Research* 24, no. 6 (2010): 905–912.

78. S. Singh et al., "Boswellic Acids: A Leukotriene Inhibitor Also Effective Through Topical Application in Inflammatory Disorders," *Phytomedicine* 15, nos. 6–7 (2008): 400–407.

79. M. Houssen et al., "Natural Anti-Inflammatory Products and Leukotriene Inhibitors as Complementary Therapy for Bronchial Asthma," *Clinical Biochemistry* 43, nos. 10–11 (2010): 887–890.

80. A. Amer and H. Mehlhorn, "Larvicidal Effects of Various Essential Oils Against *Aedes, Anopheles,* and *Culex* Larvae (*Diptera, Culicidae*)," *Parasitology Research* 99, no. 4 (2006): 466–472.

81. M. Frank et al., "Frankincense Oil Derived from *Boswellia carteri* Induces Tumor Specific Cytotoxicity," *BMC Complementary and Alternative Medicine* 18, no. 9 (2009): 6.

82. X. Pang et al., "Acetyl-11-keto-beta-boswellic Acid Inhibits Prostate Tumor Growth by Suppressing Vascular Endothelial Growth Factor Receptor 2–Mediated Angiogenesis," *Cancer Research* 69, no. 14 (2009): 5893–5900.

Relationship-Centered Care and Healing Initiative in a Community Hospital

Pamela Steinke and Nancy Moore

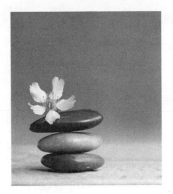

Nurse Healer

OBJECTIVES

Theoretical

- Describe the healing healthcare philosophy.
- Identify nursing theorists who support the healing healthcare philosophy.
- Describe key elements of a healing environment and their application in a tertiary medical center.

Clinical

- Describe key elements of therapeutic presence.
- Identify noninvasive methods for anxiety and pain management.
- Identify nursing interventions in providing care to patients and their families in the dying process.
- Describe how arts in the hospital can help the healing process.
- Identify research studies that support the healing healthcare philosophy.

Personal

- Discuss how nurses themselves are instruments of healing.
- Explore the ethical responsibility for self-care.
- Explore the importance of caring relationships at all levels (e.g., provider–patient, provider–provider, provider–community).

DEFINITIONS

Healing health care: The healing healthcare philosophy is an applied philosophy that facilitates and promotes the healing of the whole person—body, mind, and spirit. It responds to and serves the unique needs of individuals, groups, organizations, communities, and cultures. A healing healthcare project demonstrates the vision of healing health care, which is to heal ourselves, our relationships, and our communities.

Therapeutic presence: Therapeutic presence is the conscious intention to be present for another in a helping or healing way. Therapeutic presence is more an intention than it is a technique. Awareness of how we move into a person's personal space, the tone of our voice, and the way we make contact with our touch are all parts of therapeutic presence.

■ THEORY AND RESEARCH

The healing healthcare philosophy is a foundation that guides all activities at St. Charles Medical Center (SCMC). This philosophy was adopted in the early 1990s to develop an intentional culture and to serve as a guide to enhance the hospital's healing mission during the chaos of a rapidly changing healthcare environment. Healing healthcare is based on the belief that the essence of healing is in relationships; that we must care for the wholeness (body, mind, and spirit) of our patients and one another; and that everything in the environment has an effect on recovery and well-being, either enhancing or impairing the healing process. This philosophy incorporates the ethic of the national Association of Healing Healthcare Advocates—healing ourselves, our relationships, and our community—and is rooted in the healing service of the founders of SCMC, the sisters of St. Joseph of Tipton, Indiana. Healing Healthcare is an applied philosophy that is supported and enriched by the following nursing theorists:[1]

- Jean Watson, Transpersonal Caring Nursing Science
- Martha Rogers, Science of Unitary Human Beings
- Margaret Newman, Model of Health as Expansion of Consciousness

The following are examples of research studies that support the healing healthcare philosophy.

Cooke and colleagues conducted a randomized controlled study in 2005 of 240 patients to assess anxiety before and after listening to patient-preferred music. The study found that music statistically reduced the state of anxiety. The findings support the use of music as an independent nursing intervention for preoperative anxiety in patients having single-day surgery.[2]

Dayton and Henriksen reported in 2007 in the *Joint Commission Journal on Quality and Patient Safety* that communication, although taken for granted as a human activity, is recognized as important once it has failed and that communication failures are a major contributor to adverse events in health care.[3]

Dijkstra, Pietrerse, and Pruyn conducted a meta-analysis in 2006 focused on the developing interest of the impact of the physical environment on patients and healing. In more than 500 studies, it was concluded that there are positive effects on patients from the creation of a healing environment using sunlight, windows, odor control, and seating arrangements. There are three relevant aspects of a healing physical environment that include architectural features, interior design inclusive of color, and ambience. These aspects of the physical hospital environment do have an effect on the well-being of patients

evidenced in the reported metrics of decreased length of stay, the number and strength of analgesics used each day, and lessened anxiety.[4]

Good and colleagues conducted a randomized clinical trial in 2005 to determine the efficacy of relaxation in facilitating pain relief involving 167 patients following intestinal surgery. As a result of their findings, they recommend the use of three nonpharmacologic relaxation techniques (jaw relaxation, intentional breathing, thought stopping), sedative music, and instructions on how to splint the incision while getting out of bed, along with analgesics for greater postoperative relief without additional side effects.[5]

Kennedy and colleagues conducted a randomized controlled study in 2007 of the effectiveness and cost effectiveness of lay-led (nonprofessional) self-care support programs for patients with chronic conditions. They found that although the well-being of people with chronic diseases tends to decline, about one-third of the group participants from a wide range of backgrounds showed substantial improvements in a range of skills that enabled them to self-manage. These data support the application of self-management courses, indicating that they are a useful adjunct to usual care for a modest proportion of attendees.[6]

Lorenz provides an integrative review of research in 2007 on the potential for the patient room to have a positive influence on patients and nurses. The creation of a healing environment is described as the physical and cultural surroundings that are designed to support patients, families, and staff. Five factors were identified in healthcare environmental design that affect patient outcomes. These include psychologically supportive environments, patient control of the environment, social support, availability of positive distractions, and reduction of negative distractions such as noise and odors. Most specifically addressed was the design of the patient room to provide privacy, noise reduction, family interaction, and a sense of control. These factors affect patients' length of stay, prevent adverse events, and reduce infection.[7]

Pacheco-Lopez and colleagues cited in 2006 that recent experimental data indicate that healthcare providers are well advised to further consider placebo effects in therapeutic strategies, with better knowledge now available of their potency, psychological basis, and underlying neurological mechanisms. Current research has uncovered some of the potential neurobiological mechanisms of placebo effects. Thus, placebo effects can benefit organ functioning and the overall health of the individual through positive expectations and behavioral conditioning processes.[8]

In 2004, Ulrich et al. compiled 600 rigorous studies in a landmark analysis that documented the potential for new design concepts to make hospitals safer, more healing, and better places in which to work. They found that not only is there a very large body of evidence to guide hospital design, but a very strong one. Growing scientific literature is confirming that the conventional ways that hospitals are designed contribute to stress and danger; or more positively, that the current level of risk and stress is unnecessary. Improved physical settings can be an important tool in making hospitals safer, more healing, and better places in which to work.[9]

Kshettry and colleagues conducted a randomized study in 2006 of 104 heart patients undergoing open heart surgery who were receiving either complementary therapy (i.e., preoperative guided imagery training with gentle touch or light massage and postoperative music with gentle touch or light massage and guided imagery) or standard care. The conclusions of the study were that the complementary medical therapies protocol was implemented with ease in a busy critical care setting and was acceptable to the vast majority of patients studied. Complementary medical therapy was not associated with safety concerns and appeared to reduce pain and tension in the early recovery from open heart surgery.[10]

■ ST. CHARLES MEDICAL CENTER

Integrating a Healing Philosophy into the Hospital's Strategic Initiatives

St. Charles Medical Center (SCMC) in Bend, Oregon, is a 261-bed tertiary medical center serving central and eastern Oregon. It is the only tertiary medical center within its 33,000-square-mile service area. It offers a broad scope of services, from open heart surgery to rehabilitation, and averages a 4.0-day length of stay. It is a Level II trauma center and has a Level III neonatal intensive care unit. In 2001, St. Charles was the cornerstone of a newly formed health system,

Cascade Healthcare Community, which changed to St. Charles Health System (SCHS) in 2010. SCHS now includes St. Charles Medical Center in Bend, St. Charles Medical Center in Redmond, a 50-bed community hospital, Pioneer Memorial Hospital in Prineville, a 25-bed critical access hospital, and one additional managed critical access hospital. There are also a number of physician clinics and partnerships in the region.

St. Charles has had a history of notable national recognition since 1993 when it was awarded the Healing Healthcare Projects' organizational award for its vision and implementation of healing healthcare and the patient-centered approach. In 2000, St. Charles Medical Center was honored with the Norman Cousins Award for relationship-centered care and noted by the selection committee as "the best hospital in the country with regard to the sacredness of care."[11] St. Charles continues to be highly rated for clinical excellence, patient safety, emergency medicine, women's health, coronary intervention, critical care, and orthopedic and spine surgical excellence. St. Charles Medical Center was further recognized by Thompson Reuters (formerly known as Solucient), a leading source of healthcare intelligence, as a top 100 hospital in areas of quality of care, financial performance, operational efficiency, and adaptation to the environment.[12] Again in 2009, 2010, and 2011, SCHS was rated in the top 50 health systems in the nation for quality and service by Thompson Reuters.

St. Charles, like many hospitals, strives to keep pace with change and address the needs of the rapidly changing healthcare environment in the United States. The healing healthcare philosophy foundation has helped to guide the hospital in intentionally preserving and enhancing its mission during chaotic times. The senior leadership and CEO James Diegel recognize that applying the philosophy is not only the right thing to do, as it enhanced the hospital's mission—to improve the health of those it serves in a spirit of love and compassion—it is also the smart thing to do. People choose SCHS because of the healing nature of its service. The philosophy helps recruitment and retention because caregivers prefer to work in an environment that supports healing. When the environment is healing for patients, it is also healing for the people providing the care. The differentiation of service and care through the healing healthcare philosophy is now considered the system's historical icon and cultural strength. The main applications of the philosophy are healing ourselves, our relationships, patient-focused and family-focused care, environmental design, life skills, life–death transition, arts in the hospital, healing our community, and a principle-based care model.

Healing Ourselves and Our Relationships

Embracing a healing philosophy and integrating it into organization culture takes intention, time, and patience. It also takes a willingness to learn and change continuously based on current climate and learnings. Early in the healing healthcare philosophy implementation, it was believed that St. Charles needed to create something tangible so that people could easily understand the philosophy.

Nancy Moore, the St. Charles chief nursing officer and inspirational leader for nearly 30 years, recalls a pivotal moment that dramatically informed St. Charles's understanding of healing. She was working with the design task force, leading them toward a decision to create a wellness program. A nurse held up her hand and said, "What about us?" In her wisdom at the time, she replied, "Oh, we will get to us, but first we have to take care of the patients." Given all the turmoil and emotions of a major restructuring effort, it became clear that it would not matter what was done for the patients if the caregivers themselves were not cared for in the process. A state-of-the-art wellness center could be created and change the organization to bring each of the disciplines involved in a patient's care to the bedside, but if the caregivers themselves were not healed in the process, it would be an empty shell. No one would want what was created.

It became crystal clear that the essence of healing is in our relationships. This is a human service; who we are and how we work together is what our patients and their families receive. We use technology, but, by and large, it is an extension of ourselves that affects healing. At that time, the group also recognized that many of us did not learn from our family of origin, or during our formal education, the skills and attitudes necessary for healthy relationships.[13] As a result, St. Charles developed personal growth and development workshops, initially called People-Centered Teams: Healing Our Workplace that has evolved to training called People Skills. These workshops provide an opportunity for participants to reflect on what is most important to them and identify belief systems and behaviors that can support them in getting more of what they want. Participants learn to create healthier relationships through improved personal awareness, listening, and differentiated communication. They explore how broadening their personal "comfort zone" can increase individual flexibility and internal resourcefulness. Participants also discover ways to contribute their unique talents, skills, and experience more fully to the work they do and the people they serve. Participants report that the skills help them not only in their work, but also in their personal lives.

In recognition of the increasingly stressful work environment, St. Charles Health System offers a workshop in collaboration with HeartMath LLC, based on research from the Institute of Heart Math. The workshop, called Transforming Stress, provides an opportunity for caregivers to learn the tools of "inner quality management," based on utilizing positive emotion to affect the physiologic response to stress. Caregivers learn to achieve a state of "coherence," which supports them in detaching from stress, thinking clearly, listening more effectively, and improving resiliency and renewal.[14] Since 2005, nearly 680 caregivers have completed our HeartMath workshop. **Figure 26-1** shows the result of studies conducted at the Institute of HeartMath with data provided from St. Charles caregivers who completed preworkshop and postworkshop assessments. The standardized scales on this page are coded so that the desirable end of the graph is toward the top, where substantially above average would be a commendable result and substantially below average would be a poor result. As illustrated, St. Charles caregivers have experienced improvement in perception of well-being and health, stress level, reported depression, and sense of peacefulness after participating in the HeartMath workshop.

St. Charles nurses who are certified to provide therapeutic touch find HeartMath tools useful in centering both the patient and themselves prior to delivering therapeutic touch. In 2011, the workshop was updated to include a greater

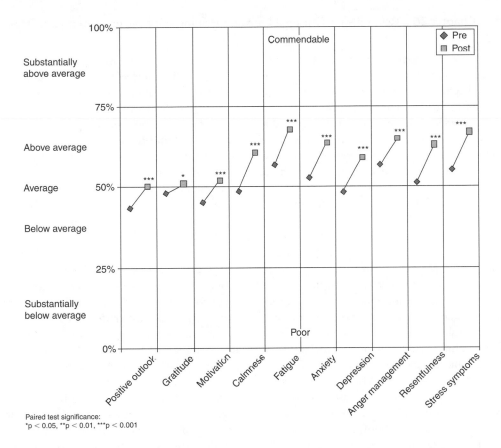

Paired test significance:
*p < 0.05, **p < 0.01, ***p < 0.001

FIGURE 26-1 Healing Ourselves and Our Relationships: HeartMath Study
Source: Copyright © 2011, St. Charles Health System.

focus on caregiver resiliency and genuine caring in the healing environment.

Other resources to support healing ourselves and our relationships include our caregiver assistance program (CAP) and critical incident stress debriefings. CAP offers confidential counseling that is available to caregivers and their family members free of charge, as well as assessment and referral to appropriate resources. The critical incident stress debriefings are available through social services for teams or individuals experiencing unusual amounts of stress, such as caring for many critical patients for a prolonged period of time or helping in a trauma or intense response to an incident.

Patient-Focused and Family-Focused Care

Research indicates that the most effective way to promote healing is for patients to become actively involved in their care.[15-17] Patient-focused and family-focused care actively involves patients and family members or significant others, as the patient desires, in the care process.

This type of care provides services based on the patient's needs. A 2005 study of family members' contribution to care of patients in ICU identified that it was through contact with the family that ICU nurses come to know more about the person for whom they are caring. Family provides a vital source of emotional support to the patient and, in fact, reduces patient anxiety.[18]

When SCMC designed and built the initial electronic medical record (EMR) in 2003, the intention was to utilize the technology to cue nurses to think about family involvement in care. The transition to new technology in 2009 continued to focus on building prompts to cue nurses to focus on patient and family needs. The admission history includes questions about patient and family preference for involvement in hygiene, meals, overnight stay, and sitting with confused patients.

St. Charles Medical Center also identified that one of the major sources of nurse burnout is that nurses often work from their assumptions of what the patient needs. This can lead to unsatisfied patients as well as burned-out nurses. Most nurses are conditioned to try to meet all of the needs they can identify for the patient whether the patient identifies them as needs or not. When nurses were students, they learned that if they missed a patient's need in developing the care plan, it often meant a lower grade. Nurses transfer this learning to the work setting. Every day nurses would go home feeling frustrated and angry because they couldn't meet all of the needs they identified for their patients. There is always more work to do than time to do it. Prioritizing care based on the patient's needs as identified by the patient is one of the most important nursing skills. St. Charles introduced a consistent service standard, Sharon K. Dingman's the Caring Model, to address this need and because of the success continues to use this model. The Caring Model consists of five behaviors that are part of an organization-wide or nursing department change initiative.[19] **Exhibit 26-1** lists the Caring Model behaviors.

Nurses are one of the most important therapeutic interventions. Nurses are people caring for people. They use technology, but it usually is as an extension of themselves. During orientation, all new caregivers are introduced to the Caring Model and asked to reflect on their own experiences as a patient and to identify what helped and what impaired the healing process. The most commonly mentioned factor is almost always the attitude and communication of the nurses. Where healing was enhanced, the nurse's attitude was described as caring, procedures were explained in advance, and education was integrated into care. This realization, and the need for enhanced anxiety and pain management, led to the development of the workshop Pain and Anxiety Management: Integrating Healing HealthCare Principles.[20] Key among these core competencies is therapeutic presence, which is outlined in **Exhibit 26-2**.

Additional pain and anxiety management competencies include several modalities that can be offered and taught to patients. The intention is to assist patients in accessing their own natural healing abilities. These methods enhance rather than replace conventional medical interventions, helping patients to help themselves and heal faster. **Exhibit 26-3** describes the performance criteria and validation methods for these competencies. Clinical caregivers (nurses and nonnurses) are required to complete an initial competency validation when hired, and an annual refresher is required via a computer-based learning module. A checklist form is built into the electronic medical record so that clinical caregivers may simply check a box when they have administered one of the healing modalities learned in the pain and anxiety management competence workshops, such as therapeutic touch, guided imagery, intentional breathing, and progressive muscle relaxation.

Patient-focused and family-focused care also requires attention in architectural and environmental design. Healing design is design with intent to give as much control to the patient as possible (temperature, lighting, etc.) and to create a home-like environment with access to natural light and views of nature.[9] Prior to implementing the healing healthcare philosophy at St.

EXHIBIT 26-1   St. Charles Medical Center Caring Model

1. Introduce yourself to patients and explain your role in their care or service today.
2. Call the patient by his or her preferred name.
3. Caregivers giving direct patient care should sit at the bedside for at least 5 minutes each shift to plan and review the patient's care and outcomes.
   - Nondirect caregivers should sit, if possible, to discuss procedures, processes, and services involved in attaining desired outcomes.
4. Use appropriate touch, such as a handshake or touch on the arm.
5. Use the mission, vision, and value statements in planning patient care (i.e., what is the most important thing the patient would like to have accomplished today).

Source: Sharon K. Dingman, consultant with Creative HealthCare Management. Used with permission of Sharon K. Dingman.

EXHIBIT 26-2   Therapeutic Presence Core Competency

The concept of therapeutic presence is based on the premise that how we are with our patients is as important as what we do to them. It is defined as the conscious intention to be present for another in a helpful or healing way. (For clarification and the sake of convenience, when the word *patient* is being used, it is also inclusive of family, friends, and significant others.)

The goal of this concept is not to teach you a canned formula for how to be with your patients, but to revisit some useful tools and to rediscover the therapeutic potential of your unique personality. Being therapeutically present is not so much about a technique as it is about an intention. This means making a conscious choice to focus our attention on one individual human being even though we might be busy or feeling rushed by all the tasks that still need to be done.

Suggestions for Becoming Therapeutically Present

Therapeutic presence is a composite of several personal skills that enhance our awareness of how we move around and into our patient's personal space, the tone of our voices, and the way we make contact with our touch. It also means being attentive to how and why our patients may be reacting successfully or unsuccessfully to their environments and taking action to make the necessary changes regarding those environmental factors.

Therapeutic presence can be viewed as a form of art, and, like all forms of art, several basic ingredients can be combined in infinite combinations to express your unique style. Through self-evaluation, feedback, and continued practice, we are asking that you commit to the ongoing process of learning to use a colorful palate of interpersonal and observational skills in your daily interactions with patients. We all want our jobs to feel rewarding, and, in this work setting, often those rewards come from our patients responding with an increased sense of trust, security, and appreciation of what we do. The following are just a few of the basics to remember when you are applying your palette of skills to daily patient interactions.

Caring model. Using the caring model (Exhibit 26-1) can help you develop a therapeutic relationship with your patient.

You only get one first impression. Your initial contact with your patient is critical in creating an atmosphere of trust, and it is a good opportunity to start building rapport. It sets the stage for having your patient's support and cooperation in doing all the things you need to do with that individual.

Inform but don't overwhelm. Explain your intentions, roles, procedures, and medications. Be clear about your expectations of what you need the patient to do. Information given in a patient's own terminology and in a timely fashion can demystify what is happening. Patients tend to be less anxious, less fearful, more cooperative, and better able to participate in their own care.

Be congruent. All communication interactions have both a verbal message (what is being said) and a nonverbal message (the way it is being delivered). If the nonverbal message conflicts with the verbal content, it confuses the patient and often increases his or her fear and distrust. Being congruent means making sure your verbal content matches your body language. Remember, however, that your nonverbal message is speaking about eight times louder than your verbal message. To ensure that your message is received as intended, consider your body posture, level and angle of eye contact, and your tone of voice.

Make eye contact. Making eye contact with your patient can be a powerful tool for establishing trust. It can convey that you are being attentive, concerned, and that you acknowledge his or her existence. Be aware, however, that the way each person interprets eye contact may be different based on gender, age, and cultural values.

Use attending actions. Attending actions such as "uh-huh," "yah," "um," nodding, and smiling can demonstrate interest if used carefully. If you skillfully place them in the right moments in a conversation, they encourage a patient to express his or her needs more freely because you appear more attentive.

Avoid listening blocks. Improving your listening skills can be enhanced by developing a commitment to listening quietly, avoiding distractions, waiting before responding, and suspending judgments. Avoid rushing someone through the communication process by trying to get just the facts or thinking about

(continues)

EXHIBIT 26-2   Therapeutic Presence Core Competency *(continued)*

what you should do or say next. You can miss a lot of the content and meaning of what the patient is trying to convey to you or appear rude, disinterested, and too busy. Refrain from developing mind-sets based on past experiences with other patients or forming judgments about the person's lifestyle and manner of behaviors. Perceived expectations can sometimes limit your ability to recognize a patient's unique differences, differences that are critical in implementing care. Last but not least, refrain from thinking about alternatives and solutions for the patient while he or she is still talking. This can deny the patient a chance to convey needs and work toward finding solutions.

Set the environmental stage. The human body is amazing. We are predominantly driven by our nervous systems, which are constantly trying to make sense of our internal and external environments so that we can adapt and survive. This is why we act and behave the way we do. Therefore, when we are chronically or acutely ill, our nervous systems are working overtime trying to make sense and adjust our inner worlds. This leaves us with very few reserves, if any, for coping with external demands. We are capable of perceiving, and constantly trying to interpret, the following stimuli: visible light (sight); vibrations in the air (hearing); tactile contact (touch); chemical molecular (taste); olfactory molecular (smell); kinesthetic geotropic (balance and movement); repetitious movement (vestibular); molecular motion (temperature); nociception (pain); neuroelectric image retention (eidetic imagery); ferromagnetic orientation (magnetic); long electromagnetic waves (infrared); short electromagnetic waves (ultraviolet); airborne ionic charges (ionic); pheromonic sensing (vomeronasal); physical closeness (proximal); surface charge (electrical); atmospheric pressure (barometric); and sensing mass differences (geogravemetric). Overwhelmed just trying to read this list? So are most of our patients when they are ill and trying to adapt in an unfamiliar, high-stimulus, work-oriented environment. Their nervous systems cannot regenerate if they are constantly being bombarded with stimulation.

Being highly skilled at observing and assessing a patient's reaction to the amount of stimulation received is a very important caregiver skill. Often our patients are experiencing overstimulation in the areas of pain, noise, noxious smells and tastes, invasions of personal space and time, and exposure to artificial lights and air. They are almost always understimulated in the areas of comforting touch and movement. Take the time to be attentive. Stop, look, listen, and feel what is going on in your patient's environment. Use the TV sparingly. Talk quietly outside a patient's room. Keep rooms organized and free of clutter. Control the number of visitors and the length of visits. Adjust the blinds to allow for natural, nonglaring light. Monitor the room temperature. Learn and use a wide range of positioning techniques. Get patients up and out of bed more frequently, but for a shorter duration. Make sure their physical environment encourages active participation.

Use caring touch. If properly used, a comforting touch is probably one of the single most valuable, but underutilized, tools we can apply in the daily care of our patients. Volumes of literature and research show how gentle, caring touch, for even a brief moment, can put a patient's mind at ease and decrease perception of pain. Touch can convey caring, acceptance, confirmation of self-worth, and relatedness to others. It can decrease heart rate, respiration rate, blood pressure and can initiate a relaxation response. Often there is little or nothing you can say with words to comfort a patient, but there is always a great deal you can say with your hands. Begin and end any physical task or procedure for a patient with a mindful, caring touch. Massaging the hands, feet, or back can go a long way in creating patient comfort. A 5-minute massage can increase blood flow to an area of the body by 60%, and the effects last for up to 3 hours afterward. Those are big payoffs for the amount of time invested.

Be a role model. When a patient's behaviors show that he or she is becoming hysterical, and anxiety and pain are escalating, it is important to remain calm. Model correct breathing, a quiet tone of voice, listening skills, nonthreatening body language, and rational problem solving for the patient. Also, become a valued role model for your coworkers by weaving in and out of your daily interactions in a mindful, observant, and respectful way.

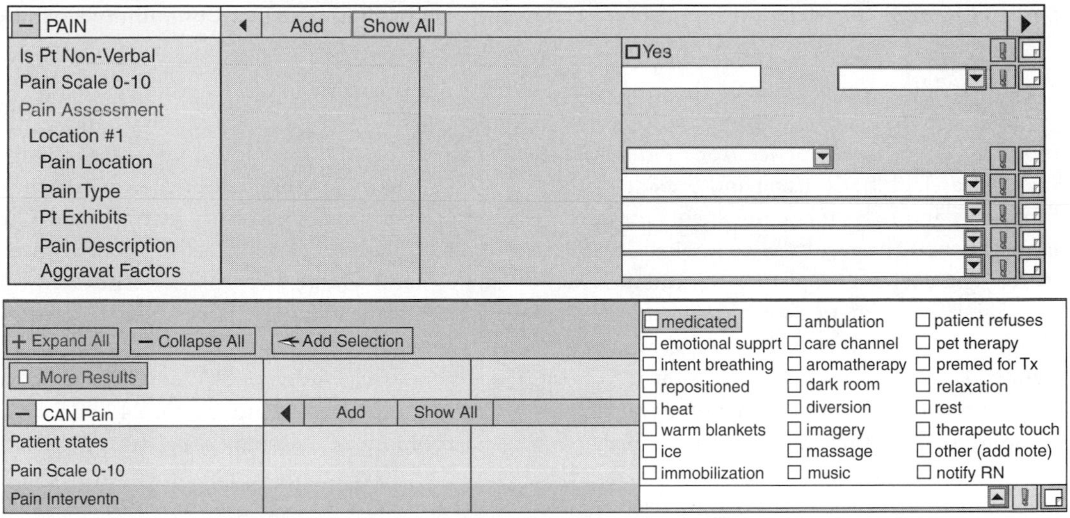

FIGURE 26-2 St. Charles Electronic Pain Assessment and Interventions
Source: Copyright © 2011, St. Charles Health System.

EXHIBIT 26-3 Nursing Care Delivery Skills in Pain and Anxiety Management

Orientation Competence and Skill Assessment Evaluation Tool

Performance Criteria	Validation Methods
Demonstrates knowledge of physiology of pain and assessment of pain/anxiety interventions	Written quiz with a score of 80% or greater
Assesses patient for pain, anxiety, and discomfort	Demonstration or role-play Documentation in patient record (EMR)
Demonstrates creation of therapeutic presence and therapeutic healing environment (caring model)	Demonstration or role-play Documentation in patient record (EMR)
Demonstrates application of: ■ Intentional breathing ■ Progressive muscle relaxation ■ Imagining a pleasant place	Demonstration or role-play Documentation in patient record (EMR)
Administers appropriate pain medications as prescribed	Written quiz score of 80%
Describes options to potentiate/enhance pain medication	Written quiz Demonstration
Demonstrates use of comfort measures: ■ Back rub ■ Ice ■ Positioning ■ Music ■ CARE channel/relaxation tapes	Demonstration and discussion
Accesses pain and anxiety management resources: ■ Therapeutic touch ■ Rehabilitation services ■ Spiritual care	Written quiz
Evaluates effectiveness of pain and anxiety interventions and revises plan as necessary	Written quiz Demonstration and documentation

Charles Medical Center, one of the most common patient complaints was concerning the quality of the food. Best practices for food services were researched, both inside and outside of the healthcare industry, including such sites as the Ritz Carlton. The results were applied in 1999 by hiring a chef and implementing room service 24 hours a day, 7 days a week. Today room service is provided so that patients select what they want to eat and when they want to eat it from a bedside menu. Special diets are noted through a computerized system and patients are helped with their choices if they choose an excluded item. The meals are delivered within 15 minutes. This practice has saved thousands of dollars in food waste and enhanced patient satisfaction. St. Charles was the benchmark for food service satisfaction for more than five years and hosted many site visits for other hospitals that have since adopted room service as a best practice. St. Charles remains in the top 15 percent of the comparison group with satisfaction of the quality of food services.[21] In 2009, SCHS also initiated a summer farmers market on the hospital grounds, inviting local growers to offer organic fruits and vegetables to the community and caregivers. It is a tribute from the community that the hospital café and cafeteria are a gathering place for lunch, meetings, and catered conferences.

To better support the patient's control of his or her environment, the semiprivate rooms were remodeled into private rooms in the areas where patients experience longer lengths of hospital stay and brought in sleeper sofas to allow family members to stay with their loved one, offering support as well as learning about the care that will need to continue when they return home. Our recent facilities expansion added 45 new rooms at the Bend site and completely renovated the Redmond site, including larger, acuity-adaptable patient rooms, with zones for the nurse, patient, and family (see **Figure 26-3**). Our visitation policy has been expanded to provide for 24-hour access and rooming in. As many other hospitals have done, we have added "quiet times" in ICU and mother–child services to provide teaching and rest times. Overhead paging is also limited to essential messages and emergency responses to reduce the noise distractions for patients and families.

St. Charles also has an active pet program with therapy dogs as well as a policy to allow appropriate pets to visit their family members who are patients. Our canine "volunteers" make regular visits to those patients who would like to participate. The 2006 addition of a traveling art cart and hospitality cart manned by volunteers delivering newspapers and visiting with patients, along with televised bingo, has helped our patients and families pass the time between nurse visits. Volunteers also round on patients daily to provide support and feedback to nurses for immediate service recovery when necessary.

Resources are provided to support patients and families in becoming informed and active

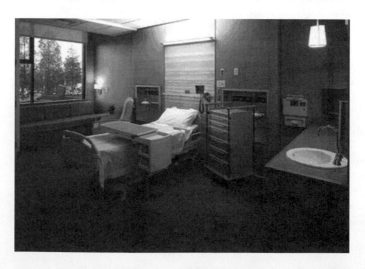

FIGURE 26-3 Nurse and Family Areas in Patient's Room
Source: Copyright © 2010, St. Charles Medical Center.

participants in their care. This includes printed materials as well as DVD players in each room for viewing entertainment and educational videos. Family and patient visiting rooms located on each patient unit offer a relaxing atmosphere, with access to an audiovisual library and computers that provide Internet access and web-based information on medications and diseases.

Life Skills

In 2002, what started as a simple handout for patients advising them of health risks and what they can do about them became the Center for Health and Learning (CHL). The CHL, funded primarily from community and caregiver donations, is now at the front door of St. Charles Medical Center. As noted in an editorial from the *Bulletin*, the local newspaper:

> The new space . . . surely accomplished all that they had hoped it would, and in a beautiful fashion to boot. The commitment to education and prevention is visible. . . . The subtle message: Stop here, learn to take care of yourself properly and, one hopes, spare yourself a stay upstairs someday. . . . A hospital all too often is a terrifying place, both for patients and those who come to call on them. The small touches—the fountain, the color scheme, and the like—help take some of that anxiety away. They're worth the price.[22]

The educational services include support groups, lifestyle-change programs, health and fitness classes including meditation and yoga, disease-specific educational programs, and personal growth and development workshops. The signature lifestyle-change programs incorporate a body-mind-spirit approach to making and sustaining lifestyle and behavior changes in support of optimal wellness. These programs are based on research that defines the components necessary to support successful lifestyle change:[23-24]

- Education
- Nutrition
- Mind and body medicine through stress management and relaxation response
- Exercise and body work
- Psychosocial support
- Spirituality or sense of purpose

Living a Healthy Life with Chronic Conditions

This 6-week program is licensed by Stanford Patient Education Research Center. Information about the program can be accessed through the Center's website, http://patienteducation.stanford.edu. The program applies 24 years of development and testing to create evidence-based self-management programs for people with chronic diseases. The facilitators for the program are persons with chronic health problems of their own. They are certified after attending four days of training given by the Stanford Center. The workshops are highly interactive and focus on building new skills, sharing experiences, and giving support. The participants conduct homework assignments between the sessions. This program has been well re-ceived by the community and is now partnering with the Deschutes County Health Department and the Volunteers in Medicine Clinic to expand the program.

Because of an underutilized Health Coach program, St. Charles has sought other ways to offer better health to the community. In 2010, a new programmatic approach to health education called Joint Camp was initiated. It is not uncommon for patients coming to SCMC to drive four hours for their care, which brings challenges for discharge planning and follow-up care. This program provides preparation for the lifestyle changes and impact from joint replacement surgery. The program outcomes have had positive impacts on patient outcomes and satisfaction. The Joint Camp class is open to patients and families in preparation for surgery and offers one-on-one support to individuals by a nurse encompassing risk factors and other aspects of a patient's health care.

Life–Death Transition

We live in a death-denying society. How do we allow ourselves to come into the inevitable unknown with openheartedness and courage? How do we support others in their grieving time, to allow the full and personal expression of their aliveness, including their denial, anger, sadness, joy, and final acceptance? How do we support nurses to focus on the dying patient's needs while managing organizational demands?[25] St. Charles is committed to the continual development of the skills and presence necessary to assist dying patients and their families. When Oregon passed the nation's first physician-assisted suicide legislation, the SCMC board of directors viewed this act by the people of Oregon as a message that health care, in general, has failed in supporting people through the dying process. As a result, the board directed the hospital staff to improve end-of-life care. Cancer Services Director Peggy Carey, RN, took on the challenge with gusto. She formed a task force and performed a community assessment. The survey found that people want sovereignty over self, including control over decisions at end of life and choice in how and where they die. They also feared becoming a burden and did not want to die in pain. They wanted care that supports their comfort. The task force evolved into two tracks: hospital-based palliative care program and a community-based program, through the Deschutes County Coalition for Quality End-of-Life Care.

St. Charles Palliative Care Program

The St. Charles Palliative Care Services raises the standard of care for dying patients by focusing on the quality of life. The program goals encompass the following:

- Care at any stage of a serious chronic illness along with all other appropriate medical treatment

- Expert management of pain and other symptoms
- Focus on the whole person: body, mind, and spirit
- Educate patients and families about healthcare options, establish care goals, and identify community resources to meet those goals
- Facilitate communication between patient, family members, and healthcare providers
- Ease transitions between care settings
- Use an interdisciplinary team approach to care

St. Charles has a case management registered nurse assigned to work with the palliative care program patients, as well as an interdisciplinary team including palliative care physicians, pharmacists, spiritual care, social services, nursing, volunteer musicians, and others as needed, as shown in **Figure 26-4**. Services are accessed through a physician's order, although the nurse is available to all staff to assist with determining whether the consult service is appropriate. The team develops an education plan, policies and procedures, and orders, and consistently works to support physicians and caregivers in caring for their patients and families in the dying process. **Exhibit 26-4** shows the comfort care patient checklist.

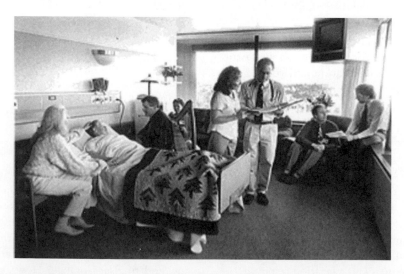

FIGURE 26-4   Patient and Comfort Care Team (Nurses, Physician, Pastoral Care, Social Service, and Harpist)
Source: Copyright © 2010, St. Charles Medical Center.

Because of the commitment of the staff involved in the program and the exceptional quality of their services, the service grew quickly and is a great success. The service helped reduce costs because physicians became more conscious of when heroic treatments are futile and that there are effective measures that can help patients in the dying process. The electronic medical record careset (group of electronic orders) emphasizes comfort measures and eliminates unnecessary testing and treatments. With changes to the program in 2011, Palliative Care Services participates in the National Palliative Care Registry and implements tracking of symptom management, length of stay, resource utilization, and patient and physician satisfaction.

Healing Has Many Dimensions

Healthcare futurist and advisor Leland R. Kaiser has been a mentor to many of the St. Charles leaders. Leland once told retired CNO Nancy Moore, "Nancy, a hospital is a sacred place. The hospital is where people most often come into life and it is also the place where they leave life. People are in the hospital during their most significant life experiences." The reality of the hospital as a sacred place and space made a significant impact on how caregivers view their work and the setting. Martha Rogers's concept that healing is pandimensional (having many dimensions) certainly supports this view.[1]

A major principle of our healing healthcare philosophy is that everything a person experiences can be used to enhance healing and the recovery process. This principle guides all of our architecture and design. Unfortunately, since the 1900s, most hospitals have been designed as functional and efficient medical workshops rather than centers for integrating the power of the body, mind, and spirit to accelerate the healing process. Research has shown that design

EXHIBIT 26-4   Comfort Care Patient Checklist

1. Place order for comfort care in the EMR.
2. Enter comfort care orders in the EMR. Make sure doctors have discontinued all labs, diagnostic procedures, and intravenous fluids.
3. Verify and complete Physician's Orders for Life-Sustaining Treatment (POLST), do-not-resuscitate comfort measures.
4. Notify case manager and spiritual care.
5. Call the donor bank for patient's eligibility as a donor. If eligible, contact a designated requester so that the patient or family can be approached.
6. Diet entered in EMR should indicate that the diet is whatever the patient desires to eat.
7. Review cafeteria hours with patient and family.
8. Give information about chapel and locations for prayer and privacy. Page spiritual care when needed for patient or family.
9. Medicate on schedule and turn patient every 2 hours. Take vital signs once per shift. If taking a blood pressure (BP) is too uncomfortable for the patient, it may be just respiratory and heart rate. Do not call the physician with readings. This monitoring is to have an awareness of a downward trend and the need for pain and anxiety interventions.
10. Make sure adequate charting is done regarding interactions you have with patient and family about emotional state, how are they feeling about the pending death, and family issues that need to be healed.
11. Encourage use of music and, if appropriate, therapeutic touch, relaxation therapies, and aromatherapy.
12. Acknowledge and support the patient's wishes. Are there phone calls that the patient wants to make or letters that the patient wants to write to say goodbye to anyone who can't be there?

that ignores people's psychological and spiritual needs contributes to anxiety and stress. Conversely, a warm, nurturing environment with access to natural light enhances recovery and healing, leading to a shorter length of stay in the hospital and a decrease in the need for pain medication.[9] It is important to integrate the need for functionality and efficiency with the need for a warm and nurturing environment. The impact of environment is significant for patients and their families, as well as caregivers.

The goal has been to create spaces to allow time for caregivers to provide relationship-based care, as well as areas for team work and the care team to engage with each other, patients, and family. This environment supports openness and learning. Nurse-architect Kerrie Cardon, who worked with SCHS on its facility expansion, expressed the important role of healing intention in architecture during an interview for *NurseWeek* magazine:

> Creating a total healing environment is a long-term design goal of many facilities, including St. Charles Medical Center in central Oregon, where patients can relax by a cozy lava fireplace, enjoy a piano concert in the lobby, and even fish for bass in a well-stocked pool. The emphasis isn't only on patient comfort; it's also on creating a warm, efficient environment for nurses that reduces stress and replenishes their spirit. With every project, I envision myself in the spaces I'm designing, and really draw on my nursing experience to assure the needs of nurses are met.[26]

The main SCMC facility was designed in the mid-1970s. The design supports nurses in being with their patients through a decentralized nursing concept, including nurse server stations containing all of the needed supplies at each patient room and a central communications system that literally did away with a central nursing station. All patient rooms have panoramic views of the high desert and the Cascade Mountain range, and careful attention was paid to detail to ensure healing in the use of colors and design.

Each time there is an opportunity for expansion and remodeling, we have applied this prin-

ciple to enhance the healing environment. For example, when we expanded our Redmond facility in 2006 we added full-length windows in each room, skylights in the center hallway with no center core walls, views of nature, and a color scheme that made the patient room a continuum of the high desert and Cascade Mountain range. The nurses played an integral part in design and reported that after moving into the new unit, patients experienced less anxiety and called on nurses less for pain and confusion because they now have access to natural light and family social spaces. See **Figure 26-5**.

When the lobby needed to be remodeled, large windows and a natural wood staircase were added. (See **Figure 26-6**.) We also enhanced the nondenominational chapel as a result of focus groups with people of all religions and belief systems. The chapel is circular with stained-glass windows, a variety of religious symbols, and includes elements of Earth, water, fire, and air. Intentional architecture and design can act as

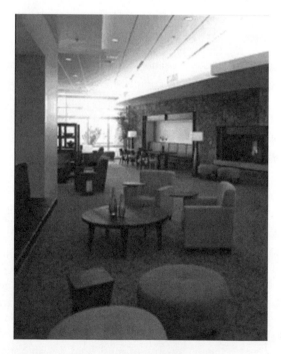

FIGURE 26-5 Family Waiting Room at St. Charles Redmond
Source: Copyright © 2010, St. Charles Health System.

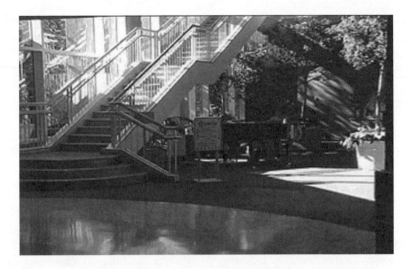

FIGURE 26-6   Window and Staircase of the Main Lobby
Source: Copyright © 2010, St. Charles Medical Center.

symbolic representations of significance and meaning. When a local physician passed away, the nurses and physicians wanted to contribute to a memorial. This memorial became Lynn's Garden, shown in **Figure 26-7**. It was funded entirely by donations; it has a fountain and pool with a sculpture and plants. It is a popular site for patients and caregivers to go for reflection and peace in the beauty of nature.

Creating a healing environment does not have to be expensive. Little things can make a big difference. Perhaps one of the most effective ways to enhance healing is through providing a safe, clean, quiet environment. These are things that require each person's awareness, and simple acts such as picking up a piece of trash that is on the floor can mean a lot in enhancing the healing environment.

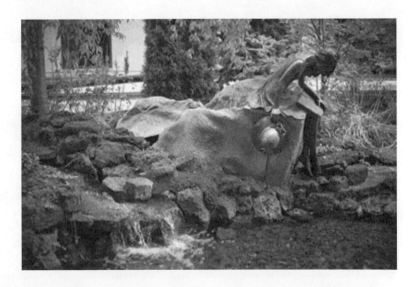

FIGURE 26-7   Lynn's Garden
Source: Copyright © 2011, St. Charles Medical Center.

■ ARTS IN THE HOSPITAL

Curing is for the body. Caring is for the soul. The arts speak to the soul. The environment is a mirror of the individual and of the culture. It echoes the values of the culture. Art enriches the environment and can connect people to purpose and meaning by representing the organization's unique mythology. Perhaps most important in the hospital setting, art can influence healing and recovery.[27] The St. Charles Arts in the Hospital program includes art, music, and humor.

Art

The significance of art in the hospital is highlighted in the hospital's practices. The following is an example of how bringing art into the hospital setting facilitates healing. Brooke isn't having a very good day. Her blood pressure is running low and she is not feeling well. It isn't the first time her daily routine seems overwhelming since a recent car accident left her in a wheelchair.

"I've got something for you," says Arts Coordinator Marline Alexander, beaming broadly at Brooke. She has a lump of bright yellow clay in her palm and a twinkle in her eye that affects Brooke almost instantly.

Just like a light turning on, Brooke's blue-gray eyes brighten. Within five minutes, she's laughing as she rolls the clay beneath the heel of her hand, intent on making the colorful beads pictured in her book.

The three galleries, the Alexander Gallery in the Cancer Treatment Center, the Family Birthing Center Gallery, and the Second Floor Gallery, display work created by local artists and patients. The purpose of the galleries is to enhance the healing environment and for patients and families to have something interesting to view. The hospital also sells art, and 30% of the proceeds directly benefit the arts program.

St. Charles uses art to express its symbology and historical roots. Sister Catherine, SCMC president emeritus, commissioned a sculptor to come to the hospital, experience its community, and create a sculpture representing the hospital's mythology. The sculptor met with caregivers, physicians, and community members, and then left to manifest the spirit of this experience. The fruits of this endeavor resulted in the Yoke of Compassion, shown in **Figure 26-8**. The Yoke of Compassion, which graces the garden off the hospital lobby, evokes a fundamental image of simple human caring. It has become the symbol of the healing role St. Charles plays for the people of central and eastern Oregon. It represents the sacredness of care, in that you cannot at first tell which figure is holding the other figure. We

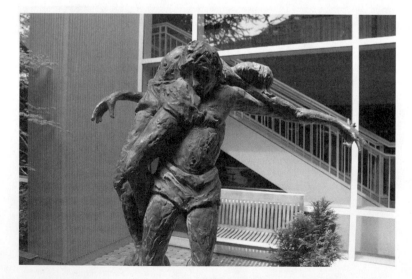

FIGURE 26-8   The Yoke of Compassion, by Father David Kocka.
Source: Copyright © 2011, St. Charles Medical Center.

are blessed in health care in that as we give, we also receive the gift of helping others. Small replicas of this symbolic statue have been used to acknowledge very special caregivers that have made significant contributions to St. Charles in the spirit of the healing healthcare philosophy.

Music

Everything in the environment has an effect on healing; very little is just neutral. Hospitals are not an implicitly relaxing environment. This is certainly true when it comes to the sound environment and disruption of healing by undesirable noise. Most people would agree that rest is a vital component of healing. Yet most would also agree that a hospital is the last place anyone would go to for rest. One of the most frequent patient complaints and notations on patient satisfaction surveys was inability to rest because of environmental noise. SCHS worked though Healing HealthCare Environmental Standards to address this concern. It began with an experiential workshop, Music: A Life-Altering Decision, by Susan Mazer and Dallas Smith, developers and owners of Healing HealthCare Systems. This workshop develops an experiential knowledge of music as a tool in the design of healing healthcare environments. Most important, the workshop heightens awareness of the sound environment and the power of intention in creating a healing environment. An intentional healing healthcare environment extends the therapeutic presence of the caregiver during and in the absence of their presence. It creates a caring sensory environment that envelops the patient.

Looking to create a better environment, St. Charles implemented the use of Continuous Ambient Relaxation Environment (CARE) on an internal television channel that is operational at the Bend and Redmond hospital campuses. This TV channel is programmed for the day–night life cycle, providing a nurturing sound and visual environment while screening out most of the ambient environmental noise. The CARE channel offers patients a tool to control their visual and auditory environment while offering nurses a therapeutic tool for alleviating patients' pain and anxiety. The channel also works as a welcoming notice to new patients and families because it is turned on in each patient room and waits for them upon admission. To enhance the overall experience St. Charles worked with Healing HealthCare Systems to create an additional channel that includes hourly segments of guided imagery exercises for relaxation and meditation. Voices of Rosemary Johnson, an oncology center nurse, and Dallas Smith of Healing HealthCare Systems guide the listener through a healing journey with loving and healing intention.

Healing HealthCare Systems also provides St. Charles with custom music in lobbies and waiting areas. This music helps reduce the actual and perceived noise levels, protects confidentiality, and relieves the typical sense of isolation in long corridors and halls.

Community musicians and artists are a vital component of the healing environment. When they became aware that the hospital was open to the use of music and art in healing, volunteers have eagerly offered their time and love of music to enhance the hospital environment. These volunteers range from a barbershop quartet to harpists and employees who play the lobby's baby grand piano during their breaks. The hospital provides support through assisting with funding education and some travel expenses for these volunteers.

The harpists personally sought funding from the community to purchase harps that now remain at the hospital. One of the harps is designed so that patients can hold it while learning to express their feelings through stroking the strings. St. Charles Hospitalist Dr. John Zachem reports that the harp specifically helps bring the level of stress down and eases tension. Most often, Donna Rustand, a certified harp therapist, plays the harp at St. Charles (**Figure 26-9**). Certified harp therapists learn how to use the harp to make patients feel better through understanding the psychology of illness. Through training and experience the musicians can help patients relax, ease pain, or, as is often the case for comfort care patients, help them to let go and die peacefully. Testimonials from patients indicate that relaxation can decrease the need for pain medication and allow them to rest and heal.

Humor

Just as stress can have negative effects, humor can have beneficial effects. Humor can increase

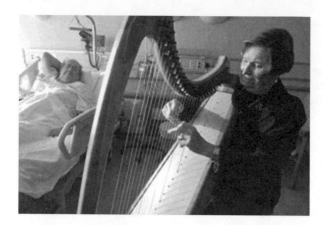

FIGURE 26-9 Volunteer Harpist and Patient
Source: Copyright © 2011, *The Bend Bulletin*.

communication, decrease anger and conflict, change perceptions, create a sense of well-being, allow detachment, and facilitate learning.[28]

Connecting humor is also a vital part of creating a healing environment in the workplace. Every one of the hospital's teams identifies humor as one of the key success factors for achieving their vision. Nurses JoAnn Miller-Watts and Karen McGuire, shown in **Figure 26-10**, have emerged as particularly gifted in

this arena. They routinely use humor to enhance education and support the healing environment of teams throughout the hospital. Sometimes St. Charles management and staff start taking themselves too seriously. Karen and JoAnn are quick to design a song or a skit that reflects the hazards of caregiver perfectionism and helps them laugh at themselves. This wonderful service always serves as a release for tension and opens up new and more beneficial perspectives.

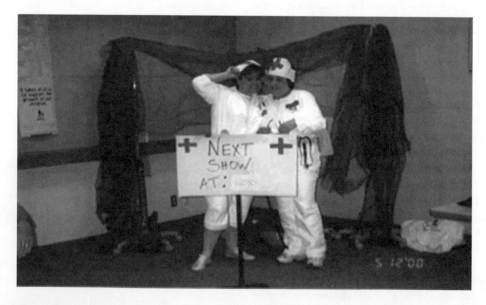

FIGURE 26-10 Karen McGuire and JoAnn Miller-Watts, Nurse Humorists
Source: Copyright © 2010, St. Charles Medical Center.

◼ HEALING OUR COMMUNITY

To improve the health of those we serve
in a spirit of love and compassion.

—*St. Charles Medical Center Mission*

In 1995, Jim Lussier, CEO of St. Charles Medical Center, formed the Central Oregon Health Council (COHC) as a resource for accomplishing our mission. In 2010, the council has grown to 35 member agencies, including such agencies as the Bend-La Pine School District, the Commission on Children and Families, Oregon Health Authority, Pacific Source, the region's safety net clinics, and representatives from Deschutes, Crook, and Jefferson County Commissions. The COHC, in partnership with the Oregon Health Authority (OHA), seeks to achieve the Institute for Healthcare Improvement Triple Aim: to improve health outcomes, increase satisfaction with our health system, and reduce costs. The goal is to manage resources efficiently and effectively, in collaboration with local and state governments, our hospital system, local providers, private insurers, health collaborative(s), and, most important, our community and the people we serve. The partnership defines, implements, measures, and leads the regional Health Improvement Plan—a collaborative community plan. There is also a proposed timeline for implementation that would result in the formation of the COHC in 2011 for regional planning purposes, with implementation of contract authority for the Oregon Health Plan by 2013 and full implementation of Central Oregon Health Council by 2014. The plan is grounded in baseline health and economic data and focused on Triple Aim metrics to measure outcomes and guide decisions that will best serve the health of the population of Central Oregon. Our goal is to make Central Oregon the healthiest region in the nation and is in alignment with the SCHS vision to achieve the Triple Aim.

The COHC developed a mission statement, community health values, and benchmarks for measurement. COHC focuses on five methods of creating a healthy community:

- Public education focusing on health
- Developing new public–private partnerships
- Resource development and alignment
- Monitoring progress of benchmarks and reporting to the community
- Influencing public policy

One example of the COHC's work is the formation of an unprecedented public–private partnership, the Central Oregon Partners for Healing Environments (encompassing Deschutes County, the Central Oregon Regional Housing Authority, and St. Charles Medical Center) to address the mental health needs of central and eastern Oregon. To meet this need, the partners contributed their experience and expertise to the development of the Healing Health Campus. The Healing Health Campus includes Sage View, a 15-bed adult psychiatric residential treatment center designed to assess, stabilize, and treat adults who are experiencing a mental or emotional crisis, and Horizon House, a 14-unit transitional housing facility. Transitional housing fills a critical gap in the continuum of care for patients with mental illnesses and often is the bridge between failure and success in returning clients to independent living.

Other examples of healing our community include the Sara Fisher Breast Cancer Project, Kids @ Heart, and the Stepping Stones Program. The Sara Fisher Breast Cancer Project, formed in 1991 in memory of Sara Fisher, is a community coalition of volunteers, physicians, and community sponsors led by Cancer Services Director Peggy Carey. This project seeks to improve women's health through aggressive prevention, research, education, and outreach with an emphasis on early detection of breast cancer. Through a combination of community fund-raising and grants, they have developed the following services:

- Community education and outreach, including programs to promote early detection, such as an annual low-cost mammogram program
- The navigator program, a partnership with community volunteers and professional counselors providing peer support for women newly diagnosed with breast cancer
- Breast cancer research, involving breast cancer studies to determine effectiveness of medications for prevention and treatment of breast cancer

- A community breast cancer case manager, who is an RN acting as a patient advocate, coordinating seamless care for women diagnosed with breast cancer
- Massage and relaxation series, offering participants opportunities to explore complementary therapies and education on health-related topics
- Emotional and educational first aid kits, developed by navigators and distributed by physicians to help newly diagnosed women progress to the decision-making phase of care
- Sara's Sisters sponsorships, to ensure that newly diagnosed women continue to receive services and have transportation to treatment

Central Oregon's rate of detecting cancer in situ (at the site only, meaning no metastasis) and local stage is 76%, whereas the national average is reported at 49%.

Stepping Stones is a foundation-supported program including HealthyStart Prenatal Services, newborn hearing screening, and follow-up clinics for new mothers. HealthyStart provides prenatal care to low-income women. HealthyStart's goal is to prevent low-birth-weight babies. It is a unique partnership of local physicians, the county health department, St. Charles Medical Center, and the St. Charles Medical Center Foundation. It provides a broad range of services including prenatal through delivery and postpartum care; parenting education; alcohol, drug, and tobacco education; and referral services. The program is a great success. In 2010, Deschutes County had a rate of 81.5% for first trimester prenatal care compared to the Oregon state average of 73%. In addition, for 2010 there was only one walk-in delivery with no prenatal care, 316 mothers enrolled in the program, and a cesarean section rate of only 17%. Hearing screening is a service that provides for early detection of hearing loss, to make sure every child has the hearing ability needed to develop language and social skills. Interested mothers can take advantage of a follow-up clinic that provides checkups, referrals, and nurse support within a week of birth.[29]

■ PRINCIPLE-BASED CARE MODEL

The healing healthcare philosophy, along with the collective vision of both management and staff nurses, guided the revision of the St. Charles care model, called the health management model. The health management model shown in **Figure 26-11** is guided by our healing healthcare philosophy and is focused on the patient and family. Our care is relationship centered, resource based, and outcomes focused. Those we serve access our care through prevention, wellness, and intervention services. Prevention and wellness services are provided through the Center for Health and Learning. Intervention services (inpatient and outpatient care) are provided by nursing and case management (including RN case managers and social services) in partnership with our community providers, the hospitalist, the attending physician, and the interdisciplinary team, as needed. The identified nurse or case manager is responsible for establishing a therapeutic relationship with the patient and a professional relationship with the physician and interdisciplinary team to develop,

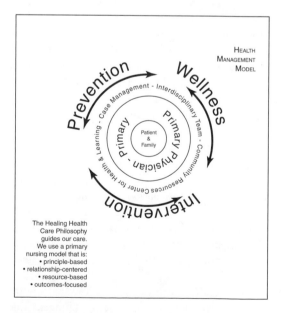

FIGURE 26-11   Health Management Model

Source: Copyright © 2010, St. Charles Medical Center.

implement, and document the plan of care, including discharge planning. The admitting or discharging nurse may be the identified nurse for patients with less than a 48-hour length of stay. The relationship is known to the patient, family, and staff. The identified nurse or case manager performs a holistic assessment of needs and resources to develop the plan of care. This person also facilitates patient control and advocates for the patient with focused attention on communication and handoffs to caregivers between departments and shifts. When patients are discharged, they are referred to community resources and the programs of the Center for Health and Learning as appropriate. The identified nurse or case manager also partners with physicians in continuous self-improvement, including ensuring appropriate diagnosis-related group (DRG) documentation compliance and following best practice guidelines, including core measures.

Examples of desired outcomes include reduced length of stay, reduced cost per discharge, improved discharge procedures, reduced readmissions, improved patient satisfaction, improved interaction between multidisciplinary caregivers, and core measures compliance.

We identified two key success factors in achieving the goals of the health management model: front-line caregiver engagement and a high degree of integration in the "next line" of support, which includes social work, case management, and utilization management. As part of the professional nursing practice enhancement initiative, unit-based practice committees (UPCs) were chartered with a clearly defined set of principles that guide each unit in creating its plan. The UPCs, which comprise staff nurses and other relevant disciplines, are responsible for assessing, designing, implementing, and continuously evaluating their unit's care plan based on the care model principles. UPCs are active champions in using current lean process improvement principles to reduce waste in their processes and to find ways for a nurse to have more time at the bedside in relationship with their patient. (See **Exhibit 26-5**.)

We are convinced that strengthening the nurse–patient relationship is a critical success factor in preparing for a more challenging future. Resources for care are not infinite and will always

be, to various extents, limited. Nurses are continuously making decisions of how best to use their resources. Ideally, these decisions are made within a therapeutic relationship with patients, and with the knowledge of what patients identify as their most important needs. The caring model provides a structure for our nurses to learn their patients' story, as Margaret Wheatley points out, "One of the easiest human acts is also the most healing, and it is to listen to someone."[30] Resource-based care—intentional decision making based on patient needs and time available—must include a therapeutic relationship with the patient.[31] To assist nurses in the development of resource-based decision making, we have added unit-based educators and are developing our system's capacity to support nurses in making care decisions while "owning" their time. We believe that when nurses have a therapeutic relationship with their patients and truly own their time, they will set appropriate care priorities based on patient needs, as articulated by the patient, and available time and resources. Nurses thus can be empowered to say what will and will not be done. By doing so, they create a real-life scenario in which they truly can provide better care and experience greater autonomy and satisfaction, even in the midst of difficult times.

■ CONCLUSION

Sustaining a culture of healing requires the intention and commitment of all members of an organization. It also requires a clearly defined process and the discipline to manage and continuously improve the process. As shown in the St. Charles Quality Management Model, **Figure 26-12**, our mission, vision, values, and the quality process guide the health system. The board of directors developed the nature of care policy that provides goals for the design and character of the system's care.

To ensure that the nature of care policy goals are implemented, department leadership is responsible for meeting department requirements. Department requirements include performance quality; customer, skill, and resource assessments; and identifying the department's scope of service. This responsibility begins with

EXHIBIT 26-5 Care Model Principles

1. ***Healing healthcare philosophy:*** Healing ourselves, our relationships, our communities. Our intention is to create an environment that supports healing: healing for our patients, their families, and caregivers. We understand that a truly healing environment exists only to the extent that our caregivers themselves have found healing. Healing for each of us is enhanced when we care for ourselves and our team members as well as the people we serve. We are a human service. Who we are and how we work together are what our patients and their families receive. People are indivisible; they are more than the sum of their parts. We care for the wholeness (body, mind, and spirit) of our patients and one another. We use technology appropriately and recognize that healing is enhanced in caring relationships. Everything in the environment has an effect on healing. Very little is simply neutral. It either enhances or impairs the healing process. This includes all sensory experience (sight, hearing, smell, and touch).

2. ***Responsibility for therapeutic relationship and plan of care.*** The identified nurse or case manager is responsible for establishing an individualized therapeutic relationship and a plan of care with a patient and family throughout the patient's length of stay on the unit or service. The admitting or discharging nurse may be the primary nurse for patients with less than a 24-hour length of stay. The relationship is known to the patient, family, and staff. Care planning includes assessment of patient expectations, patient level of knowledge and skill at managing own health, and presence of significant other and support systems. The plan is based on a holistic, individualized assessment of needs and resources and is evidence-based. The identified nurse or case manager and all nurses facilitate patient control over healthcare decisions and advocate for the patient. Outcomes are patient driven. The plan of care is specific to the disease process (standardized) and customized to the patient's unique needs and involvement

(individualized). The identified nurse or case manager works in partnership with peer registered nurses, physicians, social work, and other disciplines in implementing the plan of care. All nurses and other caregivers respect and follow the plan of care. They contribute to the plan of care as appropriate to changing conditions of the patient. All caregivers are responsible for the caring model and therapeutic presence in implementing the plan of care.

3. ***Work allocation and assignments.*** Assignments are based on patient need and provide for efficient workflow as well as continuity and consistency. Assignments and delegation of activities of care are based on the nurse's assessment of patient needs and are congruent with the caregiver's knowledge and skill.

4. ***Communication.*** Communication and documentation are patient focused, direct, and specific to the plan of care as to meeting patient safety, standards of care, and regulatory standards such as the Joint Commission standards. All members of the care team are expected to question care decisions or allocation of resources that appear to threaten patient safety. Focused attention is given to communication of a patient's individualized plan of care across the continuum, that is, in "handoffs" between shifts, service areas, departments, and caregivers. Communication is direct between caregivers and collaborative with the interdisciplinary team. Case managers partner with physicians and ER in documentation of the primary and secondary diagnoses, complications, and comorbidities to ensure an accurate reflection of the severity of illness, intensity of service and resource consumption, treatment complexity, ICD-9-CM coding, and DRG assignment.

5. ***Resource-based care decision process.*** Care decisions are made by utilizing the resource-based care decision process. This process includes the patient's identified needs, using evidence-based practice and our values to guide the prioritization of what will and will not be

EXHIBIT 26-5   Care Model Principles *(continued)*

done in the plan of care. It also includes appropriate delegation to other team members and referral to other disciplines and services.

6. ***Leadership.*** Leaders have interlocking accountability within the context of stewardship and the healing healthcare philosophy. Leaders manage the caregivers who manage patient care and provide resources, support, and insight in navigating system issues. Leaders support and mentor nurses in resource-based decision

making. Based on mutual respect, shared vision, and values, leaders are cognizant of the diversity of the workforce and promote the growth and development of staff. Leaders promote recruitment and retention by modeling the St. Charles Health System (SCHS) values and engaging in relationship-centered, resource-based leadership. Leaders delegate decisions appropriately to the nursing staff and articulate the decision-making model to the team.

Source: Copyright © 2009, St. Charles Medical Center and Creative HealthCare Management.

completing a quality assessment that includes how the department is performing in relation to organization-wide quality objectives, internal and external audit results, and regulatory requirements. Scope of service includes defining aspects of service, developing a department vision, and creating success factors for achieving the vision, as well as managing key processes. Customer needs assessment is performed through surveys and focus groups. Skill assessment includes assessing caregiver learning needs and developing an education plan. Resource

assessment marries the department requirements with the budgeting process, including labor, capital, and technological needs. Leaders are expected to benchmark with other facilities both inside and outside of the area of health care to ensure that they are meeting or exceeding national as well as local standards.

Continuous improvement involves addressing opportunities for improvement related to the department requirements, as well as preventive and corrective actions. Preventive and corrective actions are identified through internal and

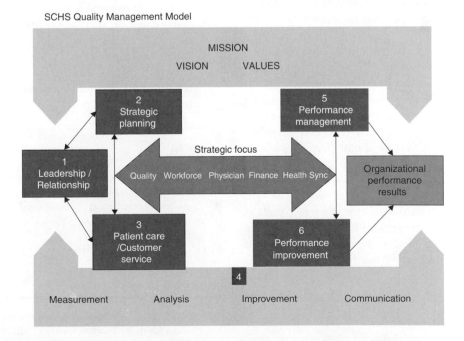

FIGURE 26-12   Quality Management Model
Source: Copyright © 2009, St. Charles Medical Center.

external surveys and audits as well as by addressing variances in quality indicator monitors.

Relationship-centered service is achieved through creating a culture of healing and accountability, implementing service standards, and designing the hospital around patient needs. It also requires a process for selecting caregivers who are compatible with the hospital's values and philosophy of care, as well as ensuring caregiver competency. Relationship-centered service requires a commitment to the ongoing development of caregivers and their teams. People Skills workshops provide an experiential learning setting for the development of communication and relationship-building skills. In addition, each team develops their own vision focused on how they support the mission and interaction agreements that describe their intention for their team and agreements on how they will work together to achieve the work environment they desire.

As with any document, this process is just words on a page unless it rests on a solid foundation of each person's participation and teamwork, as well as the hospital's commitment to the ongoing investment in the caregiver's personal growth and development.

In conclusion, at St. Charles it does not matter what position you are in or role you play—you may be a CEO responsible for strategic planning, a nurse caring for a patient at the bedside, or a housekeeper cleaning the room—you are a caregiver. Whether we directly touch the patient or not, we are all caregivers, everyone affects our patients. Patient care is our core business; we are all there to serve. It is important that each caregiver brings a focused intention to his or her work, an intention of healing. Creating a healing environment happens in large ways, such as designing a new hospital, and it happens in simple acts of everyday work as people pick up a piece of trash on the floor, hold a hand, smile at a patient, or help a visitor find the way. We have learned that implementing relationship-centered care and the healing healthcare philosophy is really a lifelong work. It starts with the intention to provide a healing environment and requires a commitment to personal growth and continuous learning. It also requires everyone's participation and is best sustained when it is a strategic initiative of the hospital supported by the board of directors and management.

Directions for
FUTURE RESEARCH

1. Further explore understandings of the role of relationships in health and healing.
2. Investigate how the arts can be used to help the healing process.
3. Research the effect of intention in healing.
4. Explore the many dimensions of healing and how they apply in your own environment.
5. Explore ways you can utilize a principle-based care model.
6. Explore ways to imbed a resource-based, waste reduction approach in care at the bedside.

Nurse Healer
REFLECTIONS

After reading this chapter, the nurse healer will be able to answer or to begin the process of answering the following questions:

- How does the environment affect my own healing?
- After reflecting on a recent time when I felt most helpful to a patient, what do I think contributed to this experience? Ask myself *why* at least five times.
- What can I do now in my work environment to better support healing?
- What does the ethic of the healing healthcare philosophy—healing ourselves, our relationships, and our communities—mean to me personally?

 For a full suite of assignments and additional learning activities, use the access code located in the front of your book to visit this exclusive website: http://go.jblearning.com/dossey. If you do not have an access code, you can obtain one at the site.

NOTES

1. K. Blais et al., *Professional Nursing Practice* (Upper Saddle River, NJ: Pearson Prentice Hall, 2006).
2. M. Cooke et al., "The Effect of Music on Preoperative Anxiety in Day Surgery," *Journal of Advanced Nursing* 52, no. 1 (2005): 47–55.

3. E. Dayton and K. Henriksen, "Teamwork and Communication: Communication Failure: Basic Components, Contributing Factors, and the Call for Structure," *Joint Commission Journal on Quality and Patient Safety* 33, no. 1 (2007): 34–47.

4. K. Dijkstra et al., "Physical Environmental Stimuli That Turn Healthcare Facilities into Healing Environment Through Psychologically Mediated Effects: Systematic Review," *The Authors, Journal* compilation 2006. Blackwell Publishing LTD (2006): 166–181.

5. M. Good et al., "Relaxation and Music Reduce Pain Following Intestinal Surgery," *Research in Nursing & Health* 28 (2005): 240–251.

6. A. Kennedy et al., "The Effectiveness and Cost Effectiveness of a National Lay-Led Self-Care Support Programme for Patients with Long-Term Conditions: A Pragmatic Randomised Controlled Trial," *Journal of Epidemiology and Community Health* 61, no. 3 (2007): 254–261.

7. S. G. Lorenz, "The Potential of the Patient Room to Promote Healing and Well-Being in Patients and Nurses: An Integrative Review of the Research," *Holistic Nursing Practice* (September/ October 2007): 263–277.

8. G. Pacheco-Lopez et al., "Brain Mechanisms of Placebo: Expectations and Associations That Heal: Immunomodulatory Placebo Effects and Its Neurobiology," *Brain, Behavior, and Immunity* 20 (2006): 430–446.

9. R. Ulrich et al., "Role of the Physical Environment in the Hospital of the 21st Century: A Once in a Lifetime Opportunity," Center for Health Design (2004). http://www.healthdesign.org/chd /research/role-physical-environment-hospital-21st-century.

10. V. Kshettry et al., "Complementary Alternative Medical Therapies for Heart Surgery Patients: Feasibility, Safety, and Impact," *Society of Thoracic Surgeons* 81 (2006): 201–206.

11. D. Sluyter, *Relationship-Centered Care Newsletter* (Kalamazoo, MI: Fetzer Institute, 2000).

12. Thomson Reuters, *Top Health Systems* (news release) (Ann Arbor, MI, 2009, 2010, 2011).

13. C. P. Tresolini and the Pew-Fetzer Task Force, *Health Professions and Relationship-Centered Care* (San Francisco, CA: Pew Health Professions Commission, 1994).

14. D. Childre and B. Cryer, *From Chaos to Coherence* (Boulder Creek, CA: Planetary, A Division of HeartMath LLC, 2000).

15. K. McCauley and R. Irwin, "Changing the Work Environment in ICUs to Achieve Patient-Focused Care: The Time Has Come," *CHEST* 130, no. 5 (2006): 1571–1578.

16. N. Moore and H. Komras, *Patient-Focused Healing: Integrating Caring and Curing in Health Care* (San Francisco, CA: Jossey-Bass, 1994).

17. N. Moore, "Relationship-Centered Service: St. Charles Medical Center and Perspective: How You Can Become Involved," in *Integrating Complementary Medicine into Health Systems*, ed. N. Faass (Gaithersburg, MD: Aspen Publishers, 2001).

18. C. Williams, "The Identification of Family Members' Contribution to Patients' Care in the Intensive Care Unit: A Naturalistic Inquiry," *Nursing in Critical Care* 10, no. 1 (2005): 6–14.

19. S. Dingman et al., "Implementing a Caring Model to Improve Patient Satisfaction," *Journal of Nursing Administration* 29, no. 12 (1999): 30–37.

20. B. Dossey, L. Keegan, and C. Guzzetta, *Holistic Nursing: A Handbook for Practice*, 4th ed. (Sudbury, MA: Jones and Bartlett, 2005).

21. Press Ganey Associates, *Press Ganey Satisfaction Measurement, St. Charles Medical Center, Bend, Oregon, 2000–2010* (South Bend, IN: Press Ganey Associates, 2000–2010).

22. J. Stephens, "St. Charles Improvements Will Serve the Community," *Bulletin* (November 14, 2002).

23. N. Faass, ed., *Integrating Complementary Medicine into Health Systems* (Gaithersburg, MD: Aspen Publishers, 2001).

24. H. Benson and E. Stuart, *The Wellness Book: The Comprehensive Guide to Maintaining Health and Treating Stress-Related Illness* (New York, NY: Simon and Schuster, 1992).

25. J. Costello, "Dying Well: Nurses' Experiences of 'Good' and 'Bad' Deaths in Hospitals," *Journal of Advanced Nursing* 54, no. 5 (2006): 594–601.

26. J. Leighty, "Healing by Design," *NurseWeek* (April 28, 2003).

27. M. Lane, "Creativity and Spirituality in Nursing," *Holistic Nursing Practice* 19, no. 3 (2005): 122–125.

28. Deschutes County Health Department, Healthy Start Program news release (March 1, 2011).

29. N. Cousins, *Anatomy of an Illness as Perceived by the Patient: Reflections on Healing and Regeneration* (New York, NY: Bantam Books, 1979).

30. M. Wheatley, *Turning to One Another: Simple Conversations to Restore Hope to the Future* (San Francisco, CA: Berrett-Koehler, 2002).

31. M. Manthey, "Leadership for Relationship-Based Care," *Creative Nursing* 1 (2006): 10.

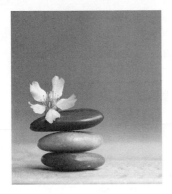

Chapter 27

Exploring Integrative Medicine: The Story of a Large, Urban, Tertiary Care Hospital

Lori L. Knutson

Nurse Healer

OBJECTIVES

Theoretical

- Discuss the integrative approach to health care.
- Analyze the components of a healing environment assessment.

Clinical

- Integrate holistic nursing in the acute care hospital setting.
- Initiate practice changes that integrate holistic therapies into the care of patients.
- Determine the relationships required for successfully changing the culture of the hospital environment.
- Model relationship-centered care in professional partnerships and in the care of the patient.

Personal

- Determine whether you can approach leadership in a changing organizational culture with passion and fearlessness.

DEFINITIONS

Integrative medicine: A philosophy of healthcare practice that emphasizes the "whole person" view of health and healing and, in practice, blends conventional, alter-

native, and complementary interventions to optimize curing and healing.

Integrative nurse clinician (IM nurse clinician): A certified holistic nurse who performs needs assessments of patients and the clinical environment and initiates appropriate healing interventions to enable positive changes in health. An IM nurse clinician is certified as a holistic nurse through the American Holistic Nurses Certification Corporation (AHNCC)[1] by completing training in a healing modality, spending a minimum of 5 years in conventional acute care nursing practice, and learning a dedication to personal self-care. The responsibilities of the IM nurse clinician include the following:

- Inpatient holistic health assessments
- Patient, staff, and community education
- Providing healing therapies for inpatients
- Quality initiatives and program development

■ INTRODUCTION

Changing the healthcare environment is an endeavor to change the culture of a tertiary hospital. Whether we speak about the internal or external elements, or the physical or psychological elements, the foundation of change is based on the interconnectedness of relationships, with the primary focus on the balance of healing and curing. Abbott Northwestern Hospital in Minneapolis, Minnesota, is redefining its culture to embrace changes that best serve the patients and support the practice of the health professionals involved in that care. The dynamics of changing a culture are continuous and require an openness to honor both the successes and the perceived failures. Blending the multiple responsibilities of the acute care hospital with the concepts of healing and utilizing a broad range of nonmedical services is based in simple relationships. The interconnectedness of relationships is the foundation of all transformative efforts. One strategic initiative that stimulated the change of culture was the development of an integrative medicine department in this hospital.

■ THE SETTING: A LARGE, URBAN, TERTIARY CARE HOSPITAL

Abbott Northwestern Hospital is the largest not-for-profit hospital in the Minneapolis area. Each year, the hospital provides comprehensive health care for more than 200,000 patients and their families from the Twin Cities area and throughout the upper Midwest. More than 5,000 nonmedical employees, 1,600 physicians, 2,000 nurses, and 550 volunteers work as a team for the benefit of each patient. Abbott Northwestern Hospital is a part of Allina Hospitals and Clinics, a family of hospitals, clinics, and care services in Minnesota and western Wisconsin. The services available at Abbott Northwestern Hospital include the following:

- Complete medical, surgical, and critical care for patients age 12 years and older
- Twenty-four-hour emergency services
- Multispecialty care and clinical expertise in behavioral health services, cardiovascular services, medical and surgical services, neuroscience, oncology, orthopedics, rehabilitation, spine care, and women's health
- Outpatient care in more than 50 specialty areas
- Innovative and individual pain treatment
- Education programs, support services, and public health screenings
- Outreach programs to improve the health of the community

■ INITIATING THE CHANGE OF CULTURE

The nurturing of relationships provides a catalyst for change and is essential to renewing and enhancing the spirit within the hospital. To strengthen and heal relationships, three components of holistic philosophy were introduced to staff: (1) relationship-centered care; (2) presence and intention; and (3) psychoneuroimmunology. The initial focus for education was with the nurses, who by virtue of their role and sheer number have the greatest impact in changing the organic aspects of the environment.

Relationship-centered care (see Chapter 1) serves as a guideline for addressing the bio-psycho-social-spiritual dimensions of individuals in integrating caring, healing, and holism into health care.[2] The framework, which consists of patient–practitioner relationship, community–practitioner relationship, and practitioner–practitioner relationship, provided the concrete criteria that staff could begin to integrate into practice. The introduction of the concepts of presence and intention to the nursing staff engaged them in revisiting their purpose, reminded them of their personal impact on the healing process of the patient, and provided them with skills in mindfulness.[3] The science of psychoneuroimmunology was incorporated to provide a scientific basis to the power of thought and its impact on their personal self-care.

Developing a common language is one of the first steps in success. The two most important concepts to understand are integrative medicine and holistic nursing.

Integrative Medicine

Integrative medicine is a comprehensive, primary care system in which wellness and healing of the whole person are the major goals, as opposed to the basic suppression of symptoms of disease.[4] However, integrative medicine is not CAM (complementary and alternative medicine). Integrative medicine is patient-centered, healing-oriented care that emphasizes the patient–caregiver relationship. It focuses on the least invasive, least toxic, and least costly methods to promote health by blending the practices of CAM and conventional Western medicine. Central to integrative medicine is the view of the whole person as a dynamic being interrelating with his or her environment, both internal and external, with this interrelationship as the key to health and well-being. The goal is to move medicine to include not only its fundamental platform of science but to create a health system that broadly focuses on the well-being of our patients as well as its practitioners.[5]

■ EMBEDDING CULTURAL CHANGE

The Integrative Medicine Initiative at Abbott Northwestern Hospital is a demonstration of the process involved in embedding change into a system. **Exhibit 27-1** lists the key embedding components in this model developed by Schein and described by Nellen.[6]

As the largest hospital-based program of its kind in the country, the Penny George Institute for Health and Healing is setting national standards for enhancing health care through an integrative health approach as follows:

- Blending complementary therapies, integrative medicine, and conventional Western medicine
- Providing services to inpatients and outpatients
- Educating healthcare professionals
- Teaching community members about health promotion and self-healing practices

- Conducting research to identify best practices of integrative health and the impact of these services on healthcare costs[5]

At Abbott Northwestern Hospital, there were very specific steps that led to the successful development of the integrative medicine program. Although the steps are not always sequential, each was approached with specific strategies. Key changes were made through inspired and gifted leadership and presence in all areas of the hospital functions. The administrator was not only an administrator for this department, but played key roles in the overall administration of other hospital functions and services. By becoming as essential to hospital functions as others in her job class, the administrator developed a position of influence and credibility from which she could nurture the concept of integrative medicine and bring it to fruition. One of the most important aspects of her work was to weave the integrative services into the daily functions of nurses within the hospital. Nurses were seen as the key to significant cultural change in the organization. The key members of the initial team of the department were integrated medicine (IM) nurse clinicians. The IM nurse clinicians also followed the model by communicating with other services within the hospital and serving on committees and activities that directly affect nursing practice within the hospital.

EXHIBIT 27-1   Culture-Embedding Mechanisms

Primary Embedding Mechanisms	Secondary Articulation and Reinforcement Mechanisms
What leaders pay attention to, measure, and control on a regular basis	Organization design and structure
How leaders react to critical incidents and organizational crises	Organizational systems and procedures
Observed criteria by which leaders allocate scarce resources	Organizational rites and rituals
Deliberate role modeling, teaching, and coaching	Design of physical space, facades, and buildings
Observed criteria by which leaders allocate rewards and status	Stories, legends, and myths about people and events
Observed criteria by which leaders recruit, select, promote, retire, and excommunicate organizational members	Formal statements of organizational philosophy, values, and creed

Key to the development of these new concepts was a mission statement. The mission chosen was and is to enhance the health of individuals, families, and communities by stimulating and supporting integrative medicine at Abbott Northwestern Hospital, its related institutions, and in the broader field of health care, through patient services, education, and research.

The Integrative Medicine Department

The design of the department included multiple steps. The following were some elements included in the process:

- Descriptions of the roles and responsibilities of staff within the department
- Identification of programs and services for patients and employees
- Financial viability
- Quality measures to support enhanced patient care and outcomes
- Interdepartmental partnerships to establish dynamic working relationships
- A focus on the self-care of the healthcare professional

The leadership of Abbott Northwestern Hospital's integrative medicine department is based on servant–leadership principles. "Servant–leadership is a practical philosophy which supports people who choose to serve first, and then lead as a way of expanding service to individuals and institutions. Servant–leadership encourages collaboration, trust, foresight, listening, and ethical use of power and empowerment."[7]

■ THE INTEGRATIVE MEDICINE DEPARTMENT

Key to the ongoing management of the department is the physician advisory committee with members who represent each of the areas of excellence or specialty within the hospital. The integrative medicine team as described in **Figure 27-1** consists of a team of practitioners linked to administrative staff. The following are the roles and responsibilities within this team:

- *Executive director:* Overall accountability, physician relationships, philanthropic initiatives, national trending, and external partnerships.
- *Director of strategy and development:* Strategic plan and financial accountability, personnel and human resource (HR) activities, performance improvement, stakeholder relationships, executive leadership for patient

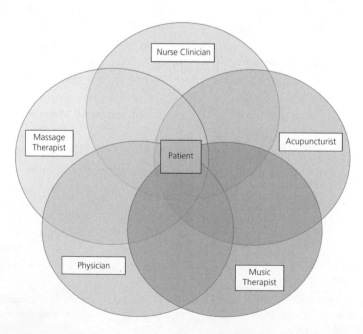

FIGURE 27-1   Integrative Medicine Inpatient Care Team

care communities, and partner with nursing leadership.

- *Director of research:* Manages research projects that address both outcomes research and specific therapy-centered efficacy studies.
- *IM nurse clinician:* Provides integrative medicine patient consultations, participates in program development, staff education and training, facilitates and manages the continuum of care, and partners in research projects and quality initiatives.
- *IM practitioner:* Provides specific alternative and complementary services; practitioners employed have a primary specialty service (e.g., massage therapy) but are trained to provide other services (e.g., guided imagery, healing touch) as well. Figure 27-1 demonstrates the interlinking of the practitioners. True to the philosophy of the department, the patient is the center of caring.

Several principles were key to sustaining the focus of the department. These include the following:

- Relationship-centered care
- Partnerships
- Whole-person view
- Focus on healing
- Emphasis on self-responsibility
- Prevention
- Blending of conventional and nonconventional healthcare practices

As the integrative medicine department began to unfold, each decision was based on the principles outlined in **Exhibit 27-2**.

EXHIBIT 27-2   Key Program Development Principles

- The program will have solid objectives.
- The program will be evidence based.
- Outcome measures will be developed.
- Productivity standards will be clearly stated and regularly evaluated.
- The program will be fiscally responsible.
- Quality assurance will be a continuous process.

Functions of Integrative Medicine at Abbott Northwestern Hospital

The integrative medicine department has focused on its threefold mission of service to patients in the areas of clinical services, education, and research.

Clinical Services

The department provides programs and services that enhance the innate healing of patients and staff. New programs and services have been developed to integrate into the hospital environment, including those provided by specialists and those provided by nurses as part of their established scope of practice. Specialty services include massage therapy, acupuncture and acupressure, reflexology, healing touch and therapeutic touch, mind–body therapies, and the services of IM nurse clinicians.

The services are provided to patients in their hospital rooms and are initiated by the nursing staff providing direct care for the patient. Including the nursing order for these services in the hospital electronic medical record (EMR) system facilitates the referral to which the integrative medicine staff respond. All the services are documented using the hospital's EMR system, which has embedded templates for the integrative medicine assessments and ongoing progress notes. Practitioners who are not nurses are identified as integrative medicine providers. Currently, the integrative medicine department staff provide an average of 1,500 visits per month (900 inpatient visits), varying with the hospital census, and 700 outpatient visits.

Education

Education is a key component of the department's mission. This education includes the education of staff nurses, nursing students, CAM practitioner students, physician fellows in medicine, and ongoing education of the community.

The education of the staff nurses is of key importance to initiate and sustain the culture change within the hospital. Nurses are the key to cultural change in the tertiary care facility. The culture of the acute care hospital has been known to make it difficult for nurses to transfer the concepts of their education in holistic nursing practices to the environment of the hospital. The key to changing nursing practice is to embrace a holistic approach that allows institutions to flourish and where healing emerges resulting in creative delivery models.[8] To change the care of patients, an educational initiative has been implemented.

The IM nurse clinicians created a 48-hour educational intervention for nurses, provided for staff nurses from each specialty area in the hospital. The program includes education to transform nursing practice by incorporating the principles of healing and holistic nursing. The program also presents a primer on mind–body therapies, traditional Chinese medicine, massage, and stress management techniques. This education program emphasizes nurse self-care to promote each nurse's health and well-being. A unique component of this program is a mentorship by the IM nurse clinician of each nurse on the unit for at least one shift.

In addition, the IM nurse clinicians participate in other valuable forums that promote excellence in nursing practice including nursing staff orientation, professional development days, and targeted educational programs for specific units. Nursing students in the hospital for a nurse internship are rotated through the department. Each nurse intern spends at least one shift with the nurse clinicians. The department has a partnership with Northwestern Health Sciences University, in Bloomington, Minnesota. The department provides internships for both the students of and traditional Chinese medicine and massage. This clinical rotation provides an opportunity for the students to develop the skills necessary to care for hospitalized patients.

The Transformative Nurse Training (TNT) Program is one example of the Penny George Institute for Health and Healing Abbott Northwestern commitment to excellence in nursing. The program brings nurses back to the essence of nursing practice and teaches the foundations and principles of holistic nursing.[5] Over the course of 6 day-long sessions, nurses acquire practical skills to promote and enhance self-care and care for patients, including massage, guided imagery, physiologic relaxation response, meditation, Oriental medicine, nutrition, and much more.

An important and unique component of the program is mentorship. After completing the course, participants have the opportunity to work with an integrative health nurse clinician to integrate what they have learned into their own lives and use it to enhance patient care. This has led to increased nurse engagement and patient satisfaction and has improved patient outcomes.

Researchers are evaluating the changes in nurses' attitudes and their knowledge and application of therapies that are addressed in the transformative nurse training program. Since it was established in 2006, 192 nurses from Abbott Northwestern and other healthcare organizations (including Courage Center, Children's Hospitals and Clinics of Minnesota, Ridgeview Medical Center, United Hospital, Walker Methodist Health Center, and Waseca Medical Center) have participated in the 48-hour training program. The program has also been provided to nurses at two Department of Veterans Affairs hospitals in California as part of a scientific study.

Research

The research department is engaged in several different types of research. Outcomes research is being completed in partnership with the Samueli Institute of Washington, D.C. The researchers are examining patient outcomes utilizing the database maintained by the department.

Therapy-specific research is being implemented by the IM nurse clinicians in specific units of the hospital, measuring the effect of aromatherapy on patients' sleep. The acupuncturists are working with a university professor measuring the effect of acupuncture on tachycardia following cardiac procedures.

The effect of the education program on nurses' beliefs and practices is being measured at the program's conclusion, at 3 months and 6 months. Directions for future research are being developed as the environment of delivering care changes and funding becomes available.

■ CONCLUSION

We are in unprecedented times in the delivery of health care by hospitals. Patients, practitioners, and hospital leadership are recognizing the need to engage in an integrative approach to health and healing. Including integrative medicine principles and practices will require changes in the culture of the hospital and of nursing. We have briefly described some of the components of this change process. Each organization approaches change with its own unique solutions and staff. By making patient care the most important focus, the changes organizations make will be profound.

Directions for
FUTURE RESEARCH

1. Evaluate the effectiveness of integrative health care as a catalyst in the transformation of hospitals as healing environments.
2. Determine the impact of the role of holistic nursing in the hospital setting.
3. Evaluate the effect of interdepartmental partnerships based on relationship-centered care in the healing of patients and staff.
4. Determine the financial impact of a healing environment on the hospital system.

Nurse Healer
REFLECTIONS

After reading this chapter, the nurse healer will be able to answer or to begin a process of answering the following questions:

- How do I contribute to the healing environment of a hospital?
- How can I cultivate knowledge, skills, and intuition in the manifestation of professional healing relationships?
- Do I feel confident to champion the evolution of integrative health care in the hospital environment?
- Is my spiritual practice one that supports my ability to initiate change in the hospital setting?

 For a full suite of assignments and additional learning activities, use the access code located in the front of your book to visit this exclusive website: http://go.jblearning.com/dossey. If you do not have an access code, you can obtain one at the site.

NOTES

1. American Holistic Nurses Certification Corporation, "Certification Process." http://www.ahncc.org/certificationprocess.html.
2. J. E. Koerner, *Healing: The Essence of Healing*, 2nd ed. (New York, NY: Springer, 2011).
3. D. Rakel, *Integrative Medicine*, 2nd ed. (Philadelphia, PA: W. B. Saunders, 2007).
4. Penny George Institute for Health and Healing, *Overview and Outcomes Report 2010* (Minneapolis, MN: Penny George Institute for Health and Healing, 2010). http://abbottnorthwestern.com/ahs/anw.nsf/page/ANW_PGIHH_Outcomes_FNL-1.ForWeb.pdf/$FILE/ANW_PGIHH_Outcomes_FNL-1.ForWeb.pdf.
5. E. Schein, "Organizational Culture and Leadership" (October 1997). http://www.tnellen.com/ted/tc/schein.html.
6. Greenleaf Center for Servant Leadership, "What Is Servant-Leadership?" http://www.greenleaf.org/whatissl/.
7. J. Crawford and L. Thornton, "Why Has Holistic Nursing Taken Off in the Last Five Years? What Has Changed?" *Alternative Therapies in Health and Medicine* 16, no. 3 (2010): 28–30.

Holistic Communication, Therapeutic Environment, and Cultural Diversity

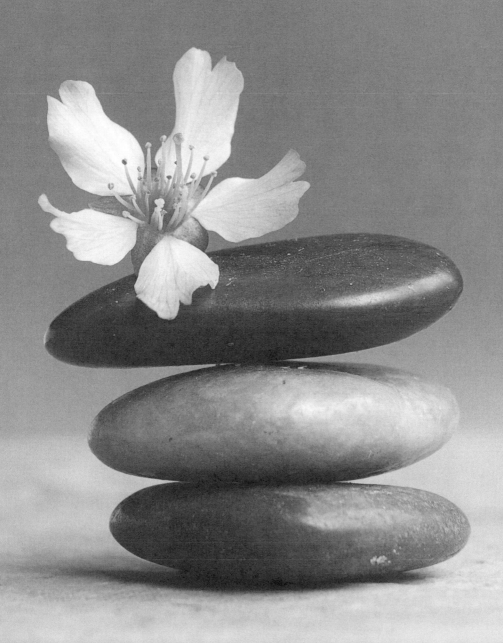

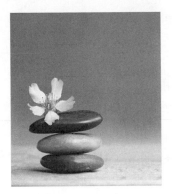

Chapter 28

Evolving from Therapeutic to Holistic Communication

Lucia Thornton and Carla Mariano

Nurse Healer
OBJECTIVES

Theoretical

- Identify foundational theories and concepts in the development of therapeutic communication.
- Describe contemporary nursing theories and concepts foundational in the development of holistic communication.
- Identify and describe the concepts that distinguish holistic communication.

Clinical

- Integrate foundational holistic communication processes into clinical practice.
- Integrate and utilize intention, centering, grounding, caring, healing, transcendent presence, and intuition in establishing a caring-healing field of communication.

Personal

- Engage in reflective practices to increase self-awareness and personal growth.
- Integrate and utilize intention, centering, presence, caring, and intuition in creating and maintaining a healing field of communication in daily life.

DEFINITIONS

Energy field: The fundamental unit of the living and nonliving. *Field* is a unifying concept. *Energy* signifies the dynamic nature of the field; a field is in continuous motion and is infinite.[1]

Holistic communication: A caring-healing process that calls forth the full use of self in interacting with another. It incorporates the constructs and processes of therapeutic communication within a framework that acknowledges the infinite, spiritual, and energetic nature of Being, the centrality of being heart centered, and the importance of intention, self-knowledge, transcendent presence, and intuition in our interactions.[2]

Person: An energy field that is infinite and spiritual in essence and is in continual mutual process with the environment. Each person manifests unique physical, mental, emotional, and social or relational patterns that are interrelated, inseparable, and continually evolving.[3]

Therapeutic communication: A goal-directed form of communication used to achieve goals that promote client health and well-being.[p15] Empathy, unconditional regard, genuineness, respect, concern, caring, and compassion are conveyed through active listening, active observing, focusing, restating, reflecting, and interpreting.[2p533]

■ THEORY AND RESEARCH

Pioneers in Therapeutic Communication

Therapeutic communication is a field of study that has been influenced by theorists, researchers, and clinicians from a multitude of professions including nursing, psychology, sociology, and physics. These early pioneers created a rich foundation of ideas and constructs, many of which were holistic in nature. It is important to understand these perspectives to gain a greater understanding of how this work has evolved and its usefulness in holistic practice. Some of the significant contributions of nurse theorist Hildegard Peplau and those of Martin Buber, Carl Jung, Harry Stack Sullivan, and Carl Rogers are presented.

Peplau: A Visionary in Relationship-Based Caring

Peplau, the "mother of psychiatric nursing," was the first to emphasize the nurse–client relationship as being the foundation of nursing practice.

The concept of partnership between nurse and client originated in Peplau's interpersonal model. The idea that the nurse helps guide the patient and the patient takes an active role in the treatment plan was indeed revolutionary in 1952 and was in opposition to mainstream thinking, which promoted a role in which the client was dependent on the nurse.

The essence of Peplau's work revolved around the concept of the shared experience. She shifted the focus of nursing practice from one that was based on medical intervention to an interpersonal model in which the nurse became the therapeutic agent. Peplau identified nursing roles during the course of the nurse–client relationship. The roles include *Stranger*, providing acceptance and trust; *Resource*, answering questions and giving information; *Teacher*, giving instruction and analyzing the learner experience; *Counselor*, helping the client derive meaning from the current experience; *Surrogate*, advocating for the client and clarifying dependence, independence, and interdependence; and *Leader*, assisting the client to assume maximum responsibility for meeting goals that are mutually established.[4p89]

Peplau's concepts provided a bridge between the old paradigm in which the client was dependent on the healthcare system to one in which the client was an active participant in treatment and care. Her ideas paved the way for communication that involved the whole person.

Cogent Concepts from Other Disciplines

In the field of therapeutic communication, many rich ideas and constructs originated with psychotherapists. Concepts and ideas from Buber, Sullivan, Rogers, and Jung are similar to concepts that are foundational to holistic communication.

Martin Buber introduced the idea that the therapeutic process involves mutual discovery and emphasized the importance of mutual respect in the client–therapist interaction. He coined the term *I-Thou relationship*, which reflects a reverence in the client–therapist relationship. In this orientation, the therapist consciously creates a transcendent space in the relationship, fostering shared authenticity and compassion.

Harry Stack Sullivan was a contemporary of Peplau and influenced the development of her interpersonal model. Sullivan introduced the idea of the therapeutic relationship and described it as being a human connection that heals. Carl Rogers saw the therapist as an agent of healing. Rogers's hallmark characteristics that he identified as being essential to the client-centered relationship were unconditional regard, empathy, and genuineness. Carl Jung examined the complexity of gender roles and our universal heritage as human beings. He described the first half of life as a search for self and the second half of life as a search for soul.[4pp9-13]

All of these therapists, and many others not mentioned, have contributed ideas that have significantly influenced the effectiveness of the therapeutic communication process. The concepts of partnership, healing, reverence, unconditional regard, empathy, genuineness, spirituality, and many more first found their place in therapeutic communication before being embraced by holistic nursing.

■ NURSING THEORY RELATED TO HOLISTIC COMMUNICATION

The nursing theorists whose theories and concepts have facilitated the evolution of therapeutic communication toward holistic communication are Martha Rogers, Margaret Newman, and Jean Watson. Concepts related to holistic communication are explicated and briefly discussed. For an overview of these theories, see Chapter 5.

Martha Rogers

Rogers uses the term *unitary human being* in place of *person* and defines who we are as "an irreducible, indivisible, pan-dimensional energy field identified by pattern and manifesting characteristics that are specific to the whole and which cannot be predicted from knowledge of the parts."[1p7] Rogers further defines energy field as "the fundamental unit of the living and the nonliving. Field is a unifying concept. Energy signifies the dynamic nature of the field; a field is in continuous motion and is infinite."[1p7]

The nature of therapeutic communication changes when Rogers's definitions are applied. How does one communicate with an energy field that is infinite in nature? Also, if we accept Rogers's definitions, then communication shifts from being a linear or circular process to a pan-dimensional energetic process. Accepting Rogers's definition also shifts our thinking to view communication as a field phenomenon. And finally, Rogers's definition invites us to entertain the idea that our interactions can extend beyond the realm of this physical universe, beyond the space–time continuum and into dimensions that are infinite.

Rogers's Principle of Integrality also has implications for the nature of holistic communication. Rogers defines integrality as a "continuous mutual human field and environmental field process."[1p8] Rogers describes person and environment as "open systems" and states that "man and environment are continuously exchanging matter and energy with one another."[5] This implies that *all* that we are—our thoughts, behaviors, emotions, that which is conscious, and that which is unconscious—interacts and affects everything and everyone in our environment. Likewise, everyone and everything that exists in our environment are continuously exchanging matter and energy with us. Integrating this concept into our lives challenges us to transform our lives and our way of being. If we are to act in a way that is therapeutic, in a way that promotes healing, we ourselves must be whole and healed.

This concept reinforces the importance of self-awareness and self-knowledge.

Margaret Newman

The task of nursing intervention, according to Newman, "is not to try to change another person's patterns but to recognize it as information that depicts the whole and relate to it as it unfolds."[6] The nurse must first be able to recognize her own patterns before entering into this process with a patient. Again, self-knowledge is paramount for the nurse to be effective in a caring, healing relationship.

The responsibility of the nurse is not to make people well or to prevent their getting sick, but to assist people in recognizing the power that is within them to move to higher levels of consciousness. The nurse's awareness of being rather than doing is the primary mechanism for helping. Newman quotes Thomas Moore to emphasize the importance of staying fully present to all that life offers, without trying to fix or intervene: "By doing less, more is accomplished . . . what is needed is not taking sides when there is a conflict at a deep level. It may be necessary to stretch the heart wide enough to embrace contradiction and paradox."[7]

Newman illuminates the concepts of pattern recognition, being fully present, and the importance of self-awareness and transformation in the holistic communication process.

Jean Watson

Watson defines person as "an embodied spirit; a transpersonal, transcendent, evolving consciousness; unity of mind-body-spirit; person-nature-universe as oneness, connected."[8] Watson is the first nursing theorist to address the concept of soul, as in the following passage:

> My conception of life and personhood is tied to notions that one's soul possesses a body that is not confined by objective space and time. . . . Notions of personhood, then, transcend the here and now, and one has the capacity to coexist with past, present, future, all at once. As a result of this view, there is a great deal of regard, respect, and awe given to the concept of a human soul (spirit, or higher sense of self) that is

greater than the physical, mental, and emotional existence of a person at any given point in time.[9p45]

How does one address the soul in the process of therapeutic communication? Watson's answer to this is the transpersonal caring relationship. Engaging with another at the transpersonal level is not a technique that can be learned. Rather, it is the ability of the person to access the higher self and move from that place of higher consciousness in interactions with another. This process calls for the "full use of the self."[9p69] Watson's description of the art of transpersonal caring also serves as a description of the caring-healing process of holistic communication.

> The nurse is able to form a union with the other person on a level that transcends the physical, and that preserves the subjectivity and physicality of persons without reducing them to the moral of objects. . . . The union of feelings can potentiate self-healing and discovery in his or her own existence. That is the great attractive force of the art of transpersonal caring in nursing.[9p68]

Another concept that Watson expanded on and that has significance in the application of holistic communication is that of the phenomenal field.

> The phenomenal field incorporates consciousness along with perceptions of self and others; feelings, thoughts, bodily sensations, spiritual beliefs, desires, goals, expectations, environmental considerations, meanings, and the symbolic nature of one's perceptions—all of this based upon one's life history and the presenting moment as well as the imaged future.[9pp55–56]

From Watson's perspective, "an event or actual caring occasion" occurs when two persons come together with their unique life histories and their phenomenal fields.[9p58] When people come together they share a phenomenal field, which becomes part of the life history of both and alters the dynamics of the present and the future. From this perspective, holistic communication can be viewed as a field experience.

This is consistent with Rogers's Principle of Integrality in relation to the open and infinite nature of energy fields, where person and environment are in continuous mutual interaction. Watson, through her descriptions of her model, shows how Rogers's Principle of Integrality can be applied.

A field perspective adds a richer and more holistic approach to therapeutic communication, wherein the gestalt of one person interacts with another. It challenges us to develop ways of being and ways of interacting that embrace the whole.

■ THERAPEUTIC COMMUNICATION SKILLS: A PREREQUISITE FOR HOLISTIC COMMUNICATION

Traditional models of therapeutic communication do the following: define and prescribe various stages or phases, delineate various roles for the nurse or therapist, identify verbal and nonverbal communication skills, and identify therapist characteristics that are essential to creating a therapeutic milieu.

It is important for nurses to be familiar with the various stages of relationship formation and to develop and refine communication skills. It is also important for nurses to understand and integrate the qualities and attributes that are important in creating a therapeutic exchange. Empathy, unconditional regard, genuineness, respect, concern, caring, and compassion are vital and essential attributes for therapeutic communication. Developing and refining communication skills, including active listening, active observing, focusing, restating, reflecting, and interpreting, are also important in facilitating the therapeutic process. The aforementioned knowledge, skills, techniques, and attributes are foundational to the therapeutic communication process and are prerequisites to engaging in the caring, healing exchange that characterizes holistic communication. Acquiring these skills takes time and is enhanced by experience. Mastering these skills is a lifelong process that is facilitated by reflective practices, guidance, sage mentoring, and a commitment to self-knowledge and awareness.

The next step is to identify how a holistic approach to therapeutic communication would manifest itself. It is important to consider the distinguishing characteristics of holistic communication and how can we integrate these to create a caring, healing environment.

■ DISTINGUISHING CHARACTERISTICS OF A HOLISTIC ORIENTATION TO COMMUNICATION

Preaccess and Assessment Phase

The holistic communication process acknowledges the importance of being centered and creating an intention before engaging in a caring-healing interaction with another. These two processes, being centered and creating intention, constitute the preaccess phase involved in holistic interactions. This phase lays the foundation for caring, healing communication and occurs before any person-to-person interaction takes place. As the nurse stays present to the moment, to self, and to the person, a healing environment is maintained. Consciously creating a healing environment, no matter where one is working, nurtures both the client and the self at a deep level.[2p537]

It is useful to note the distinction between *accessing* and *assessment*. The word *accessing* is preferred because it has the connotation of being open to receiving information in a nonjudgmental way. The term *assessment* implies appraising, evaluating, and judging. An essential characteristic of holistic communication is the mutuality inherent in the experience—this means that both the nurse and client participate equally in the process. Utilizing language that supports the concept of partnership reinforces a commitment to mutuality.

Acknowledgment of the Infinite and Sacred Nature of Being

Holistic nursing acknowledges that people are infinite, sacred, and spiritual beings. Florence Nightingale spoke of human beings as a "reflection of the Divine with physical, metaphysical, and intellectual attributes." Jean Watson teaches that we are "sacred beings," and Martha Rogers speaks of unitary human beings as "energy fields that are infinite in nature." The Model of Whole-Person Caring™ combines these concepts to define person as "an energy field that is open, infinite, and spiritual in essence and in continual mutual process with the environment. Each person manifests unique physical, mental, emotional, and social or relational patterns that are interrelated, inseparable, and continually evolving."[10] Thus, from the perspective of holistic nursing theorists and models, people are infinite and sacred in nature. This orientation makes a difference in how we approach each other. It shifts how we speak, how we listen, how we relate, and how we interact. When we perceive human beings as sacred, our words, actions, and behaviors are significantly affected.

Moreover, when we view ourselves and others as spiritual, infinite beings with finite bodies, our relationship to illness, diseases, and death shifts dramatically. Communication may be oriented to soul's purpose in addition to symptom relief. This orientation creates a potential to explore and derive meaning from life's challenges and create a healing environment even in the face of death and terminal illness. Often nurses have trouble dealing with patients with a terminal illness or who are facing imminent death. When one understands that this physical life is a small part of the infinite journey, the stigma of death becomes obsolete and allows the nurse to be fully present to persons with terminal illnesses and facing death.

Heart-Centering, Heart Coherence, and the Intuitive Heart

Heart-centering is one of the first processes the nurse engages in prior to any interaction. This process involves the nurse focusing her or his attention on the heart, setting aside concerns and thoughts, and connecting with feelings of love and compassion.

Maintaining this heart-centeredness throughout interactions has many positive effects for the nurse. Research conducted at the Institute of HeartMath shows that the resultant feelings of caring and appreciation from heart-centering creates coherence in the electromagnetic energy field; balances heart rhythms; increases IgA (immunoglobulin A) levels and natural killer cell levels; increases mental clarity and problem solving; and reduces sleeplessness, body aches, fatigue, anger, sadness, hypertension, and other chronic problems.[11] Heart coherence, also referred to as physiologic coherence, cardiac coherence, or resonance, is a functional mode measured by heart rate variability (HRV) analysis wherein a person's heart rhythm pattern becomes ordered.[12]

In addition to the positive mental, psychological, and physiologic effects, coherence may help to connect people with their intuitive inner guidance. Research suggests that the heart's energy field (energetic heart) is coupled to a field of information that is not bound by the classic limits of time and space. This evidence comes from a rigorous experimental study that investigated the proposition that the body receives and processes information about a future event before the event actually happens.[13] McCraty and Childre explain that the intuitive heart or heart intelligence is coupled to a deeper part of oneself, what some may call their "higher power" or their "higher capacities." When we are heart-centered and coherent, we have a tighter coupling and closer alignment with our deeper source of intuitive intelligence.[12pp15-16]

Research also shows that the positive mental and physiologic effects experienced by the nurse can be transmitted to the person. When a person maintains a coherent electromagnetic field through the process of centering, that person's energy field positively affects those in the surrounding environment. Morris reports that a coherent energy field can be generated and/or enhanced by the intention of small groups of participants trained to send coherence-facilitating intentions to a target receiver.[14] It is believed that information about a person's emotional state is encoded in the heart's electromagnetic field and is communicated into the external environment.[12p20] When the nurse becomes heart-centered a caring-healing field is created in which the person feels safe, nurtured, and loved and is in an optimal environment for healing communication to occur.

Grounding

Grounding is the process of connecting to the Earth and the Earth's energy field to calm the mind and focus one's inner flow of energy as a means to enhance healing endeavors.[15] Centering and grounding may be considered a single continuous process because one flows into the other. As such, grounding can also be viewed as part of the preaccess phase of the holistic communication process.

Often, communication can bring up many feelings and thoughts that are emotionally charged and difficult for the nurse to deal with. Grounding provides the nurse with a steady physical, psychological, and energetic platform on which to anchor the communication process. In physical terms, grounding provides a connection between an electric circuit and the Earth. In psychological terms, grounding helps establish a feeling of self-awareness and provides a connection to the consciousness of one's own self. Energetically, grounding establishes an awareness of the unity of body, mind, and spirit, as stated by McCartney:

> The practice of grounding connects you with your spiritual intelligence, which opens a cornucopia of wisdom tools for creating health and keeping you in emotional balance and harmony. To heighten this experience, visualize your spiritual intelligence as energy or light. To ground your spiritual intelligence into your body, visualize this light in the center of your head expanding straight down your body and anchoring into the earth. In this way you are affirming "I am a spirit grounded in my body and anchored to the earth."[16]

Creating Intention

Creating an intention ideally precedes interaction with a person and is part of the preaccess phase of the holistic nurse caring process. Intentionality is interpreted in different ways. McKivergin defines intent as "the conscious alignment with creative essence and divine purpose that allows the highest good to flow through a healing intervention or through life itself."[17]

Creating an intention is a process that affects not only the mental and emotional realms, but also the physical world. Tiller demonstrated that conscious intent can be imprinted in materials that can be shipped to a distant laboratory, where they bring out the intentional effect that is imprinted on them. Recent advances in theoretical physics suggest that the space between atoms and molecules is not inert. Tiller and Dibble speculate that "this 'vacuum' may be where the intent is imprinted."[18]

Thus, creating an intention is a powerful way for the nurse to create an optimal environment for a caring-healing interaction. Examine the following intention: "I am here for the greater good of this person. I set aside my own concerns and worries and am fully present to the person here and now." With this intention the nurse is consciously setting aside her own concerns and focusing on the patient; she has set into motion the dynamic that this interaction will be "for the greater good of this person." She is also making a conscious decision to be fully present. The nurse, through this intention, creates an environment that promotes and sustains a caring-healing interaction.

Caring-Healing, Transcendent Presence

Presence has been defined as a way of being, a way of relating, a way of being with, and a way of being there. These perspectives each speak to different facets of the quality and characteristics of the attention that one person gives to another in a relationship.

Osterman and Schwartz-Barcott characterize four ways of "being there" as presence, partial presence, full presence, and transcendent presence.[19] McKivergin describes three levels of presence as physical presence, psychological presence, and therapeutic presence.[17p724]

What distinguishes holistic communication from other types of communication is the depth and profound quality of presence. Watson speaks of the full use of self in the transpersonal caring process. When the nurse becomes heart-centered, she has the capacity to resonate with the person at a heart and soul level. At this level, the nurse connects with the person at a deep psychosocial, heart-felt, and spiritual level. This is a difficult concept to describe and remains more of a felt experience. The nurse must be able to access and rest in the depth of her own Beingness before she can bring this caring, healing, transcendent presence into a relationship.

Being able to communicate from more profound levels of presence is the result of experience and engaging in processes of deep reflection and inquiry. However, cultivating this type of presence is something that also can be taught through experiential techniques and role modeling. Various self-reflective practices such as journaling, meditation, relaxation, contemplation, dream analysis, narrative, and storytelling in one's personal daily practice can help cultivate a deeper relationship with the essence of one's existence that can then be brought into a relationship with another. The nurse must be able to connect with her own heart, soul, and transcendent nature before she can establish that connection with others.

Intuition

Intuition is a useful and foundational element in the holistic communication process. It is defined as "a perceived inner knowing and insight into things and events without the conscious use of rational process; the ability to be present to another dimension of knowing."[17p722] The usefulness of intuition in the nursing process is well researched and documented. Although intuitive knowing is something that occurs more readily with the experienced nurse, it can be consciously cultivated through various practices.

Ways to cultivate intuition are listening to music, engaging in relaxation techniques, and journal writing, which can be useful in increasing one's intuitive and spiritual development. Meditation also increases one's intuitive knowing. Regular meditation practice enables one to enter the intuitional state at will.[2p539]

When the nurse utilizes intuition she engages the full use of self, which is essential in accessing and communicating with the whole person. Intuition allows the nurse to access the subtle energies and the conscious and unconscious fields that are not readily perceived. This process allows the nurse to sense the Being of another and communicate at levels where profound healing occurs.

■ TOOLS AND PRACTICES TO ENHANCE HOLISTIC COMMUNICATION

Knowing Self

Awareness and understanding of one's self and one's values, beliefs, motivations, goals, feelings, and actions are imperative in relating in a caring-healing manner. When we are aware of ourselves and understand who we are and the basis for our own attitudes, preconceptions, and reactions, we are in a much better position to empathize, appreciate other people's differences and uniqueness, and encourage their self-revelations. To nurture caring-healing communication and relationships, we need to conduct assessments of ourselves as individuals, as well as our communications, spirituality, and cultural beliefs and traditions. All of these factors influence behavior and without a thoughtful reflection and understanding of them, we deny the very people we care for the opportunity to understand themselves.[20]

Meditation

Meditation is a quiet turning inward—the practice of focusing one's attention internally to achieve clearer consciousness and inner stillness. Meditation is both a state of mind and a method. The state is one in which the mind is quiet, open, and receptive. The meditator is relaxed but alert. The method involves the focusing of attention on something such as the breath, an image, a word, or action such as tai chi or qi gong. There is a sustained concentration, but it should be effortless. Meditation allows a better understanding of the self and increased receptivity to insights arising from one's deeper being. There are numerous methods and schools of meditation. However, all methods believe in emptying the mind and letting go of the mind's chatter that preoccupies us.[21] Various forms of meditative practice can be found in Chapter 16.

Benor says the following about meditation:

> Meditation is healing in and of itself. Meditation is a gateway into spiritual awareness and healing. By quieting our mind we can access dimensions in which spiritual healing can occur. Meditation allows us to quiet the mind from its chatter and its focus on everyday, outer-world matters. It helps us open into transcendent awareness.[22]

John Kabat-Zinn, a teacher of mindfulness meditation, describes his practice in the following way:

> It has everything to do with waking up and living in harmony with oneself and with the world. It has to do with examining who we are, with questioning our view of the world and our place in it, and with cultivating some appreciation for the fullness of each moment we are alive. Most of all, it has to do with being in touch.[23]

Meditation is perhaps the single most useful reflective practice to help gain self-awareness, self-knowledge, increase intuition, and enhance one's spiritual development. Because self-awareness, self-knowledge, and intuition are foundational to creating a caring-healing presence, meditating regularly is an important practice to engage in.

Like any reflective and contemplative process, it takes discipline and practice to reap the benefits of meditation. When nurses first begin to meditate, they can start with 5-minute sessions, and then increase to 10 minutes over a couple of weeks. Setting aside time to meditate in the morning to begin the daily routine is a wonderful way to start the day. Meditating first thing in the morning allows one to access one's spiritual essence and to approach life from a place of peace and equanimity.

Engaging Your Observer

Engaging your Observer is a process that is useful when confronting a situation or communication that is particularly difficult and emotionally charged. It also helps the nurse be present to a person or situation with clarity and without bias. This practice has its roots in Buddhist psychology.

The nonjudgmental aspect of your self is called the Observer or Witness. Some perceive this aspect as our higher Self. It can be likened to a wise grandparent that looks lovingly on the thoughts and reactions of our childlike minds. The Witness is our ability to observe life without engaging our past patterns of reacting and becoming emotionally charged. The Observer acts as a third party that allows the nurse to separate from difficult emotions and feelings in situations so that communication occurs from a space of clarity and wisdom. Utilizing this technique enhances self-knowledge and self-awareness because it provides constant feedback related to one's responses and reactions to situations. The Observer is able to transcend the ego while embracing the whole of the moment so that one responds with wisdom rather than reacting from conditioned response.[24]

Engaging the Observer involves centering, being aware of internal reactions, gratefully acknowledging these reactions, and responding from the higher Self. This is a technique that allows one to access the higher Self and move from that place of higher consciousness in interactions with another. This is central to the transpersonal caring process and communicating from a holistic perspective.[25] (See **Table 28-1**.)

CLEAR Communication

Sometimes it is useful to use an acronym when acquiring or trying to remember new skills. Nurses use the following acronym to help remember some of the processes involved in holistic communication. Being CLEAR in communication stands for Center, Listen, Empathize, Attentiveness, Respect.[26] (See **Table 28-2**.)

Drawing Out the Person's Story

We as humans ascribe unique meanings to our experiences. A person's perception of meaning is related to all factors in health-wellness-disease-illness and can influence his or her response to it. If these are not clearly articulated, either because the person is unable or, more commonly, is not given the opportunity to express comprehension and feelings about the situation—be it the illness, treatment, responses, or reason for his or her actions—meaning is then left up to the interpretation or preconceived ideas of the helper. A cornerstone of holistic communication is assisting individuals to find meaning in their experience, meanings such as the person's concerns in relation to health and family economics, as well as to deeper meanings related to the person's purpose in life. Nurses need to ask clients, patients, and families to share what meaning something has for them (e.g., symptoms, illness, treatment, outlook, fears). Only then will we truly glean an understanding of the individual's experience as he or she sees it and shape our interventions to meet the person's needs.

One of the best ways to understand what the person is most concerned about and the meaning something has for that person is through the use of narrative and story. Client narratives, whether they arise from individuals, families, or communities, provide the context of the experiences and are used as an important focus in understanding the person's situation. The nurse first ascertains what the individual thinks or believes is happening to him or her, and then assists the person to identify what will help the situation. The assessment

---

TABLE 28-1   Engaging Your Observer in a Difficult Situation

Situation: A patient's family member approaches you angrily, accusing you in a very loud voice of neglecting to administer a medication on time.

- *Center yourself and create an intention:* Take a breath and bring your consciousness or attention to the area around your heart; connect with a feeling of love and compassion. Say to yourself silently, "I am here for the greater good of all."

- *Your personal Observer relates your internal reactions—emotionally, mentally, and physically:* "This person really scares you. You want to run away from this person. Your chest is starting to feel constricted and your heart is starting to race."

- *Gratefully acknowledge these reactions, set them aside, and engage your higher Self:* "Yes, anger makes me feel really uncomfortable, thank you for these insights." Take another deep breath and upon exhalation silently repeat, "I release these thoughts and feelings, I am here for the greater good of all."

- *Focus on the person or situation:* Be fully present to the person or situation from a place of wisdom and compassion.

This entire process takes about 5 seconds and allows the nurse to set aside thoughts and feelings that interfere with a caring, healing interaction.

Source: L. Thornton, "Transcending Differences; a Holistic Approach," *Imprint* 55, no. 5 (2008): 47.

TABLE 28-2 Holistic Communication: Be Clear

Center Yourself
- Pause for a moment.
- Breathe deeply.
- Connect with a feeling of love and compassion.
- Create a silent intention that your thoughts, words, and actions will be for the greater good.

Listen Wholeheartedly
- Set aside your own thoughts, emotions, and feelings.
- Focus on the person's agenda.
- Don't judge or analyze.
- Open your heart to what is being communicated.

Empathize
- Come from a place of genuine concern.
- Have the ability to feel with a person, not sorry for.
- Empathy involves an understanding that comes from sensing into the being of another.

Attention: Being Fully Present
- Be aware of what you are feeling and sensing. Stay present to yourself.
- Bring the fullness of yourself to every moment: emotionally, mentally, physically, and spiritually.

Respect
- Respect all that is.
- Respect yourself: set boundaries if needed.
- Respect person: honor cultural, social, ontological, and ideological differences.
- Welcome diversity.

Source: L. Thornton, *Creating a Healing Environment. Course I: The Model of Whole-Person Caring* (Fresno, CA: self-published, 2010): 68.

begins from where the individual is. Space and time are allowed for exploration. Each person's health encounter is truly seen as unique. This requires a perspective that the nurse is not "the expert" regarding another's health/illness experience.[27] By simply asking, "What do you think is going on with you (or is happening to you)?" and "What do you think would help?" allows patients time to tell their story and give their perspective. The same principle applies to cultural competence. Asking, "What do I need to know about you culturally (or your culture) to care for you?" provides much more individualized and useful information about various cultures, their health beliefs and practices, and needs.[28] The nurse then discusses options, including the person's choices, across a continuum, including possible effects and implications of each.

Listening to the patient's story provides a holistic perspective and allows the nurse to get an overall sense of what the person is experienc-ing. This is more than simply using therapeutic techniques such as responding, reflecting, and summarizing. This is deep listening or, as some say, "listening with the heart and not just the ears." It is done with conscious intention and without preconceptions, busyness, distractions, or analysis. Using active listening responses, such as "Uh huh . . . uh huh," "Oh," "I see," and "Can you tell me more?" indicate that the nurse is listening, gives the person permission to continue, and keeps the patient focused on the story. It takes place in the "now" within an atmosphere of shared humanness, that is, human being to human being. Through presence or "being with in the moment," nurses provide each person with an interpersonal encounter that is experienced as a connection with one who is giving undivided attention to the needs and concerns of the individual. Using unconditional positive regard, nurses convey to the individual receiving care the belief in his or her worth and value as a human being, not solely the recipient of medical and nursing interventions.[27p57]

■ CARING-HEALING RESPONSES TO FREQUENTLY ASKED QUESTIONS AND STATEMENTS

Following are some of the questions clients, patients, and families regularly ask nurses. A brief description of the underlying dynamic of the question or statement, ineffective responses, and caring-healing responses are identified.[29]

1. "Am I dying?"
   - *Dynamic:* Request for information, reassurance.
   - *Ineffective responses:* "I really am not able to discuss that. You should talk with your doctor" or "You always have to keep hope" or "Don't say that, look how you are improving every day."
   - *Caring-healing response:* In a very gentle voice, "Do you think you are dying?" "Can you tell me why you think you are dying?" Follow up with, "What does death mean to you?"

2. "Why did God (or whomever one believes in) do this to me?" and "I don't want to go on living."
   - *Dynamic:* Spiritual distress.
   - *Ineffective responses:* "Sometimes in life, bad things happen to people who don't deserve them," or "Don't feel that way. God has not abandoned you," or "We can't always understand why things happen, but there is a reason."
   - *Caring-healing response:* Be silent. If acceptable, hold the person's hand and let them know by your full attention and presence that you are willing to bear witness to their deepest despair and sorrow. "This seems to be a very difficult time for you on many different levels." Wait for a response. If none, gently ask, "Can you explain that to me so that I can understand?"

3. "Don't tell anybody else what I am telling you."
   - *Dynamic:* Can I trust you?
   - *Ineffective responses:* "You can trust me not to tell anyone else" or "Your request makes me really uncomfortable."

   - *Caring-healing response:* "Is there a particular reason why you do not want me to share this information?" Wait for a response. Depending on the answer, "I understand your wish to keep this between us, but others may need to know this information to provide you with (what you need, or the best care possible, or to help you make a decision, etc.)" or "If it is not imperative for anyone else to know, certainly I will keep it confidential."

4. Repeated requests for the nurse's personal information.
   - *Dynamic:* A need to be connected.
   - *Ineffective responses:* "I don't talk with clients or patients about my personal life" or answering every question that the individual asks.
   - *Caring-healing response:* "Is there a reason why you would like to know about (the topic asked about)?"

5. Silence.
   - *Dynamic:* Individual is thinking, processing, feeling, cannot put thoughts and feelings into words, or is physically or emotionally exhausted. Silence is a form of communication and has a great deal of meaning.
   - *Ineffective responses:* Filling the silence with any words to keep conversation alive or "I can see that you do not want to talk now, I will come back later."
   - *Caring-healing response:* "You seem quiet." Wait for a response. "Would you like to talk or would you just like me to sit here with you for a while?" Get in touch with your own discomfort if this is an issue for you, relax into the silence, understanding that this is what the person needs at this time. Communicate through presence and intent that you are there for this person.

6. "What should I do? What would you do?"
   - *Dynamic:* Insecurity about decision, lack of knowledge, second guessing, too much input.
   - *Ineffective responses:* "Well, I would ____," or "When this happened to (me, my brother/friend/another patient), I/she/he did ____," or "I think you should discuss this with your doctor."

- *Caring-healing response:* "First, tell me what you understand about your illness and treatment." Wait for a response. Then, "Tell me what you think you should do or what you feel would be best or most helpful for you." The nurse is an option giver, not the prescriber. Discuss options, implications of each option, and the individual's thoughts, feelings, beliefs, and concerns about each option so that the person has sufficient information to make an informed decision with which he or she is comfortable.

7. Anger.
   - *Dynamic:* Powerlessness.
   - *Ineffective responses:* "Don't get angry at me, I am just trying to help you," or "I don't have to take this from (a patient, a colleague, a family, the doctor, etc.)," or "Call security."
   - *Caring-healing response:* Stop and center, and then send peace. Visualize the person as he or she was as an innocent, precious baby. The energy tends to change immediately when we image babies because they connect with our joy. Wait calmly until the angry person completes the attack, and then begin the discussion.

8. Fear.
   - *Dynamic:* Projection, misperception. Fear and worry are the most common form of imagery.
   - *Ineffective response:* "Don't worry, everything will work out."
   - *Caring-healing response:* "Can you share with me what your understanding of ____ is or what you think is going to happen?" Then, reality test by gently asking, "What do you think is the worst that can happen?" and "What might be a positive that can happen in this circumstance?"

9. Anxiety
   - *Dynamic:* Projection, unknowing, too much input, inability to stay in the present or listen to and trust one's own inner wisdom.
   - *Ineffective responses:* "Constantly thinking or worrying about this is not going to help, it will only make it worse" or "Try to get your mind off of it."

- *Caring-healing response:* "It sounds like a lot is going on, so let's see if we can focus on ____ right now and deal with ____ after that" or "What do you think is best or necessary for you? What is your body, mind, and gut telling you?"

10. "It's all my fault."
    - *Dynamic:* Guilt often rooted in shame.
    - *Ineffective responses:* "Of course you are not to blame" or "Well, it was going to happen some time or another, it's not your fault."
    - *Caring-healing response:* "Can you tell me why you think you are responsible for (or are to blame for) ____?"

11. "I am such a burden (e.g., bothering you, having you see me like this, having to clean me up, can't do anything for myself)."
    - *Dynamic:* Guilt as an assault on one's assumptions and beliefs about oneself and what one wants others to believe about him or her, creating vulnerability and exposure.
    - *Ineffective response:* "Oh, I've seen (or dealt with) worse. You're not so bad."
    - *Caring-healing response:* "It is a gift to care for you and share this part of your journey (your experience) with you" or "It is my pleasure."

■ CONCLUSION

Holistic communication is a caring-healing process that calls forth the full use of self in interacting with another. The elements that distinguish holistic communication are acknowledgment of the infinite and sacred nature of Being; the use of centering, grounding, intention, and intuition; and caring-healing, transcendent presence. Holistic communication can be viewed as a field experience in which there is constant mutual exchange between the nurse's field and the patient's field. Communication is constantly occurring on physical, mental, emotional, and energetic levels. We are never not communicating.

Self-knowledge and self-awareness are foundational to the process of holistic communication. Tools and practices that help the nurse gain a greater understanding and awareness of self include journaling, dream analysis, relaxation techniques, self-reflective practices, and meditation. Growing in self-knowledge and self-awareness increases the nurse's effectiveness as an instrument in the caring-healing process. Holistic communication invites us to engage our higher Self as we meet another in that transcendent space where profound healing occurs. When this happens, a "healing field of communication" is created in which both the nurse and person are enriched and nurtured.

Directions for
FUTURE RESEARCH

1. Explore research findings related to holistic communication.
2. Examine how various aspects of holistic communication are implemented in nursing settings.
3. Explore ways in which cultural learning can be incorporated into nurses' practice to influence the effectiveness of holistic communication.

Nurse Healer
REFLECTIONS

After reading this chapter, the holistic nurse will be able to answer or begin a process of answering the following questions:

- How does being centered and creating an intention affect the quality of my communication?
- When I view another as sacred, how does this affect the quality of my interaction?
- What are my attributes as a holistic communicator?

> *For a full suite of assignments and additional learning activities, use the access code located in the front of your book to visit this exclusive website: http://go.jblearning.com/dossey. If you do not have an access code, you can obtain one at the site.*

NOTES

1. M. Rogers, "Nursing: Science of Unitary, Irreducible, Human Beings: Update 1990" in *Visions of Rogers' Science-Based Nursing*, ed. E. A. M. Barrett (New York, NY: National League for Nursing, 1990): 7.
2. L. Thornton and C. Mariano, "Evolving from Therapeutic to Holistic Communication" in *Holistic Nursing: A Handbook for Practice*, 5th ed., ed. B. Dossey and L. Keegan (Sudbury, MA: Jones and Bartlett, 2009): 533.
3. L. Thornton, "Where Heart and Soul Meet the Bottom Line: Using the Model of Whole-Person Caring to Promote Health and Wellness in Your Organization," *LOHAS Journal* 12, no 1 (2011): 31–33.
4. E. Arnold and K. Underman-Boggs, *Interpersonal Relationships: Professional Communication Skills for Nurses*, 6th ed. (St. Louis, MO: Saunders Elsevier, 2011).
5. M. Rogers, *An Introduction to the Theoretical Basis of Nursing*, 7th ed. (Philadelphia, PA: F. A. Davis, 1977): 54.
6. M. Newman, *Health as Expanding Consciousness*, 2nd ed. (New York, NY: National League for Nursing Press, 1994): 13.
7. T. Moore, *Care of the Soul* (New York, NY: Harper Collins, 1992): 10.
8. J. Watson, *Postmodern Nursing and Beyond* (New York, NY: Churchill Livingston, 1999): 129.
9. J. Watson, *Nursing: Human Science and Human Care, a Theory of Nursing* (Sudbury, MA: NLN Press/Jones and Bartlett, 1999).
10. L. Thornton, "A Spiritual and Energetically-Based Model Supporting the Practice of Healing Touch" *Energy Magazine*, no. 45 (2010): 15.
11. R. McCraty and R. Reese, *The Central Role of the Heart in Generating and Sustaining Positive Emotions*, Institute of HeartMath, Publication No. 06-022 (Boulder Creek, CA: HeartMath Research Center, 2009).
12. R. McCraty and D. Childre, "Coherence: Bridging Personal, Social, and Global Health," *Alternative Therapies* 16, no. 4 (2010): 12.
13. R. McCraty, M. Atkinson, and R. T. Bradley, "Electrophysiological Evidence of Intuition: Part 1. The Surprising Role of the Heart," *Journal of Alternative and Complementary Medicine* 10, no 1 (2004): 133–143.
14. S. Morris, "Achieving Collective Coherence: Group Effects on Heart Rate Variability Coherence and Heart Rhythm Synchronization," *Alternative Therapies* 16, no. 4 (2010): 62–72.
15. C. Jackson and L. Keegan, "Touch," in *Holistic Nursing: A Handbook for Practice*, 5th ed., ed. B. Dossey and L. Keegan (Sudbury, MA: Jones and Bartlett, 2009): 348.

16. Personal communication, F. McCartney, May 2, 2011.

17. M. McKivergin, "The Nurse as an Instrument of Healing," in *Holistic Nursing: A Handbook for Practice*, 5th ed., ed. B. Dossey and L. Keegan (Sudbury, MA: Jones and Bartlett, 2009): 722.

18. W. Tiller and W. Dibble, "A Brief Introduction to Intention-Host Device Research" (white paper, William A. Tiller Foundation, 2009). http://www.tiller.org.

19. P. Osterman and D. Schwartz-Barcott, "Presence: Four Ways of Being There," *Nursing Forum* 31, no. 2 (1996): 23–30.

20. C. Mariano, "Holistic Nursing as a Specialty: Scope and Standards of Practice," *Clinics of North America* 42, no. 2 (2007): 165–188.

21. C. Mariano, "Holistic Integrative Therapies in Palliative Care," in *Palliative Care: Quality Care to the End of Life*, 3rd ed., ed. M. Matzo and D. Sherman (New York, NY: Springer, 2010): 44–45.

22. Personal communication, D. Benor, May 17, 2011.

23. J. Kabat-Zinn, *Wherever You Go There You Are: Mindfulness Meditation in Everyday Life* (New York, NY: Hyperion, 1994): 3.

24. L. Thornton, "Self-Compassion: A Prescription for Well-Being," *Imprint* 58, no. 2 (2011): 43.

25. L. Thornton, "Transcending Differences; a Holistic Approach," *Imprint* 55 no. 5 (2008): 47.

26. L. Thornton, *Creating a Healing Environment: The Model of Whole-Person Caring*™ (Fresno, CA: self-published, 2010): 68.

27. C. Mariano, "Holistic Nursing: Scope and Standards of Practice," in *Holistic Nursing: A Handbook for Practice*, 5th ed., ed. B. Dossey and L. Keegan (Sudbury, MA: Jones and Bartlett, 2009): 54.

28. C. Mariano, "Why Am I Here? The Koan of Our Journey" (keynote address, Birchtree Center for Healthcare, NJ, 2010).

29. C. Mariano, "Therapeutic Interactions" (adapted course materials, New York University, 2007, and Pacific College of Oriental Medicine, 2011).

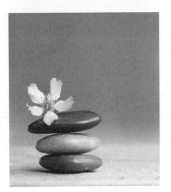

Chapter 29

Environmental Health

Susan Luck and Lynn Keegan

Nurse Healer
OBJECTIVES

Theoretical

- Identify three principles that can direct human endeavors toward a sustainable future.
- Describe three characteristics of a sustainable community.
- Describe four ways in which substantive systems changes can diminish toxic exposures in life.

Clinical

- Examine environmental hazards, and make a commitment to reducing these hazards in your home, community, and workplace.
- Examine systems changes that can reduce toxic exposures in the hospital or health-care environment where you work.
- Subscribe or arrange to have consistent access to periodical literature specific to clinical application of environmental principles (e.g., *Health Care Without Harm Newsletter, Physicians for Social Responsibility*) and website information (Environmental Working Group, www.ewg.org).
- Identify and act on ways to influence environmental accountability in the workplace.

- Commit to joining an organization created to influence the direction of future sustainability in health care.
- Become sensitive to the environmental space in the institution, health agency, or clinic.
- Explore with other staff possibilities for creating healing environments in the workplace.

Personal

- Increase knowledge of the relationship between health and the environment.
- Assess the health of your personal environment.
- Increase awareness on how to reduce your environmental imprint (i.e., recycling).
- Volunteer and join local groups and organizations to support environmental efforts in your community.
- Explore what is essential about environmental relationships in your life.
- Eliminate unhealthy exposures in your personal environment (e.g., stale air, artificial lighting, subliminal noises, chemicals) whenever possible.
- Experiment with healing colors, scents, textures, sound, and lighting in your personal environment.

DEFINITIONS

Ambience: An environment or its distinct atmosphere; the totality of feeling that one experiences from a particular environment.

Anthropocentrism: The worldview that places human beings as the central fact or final aim of the universe.

Bisphenol A (BPA): An organic compound with two phenol functional groups. It is used to make polycarbonate plastic and epoxy resins, along with other applications, and since the mid-1930s is known to be estrogenic.

Chaos Theory: Sometimes called the "new science," this theory offers a way of seeing order and patterns where formerly only the random, the erratic, and the unpredictable had been observed.

Detoxification: The metabolic process by which the toxic qualities of a poison or toxin are reduced or eliminated from the body.

Earth jurisprudence: Earth law recognizes the Earth as the primary source of law that sets human law in a context that is wider than humanity

Ecology: The scientific study of interrelationships between and among organisms, and among them and all aspects, living and nonliving, of their environment.

Ecominnea: The concept of an ecologically sound society.

Electromagnetic fields (EMFs): The field force in motion coupled with electric and magnetic fields that are generated by time-varying currents and accelerated charges.

Endocrine disruptors (xenoestrogens): Synthetic hormone-mimicking compounds found in many pesticides, drugs, plastics, and personal care products.

Environment: Everything that surrounds an individual or group of people: physical, social, psychological, cultural, or spiritual characteristics; external and internal features; animate and inanimate objects; climate; seen and unseen vibrations, frequencies, and energy patterns not yet understood.

Environmental ethics: A division of philosophy concerned with valuing the environment, primarily as it relates to humankind, secondarily as it relates to other creatures and to the land.

Environmental justice: A subbranch of ethics examining the innate and relational value among organisms and all aspects of their environment.

Epistemology: The branch of philosophy that addresses the origin, nature, methods, and limits of knowledge.

Ergonomics: The study of and realization of the importance of human factors in engineering.

Permaculture: An approach to designing human settlements and agricultural systems that are modeled on the relationships found in natural ecologies.

Persistent organic pollutants (POPs): Chemical substances that persist in the environment, bioaccumulate through the food web, and pose a risk of causing adverse effects to human health and the environment.

Personal space: The area around an individual that should be under the control of that individual, including air, light, temperature, sound, scent, and color.

Phthalates: Classified as "plasticizers," a group of industrial chemicals used to make plastics such as polyvinyl chloride (PVC) more flexible or resilient. They are also known to be endocrine disruptors.

Precautionary principle: When an activity raises threats of harm to human health or the environment, precautionary measures shall be taken, even if some cause-and-effect relationships are not fully established scientifically.

Restorative justice: An ethical perception that directs that environmental damages not only be curtailed, but also repaired and recompensed in some meaningful way.

Superfund sites: Hazardous waste landfills or abandoned manufacturing sites, names of which appear on the Environmental Protection Agency's National Priorities List.

Sustainable future: Meeting the needs of the present without compromising the needs of future generations.

Toxic substance: A substance that can cause harm to a person through either short- or long-term exposure, as by (1) inhalation;

(2) ingestion into the body in the form of vapors, gases, fumes, dusts, solids, liquids, or mists; or (3) skin absorption.

■ THEORY AND RESEARCH

To engage successfully with life in modern times, we are challenged to increase awareness of how our external environment affects our health and the health of our clients/patients, families, communities, and the planet. In the spirit of Florence Nightingale, as healthcare providers and holistic nurses, how can we develop self-awareness and self-care practices that support our own inner and external healing environments? How can we integrate environmental assessment tools, education, and strategies into our professional practice and commit ourselves as Earth dwellers and Earth citizens, to the following:

- Recognize that we are the microcosm of the macrocosm; a world of vast complexity and unpredictability; understanding that our health and the health of our planet are inextricably interwoven.
- Engage in practices that create healing environments in our home, workplace, and community.
- Take the risk to challenge the existing structures and maintain values and convictions to create healthier environments.
- Reside in knowing that each individual makes a difference toward healing the global community beginning with individual actions.
- Experience the fullness of life and the wonders of the natural world.

Environmental Leadership in Holistic Nursing

In its broadest sense, the term *environment* can mean everything, both within and external to each person. As a result, it is a challenge to determine for ourselves and others what constitutes a healing environment. In defining the constellation of environment in a grand way, five themes can be used to form a constellation—a mental map—to conceptualize the environmental world and the human place in it: (1) sharing, listening, and learning through our personal and collective life stories; (2) increasing self-awareness and self-care when living in a toxic world; (3) choos-

ing a sustainable future; (4) building communities that support learning and positive actions for creating change: *start local, think global*; and (5) working from the inside out: healing our internal and external environments.

Telling Our Story: Local to Global

Each nurse, and each client, has a unique and personal story to tell. Everyone has an explanatory narrative that encompasses the multidimensional layers of being human. Listening to our own story and the story of others reveals the storyteller's beliefs and worldview and opens doors to exploring and expanding possibilities for growth and change in our movement toward wholeness. Within our holistic nursing worldview, we embrace the interconnectedness of body, mind, and spirit, knowing that when there is disharmony or disruption in our internal or external environment, we are out of balance. As living beings, we are a reflection of our world, and any environmental assault directly affects our energetic patterns and well-being.

When considering the environment, it is imperative to listen and respond to a larger story, not only as practitioners, but also as members of humankind. This reaffirms what we deeply know through all the senses as we ask ourselves, "What does it mean to be human? What does it mean to be an Earth citizen? What are our beliefs about health when we tell our story? Do we consider all of the possible influences that affect our daily lives, and those with whom we live and work? How can we face the great ecological crises of our time (as recently witnessed and experienced in Japan)? How does each of our stories contribute to the larger story? How does changing our own story lead to planetary change?" When we embrace the matrix of our own being, we can understand, respond to, and participate in positive actions, raising the level of consciousness of our oneness with the universe. Richard Tarnas, a philosopher and historian of Western thought, helped bring this existential human predicament into consciousness.[1]

There are two versions of the evolution of human consciousness. Both are basic truths and deep patterns in the psyche that inform an individual's day-to-day experience in various ways. One is progress and heroic advance, characterized by gradual, progressive, and familiar milestones of discovery and accomplishment: the harnessing of electricity and nuclear fission, for example. Generally, this equates with ever-increasing and refined knowledge and is thought to bring a sense of fulfillment and well-being. The scientific mind is the apex of this worldview, having its roots in ancient Greece and a flourishing in the European Enlightenment of the 1700s. The modern mind is known for individualistic democracy, power, and emancipation. Inventiveness, endurance, will to succeed, and adventuresome spirit are sources for pride. The "miracles of modern medicine" are found here.

The second version of the evolution of human consciousness is the fall and tragic separation, which is a deep wounding or schism that separates humankind from nature. Manifestations of this version include exploitation of the natural environment, devastation of indigenous cultures, and an increasingly unhappy state of the human soul. Through the lens of tragic separation, humanity and nature are seen as having suffered grievously under an increasingly dualistic domination of thought and society. The worst consequences of this development are directly derived from the hegemony of modern industrial society and empowered by science and technology.

All individuals are challenged, although they may not recognize it, to reconcile these perspectives in their day-to-day lives. The two perspectives are both occurring simultaneously although not always at the level of awareness. For example, it is possible for a family to decide to maintain heroic life support systems, beyond all parameters of the natural dignity of dying, while their deeper desire is that their loved one be at peace. Both are apprehensions of a deeper, larger, and more complex story. Gain and loss have been working together simultaneously. As nurses, we are aware of pervasive and intense suffering, not only in our own inner work, but beyond, to the transpersonal and collective unconscious. Currently, the whole planet is in a transformative crisis.

Several core elements drive the multidimensional crisis. The modern mind—the mind of progress—originates in the worldview that there is a radical and irreconcilable distinction between the human self as subject and the world as object. In contrast, the primal worldview is that spirit or soul permeates the entire universe, within which the soul is embedded. The modern mind condemns this as a naive epistemologic error—childish, immature, and to be outgrown. The wisdom of the modern mind asserts that the human self is the exclusive repository of conscious intelligence; all meaning in the universe comes from the human subject. This is the classic existentialist assumption that, without humankind, the universe is meaningless.

Typically, a modern person's allegiance is to science, in the belief that science rules the cosmos and objective world, while poetry, music, and spiritual strivings inhabit the internal world. Our cherished Western autonomy, offspring of the progress perspective, has been purchased at a staggering price: gradual dilution and diminution of soul, meaning, and spirit. Thus, the purpose of the entire world is exclusive to the human self. Everything else is "out there," resulting in the demise of the metaphysical world and the disenchantment of the cosmos. Whether in conscious awareness or not, the greatest demand of modern time is to reconcile the imperatives of the two versions of what it means to be human. Must everyone choose and align themselves with one or the other? Must everyone consign themselves to an existence where "progress" is purchased with the coin of soul loss?

Modern culture itself is immersed in a rite of the most epochal and profound kind: the entire path of human civilization has taken humankind, the planet, and all its members into a trajectory of complete alienation that is part of the mythic death and rebirth story. Something new is being formed, however, that is a new participative and holistic vision of the universe amply reflected by contemporary scientific and philosophic insights. In this emerging view, the human self is both highly differentiated, yet reembedded in a participatory, meaning-laden universe. Throughout human history, all cultures have embedded within their collective psyche a connectedness to nature for survival of not only the human species but for the life of planet Earth.

Holistic nursing honors human history as part of our collective story that we carry in our cellular memory, with all its triumph and vulnerability. Holistic nurses strive for clarity of meaning, values, beliefs, and relationships.

The roots and intention of nursing in caring for others is to honor the totality of the individual and support creating environments that promote healing. Florence Nightingale, through her 13 canons, gave the most basic instruction of all: "The art of nursing requires us to alter the environment safely."[2] In *Notes on Nursing*, Florence Nightingale wrote, "No amount of medical knowledge will lessen the accountability for nurses to do what nurses do, that is, manage the environment to promote positive life processes." This is our collective story as nurses, and it is the foundation on which nursing stands. Today, we are being called on and guided as 21st-century Nightingales to reclaim our highest aspirations, values, ethics, thought, and activity, to lead the way on this highest calling to heal our planet and all that dwell here today and for any foreseeable future.

Florence Nightingale as Environmentalist

Florence Nightingale, the founder of modern nursing, understood what we recognize today as ecological medicine and environmental health, involving the health of not only humans, but of all species and ecosystems with which we are connected physically, psychologically, and spiritually. Nurses have always been sensitive to environmental issues. Historically, nurses have been primarily concerned with health promotion, sanitation, and improvement in the quality of life for all people. Our modern world raises new issues and concerns for nurses, ranging from the use of increasingly toxic substances to high-technology machinery.

Dossey, in her seminal, scholarly works on Nightingale, delineates many of Nightingale's tenets. One of these was "the precautionary principle." It implies that when an activity raises threats of harm to human health or the environment, precautionary measures shall be taken, even if some cause-and-effect relationships are not fully established scientifically. The precautionary principle boils down to "better safe than sorry." Nightingale wrote specifically on observations of hazards in the environment and the nurse's responsibility: "If you think a patient is being poisoned by a copper kettle, cut off all possible connection to avoid further injury."[3] The essence of the precautionary principle is if there is a suspicion about a harmful environment or

exposure, even though all of the evidence is not in, remove the person from the situation or stop the use of suspected harmful exposures.

Nightingale understood that nurses have a duty as well as an ethical and moral responsibility to take anticipatory actions to prevent harm; the burden of proof for a new technology, process, activity, or chemical lies with the proponents, not with the public. The precautionary principle always inquires about alternatives. Precautionary decision making is open, informed, and democratic and must include all affected parties. The first sentence of the Preface in Nightingale's third edition of *Notes on Hospitals* (1863) reads as follows:

> It may be a strange principle to enunciate as the very first requirement in a Hospital that it should do the sick no harm. It is quite necessary nevertheless to lay down such a principle, because the actual mortality in hospitals, especially in those of large crowded cities, is very much higher than any calculations founded on the mortality of the same class of patient treated out of hospitals would lead us to expect.

Dossey goes on to tell us that Nightingale doesn't say a little harm or negligible harm; she says *no* harm. This anticipates the precautionary principle, which emphasizes that zero tolerance for the contamination of our environments is acceptable, not minimal or moderate contamination.[4]

Nightingale focused not only on problems, but sought solutions that guide us today. Nightingale engaged in what we today call risk assessment and on facts on which we base environmental decisions. Nurses are working with others to determine the degree of risk that is acceptable and asking questions such as "What is considered safe drinking water in hospitals and in homes?" "How much atmospheric pollution is safe in urban environments?" However, we must remember that the precautionary principle advocates zero degradation of the environment because of the uncertainty of risk assessment.[5] Precautionary principle proponents and health policy analysts today advocate that it is incumbent on those introducing a new chemical or technology to demonstrate that it is safe, and not for the rest of us to prove it is harmful.[6]

Environmental initiatives and movements are part of a general societal intention to have a habitable planet, now and in years to come. These movements remain largely grassroots, or citizen driven, addressing impacts as they relate to humankind and Earth jurisprudence. Any benefit for the rest of the biotic community is a by-product from that frame of reference. The holistic outlook, as has been stated, recognizes all systems as interacting. If one part is affected, change of a greater or lesser magnitude occurs everywhere.

The roots of the environmental movement in the United States can be attributed to Native American cultures and traditions deeply honoring the feminine nurturing Earth for sustaining life for present and future generations. The conservation movement of the 1800s continued this tradition and was inspired by writers and artists such as Henry David Thoreau and Ralph Waldo Emerson to preserve indigenous territories and the wilderness from the expansion of the times. As the vast American wilderness began to be explored, settled, and exploited, the idea that some wild spaces had to be preserved for future generations began to take on great significance. The national park system arose from this new awareness and declared land that could remain pristine as well as promote tourism. By 1916, the Interior Department was responsible for 14 national parks. There was not much societal activity for more than 50 years until the 1960s and 1970s, when activists elucidated the dangers of DDT and other hazardous materials—polychlorinated biphenyls (PCBs), mercury, lead, and other heavy metals. In 1976, the Environmental Protection Agency was established and environmental legislation and state and federal protection agencies widened the focus from preservation to protection and banned the pesticide DDT, what would later be classified as a "hormonal disruptor" and a carcinogen, and removed lead from paint in 1978.[7]

■ ENVIRONMENTAL CONDITIONS AND HEALTH

Since the 1970s, national attention has focused on efforts to clean up the nation's environment and to ensure workers' safety. Two federal agencies, the Environmental Protection Agency (EPA) and the Occupational Safety and Health Administration (OSHA), were formed to monitor environmental concerns. In the 1980s, several states enacted right-to-know laws that require employers to notify employees of health hazards, to provide formal education regarding the safe use of toxic substances, and to keep medical records of those workers routinely exposed to specific toxic substances. Federal agencies were fully involved in public safety amid concerns about the fires and suspected presence of toxic materials in the rubble pile following the collapse of the World Trade Center (WTC) buildings on September 11, 2001.[8] In addition, natural disaster environmental effects on health and established disaster management systems in place have been and continue to be evaluated and critiqued by diverse national agencies, including the Federal Emergency Management Agency (FEMA) and Office of Homeland Security.

In the early 1980s, the United States projected national health objectives for every decade. The latest of these documents, titled *Healthy People 2020*, is a set of health prevention goals that challenges health providers to strongly consider the environment's effect on several health indicators. The environment can influence several of the indicators being targeted, and these include asthma, work-related assaults, lead exposure, needlestick injuries, noise-induced hearing loss, and worksite stress.[9] These have implications for occupational risk exposure and possible prevention strategies.

Environmental concerns range from eating contaminated poultry, hormone-fed beef, and irradiated fruits and vegetables to living near high-voltage power lines, understanding the Antarctic atmospheric ozone hole, the threat of nuclear power plants, and coping with other new high-technology hazards that we now fully acknowledge (**Figure 29-1**). Noise, lighting, air quality, space allocation, and workplace toxins have gained increasing attention as chronic stressors.

In the 1980s, the discovery of the hole in the ozone layer over Antarctica, along with escalating concern over global warming and climate change, introduced another phase of environmentalism, one that emphasized sustainability and an awareness in protecting future generations from the dangers of exceeding nature's ability to restore itself. Many people began to leave the cities, and a "back to the land" movement flourished. Other evolving perspectives addressed environmental justice and environmental ethics.

Today, a new environmental movement is rising up following 50 years of "better living through chemistry" and is gathering momentum as baby boomers, exposed to chemicals over the course of their lifetime, are exhibiting epidemic rates of cancers and Alzheimer's while those just beginning life are being plagued with learning disabilities, childhood cancers, and record rates of asthma and obesity. Chemicals are the basic building blocks that make up all living and non-living things on Earth. Many chemicals occur naturally in the environment, and many more are man-made. Chemicals can enter the air, water, and soil when they are produced, used, or disposed. Chemicals are of concern because they can work their way into the food chain and accumulate and/or persist in the environment and in our bodies for many years.

Living in a Toxic World

In June 2006, the World Health Organization (WHO) issued a report *Preventing disease through healthy environments— towards an estimate of the environmental burden of disease*, the most comprehensive and systematic study yet undertaken on how *preventable* environmental hazards contribute to a wide range of diseases and injuries. By focusing on the environmental causes of disease, and how various diseases are influenced by environmental factors, the analysis breaks new ground in understanding the interactions between environment and health. The estimate reflects how much death, illness and disability could be realistically avoided every year as a result of better environmental management.

The report stated that nearly one-quarter of global disease is caused by environmental exposures, and "well targeted interventions can prevent much of the environmental risk," saving suffering and millions of lives every year.[10]

Over the past century, humans have introduced a large number of chemical substances

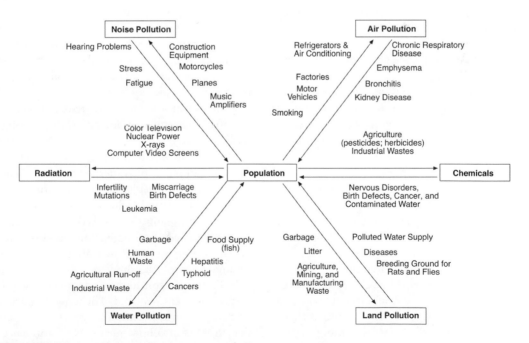

FIGURE 29-1 Current Environmental Concerns

Source: Reprinted with permission from the *Journal of Health Education*, August/September 1986, pp. 26–27. The *Journal of Health Education* is a publication of the American Alliance for Health, Physical Education, Recreation and Dance, 1990 Association Drive, Reston, VA 20191.

into the environment; with the intention of creating "better living through chemistry". Many of these substances are by-products of waste from industrial and agricultural processes. Today, chemical compounds are ubiquitous in our food, air, and water and have now found their way into every person and species. The bioaccumulation of these compounds is fueling metabolic and systemic dysfunctions and disease states. The systems most affected by these toxic compounds include the immune, neurological, and endocrine systems. This toxic "body burden" can trigger autoimmune reactivity, asthma, allergies, cancers, cognitive deficits, mood changes, neurological illness, reproductive dysfunction,[10] glucose dysregulation, and obesity.[11]

We can no longer deny or avoid the environmental chaos that is occurring on a planetary level in these times. We read daily about nuclear disasters, global water crises, famines from loss of land, disappearance of the Earth's rain forests, coastal devastation from toxic waste, climate change, and the long list of endangered species that could include humans, if actions are not taken soon.

To make a list of problems or to dwell on the environmental global crises is not a solution; a more life-affirming exercise is to clarify individual and collective goals for healing our planet, beginning with our individual actions and working toward attainable goals for oneself, family, and community. Human beings are characterized by the ability to choose and change; the same minds that have created the technology and our modern world can create new solutions. Rather than continue down our current environmental path, the past need not be perpetuated. Human beings can elect and select life-affirming ways, use their inventive genius to reinvent a world that can sustain present and future generations, nurturing ourselves physically, mentally, and spiritually.

A very different world could be created by using alternative strategies and technologies that could offer the same essential services that chemicals and current energy sources provide.

Our Environmental Story

In less than one lifetime, production of synthetic organic chemicals (e.g., dyes, plastics, pesticides, and solvents) has increased more than 1,000-fold in the United States alone. According to the National Toxicology Program, more than 80,000 chemicals are registered for use in the United States. Each year, an estimated 2,000 new ones are introduced for use in such everyday items as foods, personal care products, prescription drugs, household cleaners, and lawn care products, and most are never tested for their impact on human health. In addition, many chemicals are emitted as by-products of production or incineration (particularly relevant to the hospital industry). Some chemicals, such as life-saving medications, can have direct health benefits. Others, such as pesticides and herbicides, are designed to be usefully lethal. The most pernicious and pervasive were not meant to come into human contact. When PCBs were created in 1929, for example, they were intended for use only in electrical wiring, lubricants, and liquid seals. Although many chemicals, including DDT and PCBs, have been banned by the Environmental Protection Agency since 1978, they can still be found in human blood samples today along with 250 other synthetic chemicals in the bodies of almost everyone in the industrial world. A recent study by the Centers for Disease Control and Prevention conservatively estimates that Americans of all ages carry a body burden of at least 148 chemicals, some of them banned for decades.[12]

Many chemicals in use today have not yet been classified as harmful to human health, although recent reports based on current research are sounding the alarm and many organizations are hopeful that consumer activism will gain momentum and fuel legislation for formulating a new environmental and public health policy.

One of the reasons that it is difficult to study the link between environmental conditions and illness or disease is that there are so many intervening variables. Hundreds of substances along with lifestyle factors and individual genetic predispositions are involved. The emerging scientific inquiry in the field of epigenetics provides new insights into how our genes are influenced to express themselves under environmental stress. Furthermore, not all toxic substances and environmental conditions induce immediate untoward reactions; many toxins seem to cause disease later, perhaps years after the initial exposure. Many chemical substances do not appear harmful at low-level exposures, but it is not well understood how small amounts of repeated chemical exposures when combined with other substances work synergistically over time. Breathing asbestos fibers, for example, seldom causes immediate symptoms, but often has resulted in serious chronic disease many years later. Environmental elements known to be hazardous include lead, cigarette smoke, silica, benzene, mercury, chlorine, formaldehyde, poor lighting, stress, and noise. Converging themes from the fields of environmental health and human ecology and health highlight opportunities for innovation and advancement in environmental health theory, research, and practice.[13]

The *Fourth National Report on Human Exposure to Environmental Chemicals 2009* and the *Updated Tables*, released in February 2011, together are the most comprehensive assessment of environmental chemical exposure in the U.S. population. The *Fourth Report* includes the findings from national samples for 1999–2000, 2001–2002, and 2003–2004. The blood and urine samples were collected from participants in the CDC's National Health and Nutrition Examination Survey (NHANES), which obtains and releases health-related data from a nationally representative sample in 2-year cycles. For the first time, the CDC has tracked national exposure levels of the U.S. population for 27 different substances—some to be proven carcinogens. The CDC report expresses hopes the data will help public health officials better understand the relationship between chemical exposures and health consequences—and to ultimately help legislate for more effective public policy decisions.[14]

In June 2011, the U.S. Department of Health and Human Services added formaldehyde, styrene, and six other substances to its *Report on Carcinogens* after scientists discovered that exposure to the substances can increase the risk of developing certain cancers. Formaldehyde is a colorless, flammable, strong-smelling chemical widely used to make resins for household items, such as composite wood products, paper product coatings, plastics, synthetic fibers, and textile finishes. It is also commonly used as a preservative in medical laboratories, mortuaries,

and some consumer products, including hair-straightening products.

A number of cohort studies involving workers exposed to formaldehyde have recently been completed. One study, conducted by the National Cancer Institute (NCI), looked at 25,619 workers in industries with the potential for occupational formaldehyde exposure and estimated each worker's exposure to the chemical while at work . The results showed an increased risk of death due to leukemia, particularly myeloid leukemia, among workers exposed to formaldehyde.[15]

Children's Health

> We do not inherit the Earth from our ancestors, we borrow it from our children.
>
> *Native American Proverb*

Childhood is a sequence of life stages from conception through fetal development, infancy, and adolescence, as defined by the Environmental Protection Agency. Children are the most vulnerable to environmental exposures for the following reasons:

- Their bodily systems are still developing.
- They eat more, drink more, and breathe more in proportion to their body size.
- Their behaviors can expose them more to chemicals and organisms (e.g., crawling on the ground).

Dr. Phillip Landrigan, director of the Children's Environmental Health Center, dean for Global Health, chair of Preventive Medicine, professor of Pediatrics at Mount Sinai School of Medicine, and an international leader on children's health and the environment, has written extensively and advocated for updated federal regulation of pesticides in food. He has repeatedly expressed that the public is rightly concerned about possible health impacts from frequent exposures through our food supply. He reports on a trio of peer-reviewed studies published June 2011 that found children exposed in the womb to high levels of a class of pesticides known as organophosphates had lower average intelligence than other children by the time they reached age 7 years. Researchers found that exposure during pregnancy may impair a child's cognitive development. "If exposure to pesticides are harming children, it doesn't matter if the levels are below the legal limit set by the government," says Landrigan, whose research in the 1990s compelled the federal government to tighten pesticide standards significantly.[16] Since that time, new and more potent pesticides have been introduced to the global market, including a new generation of pesticide-induced genetically modified organisms to "protect" crops from external threats. Research on the threat to the health of humans and other species with this new technology has many researchers and scientists apprehensive about the potential deleterious effects.[17] Dr. Landrigan and Lynn R. Goldman, dean of the School of Public Health at George Washington University, have proposed a three-pronged approach to reduce the burden of disease and rein in the effects of toxic chemicals in the environment:

- Conduct a requisite examination of chemicals already on the market for potential toxicity, starting with the chemicals in widest use, using new, more efficient toxicity testing technologies.
- Assess all new chemicals for toxicity before they are allowed to enter the marketplace, and maintain strictly enforced regulation on these chemicals.
- Bolster ongoing research and epidemiologic monitoring to better understand, and subsequently prevent, the health impact of chemicals on children.

Pesticide exposure in our food supply is not only associated with neurological and learning disabilities. Increasingly, research studies show increased risk of several types of cancers from airborne exposure via pesticide drift, including brain cancer from home pesticide and insecticide use, leukemia from home and garden pesticides, and nonlymphocytic leukemia from extermination use.[18] The authors report positive associations with exposures during pregnancy to pesticides, insecticides, and herbicides, and positive associations with childhood exposures to pesticides and insecticides. It has long been established that many pesticides cause cancer in animals. A new study finds that children who live in homes where their parents use pesticides are twice as likely to develop brain cancer versus those who live in residences in which no pesticides are used. It appears to cause an elevated risk for certain types of cancers and positive associations with exposures during pregnancy to pesticides, insecticides, and herbicides, and positive associations with childhood exposures to pesticides and insecticides, and leukemias.[19] The risk of childhood brain cancer increases with exposures received from either parent. Studies show that risk was significantly lower with fathers who washed immediately after the pesticide exposure or wore protective clothing versus those who never or only sometimes took precautions. The parents assessed in this study were generally in contact with the pesticides through residential exposure, including lawn and garden care.[20-22]

In an earlier study spearheaded by the Environmental Working Group (EWG) in collaboration with the American Red Cross, two medical laboratories found an average of 200 industrial chemicals and pollutants in the umbilical cord blood of 10 babies born in U.S. hospitals between August and September 2004. Tests revealed a total of 287 different chemicals in the group. The umbilical cord blood of these 10 children, collected by Red Cross after the cord was cut, harbored pesticides, consumer product ingredients, and wastes from burning coal, gasoline, and garbage. This study represents the first reported cord blood tests for targeted chemicals and the first reported detections in cord blood for multiple compounds. Among those found were eight perfluorochemicals used as stain and oil repellents in fast-food packaging, clothes, and textiles—including the Teflon chemical PFOA, recently characterized as a likely human carcinogen by the EPA's Science Advisory Board—; dozens of widely used brominated flame retardants and their toxic by-products; and numerous pesticides and plastics including bisphenol A. Of the 287 chemicals detected in umbilical cord blood, 180 have been shown to cause cancer in humans or animals, 217 are toxic to the brain and nervous system, and 208 cause birth defects or abnormal development in animal tests. The dangers of pre- or postnatal exposure to this complex mixture of carcinogens, developmental toxins, and neurotoxins have never been studied.[23,24]

Endocrine Disruptors

Human beings and animals are most vulnerable to hormonal disruption during prenatal development when a fetus is undergoing rapid, hormonally orchestrated change. Other critical windows of development when the endocrine system is particularly sensitive to hormonal disruption include early life, puberty, pregnancy, and lactation.[25]

According to the National Institute of Environmental Health Sciences (NIEHS), endocrine disruptors are chemicals that may interfere with the body's endocrine system and produce adverse developmental, reproductive, neurological, and immune effects in both humans and wildlife. Endocrine disruptors may pose the greatest risk during prenatal and early postnatal development when organ and neural systems are forming. Diethylstilbesterol (DES), a drug with strong estrogenic properties administered to pregnant women until 1971 to prevent miscarriages, is a tragic example. Female children of mothers who took DES during pregnancy have a higher incidence of certain forms of ovarian, cervical, and vaginal cancer.[26]

A wide range of substances, both natural and man-made, is thought to cause endocrine disruption, including pharmaceuticals, polychlorinated biphenyls, DDT, dieldrin, atrazine and other pesticides and herbicides, and plasticizers such as bisphenol A and phthalates. Endocrine disruptors are found in many everyday products, including plastic bottles, metal food cans, detergents, flame retardants, food, toys, cosmetics, pesticides, and industrial chemicals and by-products such as polychlorinated biphenyls (PCBs), dioxins, and phenols. Many endocrine disruptors affect sex hormone function and reproduction, according to the findings of multigeneration animal studies. The full effects of endocrine disruptors are not completely understood because they have been around only for a few generations. A recently published article in *Environmental Health Perspectives* reports the conclusions of an international research team on the current science related to early-life environmen-

tal exposures and mammary gland development, preconception, in utero development, childhood, and reproductive years.[27]

In 2009, at its 91st annual meeting, the Endocrine Society, a research-based medical association, issued a strong statement citing the science on the adverse effects of endocrine-disrupting chemicals and offered guidelines and recommendations intended to educate and increase awareness. According to Robert M. Carey, president of the Endocrine Society and professor of medicine at the University of Virginia, "Endocrine-disrupting chemicals interfere with hormone biosynthesis, metabolism and action resulting in adverse developmental, reproductive, neurological and immune effects in humans and wildlife. Endocrine disrupting chemicals include substances in our environment, food and consumer products."[28]

One such chemical described in the statement, bisphenol A, a chemical that permeates our lives, is widely used in the manufacturing of plastics including baby bottles, toys, and metal cans. According to the U.S. Centers for Disease Control, 95% of Americans have detectable levels of bisphenol A in their bodies. In a recent CDC study, the observed BPA levels detected—0.1 to 9 parts per billion (ppb)—were at and above the concentrations known to reliably cause adverse effects in laboratory experiments

The evidence of the mechanisms of action and the effects of endocrine-disrupting chemicals on male and female reproduction, thyroid function, metabolism, and obesity are well documented.[28]

Known to be estrogenic since the mid-1930s, BPA serves as a chemical building block and a polycarbonate plastic and epoxy resin in technology applications, paints and adhesives, and as a protective coating in many products. For more than 20 years, researchers in the scientific community have expressed concerns about its safety in consumer products.[29] In September 2010, Canada and, soon thereafter, the European Union declared BPA a toxic substance and banned BPA use in baby bottles, expressing fears that it may harm the health of children.[30] Numerous studies indicate that the chemical leaches into food and disrupts hormones. States including Maine, New York, and Minnesota have introduced legislation to ban children's products containing BPA. The U.S. Department of Health and Human Services released information to help parents reduce children's BPA exposures. In 2010, in response to consumer concerns, Walmart banned BPA plastic baby bottles, and General Mills, a major corporation in the food industry, is currently seeking new technology to make canned food products without BPA.

After being pressed to reevaluate its position by the National Toxicology Program, in January 2010, the FDA expressed "some concern" about the potential effects of BPA on the "brain, behavior, and prostate gland in fetuses, infants, and young children." The agency states that it will not issue a ban on BPA. The American Chemistry Council (ACC) position supports the FDA's decision, insisting that a ban on BPA is unnecessary. According to the ACC, research indicates that BPA is "perfectly safe."[31]

Prenatal exposure of rats to BPA results in increases in the number of precancerous lesions and in situ tumors (carcinomas) as well as increased number of mammary tumors following adulthood exposures to subthreshold doses (lower than that needed to induce tumors) of known carcinogens. Epigenetic changes in mammary tissue were measured following several generations. Exposures to BPA in adulthood also enhance the rate of growth and proliferation of existing hormone-sensitive mammary tumors, suggesting multiple mechanisms by which BPA may affect breast cancer development. This suggests that exposures to bisphenol A in utero is a predictor of breast cancer in adulthood.[32]

Women's Health

Over the past few years, leading researchers specializing in issues related to hormone disruption and women's reproductive health have convened to address why conception rates fell 44% in the United States between 1960 and 2002.[33] Hormone disruptors can affect both parents, and scientists have linked fertility problems to exposure to BPA, DDT, DES, cigarette smoke, and PCBs.[34] Early puberty, known as precocious puberty in the scientific literature, is another growing concern. The onset of the age of puberty has declined over the last half century, and girls today begin to develop breast buds 2 years earlier than they did 40 years ago. Girls who go through puberty early have

increased risk for depression, obesity, polycystic ovarian syndrome, breast cancer, and experimentation with sex and drugs at a younger age. The hormonal cues that initiate the onset of puberty are sensitive to a variety of environmental influences.[35] Prepubertal stages of development, such as in the womb and early life, are thought to be vulnerable windows for triggers of hormonal disruption. In human studies, early puberty is linked to greater cumulative estrogenic exposure to multiple contaminants, such as phthalates, BPA, and organochlorine pesticides among others.[36]

Pesticides Permeate Our World

Atrazine, a potent endocrine disruptor chemical, is the most common herbicide used globally. In the United States, 34 million kilograms of atrazine are used yearly, mostly on cotton, corn, sorghum, sugarcane, pineapple, Christmas trees, and golf course greens. Atrazine poses serious health safety concerns, and the chemical has been banned by the European Union, and even Switzerland, where atrazine's leading manufacturer is headquartered. Atrazine is an organic compound in the triazine family of herbicides. It has been shown to inhibit electron transport, which then blocks photosynthesis. Increased concern about the safety of atrazine arose after monitoring programs found the chemical in drinking water and several scientific studies demonstrated the pollutant's ability to emasculate amphibians and fish. Male frogs were found to have egg sacs and other abnormal sexual characteristics. More recent studies have shown an association with birth defects in male newborns including hypospadias. In view of several compelling scientific studies, the EPA is reinvestigating atrazine, although the industry denies all reports. In 2009, the National Resource Defense Council (NRDC) analyzed results of surface water and drinking water monitoring data for atrazine and found pervasive contamination of watersheds and drinking water systems across the Midwest and southern United States.[37]

Early Child Development

Environmental factors during pregnancy might play a larger role than genetics in the development of autism spectrum disorders, according to two studies in the *Archives of General Psychiatry*. In one study, researchers at Stanford University and the University of California at San Francisco found that genetics account for about 38% of the risk of autism and that environmental factors account for about 62%. In a second study, researchers from the Kaiser Permanente Northern California system found that children faced a higher risk of autism if their mothers took antidepressants during the year prior to giving birth. According to the Centers for Disease Control and Prevention, approximately 13% of children have a developmental disability, ranging from language and speech impairments to serious developmental problems classified along the autism spectrum disorder.

The role of environmental factors in the development of autism is a crucial area of study. Along with genetics, the increase in autism cases has generated extreme concern over potential epigenetic changes when prenatal exposures are combined with specific genetic codes.

A recent study conducted by Harvard School of Public Health and published in the journal *Pediatrics* links dietary pesticide exposure to attention deficit disorders in children. The study followed more than 1,000 children and found 94% of them had pesticide residues in their urine. Those with the highest levels were nearly twice as likely to have attention deficit hyperactivity disorder (ADHD).[38] The pesticide class analyzed was the common and widely used organophosphates (OPs), known to be toxic because they work by disabling a nerve chemical used to transmit signals.[39] In the study, the fruits with the highest concentration of pesticides included commercial strawberries, raspberries, and frozen blueberries. Researchers write that this study is important for two reasons. First, it examined children with average exposure (not those with increased exposure such as children of farm workers); second, it shows that even small and allowable amounts of pesticides can have significant effects on a young person's brain. Children are at increased risk because they are exposed to higher levels of chemicals relative to their body size and their detoxification abilities are less developed. Dr. Susan Kegley, consulting scientist with Pesticide Action Network, explains:

> When it comes to pesticides, children are among the most vulnerable—pound for pound, they drink 2.5 times more

water, eat 3–4 times more food, and breathe twice as much air as adults. They also face exposure in the womb and via breast milk. Add to this the fact that children are unable to detoxify some chemicals and you begin to understand just how vulnerable early childhood development is. We've known for a long time that OP's poison farm workers at higher doses, and now we have a window into their lower-dose effects on the broader population.[40]

In May 2011, U.S. pediatricians called for Congress to overhaul a failed federal law that has exposed millions of children, beginning in the womb, to an untold number of toxic chemicals. In its statement, *Chemical-Management Policy: Prioritizing Children's Health*, the American Academy of Pediatrics recommends that the 1976 Toxic Substances Control Act be "substantially revised" because it has "been ineffective in protecting children, pregnant women, and the general population from hazardous chemicals in the marketplace."[41-43]

As researchers study the impact of pesticides on health and the environment, analysts and consumers demand safer food products. The U.S. Department of Agriculture issues an annual report on the amount of pesticide residue it detects in samples of fresh fruits and vegetables around the country. The Environmental Protection Agency uses the data to monitor exposure to pesticides and enforce federal standards designed to protect infants, children, and other vulnerable people. But the 200-page annual report has become a target of a lobbying campaign by the commercial produce industry, which worries that the data are being misinterpreted by the public. Eighteen produce trade associations have written to complain that the data have "been subject to misinterpretation by activists, which publicize their distorted findings through national media outlets in a way that is misleading for consumers and can be highly detrimental to the growers of these commodities."[44] In 2010, sales of organic fruits and vegetables, which are grown without synthetic chemicals, increased rapidly. Organic produce purchases now make up 12% of all U.S. fruit and vegetable sales, according to the Organic Trade Association. Even during the economic downturn, organic fruit and vegetable sales reached nearly $10.6 billion in 2010, up nearly 12% from 2009.[44]

Breast Cancer

Breast cancer incidence rates in the United States increased more than 40% between 1973 and 1998. In 2008, a women's lifetime risk of breast cancer was 1 in 8. Breast cancer arises from genetic, lifestyle, and environmental causes, several of which relate to lifetime exposure to hormones.[44]

Contrary to popular belief, only about 5% of women diagnosed with breast cancer have a link to the "breast cancer gene." Contributing factors that increase breast cancer risk include having children late in life and early onset of puberty. Exposure to radiation from chest x-rays during childhood and taking hormone replacement therapy are also known risk factors, along with alcohol abuse, tobacco exposure, and second-hand smoke exposure. Breast cancer rates are higher in women who are obese and women who gain excess weight during adulthood. Yet, the vast majority of women will never know the cause of their disease. The degree of alarm within the scientific community concerning the dangers of hormone-disrupting environmental pollutants as major contributors to breast cancer in younger women was evident when Health and Environment Alliance (HEAL), a European umbrella group of nongovernmental research organizations, released a report in 2010 stating, "We will not be able to reduce the risk of breast cancer without addressing preventable causes, particularly exposure to chemicals."[45]

Prevention is a solution that requires addressing the real issues surrounding the global increase in breast cancer and all cancers. Public health education, corporate responsibility, and governmental regulation of harmful chemicals must be included in addressing rising rates of cancer. According to the latest research, cumulative toxic exposures often beginning in utero show clear links to increased risks for breast cancer later in life.[46]

Research also links the role of the environment to the rise in testicular and prostate cancers in men.[47] To compound the problem of our toxic environment, we refine and process away much of the nutritional value in our food supply and replace it with imitation foods lacking protective phytonutrients that can filter, neutralize, and detoxify many of these potentially harmful chemicals. Products too often are filled with artificial colorings, preservatives, flavorings, and many unlisted industrial ingredients. Our modern poor-quality diet, combined with agricultural pesticides and animals being raised on antibiotics, chemical feed, and growth hormones, may dispose many of us to a toxic body burden, stressing the body's ability to detoxify and eliminate these products. According to Dr. Walter Willett at the Harvard School of Public Health and the American Institute for Cancer Research, a review of 4,500 scientific studies on diet and nutrition concludes in a 650-page report that 40% of cancers are avoidable. The document states, "The bottom line: eat a plant based diet, maintain moderate weight throughout life, and get some exercise."

The most challenging aspect to creating healthier environments includes discovering how to eliminate many of these compounds from the environment. The good news is that cancer and other health problems can be reduced by lifestyle interventions that can lower exposures to environmental toxicants and enhance our innate immune surveillance systems, increasing cellular energy for healthy metabolism and improving detoxification pathways through nutrition, stress reduction, and exercise.[47,48]

The following list shows the everyday products that contain endocrine disruptors that people can try to avoid or eliminate from their lives when possible:

- Pesticides, herbicides, including pesticide residues in soil
- Dry cleaning chemicals
- Solvents: paints, varnishes, cleaning fluids
- Spermicidal contraceptives and treated condoms
- Perfume fragrances, air fresheners, cleaning fragrances
- Car exhaust, car interiors—especially that "new car smell": (off-gassing)
- Plastics, plastic baby bottles, plastic food storage containers, Styrofoam, tin cans (BPA lining)
- PVC plumbing pipes

- Pharmaceutical runoff in the water supply
- BHA and BHT, common food preservatives
- FD&C Red No. 3, a common food dye (erythrosine)
- Personal care products that contain parabens, phthalates

Scientists and advocacy groups are informing the public and advocating for the precautionary principle while demanding health policy actions and regulation of the chemical industry.

Following is a review of the prevention strategies that can be implemented:

- Choose your food wisely; eat organically grown and raised foods when possible.
- Limit intake of animal fats because endocrine disruptors and heavy metals accumulate in the food chain and are stored in fat. The higher the intake of commercially raised animal products, the greater the potential for increasing toxic load.
- Choose seasonal and local foods.
- Monitor fish consumption. Large, deep-water "fatty" fish such as tuna and swordfish may contain higher levels of synthetic chemicals and heavy metals, so eat them infrequently. Better choices are wild-caught salmon, sardines, cod.
- Avoid pesticides. If you can't buy all organic food, try to pick and choose. Certain crops are more heavily treated than others are. The Environmental Working Group database (www.ewg.org) offers guidelines on the fruits and vegetables containing both the highest pesticide residues and the lowest. Produce containing the highest pesticide levels include peaches, apples, bell peppers, celery, nectarines, strawberries, cherries, lettuce, grapes, pears, spinach, and potatoes. Wash all fruits and vegetables thoroughly before consuming, or peel them if they are not organically grown.
- Support your body's natural ability to detoxify by exercising and sweating on a regular basis. Use a sauna or steam bath. Get regular sleep (you detoxify at night) and drink plenty of clean or filtered water.
- Consume plenty of fiber, which is found in whole grains, beans, vegetables, fruits, seeds (flax), and nuts.

- Drink beverages such as green tea that contain antioxidants and phytonutrients that can assist the body to rid itself of toxins.
- If planning a pregnancy or breastfeeding, be vigilant about chemicals and eliminate as many as possible for 1 year prior to conception. Guidelines for pregnant women on eating fish are listed at www.americanpregnancy.org/pregnancyhealth/fishmercury.htm.
- Become an environmental detective. Investigate the chemicals in your home, work, and community environments.
- Know your water supply. Find out whether your local community's water testing program checks for hormone-disrupting chemicals and heavy metals. Not all household filters work effectively on chemicals and, unfortunately, not all bottled water is checked either. Read water quality reports. If you drink purified water out of plastic bottles, do not leave the bottles in the car or the hot sun for any length of time; heat activates the molecules in the plastic, which increases the rate at which the polycarbons leach into the water.
- Avoid using plastics. If you do use plastics, the safest plastics are marked with the recycling codes 2, 4, and 5. Never let infants chew on soft plastic toys and never microwave food in a plastic bowl or covered in plastic wrap. A good rule of thumb is that the softer the plastic, the more chemicals it contains. Buy in bulk and store foods in glass jars. Limit use of plastic bags and cling-wrap products on your food. Assess the amount of plastic in your life and try to reduce it by five. For example: bring a reusable mug to the local coffee stop. Buy a refillable glass or earthenware water jug. Invest in glass food storage containers that can be washed and reused for a lifetime. Use reusable cloth totes for groceries.
- Exercise your rights as a consumer—never doubt the power of consumer demand. Ask for green products when you don't see them in your neighborhood stores. If you have a talent for organizing and recruiting people, use it to develop community groups and work with public officials to

develop ordinances regarding the use of chemicals in public places. It took a while to legislate no-smoking areas; hopefully "chemical-free" will not be far away. Encourage youth to learn more about environmental issues and to pursue research into redesigning our future.

- Become a community advocate. Support local and federal clean air and water initiatives. Write to your local and state representatives and encourage them to vote for a healthy future. Support elected officials who make a clean environment their priority. Join national campaigns to support health policy change.
- Together, we can create a healthier future for us all.

■ THE WATER WE DRINK

The majority of the planet is composed of water. Ninety-seven percent of this water is saltwater; the fresh water used to sustain life is only 3% of the total amount of water on Earth. Whereas the world's population tripled in the 20th century, its need for water resources has grown sixfold. The Earth has a limited supply of fresh water, stored in aquifers, surface waters, and the atmosphere. Within the next 50 years, the world population will increase by another 40–50%. This population growth, coupled with industrialization and urbanization, will result in an increasing demand for water and will have serious consequences on human health and the environment. We cannot live without water. Currently, there is a global water shortage crisis and futurists predict that water will trigger new wars for access. Globally, we are seeing this in the Horn of Africa, where millions of people are suffering from droughts and barren soil and no water. Here in the Western world, we face another water crisis. Chemicals leach into our urban and rural water supplies in municipalities and in wells.

A recent report by the U.S. Government Accountability Office titled *Safe Drinking Water Act: Improvements in Implementation Are Needed to Better Assure the Public of Safe Drinking Water* gave testimony to the Environmental Protection Agency, stating that requirements for determining whether additional drinking water contaminants warrant regulation must be implemented.

The number of potential drinking water contaminants is vast—tens of thousands of chemicals are used across the country, and the EPA has identified more than 6,000 chemicals that it considers to be the most likely source of human or environmental exposure. The potential health effects of exposure to most of these chemicals, and the extent of their occurrence in drinking water, are yet unknown.[49]

In early 2011, the EPA announced the agency's new Drinking Water Strategy (DWS), which aims to find ways to strengthen public health protection from contaminants in drinking water. Throughout the summer of 2010, the EPA listened and shared information with stakeholders as part of a national conversation to identify which factors were important for grouping contaminants and which contaminant groups might be important to address. After careful consideration, the EPA decided to address carcinogenic volatile organic compounds (VOCs) as a group. The new vision was intended to streamline decision making, expand protection under existing laws, and promote cost-effective new technologies to meet the needs of rural and urban communities. Since March 2010, there has been progress in addressing each of the four goals identified under the Drinking Water Strategy plan. The EPA is investing significant resources to conduct key studies of the environmental technology available for making drinking water safer so that these processes and technologies can be developed, tested, and marketed. Effective methods must meet the following standards:

- Are sustainable and water and energy efficient
- Are cost-effective for utilities and consumers
- Address a broad array of contaminants
- Improve public health protection

Some of the key accomplishments for each of the four goals are noted in **Table 29-1**.

■ THE AIR WE BREATHE

The number of people diagnosed with asthma in the United States grew by 4.3 million between 2001 and 2009, according to a new Vital Signs report released recently by the Centers for Disease Control and Prevention. In 2009, nearly

1 in 12 Americans were diagnosed with asthma. In addition to increased diagnoses, asthma costs grew from about $53 billion in 2002 to about $56 billion in 2007, about a 6% increase. Asthma is an increasingly common chronic disease among children in the United States. In 2006, 9.9 million children younger than 18 years of age were reported to have ever been diagnosed with asthma.[51]

Since 1970, the EPA has protected public health by setting and enforcing standards to protect the quality of the air we breathe and the water we drink. Today, many older power plants and industrial facilities employ loopholes in the current regulations to allow them to pollute at much higher levels than recommended. To protect public health from these polluting plants, the EPA must require that all facilities meet the same cleaner standards. There is much resistance in government and industry to create legislation to address global warming and pollution. In 2011, diverse business organizations lobbied members of Congress to stop the EPA from doing its job of protecting public health by rolling back existing public health laws such as the Clean Air Act and blocking needed clean

air and clean water protections. Despite the EPA and the Clean Air Act's success, air pollution continues to be a health problem, with many types of pollution and sources of pollution left unaddressed because of loopholes or political pressure or delays. Industry and special interests must not put profits before public health, and Congress must mandate that the EPA do its job to ensure healthy air for all Americans.

■ CLIMATE CHANGE: REDUCING GLOBAL WARMING

Under the Clean Air Act, the pollution that causes global warming and climate change must be treated like any other air pollution. The Supreme Court affirmed this view in its landmark 2007 decision *Massachusetts v. EPA* and ordered the EPA to decide, based on the best available science, whether these pollutants pose a danger to public health or welfare. In December 2009, the EPA responded to the Supreme Court by issuing an "endangerment finding" determining that carbon dioxide and five other greenhouse gases are dangerous to both health and welfare. This finding enables the EPA to use its

TABLE 29-1   Safe Drinking Water

Drinking Water Strategy Goal	Accomplishment(s)
Address contaminants as groups rather than one at a time so that enhancement of drinking water protection can be achieved cost-effectively.	In January 2011, identified carcinogenic volatile organic compounds as the first group that the agency plans to address
Foster development of new drinking water technologies to address health risks posed by a broad array of contaminants.	In January 2011, promoted the formation of a Regional Water Technology Innovation Cluster to bring together public and private partners to focus on finding new ways to simultaneously treat multiple contaminants in drinking water
Use the authority of multiple statutes to help protect drinking water.	Currently developing pesticide health benchmarks that can be used as tools in assessing the occurrence of contaminants in drinking water (when regulatory values are not available)
Partner with states to develop shared access to all public water systems (PWS) monitoring data.	In 2010, developed a Memorandum of Understanding between EPA and state partners to facilitate sharing of drinking water monitoring data

Source: Environmental Protection Agency, *Drinking Water Strategy Fact Sheet*, EPA 815-F-10-001 (Washington, DC: EPA, March 2010).[50]

authority to develop standards to reduce global warming pollution.

In April 2010, the EPA took its first steps to develop standards for vehicles, setting in motion standards for cars and light-duty trucks and separate standards for medium- and heavy-duty trucks.

Some key public health standards that must be legislated for public health safety can have the following effects:

- Standards to reduce toxic pollution from the thousands of power plants nationwide could save as many as 17,000 lives a year, prevent respiratory and cardiovascular diseases, and reduce the exposure of children to mercury and lead.
- Improving emissions performance in cars and light trucks would reduce heat-trapping carbon pollution that causes global warming while saving consumers billions of dollars and cutting oil use.
- The first-ever standards to cut carbon dioxide emissions and improve fuel efficiency in medium- and heavy-duty trucks would reduce global warming pollution, save 500 million barrels of oil over the lifetimes of the trucks sold during model years 2014 to 2018 and save truck operators $49 billion over the life of the vehicles.
- Instituting standards to reduce global warming pollution from power plants would help reduce the pollution that is increasing deaths and illnesses from heat waves, air pollution, infectious diseases, and severe weather events.[52]

■ INCREASING AWARENESS FOR CHANGE

Clearly, the hazards that began to be identified 50 years ago have grown exponentially. They continue to live among us despite vast concern, attempted legislation, and grassroots actions by many people and organizations. Probably the best-known contemporary author and activist is Al Gore. In his first work in 1992, *Earth in Balance: Ecology and the Human Spirit*, Gore argued that only a radical rethinking of our relationship with nature can save the Earth's ecology for future generations. This book was an urgent

call to action to America's citizens to wake up to the crisis and work together to save our seriously threatened climate, water, soil, diversity of plant and animal life, and indeed our entire living space.[53]

His second book in 2006 was another call to action. *An Inconvenient Truth* brings together leading-edge research from top scientists around the world; photographs, charts, and other illustrations; as well as personal anecdotes and observations to document the fast pace and wide scope of global warming.[54] In 2007, in his third work, *The Assault on Reason*, Gore argues that the marketplace of reasoned debate our country was founded on is being endangered by a variety of forces: the use of fear and the misuse of faith, the distractions of our entertainment culture, and the concentrations of power in the national media and the executive branch. All of these things divert us from our needed focus on the serious nature of Earth's environment and our very existence.[55] A way of life—a conscious choice—is possible only if we are willing to work, really work, to change from the industrial growth society to a life-sustaining society. It is possible to meet our needs without destroying our life support system.[56]

■ LIFE SUPPORT TRENDS

As consumer awareness and knowledge expands, so does the public's influence on industry as well as retail outlets. Public awareness, especially if it is organized, can revolutionize both industry and the marketplace as demonstrated by the health food industry, which thrives in cities and small towns across the United States. Whole Foods Market, the organic food supermarket chain, reported a sales profit that more than doubled in 1 year from 2009 to in 2010. Major big box stores including Costco and Walmart now carry organic food and safe cleaning products in response to consumer demand.[57]

Community Gardens

More than 1 million acres of farmland are lost each year to urban development. The average age of the farmers in this country is older than 50 years. Over the next decade, as much as 80% of the nation's farmland will turn over, with much of it going to people who won't live on the land. At the same time, resourceful communities are creating local community gardens and farms. Perhaps inspired by Michelle Obama's organic White House garden initiative, school-based gardens for students are a national trend that allows access to affordable organic fresh fruits and vegetables in urban communities where access has been limited, if not absent. A diverse consumer movement holds a shared philosophy that healthy soil means healthy food and healthier individuals, families, and communities. Healthy soil is soil in which no herbicides, pesticides, or artificial fertilizers are used and the consequences of ground water pollution and toxic residues on food are avoided. There is a growing awareness that the Earth is a living Being and the actions of every individual have an effect on the whole. The quality of the soil and water are the basis of all human life, and the quality of caring for the Earth and the resulting health benefits will not only affect the people who eat the food grown sustainably today, but also those who will depend on the soil in the future. The proper tending of the environment is the concern and responsibility of every individual. The positive public health consequences of sustainable gardening and farming affect the long-term health of future generations.

Community workers, public health officials, and urban planners are increasingly concerned about the declining levels of physical and psychological health of city dwellers. The reasons behind this alarming trend are complex. Much of the focus is on the changing environment and factors such as car dependency, long commuter distances, polluted and unsafe environments—all of which make it difficult for people to undertake the physical exercise needed to prevent many serious health issues. Poor nutrition, particularly overconsumption of processed and refined foods and underconsumption of clean plant-based foods, is a significant factor in poor health, especially in disadvantaged communities where fresh produce is often hard to find and expensive.

Urban planners, citizens, and health professionals must work together to better understand these issues if workable solutions are to be found. As community-supported agriculture gains ground everywhere, small farmers and citizens can grow high-quality, nutritious food while preserving the health and quality of the land. At the same time, resourceful communities are creating local community gardens and soil. Inherent in this movement is the understanding that the Earth and its inhabitants all benefit; as the Earth heals, so do we. At the same time, the individual becomes reconnected and reintegrated into the community, healing much of the isolation and alienation experienced in modern society.

Research has found that in urban settings sustainable garden projects result in a broad range of positive physical and psychological well-being outcomes for public housing tenants. These include providing opportunities for individuals to relax, undertake physical activity, socialize and mix with neighbors, and share across culturally different backgrounds and religions. Changing one's neighborhood and community environment can improve health, according to a recent study in the *New England Journal of Medicine*.[58]

Community gardens also afford people opportunities to learn about horticulture and sustainable environmental practices, such as composting and recycling, as well as are an important source of low-cost, fresh produce for a healthy diet. Community gardens around the world have been credited with an array of beneficial outcomes for participants. These include local political activism; environmental education where participants learn about sustainable urban agriculture, biodiversity, and improved waste management; and opportunities for training, employment, and local economic development in the form of markets and food cooperatives Nevertheless, the most significant and widely reported benefits are associated with individual and community health and well-being.[58]

Sustainable Health Care

In the past several years in the healthcare sector, a nurse-inspired environmental health movement has emerged with outreach efforts, local to global. Health Care Without Harm (HCWH), along with its sister organizations, has been in the forefront to transform the way hospitals are designed, built, and operated and be involved with the greening of health care.

According to its mission, environmentally responsible health care and its sustainable development is a concept vital to all healthcare partners: as major users of natural resources and toxic materials, hospitals make a dramatic contribution to society's ecological footprint. By using excessive amounts of energy; polluting the environment with medical supplies and materials made from plastics that include phthalates, mercury, and a multitude of other toxic chemicals; and producing waste that is burned instead of recycled, health care is ultimately compromising public health and damaging the ability of future generations to be healthy.

Hospitals all over the world are discovering that energy use can be drastically reduced, that mercury can be eliminated, and better quality food for patients can be sustainably sourced. Because the purchasing power of healthcare systems is enormous, the decisions healthcare institutions make as a living cultural system can have a substantial impact on public and environmental health.

Issues to be addressed in environmentally responsible health care include waste management; elimination of toxic materials; safer cleaners, chemicals, and pesticides; healthy food systems; cleaner energy; and safe disposal of pharmaceuticals. HCWH promotes adopting food procurement policies that are environmentally sound and socially responsible. The foods that employees and patients consume often are the very foods that the public is being warned to avoid. Adopting policies that include protecting the health of workers, patients, and communities and, by example, having a positive impact on the ecological health of the planet are moral and ethical imperatives of a healthcare model. Toward that goal, HCWH is working with hospitals to adopt food procurement policies that provide nutritionally improved food for patients, staff, visitors, and the general public and support and create food systems that are ecologically sound, economically viable, and socially responsible.[59]

■ CHOOSING A SUSTAINABLE FUTURE

In 1993 in the United States, the President's Council on Sustainable Development was convened to find ways to meet people's needs without jeopardizing the future. In its vision statement, the 30-member council stated:

> Our vision is of a life-sustaining Earth.
> We are committed to the achievement

of a dignified, peaceful, and equitable existence. A sustainable United States will have a growing economy that provides equitable opportunities for satisfying livelihoods, and a safe, healthy, high quality of life for current and future generations. Our nation will protect its environment, its natural resource base, and the function and viability of natural systems on which all life depends.[60]

The fact is that growth, demographic or economic, is ultimately unsustainable; perpetual growth is mathematically impossible in a finite space such as the Earth. Sustainability demands a redefinition of consumption goals, such as use of renewable resources at a rate that does not exceed their rates of regeneration and use of nonrenewable resources at a rate that does not exceed the rate at which sustainable, renewable substitutes are developed. The task is to confine human activity so that it can be pursued without damage to the natural systems. No goal, including sustainability, is absolute, however. For every contemplated policy or action, it is essential to consider what the threat to sustainability is and whether the anticipated gains are so overwhelming that they justify the action.

Part of being a sustainable and resilient community is the conscious intent to bring all stakeholders into future planning. On one university campus, a full design team was engaged from the inception of an idea for a new ecologic center building. Students, faculty, and administrators, as well as architects, were integral to this rich, real-life experience of planning and implementation. The basic building program emerging from a 1-year planning phase demonstrates decisions based on principles of sustainability. Most, if not all, of the project goals can be applied to other building or renovation projects as well.[60] The building:

- Discharges no waste water (i.e., "drinking water in; drinking water out")
- Generates from sunlight more electricity in the course of a year than it uses
- Uses no material known to be carcinogenic, mutagenic, or an endocrine disruptor
- Uses energy and materials efficiently

- Uses products or materials grown or manufactured sustainably
- Is landscaped to promote biological diversity
- Promotes analytic skills in assessing full costs over the lifetime of the building
- Promotes ecologic competence and mindfulness of place
- Is genuinely pedagogical in its design and operations
- Meets rigorous requirements for full cost accounting

Today, organizations and industry are leaders in designing, developing, and regulating green sustainable communities. The Leadership in Energy and Environmental Design (LEED) Council is an internationally recognized green building certification system, providing third-party verification that a building or community was designed and built using strategies intended to improve performance in metrics such as energy savings, water efficiency, CO_2 emissions reduction, improved indoor environmental air quality, and stewardship of resources and sensitivity to their impacts.[61]

The Sustainable Industry Council exemplifies national industry leadership in defining the concept of high performance that focuses on the full range of sustainable/green strategies. The council is now moving to the next phase of this evolutionary process to create facilities that integrate an even more comprehensive range of design objectives into high-performing, whole system buildings. Such buildings, whether they are residential or commercial, privately or publicly owned, favor sustainability as a prominent characteristic, but also are architecturally stimulating, cost-effective, functional, operational, respectful of historic resources, safe, and secure.

Green Job Networks and other national organizations provide meaningful employment and training opportunities. They also connect people seeking and offering jobs that focus on environmental and social responsibility. Such organizations offer opportunities and resources and provide renewed hope for the environment in the future.

Environmental efforts are part of a general societal impetus to have a habitable planet, now and in years to come. Many of these efforts, in the aggregate, are pragmatic and based on economic interests; others are derived from a philosophic outlook such as environmental justice. Many, if not most, of the movements remain human centered, addressing impacts as they relate to humankind. Any benefit for the rest of the biotic community is a by-product from that frame of reference. The holistic outlook, as has been stated, recognizes all systems as interacting. If one part is affected, change of a greater or lesser magnitude occurs everywhere. This way of thinking is to weave the human economy back into the Earth economy. Cowan, a building and landscape architect, notes that toxicity, waste, and extravagant resource use are all symptoms of poor design and production processes.[62]

Around the world, innovative companies and product designers are taking ecology as the basis for design, thus phasing out toxicity, cutting waste, and increasing resource efficiency. Cowan proposes strategic questions for use in evaluating which products, companies, and initiatives will lead to a less toxic world. The four major categories of questions, as shown in **Exhibit 29-1**, can be asked when potential products are considered for use: substitution, stewardship, ecology, and simplicity.

For shelter, humankind originally constructed mud huts or simple structures made of found natural materials structures. Today, it is beyond imagination the devastation that has been inflicted on the Earth by the construction industry: sand and water are sucked from the rivers, stones are taken from the mountains, cement is manufactured from resources dug from the ground. In addition, carbon emission from the buildings and manufacturing of construction materials warm the air and space. To address these problems, the concept of Green Buildings has arrived. Green Buildings take a new approach to save water, energy, and material resources in the construction and maintenance of the buildings and can reduce or eliminate the adverse impact of buildings on the environment and occupants. Green communities are planned, designed, and created to reestablish balance. Although it originally referred to restoring balance in natural ecosystems, the term *permaculture* has come to mean any system, natural, political, or cultural, that can be structured to be more self-sustaining, cooperative,

EXHIBIT 29-1   Strategic Questions to Evaluate Products, Companies, and Initiatives for a Less Toxic World

1. Substitutions of materials
   - Is it synthetic? Does it biodegrade? Does it accumulate in living tissues?
   - Is it a known carcinogen, mutagen, teratogen, endocrine disruptor, or acute toxin?
   - When it degrades, off-gases, combusts, or reacts, does it pose any of the preceding threats?

2. Substitution of less toxic or nontoxic products
   - How toxic is this product during its extraction, manufacturing, use, recycling, or disposal?
   - Is this product durable, easy to maintain, repair, reuse, remanufacture, or upgrade?
   - Does it have replaceable or reusable components, parts, and materials?
   - Will the manufacturer take responsibility for this product and packaging?
   - Will the manufacturer completely recycle the product and packaging?
   - Can the benefits of this product best be provided by turning it into a service product?

3. Industrial ecology
   - If "waste equals food," what processes does this chemical or product feed during its entire life cycle?
   - Can this entire class of chemicals or products be phased out by reconfiguring industrial ecosystems?
   - At the most basic level, what services does this product provide?
   - Can these services be provided by healthy ecosystems instead?

4. Voluntary simplicity
   - Despite all efforts, does this product remain unacceptably toxic? If so, is it truly essential?
   - Does the product have other purposes? Does it meet basic needs?
   - What level of this product or service genuinely contributes to the quality of my life?
   - Can this level of service be best supplied through my own initiative and that of my local community?

and resilient. Permaculture can be applied to sustainable, human living systems.

Green Buildings Are Eco-Friendly Structures

The idea of Green Buildings evolved from an initial focus on building energy use to a broader focus on the full range of sustainable/green strategies. The Sustainable Industry Council is now moving to the next phase of this evolutionary process: going Beyond Green to create facilities that integrate an even more comprehensive range of design objectives into high-performing, whole buildings.

Green Engineering

Green engineering advances the sustainability of manufacturing processes, construction, and infrastructure and supports research on envi-ronmentally benign manufacturing and chemical processes. Environmental sustainability encompasses consideration of more than one chemical or manufacturing process. It takes a systems or holistic approach to engineering infrastructure and buildings. Improvements in distribution and collection systems that advance smart growth strategies and ameliorate effects of growth are research areas that are supported by environmental sustainability. Innovations include management of storm water, recycling and reuse of drinking water, and other green engineering techniques to support sustainable construction projects.

Ecological Engineering

Ecological engineering focuses on the engineering aspects of restoring ecological function to natural systems. Many communities are involved in stream restoration, revitalization of urban rivers, and rehabilitation of wetlands that require engineering input. This area addresses what fundamental engineering knowledge is necessary for ecological engineering to function sustainability.

Earth Systems Engineering

Earth systems engineering considers large-scale engineering projects that involve mitigation of greenhouse gas emissions, adaptation to climate change, and other global-scale concerns.

Although government provides guidelines and safeguards for the environment, these are frequently diluted or diverted by partisan or special interest groups, as demonstrated recently by challenges to the environmental protection guidelines for human health by powerful industry lobbying efforts.

An environmentally responsible citizen movement in all sectors is organizing to present a clear vision with zest, care, and drive to see a more sustainable and inhabitable world for present and future generations. Because the emerging world paradigm is a participative one, a community's environmental sustainability depends in large measure on how well it is able to recruit, mobilize, and retain citizen involvement at all levels.[63]

Effective citizen involvement has the following characteristics:

1. Political, corporate, and civic leadership listens to all voices in the community.
2. Community activists focus on the common good.
3. Media (print, television, radio, and Internet) value and commit resources to building community.
4. Technology, hardware, and software are of sufficient quantity and quality to enable community and regional deliberation processes.
5. Projects reflect natural ecologic and economic regions; they are not bound by traditional political jurisdictions.
6. Citizen involvement in a project can continue for the long term.
7. Resources are committed to enhancing community members' skills for the short and long terms.
8. There is an established sense of trust and mutual valuing among community members.
9. Leaders recognize that needed changes are systemic, not isolated, and that both individuals and institutions are responsible for making them.

The concept of sustainability is complex and intertwined because it has to do with interrelated systems. The bottom line is wonderfully simple and straightforward, however: to live as if we belong here and are planning to stay a while.

Cultivating Healing Environments

Optimizing a healing environment in the acute care setting has been a prevalent goal for many years. Molter suggests that the healing environment in the critical care setting is a synergistic integration of components of a holistic intention in care. This integration offers complementary alternative therapies with family and patient-centered interventions and an aesthetic setting with administrative support of health professionals who value a body-mind-spirit approach. Multiple driving forces are leading the way to the development of healing environments, such as the increased utilization of complementary and alternative therapies by the general public[64] and nurses,[65] steady increase of persons living with chronic illness, and the holistic movement toward care versus cure.

In 1990, the American Association of Critical Care Nurses initiated a consensus panel to establish guidelines for creating a healing and humane environment in the critical care setting. The organization has just published its second edition of the *AACN Protocols for Practice: Creating Healing Environments* that summarizes interventions that are evidence based.[64] The interventions focus on environmental design and strategies, family needs interventions and presence, family visitation and partnership, family pet visiting and animal-assisted therapy, spiritual and complementary therapies, and pain management—all supported by evidence-based knowledge.

A number of contemporary nurses have modeled and evolved the Nightingale tenets. For example, at one Oregon hospital use of a theoretical Model of Whole-Person Caring resulted in quantifiable and sustainable results in the areas of increased patient and employee satisfaction and decreased nursing turnover, and now serves as the foundation for a comprehensive healing environment.[66]

The American Association of Critical Care Nurses began promoting its Healthy Work Environment standards in 2005. These standards address how the organization should promote employee communication skills, true collaboration, effective decision making, appropriate staffing, meaningful recognition, and authentic leadership to promote quality outcomes for patients as well as nurses. This move is essential in creating an environment where nurses can effectively care for persons with healthcare needs, while doing so with "infrastructures that are healing sanctuaries." Authentic nurse leaders are needed to implement these guidelines. The benefits will be a satisfied nursing staff, a joyful workplace, and a learning organization.[67]

Creating Optimal Healing Environments

More and more hospitals are implementing "healing initiatives" that can have a transformative effect on the healthcare system. They are creating a framework of actionable practices and evaluation methods that, when implemented, lead to more cost-effective, efficient organizations in which the environment truly facilitates healing and where care providers are fully supported to reconnect to the mission at their professional roots—the mission of caring. Samueli Institute's Optimal Healing Environments (OHE) program seeks to build the knowledge base of healthcare practices that influence the healing process of recovery, repair, and return to wholeness. OHE is unique in that it is a comprehensive approach to health care that encompasses all of the social, psychological, organizational, behavioral, and physical conditions that contribute to healing and achievement of wholeness. OHE research is conducted in real-world settings, including hospitals, outpatient clinics, workplaces, and among specialized populations, to demonstrate how healing translates directly into current healthcare practices.[68] Optimal healing environments are created through eight domains that include the inner environment of the patient and caregiver, the interpersonal environment of relationships and healing

practices, and the external environment of healing spaces and sustainable communities.[69] The eight domains of an optimal healing environment are the following:

- Developing healing intention
- Experiencing personal wholeness
- Cultivating healing relationships
- Creating healing organizations
- Practicing healthy lifestyles
- Applying integrative health care
- Building healing spaces
- Fostering ecological sustainability

With this increasing awareness of how the external environment affects the internal healing process, there is a growing movement coming from the healthcare sector and from industry to rethink how institutions that care for people can create greener sustainable buildings, including hospitals. Some of the newest technology being studied and researched to create sustainable communities include that discussed in the following subsections.

Building Learning Communities

A learning community is a group of people who choose to enter into a discovery mode, meaning that each person is willing to teach or learn, depending on what he or she has to contribute. Characterized by safety, support, and openness, the learning community focuses on personal and societal learning. Within the context of seeking a sustainable future, the search for humankind's rightful and responsible place in the natural world fuels learning.

The community bond for many groups is the opportunity to honor deeply held values that integrate personal, social, and spiritual lives. Members enrich their inner lives while selectively engaging in some form of service work. These small grassroots efforts are conducting much of future sustainability work.

In some select instances, business communities are assuming leadership in striving toward sustainability. The trend engenders a different type of learning community, one that is integral to the preferred corporate image. Perhaps the most remarkable contemporary example is Interface, a global manufacturing enterprise that produces 40% of the world's carpeting. Because of a personal, radical commitment to sustainability, its founder and chief executive officer Ray Anderson committed his company to becoming a zero-waste enterprise. It is well on its way to realizing this goal. To accomplish this immense task, involving 26 manufacturing sites delivering to 110 outlets worldwide, a very specific educational process has been initiated to engage the conscious commitment of employees at all levels over time, as well as that of stockholders. Increasingly, businesses are seeing that "green is good"—economically, socially, and sustainably.

Many facilitative and reliable resources are available to seekers and learners, from neighborhood "wise persons" to the Internet. Highly authoritative avenues for learning and practicing sustainability include, but are not limited to, the three named here because of their excellence and widespread recognition over time: (1) Co-op America, an organization dedicated to creating a just and sustainable society through economic means;[70] (2) Worldwatch Institute, which provides in-depth analysis of environmental issues and trends, providing information on how to build a sustainable society (www.worldwatch.org);[71] and (3) *Yes! A Journal of Positive Futures* (www.yesmagazine.org) which fosters the evolution of a just, sustainable, and compassionate future.[72] The National Resource Defense Council, a nonpartisan international environmental advocacy group, works to protect wildlife and wild places and to ensure a healthy environment for all life on Earth (www.nrdc.org), and the mission of the Environmental Working Group (EWG) is to use the power of public information to protect public health and the environment (www.ewg.org).

Sustainability includes a resolve to live in harmony with biological and physical systems and to work to create social systems that can enable us to do that. It includes a sense of connectedness and an understanding of the utter dependence of human society on the intricate web of life, a passion for environmental justice and ecological ethics, an understanding of dynamic natural balances and processes, and a recognition of the limits to growth resulting from finite resources. Our concern for sustainability recognizes our responsibility to future generations, to care for the Earth as our own home and the home of all who dwell herein. We seek a relationship between human beings and the Earth that is mutually enhancing.

Working from the Inside Out

As holistic nurses who are acutely sensitive to environmental issues, we know that the most important tool we have to offer is modeling the way we live our lives. The way we live is crafted and emerges from our day-to-day choices.

We live in a world of vast complexity and diversity. Our choice is to do whatever it takes to commit to and maintain our basic values, whatever we determine them to be. Only we can arrive at the personal meanings and understanding of relationships that provide coherence to our existence. Although we may have models, support, and assistance, each of us is called to make this determination. In our holistic practice, we assist others in examining their options and encourage them to make life-affirming choices. Our primary task is to be with our clients within their life circumstances. Often, our greatest contribution is to walk freely with our clients as they face their ordeals, joys, and transitions.

As we deepen our awareness, we engage in our own grief work. We acknowledge and choose to make amends for our complicity, whether conscious or unintended, in the seemingly insurmountable environmental degradation observed today. We are not immobilized or demoralized by grief, however. We use it to fuel our resolve to "make it right." Because humankind has brought us to today's apparent impasse, we freely claim accountability and acknowledge our own vulnerability as planetary citizens. We have a heightened sense of belonging as we walk this path, for we know in some way that the ills we see through our nursing lens derive in large measure from the pervasive sense of vulnerability of our clients and, indeed, of communities and larger societies. We have a heightened awareness that the consequences of "not belonging" and of feeling isolated and alienated from families and communities give rise to depressive disorders and disease states with innumerable manifestations.[73]

We risk everything through the clarity of our values and convictions. Being human is not for the fainthearted. Before we can take a stand or set a direction on an issue, we must reflect long and carefully about what gives meaning and brings a sense of purpose to our lives. One approach is to seek clarity, within ourselves, about our purpose for existence. Holistic nurses are uniquely positioned to access the fountainhead of wisdom and strength within ourselves and to assist others to reclaim their own inner strength. The work, as in all authentic endeavors, is born in silence and stillness. Striving with joy and equanimity for an environmentally conscious life means aspiring to be part of a larger whole, our inner life as a reflection of its outer manifestation.

■ NOISE AND THE STRESS RESPONSE

> In dwelling on the importance of sound observation, it must never be lost sight of what observation is for. It is not for the sake of piling up miscellaneous information or curious facts, but for the sake of saving life and increasing health and comfort.
>
> —*Florence Nightingale*

Noise pollution may be the most common modern health hazard. A growing body of data suggests a link between noise pollution and adverse mental and physical health. Elevated workplace or other noise can cause hearing impairment, hypertension, ischemic heart disease, annoyance, and sleep disturbance. Changes in the immune system and birth defects have been attributed to noise exposure, but evidence is limited. Early studies show that noise causes changes in blood pressure, sleep patterns, and digestion, all signs of stress on the body. Studies have been looking at the relationship among stress and noise pollution and public health for many decades

The United Kingdom and Japan national laws enacted in 1960 and 1967, respectively, and the Noise Control Act of 1972 in the United States were the direct result of early scientific studies showing the extreme havoc noise causes for humans. In recent times, the federal government has limited its responsibilities with respect to noise control after an initial interest in the 1970s, when legislation was passed promising to protect the American people from the harmful effects of noise. However, stress and noise pollution are far worse than originally thought

because science now shows that noise raises stress levels to the point of causing heart and immune system problems and can alter brain chemistry in harmful ways.

The danger posed by noise pollution is a function of the volume of sound heard over a period of time. Sound and its intensity are measured in decibels, abbreviated dB (**Table 29-2**). The European Union (EU) now considers living near an airport to be a risk factor for coronary heart disease and stroke because increased blood pressure from noise pollution can trigger these more serious maladies. The EU estimates that 20% of Europe's population—or about 80 million people—are exposed to airport noise levels it considers unhealthy and unacceptable. Airport noise can also have negative effects on children's health and development. A 1980 study examining the impact of airport noise on children's health found higher blood pressure in kids living near the Los Angeles LAX airport than in those living farther away.[74]

| TABLE 29-2 | Decibel Levels of Various Sounds |

Decibel (dB) Level	Generating Sound
120–140	Jet engine at take-off Amplified rock band at close range
100–110	Power lawn mower Oncoming subway train Chain saw Jackhammer
80–100	Alarm clock Screaming child Truck traffic at close range Cocktail party
60–80	Electric kitchen aids Washing machine
40–60	Normal conversation Refrigerator hum
20–40	A cat's purr
0–10	Threshold of hearing

In the United States, antinoise activists have been working arduously to urge the federal government to take an active role once again in abating and controlling noise. They have also been enlisting more citizens to their cause as they educate them to the hazards of noise.

Even low-frequency noise appears to be a problem. One study found that low-frequency noise interfered with a proofreading task by lowering the number of marks made per line read. The subjects reported a higher degree of annoyance and impaired working capacity when working under conditions of low-frequency noise. The effects were more pronounced for subjects rated as highly sensitive to low-frequency noise, while somewhat different results were obtained for subjects rated as highly sensitive to noise in general. The results suggest that the quality of work performance and perceived annoyance may be influenced by a continuous exposure to low-frequency noise at commonly occurring noise levels. Subjects categorized as highly sensitive to low-frequency noise may be at highest risk.[75]

The auditory system is permanently open—even during sleep. Its quick and overshooting excitations caused by noise signals are subcortically connected via the amygdala to the hypothalamic-pituitary-adrenal axis (HPA axis). Thus, noise causes the release of different stress hormones, such as corticotropin releasing hormone (CRH) and adrenocorticotropic hormone (ACTH), especially in sleeping persons during the vagotropic night/early morning phase. These effects occur below the waking threshold of noise and are mainly without mental control. The widespread extrahypothalamic effects of CRH and ACTH have the potential to influence nearly all regulatory systems, causing, for example, stress dysmenorrhea, a sign of disturbed hormonal balance.[76] As part of a 5-year study, researchers at Georgia Institute of Technology, Emory University, and the Atlanta Veterans Administration Medical Center collected data from 92 nursing home residents. Even modest increases in noise above the background level disturbs sleep of seniors in nursing homes, the study reports.

Researchers are now testing the effectiveness of several noise-reducing environmental interventions to reduce sleep disturbances among nursing home residents. The ultimate goal is to improve the residents' health and quality of life.

Considerable empirical evidence supports the claim that advances in hospital technology have led to increased sound levels in the critical care unit. In one study, 70 patients were randomly assigned to a noise- or quiet-controlled environment while attempting to sleep overnight in a simulated critical care unit. Researchers sought to determine whether the sound levels suppress rapid eye movement (REM) sleep. Subjects in the noise group heard an audiotape recording of critical care unit nighttime sounds. These subjects showed poorer REM sleep on 7 of 10 measures. Thus, there appears to be a causal relationship between critical care units and suppression of REM sleep.[77]

The biological plausibility for noise stress–related cardiovascular responses is well established. Epidemiologic studies on the relationship between transportation noise and ischemic heart disease suggest a higher risk of myocardial infarction in subjects exposed to high levels of traffic noise. One study determined the risk of road traffic noise for the incidence of myocardial infarction (MI). Patients (n = 1,881), age 20–69 years, with confirmed diagnosis of MI from 1998 through 2001 were matched with controls (n – 2,234) according to sex, age, and hospital. Outdoor traffic noise level was determined for each study subject based on noise maps of the city. Standardized interviews were conducted to assess possible confounding factors and the annoyance from various noise sources. The adjusted odds ratio for men exposed to sound levels of more than 70 dBA during the day was 1.3 with those where the sound level did not exceed 60 dBA. In the subsample of men who lived for at least 10 years at their present address, the odds ratio was 1.8. The results support the hypothesis that chronic exposure to high levels of traffic noise increases the risk for cardiovascular diseases.[78]

One review provides an overview of epidemiologic studies that were carried out in the field of community noise and cardiovascular risk. Risk estimates derived from the individual studies are given for five dBA categories of the average A-weighted sound pressure level during the day. The noise sources considered in the studies are road and aircraft noise with the health endpoints being mean blood pressure and hypertension and ischemic heart disease, including myocardial infarction. There is strong evidence of an association between transportation noise and cardiovascular risk that has increased since the previous review published in *Noise and Health* in the year 2000.[78] Theoretical models are needed to change noise levels in healthcare institutions because the literature demonstrates EPA-recommended noise levels are notoriously high.

■ RADIATION EXPOSURES: LIVING IN THE MODERN WORLD

We live in a radioactive world—and always have. Radiation is part of our natural environment. We are exposed to radiation from materials in the Earth itself and from the sun. With the recent nuclear disaster in Japan, renewed concerns over the long-term risks of radiation exposure are again in the minds of people around the world. The question becomes, How can we reduce our exposures over the course of a lifetime?

Living in today's world, we are all exposed to far more radiation than ever before, and we are only beginning to calculate the impact on our health. Estimates have been that we receive up to 100,000 times more radiation than our great-grandparents did. We receive radiation exposure from routine diagnostic medical testing including dental and chest x-rays and mammograms. We get it from background radiation in everyday life from electromagnetic fields, microwaves, flying in airplanes at high altitude, and the latest technology toys. We all carry very small amounts of naturally occurring radioactive materials in our bodies.

Radiation in Tobacco Leaves

Former U.S. Surgeon General C. Everett Koop stated that tobacco radiation is probably responsible for 90% of tobacco-related cancer. Dr. R. T. Ravenholt, former director of World Health Surveys at the Centers for Disease Control and Prevention, states, "Americans are exposed to far more radiation from tobacco smoke than from any other source." Second-hand smoke is harmful to nearby nonsmokers, especially children.

Naturally occurring radioactive minerals accumulate on the sticky surfaces of tobacco leaves as the plant grows, and these minerals remain on the leaves throughout the manufacturing pro-

cess. Additionally, the use of the phosphate fertilizer Apatite—which contains radium, lead-210, and polonium-210—also increases the amount of radiation in tobacco plants. The radium that accumulates on the tobacco leaves predominantly emits alpha and gamma radiation. The lead-210 and polonium-210 particles lodge in the smoker's lungs, where they accumulate for decades (lead-210 has a half-life of 22.3 years). The tar from tobacco builds up on the bronchioles and traps even more of these particles. Over time, these particles can damage the lungs and lead to lung cancer.[79] Conservative estimates put the level of radiation absorbed by a pack-and-a-half-a-day smoker at the equivalent of 300 chest x-rays every year. The Office of Radiation, Chemical and Biological Safety at Michigan State University reports that the radiation level for the same smoker was as high as 800 chest x-rays per year. Another report argues that a typical nicotine user might be getting the equivalent of almost 22,000 chest x-rays per year.[80]

Microwave Cooking

According to research, cooking food in a microwave may alter the physical makeup of the food. It is known that the irradiation process breaks up the molecular structure of food and creates a whole new set of chemicals, known as unique radiolytic products (URPs). These URPs include benzene, formaldehyde, and a host of known mutagens and carcinogens. This fact alone has obviously caused considerable controversy over the potential hazards of eating irradiated foods of any kind.

Food Irradiation

Food irradiation is a process whereby food is exposed to a controlled source of ionizing radiation to prolong shelf life and reduce food losses, improve microbiologic safety, and/or reduce the use of chemical fumigants and additives in controlling organisms. It is used to reduce insect infestation of grain, dried spices, and dried or fresh fruits and vegetables; inhibit sprouting in tubers and bulbs; retard postharvest ripening of fruits; inactivate parasites in meats and fish; eliminate spoilage microbes from fresh fruits and vegetables; extend shelf life in poultry, meats, fish, and shellfish; decontaminate poultry and beef; and sterilize foods and feeds.[81] Irradiating food has been practiced in the United States since the 1960s, when the Food and Drug Administration approved the irradiation of wheat and white potatoes. During the 1980s, the FDA approved petitions for irradiation of spices, herbs and seasonings, pork, fresh fruits and vegetables, and dry or dehydrated substances such as enzymes. Poultry received approval in 1990. The FDA approved irradiation for unfrozen red meat in 1992, frozen red meat in 1999, and eggs in 2000.[82] Gamma energy penetrates the food and its packaging, but most of the energy simply passes through the food, similar to the way microwaves pass through food, leaving no residue. From a nutritional aspect, irradiation of food can destroy 20–80% of several essential nutrients including vitamin A; thiamine; vitamins B_2, B_3, B_6, B_{12}; folic acid; and vitamins C, E, and K. Some essential fatty acids may also be affected. Irradiation also kills friendly bacteria and enzymes, effectively rendering the food "dead." In the words of Donald R. Louria, chairman of the Department of Preventive Medicine and Community Health for the University of Medicine and Dentistry of New Jersey:

> The supporters of food irradiation treat the potential damage to the nutrient value of food as if it were unimportant or nonexistent. That is a major mistake. If the nutrient value of food is reduced, then the argument for food irradiation prolonging shelf life is undercut. Surely, it would not make sense to prolong shelf life if the foods are nutritionally defective.[80]

In the United States, food growers and manufacturers must mention on the label that the food is irradiated, so avoidance of irradiated foods is possible if one shops carefully. (The package symbol for irradiated food is a green flower-like graphic.) Currently, there are strong lobbying efforts by the food industry to allow foods to be irradiated without informing the public. One of the concerns voiced by health advocates is that the need to irradiate meats masks the unsanitary conditions of factory farms. According to the Center for Food Safety, a Washington consumer

protection organization, radiation is an after-the-fact "solution" that does nothing to address the unsanitary conditions of factory farms and actually creates a disincentive for producers and handlers to take preventative steps in production. The longer shelf life created by irradiation (affording longer shipping distances) also provides greater opportunity for posttreatment contamination via shipping and handling. Additionally, irradiation does not work to stop toxins produced by some bacteria (such as botulism); viruses, including foot and mouth disease and hepatitis, all resistant to the irradiation doses used in food; prions (thought to be the cause of BSE, or Mad Cow disease) are resistant as well. It is clear that food irradiation, although protecting parts of the food supply, has not been adequately tested on humans and more research is needed.[81]

Diagnostic Radiation

The average lifetime dose of diagnostic radiation has increased sevenfold since 1980, mostly through the use of x-rays. X-rays are energy in the form of waves, identical to visible light, the difference being that light doesn't have enough energy to go through the body. Some advances in equipment design reduce the radiation exposure from previously, such as dental x-rays. A typical dental x-ray image exposes the patient to only about 2 or 3 millirems. However, diagnostic scans are being used more routinely than ever before, especially in emergency rooms; sometimes they are ordered before the doctor has even examined the patient.

CT Scans

Whole-body scans of healthy patients looking for hidden tumors or other illnesses are also becoming more common. In many states, people in search of "early diagnosis" do not need a health practitioner to order a whole-body scan and can schedule their own. The irony is that by exposing healthy people to radiation, the scans may be creating more problems than they solve. Two recent studies concerning radiation exposure associated with computed tomography (CT) scans have raised concerns about long-term cancer risks. Both studies were published in the *Archives of Internal Medicine*.[83]

CT scans are an important diagnostic tool that help physicians and healthcare providers to evaluate trauma, abdominal pain, chronic headaches, and other ailments. The fast, noninvasive CT scan offers a painless way to get three-dimensional images of the inside of the body. Use of the technology since it was introduced in 1980 has jumped from about 3 million scans to 70 million scans in 2007. CT technology, especially in vascular and cardiac imaging, increasingly exposes individuals to a type of radiation that has long been associated with the development of cancer. Researchers are concerned that the growing use of scanning exposes a patient to much higher doses of radiation than does a conventional x-ray. For example, one chest CT scan results in more than 100 times the radiation dose of a routine chest x-ray. CT scans provide exceptionally clear views of internal organs by combining data from multiple x-ray images. But the price for that clarity is increased exposure to x-rays, which cause mutations in DNA that can lead to cancer. When the screening is used for diagnostic purposes, the benefits outweigh the risks, most experts agree, though the toll increasingly can't be ignored.

Scanner manufacturers are designing instruments that use lower doses of radiation, but many older machines rely on higher doses. Machine settings for particular procedures are not standardized, and individual radiologists use the technology differently for different patients, leading to wide variance in doses delivered to the subjects. The recent episodes of unusually high radiation doses delivered to patients at Cedars-Sinai Medical Center in Los Angeles and Glendale Adventist Medical Center were particularly egregious examples that involved inadvertently inappropriate settings on the instruments, and such cases were not included in the new analyses.

The highest doses of radiation are routinely used for coronary angiography, in which cardiologists image the heart and its major blood vessels to look for blockages or other abnormalities.[83] Under the normal dosages of radiation for the procedure, about 1 in 270 women and 1 in 600 men who receive it at age 40 years will develop cancer as a result, reports Dr. Rebecca Smith-Bindman, a professor of radiology and epidemiology at University of California at San Francisco. Smith-Bindman and her colleagues studied the radiation doses received by 1,119 adult patients at four San Francisco Bay Area hospitals between January 1 and May 30, 2008. Taking into account the cancer mortality rate from radiation exposure, plus the age of the population undergoing such scans, the researchers estimated that the cases would result in 14,500 deaths per year. "For 20-year-old patients, the risks were approximately doubled," the researchers wrote.[84]

"This study is being taken very seriously by radiologists," Dr. Alec Megibow, a professor of radiology at New York University Langone Medical Center, said in a statement. He cautions that careless use of scanners can lead to high doses of radiation, but argues that, with proper use, "the benefits of a CT scan far outweigh the risks."

In a separate paper, epidemiologist Amy Berrington de Gonzales and her colleagues at the National Cancer Institute constructed a computer program to estimate the risks associated with CT scans. They concluded that about 29,000 future cancers could be related to CT scans performed in the United States in 2007 alone. That includes 14,000 cases resulting from scans of the abdomen and pelvis, 4,100 from chest scans, and 2,700 from heart scans. Two-thirds of the cancers would be in women, who are more vulnerable to radiation. And the younger a patient is at the time of the scan, the higher is the risk of cancer eventually developing.[85]

For women, the most frequent source of radiation exposure is the annual mammogram. Yearly mammograms have been recommended for women age 40 years and older. In November 2009, the U.S. Preventive Services Task Force recommended that women without risk factors for breast cancer wait until their 50s before going in for regular mammograms, and then only every other year; this remains controversial.[86]

Although studies have shown no increased risk of cancer among people experiencing as many as 1,000 millirems per year of background radiation, these dosage figures are for environmental radiation on the whole body. When diagnostic tests or radiation treatments are run, radiation is delivered to specific body parts and can potentially have a greater effect. Tissues that grow new cells more rapidly, such as bone marrow or the thyroid gland, are most vulnerable. In the breast, the rate of cell growth varies with the amount of estrogen. Younger women who have more estrogen are more susceptible, and postmenopausal women are less so.

Weighing the benefits and risks of diagnostic tests has always been an issue. Mammograms do reduce the risk of dying from breast cancer by about 15% for women in their 40s and 50s, the task force says. But their absolute benefit for younger women, whose risk of cancer is very low, is much smaller. Doctors would have to screen 1,904 women ages 39–49 years for a decade to prevent one death versus 1,339 women aged 50–59 years and 377 women aged 60–69 years, according to a study accompanying the recommendations in the *Annals of Internal Medicine*.[87]

Airport Scanners

Recently mandated as part of the enhanced screening for travelers from selected countries, body scanners are in use at many U.S. airports. The number is expected to skyrocket over the next few years. Currently, the Transportation Security Administration (TSA) is using two types of screening machines. The millimeter wave imaging machine uses radiofrequency energy to image the body. According to TSA, these scanners deliver 10,000 times less energy than a cell phone does. The other type of machine is a backscatter x-ray, which can render a three-dimensional image of people by scanning them for as long as 8 seconds and produce a ghostly naked image. These x-rays are very low level because they bounce radiation off the skin, not penetrating organs, and back to the machine, allowing authorities to scan for dangerous items under someone's clothes. This functionality is unlike a medical x-ray, which is a higher level of radiation penetrating the skin to see bones and other tissues. Most airport scanners deliver less radiation than a passenger is likely to receive from atmospheric radiation while airborne.

In a study in the journal *Lancet*, airline pilots and cabin crews were found to have a significant incidence of leukemia and skin and breast cancer as a result of chromosomal damage from ionizing cosmic radiation encountered during years of flying at high altitudes. The American Cancer Society stated recently that it does not antici-

pate airport scanners to be a serious issue for infrequent travelers. The topic remains controversial, and if made mandatory, passengers and airline crews could pass through airport screening checkpoints in the United States frequently, and some fliers could be scanned several times in one day. Frequent fliers could get hit hundreds of times each year. Pregnant women, infants, chronically ill and immune-suppressed persons would also be exposed.

The Inter-Agency Committee on Radiation Safety recently issued a report that is restricted to the agencies concerned and not meant for public circulation. The committee, which includes the European Commission, International Atomic Energy Agency, Nuclear Energy Agency, and the World Health Organization, recommends that air passengers be made aware of the health risks of airport body screenings and that governments must explain any decision to expose the public to higher levels of cancer-causing radiation. It also concludes that pregnant women and children should not be subjected to scanning, even though the radiation dose from body scanners is "extremely small."

Cell Phones

The number of cell phone users has increased rapidly since 2000. In 2010, there were more than 303 million subscribers to cell phone services in the United States, according to the Cellular Telecommunications and Internet Association. This is an increase from 110 million users in Globally, the number of cell phone subscriptions is estimated to be 5 billion, according to the International Telecommunication Union (ITU) and stated by ITU Secretary-General Dr. Hamadoun Toure at the Mobile World Congress in Barcelona in 2010.

Cell phones emit radiofrequency energy. Concerns have been raised that this energy from cell phones may pose a cancer risk to users. Radiofrequency energy is a form of nonionizing electromagnetic radiation; exposure depends on the technology of the phone, distance between the phone's antenna and the user, the extent and type of use, and distance of the user from base stations. Researchers are studying tumors of the brain and central nervous system and other sites of the head and neck because cell phones are typically held next to the head when used. They have focused on whether radiofrequency energy can cause malignant (cancerous) brain tumors, such as gliomas, as well as benign (non-cancerous) tumors, such as acoustic neuromas (tumors in the cells of the nerve responsible for hearing), meningiomas (tumors in the meninges, membranes that cover and protect the brain and spinal cord), and parotid gland tumors (tumors in the salivary glands). Researchers have investigated the possible role of cell phones or other sources of radiofrequency exposure and cancer risks in humans and animals. Studies have not shown a consistent link between cell phone use and cancer.[88]

The Interphone Study, a 13-country consortium of case-control studies of cell phone use and risk for malignant or benign brain tumors, is the largest study of long-term cell phone use. Published in 2010, the study found that, overall, cell phone users are at lower risk for two of the most common types of brain tumor—glioma and meningioma—compared to nonusers. Interphone researchers also found no evidence of increasing risk with progressively increasing number of calls, longer call time, or years since beginning cell phone use. The small proportion of study participants who reported spending the most total time on cell phone calls (13% of people with brain tumors and 8% of those without tumors) experienced a statistically significant, albeit modest, increase in risk of glioma. There was some indication that the association with glioma among heaviest users of cell phones was more apparent for phone use on the same side of the head as the tumor, but the authors noted that this could have been the result of reporting bias. However, if the relationship is causal, it would translate into an increase from the current age-adjusted incidence rate of brain cancer in the United States of about 6.5 cases per 100,000 people to about 9 cases per 100,000. The Interphone researchers considered this finding inconclusive because of the implausible levels of use reported by a subset of the heaviest users. Interphone was coordinated by the International Agency for Research on Cancer (IARC) and included European brain cancer patients and 646 control subjects between the ages of 7 and 19 years. Children with brain tumors were

not more likely to have been regular cell phone users than control subjects.

Devra Davis, president of the Environmental Health Trust, in reviewing these findings, questions the accuracy of the report:

> This report represents an astonishing, disturbing and unwarranted conclusion. Of course, the researchers found no link between children's brain tumors and their reported cell phone use. Brain tumors can take ten years to form and young children certainly have not been heavy cellphone users for very long. There has been a quadrupling of cell phone use in the past few years that this study could not possibly capture.[89]

She does note, however, the inconsistency as the researchers advocate implementing simple precautions including the use of a headset and speakerphone when using a cell phone. Further research is needed to investigate possible health effects in children and persons who have used cell phones heavily for many years.[89]

Electromagnetic Fields

Every year, more research is published about the hazards of electromagnetic pollution, and more evidence is collected and large epidemiologic studies are conducted. The conclusion is that electromagnetic fields (EMF) can adversely affect health, and it is important to reduce exposure to electromagnetic radiation whenever possible.

An important formula for EMF protection, and often the easiest to apply, is to know how much to increase distance from the source depending on the type of EMF hazard. For example, to halve the field intensity, a person might have to move farther away from the source of the EMF by the following distances:

25 meters (27 yards) for power lines and cell towers

30 centimeters (15 inches) for CRT computer monitors

5 centimeters (2 inches) for electric clocks

2.5 centimeters (1 inch) minimum for cell phones

To calculate exposures and risks, see www.ans.org/pi/resources/dosechart.

The following is a list of ideas on how people can protect themselves from radiation exposure:

- Maintain and review a personal history of diagnostic x-ray exposures to calculate risk and make informed choices moving forward:
  - Request minimal amount of x-ray during any treatment and ask for a lead shield for susceptible body parts not being scanned when possible.
  - Avoid CT scans if x-rays, magnetic resonance imaging (MRI), or other diagnostic procedures are available.
- Avoid microwaved foods (and do not stand in front of the microwave while it is on; do not use plastic in the microwave).
- Keep a distance from big-screen TVs.
- Request a patdown at the airport instead of scan if you are a frequent flyer.
- Take action and make your concerns known. TSA's consumer e-mail address is TSAContactCenter@dhs.gov.
- Do a radiation assessment and calculate your annual dose and risk.

■ SMOKING

Everyone, including the at-risk population of nonsmokers, is aware of the health hazards related to smoking tobacco products. Worldwide, though, it seems that women are the group most at risk. Smoking prevalence is lower among women than men in most countries, yet there are about 200 million women in the world who smoke, and in addition, there are millions more who chew tobacco. Approximately 22% of women in developed countries and 9% of women in developing countries smoke. Unless effective, comprehensive, and sustained initiatives are implemented to reduce smoking uptake among young women and increase cessation rates among women, the prevalence of female smoking in developed and developing countries is likely to rise.

Even if prevalence levels do not rise, the number of women who smoke will increase because the population of women in the world is predicted to rise. Thus, whereas the epidemic of tobacco use among men is in slow decline, the epidemic among women will not reach its peak until well into the 21st century. This will have enormous consequences not only for women's health and economic well-being, but also for that of their families. The health effects of smoking for women are more serious than for men. In addition to the general health problems common to both genders, women face additional hazards in pregnancy, female-specific cancers such as cancer of the cervix, and exposure to passive smoking.

In Asia, although there are currently lower levels of tobacco use among women, smoking among girls is already on the rise in some areas. The spending power of girls and women is increasing so that cigarettes are becoming more affordable. The social and cultural constraints that previously prevented many women from smoking are weakening, and women-specific health education and quitting programs are rare. Furthermore, evidence suggests that women find it harder to quit smoking. The tobacco companies are targeting women by marketing light, mild, and menthol cigarettes and introducing advertising directed at women. The greatest challenge and opportunity in primary preventive health care in Asia and in other developing areas is to avert the predicted rise in smoking among women.[90]

Breathing secondhand smoke (SHS) causes heart disease and lung cancer in adults and increased risks for sudden infant death syndrome, acute respiratory infections, middle ear disease, worsened asthma, respiratory symptoms, and slowed lung growth in children. No risk-free level of exposure to SHS exists. The Global Youth Tobacco Survey (GYTS), initiated in 1999 by the World Health Organization (WHO), the Canadian Public Health Association, and CDC, includes questions related to tobacco use, including exposure to SHS. This report examines data collected from 137 jurisdictions (i.e., countries and territories) during 2000–2007, presents estimates of exposure to SHS at home and in places other than the home among students aged 13–15 years who had never smoked, and examines the association between exposure to SHS and susceptibility to initiating smoking. GYTS data indicate that nearly half of never smokers were exposed to SHS at home (46.8%), and a similar percentage was exposed in places other than the home (47.8%). Never smokers exposed to SHS at home were 1.4–2.1 times more likely to be susceptible to initiating smoking than those not exposed. Students exposed to SHS in places other than the home were 1.3–1.8 times more likely to be susceptible to initiating smoking than those not exposed. As part of their comprehensive tobacco control programs, countries and companies should take measures to create smoke-free environments in all indoor public places and workplaces.[91]

■ DETOXIFICATION

Internal biochemical processes combined with man-made chemicals can overwhelm the body's detoxification pathways and accumulate and get stored in tissues, particularly body fat. The good news is that research in the fields of human genomics, nutrition, and lifestyle choices provides new and intriguing information about how to minimize exposures and prevent toxins from wreaking havoc on immune systems and overall health.

The body has efficient mechanisms in place to detoxify harmful toxins including the lymphatic system and the most important cleansing organ, the liver. Other eliminative channels are the bowels, kidneys, skin, and lungs. When the body is doing its job and is not overburdened, the blood carries toxins to the liver, which uses enzymes, amino acids, and phytonutrients to detoxify and neutralize harmful substances, rendering them harmless by converting them into a water-soluble form to be eliminated via the urine or feces.

Carrying a large toxic body burden can stress the ability of this system, built for natural toxins and biochemical by-products, not the man-made ones people have to deal with in these modern times. If detoxification pathways in the liver are impaired, the breakdown of toxins can form intermediary metabolites that are often more toxic than the original item.

Optimizing the body's ability to detoxify, it is essential for individuals to maintain good elimination patterns, consume a whole-food diet, avoid chemicals in the food chain, and receive fresh air, natural sunlight, and exercise to support vitality and health. As a hardy and resilient species, changes we make in our lifestyles today can affect our long-term health.

■ HOLISTIC CARING PROCESS

Holistic Assessment

In preparing to exercise environmental control, the nurse assesses the following parameters as they apply to the client:

- Personal space for comfort, lighting, noise, ventilation, and privacy
- Other people or troublesome objects that may induce anxiety
- Awareness that environmental concerns affect individual and family coping skills
- Awareness of objects or other environmental factors in the physical space that induce comfort or discomfort
- Environmental concerns about impact on health as well as the family's environmental concerns
- Possible environmental fears (e.g., a feeling of claustrophobia from being confined to a hospital intensive care bed or intravenous lines, or a fear of death because the patient in the next bed just died)
- Grief and its relationship to environmental factors: Is the client in the same home atmosphere in which the spouse just died? Are others around the client sad and depressed? Are the colors in the environment dark and heavy?
- Personal health maintenance in relation to environmental factors: Can the client easily reach self-care hygiene items? Are throw rugs anchored? Are sunglasses worn outside to prevent glare?
- Ability to maintain and manage his or her own home
- Risk of injury associated with factors in the environment
- Activity deficits as a result of environmental factors
- Home environment for its potential impact on effective parenting
- Potential noncompliance because of environmental factors
- Risk of impairment in physical activity because of environmental factors
- Risk of impairment in respiratory function because of environmental factors, such as feather pillows, polluted or stale air, cigarette smoking, known or suspected

allergens, or overexertion with chronic respiratory conditions

- Possible sleep deficit because of agents in the environment, such as lighting, noise, overstimulation, overcrowding, or allergenic pillows
- Alterations in thought processes that may be influenced by environmental factors, such as sensory bombardment with noise, lack of sleep, and transient living patterns

Identification of Patterns/ Challenges/Needs

The following patterns/challenges/needs (see Chapter 7) are compatible with environmental interventions:

- Potential for ineffective choices
- Altered self-care

- Altered growth and development
- Potential for sensory perceptual alteration
- Impaired environmental interpretational syndrome
- Potential for knowledge deficit
- Altered comfort
- Altered role performance

Outcome Identification

Table 29-3 guides the nurse in client outcomes, nursing prescriptions, and evaluation for the use of the environment as a nursing intervention.

Therapeutic Care Plan and Interventions

Before the session:

- Become aware of personal thoughts, behaviors, and actions that may contribute to the coaching, teaching, counseling, or caring environment.

TABLE 29-3   Nursing Interventions: Environment

Client Outcomes	Nursing Prescriptions	Evaluation
The client will demonstrate awareness of environment.	Assist the client in shaping his or her own personal space environment.	The client personalized his or her own environment.
	Assist the client with choices that contribute to a positive, safe environment for those who share his or her personal and community space.	The client monitored and controlled the noise that he or she contributed to the surrounding area.
	Coach the client on creative strategies and action steps for optimizing his or her personal healing environment.	The client respected the rights of others by not polluting air, water, and public places with wastes.
		The client did not violate the personal space of others with tobacco smoke.
	Provide the client with information that helps in expanding concern for the concept of a healthy global environment.	The client participated in discussions, committees, or programs to work for a safe global environment.
The client will avoid contact and exposure to toxic substances and/or hazardous materials.	Give the client ideas for how to participate in safety education programs at his or her place of employment.	The client participated in his or her workplace offerings of environmental safety programs.
	Teach the client the importance of not unnecessarily handling toxic substances.	The client did not handle unnecessary toxic substances and educated himself or herself about the dangers of hazardous materials.

- Prepare the physical environment for optimal lighting, seating, air quality, and noise control.
- Consider your internal environment. Is it calm, centered, and ready to interact with others?
- Clear your mind to be fully present when meeting with the client.

Beginning the session:

- Take a moment to center with the client.
- Allow the client to express specific environmental concerns.
- Offer the client an environmental assessment tool. See pp. 175–176.
- Review the assessment with the client to discover areas of concern.
- Explore how the personal environment may affect well-being (positively or negatively).
- Encourage the client to write down areas of concern or areas for improvement.

During the session:

- Encourage the client to initiate specific intervention ideas in his or her personal or professional work environment.
- Explore workplace issues and possibilities for affecting change, serving on the environmental control committee, or initiating meetings with coworkers to form a committee to improve the workplace environment, including creating a healing room for staff.
- Guide the client to consider changes that would improve his or her personal and/or work environment.
- Increase awareness of sound (e.g., noise, music, machinery), air (e.g., quality, smell, circulation), and aesthetics (e.g., art, color, design, texture), as well as other areas specific to the client's overall environment.
- Educate hospitalized clients about the deleterious effects on their healing process of too much noise.
- Encourage hospitalized clients to limit the time spent watching television and instead listen to their own personal cassette players with headphones.
- Create mechanisms whereby music, imagery, relaxation, colors, aromas, and lighting can be introduced into workplace settings.

At the end of the session:

- Coach clients to learn practical ways to cope with hazards in the environment (**Table 29-4**).
- Coach the client to write down environmental goals, action steps, and target dates.
- Provide handout materials to support established goals.
- Schedule follow-up sessions.

Specific Interventions

Personal Environment

Strategies to heal the environment abound on both a personal and a professional level. Personally, we can begin to modify our own internal environment. The ability to regulate our state of consciousness, thought patterns, and reactive behaviors gives us the power to move smoothly through external crises both at work and at leisure. Approaching a hectic external environment with internal composure and tranquility makes it possible to transform crises into manageable situations. Nurturing our internal environment with food, quality sleep, supportive relationships, and joy can influence all the external environments in which we work and live.

As we develop the optimal workplaces and living areas to foster self-actualizing conditions and maximize body–mind responses, we must continue to stay aware and informed of the impact of all aspects of the environment on human health. Many nurses find that the following exercise increases their sensitivity to the environment and its impact on their lives:

- At different times during the day, close your eyes, and take a few moments to listen carefully to all the sounds in your environment.
- Jot down the many different sounds you hear, noting which are pleasant and which are distracting or disturbing noises.
- Become aware of all the sounds that you ordinarily hear, such as the air conditioner, radios and televisions, the hum of fluorescent lights, the beeping and buzzing of hospital machinery, or the background music that some institutions play over the speaker system.
- Notice new smells, feelings of temperature, and so forth. There will be many sounds, smells, and sensations of which you may not previously have been aware.

TABLE 29-4   Coping with Environmental Hazards

Problem	Solution
Too much noise	1. Turn off radios and televisions.
	2. Lower your voice.
	3. Ask your colleagues to quiet down.
	4. Ask to serve on the agency's environmental control committee.
Inadequate lighting	1. Add more lights.
	2. Use incandescent bulbs instead of fluorescent tubes whenever possible.
	3. Open curtains and blinds whenever possible.
	4. Go outdoors for full-spectrum light breaks, rather than taking cafeteria coffee breaks.
Stale air	1. Make sure agency ventilation systems work.
	2. When doing home health visits, open the doors and windows and get fresh air and natural light in the home when appropriate.
	3. Request that broad-leaf green plants be stationed in the workplace. They are aesthetically pleasing and give off oxygen.
	4. Wear masks or protective gear if there is any risk of toxic inhalants.
Long periods at computer	1. Use a shield that cuts down glare and radiation and grounds the field of electrostatic charge.
	2. Learn some relaxation exercises to do at your desk.
	3. Ask your institution or agency to have short massage sessions available on the premises.
	4. Take frequent eye and movement breaks away from the computer screen.
	5. Use properly designed chairs.
Space allocation	1. Try to find some personal space in the workplace.
	2. Respect others' personal space. Ask before entering the client's room, closet, or dresser.
	3. Make the space you are allocated as pleasant as possible. Decorate with colorful objects, soothing scents, and aesthetic objects.

Noise seems to be a major area of environmental concern that nurses can control. It is the accumulation of noises that adds up the decibels and can cause stress. By becoming increasingly sensitive to all potential environmental stressors, the nurse becomes more attuned to coaching opportunities and for offering specific interventions.

Some specific recommendations to reduce workplace noise are as follows:

- Developing staff education programs about noises, their source, and ways to quiet them

- Setting telephones and alarms to low volumes, or replacing sound devices with flashing lights
- Installing buffers in open space areas to minimize impact noise
- Closing the patients' doors whenever feasible
- Using bedside chairs with wheels in patient rooms with hard floors
- Choosing quieter equipment
- Placing computer printers away from patient rooms and/or installing soundproof covers

- Giving patients headphones to listen to television or radio so that they do not disturb others
- Speaking in a softer voice

Planetary Consciousness

Schuster suggests there is an impetus and underlying reason for our developing environmental consciousness. She notes that we are all hoping to foster and sustain our fullest conscious participation in the ongoing web of interrelationships.[92] Two points emerge as most salient within the context of nursing in general and holistic practice in particular:

1. It is important to address the nature of being human and, in our Western mode, the pervasive influence of the self–other dichotomy.
2. We must be aware that we have viable choices of how we want to be and how we represent ourselves in the world.

An integration of items 1 and 2 develops a personal orientation to all environmental concerns. With such an orientation, we can act from internal conviction and relatedness, rather than from institutional directives.

The most enduring and far-reaching environmental work originates with individuals as consumers and practitioners, not with organizations, however enlightened they may be.[93] Thus, it is up to each of us to develop an environmental sensitivity in our daily lives and become increasingly cognizant of our opportunities to institute positive change.

CASE STUDY (IMPLEMENTATION)

Setting: Outpatient clinic, or private visit

Client: A. B., a 55-year-old married man

Patterns/Challenges/Needs:

1. Altered comfort related to recurrent headaches
2. Ineffective individual coping related to environmental stress

A. B. visited the occupational health nurse because of recurrent headaches and chronic fatigue.

A physical examination and laboratory tests revealed no pathology or disease, but his subjective declaration of feeling stress in the workplace warranted a closer examination of his workplace environment. A detailed history of his work hours, commuting travel, and work setting yielded evidence of environmental imbalance.

A. B. began his day with a 45-minute automobile commute through a suburban area to the inner city; he finished the day the same way. He had made this commute for years, but the traffic had lately increased and road repairs frequently slowed his pace. When he arrived at work, he went to his office, an interior room with no windows and fluorescent ceiling lights. The office walls were the standard institutional beige color; A. B. had done nothing to decorate or personalize his office. Instead of a secretary outside his office, he now had his own computer inside his office. During the company's modernization process, middle managers had been taught computer skills, and many secretarial positions had been eliminated. Each manager was now responsible for developing reports and interacting with others via personal computer terminals.

A. B.'s work routine had little variation. It consisted of meetings, telephone work, and online computer time. He kept an air freshener in his office to mask the smell of the floor cleaners that were used daily. He rarely took lunch hour and kept a large bowl of multicolored jelly beans on his desk to fuel him throughout the day.

This information suggested that A. B. was experiencing environment-related stress, and the nurse worked with him to develop a seven-step plan of action:

1. Vary the commuting time. Begin the commute 15 minutes earlier to decrease the rushed feeling of getting to work on time. Join a health club in the city, and stay after work to exercise. The traffic would be considerably less 1 hour later, and the commute would then take only 30 minutes. Total morning and evening commute time would remain the same as before, but more would have been accomplished with less environmental stress.
2. Implement and practice computer protection skills (see Table 29-4).

3. Use a cordless earphone to prevent neck strain after long periods on the telephone. Use a headset on his wireless phone.
4. Personalize the office with soft, soothing colors. Add a wall picture of a mountain valley and stream that have personal significance.
5. Put an incandescent lamp on the desk, and use that rather than the overhead fluorescent lights for desk work.
6. Schedule regular lunch hour time. Replace jelly beans with healthier snacks.
7. Begin using natural aromatherapy in his office to relax him and add fragrance.

A copy of this plan was posted in a prominent place in A. B.'s home. Along with a plan for exercise and weight management (see Chapters 13 and 14) and a plan for the development of relaxation and imagery skills (see Chapters 16 and 17), this program incorporated A. B.'s need for motivation, lifestyle change, and values clarification.

When A. B. returned for his follow-up visit 2 months later, his headaches had abated, and he had made some progress toward his weight loss goals. He and his wife had redecorated his office, and on his own he had added a small cassette player to play his favorite classical music. He was bringing a healthy lunch to work and had replaced the jelly beans with a mix of nuts and dried fruit.

Six months later, A. B. was free of headaches. He had spearheaded a no-smoking policy for his workplace and asked the company director to install full-spectrum lights on all ceiling overhead panels. He also requested that nonfragrant and more "natural" cleaners be brought onto the unit. He felt he had regained some sense of control over his environment and was working on improvement in the other areas for which he and the nurse had developed plans.

Evaluation

How do we evaluate, for example, what may have triggered A. B.'s headaches? And what alleviated them? Could it have been a combination of factors or one specific action taken? Could his feeling empowered and supported in making changes contribute to his overall feeling of well-being and alleviation of his headache symptoms?

Trusting the client's inner wisdom, the nurse as coach can explore the chosen interventions

and document changes and listen to the client's beliefs to guide future actions. For example, the nurse could ask A. B. to keep a journal to record any health changes or headache recurrence that he can relate to his environment and any alteration in the environment, including foods, stress, exercise, sleep, and any other areas that might trigger this pattern.

Each environmental intervention should be measured. The nurse can evaluate with the client the outcomes established before the implementation of any interventions (see Table 29-3). To evaluate the results further, the nurse can explore the subjective effects of the experience with the client, based on the evaluation questions in **Exhibit 29-2**. Last year's methods of handling laboratory specimens and chemotherapy preparations, for example, may be outdated next year. Nurses keep abreast of the changing face of the environment to equip themselves with the newest strategies to counteract hazards. Future nurses would be well advised to remember and recall some of the basic nursing tenets of yesteryear that are still most relevant today. These interventions include fresh air, a comfortable climate, calming colors, and noise reduction.

Much of how we relate to and what we do about environmental issues is based on the development of our personal philosophy. We continue to become increasingly aware that each of the small things that we do for or against the environment has short- and long-term ramifications. Nurses want to be alert for ways to contribute to positive environmental changes for their own lives, their clients' lives, and the overall health of the planet. Environmental concerns are important to all of us, and one person's actions can have a ripple effect on many other lives. Nurses can be key agents to ensure that the environment is held sacred, supported, and tended as it supports and gives life to all of the Earth's people.

As Larry Dossey states, "The hour is late and the task is great. Think globally, act nonlocally." What we do to the world, we do to ourselves.[94] Full realization of this fact can lead to a reformulation of the Golden Rule—from "Do unto others as you would have them do unto you" to "Do good unto others because in some sense they are you." The extraordinary healing power of ordinary things is immense.[95]

EXHIBIT 29-2   Evaluating the Client's Subjective Experience with Environmental Concerns

1. Were you aware that noise, lighting, air quality, space allocation, and workplace toxins could be chronic stressors?

2. Are there any of these potential stressors in your environment? If so, can you do anything to reduce or remove them?

3. Do you realize that you can contribute to a healthier planet by virtue of changing elements in your own personal space?

4. Do you have an environmental sensitivity group at your workplace? If one existed, would you like to be a part of it?

5. Do you feel empowered to be the person who initiates change in your work setting?

6. What are some specific things that you would like to do to create a healthier environment in your personal space or work setting?

7. What is your next step (or your plan) to integrate these changes in your life?

Directions for
FUTURE RESEARCH

1. Evaluate the perception of quality of rest by subjects with different types of auditory stimulation.

2. Study the relationship between environmental hazards (e.g., artificial lighting, working on video display terminals, unventilated air, shift work, high noise levels) and the rise in infertility, miscarriages, and neonate abnormalities.

3. Using an environmental assessment tool, research the health of nurses, their work environments, and health risks associated with endocrine disruptors and women's health.

4. Investigate the use of tactile, auditory, or olfactory stimuli on wound healing, rate of complications, length of recovery, and other health-related factors.

5. Study the effect of the environment on the reduction of stress and anxiety in ambulatory clients.

Nurse Healer
REFLECTIONS

After reading this chapter, the nurse healer will be able to answer or to begin a process of answering the following questions:

- How does the environment affect my job satisfaction?

- How does my work environment affect my health?

- What are the environmental stressors at work and at home?

- What strategies can I incorporate in my environment to be healthier?

- What things can I do to improve my own personal and workplace environment?

- How can I be involved with environmental issues at work and in my community?

> *For a full suite of assignments and additional learning activities, use the access code located in the front of your book to visit this exclusive website: http://go.jblearning.com/dossey. If you do not have an access code, you can obtain one at the site.*

NOTES

1. R. Tarnas, "The Great Initiation," *Noetic Sciences Review*, no. 47 (1998): 24–31, 57–59.

2. B. M. Dossey et al., *Florence Nightingale Today: Healing, Leadership, Global Action* (Washington, DC: NurseBooks.org, 2005).

3. Florence Nightingale, *Notes on Nursing: What It Is, and What It Is Not* (London, England: Harrison and Sons, 1860): 70.

4. H. Frumkin, ed., *Environmental Health: From Global to Local*, 2nd ed. (San Francisco, CA: John Wiley, 2010).

5. B. M. Dossey et al., *Florence Nightingale Today: Healing, Leadership, Global Action* (Washington, DC: NurseBooks.org, 2005).

6. R. Morello-Frosch, "Integrating Environmental Justice and the Precautionary Principle in Research and Policy Making: The Case of Ambient Air Toxics Exposures and Health Risks Among Schoolchildren in Los Angeles," *Annals of the American Academy of Political and Social Science*, 584, no. 1 (November 2002): 47–68.

7. Agency for Toxic Substances and Disease Registry "Toxicological Profile for DDT, DDE, and DDD" (September 2002). http://www.atsdr.cdc.gov/toxprofiles/tp.asp?id=81&tid=20.

8. "Occupational Exposures to Air Contaminants at the World Trade Center Disaster Site—New York, September–October, 2001," *Morbidity and Mortality Weekly Report* 51, no. 21 (May 31, 2002): 453–456.

9. K. Olszewski, C. Parks, and N. E. Chikotas, "Occupational Safety and Health Objectives of *Healthy People 2010*: A Systematic Approach for Occupational Health Nurses, Part II," *American Association of Occupational Health Nurses Journal* 5, no. 3 (2007): 115–125._

10. D. C. Luccio-Camelo and G. S. Prins, "Disruption of Androgen Receptor Signaling in Males by Environmental Chemicals," *Journal of Steroid Biochemistry and Molecular Biology* 127, nos. 1–2 (April 13, 2011): 74–82.

11. O. A. H. Jones, M. L. Maguire, and J. L. Griffin, "Environmental Pollution and Diabetes: A Neglected Association," *Lancet* 371, no. 9609 (January 26, 2008): 287–288.

12. Department of Health and Human Services, Centers for Disease Control and Prevention, *Fourth National Report on Human Exposure to Environmental Chemicals 2009* (Atlanta, GA: CDC, 2009).

13. M. E. Northridge et al., "Environmental Equity and Health: Understanding Complexity and Moving Forward," *American Journal of Public Health* 93, no. 2 (February 2003): 209–214.

14. *Fourth National Report on Human Exposure to Environmental Chemicals 2009*. Centers for Disease Control and Prevention 1600 Clifton Rd. Atlanta, GA 30333, USA

15. L. Beane Freeman, A. Blair, and J. H. Lubin et al., Mortality from lymphohematopoietic malignancies among workers in formaldehyde industries: The National Cancer Institute Cohort, *Journal of the National Cancer Institute* 101, no. 10 (2009): 751–761.

16. M. F. Bouchard et al., "Prenatal Exposure to Organophosphate Pesticides and IQ in 7-Year-Old Children," *Environmental Health Perspectives* 119, no. 8 (August 2011).

17. G.-E. Séralini et al., "How Subchronic and Chronic Health Effects Can Be Neglected for GMOs, Pesticides or Chemicals," *International Journal of Biological Sciences* 5, no. 5 (2005): 438–443.

18. F. Vinson, M. Merhi, I. Baldi, H. Raynal, and L. Gamet-Payrastre, "Exposure to Pesticides and Risk of Childhood Cancer: A Meta-Analysis of Recent Epidemiological Studies," *Occupational and Environmental Medicine* (May 23, 2011).

19. G. Van Maele-Fabry, A. C. Lantin, P. Hoet, and D. Lison, "Review. Residential Exposure to Pesticides and Childhood Leukaemia: A Systematic Review and Meta-Analysis," *Environment International* 37, no. 1 (January 2011): 280–291.

20. G. Van Maele-Fabry, A. C. Lantin, P. Hoet, and D. Lison, "Childhood Leukemia and Parental Occupational Exposure to Pesticides: A Systematic Review and Meta-Analysis," *Cancer Causes and Control* 21, no. 6 (June 2010): 787–809.

21. D. T. Wigle, M. C. Turner, and D. Krewski, "A systematic review and meta-analysis of childhood leukemia and parental occupational pesticide exposure," *Environmental Health Perspectives* 117, no. 10 (2009): 1505–1513.

22. A. L. Hernández-Morales, A. Zonana-Nacach, and V. M. Zaragoza-Sandoval, "Associated Risk Factors in Acute Leukemia in Children. A Cases and Controls Study," *Revista Medica del Instituto Mexicano del Seguro Social* 47, no. 5 (September–October 2009): 497–503. (Spanish)

23. Environmental Working Group, "Body Burden—the Pollution in Newborns: A Benchmark Investigation of Industrial Chemicals, Pollutants and Pesticides in Umbilical Cord Blood" (July 14, 2005). http://www.ewg.org/reports/bodyburden2/execsumm.php.

24. W. J. Rogan and N. B. Ragan, "Evidence of Effects of Environmental Chemicals on the Endocrine System in Children," *Pediatrics* 112, no. 1 Pt. 2 (July 2003): 247–252.

25. D. A. Crain and S. J. Janssen, "Female Reproductive Disorders: The Roles of Endocrine Disrupting Compounds and Developmental Timing," *Fertility and Sterility* 90 (2008): 911–940.

26. R. R. Newbold and E. Padilla-Banks, "Adverse Effects of the Model Environmental Estrogen Diethylstibesterol Are Transmitted to Subsequent Generations," *Endocrinology* 147, no. 6 (2006): S11–S17.

27. J. G. Brody, R. A. Rudel, and M. Kavanaugh-Lynch, "Testing Chemicals for Effects on Breast Development, Lactation, and Cancer," *Environmental Health Perspectives* 119 (August 2011): a326–a327.

28. Endocrine Society, *Endocrine-Disrupting Chemicals* (Chevy Chase, MD: Endocrine Society, 2009). http://www.endo-society.org/journals/scientific-statements/upload/edc_scientific_statement.pdf.

29. J. C. O'Connor and R. E. Chapin, "Critical Evaluation of Observed Adverse Effects of Endocrine

Active Substances on Reproduction and Development, the Immune System, and the Nervous System," *Pure and Applied Chemistry* 75, nos. 11–12 (February 28, 2007): 2099–2123.

30. K. Kelland, "Experts Demand European Action on Plastics Chemical," Reuters (June 22, 2010). http://www.reuters.com/article/2010/06/22/us-chemical-bpa-health-idUSTRE65L6JN20100622.

31. U.S. Food and Drug Administration, "Update on Bisphenol A for Use in Food Contact Applications: January 2010" (January 15, 2010). http://www.fda.gov/newsevents/publichealthfocus/ucm197739.htm.

32. K. W. Lozada and R. A. Keri, "Bisphenol A Increases Mammary Cancer Risk in Two Distinct Mouse Models of Breast Cancer," *Biology of Reproduction Papers* (June 2, 2011). doi:10.1095/biolreprod.110.090431

33. B. E. Hamilton and S. J. Ventura, "Fertility and Abortion Rates in the United States, 1960–2002," *International Journal of Andrology* 29 (2006): 34–35.

34. D. C. Luccio-Camelo and G. S. Prins, "Disruption of Androgen Receptor Signaling in Males by Environmental Chemicals," *Journal of Steroid Biochemistry and Molecular Biology* (April 13, 2011).

35. S. Steingraber, *The Falling Age of Puberty in U.S. Girls: What We Know, What We Need to Know* (San Francisco, CA: Breast Cancer Fund, 2007). http://www.breastcancerfund.org/assets/pdfs/publications/falling-age-of-puberty.pdf.

36. J. R. Chakraborty and T. R. Chakraborty, "Estrogen-like Endocrine Disrupting Chemicals Affecting Puberty in Humans—a Review," *Environmental Science and Technology* 43, no. 9 (May 1, 2009): 2993.

37. F. Fack et al., "Effects of the Endocrine Disruptors Atrazine and PCB 153 on the Protein Expression of MCF-7 Human Cells," *Journal of Proteome Research* 8, no. 12 (December 2009): 5485–5496.

38. B. Weiss, "Endocrine Disruptors as a Threat to Neurological Function," *Journal of Neurological Science* 305, nos. 1–2 (June 15, 2011): 11–21.

39. B. M. Kuehn, "Increased Risk of ADHD Associated with Early Exposure to Pesticides, PCBs," *Journal of the American Medical Association* 304, no. 1 (July 7, 2010): 27–28.

40. M. F. Bouchard, D. C. Bellinger, R. O. Wright, and M. G. Weisskopf, "Attention-Deficit/Hyperactivity Disorder and Urinary Metabolites of Organophosphate Pesticides," *Pediatrics* 125, no. 6 (June 2010): e1270–e1277.

41. C. A. Riccio, L. Avila, and M. J. Ash, "Pesticide Poisoning in a Preschool Child: A Case Study Examining Neurocognitive and Neurobehavioral Effects," *Applied Neuropsychology* 17, no. 2 (April 2010): 153–159.

42. S. K. Sagiv et al., "Prenatal Organochlorine Exposure and Behaviors Associated with Attention Deficit Hyperactivity Disorder in School-Aged Children," *American Journal of Epidemiology* 171, no. 5 (March 2010): 593–601.

43. G. Panzica et al., "Effects of Xenoestrogens on the Differentiation of Behaviorally-Relevant Neural Circuits," *Frontiers in Neuroendocrinology* 28, no. 4 (2007): 179–200.

44. Willer, Helga and Kilcher, Lukas (Eds.), *The World of Organic Agriculture-Statistics and Emerging Trends 2011*. (Bonn: Research Institute of Organic Agriculture in cooperation with the International Federation of Organic Agriculture Movements (IFOAM), 2011).

45. A. M. Soto and C. Sonnenschein, "Environmental Causes of Cancer: Endocrine Disruptors as Carcinogens," *Nature Reviews Endocrinology* 6, no. 7 (2010): 363–370.

46. A. Soto, L. Vandenberg, M. Maffini, and C. Sonnenschein, "Does Breast Cancer Start in the Womb?" *Basic and Clinical Pharmacology and Toxicology* 102, no. 2 (2008): 125–133.

47. World Cancer Research Fund and American Institute for Cancer Research, *Second Expert Report: Food, Nutrition, Physical Activity, and the Prevention of Cancer: A Global Perspective* (London, England: World Cancer Research Fund, 2007).

48. B. Sung, S. Prasad, V. R. Yadav, A. Lavasanifar, and B. B. Aggarwal, "Cancer and Diet: How Are They Related?" *Free Radical Research* 45, no. 8 (August 2011): 864–879.

49. U.S. Government Accountability Office, *Safe Drinking Water Act: Improvements in Implementation Are Needed to Better Assure the Public of Safe Drinking Water*, GAO-11-803T (Washington, DC: U.S. GAO, July 12, 2011). http://www.gao.gov/new.items/d11803t.pdf.

50. Environmental Protection Agency, *Drinking Water Strategy Fact Sheet*, EPA 815-F-10-001 (Washington, DC: EPA, March 2010).

51. Centers for Disease Control and Prevention, National Center for Health Statistics, "National Health Interview Survey Raw Data, 2009" (analysis by the American Lung Association Research and Program Services Division Asthma Statistics CDC, May 3, 2011).

52. L. McKelvey, "Background on National Emission Standards for Industrial, Commercial, and Institutional Boiler and Process Heaters; and Commercial/Industrial Sold Waste Incineration (CISWI) Units" (webinar, June 2010). http://www.epa.gov/ttn/atw/129/ciwi/20100609combustion.pdf.

53. A. Gore, *Earth in Balance: Ecology and the Human Spirit* (New York, NY: Plume, 1992).

54. A. Gore, *An Inconvenient Truth* (New York, NY: Rodale Press, 2006).

55. A. Gore, *The Assault on Reason* (New York, NY: Penguin Group, 2007).

56. J. Ludwig, L. Sanbonmatsu, L. Gennetian. E. Adam, G. J. Duncan, L. F. Katz, et al., "Neighborhoods, Obesity, and Diabetes—A Randomized Social Experiment," *New England Journal of Medicine,* 365, no. 16 (2011):1509–1519.

57. J. Litt, "New Research Reveals Emotional and Physical Health Benefits of Community Gardening," *University of Colorado School of Public Health* (June 28, 2011).

58. S. Kaplan, P. Orris, and R. Machi, *A Research Agenda for Advancing Patient, Worker and Environmental Health and Safety in the Health Care Sector* (Chicago: Health Care Research Collaborative, October 2009).

59. D. Orr, *Transformation or Irrelevance: The Challenge of Academic Planning for Environmental Education in the 21st Century* (address to the North American Association for Environmental Education, Florida Gulf Coast University, March 4–8, 1998).

60. *The President's Council on Sustainable Development, Sustainable America: A New Consensus for Prosperity, Opportunity and a Healthy Environment* (Washington, DC: U.S. Government Printing Office, 1996), iv.

61. G. H. Kats, *Green Building Costs and Financial Benefits* (Boston: Massachusetts Technology Collaborative, 2003). http://www.sfenvironment.org /downloads/library/costs__financial_benefits_of_ green_building.pdf.

62. S. Cowan, "A Design Revolution," *Yes! A Journal of Positive Future,* Summer, no. 6 (1998): 27–30.

63. R. Lindquist et al., "Regional Use of Complementary and Alternative Therapies by Critical Care Nurses," *Critical Care Nurse* 25, no. 2 (2005): 63–64, 66–68, 70–72.

64. R. Lindquist, M. F. Tracy, and K. Savik, "Personal Use of Complementary and Alternative Therapies by Critical Care Nurses," *Critical Care Nursing Clinics of North America* 15, no. 3 (2003): 393–399.

65. N. C. Molter, "Creating a Healing Environment for Critical Care," *Critical Care Nursing Clinics of North America* 15, no. 3 (2003): 295–304.

66. L. Thornton, "The Model of Whole-Person Caring: Creating and Sustaining a Healing Environment," *Holistic Nursing Practice* 19, no. 3 (2005): 106–115.

67. M. Shirey, "Authentic Leaders Creating Healthy Work Environments for Nursing Practice," *American Journal of Critical Care* 15, no. 3 (2006): 256–267.

68. K. Firth, K. Smith, and K. Gourdin, "The Nature and Prevalence of Healing and Wellness Initiatives in American Hospitals," *Wellness Management* Fall (2010).

69. S. Ananth, "Optimal Healing Environments: Creating Healing Organizations," *Explore* 5, no. 1 (2009): 59–60.

70. Co-op America Quarterly, #64, Fall 2004. 1612 K Street, #600, Washington, DC, 20006.

71. Worldwatch Institute, 1776 Massachusetts Avenue, N.W., Washington, DC, 20036. http//:www .worldwatch.org.

72. *Yes! A Journal of Positive Futures*, P.O. Box 10818, Bainbridge Island, WA, 98110.

73. B. H. Morris, L. M. Bylsma, and J. Rottenberg, "Does Emotion Predict the Course of Major Depressive Disorder? A Review of Prospective Studies," *British Journal of Clinical Psychology* 48, Pt. 3 (September 2009): 255.

74. W. Passchier-Vermeer and W. F. Passchier, "Noise Exposure and Public Health," *Environmental Health Perspectives* 108, Suppl. 1 (2000): 123–131.

75. W. Babisch, "Guest Editorial: Noise and Health," *Environmental Health Perspectives* 113 (2005): A14–A15.

76. M. Spreng, "Possible Health Effects of Noise-Induced Cortisol Increase," *Noise and Health* 2, no. 7 (2000): 59–64.

77. A. White and M. Burgess, "Strategies for Reduction of Noise Levels in ICUs," *Australian Journal of Advanced Nursing* 10, no. 2 (1992–1993): 22–26.

78. W. Babisch, "Transportation Noise and Cardiovascular Risk: Updated Review and Synthesis of Epidemiological Studies Indicate That the Evidence Has Increased," *Noise and Health* 8, no. 30 (2006): 1–29.

79. K. M. Shea and the Committee on Environmental Health Technical Report, "Irradiation of Food, Committee on Environmental Health," *Pediatrics* 106, no. 6 (December 2000): 1505–1510.

80. RadTown USA, "Radiation in Tobacco" (2010). http://www.epa.gov/radtown/tobacco.html.

81. D. Malmo-Levine, "Radioactive Tobacco" (American Computer Science Association, January 2, 2002). http://www.acsa2000.net/HealthAlert /radioactive_tobacco.html.

82. Center for Food Safety, "Food Irradiation" (2011). http://www.centerforfoodsafety.org/campaign /food-irradiation.

83. R. Smith-Bindman et al., "Radiation Dose Associated with Common Computed Tomography Examinations and the Associated Lifetime Attributable Risk of Cancer" [abstract], *Archives of Internal Medicine* 169, no. 22 (December 14/28, 2009): 2078–2086.

84. www.usda.gov

85. J. Hausleiter et al., "Estimated Radiation Dose Associated with Cardiac CT Angiography," *Journal of the American Medical Association* 301, no. 5 (February 4, 2009): 500–507.

86. E. Dougeni, K. Faulkner, and G. Panayiotakis, "A Review of Patient Dose and Optimisation Methods in Adult and Paediatric CT Scanning," *European Journal of Radiology* (June 16, 2011).

87. L. Xu and Z. Zhang, "Coronary CT Angiography with Low Radiation Dose," *International Journal of Cardiovascular Imaging* 26, Suppl. 1 (February 2010): 17–25.

88. H. Bryant and V. Mai, "Impact of Age-Specific Recommendation Changes on Organized Breast Screening Programs," *Preventive Medicine* (June 24, 2011).

89. D. Salas et al., "Effect of Start Age of Breast Cancer Screening Mammography on the Risk of False-Positive Results," *Preventive Medicine* 53, nos. 1–2 (July–August 2007) : 76–81.

90. A. Ahlbom et al., "Epidemiologic Evidence on Mobile Phones and Tumor Risk: A Review," *Epidemiology* 20, no. 5 (2009): 639–652.

91. International Agency for Research on Cancer, the INTERPHONE Study Group, "Brain Tumour Risk in Relation to Mobile Telephone Use: Results of the INTERPHONE International Case-Control Study," *International Journal of Epidemiology* 39, no. 3 (2010): 675–694.

92. J. Mackay and A. Amos, "Women and Tobacco," *Respirology* 8, no. 2 (2003): 123–130.

93. Centers for Disease Control and Prevention, "Exposure to Secondhand Smoke Among Students Aged 13–15 Years—Worldwide, 2000–2007," *Morbidity and Mortality Weekly Report* 56, no. 20 (2007): 497–500.

94. L. Dossey, "Think Globally, Act NonLocally: Consciousness Beyond Space and Time," in *Ecological Medicine: Healing the Earth, Healing Ourselves*, ed. K. Asubel (San Francisco, CA: Sierra Books, 2004).

95. L. Dossey, *The Extraordinary Healing Power of Ordinary Things* (New York, NY: Harmony, 2006): 209.

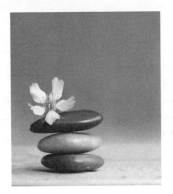

Chapter 30

Cultural Diversity and Care

Joan C. Engebretson

Nurse Healer
OBJECTIVES

Theoretical

- Compare common value orientations associated with culture.
- Describe the influence of technology on cultural development and communication systems.
- Analyze components of cultural diversity.
- Describe the components and principles of cultural competence.
- Discuss cultural influences on beliefs and explanatory systems related to health and illness.

Clinical

- Discuss the role of culture in interactions with clients.
- Use components of transcultural assessment in caring for clients.
- Identify appropriate patterns, challenges, and needs of clients in the cultural domain.
- Explore interventions that reflect cultural competence.
- Discuss ways in which nursing interventions may be evaluated in relation to cultural competence.

Personal

- Clarify your own values, beliefs, and ideas related to your cultural heritage.

- Identify barriers in your own life to acceptance of cultural diversity.
- Explore activities that will increase your awareness and acceptance of cultural differences.

DEFINITIONS

Acculturation: The process of the adaptation or accommodation of an individual immigrant or immigrant group to a new culture.

Culturally competent health care: Health care delivered with knowledge of and sensitivity to cultural factors that influence the health and illness behaviors of an individual client, family, or community.

Culture: The values, beliefs, customs, social structures, and patterns of human activity and the symbolic structures that provide meaning and significance to human behavior.

Ethnicity: Designation of a population subgroup sharing a common social and cultural heritage.

Ethnocentrism: A worldview that is based to a great extent on the socialization of individuals within their own culture, to the extent that such individuals believe that all others see the world as they do.

Race: A social classification that denotes a biological or genetically transmitted set of distinguishable physical characteristics.

Stereotyping: Consigning cultural attributes to a group of people based on assumptions, opinions, or attitudes.

Xenophobia: An inherent fear or hatred of cultural differences.

■ THEORY AND RESEARCH

Culture is the combination of ideas, customs, skills, arts, and other capabilities of a people or group, although as a whole, it is more complex than any one of these elements. Culture is learned from birth through language acquisition and socialization and is the process by which an individual adapts to the group's organized way of life. This process also provides for the transmission of culture from one generation to another. Members of the cultural group share cultural values, beliefs, and patterns of behavior that create and reflect a group identity. This has a powerful influence on behavior, usually on a subconscious level. Culture is largely tacit, meaning it is not generally expressed or discussed at a conscious level. Most culturally derived actions are based on implicit cues rather than written or spoken sets of rules.

Although many of the underlying beliefs and value systems of a culture are stable, all cultures are inherently dynamic and changing; therefore, it is difficult to generalize from one person, situation, or time to another. Cultural practices are continually adapting to the environment, historical context, technology, and availability of resources. As a result, the context in which people live influences, and is influenced by, cultural practices.

Anthropology, the study of cultures, and nursing are both based on a holistic perspective that incorporates the issues of context. Culture has a significant impact on health and illness behaviors, as well as patterns of response to illness or medical care. It directly influences health behaviors such as diet and exercise. Cultural beliefs and practices also affect the types of health problems that are attended to and the actions taken to deal with them. Activities taken to promote, maintain, or restore health are all performed in a cultural context. Therefore, an understanding of the client's perceptions and the context in which he or she lives is necessary for optimal client care.

Culture also determines much of the relationship and type of communication between a client and a healthcare provider. Given that the United States is a culturally diverse nation, nurses and other healthcare providers encounter individuals and groups whose habits of health maintenance, reactions to illness or disease, and use of healthcare services may differ from their own. An awareness of and accommodation to the cultural aspects of health and illness behaviors enables one to promote health by skillfully blending professional knowledge with knowledge of the individual's or group's beliefs. Culturally competent care is the delivery of health care with skill, knowledge, and sensitivity to cultural factors. With the increase of cultural pluralism in North America, it is essential that nurses develop cultural competency to deliver holistic care.

Cultural Competency

With increasing diversity in the population, and the recognition that health disparities exist across ethnic groups, healthcare regulatory agencies recommend that cultural competency become a goal in the provision of health care. The Office of Minority Health developed standards and recommendations that apply to the institutional level as well as to the individual provider.[1] Institutions are mandated to provide adequate translation, and individual providers are encouraged to develop more culturally appropriate care.

The idea of developing cultural competence has been increasingly discussed in the literature. The National Center for Cultural Competency at Georgetown University developed an often cited conceptual framework created by Cross, Barzon, Dennis, and Issacs that describes a continuum from cultural destructiveness to cultural competency.[2] This continuum positions cultural destructiveness at the lowest level, with four intermediary steps to cultural proficiency at the top. This continuum can be viewed as corresponding to well-established values in medicine. **Figure 30-1** illustrates this continuum along with parallel values in biomedicine with a recent value of evidence-based practice superimposed on the model.[3]

Cultural destructiveness, the lowest level of the continuum, corresponds to maleficence in medicine and this is countered through laws such as the Civil Rights Act of 1964 (Title VI), which mandates that healthcare providers do not discriminate according to race, ethnicity, or creed. The ethic of nonmaleficence, or "do no harm," also addresses this basic level. The second level of the continuum, cultural incapacity, corresponding to incompetence, refers to nonintentional practices that may be harmful to clients through ignorance, insensitive attitudes, or improper allocation of resources. Cultural blindness, the third level that corresponds to standardization, is exemplified by treating all patients alike without accommodating or recognizing cultural differences. Precompetence, corresponding to outcomes-focused care, is the next step toward cultural competence and proficiency. Providing translators, developing health education aimed at specific cultural groups, and creating programs that address diverse groups' access to care are good examples of cultural precompetence, which is level 4. Cultural competence, level 5, is best described as an ongoing learning process for the provider, who can integrate cultural knowledge into individualized client-centered care. This eventually leads to the highest level of the continuum, cultural proficiency. These two levels correspond to the movement to patient-centered care, or what holistic nurses would identify as individually focused holistic care.

Evidence-based practice has been an important issue in healthcare delivery. It grew out of the outcomes-focused value, as an effort to incorporate the best research evidence in healthcare delivery. In the focus on applying these findings, many revert back to standardized care or cultural blindness. According to some of the leaders in the evidence-based practice field, practicing in a culturally competent manner incorporates three aspects of evidence-based practice (EPB): best evidence from valid and clinically relevant research, provider's clinical expertise, and the client's values, unique preferences, and situation.[4] The emphasis on the client's values, preferences, and situation moves EBP into cultural competence and proficiency. Much of the literature in cultural competency also tends to focus only on the evidence or the studies or the literature that describes particular ethnic groups. It is important for holistic nurses to recognize that applying that information to clients of a specific ethnic group is only at the precompetence level at best. However, at the individual patient–provider encounter, it must be individually based and patient-centered.

Culturally competent health care must be provided within the context of a client's cultural

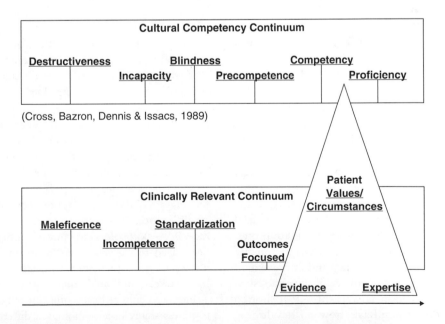

FIGURE 30-1   Cultural Competence in the Era of Evidence-Based Practice
Source: J. Engebretson, J. Mahoney, and E. Carlson, "Cultural Competence in the Era of Evidence-Based Practice," *Journal of Professional Nursing* 24, no. 3 (2008): 172–178.

background, beliefs, and values related to health and illness to attain optimal client outcomes. To enhance one's understanding of cultural issues, it is therefore important for nurses to continue their understanding of cultural diversity. In addition to the Transcultural Nursing Society, there is a corpus of literature in nursing about cultural competence.[5-10]

A plethora of sensitivity training and educational programs has been implemented, and curricula have been developed in nursing and other healthcare professions. Lipson and Desantis recently reviewed a number of approaches in nursing education and concluded that there is a lack of consensus on what should be taught and how it should be integrated into the curricula.[11] A recent systematic review of healthcare provider education was also conducted, concluding that cultural competence training shows promise for improving knowledge, attitudes, and skills of the healthcare professionals. However, there was little evidence in client outcomes.[12] Most educational approaches have addressed knowledge, attitudes, and skills. Knowledge has often focused on facts and characteristics about specific cultures. This "cookbook" approach has been criticized as leading to stereotyping. The approach of cultural sensitivity training attempts to address attitudes. What seems to be more valuable is for providers to learn a set of skills that enables them to provide high-quality client care to everyone.

In a literature review of cultural competence and the clinical encounter, Betancourt concludes that healthcare providers develop the skills for a client-centered approach that does the following: (1) assesses core cross-cultural issues, (2) explores the meaning of the illness to the patient, (3) determines the social context in which the patient lives, and (4) engages in a negotiation process with the patient.[13] Cultural competence represents an important element of clinical care and skills that are central to professionalism across disciplines. The relationship between cultural competency and improvement in health outcomes is not yet firmly established and more research is warranted.[14] Although there is much emphasis now on developing cultural competency, there is also a developing awareness that competency is always a growth process, which means that it requires more than an accumulation of facts about different cultures.[15] The clinical encounter, in which cultural competency is most demanding, requires individual- or family-centered care.[16]

Cultural Diversity and Health Disparities

Despite the fact that human beings are 99.9% identical at the DNA level, there are differences in prevalence of illness between groups. This may be explained by genetic differences; dietary, cultural, environmental, and socioeconomic factors; or combinations thereof.[17] Health disparities in the United States exist for multiple health outcomes. For example, in the United States, infant mortality is inversely related to the mother's educational level. It is also highest for infants of non-Hispanic black mothers and is lowest for those of Chinese mothers.[18] According to a recent Centers for Disease Control and Prevention (CDC) report, some of the key social determinants of health include education and income, inadequate and unhealthy housing, unhealthy air quality, and health insurance coverage.[19] Socioeconomic status underlies three major determinants of health: access to health care, environmental exposure to health-related agents, and health behaviors.[20]

Race and Ethnicity

Ethnicity refers to values, perceptions, feelings, assumptions, and physical characteristics associated with ethnic group affiliation. Often, *ethnicity* refers to nationality—a group sharing a common social and cultural heritage. In contrast, *race* typically refers to a biological, genetically transmitted set of distinguishable physical characteristics. In some literature, however, *race* has often been misused to describe differences in people that have no basis in biology or science. Demographic data are commonly gathered with no differentiation of ethnicity or definitions of race. Both skin color and country of origin have been used to classify race. For example, many natives of India (considered racially Caucasian) have darker skin than do many natives of Africa.

Race and culture have significant relationships to illness states because biological differences can make certain groups of people vulnerable to specific diseases. For example, genetic predisposition for sickle cell disease affects people of African and Mediterranean descent; predisposition for Tay-Sachs disease affects Ashkenazi Jews. Also, certain diseases that may be attributable to a combination of genetic predisposition and lifestyle, including nutritional patterns, are more prevalent in some groups. One example is the disproportionately high prevalence of diabetes in Native Americans and Hispanics. Some diseases are connected to lifestyle risks, such as substance abuse and human immunodeficiency virus (HIV) infection, which are related to particular social behaviors. An emerging body of information on the differences in response to pharmaceuticals by ethnic and racial groups has led to a new field of pharmacogenomics.[21] Cultural subgroups can be identified by virtue of shared experiences or circumstances that may influence values, beliefs, and behaviors. Ethnicity is the most common cultural demarcation, but intraethnic variations may be more pronounced than interethnic variations, especially in a culturally pluralistic society. Other variables that have been proposed as influencing cultural groupings are religion, socioeconomic status, geographic region, age, common beliefs, and professional orientation, such as nursing and medicine.

Factors Related to Culture

Along with ethnicity, religion is an important factor in determining the values and beliefs of a culture.[22] Religion, an organized system of beliefs, is differentiated from spirituality, which is born out of each individual's personal experience in finding meaning and significance in life. Religious faith and the institutions derived from that faith have a powerful influence over human behavior. All religions have experiential, ritualistic, ideological, intellectual, and consequential dimensions. Religious views have historically served as a unifying force for groups of people with a set of core values and beliefs.

Socioeconomic status refers to an individual's social status, occupation, education, economic status, or a combination of these. Socioeconomic explanations are often discounted when determining the relationships between ethnicity or race and health status or health. It is necessary to distinguish between cultural identification and the common experience of being poor

in our society. By illustration, the experience of being poor in our society is different from that of being Hispanic, and also must be further distinguished from being both poor and Hispanic. The impact of socioeconomic status on both morbidity and mortality measures of specific groups is highly significant and is related to health disparities; lower socioeconomic status groups have higher morbidity and mortality rates for various diseases.[23]

The local or regional manifestations of the larger culture bring up such distinctions as rural, urban, southern, or midwestern. For example, African Americans living in the southern region of the United States may have beliefs and behaviors different from those in the northern region, based somewhat on their heritage of slavery and exposure to the civil rights movement.

Age of the individuals within a cultural group has a profound influence on their beliefs and behaviors as well. Value systems are tied to historically shared events that occur in childhood; therefore, each generation develops a unique value system. For example, there is much in the popular literature about the differences between the baby boomers (people born in the late 1940s and 1950s), generation X (those born in the 1960s and 1970s), and generation Y (folks born in the late 1970s and 1980s).

Common beliefs or ideologies may unite a cultural group or subculture, as well as differentiate that group from the larger culture. These value systems may be related to religion (e.g., the Amish), lifestyle (e.g., communal groups), sexual orientation (e.g., gay and lesbian groups), or political ideologies (e.g., feminist separatist groups). Social or professional orientations often constitute a type of cultural grouping. Medical anthropologists have described the biomedical system as a cultural system.[24] The biomedical culture of many hospitals constitutes an unfamiliar culture for many laypeople. Healthcare professionals use unique and esoteric language, as well as rituals, roles, expectations, patterns of behavior, and symbolic communication that are often alien to the layperson.

Common Myths and Errors

Errors of stereotyping are common among those who define the world by strict categories of ethnicity or race. It is also problematic to presume that all members of another culture conform to a common pattern without regard to individual characteristics or the variety found within one cultural grouping. For example, some people assume that all African Americans eat soul food or that all Hispanics are Catholic. Failure to recognize that values from a particular cultural group can vary across time and location leads to stereotyping cultures with values that no longer guide the group's or the individual's thinking or behavior. Stereotyping is less obvious in some cases, such as a nurse manager assigning all Hispanic clients to the Mexican American nurse. Such action does not take into account the differences within the Hispanic group, presumes that all Hispanics are alike, and disregards the individual.

The heterogeneity of ethnic groups is often underestimated, but as mentioned earlier, the variations within ethnic groups may be as great or greater than those between ethnic groups. For example, the Hispanic culture includes persons of Puerto Rican, Cuban, Spanish, and South and Central American origins. These people are from many different socioeconomic backgrounds and represent the Caucasian, Mongoloid, and Negroid racial groups. Sometimes Asians from different countries and backgrounds are grouped together and treated as generic Asians, an attitude that totally ignores the historical differences among Asians. Kipnis relates a clinical incident that occurred in Hawaii in which a Korean client with a serious medical condition refused a treatment that promised a better than 50% recovery with minimum risks.[25] Clinical staff were puzzled by his refusal of treatment coupled with his request for life support if he experienced cardiopulmonary arrest. On further investigation, he mentioned that all his physicians were Japanese. In the early 1900s, Japan had ruthlessly tyrannized Korea, much as the Nazis in Germany tyrannized Poland prior to and during World War II. Thus, the Korean gentleman very much wanted to live, but his cultural history caused him to refuse treatment directed by the Japanese physicians.

Ethnocentrism is the tendency, usually unconscious, for individuals to take for granted their own values as the only objective reality and to look at everyone else through the lens of their own cultural norms and customs. Ethnocentric views often result from a lack of knowledge of other cultures and the presumption that one's own behavior is not influenced by culture. Many people of the dominant culture falsely assume that they have no cultural practices and beliefs. This restrictive view of the world perceives people and cultures with different beliefs and behaviors as culturally inferior. An extreme and more conscious form of ethnocentrism is xenophobia, an inherent fear of cultural differences, which often leads people to bolster their security in their own values by demeaning the beliefs and traditions of others. This attitude often takes the form of prejudice or racism.

Cultural imposition is the perception that successful cultural adaptation involves a change to the cultural views of the dominant group, regardless of an individual's cultural heritage. This posits an inherent view that the dominant culture is superior, and its values are imposed on others.

Often disguised as equal treatment for everyone, cultural blindness ignores cultural differences as if they did not exist. This view overlooks real diversity and the importance of other perspectives. The concept of the "melting pot" assumes that, in the process of acculturation and assimilation, everyone takes on significant aspects of the dominant culture such that the original culture is largely lost. This assimilation or melting pot view is challenged by concepts of heritage consistency, which is the degree to which one maintains practices and beliefs that reflect one's own heritage.

Development of Cultural Patterns and Behaviors

Anthropologists have studied practices among cultures in relation to the universal experience of being human. Their major focus has been on the variation of ways that humans organize and structure their social world. Some of the factors that contribute to the development of cultural patterns and behavior are geography and migration, gender-specific roles, value orientations and cultural beliefs, and technological development.

Geography and Migration

Social groups evolve through interaction with the climate, as well as in conjunction with the availability of food and resources. The persistence of dietary patterns reflects the types of food available in a particular region. For example, fish constitutes a large portion of the traditional diet of people from Norway and the Philippines, whereas dairy products and meats are dominant in the food patterns of Finland and Germany.

Social organization falls in line with these geographic patterns. For example, the social structure of a fishing village differs from that of a nomadic group that hunts for food, and from that of a settled agrarian culture. Urbanization and industrialization are also important for the way society organizes and social roles develop. Social roles become patterned and often institutionalized into hierarchical structures that reflect social, economic, and political power. These social structures and roles greatly alter people's daily lives and the economics of providing for families.

Climate, environmental conditions, and political and economic factors are very important in migration patterns. Climate change, famine, political upheaval, and overpopulation have all been responsible for migration. For example, a large wave of Irish immigrants came to the United States in the late 1840s following a potato famine that was causing starvation, disease, and death in Ireland. Many immigrants came to the United States to flee political unrest in El Salvador in the 1980s. Many Vietnamese and Southeast Asians sought political refuge and opportunities in the United States following the Vietnam War. A large number of nurses seeking professional and economic opportunities moved to the mainland United States from the Philippines in the 1980s. Even in the 1990s and the early 21st century, a large number of immigrants have steadily come to the United States seeking economic opportunities.

Cultural patterns change through the sharing of ideas, beliefs, and practices that follow trade or migration. Immigrants bring cultural patterns, values, and beliefs with them. Along with their adaptation to the new host culture, they expose the host culture to a different set of cultural beliefs and practices. Both cultures assimilate aspects of the other.

The historical context of immigration is important and varies among groups. Many African Americans arrived involuntarily and endured a lengthy history of slavery. Hispanics may be immigrants seeking economic opportunity, refugees from political upheavals, or descendants of people living in the Southwest before it became a part of the United States. The fact that many Asian immigrants find it necessary to take a job with lower status than they had in their country of origin creates cultural and economic hardship for the family. In many Hispanic families, the father immigrates alone to establish a better economic future for the family. Estranged from the family, he may be at risk for such behavioral health risks as AIDS and alcohol abuse. Health issues may also arise because of low income and low self-esteem.

Acculturation is an important process in the adaptation, assimilation, or accommodation of immigrant groups to a new culture. This is sometimes referred to as hybridization. This is because in the process of adapting to a new culture, immigrants integrate the new culture into their beliefs and lifestyle and yet retain heritage consistency, maintaining pride in and adhering to their parent culture. According to the Theory of Orthogonal Cultural Identification, this process does not take place along a single continuum, but rather has numerous dimensions that operate independently from each other.[26] Intergenerational gaps frequently develop because the youth become more quickly acculturated to the dominant society, and they may challenge the more traditional values, beliefs, and customs of their parents. This, in turn, may threaten the integrity and lines of respect in the family and roles within the family and society, particularly the role of women. Conflicts that arise from intergenerational gaps can lead to the alienation of young people and families from both the ethnic culture and the general dominant culture.

Gender Roles

All cultures develop socially sanctioned roles for respective genders. Over the past century, the social role for women in the United States has undergone many changes. The role of women has expanded from its traditional focus on childbearing and child rearing to include participation in the workplace and marketplace. The feminist movement has championed this expanded role and has heightened consciousness about opportunities consistent with the American values of individualism, equality, and political freedom. Furthermore, the feminist movement has challenged the values and structures developed by elite, masculine power, such as competition, strong focus on objectives and goals, the harnessing and control of nature, principle-based ethics, and productive activities. Feminists have promoted cultural practices and organizations that espouse more feminine values such as teamwork, focus on social process, working in harmony with nature, relationship-based ethics, and social connections. As people from other cultures move into the United States, these differing values and expanded roles for women may challenge the traditional family roles. In some cases where women's roles take a more traditional position, a woman may need to get her husband's or father's permission prior to receiving medical care for herself or her children.

Women have played significant roles in the healing arts as well. Historically and cross-culturally, women have discovered and preserved information about healing herbs and plants. In the Middle Ages, women were often persecuted for their knowledge of plants and other healing arts, which were deemed mysterious and suspicious. As medicine became more scientific and moved into a professional and scientific status, women were disengaged from the official healing roles.[27] Women were associated with nature, and men with developing technology to tame and control nature. Women's roles in the healing arts reflected this dichotomy. With the establishment of medical professions, women's roles even in midwifery—a traditional role for women—were reduced, and physicians took over the practice and moved childbirth into hospitals. Women who worked in medical professions were often in nonphysician roles or positions of lower power and social status, such as nurses, social workers, and physical therapists. However, women have a strong presence among complementary healers and users of complementary therapies.[28]

Basic Value Orientations and Beliefs

All cultures hold certain value orientations that are central to their cultural patterns of behavior. These values can be both implicit and explicit. They influence an individual's perception of others, direct that individual's responses to others,

and reflect his or her identity. These values are the basis for understanding oneself and one's social relationships, political and economic structures, and direct and motivate behavior. These values are generally quite stable and do not change quickly. In a classic work on cultural orientations, Kluckhohn identifies five categories by which cultures address universal concerns of human nature:[29]

1. Innate human nature as being good, evil, or mixed
2. Humans' relationship to nature as being subjugated to the forces of nature, harmonious coexistence with nature, or using human abilities to master nature
3. Relationship to time as past oriented, present oriented, or future oriented
4. Purpose of being seen as focused on self-realization or a more action-orientation focus on doing
5. Relationship to other persons is expressed in individual, familial, or communal orientations

In Western culture and in particular the United States, these value orientations are reflected in a strong emphasis on individualism, mastery over nature, future-focused time orientation, and an action orientation to being. This can be seen in health care when we see the individual as the client and often ignore the family. Our mastery over nature is illustrated in our efforts to understand and cure disease and control health issues. Future orientation is reflected in our goal orientation and an emphasis on the effect our actions may have on the future. Both healthcare providers and clients expect some type of action or treatment from the clinical encounter. This reflects the shared value of an action-oriented culture. The healthcare system both influences and is influenced by the general cultural orientations. Cultural conflicts may occur when we fail to recognize that our clients hold differing value orientations.

Worldviews and cosmologies essential to Western Judeo-Christian-Islam beliefs differ from those of other world religions. Three dominant cosmology assumptions foundational to Western Judeo-Christian-Islam beliefs are monotheism, transcendence, and dualism.[30] Monotheism, the belief in one God or Creator, who is separate from humans, contrasts with the beliefs common in many agrarian societies, whose members believe in polytheism (i.e., multiple gods with different attributes) or pantheism (i.e., the locus of the sacred in all living things). The Western view of transcendence, or relating to God as separate from humans and knowing God through prayer, supplication, and rituals, can be contrasted with the Eastern view of immanence, or finding God by looking inward and doing other spiritual exercises to discover the sacred. Finally, Western dualism, separation of material from nonmaterial aspects of being, is in contrast to monism, or the essential unity found in both the pantheistic and Eastern belief systems. Many "new age" perspectives are exploring these issues as they are exposed to different cultural beliefs.

Technology and Culture

In contemporary Western culture, as well as in much of the world, technology is widely expanding. The development of technology affects values, religion, politics, and the arts and sciences. Medical technology in particular has progressed in its development of intricate instruments that allow for more complex procedures, such as computer-based imaging, microsurgery, gene mapping, targeted therapies, and pharmacogenomics. The development of these technologies poses new ethical and cultural questions related to the human and social impact this technology may have. Often the use of these technologies challenges existing cultural values. Once the technology is available for use, it often becomes the fuel for ethical debates related to such issues as allocation of resources, fetal tissue transplantation and right to life, and genetic testing and right to privacy.

Technology has also held a powerful influence on culture through its use in communication, which affects not only how information is conveyed, but also what type of knowledge is valued.[31] Traditionally, knowledge was passed on by oral means in stories, parables, and poetry. Essential knowledge (i.e., cultural wisdom associated with oral tradition) was preserved through memory, often aided by rhythm and rhyme. Many cultures today have their roots in oral traditions.

With the advent of written communication, the Western world became a different culture based on the type of knowledge that was conveyed and developed. Printed materials recorded information with detail, precision, and accuracy in a way that oral speech could not. The ability to read this information also facilitated discussions and formation of complex thoughts. Thus, scientific and factual information gained value, giving rise to the development of modern scholarship.

Today's electronic culture, dependent on telephones, radio, television, and computers to communicate information, has an enormous impact on the beliefs, values, and behaviors of contemporary society. In relation to health care, clients have access to a plethora of health-related information from multiple sources. This has presented new challenges for healthcare providers to help clients interpret information and make appropriate choices.

Changing Beliefs and Values

In the late 20th century, people in the developed and industrialized world have been exposed to a number of different cultures, as a result of both immigration and electronic technology. Electronic media, allowing for fast and more universal dispersal of information, has promoted intercultural communication throughout the world as never before. Such communication has led to unprecedented exposure to different cultures, with results ranging from attempts to integrate diverse ideas to overt conflict and violence. Scientific and technologic advances, as well as global, political, social, and economic changes, have challenged existing cultural systems and increased the velocity of cultural change.

A large marketing survey indicated that the U.S. population could be divided into three groups according to values. Ray identified one of these groups, cultural creatives, as those who are on the leading edge of change, comprising nearly one-quarter of the population.[32] This group holds a holistic philosophy of health; values ecologic preservation, spirituality, relationships, and self-actualization; and expresses interest in other cultures and new ideas. The largest group identified (47%), the moderns, places a high value on success, consumerism, materialism, and technologic rationality. The third group (29%), the traditionalists, or heartlanders, believes in the nostalgic images of small towns and strong churches that define the "good old American way."

In a survey of more than 1,000 adults, Astin found that those who use alternative and complementary therapies generally have a higher education level, have a more holistic orientation to health, and often have been through a transformational experience that changed their worldview. They also were more likely to have had a chronic health problem or other recent illness.[33] This group expressed a set of values, beliefs, and philosophic orientations that included commitment to environmentalism and feminism and an interest in spirituality and personal growth. Other studies have described these consumers as generally well educated and affluent members of the middle class.[34] The use of complementary therapies and the search for holistic approaches to health care are consistent with the cultural beliefs of the cultural creatives. This percentage of the population is substantial and, according to Ray, is growing, whereas individuals in the traditionalist groups are generally older and this group is not growing as quickly.

■ ETHNIC GROUPS IN NORTH AMERICA

Culturally diverse groups in the United States have grown to substantial proportions of the population. In their practice, nurses are likely to encounter representatives of different cultures. General descriptions about these various ethnic groups may provide helpful orientations to the group. It is important to remember that there is much diversity within ethnicities and that in the processes of globalization and exposure to other cultures, these cultural beliefs are dynamic. Therefore, it is extremely important for nurses to avoid stereotyping. Reading about and engaging in discussions and activities with members of these cultural groups can help to avoid stereotypic interpretations of these groups and aid in developing cultural competency. The compiled U.S. Census data give estimates for 2009.[35]

American Indian and Alaska Natives

According to the census data, American Indians and Alaska Natives (AIAN) are classified as AIAN alone or AIAN mixed with another race. The combined group represents 4.9 million, or 1%, of the total population, with the percentages rising.[35] They have a higher rate of poverty than does the population as a whole. They often cluster in tribal groups, with the largest concentrations located in the Pacific and western mountain regions of the United States. There is considerable variation among the tribes regarding language, beliefs, customs, health practices, and rituals. Tribes or clans constitute a social unit in which members may or may not be blood relatives, and both family and clan are powerful sources of the Native American's identity and support. Largely because of the respect for the wisdom accrued with aging, elders are typically the community leaders. Value orientations center on harmony with nature, a present-time orientation, and an integration of rituals and religion into everyday life. Many Native Americans still adhere to folk healing practices, seeking out local healers before going to a healthcare clinic. Folk healing practices may fall into the shamanic category or often are understood in a supranormal paradigm. Common health problems include diabetes, obesity, infectious disease, alcohol abuse, and diseases associated with poverty. Years of racism, dehumanization, and oppression have left a legacy in which many Native Americans may mistrust Caucasian healthcare providers.

European Americans

The largest ethnic group in North America is made up of European Americans. According to the Census Bureau, they constitute the dominant culture and comprise approximately 79.6% of the population of the United States. However, that percentage is declining. White persons, not Hispanic constitute 65.1% of the population.[36] The largest emigrations from various regions in Europe occurred in the late 1700s, all through the 1800s, and into the first half of the 20th century. Many immigrants to the United States carried the European ideas of the Age of Reason, dominance over nature, and the belief in progress and technologic advancement. Their quest for freedom enhanced an abiding value of individualism. They are generally action oriented, future directed, and focused on progress and productivity. Families are an important social unit among European Americans, but the value of individualism is pervasive. Although this group is diverse, the values are usually consistent with dominant values of the culture. Therefore, members of this group may not be as aware of the role that culture plays in their lives as the members of other cultural groups are.

African Americans

The 2008 Census estimates the number of African Americans (AA), also classified as AA alone or combined with another group, in the United States to be 41.1 million, or almost 14% of the population.[35] This number and proportion have grown since the 2000 census. The highest concentrations of African Americans are in the South and on the East Coast. One-third of this population was younger than age 18 years in 2000. This group is very heterogeneous and varies in economic status, religion, education, and regional background. Many African Americans are descendants of slaves who were brought to the United States; others are recent immigrants from Africa and the Caribbean Islands. Within the social structure of slavery, families were dispersed and individuals were not allowed to read. Thus, a tradition of strong matriarchal family units with a rich oral tradition developed. Social organization centers on the family, kinship bonds, and the church. Some of the health disparities among African Americans may be related to the disproportional rate of poverty. Many African Americans have absorbed much of the dominant culture, but some adhere to ancestral beliefs of illness as disharmony with nature and supranormal healing rituals or folk healing. The history of slavery and the Tuskegee atrocities have made some African Americans mistrustful of receiving professional health care or participating in clinical research studies.

Asian Americans

Constituting 4.6% of the total U.S. population, or approximately 15.5 million people in 2008,[35] Asian Americans are expected to represent 9% of the population by 2050. Approximately two-thirds reside in the western part of the United States. This group is composed of immigrants and refugees from the Pacific Rim countries, such as China, Japan, Korea, Thailand, Laos, Vietnam, Cambodia, the Philippines, and other Asian countries. People from India are often included in this group as well. There is wide diversity in language, customs, and beliefs in this group. Traditional Asian families tend to be patriarchal, revere their elders, and value achievement and honor. Certain infectious diseases, such as tuberculosis and hepatitis, are common among Asian Americans, depending on the country from which they emigrated. Stress-related diseases and suicides are high, as many do not seek mental health care because of an associated stigma and a threat to honor. Asians' traditional health practices often are oriented around the balance paradigm in which health is equated with balance and unimpeded flow of energy, or *chi*. Traditional healing includes the use of herbal preparations, and many families practice traditional dermabrasion procedures such as coining, pinching, or rubbing.

Pacific Islanders and Native Hawaiians

The Native Hawaiian and Other Pacific Islander (NHPI) population constituted 1.1 million individuals, or 0.2% of the U.S. population, in the 2008 census.[35] Native Hawaiians are the largest subgroup (58%), although the majority of this group reported one or more other races as well. Nearly three-fourths of this population lives in the West, with more than half living in California and Hawaii combined. There is great diversity in beliefs and customs. As an aggregate group, NHPIs are socioeconomically disadvantaged and underserved in terms of access to social and health services. Pacific Islanders have high rates of health-related risk behaviors, such as smoking, heavy alcohol consumption, and high fat and caloric intake, which leads to obesity.

Hispanics

The Hispanic population in the United States included more than 35 million people, or constituted 12.5 5% of the U.S. population in 2000, and is predicted to reach 24% by 2050.[36] The majority of these immigrants come from Mexico, with others from Puerto Rico, Cuba, and Central and South America. This is the fastest growing group in the United States. Although the Spanish language is a common factor, there is much diversity in dialects and cultural practices. This group comprises indigenous peoples of the Americas, Spanish and other European settlers, and some African-Caribbean groups. Predominant religions are Catholicism and Pentecostalism. The family and extended family are important, and the family unit is traditionally patriarchal. Many believe that illness may be punishment for sins or the result of witchcraft or *brujería*, meaning the "evil eye." Traditional health beliefs regarding hot and cold remedies for various maladies reflect humeral balance beliefs. Healing also incorporates many spiritual elements, such as worship of saints and use of talismans.

■ IMPACT OF CULTURE ON HEALTH CARE

Concepts of health and healing are rooted in culture. The concept of disease generally refers to the diagnostic label or categorization of a disorder that medicine treats, whereas the concept of illness incorporates the personal, social, and cultural aspects of the experience. Cultural practices influence an individual's behavior to promote, maintain, and restore health and how, when, and with whom the individual seeks help or treatment. Cultural beliefs, values, and practices are also extremely important in birth and death.

Cultural understandings of health and illness reflect larger philosophic worldviews, or paradigms, that provide a way of understanding the body and the forces that influence health and illness. According to Andrews and Boyle, there are three major types of cross-cultural paradigms: magicoreligious, holistic, and scientific.[37] Although aspects of all three are found in most cultures, one usually predominates.

In the magicoreligious health paradigm, the fate of the world depends on God, gods, or supernatural forces. Events such as sorcery, breach of taboo, intrusion of a disease-causing spirit, or loss of soul are considered responsible for illness. This paradigm relates to a psychic or metaphysical need of humanity for integration and harmony. For example, people from some African-Caribbean cultures believe that parts of a person such as hair, fingernails, or blood represent the person and can be used in healing. Also, they may believe that lack of protection for these body parts can make the person vulnerable to illness.

In the holistic health paradigm, the forces of nature must be kept in harmony according to natural laws and the larger universe. These systems often have a strong emphasis on health rather than on the treatment of disease. In Ayurvedic medicine from India, for example, health results from being in harmony with oneself, others, and the environment. Diet and activity are adapted according to the individual's *doshas* (i.e., forces of the human body whose composition varies among individuals) and the seasonal variations in the environment. In Western culture, this idea appears in humoral theories, such as the concepts of balancing hot and cold held by Hispanic, Arab, African, Caribbean, and other societies. Holistic health care is regaining some popularity in developed countries, which are currently the bastions of the scientific paradigm, as the focus begins to shift to promoting health.

The scientific or biomedical paradigm is characterized by four main concepts:

1. *Determinism:* A cause-and-effect relationship exists for all natural phenomena.
2. *Mechanism:* The relationship of life to the structure and function of machines suggests the possibility of control through mechanical or engineered interventions.
3. *Reductionism:* The division of all life into isolated smaller parts, such as the dualism of mind and body, facilitates the study of the whole.
4. *Objective materialism:* That which is real can be observed and measured.

This paradigm is the basis for healthcare systems in Western society, where disease is viewed as the "enemy," the body is the "battlefield," and the physician is the "general." Great effort, expense, and technology are invested in determining the underlying cause of disease. The "system at fault" is isolated, and the most medical attention is directed toward measuring the functions of, and repairing, this faulty part. Persons are often placed in foreign environments (e.g., hospitals) in which limited attention is given to individual needs and cultural beliefs. Anthropologists have also described the healthcare system as a culture with its historical underpinnings in the scientific approach, mind–body dualism, and reflecting American or Western capitalism.[38]

Kleinman, a much referenced medical anthropologist, has described three sectors of health care that are common in all healthcare systems: professional, popular, and folk.[39] Cultures vary widely in the way that they combine these three systems. Usually, one is dominant, although simultaneous use is common. In the United States, the *professional*, or orthodox biomedical, sector of health care has held a legal, political, and ideological monopoly for most of the 20th century. This sector corresponds to the scientific paradigm described earlier. Nurses and other healthcare professionals are part of this sector.

The *popular* sector includes all the personal and social networks that laypeople use to understand their health and plan their health care. Individuals, family, and social networks determine whom to consult, when to seek a consultation, whether to adhere to suggested treatments, when to switch treatments, and how to evaluate the usefulness of treatments. Nearly all persons are active in their own healthcare decisions and practice some form of private or self-prescribed health care. This is the area where the majority of health decisions are made and the one that is the least studied or understood. All secular and sacred healers that are generally outside the professional sector make up the *folk* sector. This sector also includes healing practices used to promote health and treat illness. Many of the currently popular complementary healing practices are in this sector.

Explanatory Models of Health and Illness

Kleinman also describes explanatory models as notions that individuals or groups have about understanding the causes, symptoms, and treatments of illness.[39] Culturally specific explanatory models are interpretations of the culture's worldview as it pertains to health and healing and generally provide an understanding of disease and direct treatment. Explanatory models of health and healing are used to recognize, interpret, respond to, cope with, and make sense of an illness experience. For example, a client who believes that the cause of his or her illness is related to committing a sin or breaking a taboo may not accept biomedical treatment as a cure. Some form of catharsis, forgiveness, or ritual may be necessary. Some of these explanatory models are associated with the three sectors of health care. For example, the professional sector has a particular explanatory mode that may differ from various models in the folk or popular sector.

Kleinman recommends that clinicians explore the explanatory models of their clients in an effort to promote better communication. These questions elicit a framework that allows the cli-

nician to compare the client's explanatory model of etiology, pathology, course of the disease, treatment, and possible outcomes with those of the medical model. Kleinman recommends specific questions to explore what the client calls the disorder, thinks caused it, thinks is happening, thinks will happen, and thinks might make it better or worse.

Giger and Davidhizar and many anthropologists describe explanatory models of folk medicine as classifying diseases or illnesses as natural or unnatural.[40] Natural events arise from the way that a higher power made the world and intended it to be. The basic principle is that everything in nature is connected and events can be explained in terms of this relationship. In some folk sectors, disease represents a disturbance in that relationship with nature. A natural disease or illness results from a disturbance in the person's relationship or balance with nature, and recovery requires the restoration of this relationship. This view is common among Native Americans, whose concept of medicine embraces the forces of nature. Because death is seen as part of the life cycle and a component of natural harmony, a cure for illness is not necessarily sought. Unnatural illnesses are often attributed to punishment from a higher power for one's sins or improper behavior. The origin of unnatural illnesses in folk medicine is based on the continuous battle between good and evil forces. Witchcraft and breaking of a taboo are sometimes considered the origin for unnatural illnesses.

Multiparadigm Model of Healing

As Western culture is becoming increasingly culturally pluralistic, a number of alternative and complementary healing practices and beliefs are surfacing. The word *holistic* is related to the word *health*, which stems from the root word *hale*, the same root as "to make whole." This definition would necessarily incorporate multiple approaches to support health. One effort to place diverse modalities, including biomedicine, into a unified model is illustrated in **Exhibit 30-1**.[41] Paradigms of health and healing are based in underlying philosophy, cultural beliefs, and explanatory models of health and illness. Hence, there is resonance between the biomedical model and the technologic development of modern society. In this unified model, modalities or healing

EXHIBIT 30-1   Multiparadigm Model of Healing

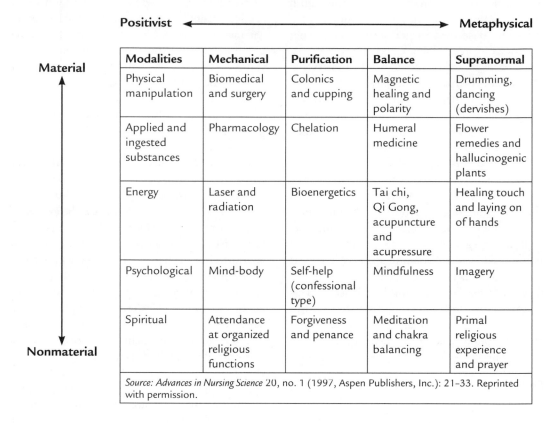

Positivist ←————————————————————→ Metaphysical

Material ↕ Nonmaterial

Modalities	Mechanical	Purification	Balance	Supranormal
Physical manipulation	Biomedical and surgery	Colonics and cupping	Magnetic healing and polarity	Drumming, dancing (dervishes)
Applied and ingested substances	Pharmacology	Chelation	Humeral medicine	Flower remedies and hallucinogenic plants
Energy	Laser and radiation	Bioenergetics	Tai chi, Qi Gong, acupuncture and acupressure	Healing touch and laying on of hands
Psychological	Mind-body	Self-help (confessional type)	Mindfulness	Imagery
Spiritual	Attendance at organized religious functions	Forgiveness and penance	Meditation and chakra balancing	Primal religious experience and prayer

Source: Advances in Nursing Science 20, no. 1 (1997, Aspen Publishers, Inc.): 21–33. Reprinted with permission.

activities are suggested based on the explanation that healers have given for their use.

The unified model illustrated in Exhibit 30-1 uses four paradigms across the horizontal axis: mechanical, purification, balance, and supranormal. The mechanical paradigm best describes the biomedical model or the professional sector, in which the prevailing views are that the body is a system of structure and function, disease is a disruption of its mechanism of action, and the purpose of treatment is to restore or replace that function. The mechanical paradigm is self-correcting and produces increasingly sophisticated understandings of the mechanics of the function of the human body.

The purification paradigm underlies many healing and religious healing practices. The general intention is to cleanse and rid the body of polluting influences. This approach to healing is evident as far back as the early Egyptians, who understood and used some of the concepts of purification in the process of mummification.

This paradigm was quite dominant in European medicine as late as the 19th century and was the rationale behind purges, bloodletting, and other cathartic treatments.

Evident in many cultures, the balance paradigm was part of Hippocratic medicine in the form of balancing the humors and still is evident in Mexican dietary patterns used to balance disorders with cold or hot foods. Balance is epitomized in many of the Oriental healing practices that balance yin and yang and the harmonious flow of chi. There is no English equivalent to the word *chi*, but it is commonly translated as energy. This may be misleading because, according to Kaptchuk, *chi* implies matter at the verge of energy or energy at the point of materializing.[42]

The final paradigm, supranormal, corresponds to some of the magicoreligious healing practices and has been used cross-culturally to explain phenomena that physical laws cannot explain. Many paradoxical healings that defy a scientific understanding of physiology may be more clearly understood from this paradigm. Many of the more mystical spiritual practices of ritual, pilgrimage, prayer, and other activities of religious discipline related to healing the mind, body, and spirit stem from this paradigm. Spontaneous healing that has no medical explanation may be attributed to divine intervention, miraculous synergy, vital energies, or capabilities of living organisms beyond the current understanding of medicine. Many of the explanations refer to abilities acquired in an altered state of consciousness by the healer, healee, or both. Several complementary modalities of healing, such as visual imagery, healing touch, or prayer, are best understood through this paradigm. This paradigm is the most distant from the mechanical paradigm, an opposition that may explain some resistance to these types of healing activities.

In the multiparadigm model, the healing activities on the vertical axis are classified as physical manipulation, applied or ingested substances, use of energy, psychological modalities, and spiritual modalities. Each of the paradigms contains all types of healing activities. However, as one moves to the right in the model (see Exhibit 30-1), all healing is conceptualized as more holistic; all activities affect the entire human. For example, a physical manipulation in the supranormal paradigm is assumed to have spiritual effects, and vice versa.

Healing activities are inserted in the model as examples; other modalities can be added. Among the examples that are useful to illustrate healing activities is the practice of cupping, which involves placing heated cups on parts of the body. The cooling of the air creates suction, causing superficial capillaries to break, and blood to collect in the cup. Cupping exemplifies physical manipulation in the purification paradigm, a healing modality that removes toxins or impurities from the body. Bach flower remedies are viewed as an ingested or applied substance in the supranormal paradigm because their action is understood through a more spiritual or essential manner than a biochemical mechanism. Acupuncture is an energy activity in the balance paradigm because it is the energy or chi that is being acted on, not the physical manipulation of the needles on the physical body.

Mindfulness is a mental discipline based on Eastern thought. This practice is a process of becoming detached and observing thoughts, feelings, and perceptions while remaining fully attentive and in the present. This is a psychological activity in the balance paradigm. Spiritual practices extend through all paradigms. Attendance at organized religious functions is an example of spiritual activities in the mechanical paradigm. Epidemiologic research indicates that attendance at religious events or membership in religious organizations has a salutary effect on health.[43] Some proposed explanatory mechanisms are that these individuals have healthier lifestyles, benefit from social support, or have better stress-coping abilities. This example illustrates the link of mental and spiritual activities to physical outcomes. This understanding has promoted the legitimacy of many of the psychological and spiritual activities that holistic nurses use in promoting physical health within the mechanical paradigm.

In many cultures, systems of healing combine many levels of activities. For example, shamanism includes physical manipulation, applied and ingested substances, use of vital energy, psychological aspects of belief, and spiritual practices that cluster in the supranormal paradigm. Contemporary complementary healers may use modalities from several paradigms. An understanding of the paradigm from which the modality was developed is important for appropriate use in conducting research.

■ NURSING APPLICATIONS

Six phenomena found in all cultural groups have variations that are relevant to the provision of culturally competent nursing assessment and care and are outlined here.[40] It is useful to understand these variations in clinical practice.

Communication: There are cultural variations in expression of feelings, use of touch, body contact, gestures, and verbal and nonverbal communication. Language shapes experiences and influences perceptions and actions. Warmth and humor are two communication factors that are interpreted differently through various cultures. For example, many Asians may not overtly express their emotions because they may fear "losing face."

Personal space: Spatial behavior refers to the comfort level related to personal space, meaning the area that surrounds a person's body. Spatial territoriality is the need to have and to control personal space. Cultures vary in the level of proximity to others that is acceptable. For example, Western culture has three zones: the intimate zone (less than 18 inches), the personal zone (18 inches to 3 feet), and social zone (3 feet to 6 feet). Cultural background also influences aspects of objects within space, such as orderliness, cleanliness, and structural boundaries of furniture and architecture.

Time: Cultures vary in their orientation toward time, both social time and clock time. *Social time* refers to patterns and orientations related to the ordering of social life, whereas *clock time* represents an objective, ordered approach of viewing time in a linear fashion that implies causality. Some cultures orient around cyclic approaches that attach time to natural events that repeat, such as seasons or migration patterns. For example, in mystical thought, magic or ritual may negate the temporal order of causality and reverse a bad event. All cultures contain the three orientations of future, present, and past, with one being dominant.

Social organization: Families, religious groups, kinship groups, workplace groups, and special interest groups are social organizations. Families vary in structure, dynamics, roles, and organizational patterns. Kinship structures and the relative geographic location of family members have cultural implications. Religious organizations provide not only social connections, but also a context in which to understand one's relationship to the world, the cosmos, and the meaning in life.

Environmental control: Different cultures have different perceptions of the ability of an individual to control nature, the environment, and personal relationships. The locus of control may be external (i.e., an event contingent on luck or fate), internal (i.e., an event contingent on one's own behavior or characteristic), or outside (i.e., an event in harmony with nature, as in some Asian cultures). In folk medicine, for example, events are perceived as natural and unnatural. Natural events have

to do with the world as God intended and the laws of nature. Unnatural events upset the harmony of nature and are outside the world of nature.

Biological variations: In a pluralistic culture, it is important to distinguish among factors that are strictly biological (i.e., genetic) and those that are ethnic adaptations related to living in a particular environment (e.g., availability of certain types of food) or in certain social conditions (e.g., socioeconomic status, lifestyle). Biological factors to be considered are body size and structure, including variations in teeth, facial features, and skin color; variations in metabolism and enzyme production that result in drug reactions, interactions, and sensitivities; and susceptibility to disease (e.g., hypertension, diabetes, sickle cell anemia). Nutritional issues, including food preferences, habits, and patterns, as well as deficiencies such as lactose intolerance, all have medical implications.

This information is a helpful guide to thinking about cultural variations. However, no amount of factual knowledge about cultural variation can replace careful individual assessment because there is more intracultural variation than intercultural variation.

Cross-Cultural Communication

Members of minority groups may distrust and fear the Western biomedical healthcare system, of which nurses are a part. Because the element of trust is essential to the formation of a therapeutic nurse–client relationship, clients need to know that nurses are receptive and nonjudgmental regarding their differences. Nurses must approach cultural competency through knowledge of self and knowledge of other cultures. To develop the ability to interact with clients appropriately, nurses should clarify their personal values, recognize the healthcare system as a culture, learn about the specific culture of each client, interact and intervene in a culturally congruent manner, and elicit feedback regularly from the client and family. Skills such as listening, explaining, acknowledging, recommending, and negotiating facilitate a nonjudgmental perspective toward the client's cultural beliefs.

Nurses and clients should validate their perceptions and discuss similarities and differences in their perceptions to formulate health-related goals and interventions.

Cultural competency is a dynamic, challenging process faced by all healthcare providers, regardless of their cultural background or association. Providers who are members of minority groups also encounter situations in which their cultural competency is desirable. Various principles are important in developing cultural competency. The process of sharing information in a straightforward manner demystifies other cultures and, for example, makes it possible for the nurse and client to find common ground and understand the context of differences. To find common ground, it is necessary to consider terminology. Many individuals may consider some terms such as *Negro*, *black*, or *foreigner* inappropriate and possibly offensive. The terms *Hispanic*, *Latino*, and *Chicano* are used to describe people from Spanish-speaking cultures. The terms may be used by the individuals themselves in some cases or, in other cases, may be considered insulting. Individuals working together in provider–client interactions need to ensure that the terminology used is mutually understood and acceptable. Researchers and scholars need to strive for consensual cultural terminology so that research findings can be appropriately applied and compared.

Professional Recommendations

A number of healthcare organizations and regulatory bodies have developed standards and recommendations. The Office of Minority Health issued the Culturally and Linguistic Appropriate Services (CLAS) standards in an attempt to synthesize cultural competency definitions and requirements into a single set of standards. The CLAS standards contain a number of regulations and recommendations for organizations regarding the use of translations and providing culturally appropriate health care. Cultural and linguistic competence has been incorporated in the curricula of medicine, nursing, and other healthcare professions and endorsed by many professional organizations. It is reflected in standards and guidelines from a number of health regulatory agencies. Some promising studies do support positive impact on health and mental health outcomes from culturally and linguistically based programs for specific populations.

Other major governmental agencies have also emphasized the importance of cultural competency in the delivery of health care. The Agency for Healthcare Research and Quality (AHRQ) has a focus on health literacy and cultural competency and reducing health disparities.[44] The Health Resources and Service Administration (HRSA) also recommends enhancing cultural competency and has recommendations for organizations and reimbursement.[45] The Joint Commission has also put forth cultural competency standards that include patient- and family-centered care.[46] It is noteworthy that a number of national sources are now linking cultural competency with patient-centered care.

The American Academy of Nursing established a Nursing Expert Panel that made the following recommendations for the development of cultural competence and reduction of health disparities:[47]

Education: The integration of knowledge, skills, and basic competencies to develop sensitivity and competence in curricula.

Practice: Healthcare organizations provide a supportive climate for culturally competent care. This includes appreciation of complementary alternative therapies.

Research: Research on diversity, disparities, and culture is necessary. Inclusion of women and minorities for representative samples and adequate funding is needed.

Policy: Education of policymakers is needed to ensure funds and care in areas that can change outcomes.

Advocacy: Advocacy is needed for vulnerable populations.

Communication

All healthcare providers of the professional sector in the United States have acculturated to the biomedical model and accompanying technology by virtue of their education and the sociology of the healthcare institution where they practice. Each institution has its own culture that defines the norms, protocols, and hierarchy, both formal and informal. Most healthcare institutions are based on the biomedical model and accept clients into the system because of a perceived physical or mental disease or illness. In contrast, healers in the folk sector are more likely to approach health from a holistic perspective, with focus on the emotional and spiritual domains, as well as on the physical domain. Such healers have become acculturated to the holistic model through education, which is often based on an apprenticeship with a more experienced practitioner.

The purposes of communication in the healthcare environment are to create an interpersonal relationship, exchange information, and allow for decision making. Specific barriers may impede the achievement of these goals. First, communication between the provider and client generally involves individuals of unequal positions, with the provider assuming a higher rank to some extent simply by virtue of greater medical knowledge. Second, communication related to health care is often not planned, involves vitally important issues, and is emotionally laden. Finally, differences in language, both verbal and nonverbal, may isolate the client and the family. Nonverbal aspects of oral communication, such as voice tone, eye contact, and body positioning, are often as significant as verbal communication. If the cultural backgrounds of the provider and the client are significantly different, these communication factors may make it difficult to obtain and provide health care without misunderstandings.

Roles in the relationship between the provider and client are frequently derived from cultural norms and can enhance or impede communication. Such roles can be seen as a spectrum of control, ranging from paternalistic to mutualistic.[48] In a paternalistic (i.e., provider-centered) relationship, the provider has the control, directs care, makes decisions about treatment, and is authoritative. A mutual, client-centered relationship involves shared decision making and is more egalitarian. Problems can arise in communication and the therapeutic relationship if the expectations of the client do not match those of the provider with respect to control and decision making. Problems can also arise if communication styles, both nonverbal and verbal, differ. Such expectations are often culturally related,

and nurses can avoid some problems by developing sensitivity to various communication styles.

Use of Translators

The increasing number of languages and dialects in the United States means that nurses, even those who are bilingual, often rely on translators or interpreters to communicate with clients. Translators play powerful roles in the exchange of valuable information between nurses and their clients. The national CLAS standards require that language services be made available for all individuals with limited English proficiency who seek services at all institutions receiving federal funds. The California Endowment published National Standards of Practice for Interpreters in Health Care.[49] These standards are aligned with the National Code of Ethics and address the ethical issues of accuracy, confidentiality, impartiality, respect, cultural awareness, role boundaries, professionalism, professional development, and advocacy.

Bilingual staff or trained on-site interpreters are preferred over family members. If interpretation is needed immediately or the language is infrequently encountered, then telephone interpreter systems should be used. Untrained interpreters may provide misinformation to the client, but also may use words, tones, or gestures that emphasize the translator's own personal preferences, omit portions of a message deemed irrelevant, or diminish the importance of the intended message. Indeed, translators may dominate the conversation. It is best to avoid using family members as translators whenever possible because they are likely to filter information based on what they want the client to hear. Also, it might be culturally inappropriate for the client to discuss some health matters with certain family members. Additionally, not all interpreters fully understand issues of confidentiality. Regardless of the source or skill of the translator, nurses should attempt to do the following when using a translator:

1. Orient the client to the process and the purpose of using a translator.
2. Orient the translator to the topics to be covered, the client's situation, and the degree of accuracy required.

3. Avoid standing; sit so that the client can observe the nurse and make eye contact; avoid placing the translator between the nurse and the client.

4. Observe the client for nonverbal communication that does not match the message intended and request clarification.

5. Slow down the communication process.

6. Encourage the translator to let the nurse know when something is difficult to translate so that it may be reworded.

7. Limit the use of medical jargon, slang, and metaphors to reduce the chance for error.

8. Consider the impact of differences in gender, educational level, and socioeconomic status between the client and translator. This is particularly important when topics of a sensitive or personal nature are to be discussed.

9. Ask translators to translate in the client's own words and ask clients to repeat the information communicated to increase accuracy.[50]

■ HOLISTIC CARING PROCESS

Interactions between the healthcare provider and client are based on the communication between the two and reflect their respective cultures. Both the provider and the client bring their personal beliefs, values, and cultural backgrounds to the interaction. These factors then affect the transfer of information, decision making, adherence to treatment, and healing outcomes. The professional nature of the encounter brings the culture of the healthcare system into the exchange, even if the meeting occurs in the client's home or a community setting. An understanding of the cultural world of the client and the cultural world of the healthcare system enables the provider to deliver culturally appropriate care. Nurses often act as cultural brokers between the client and the biomedical culture.

A midrange theory of cultural negotiation for clinical nursing was proposed.[51] (See **Figure 30-2**.) This model links the holistic perspective of nursing theories with the pragmatic elements of the nursing process. This situates the clinical

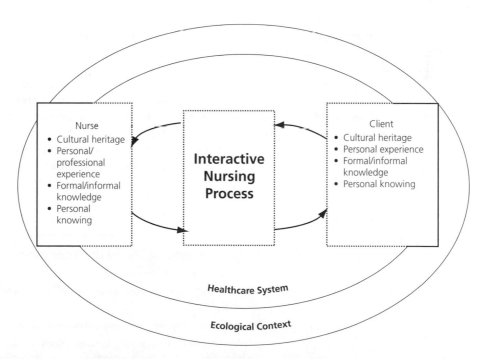

FIGURE 30-2   Cultural Negotiation Model for Nursing Practice
Source: J. Engebretson and L. Littleton, "Cultural Negotiation: A Constructivist-Based Model of Nursing Practice," *Nursing Outlook* 49, no. 5 (2001): 223–230. Copyright © Elsevier.

encounter between the patient and the clinician within the culture of the biomedical healthcare system, which is located within an ecological hierarchy of cultures reflecting the social world (e.g., Western culture). Both the nurse and the patient bring expert knowledge to this encounter. This expert knowledge includes cultural heritage, personal experiences, formal and informal knowledge, and personal knowing. Both also bring aspects of their cultural heritage and it is important that the nurse engage in some of the previously mentioned practices to become aware of these influences to better understand that of the patient. Both have a history of experiences. Patients have often had previous experiences with the healthcare system. Nurses have their professional/personal experiences as well. For example, a nurse may have experienced caring for patients from a specific culture or had personal experience as a patient, which influences her encounter with a patient. Nurses have formal knowledge that they bring to the encounter and they are responsible for applying this knowledge competently. Nurses are also exposed to a lot of informal knowledge. Currently, there is an abundance of health information available through the media. Patients also are exposed to various media and have varying levels of formal knowledge. Both nurse and patient have personal or intuitive knowledge that each bring to the encounter.

Central to this encounter is the nursing process. The nursing process is the basic problem-solving approach. Holistic nurses have long advocated that the process reflects an active

en-gagement between the patient and the clinician. This positions the patient to have more agency, or power, in the relationship than the classic nursing process in which the clinician has the agency and the patient complies. In this model the agency is fluid. For example, in a case in which the patient is too ill to exert much agency, the nurse and medical team assume more agency. In contrast, in health promotion or management of chronic conditions, the patient must assume greater agency. Consistent with this perspective, the steps in the nursing process are refigured (see **Exhibit 30-2**).

Holistic Assessment

In this model, nursing assessment becomes the exchange of expert knowledge. This focuses on the sharing of knowledge. The patient is the expert in knowledge about symptoms, history, perceptions, fears, concerns, and expectations. Nurses are experts in using technical skills, professional knowledge, and experience in the examination of the patient and incorporating information from laboratory reports and other medical data. In addition to uncovering explanatory models, the nurse could ask where the patient gets information about health issues and how the patient integrates that information into health practices.

Data from a brief assessment, including questions about ethnic background and religion, can be used to determine the need for a more in-depth assessment that focuses on specific parameters, such as nutritional patterns, social support networks, and beliefs about treatments

EXHIBIT 30-2   Nursing Process

Traditional Nursing Process Model	Negotiated Holistic Model of Nursing Process
Nursing assessment	Exchange of expert knowledge.
Nursing diagnosis	Analysis and interpretation of information from both client and nurse.
Planning	Joint decision making between client and nurse.
Intervention	Implementation of mutually derived plans for action with specific agreed upon actions for nurse and client.
Evaluation	Outcomes appraisal of goals and processes. This is also a mutual undertaking.

and coping. See **Exhibit 30-3** for some suggested areas to question patients to get a better understanding of their cultural orientations.

Nursing Diagnosis, or Analysis and Interpretation of the Information

The nurse begins to interpret and analyze the information and, at this point, brings in the use of both formal and informal knowledge and professional experience concerning problems, risks, patterns, challenges, and needs. Ideally, information is shared in this process so that the nurse can explain to and interpret medical matters for the client, begin the process of consolidating explanatory models, establish a foundation for further communication, and incorporate salient concerns of the patient.

Identification of Patterns/ Challenges/Needs

In addition to the impact of culture in the process of developing a mutual interpretation of needs and establishing common goals and plans for action, there may be specific concerns in the cultural domain. For example, a client's needs typically involve biophysical and psychological disturbances, alterations, impairments, and distresses. These patterns, challenges, and needs are largely derived from the conceptual areas of normalcy based on North American culture and heavily influenced by biomedicine. The patterns/ challenges/ needs (see Chapter 7) directly related to cultural interventions are as follows:

- Altered or impaired communication related to language differences or communication style—even with the aid of translators, language and dialect differences may exist based on the region in which the client was born (e.g., China and Mexico have multiple dialects)
- Altered or impaired social interaction related to sociocultural dissonance—difficulties in relating with members of the healthcare team may occur when there are gender, socioeconomic, or educational gaps
- Lack of adherence related to incongruent value systems between provider and client—clients may be considered noncompliant with follow-up appointments when differences in the perception of time are at the root of missed or late appointments
- Anxiety related to culturally unusual expectations for behavior and treatment; fear related to unknown environment or customs—the biomedical healthcare system may be particularly anxiety provoking for clients whose custom is to be cared for in the home during an illness

---

EXHIBIT 30-3   Suggested Areas for Cultural Assessment

Everyday health practices
- Nutritional patterns
- Exercise and physical activities
- Health and healing practices
- Sources of information about health

Family organization, structure, and role differentiation and child care practices
- Decision making: how made, who is involved, and why
- Health seeking: who, when, and how to consult about health issues
- Communication style and relationship toward authority
- Social support networks and relationships

Demographics, socioeconomic status, and employment patterns
- Spiritual beliefs, rituals, and practices
- Immigration and cultural history

Explanatory models of illness

Outcome Identification

Culturally appropriate outcomes are developed with the client. This incorporates the client's values and explanatory model expectations. This allows for accommodations of other outcomes beyond the disease treatment.

Therapeutic Care Plan and Interventions

The nurse and patient conjointly develop an approach to address the mutually identified concerns and the agreed upon goals. The patient discusses assets, barriers, and priorities, and the nurse shares expert knowledge and may suggest other resources. Based on the mutual decision making, alternative solutions and modalities may be incorporated into the plan of care. Explanatory models are often reflected in the care plan.

Cultural healing practices, unless there are clear counterindications, may be incorporated into the plan of care. Nurses should convey respect for the practice and should make every effort to acquire appropriate foods, people, artifacts, and so on, as well as to secure space and time for such practices. During this clinical process, Leininger's three modes of incorporating cultural practices may be evident:[52]

1. *Cultural preservation and maintenance* refers to professional actions that retain relevant care values to support aspects of the client's culture that positively influence his or her health care.
2. *Cultural accommodation and negotiation* refers to professional actions to bridge the gap between the client's culture and biomedicine for beneficial health outcomes, by recognizing the cultural relevance of a practice and integrating it into the treatment plan, even though the cultural practice has no scientific basis.
3. *Cultural repatterning and restructuring* refers to professional actions that assist the client in making changes in, but not discarding, practices that may be harmful to his or her well-being.

Therefore, a variety of healing modalities may be used, depending on the illness and cultural preferences. Two aspects of healing, touch and spiritual practices, have deep cultural meaning.

Touch, even as an element of communication, has culturally specific meanings. In some Arab and Hispanic cultures, male providers may be prohibited from examining or touching parts of the female body. Some Asians believe that the center of strength lies in the head, and touching the head is a sign of disrespect or threat. Thus, the process of shaving the head preoperatively may be viewed very negatively. Gentle touch may be seen as a caring gesture. Specific healing modalities using human touch are often viewed from an energetic or spiritual framework. Many cultures have traditions of "laying on of hands." Some patients may be suspicious if a nurse uses a touch therapy that is not consonant with or connected to their specific religious beliefs. Spiritual rituals or practices are associated with healing in many cultures. Rituals and practices to protect one from evil, disease, or danger include the use of amulets, talismans, ritualistic behavior, the avoidance of taboos, exorcism, and purification or cleansing rituals. Prayer and other spiritual practices are widely associated with healing. Rituals may be positive in nature, including those related to spiritual growth, redemption, and life transitions, such as birth or initiations into adulthood.[53] Often viewed as having divine gifts, healers or spiritual leaders are believed to be able to negotiate with the spiritual world through prayer, meditation, blessings, chants, and other primal religious experiences, many of which incorporate altered states of consciousness. Individuals also may seek healing forces by sacrifice, penance, and pilgrimages.

Evaluation

Together, the nurse, the client, and any member of the extended family or social group who the client feels is significant should evaluate desired client outcomes. Evaluation must be woven throughout the entire holistic caring process because it is essential to obtain validation through mutual understanding, especially when there are differences between the cultural backgrounds of nurse and client. It is important to note the purpose of the activity in evaluating its effectiveness. A massage that is given for the purpose of comfort needs to be evaluated on the basis of comfort, for example, not its medical effect on the disease process. A healing activity that is understood by the client as having multiple effects (e.g., spiritual benefits, psychological benefits, better health) should be evaluated on many levels and should not be discounted if the physical benefits are not comparable to those of a pharmaceutical product. Each component of the healthcare plan and each nursing intervention should be carefully examined to ensure that it is understandable and acceptable to the client, effective for achievement of short- and long-term goals, and appropriately revised as necessary during the evaluation process. Cultural modifications can be made upon careful evaluation.

Directions for
FUTURE RESEARCH

1. Survey patterns of usage of healing modalities from various paradigms and cultural backgrounds.
2. Develop efficient and effective ways of assessing the degree of acculturation in clients with various cultural backgrounds.
3. Analyze effective models for interaction between biomedical and traditional healthcare systems.
4. Evaluate the degree to which healthcare goals are achieved when nurses deliver culturally competent care.
5. Analyze various methods for teaching nursing students or staff how to provide culturally competent care.

Nurse Healer
REFLECTIONS

After reading this chapter, the nurse healer will be able to answer or to begin a process of answering the following questions:

- What are my values and beliefs regarding health and illness in relationship to models of healing?
- How do I feel when caring for clients whose cultural backgrounds differ from my own?
- What are my biases and attitudes toward clients with various cultural backgrounds?
- How can I determine whether I am offering culturally competent care in a holistic manner?

> *For a full suite of assignments and additional learning activities, use the access code located in the front of your book to visit this exclusive website: http://go.jblearning.com/dossey. If you do not have an access code, you can obtain one at the site.*

NOTES

1. Office of Minority Health, *National Standards for Culturally and Linguistically Appropriate Services in Health Care* (Washington, DC: U.S. Department of Health and Human Services, March 2001). http://minorityhealth.hhs.gov/assets/pdf/checked/executive.pdf.
2. T. Cross et al., *Toward a Culturally Competent System of Care*, vol. 1 (Washington, DC: CASSP Technical Assistance Center, Georgetown University Child Development Center, 1989).
3. J. Engebretson et al., "Cultural Competence in the Era of Evidence-Based Practice," *Journal of Professional Nursing* 24, no. 3 (2008): 172–178.
4. S. Strauss et al., *Evidence-Based Medicine: How to Practice and Teach EBM*, 2nd ed. (New York, NY Elsevier Churchill Livingstone, 2005).
5. J. Campinha-Bacote, "A Model and Instrument for Addressing Cultural Competence in Health Care," *Journal of Nursing Education* 38 (2001): 204–207.
6. M. Douglas, "Developing Frameworks for Providing Culturally Competent Health Care," *Journal of Transcultural Nursing* 13 (2002): 177.
7. L. Purnell and B. Paulanka, *Transcultural Health Care: A Culturally Competent Approach* (Philadelphia, PA: F. A. Davis, 1998).
8. J. Giger and R. Davidhizar, *Transcultural Nursing: Assessment and Intervention*, 5th ed. (St. Louis, MO: Mosby, 2007).
9. R. E. Spector, *Cultural Diversity in Health and Illness*, 5th ed. (Upper Saddle River, NJ: Prentice Hall, 2000).
10. M. Leininger, *Culture Care Diversity and Universality: A Theory of Nursing* (Sudbury, MA: Jones and Bartlett, 2001).
11. J. G. Lipson and L. A. Desantis, "Current Approaches to Integrating Elements of Cultural Competence in Nursing Education," *Journal of Transcultural Nursing* 18, no. 1 (2007): 10S–20S.
12. M. C. Beach et al., "Cultural Competence: A Systematic Review of Health Care Provider Educational Interventions," *Medical Care* 43, no. 4 (2005): 356–373.

13. J. R. Betancourt, "Cultural Competency: Providing Quality Care to Diverse Populations," *Consultant Pharmacist* 21, no. 12 (2006): 988–995.

14. J. R. Betancourt and A. R. Green, "Commentary: Linking Cultural Competence Training to Improved Health Outcomes: Perspectives from the Field," *Academic Medicine* 85, no. 4 (2010): 583–585.

15. G. R. Gregg and S. Saha, "Losing Culture on the Way to Competence: The Use and Misuse of Culture in Medical Education," *Academic Medicine* 41 (2006): 1–8.

16. M. Dreher and N. MacNaughton, "Cultural Competence in Nursing: Foundation or Fallacy?" *Nursing Outlook* 50, no. 5 (2002): 181–186.

17. F. Collins, "Genomics and Health Disparities," in *Disparities in Health in America: Working Toward Social Justice* (Houston, TX: Summer Workshop, 2003).

18. M. F. MacDorman and T. J. Mathews, "Infant Deaths—United States 2000-2007," *Morbidity and Mortality Weekly Report* 60, no. 1 (January 14, 2011): 49–51. http://www.cdc.gov/mmwr/preview/mmwrhtml/su6001a9.htm.

19. Centers for Disease Control and Prevention, "CDC Health Disparities and Inequalities Report—United States, 2011," *Morbidity and Mortality Weekly Report* 60, suppl. (January 14, 2011). http://www.cdc.gov/mmwr/pdf/other/su6001.pdf.

20. N. E. Adler and K. Newman, "Socioeconomic Disparities in Health: Pathways and Policies" and "Inequality in Education, Income, and Occupation Exacerbates the Gaps Between the Health 'Haves' and 'Have-nots,' " *Health Affairs* 21 (2002): 60–76.

21. V. J. Burroughs, R. W. Maxey, and R. A. Levy, "Racial and Ethnic Differences in Response to Medicines: Towards Individualized Pharmaceutical Treatment," *Journal of the National Medical Association* 94, no. 10 (2002): S1–S25.

22. A. Rundle et al., eds., *Cultural Competence in Health Care: A Practice Guide* (San Francisco, CA: Jossey-Bass, 1999).

23. T. R. Marmor,, M. L. Barer, and R. G. Evans, "*Why Are Some People Healthy and Others Not?: The Determinants of Healthy Populations*" (New York, NY: Aldine de Gruyter, 1994).

24. M. Lock and D. Gordon, *Biomedicine Examined* (Dordrecht, Netherlands Kluwer Academic Publishers, 1988).

25. K. Kipnis, "Quality Care and the Wounds of Diversity" (paper presented at the meeting of the American Society for Bioethics and Humanities, Houston, TX, November 18, 1998).

26. E. R. Oetting and F. Beauvais, "Orthogonal Cultural Identification Theory: The Cultural Identification of Minority Adolescents," *International Journal of Addiction* 5A, 6A (1990–1991): 655–685.

27. J. Achterberg, *Woman as Healer* (Boston, MA: Shambhala, 1990).

28. J. Engebretson, "Comparison of Nurses and Alternative Healers," *Journal of Nursing Scholarship* 28 (1996): 95–99.

29. F. R. Kluckhohn, "Dominant and Variant Value Orientations," in *Transcultural Nursing: A Book of Readings*, ed. P. J. Brink (Englewood Cliffs, NJ: Prentice Hall, 1976): 63–81.

30. J. Engebretson, "Considerations in Diagnosing in the Spiritual Domain," *Nursing Diagnosis* 7 (1996): 100–107.

31. N. Postman, *Technopoly* (New York, NY: Vintage Books, 1993).

32. P. H. Ray, "The Emerging Culture," *American Demographics* 19 (February 1997): 28–34. http://www.demographics.com.

33. J. A. Astin, "Why Clients Use Alternative Medicine," *Journal of the American Medical Association* 279 (1998): 1548–1553.

34. D. M. Eisenberg et al., "Trends in Alternative Medicine Use in the United States, 1990–1997," *Journal of the American Medicine Association* 280 (1998): 1569–1575.

35. U.S. Census Bureau, *2010 Census Briefs*: The Black Population 2010. http://www.census.gov/prod/cen2010/briefs/c2010br-06.pdf.

36. U.S. Census Bureau, *2000 Census Briefs and Special Reports*. http://www.census.gov/population/www/cen2000/briefs.html.

37. M. M. Andrews and J. S. Boyle, eds., *Transcultural Concepts in Nursing Care*, 4th ed. (Philadelphia, PA: J. B. Lippincott, 2002).

38. M. O. Loustaunau and E. J. Sobo, *The Cultural Context of Health, Illness, and Medicine* (Westport, CT: Bergin & Garvey Press, 1997).

39. A. Kleinman, *Patients and Healers in the Context of Culture: An Exploration of the Borderland Between Anthropology, Medicine and Psychiatry* (Berkeley, CA: University of California Press, 1980).

40. J. Giger and R. Davidhizar, *Transcultural Nursing: Assessment and Intervention*, 3rd ed. (St. Louis, MO: Mosby, 1999).

41. J. Engebretson, "A Multiparadigm Approach to Nursing," *Advances in Nursing Science* 20 (1997): 22–34.

42. T. J. Kaptchuk, *The Web That Has No Weaver: Understanding Chinese Medicine* (New York, NY: Congdon & Weed, 1983).

43. J. S. Levin, "Religion and Health: Is There an Association, Is It Valid and Is It Causal?" *Social Science in Medicine* 29 (1994): 589–600.

44. Agency for Healthcare Research and Quality (AHRQ), *Cultural and Linguistic Competency*. http://www.ahrq.gov/browse/hlitix.htm#Cultural.

45. Health Resources and Services Administration, home page. http://www.hrsa.gov.

46. Joint Commission, "Advancing Effective Communication, Cultural Competence, and Patient- and Family-Centered Care: A Roadmap for Hospitals," (2010). http://www.jointcommission.org/Advancing_Effective_Communication/.

47. J. Giger et al., "American Academy of Nursing Expert Panel Report: Developing Cultural Competence to Eliminate Health Disparities in Ethnic Minorities and Other Vulnerable Populations," *Journal of Transcultural Nursing* 18, no. 95 (2007): 95–102.

48. D. W. Sue and D. Sue, *Counseling the Culturally Different: Theory and Practice*, 4th ed. (New York, NY: John Wiley & Sons, 2003).

49. National Council on Interpreting in Health Care, *National Standards of Practice for Interpreters in Health Care* (Washington, DC: National Council on Interpreting in Health Care, September 2005). http://mchb.hrsa.gov/training/documents/pdf_library/National_Standards_of_Practice_for_Interpreters_in_Health_Care%20(12-05).pdf.

50. C. Degazon, "Cultural Diversity and Community Health Nursing Practice," in *Community Health Nursing: Promoting Health of Aggregates, Families and Individuals*, 4th ed., ed. M. Stanhope and J. Lancaster (St. Louis, MO: Mosby, 1996): 117–134.

51. J. Engebretson and L. Littleton, "Cultural Negotiation: A Constructivist-Based Model for Nursing Practice," *Nursing Outlook* 49 (2001): 223–230.

52. M. M. Leininger and M. R. McFarland, *Transcultural Nursing: Concepts, Theories, Research and Practices*, 3rd ed. (New York, NY: McGraw-Hill, Medical Publishing Division, 2002).

53. D. Kinsley, *Health, Healing, and Religion: A Cross-Cultural Perspective* (Upper Saddle River, NJ: Prentice Hall, 1996).

CORE VALUE 4

Holistic Education and Research

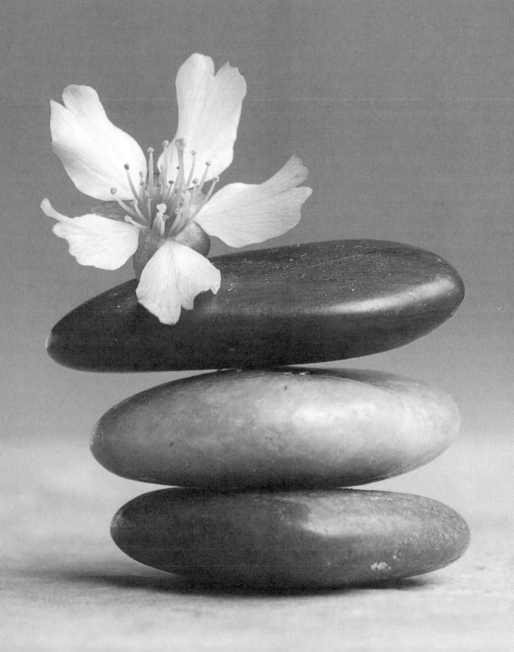

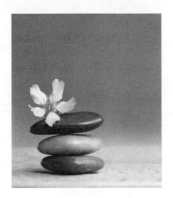

Chapter 31

The Psychophysiology of Body–Mind Healing

Genevieve M. Bartol and Nancy F. Courts

Nurse Healer
OBJECTIVES

Theoretical

- Articulate a comprehensive conceptual model of body–mind interactions.
- Interpret the application of selected models, theories, and research in the field of psychoneuroimmunology.
- Explain the interconnections of mind modulation and the autonomic, endocrine, immune, and neuropeptide systems.

Clinical

- Recognize the implications of body–mind interactions for clinical practice.
- Incorporate the knowledge of body–mind interactions in planning nursing interventions.

Personal

- Identify one's own patterns of body–mind interactions as expressed in attitudes, tensions, and images.
- Recognize the implications of one's own body–mind patterns for self-care and self-healing.

DEFINITIONS

Allostasis: The adaptation process to maintain homeostasis and well-being.

Allostatic load: Occurs when one experiences overwhelming stress or has inadequate coping skills.

Autopoiesis: The self-organizing force in living systems.

Bifurcation: A point at which transformational change occurs in a complex system; at a fork in the road of life.

Body–mind: A state of integration that includes body, mind, and spirit.

Chaos: The stable and orderly but irregular, unpredictable behavior of a complex system.

Cycles: One of the simplest nonlinear behaviors that is periodic and recurrent.

Epigenetics: The study of how genes produce their effect on the phenotype of the organism.

Information Theory: A mathematical model that helps explain the connections between consciousness and body–mind healing.

Limbic-hypothalamic system: The major anatomic modulating link connecting the brain/mind and the autonomic, endocrine, immune, and neuropeptide systems.

Mind modulation: The bidirectional interrelationships of thoughts and feelings with neurohormonal messengers of the nervous, endocrine, immune, and neuropeptide systems that support body–mind connections.

Network: Interconnected and interrelated system.

Neuropeptides: Messenger molecules produced at various sites throughout the body to transmit body–mind patterns of communication.

Neuroplasticity: The ability of the nervous system to respond to intrinsic and/or extrinsic stimuli by reorganizing its structure, function, and connections.

Neurotransmitters: Chemicals that facilitate the transmission of impulses through nerves in the body.

Psychoneuroimmunology: A branch of science that strives to show the connections among psychology, neuroendocrinology, and immunology.

Receptors: Sites on cell surfaces that serve as points of attachment for various types of messenger molecules.

Self-Regulation Theory: A person's ability to learn cognitive processing of information to bring involuntary body responses under voluntary control.

Traumatic stress response (TSR): Occurs when the normal stress response is altered as a result of overwhelming and/or ongoing stress.

■ NEW SCIENTIFIC UNDERSTANDING OF LIVING SYSTEMS

Developments in science and concomitant advances in technology continue to reveal human beings in new ways. The mechanistic view of the body–mind has given way to a holistic view. The habit of looking at persons from their component parts while ignoring interactions and contexts is misleading and creates problems of its own. The body can no longer be considered a machine powered by the mind or spirit to which healthcare practitioners apply assorted therapies to effect healing. Humans are complex, highly integrative systems embedded in and supporting other systems. As we free our scientific imagination and increase our knowledge of laws that are the opposite of mechanistic, such as the concepts of nonlocality and superposition of states in quantum physics, our understanding of living systems will continue to change.[1,2] The term *body–mind* can include the body, mind, and spirit as a unified whole.

Quantum Theory

Discoveries in quantum physics negate the old ways of viewing phenomena. Heisenberg described the changed world as a complicated tissue of events, in which connections of different kinds alternate, overlap, or combine, and thereby determine the texture of the whole.[3] In the past, the properties and behavior of the parts were believed to determine those of the whole. Now it is clear that the whole also defines the behavior of the parts.

The realization that systems are integrated wholes that cannot be understood simply by analysis shattered scientific certitude. No longer was it possible to believe that given enough time, effort, and money, all questions would have answers. Rather, all scientific concepts and theories have limitations. Scientific explanations do not provide complete and conclusive answers, but instead generate other questions.[4] The more we learn, the more we discover how much we do not know. Even one additional piece of data can change the whole configuration. It is important to remain open to all possibilities because absolute certainty is an illusion.[2pp25 26]

Increasingly, scientific findings demonstrate a changing world. Planck found radiant energy was emitted from light sources in discrete amounts or *quanta*, and that changes in the amount of radiant energy occurred in leaps, not sequential steps.[3] Bohr extended Planck's discovery to the field of subatomic particles and showed that electrons could move from one orbit of energy to another. The behavior of light does not follow one set of rules. Light possesses the qualities of both waves and particles. One explanation is not correct and the other wrong; both interpretations are useful in explaining the behavior of light in different situations.

The world is complex and unified; parts complement one another and participate in the whole. Similarly, all parts of the body work together. Health and illness are indivisible; both are natural and necessary. Hyperpyrexia (fever) may be seen as a sign of illness as well as a sign of the body's healthy response to a threat. Fever indicates that the hypothalamic setpoint of the body has changed.[5] The alteration occurs in the presence of pyrogens (e.g., bacteria, viruses).

A mild temperature elevation up to 39 degrees Centigrade (102.2 degrees Fahrenheit) stimulates the body's immune system, increases white blood cell production, and reduces the concentration of iron in blood plasma, thereby suppressing the growth of bacteria. Fever also stimulates the production of interferon, which protects the body against viruses. Using medications to lower the body temperature prematurely, particularly in the first 24 hours, may actually interfere with this important defense mechanism.

Systems Theory

The major traits of systems thinking appeared concurrently in several disciplines during the first half of the 20th century, but it was von Bertalanffy's General Systems Theory that established systems thinking as the predominant scientific movement.[6] Resultant theories and models of living systems initiated a radical shift in the understanding of human beings. It is now believed that persons and their environments make up an interconnected dynamic system in which a change at any point may effect changes at other points. The idea that the world is hierarchical, with each level organized separately, has been replaced with a new understanding of relatedness and context.

Human beings are living systems, organizationally closed and structurally open, embedded within the web of life.[7] They are *organizationally closed* because they are self-organizing; that is, they establish their own order and behavior rather than submitting to those imposed by the environment. They are *structurally open* because they engage in a continual exchange of energy and matter with their environment. Words like *feedback, integration, rhythm,* and *dynamic equilibrium* account for the continually changing components of living systems. These components do not operate in isolation from each other. A dysfunction in any one system of the body reverberates in the other systems. For example, a dysfunction of the endocrine system referred to as hypothyroidism may manifest itself by thinning hair or clinical depression.[8] Hypothyroidism, in fact, may be secondary to a dysfunction in another organ system and not represent primary failure of the thyroid gland. Thyroid deficiency may occur when the pituitary gland is malfunctioning or when there is damage to the hypothalamus. It is not possible to identify conclusively a single cause of what was formerly named a primary dysfunction. All body systems participate in the biodance; changes in one system result in changes in the other systems and, in circular fashion, changes in itself, just as the pituitary gland increases its secretion of thyroid-stimulating hormone (TSH) when the thyroid gland is underproducing thyroid hormone.

Theory of Relativity

Einstein developed a system of mechanics that acknowledges the relative character of motion, velocity, and mass, as well as the interdependence of matter, time, and space.[3] The theory is based on the principle that there is no absolute frame of reference independent of the observer. Each person views others from his or her own perspective, including his or her particular biases.

Scientists can no longer describe their work as finding a piece to a puzzle or as adding a building stone to a firm foundation of knowledge. Rather, it has become increasingly apparent that scientific knowledge is a network of concepts and models, none of which is any more fundamental than the other. All things (objects) and events (happenings) in one's life are connected and relative within the whole. The mind and body are inseparably intertwined. Whatever happens in one's life is interconnected. Thoughts, feelings, and actions influence a person's state of health and illness, as discussed in this chapter.

Koenig and associates reported that Christian persons who attend religious services at least once per week and who read the Bible or pray regularly have consistently lower diastolic blood pressure readings than those who do not.[9,10] A lower diastolic reading, which indicates the blood pressure when the heart relaxes, is associated with improved health. It is not known how these religious activities influence the blood pressure or if a specific spiritual orientation accompanies these activities and accounts for the difference.

Studies using imaging devices show that mindfulness meditation strengthens the neurological circuits that calm a part of the brain that acts as a trigger for fear and anger and increases the amount of activity in the brain associated with positive emotions. Fear and anger can provoke harmful actions. Happiness and inner balance are crucial to survival. We need to cultivate our inner development if we are to keep our destructive emotions in control.[11]

Principles of Self-Organization

The key ideas of current models of self-organizing systems were refined and extended during the 1970s and 1980s, and a unified theory of living systems emerged.[7,12] This unified theory encompassed the creation of structures and modes of behavior in the processes of development, learning, and coevolution. In the past, living systems were viewed from two perspectives: in terms of physical matter (structure) and the configuration of relationships (pattern). Structure is concerned with quantities, things weighed and measured. Pattern is concerned with qualities and is expressed by a map of the configuration of relationships. Qualities, such as color or size, were considered accidental characteristics. A bicycle may be red or green; may stand 24 or 26 inches high; may have a light or heavy frame, but remains a bicycle as long as it has the configuration of relationships consistent with a bicycle.

Systems, whether nonliving or living, are configurations of ordered relationships whose attributes are the properties of pattern. The bicycle, a nonliving system, consists of a number of components arranged to perform a particular function. The various kinds of bicycles (e.g., mountain bicycles, touring bicycles) embody the essential characteristics known as a bicycle. In brief, bicycles have a structure with specific components and operate as bicycles as long as the pattern of relationships that defines them as bicycles remains.[12p85] Living systems, however, are fundamentally different from nonliving systems. Living systems do not function mechanically and are not explained just by physical principles. The components of living systems are interconnected by internal feedback loops in a nonlinear fashion and are capable of self-organization.

Not only is the activity of living systems purposeful, but also it appears to be under the direction of an overall design or purpose.[7p40]

The pattern of organization of living systems includes a fundamental self-organizing force known as autopoiesis.[13] If the pattern of a living system is destroyed, the system dies even though all the components of the system remain intact. A living system cannot be restored simply by re-creating the pattern. However, a nonliving system, like a bicycle, will regain function if the parts are reassembled correctly. Living systems do not rest in a steady state of balance as do nonliving systems but rather operate far from equilibrium.[14] Stability in living systems embodies change. Relationships are not linear, but extend in all directions. Bifurcation occurs and generates new feedback loops.[7pp38-39] Living systems regulate and re-create themselves.

Life process (cognition) is the link between pattern and structure in a living system.[13pp150-162] Life process is "the activity involved in the continual embodiment of the system's pattern of organization."[13p162] It is related to autopoiesis, and they may be considered two distinct facets of the same phenomenon of life. All living systems are cognitive systems, and cognition indicates the existence of an autopoietic network.[15] Structure, pattern, and process are inextricably intertwined in a living system.

Organisms appear to be under the direction of an overall design or purpose and do not just function mechanically. For example, the symptoms experienced by humans represent attempts to gain health and, therefore, are signals of stability, not breakdown. The human immune system recognizes an invading organism as dangerous and quickly reacts to counter the threat. Symptoms are really signs of the inherent organization and adaptability of a living system. We cannot unerringly predict the outcome of these complex relationships among organisms—one person may become sick and die while another may be seemingly unaffected and yet infect others with whom he has contact. Even invading organisms, also living systems, learn and adapt. The ability of pathogens to modify themselves and develop resistance to antibiotics is a striking example of the ability of a living system to reorganize.

Bell's Theorem

Cause-and-effect thinking with its before, after, now, and later sequence is no longer acceptable.

According to Bell's Theorem, the whole determines the actions of the parts, and changes occur instantaneously.[7pp35-36,16] Experience teaches us that not all people respond in the same way to the same treatment. Peptic ulcers, for example, were once considered the result of excessive production of stomach acid stemming from stress. Treatment was directed toward reducing the stress with rest and counteracting the acid with a special diet. Some patients recovered after submitting to this regimen; others did not. Did those who recovered do so because of the treatment of diet and rest or did some other intervening factor bring about this change? Surely for some, the enforced rest increased their stress and the restrictive diet exacerbated the ulcer. We have since learned that peptic ulcers are associated with a common bacterium and may be healed with an antibiotic. We also learned that we can prevent the development of peptic ulcer in patients experiencing stress from trauma with prophylactic administration of ranitidine hydrochloride (Zantac).

Even a fleeting thought or a passing feeling can hasten or hinder recovery. Changes do not happen in an orderly stepwise sequence. Healing does not take time, but is dependent on hope and belief beyond time. Beliefs, thoughts, and feelings are all part of the configuration, and each affects the human states of wellness and illness. Individuals have personal preferences for coping with adverse events. Miller classifies people as monitors and blunters.[17] Monitors need information to reduce their stress whereas blunters prefer distraction. Explaining the details of upcoming surgery to a monitor can be expected to reduce stress and promote healing. Blunters prefer to trust in the skills of the caregiver and do not even want to hear how that will be accomplished.

Personality and Wellness

Researchers have unsuccessfully tried to link specific illnesses with particular personality constellations.[18] Yet, individuals with peptic ulcers have as many personality configurations as does the general population. Several researchers, however, have uncovered particular personality traits associated with wellness.[10pp713-715,15pp683-688,19] Schwartz discovered that persons who with will-

ful, mindful effort attend to symptoms, sensations, and feelings and who believe they can do something about their symptoms can alter their brain chemistry and move toward health. Kabat-Zinn found that healthy attention and meditation helped persons effectively cope with chronic illness and intractable pain. Pennebaker found that persons who admit their feelings to themselves and others have healthier psychological profiles and had fewer illnesses than those who do not.

Scientific studies of forgiveness have revealed that whenever people choose to forgive a transgression, areas in the emotional limbic center of the brain are activated.[20] The activity decreases when the person focuses on the unfairness of the situation, but increases when the person imagines forgiving the offender. Multifaceted research studies on the relationship of forgiveness and health repeatedly show that forgiveness is good for our physical, mental, and emotional well-being. Not forgiving creates a state of anger, bitterness, hostility, and possibly hatred that leads to a stress response and increases the risk of illness.

There is increasing interest in the benefits of positive emotions on the immune system.[21] Altogether, studies suggest that transient positive mood states such as humor and joy are associated with an up-regulation of components of the innate immune system among healthy volunteers and a reduction in allergic responses among allergy sufferers. Even though a direct cause-and-effect relationship between any personality factor and health or illness cannot be determined, the research suggests that developing personality strengths to protect one from the stresses of living seems to bolster one's defense against illness.

Information Theory

Patterns of communication and patterns of organization in organisms can be viewed analogously.[13] Information Theory, a mathematical model, was developed to define and measure amounts of information transmitted through telegraph and telephone lines. The theory was used to explain how to get a message coded as a signal to determine what to charge customers. A coded message (signal) is essentially a pattern of organization. Information flow (i.e., pattern of communication and pattern of organization) in human beings is able to unify physiologic, psychological, sociological, and spiritual phenomena in a holistic framework. Information flow is the missing piece that makes it possible to transcend the body–mind split because information resides in both the body and the mind. Our emotions and feelings are sources of vital information. Emotions-proper are life-regulating phenomena that help maintain our health by making adaptive changes in our body states and form the basis for feelings.[22] The information generated by these processes is designed to be protective and is more complex than reflexes.[23]

Santiago Theory of Cognition

Derived from the study of neural networks, the Santiago Theory of Cognition is linked to the concept of autopoiesis.[13] Cognition is generally defined as the process of knowing or perceiving; it is associated with the mind, implicitly with the brain and nervous system. The Santiago Theory offers a radical expansion of the traditional concept of cognition. In this new view, cognition involves the whole process of life, including perception, emotion, and behavior. Even the cells that make up the immune system perceive the characteristics of their environment and will, for example, move to the site of a wound and increase in numbers to deal with an invading organism. Despite the absence of a brain, cognition is present; in this event, it can be described as embodied action.[13p268] Perception and action in these cells are inseparable.

A living organism is an interconnected network (system) that undergoes structural change while preserving its pattern of organization as it interacts with other systems.[7] Changes in both autopoietic networks take place. In other words, one living system may trigger an autopoietic network response in the other, but does not direct or control the response. A living organism chooses which stimuli from the environment will trigger structural changes. Moreover, not all changes in an organism are acts of cognition. A person who is injured in an accident does not specify and direct those structural changes, for example. Other structural changes (e.g., perception and response of the circulatory system) that accompany the imposed changes are acts of cognition.

Fundamental shifts in our understanding of the human mind help explain how humans receive, generate, and transduce information. New ideas and events evoke body–mind changes; that is, neural pathways and consciousness couple to enable information transduction.[24] For example, a client with severe episodes of asthma that increasingly interfere with her activities may remember that her mother's asthma became more severe as she aged, and she may begin to become despondent at what she views as an inevitable decline in her health. Subsequently, a nurse teaches her how to monitor her asthma with the help of a flow meter. The client begins to see a pattern to her attacks and identifies potential triggers. She gains a new understanding of body–mind connections and uses both traditional and holistic interventions to avoid the triggers. These interventions lead to a change in the pattern of her attacks and provide her with a greater sense of control. The asthma attacks decrease in severity and frequency. The client acquired a new understanding of the interconnectedness of body-mind-spirit and used this information to transform her response.

The extent of the interactions that a living system can have with its environment outlines its "cognitive domain."[13p175] Emotions are not just an accompaniment of perception and behavior but are an inherent part of this domain. For example, a fear response to a situation initiates an entire pattern of physiologic processes. Blood goes to the large skeletal muscles, making it easier to run, while the face blanches. Freezing for a moment allows time to assess the situation and determine whether hiding might be a wiser choice. Circuits in the brain's emotional centers trigger a flood of hormones that sounds a general alert. Although experience and culture modify responses, emotions occur simultaneously with and are part of every cognitive act.

■ EMOTIONS AND THE NEURAL TRIPWIRE

The traditional view in neuroscience has been that the sensory organs transmit signals to the thalamus and from there to the sensory process areas of the neocortex, which translates the signals into perceptions and attaches meanings.[22] The signals then move to the limbic system, which sends the appropriate response to the body. This has all changed, however, with the discovery of a smaller bundle of neurons that leads directly from the thalamus to the amygdala—in addition to those that connect with the neocortex (see **Figure 31-1**). Sensory impulses go directly from the sensory organs to the amygdala, allowing for a faster response. The amygdala triggers an emotional response even before the person fully understands what is happening. Taking immediate action, the amygdala sends impulses through the brain to the body. If the stimulus is traumatic, the amygdala responds with extra strength. Key changes take place in the locus ceruleus, which regulates catecholamines; adrenaline and noradrenaline are released. Other limbic structures, such as the hippocampus and the hypothalamus, respond, and the main stress hormones bring about the typical body responses labeled *fight, flight, faint,* or *freeze.* Changes in the brain opioid system that secretes endorphins prepare the person to meet the danger. Meanwhile, the neocortex processes the impulse, and a more considered response follows. Emotions are not dispensable, but rather an integral part of the whole.

State-Dependent Memory and Recall

What people learn depends on their mood or feelings at the time of the experience.[25] Feelings are integral to human living; not just an extravagance or an annoyance. The emotion-carrying molecules or ligands, which accompany all human activity, bind to cellular receptors and send an informational message to the cell where they can be stored as memories.

Feelings and actions are intertwined. People are more likely to help others when they are in a good mood and more likely to hurt others when they are in a bad mood. Likewise, feelings and memories are intertwined. Thoughts that occur throughout daily routines are repeated patterns of memories and their associative emotional connections. Memories

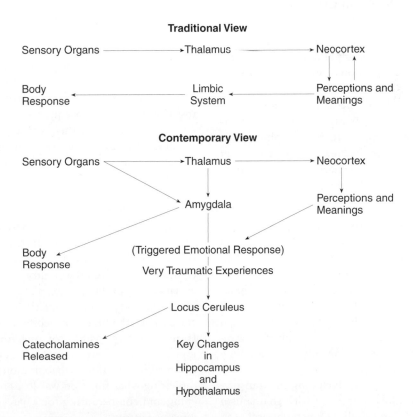

FIGURE 31-1   Emotions and the Neural Tripwire
Copyright © Genevieve Bartol.

are accompanied by emotions that, in turn, are influenced and affected by the context in which they were acquired. A particularly traumatic experience is stamped in the memory with special strength. Subsequent stimuli in new situations and emotional experiences can attach to and reawaken past memories. These reactivated thoughts and emotions direct and shape our actions in the present.

Feelings or mood also plays a major role in body–mind healing. Recent work with persons suffering from posttraumatic stress disorder (PTSD) has revealed that relearning is the route to healing. Writing therapy, bibliotherapy, body-work, art therapy, and even the traditional talk therapies are all ways of unfreezing a picture frozen in the amygdala that is capable of triggering the fight, flight, freeze, or faint response provoked by seemingly benign stimuli. Because people have network responses with the systems that they contain and those within which they nest, healing can occur from multiple directions.[26]

Location of the Brain Centers

Brain function may be best understood using the model of a hologram. A hologram is a specially processed photographic record that provides a three-dimensional image when a light from a laser is beamed through it. If any part of the hologram should be destroyed, any one of the remaining parts is capable of reconstructing the whole image. This holographic model is congruent with the new understanding of the way in which information is transmitted, received, and stored (learned).

- Memories are not stored in any specific part of the brain, but rather in multiple overlapping areas. They can be retrieved in their entirety by a stimulus to more than one area of the brain. Loss of specific memory is related more to the amount of brain damage than to the site of the injury.
- The ability to recall what was lost when gunshot wounds injure the brain, for example, often returns. The brain has the ability to grow whole new neurons.
- Paranormal events, including the transpersonal healing associated with shamanism and other approaches to metaphysical heal-

ing, involve communicating information in ways that do not conform to the current understanding of receiving, processing, and sending energy.
- Phenomena such as phantom limb sensations and auras that extend beyond the corpus challenge traditional perceptions of body image, as well as the understanding of the physical boundaries of the body.
- Mechanisms of consciousness, such as the ability of the person to reflect on the self or create and retrieve images, cannot be explained simply in terms of the structure and function of current anatomic models. Experience can change brain structure.

Viewing the brain in a holographic manner reveals its influence on psychophysiologic functioning. People who believe that they do not have the conscious ability to effect a physical change with their imagination do not try to do so. They will not explore memories and patterns formed of past experience and will continue to respond unconsciously as they always have in the past. Cognitive therapy is an example of an attempt to modify negative irrational thinking that leads to emotional distress. People are taught strategies that help them evaluate their thoughts, challenge them, and replace them with more rational responses, thereby reducing the negative consequences of stress and enhancing health. Furthermore, the revolutionary discovery of the neuroplasticity of the brain is opening new worlds of possibility in human development.[10p719,24pp137–141,27]

Neuroplasticity

It was once believed that the hardware of the brain was fixed and immutable. According to that belief, the brain virtually establishes all its connections, such as the auditory cortex and the visual cortex, in the first years of life. Depictions of the specific areas and functions of the different parts of the brain were commonly accepted. If an area responsible for one function was injured, it was believed no other area of the brain assumed its function. Rehabilitation focused on forgetting what function was lost and strengthening and compensating for whatever function remained intact.

Current neurorehabilitation efforts not only compensate for the loss of cognitive abilities, but also are directed to restore those abilities. Now we acknowledge that the brain can respond to altered sensory inputs and reprogram itself to resume previous functions. Furthermore, our brain is continuously getting rewired in keeping with the world of digital technology and the information revolution. The human brain changes throughout a person's lifetime. The changes are reflected in our new vocabulary. Consider such terms as *digital technology*, *cyberspace*, and *collective intelligence* and how they bring about neural rewiring. Reflect on how Facebook, LinkedIn, and Twitter are changing our communication patterns and making new neural connections in response to the intercultural world of the global society in which we live.[28]

Epigenetics

Furthermore, our genes are not fixed; we are not simply genetically determined. Our genes are modulated by our inner environment—the emotional, chemical, mental, energetic, and spiritual landscape—as well as our outer environment—the social and ecological systems in which we reside. Genes may be activated or deactivated by the meaning we assign to an experience. Truly we are formed and molded by the thoughts that stimulate the formation of neural pathways that either reinforce old patterns or initiate new ones.

The process by which a gene produces a result in the body is well established. Signals pass through the cell membrane to the nucleus, enter the chromosome, and activate a specific strand of DNA. Each strand of DNA is protected by a protein. The protein serves as a barrier between the information contained in the DNA and the rest of the intracellular environment. As long as the DNA is wrapped by the protein, the DNA lies dormant. When a signal arrives, the protein around the DNA unwraps and, with the assistance of RNA, the DNA molecule replicates an intermediate template molecule. At this point, the targeted gene moves into active expression where it creates other actions within the cell by constructing, assembling, or altering products. What was dormant potential is moved into active expression by a signal that comes from

outside the cell and not from the DNA. This process may take 1 second or hours.[29,30]

According to McClellen, Korosi, Cope, and Baram, epigenetic mechanisms program gene expression.[31] Key neuronal genes are fine tuned by early life experience and govern learning and memory throughout life. Enriched postnatal experience enhances spatial learning, whereas chronic early life stress may result in persistent deficits in the structure and function of hippocampal neurons. Graff, Kim, Dobbin, and Tsai note that epigenetic mechanisms are an integral part of a multitude of brain functions, including basic neuronal functions and higher-order cognitive processes.[32] Wright discusses the role of stress in the development of asthma.[33] Evidence suggests that maternal stress influences programming of integrated physiologic systems in the offspring beginning in pregnancy, suggesting stress effects may be transgenerational. Biological, psychological, and social processes clearly interact throughout life to influence the expression of strengths as well as disorders. De Sevo annotates 16 websites for readers who would like additional timely, reliable, genetic and genomic information.[34]

■ MIND MODULATION

Indirect and direct anatomic and biochemical pathways connect the neuroendocrine, nervous, and immune regulatory systems.[35] Communication among these systems is multidirectional with signal molecules and their receptors regulating the cellular outcomes. Feedback loops, up-regulation, and down-regulation of hormones and receptors function to protect the body.

Stress Response

The stress response is designed to protect against threats to well-being.[35] Threats may be physical, social, psychosocial, real, and/or simply perceived. Moreover, biochemical functions of the major organ systems are modulated by the mind.[36] Thoughts and feelings are transduced into chemicals (i.e., neurotransmitters, neurohormones, and peptides) that circulate throughout the body and convey messages to various systems within the body. The stress response illustrates the way in which various systems cooperate to protect an individual from harm.

A young man is walking to his car alone late at night when a stranger grabs his arm and attempts to rob him. His immediate response is one of fear, and his body prepares him to manage the danger by preparing him physically. The locus ceruleus (LC) with nerve endings in the forebrain instantaneously secretes norepinephrine directly into the cortex. At the same time, the sympathetic nervous system (SNS) fibers also extend into the adrenal medulla, stimulating medulla secretion of norepinephrine. The young man's body is now full of norepinephrine, and he feels the effects. Muscular tension results from neural messages and stimulation of the SNS to prepare him for physical challenges. All of this happens even before he is fully aware of the danger.

Quickly, the young man registers what is happening. The hypothalamus secretes corticotropin-releasing factor (CRF) into the hypothalamic-pituitary circulation in the brain. Within approximately 15 seconds, CRF triggers the release of the pituitary hormone adrenocorticotropic hormone (ACTH). In a matter of minutes, the adrenal cortex releases glucocorticoids. Hypothalamic, pituitary, and adrenal neuropeptides and other substances interact with the immune response, completing the multidirectional circle of communication among the nervous, endocrine, and immune systems. The young man has now experienced a full-blown psychophysiologic stress reaction to the fear of being hurt.

Physiologically, the cascade of changes associated with the stress response manifests as increased heart and respiratory rates, tightened muscles, increased metabolic rate, and a general sense of foreboding, fear, nervousness, irritability, and negative mood. Other physiologic responses include elevated blood pressure, dilated pupils, stronger cardiac contractions, and increased levels of blood glucose, serum cholesterol, circulating free fatty acids, and triglycerides. Although these responses prepare a person for short-term stress, they can lead to structure changes and clinical illness if prolonged. The memory of this experience is stored in the brain and other body cells and has psychological and spiritual effects. The individual may reexperience the stress reaction in future similar events with less intense stress, such as having a friend brush against his arm as they walk toward the car. Indeed, just thinking about this experience can initiate a stress response. **Table 31-1** contains a review of the effects of sympathetic and parasympathetic stimulation.

When the stress has been dealt with or is no longer a threat, the body returns to its normal, homeostatic state. However, when one experiences a threat so traumatic or the threat is so chronic, the normal stress response is altered, resulting in the traumatic stress response (TSR).[37] Severe traumatic threats range from childhood abuse to a near-death automobile accident or the sudden, unexpected death of a child while a chronic ongoing threat or stress could be caregiving for an elderly spouse with Alzheimer's disease or unpleasant work conditions. Initiation of the stress response that is short lived does not lead to adverse health results, whereas severe and/or long-term stress can lead to adverse health events.[38]

Homeostasis, the body's steady state, is maintained through ongoing changes in response to physical and environmental challenges. Allostasis is the process used to maintain homeostasis and well-being.[39] The general adaptation syndrome, the nonspecific physiologic stress response, is part of allostasis. The number of demands requiring adaptation determines the allostatic load. When an individual experiences overwhelming stress or has inadequate coping skill to deal with the stress, allostatic overload occurs. Allostatic overload can lead to structural changes in the body and illness.[39]

Long-term and unremitting stress can influence cardiovascular disease and gastrointestinal problems, and lead to depression, drug problems, and accidents. The long-term presence of high levels of cortisol over an extended period of time promotes lipolysis in the extremities and lipogenesis in the face and back, suppresses the inflammatory process, increases the risk of

TABLE 31-1   Effects of Sympathetic and Parasympathetic Stimulation

Structure	Sympathetic Stimulation	Parasympathetic Stimulation
Pupil of eye	Dilates	Contracts
Ciliary muscle	Relaxes, accommodates for distance vision	Contracts for close-up vision
Bronchial tubes	Dilates	Constricts
Heart	Accelerates and strengthens actions	Depresses and slows actions
Stomach muscles	Depresses activity	Increases activity
Glands	Alters secretion	Increases secretion
Liver	Stimulates glycogenolysis	
Visceral muscles of the intestine	Depresses peristalsis	Increases peristalsis
Adrenal medulla	Causes secretion of epinephrine	
Sweat glands	Increases activity	Decreases activity
Coronary arteries	Dilates	Constricts
Abdominal and pelvic viscera	Constricts	
Peripheral blood vessels	Constricts	
External genitalia	Constricts blood vessels	Dilates causing erections

Source: Copyright © Genevieve Bartol.

osteoporosis and ulcers, and leads to atrophy of immune system organs. Levels of various reproductive hormones (e.g., progesterone, estrogen, and testosterone), growth and thyroid hormones, and insulin decline during stress, probably to conserve energy.[40]

The stress response is modulated by disposition, personality, and coping skills. Psychological stressors stimulate a physiologic response and are referred to as a reactive response. Students may have a reactive response when taking an examination. Anticipatory stressors can also elicit the stress response. For example, children who have been abused by a parent may experience a physiologic response when the parent comes near. Perceived stressors begin in the area of the brain that controls cognition and emotions, the cerebral cortex and the limbic system. For example, one person may have a full-blown stress response to a damaged fingernail whereas another person may not have a stress response to the loss of a best friend. Additionally, there are individual differences in hormonal, neuroendocrine, and immunologic responses to stress.[36,40]

Three major body systems are involved with the stress response: the nervous system, the endocrine system, and the immune system. These systems work in symphony-like ways to protect the body from harm because all systems work in harmony.

Nervous System

The brain is the cognitive center. It is here that memories are stored, ideas generated, and emotions expressed.[41] Emotions that affect the body originate in the brain; the brain, then, has a powerful influence over the body and is also the link to emotions and the immune system. The interconnectedness of the central nervous system (CNS) means that frontal cortex thoughts and images are in intimate communication with the emotion-related limbic center. As the biochemicals transduced from thoughts and ideas circulate through the limbic-hypothalamic system, memory cells from past experiences affect their structure. The hypothalamus, the central control center, coordinates the biochemical cascade, integrating neuroendocrine functions by secreting both releasing and inhibiting hormones, as well as stimulating the SNS.[42] The SNS branch of the autonomic nervous system (ANS) is connected to the limbic system, has fibers extending into the adrenal medulla, and includes a pathway of nerves to the thymus, lymph nodes, spleen, and bone marrow. Hence, the connections are not only biochemical, but also anatomic. The SNS with preganglionic fibers that terminate in the adrenal medulla stimulate the secretion of epinephrine (80%) and norepinephrine (20%) that begin the physiologic stress response and result in increased heart and respiratory rates, elevated blood pressure, and increased blood to skeletal muscle. The effects of epinephrine occur within seconds.[40,42]

Integration of the stress response occurs in the CNS. Communication is dependent on neuronal pathways among the cerebral cortex, the limbic system, the thalamus, the hypothalamus, the pituitary gland, and the reticular activating system (RAS).[35] The focus of the cerebral cortex is on cognition, focused attention, and vigilance. The limbic system is the emotional center focused on feelings such as rage, anger, and fear. This system elicits an endocrine response indirectly via stimulation of neural pathways for sensory information and stimulates a central response by direct stimulation of the LC. The thalamus is the relay station. It is in the thalamus that sensory data are sorted and distributed. The hypothalamus is the coordinator of the endocrine and the ANS. The RAS is the modulator of ANS activity, skeletal muscle tone, and mental alertness. The LC, located in the brain stem, has afferent pathways connecting the hypothalamus, hippocampus, limbic systems, and cerebral cortex; it is rich with norepinephrine-producing cells, integrating the ANS response. The entire process is not only complex but also not completely clear.[35]

Understanding the psychophysiologic stress response as it affects the nervous system helps to clarify how the different holistic therapies work. It is possible to interrupt feelings of anxiety by using a relaxation technique to calm the self or a cognitive restructuring technique to change thought patterns. When patients learn to use relaxation, imagery, music therapy, or certain types of meditation training, their sympathetic response to stress decreases, and the calming effect of the parasympathetic system takes over, leading to body–mind healing. Biofeedback can reduce arousal and tension, and it is so effec-

tive that it has become a common intervention for a number of conditions induced or exacerbated by uncontrolled stimulation of the stress response.[35] To illustrate, warming the fingers by using biofeedback decreases the discomfort that accompanies Raynaud's disease. Changes in physiology change thoughts and feelings; changes in thoughts and feelings, conversely, change physiology.

Medications are used to treat conditions, such as panic attack, that consist of a hyperreaction of the SNS. Beta blockers, for example, block the alpha adrenergic receptors, producing lower heart rate and blood pressure. Patients who are taking beta blockers may not exhibit the normal reactions to threat. Also, older people often have decreased psychophysiologic stress responses because their reactions to SNS stimulation are blunted. In severe panic attacks, medications may be required but they sometimes have troublesome side effects. The use of mind–body interventions may reduce or eliminate the need for medication.

Endocrine System

The nervous and endocrine systems are so closely connected and interactive that they are referred to as the neuroendocrine system. The specific organs of the endocrine system and the stress response are the pituitary and adrenal glands. Hormones, secreted by the endocrine glands, are the specialized chemical messengers that act to modulate both cellular and systemic responses. They are always present in body fluids, but their concentrations vary. They produce both localized and generalized effects. Furthermore, one hormone can stimulate a variety of effects in different tissues, and a single function may be subject to regulation by more than one hormone. Hormones include amines and amino acids (e.g., norepinephrine, epinephrine, dopamine), peptides, polypeptides, proteins, and steroids.[43]

Each cell has a multitude of receptor molecules that can be modified or altered. Hormones act by binding to their specific receptor on target cell surfaces. Treatment with methadone is effective for heroin addicts, for example, because the methadone binds to the opioid receptor sites. A decrease in hormone levels can increase the number of receptor sites available. This is *up-regulation*. Conversely, an elevated hormone level leads to a decrease in receptors, or *down-regulation*.[43] Also, many of the hormones have a negative feedback loop that maintains the balance in serum hormonal levels. Stimuli such as circadian rhythms, the environment, and emotional and physical stressors influence the secretion of hypothalamic hormones.

The major endocrine hormones in the stress response are epinephrine from the adrenal medulla and glucocorticoids from the adrenal cortex (see next section). Other hormones associated with the stress response include pituitary hormones (growth hormone, prolactin, estrogen, and testosterone). Growth hormone (GH) and prolactin are secreted by the anterior pituitary during stress. GH affects metabolism of carbohydrates, protein, and lipids. Estrogen may attenuate the hypothalamus-pituitary-axis (HPA) effects because women tend to respond more to stressors with a greater HPA stress response. Decreased testosterone levels occur in men during stressful experiences, but more research is needed to understand the significance. The opioids (i.e., endorphins, enkephalins) are synthesized in the pituitary and other parts of the CNS. Opioids have a morphine-like effect with receptors throughout the body. These naturally occurring hormones produce the "runner's high," increase a person's pain threshold, and explain how people can "ignore" their own serious injury to save a loved one. The endorphins are secreted by immune cells during stress, leading to analgesia.[42]

Corticotropin-Releasing Factor

Corticotropin-releasing factor (CRF), a peptide and neurotransmitter, is part of the neuroendocrine stress response. CRF is found in the brain stem, hypothalamus, limbic systems, and extrahypothalamic structures. When released from the hypothalamus, CRF leads to pituitary secretion of adrenocorticotropic hormone (ACTH). ACTH induces the secretion of glucocorticoid hormones from the adrenal cortex. Cortisone helps to mediate the stress response and has a number of physiologic outcomes.[35] There is a sympathetic nervous system connection to the blood vessels supplying the immune cells,

thereby creating a direct nervous system and immune system pathway.[42]

Cortisol produces similar effects as those of epinephrine, but the effects last from minutes to days. To explain, epinephrine is secreted quickly during the alarm stage and cortisol is secreted for the long term during the resistant and exhaustion stages. Cortisol stimulates gluconeogenesis, increasing blood glucose levels and resulting in protein breakdown. This breakdown leads to loss of muscle, negative nitrogen balance, increased gastrointestinal secretion, and suppression of the immune system.[42]

Immune System

The immune, endocrine, and nervous systems communicate with hormones, neuropeptides, neurotransmitters, and products of immune cells. This communication is bidirectional.[40] Anatomically, the nervous system has direct connections to immune system organs (thymus, bone marrow, lymph nodes, and spleen). Likewise, immune system cells produce messengers that signal the nervous system.[41] There are receptors on the immune system cells for the neurotransmitters such as the opioid peptides, dopamine, catecholamines, and ACTH.[40] The nervous system has direct sympathetic innervation of immune system blood vessels.[42] The SNS pathways of norepinephrine and epinephrine secretion and the hypothalamic-pituitary-adrenal axis with glucocorticoid secretion have direct effects on immune system cells. Glucocorticoids suppress the immune system. Cortisol, for example, suppresses white blood cells, and it is even administered to suppress the immune system in people with autoimmune diseases.

Recent findings indicate that CNS and ANS neuropeptides and endocrine hormones stimulated by the nervous system directly affect immune system cells. Receptor sites located on the surface of the T and B lymphocytes have the ability to activate, direct, and modify immune function. For example, CRF suppresses monocytic macrophages and T helper lymphocytes. Lymphocytes produce the stress hormone ACTH and the brain peptide endorphin.[40] Endorphins have both enhancing and suppressing effects on immune system cells, depending on their concentration. They may elevate active T cells

718 Chapter 31 The Psychophysiology of Body–Mind Healing

whereas too many endorphins may suppress the immune system.[41,42] In turn, cytokines, that is, secretions of immune system cells, affect the nervous and endocrine systems.

Interventions to reduce the stress response can have a positive effect on the immune system. Interventions that induce the parasympathetic response have healing effects on the body. Because all systems are interconnected, holistic interventions contribute to health and healing. It is important to remember that there are individual differences in immunologic reactivity, hormonal responses, and autonomic responses to stress.[36]

Neuropeptides

With their receptors, neuropeptides help further explain body–mind interconnections and the way that emotions are experienced in the body. Circulating throughout the body, neuropeptides are considered the messengers that connect body and mind. The first neuropeptides were discovered in the intestine, which has many receptors; this may help explain those "gut feelings." Neuropeptides can be exchanged and produced by most all body tissues and even from inflammatory cells.[44]

The limbic system and hippocampus are rich with neuropeptide receptors, containing almost all of them and connecting emotions and learning. The concept of emotions as neuropeptides explains why people have trouble remembering and learning when they are experiencing psychophysiologic stress. Performance, too, is affected. Those who experience severe anxiety and panic before speaking in public or performing a concert benefit from relaxation techniques and cognitive restructuring. This ability to alter biochemicals and the consequent effects on memory and learning occur when the unconscious mind is brought into consciousness with hypnosis.

Emotions and spirituality cannot be ignored. Nurses who attend only to the body are not providing holistic care. Referrals to chaplains or therapists are positive interventions but may leave patients and families feeling uncared for, unattended, unheard, and lonely. Interventions to support and enhance coping offer another opportunity to promote healing and wholeness. We are increasingly faced with the challenges of complexity.[45]

■ CONCLUSION

New scientific understandings of living systems, such as principles of self-organization and mind modulation of the body–mind systems, provide a theoretical base for holistic healing interventions. Understanding the physiologic principles that are involved in nursing interventions helps nurses design individualized and appropriate holistic care for clients. Nurses, aware of their own wounds and sensitive to the wounds of clients, are strategically placed to lead clients in facilitating health and healing. Walking the talk is about being authentic and congruent, allowing nurses to relate to patients in authentic and congruent ways. Caring for oneself is essential for nurses to model wholeness. For, if truth be known, nurses who do not care for themselves are unable to provide holistic care for their patients. The process of becoming authentic makes one sensitive to the needs of others. Modeling is, perhaps, the strongest teaching strategy.

Clients often know more about complementary interventions than do those who care for them. It is essential, therefore, to educate nurses to empower them as well. Knowledge of the communication of the nervous, endocrine, and immune systems is necessary but insufficient for holistic nursing—neither does it explain all aspects of illness. New scientific information invalidates the idea of the dualism of mind and body. Thoughts, emotions, and consciousness do not reside solely in the brain, but are present in various body parts—the brain, the glands, and the immune, enteric, and sexual systems.

The research data overwhelmingly document the body–mind interrelationships. There are still many unanswered questions, however. Does the mind exist after the physical death? Does the soul survive death of the body? Why do some people experience phantom pain after an amputation? Nurses must continue to incorporate wholeness into their own lives while exploring effective ways to deliver holistically oriented care to their clients. The meaning of the illness, the method of giving the diagnosis, the tone of voice and the touch of the nurse, and the relationships to family and friends must all be investigated. To achieve this goal, nurses must be aware of what they focus on and what they choose to ignore.

Directions for
FUTURE RESEARCH

1. Develop instruments that accurately measure psychophysiologic responses for particular holistic nursing interventions.
2. Explore the effectiveness of holistic interventions in preventing illness and promoting health.
3. Investigate the effects of holistic nursing practice on nurses.
4. Carry out longitudinal studies to examine the effects of the regular use of holistic nursing interventions.

Nurse Healer
REFLECTIONS

After reading this chapter, the nurse healer will be able to answer or to begin a process of answering the following questions:

- Do I attend to my own body–mind communication?
- Do I provide time for self-reflection?
- How do I heighten my awareness of who I am?

> *For a full suite of assignments and additional learning activities, use the access code located in the front of your book to visit this exclusive website: http://go.jblearning.com/dossey. If you do not have an access code, you can obtain one at the site.*

NOTES

1. S. K. Leddy, *Integrative Health Promotion Conceptual Bases for Nursing Practice* (Sudbury, MA: Jones & Bartlett, 2006): 16–26.
2. L. Dossey, "The Unsolved Mystery of Healing," *Shift: At the Frontiers of Consciousness* (December 2004–February 2005): 24–26.
3. D. Lindley, *Uncertainty: Einstein, Heisenberg, Bohr, and the Struggle for the Soul of Science* (New York, NY: Doubleday, 2007).
4. B. Haisch, "Freeing the Scientific Imagination," *IONS Noetic Science Review* (September–November 2001): 24–29.
5. M. A. Boyd and M. A. Nihart, *Psychiatric Nursing* (Philadelphia, PA: Lippincott-Raven, 2003): 197–198.
6. L. von Bertalanffy, *General Systems Theory* (New York, NY: George Braziller, 1968).
7. E. Laszlo, *The Systems View of the World. A Holistic Vision of Our Time* (Cresskill, NJ: Hampton Press, 2002): 16–21.
8. M. C. Porth, *Essentials of Pathophysiology Concepts of Altered Health States*, 3rd ed. (Philadelphia, PA: Lippincott Williams & Wilkins, 2010).
9. R. Ader (ed.), *Psychoneuroimmunology*, 4th ed., Vol. 1 (New York: Elsevier, 2007): xv–xvii.
10. B. Rabin, "Stress: A System of the Whole," in *Psychoneuroimmunology*, 4th ed., Vol. 1, ed. R. Ader (New York, NY: Elsevier, 2007): 216.
11. T. Gyatso, "The Monk in the Lab," *New York Times* (April 6, 2003): opinion 26.
12. I. Prigogine, *The End of Certainty* (New York, NY: The Free Press, 1997): 9–56.
13. F. Capra, *The Web of Life* (New York, NY: Doubleday, 1996): 157–158.
14. R. Larter, "Life Lessons from the Newest Science," *IONS Noetic Science Review* (March–May 2002): 22–27.
15. H. Antoni, N. Schneiderman, and F. Penedo, "Behavioral Interventions: Immunologic Mediators and Disease Outcomes," in *Psychoneuroimmunology*, 4th ed., Vol. 1, ed. R. Ader (New York, NY: Elsevier, 2007): 675.
16. J. Kabat-Zinn, *Coming to Our Senses* (New York: Hyperion, 2005): 374.
17. G. M. Bartol, "Creating a Healing Environment," *Seminars in Perioperative Nursing* 92, no. 7 (1998): 90–95.
18. R. Glaser, "Stress and Immunity," in *Psychoneuroimmunology*, 4th ed., Vol. 2, ed. R. Ader (New York, NY: Elsevier, 2007): 705–708.
19. K. J. Karren, B. Q. Hafen, N. L. Smith, and K. J. Frandsen, *Mind/Body Health. The Effects of Attitudes, Emotions and Relationships*, 3rd ed. (New York, NY: Pearson, 2006): 251–271.
20. V. Simac, "The Challenge of Forgiveness," *Shift: At the Frontiers of Consciousness*, no. 13, (December 2006–February 2007): 29–33.
21. A. L. Marsland, S. Pressman, and S. Cohen, "Positive Effect and Immune Function," in *Psychoneuroimmunology*, 4th ed., Vol. 1, ed. R. Ader (New York, NY: Elsevier, 2007): 761–779.
22. C. B. Pert, *The Molecules of Emotion: Why You Feel the Way You Feel* (New York, NY: Charles Scribner's Sons, 1997): 261.
23. A. Damasio, *Looking for Spinosa* (New York, NY: Harcourt, 2003).
24. S. Begley, *Train Your Mind, Change Your Brain* (New York, NY: Ballantine Books, 2006).

25. D. Goleman, *Emotional Intelligence* (New York, NY: Bantam Books, 1995).

26. N. C. Frisch and L. E. Frisch, *Psychiatric Mental Health Nursing*, 4th ed. (New York, NY: Delmar, 2011).

27. J. E. Graham, L. M. Christian, and J. K. Kiecolt-Glaser, "Close Relationships and Immunity," in *Psychoneurimmunology*, 4th ed., Vol. 1, ed. R. Ader (New York, NY: Elsevier, 2007): 792.

28. S. A. Raskin (ed.), *Neuroplasticity and Rehabilitation* (New York, NY: Guilford Publications, 2011).

29. C. W. Mark, *Spiritual Intelligence and the Neuroplastic Brain* (Bloomington, IN: Authorhouse, 2010).

30. D. Church, *The Genie in Your Genes* (Santa Rosa, CA: Elite Books, 2007).

31. S. McClelland, A. Korosi, J. Cope, A. Ivy, and T. Z. Baram, "Emerging Roles of Epigenetics Mechanisms in the Enduring Effects of Early-Life Stress and Experience on Learning and Memory," *Experimental Neurology* (February 12, 2011).

32. J. Graff, D. Kim, M. M. Dobbin, and L. H. Tsai, "Epigenetic Regulation of Gene Expression in Physiological and Pathological Brain Process," *Annals of Anatomy* (March 17, 2011).

33. R. J. Wright, "Epidemiology of Stress and Asthma from Constricting Communities and Fragile Families to Epigenetics," *Immunology and Allergy Clinics of North America* (February 31, 2011): 19–39.

34. M. R. DeSevo, "Genetics and Genomics Resources for Nurses," *Journal of Nursing Education* 49, no. 8 (2010): 470–474.

35. M. C. Porth, *Essentials of Pathophysiology: Concepts of Altered Health States,* 4th ed. (Philadelphia, PA: Lippincott Williams & Wilkins, 2010).

36. R. Ader, "Integrative Summary: On the Clinical Relevance of Psychoneuroimmunology," in *Human Psychoneuroimmunology,* ed. K. Vedhara and M. Irwin (Oxford, England: Oxford University Press, 2005).

37. K. R. Wilson, D. J. Hansen, and M. Li, "The Traumatic Stress Response in Child Maltreatment and Resultant Neuropsychological Effects," *Aggression and Violent Behavior* 16 (2010): 87–97.

38. J. R. Piazza, D. M. Almeida, N. O. Dmitrieve, and L. C. Klein, "Frontiers in the Use of Biomarkers of Health in Research on Stress and Aging," *Journal of Gerontology Series B: Psychological Sciences and Social Sciences* 65B (2010): 513–525.

39. R. J. Emerson, "Homeostasis and Adaptive Responses to Stressors," in *Pathophysiology*, 4th ed., ed. L.-C. Copstead and J. L. Banasik (St. Louis, MO: Elsevier Saunders, 2010): 14–27.

40. K. L. McCance, B. A. Forshee, and J. Shelby, "Stress and Disease," in *Pathophysiology: The Biologic Basis for Disease in Adults and Children,* ed. K. L. McCance et al. (St. Louis, MO: Elsevier Mosby, 2006).

41. K. J. Karren, B. Q. Hafen, N. L. Smith, and K. J. Frandsen, *Mind/Body Health: The Effects of Attitudes, Emotions, and Relationships*, 3rd ed. (Boston, MA: Pearson, 2006).

42. L. D. Oakley, "Stress, Adaptation, and Coping," in *Pathophysiology,* 3rd ed., ed. L. C. Copstead and J. L. Banasik (St. Louis, MO: Elsevier Saunders, 2005).

43. S. E. Huether, "Mechanisms of Hormonal Regulation," in *Pathophysiology: The Biologic Basis for Disease in Adults and Children,* ed. K. L. McCance and S. E. Huether (St. Louis, MO: Elsevier Mosby, 2006).

44. N. P. M. Van der Kleij and J. Bienenstock, "Significance of Sensory Neuropeptides and the Immune Response," in *Psychoneuroimmunology,* 4th ed., Vol. 1, ed. R. Ader (New York, NY: Elsevier, 2007).

45. B. S. Barnum, *Spirituality in Nursing: The Challenges of Complexity*, 3rd ed. (New York, NY: Springer, 2011).

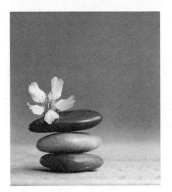

Chapter 32

Spirituality and Health

Margaret A. Burkhardt and
Mary Gail Nagai-Jacobson

Nurse Healer
OBJECTIVES

Theoretical

- Describe spirituality.
- Compare and contrast spirituality and religion.
- Discuss common elements of spirituality and their varying manifestations in different people.
- Recognize mystery, suffering, love, forgiveness, hope, peacemaking, and grace as spiritual issues.
- Discuss the interplay of spirituality and psychology.

Clinical

- Explore the efficacy and place of prayer in healing.
- Discuss listening as intentional presence.
- Incorporate different approaches to spirituality assessment into holistic care.
- Discuss the use of story in spirituality assessment and care.
- Describe approaches for responding to spiritual concerns.

Personal

- Explore the need for nurses to nurture their own spirits and ways to do so.

- Discuss ways in which ritual, rest and leisure, play, and creativity relate to spirituality.
- Explore ways of naming and nurturing important connections.

DEFINITIONS

Religion: Refers to an organized system of beliefs regarding the cause, purpose, and nature of the universe that is shared by a group of people, and the practices, behaviors, worship, and ritual associated with that system. Religion connects persons through shared beliefs, values, and practices, making clear particular belief systems that are different from other belief systems, thus defining differences between groups of persons.

Spirituality: The essence of our being. It permeates our living in relationships and infuses our unfolding awareness of who we are, our purpose in being, and our inner resources. Spirituality is active and expressive. It shapes—and is shaped by—our life journey. Spirituality informs the ways we live and experience life, the ways we encounter mystery, and the ways we relate to all aspects of life. Inherent in the human condition, spirituality is expressed and experienced through living our connectedness with the Sacred Source, the self, others, and nature.

■ THEORY AND RESEARCH

*We join spokes together in a wheel
but it is the center hole that makes the
wagon move.*

*We shape clay into a pot,
but it is the emptiness inside that holds
whatever we want.*

*We hammer wood for a house,
but it is the inner space that makes
it livable.*

*We work with being,
but nonbeing is what we use.*[1]

Spirituality is perhaps the most basic, yet least understood, aspect of holistic nursing. Spirituality often eludes the cognitive mind because it is intangible in many ways and defies quantification. A definition of spirituality is a starting point, appreciating that the mystery and human experience of spirituality cannot be fully captured by any definition. Language for expressing the experience of spirit or soul is limited, thus people speak of spirituality however they can, often with symbols, metaphor, and story.[2] The term *spirituality* derives from the Latin *spiritus*, meaning breath, and relates to the Greek *pneuma* or breath, which refers to the vital spirit or soul. Spirituality is the essence of who we are and how we are in the world and, like breathing, is integral to our human existence.

All people are spiritual. By virtue of being human, all persons, at all ages, are bio-psychosocial-spiritual beings. Attending to spirituality across the life span implies an understanding of the developmental aspects of spirituality, particularly an awareness that expressions of spirituality may vary with age. Some people describe themselves or others as not spiritual because they do not attend religious services or believe in God. This reflects the common practice of describing spirituality in terms of religious beliefs and practices. Nurses and other healthcare providers often link spiritual caregiving with determining a patient's religious affiliation and understanding the health-related beliefs, norms, and taboos of that religion. Although such knowledge is important for holistic nursing, spiritual caregiving requires an understanding that spirituality is broader than religion and a recognition that, although some people may not be religious, everyone is spiritual.

Relationship Between Spirituality and Religion

The nursing and healthcare literature continue to reflect the understanding that spirituality and religion are not synonymous.[3-6] As the essence of our being, spirituality is integral to all persons. Spirituality is a manifestation of each person's wholeness and being that is not subject to choice, but simply is. Religion per se is not essential to existence. Religion is chosen. Spirituality is expressed and experienced in many ways, both within and beyond the context of religion.

Religion refers to an organized system of beliefs shared by a group of people and the practices related to that system. Ritual, worship, prayer, meditation, style of dress, and dietary observances are examples of such practices. Because culture influences a person's values and beliefs, religious and other spiritual expressions often relate to personal culture. Religions reflect particular approaches to and understandings of spirituality. Religious precepts and practices often assist persons in attending to their spiritual selves; at times, however, these actions do little to nurture a person's true spirituality. Life issues that are spiritual in nature may or may not relate to religion. Knowledge of the histories, symbols, beliefs, practices, and languages of various religious traditions increases the nurse's ability to hear, recognize, and address religious needs of patients; however, information alone about religious affiliation and practices offers only a glimpse into a person's spiritual self.

Because religion offers a particular structure for expressing spirituality, nurses may be more comfortable discussing spiritual concerns when they arise within an identifiable religious context than when they occur within a broader perspective of spirituality. Satisfying the rites and rituals of a particular religion may or may not meet all of a patient's spiritual needs. Spiritual care and interventions need to be individualized and reflect the patient's perspectives and worldview.[7] This is of particular concern when a patient's spirituality is not expressed through an affiliation or alignment with the practices of a particular religion, and when the patient's culture and spiritual perspective are different from that of the nurse. Holistic nursing practice recognizes that religion and spirituality are different and honors the unique ways in which people express, experience, and nurture their spiritual selves.

Understanding Spirituality

One of the barriers to incorporating spirituality into holistic nursing care is the paucity of language within Western societies for discussing and expressing matters of the spirit or soul. This difficulty with the language of spirituality is evident in the nursing literature. In Western cultures, the language used for describing and expressing spirit is generally that of science or of religion derived from the Judeo-Christian tradition. Indeed, much of the discussion of spirituality within nursing and other healthcare literature reflects Judeo-Christian values and perspectives regarding the Divine, relationships with others and the world, experience of suffering, prayer, and the like. Understandings of spirituality and language describing spiritual values and experience may be different for many people in the world who do not adhere to the Judeo-Christian tradition. Because spirituality is the essence of every person and is not limited to a particular religious perspective, nurses strive to be open to, or to create a language that allows room for, each person's unique expression of spirituality.

A Western cultural bias can lead to misinterpretation of spiritual expression and concerns. Engebretson and Headley note that not all assumptions of Western Judeo-Christian-Islamic traditions (e.g., monotheism, transcendence, dualism) are shared with Eastern and Nature religious traditions.[8] Monotheism is a belief in one God that is above and beyond Nature, contrasted with a belief in the existence of many gods (polytheism) or the existence of the sacred in all living things (pantheism) found in Eastern and Nature religions. Transcendence, which means to exist above material existence, is implied in the Western view of God as separate from humanity. People from such Western traditions often seek connection with the Divine by focusing outward through ritual and prayer. Eastern and Nature traditions focus on immanence, the experience of the Divine within each person. Looking inward through meditation and spiritual exercises is a way of connecting with the Divine in these traditions. Dualism (the separation of spirit and matter) is a familiar concept in Western traditions, while reality is conceived as a unified whole in Eastern metaphysical traditions of monism. Engebretson notes that the polarization of science and religion found in the West reflects the institutionalization of dualism. She emphasizes the importance of recognizing the impact of these assumptions on perceptions, definitions, and expectations of the spiritual experience within health care. She is especially concerned about labeling spiritual issues as pathology, or not recognizing them at all because they do not fit a familiar paradigm.

Elements of Spirituality

Increased interest in spirituality and health over the past two decades has generated many definitions and descriptions of spirituality within the healthcare literature. In many ways, however, trying to define spirituality is like trying to lasso the wind. The wind can be felt and its effect on things seen, but it cannot be contained within imposed boundaries, conceptual or otherwise. The similar nature of spirituality poses a particular challenge for minds that feel more at home with phenomena that can be categorized, quantified, and measured. Understanding spirituality requires opening to many ways of knowing, including cognitive, intuitive, aesthetic, experiential, and deep inner sensing or knowing.

The healthcare literature provides no single agreed-upon understanding of spirituality. Elements of spirituality found in broad descriptions of the concept include the essence of being, a unifying and animating force, the life principle of each person, a sense of meaning and purpose, and a commitment to something greater than the self.[2,9-13] Spirituality permeates life, shapes our life journey, and is vital to the process of discovering purpose, meaning, and inner strength. Although matters of spirit transcend culture, a person's cultural perspective influences personal expressions of spirituality. Personal values are rooted in and flow from spirituality and are reflected in a cultural perspective. Spirituality helps to ground one's sense of place and fit in the world. Because it is practical and relevant to daily life, people experience spirituality in the mundane as well as in the profound, the secular as well as the sacred.

A sense of trust that people have or are given the resources needed for dealing with whatever comes their way—expected or not—is a manifestation of spirituality. These resources include both strength and guidance from within and support from sources beyond themselves. Through encountering obstacles along their life path, learning through experiences, and developing new awarenesses, people gain appreciation for the ways that spirituality shapes and gives meaning to their unfolding life journey. To reach this point, people may find it necessary to reconcile new experiences with previously held values, resulting in new values and understandings. Often, the pattern of the journey and the meaning of life events become clear only in retrospect.

A sense of peace, often described as inner peace, is a spiritual attribute. Peace in this context implies a deep confidence and an ability to remain calm in the midst of the storm, to know somehow that all is well. Spiritual peace is experienced in the space of the heart and may not make sense to the cognitive mind. In the Judeo-Christian tradition, references to "a peace which passeth understanding" flow from an awareness of life beyond immediate circumstances and unbounded by the past. In the Zen tradition, practices of mindfulness foster connection with the peace that is available in every moment within every life experience. Peace is a product of living in relationship with the Sacred Source, others, and all creation in a way that acknowledges and nurtures the soul in the midst of all that life brings.

Connectedness with the Sacred Source

Research continues to demonstrate that people express and experience spirituality in the context of relationships with the Sacred Source, Nature, others, and the self.[2,14,15] The Sacred Source may be experienced as a person, a presence, or as a mystery that is beyond words. The inadequacy of language is especially apparent when we try to discuss or describe that which is within and among us, yet beyond and a power greater than us. From before the beginning of recorded history, humanity has searched and sought to understand the mystery of the Sacred Source. Various cultures, faith traditions, individuals, and groups use names such as Life Force, Source, God, Allah, Lord, Goddess, Absolute, Higher Power, Spirit, Vishnu, Inner Light, Tao, Great Mystery, Tunkasila, the Way, Universal Love, and

the One with No Name to refer to that in which we live, move, and have our being. For this discussion, this Being or Sacred Mystery is referred to as God or the Sacred Source.

A connection with the Sacred Source is at the heart of one's being. Our rational minds cannot think or grasp God, and any descriptions or words used to speak of the Sacred Source are lacking. God is far more than anything the human mind can conceptualize. Words and descriptions are, however, tools of the rational mind that can point us toward God or the Sacred Source. Concepts of God developed by the rational mind may be personal or shared within a group. Persons find and name the Sacred Source in ways that are authentic to them, using terms and language that reflect their experiences and perspectives. Connecting with the Sacred Source may involve such things as prayer, ritual, reconciliation, and stillness. Teachings of various religious traditions offer their own perspectives and guidance on how to be in relationship with the Sacred Source. Understanding how persons seek and experience connection with the Sacred Source and the obstacles they may encounter are important in spiritual caregiving.

The concept of reverence is associated with many understandings of the Sacred Source. Reverence arises from a deep appreciation of human limitations and a sense of awe in relation to what is understood to be outside our control—God, truth, the natural world, even death. Awareness that the sacred is intrinsic and omnipresent engenders reverence toward the Sacred Source and all of life.[16] Reverence acknowledges that we are in and of God, yet, as Woodruff notes, it also keeps human beings from trying to act like gods.[17] Some persons do not claim a religion or give a name to that which they hold most sacred. However, they may experience a sense of reverence in their recognition of that which is beyond and greater than their own understanding, but with which they experience an often mysterious relationship.

Connectedness with Nature

Spirituality is frequently expressed and experienced in and through a sense of connectedness with Nature, the environment, and the universe. Relationship with creatures of the Earth, both wild and domesticated, provide meaning and joy for people of all ages. Awareness of all beings of the Earth, and their place within the natural order, is a way of connecting with the spiritual in all of life.[18] Beavers at work on a dam, red rock canyons, or bees among the flowers all illustrate the wonder of various life forms that may provide deeply spiritual experiences.

Awareness of a connectedness with the Earth and, indeed, the entire cosmos is particularly evident within indigenous spiritual traditions. A speech attributed to Chief Seattle emphasizes that all things are connected.[19] Individuals are not the weavers of the web of life; rather, each is a strand in the web. What they do to the web they do to themselves. Thus, what happens to the Earth and the environment affects them, and conversely, their choices and actions in all levels of their being affect the Earth.[16,20] Understanding the interconnectedness of spirit and matter is basic to some traditions and known at some level in all spiritual traditions, particularly among the mystics.

Many people, particularly those who live close to the land, experience a sense of connection with the Sacred Source through Nature, regardless of their religious background. Paying close attention to the natural world and living in conscious relationship with the other-than-human beings of the world is a way of attuning more to one's own soul and spirit. People often express a particular feeling of closeness to their spiritual selves while walking on a beach, sitting by their favorite tree, viewing a sunset, listening to flowing water, watching a fire, caring for plants, and otherwise experiencing the natural order. Nature can be a source of strength, inspiration, and comfort, all of which are attributes of spirituality. A sense of awe at the wonder of life and a feeling of connectedness with all things, with or without a belief in a divine being, is an experience of spirituality. For some, connection with Nature flows from a sense of finding God in all things; many experience a relationship with the Earth and all its creatures at an energetic level. Appreciating, respecting, and caring for the Earth and all its inhabitants are elements of spirituality.

Connectedness with Others

Spirituality is known and experienced in and through relationships, with the comfort, support, conflict, and strife that mark those connec-

tions. People express and experience spirituality through an appreciation of a common bond with all humanity and in their particular relationships with others. Spirituality is shaped and nurtured within one's experience of community, beginning with one's family. The many communities, both formal and informal, in which people live provide a context for spiritual expression and development. Communities provide an opportunity for sharing spiritual journeys.

People often speak of their spirituality in terms of their relationships, both harmonious and discordant. The formation, work, nurture, and healing of relationships are an important part of one's spirituality. Being with others in loving and supportive ways is an expression of spirituality, as is struggling with painful and difficult relationships with family, friends, and acquaintances. Relationships that need healing are as important to spirituality as those that provide support and comfort. Spirituality embraces both the joys and sorrows of relationships and prompts reconciliation where connections have been frayed. Lack of connections often produces a dispiriting sense of aloneness and isolation and may lead to spiritual crisis.

Spiritual connectedness with others involves both giving and receiving. Receptive openness to Love, Light, Life, and the Sacred Source is a spiritual stance. Although it is common to think of spirituality in terms of doing for another, being able to receive from others, both the gift of themselves and the things that they do or say, is also an expression of spirituality. Indeed, the genuine presence that someone shares with another, with its implicit loving honesty and intimacy, is a manifestation of spirituality.[7,21-23] Spirituality is evident in both common experiences of daily living and special times shared with others: times of joy, sorrow, ritual, loving sexuality, prayer, play, encouragement, anger, reconciliation, and concern. Relationships as a source of growth and change are integral to spirituality.

Advances in technology have brought distant and isolated countries and cultures together into a world community. As a result, understanding factors that create and support community has become essential. The ability to connect with people around the globe enables better understanding of how personal and collective decisions impact the larger human family. Social structures that provide a context for relationships with others often are instrumental in nurturing the spiritual dimensions of community life. Structures such as health care, educational institutions, faith-based services, social organizations, informal affiliations, and Internet links with others are often places that mediate and support the spiritual dimensions of life.

Connectedness with Self

Spirituality infuses the ever-unfolding awareness of who one is—of self-becoming. The ability to be in the place of awareness that flows from spirit or soul is a pivotal element of connectedness with self. Awareness opens people to the experience of living in the moment, present to their own bodymindspirit, and allows them to receive all aspects of themselves without judgment. They experience awareness through Being, the art of stillness and presence with self, others, the Sacred Source, and Nature. Being simply is. Being includes experiencing the present moment more deeply, aware from the physical experience of all levels of one's bodymindspirit energetic self in interaction with all in the environment. Being is bringing one's whole self—alert and aware—to an experience, allowing one to pay attention to the quiet place inside and find inner peace, synchrony, harmony, and openness. Attentiveness to being allows a person to attune to sources of inner strength and deepest knowing.

Spirituality manifests and is experienced in knowing, which includes cognitive, intuitive, and energetic dimensions. Knowing provides ways of understanding our multidimensional nature and our relationships to the Sacred Source, self, others, Earth, and the cosmos. Knowing flows from a stance of openness and attuning to an inner source. It involves actively seeking knowledge and insights and maintaining an openness and receptivity to the lessons life offers. Spirituality reflected in one's knowing includes appreciation of life as a gift and a sense of connectedness to all creation.

From being and knowing flows doing, the outward and more visible aspect of spirituality. Because doing is more tangible and measurable, it is the manifestation of spirituality that is most often addressed in healthcare literature. Generally, the concept of doing brings to mind activities such as attendance at religious services or ceremony, scripture study, prayer or meditation, participation as student or teacher in religious education, and spiritual reading. Spirituality can be demonstrated as well through actions such as assisting others, gardening, becoming involved in environmental concerns, attending to the sick, caring for family, spending time with friends, taking a walk, taking time to nurture one's own spirit, and creating sacred space for self and others.

The concept of sacred space applies both to one's inner being and to places in one's environment. Although to "create" sacred space suggests doing something, inner sacred space is often the result of being in awareness and stillness. Buildings such as religious edifices or monuments represent sacred space for many. Special places in Nature are often experienced as sacred. Any place can become sacred space if one intentionally brings awareness of the spirit into the setting. Words, actions, sounds, scents, colors, and objects may shape such spaces. A sacred space is a home for the spirit, providing rest, stillness, nurture, and opportunities for opening to various connections. A special plant in a sunlit space, a garden or workshop, a room for prayer or meditation, a corner of a porch with a rocking chair, family surrounding a loved one in a hospital bed—each space touched by the intention of those who arrange it—are examples of sacred spaces.

■ SPIRITUALITY AND THE HEALING PROCESS

In a holistic paradigm, bodymindspirit is an intertwined and interpenetrating unity; thus, every human experience has bodymindspirit components. In considering spirituality and healing, it is useful to remember that the words *healing*, *whole*, and *holy* derive from the same root: Old Saxon *hal*, meaning whole. This suggests that, by its nature, healing is a spiritual process that attends to the wholeness of a person. The work of healing requires recognition of the spiritual dimension of each person, including the healer, and an awareness that spirituality permeates every encounter. The shared relationship acknowledging the common humanity and connectedness between the caregiver and the receiver, which is basic to healing, is a manifestation of spirituality.

Spiritual View of Life Issues

Spiritual issues are core life issues that often draw people to look into the deepest places in their beings. These issues are not quantifiable and are more authentically expressed as questions, tentative definitions, or as mysteries that cannot be fully explained. They challenge the individual to experience life at its highest heights and deepest depths. Considerations of mystery, love, suffering, hope, forgiveness, grace, peacemaking, and prayer are all inherent in the spiritual domain.

Mystery

Discovering with others the personal and unique ways that mystery is encountered on their spiritual journeys is an important part of spiritual care. Mystery is inherent to human experience, and thus is inherent to spirituality. Mystery may be described as a truth that is beyond understanding and explanation. Many life experiences prompt questions of why and wonderings about what if. Appreciation of the mystery inherent in life events often sustains people in the unknowing. As people encounter that which is troubling and unexplainable, spirit recognizes mystery and helps them survive the unknowing. Spirituality supports and encourages them in the questioning and seeking that often emerge when they are faced with such mystery. The spiritual self helps them embrace both the darkness and the light, enabling them to appreciate the challenges and gifts of both.

Love

Loving presence is a key component of spiritual care. Love, which is the source of all life, fuels spirituality, prompting each person to live from the heart, the center where the ego is detached from outcomes. Love, like the spirit, is nonlocal, transcending place and time, enabling its energy to be shared for healing at many levels. The relationship of love to healing is a continuing source of exploration and wonder.[22,24] In its truest sense, love is a mystery that involves both choice and emotion. It often underlies acts of courage and compassion that defy explanation. Love is both personal and universal and is experienced and expressed in both giving and receiving care. Flowing from and prompting interconnectedness, love includes dimensions of self-love, divine love, love for others, and love for all of life.

Suffering

In both its presence and its meaning, suffering is one of the core issues and mysteries of life. It occurs on physical, mental, emotional, and spiritual levels. People throughout the ages have struggled to understand the nature and meaning of suffering. Their attempts to make sense of suffering have shaped cultural and religious traditions. Suffering may be a transformative experience, the nature of the transformation varying with each individual. For some, suffering enhances spiritual awareness; for others, suffering appears meaningless and engenders feelings of anger and frustration. One interpretation of burnout among healthcare professionals is that it represents the inability to find ways to tend the spirit as one suffers the suffering of another.

Sociocultural, religious, familial, and environmental factors influence an individual's response to suffering. Thus, having knowledge of personality, culture, religious traditions, and family background helps the nurse understand the nature and meaning of suffering for a particular person. In the same vein, nurses who are aware of their own responses to and understanding of suffering are less likely to confuse their perceptions with those of the patient. This awareness enables nurses to be more fully present in an intentional, healing way with those who are suffering. Such presence allows nurses to discern whether honoring another's suffering requires action, presence, absence, or a combination of these. The ability to be with another who is suffering is crucial, particularly when nurses confront suffering that cannot be alleviated and must simply be borne. Such presence supports a person's spiritual journey toward discovering transcendent meaning within the experience.[25] Listening with one's whole being as another wonders aloud and expresses deep feelings regarding some of life's unanswered questions is a critical part of being with those who suffer.

Hope

Hope, a desire accompanied by an expectation of fulfillment, goes beyond believing or wishing.

Hope is future oriented yet grounded in the present moment. The saying "hope springs eternal" reflects this energy of the spirit and prompts the anticipation that tomorrow things will be better, or at least different! There are two levels of hope: The first, specific hope, implies a goal or desire for a particular event or outcome. The second is a more general sense of hope that the future is somehow in safekeeping. Hope is a significant factor in overcoming illness and in living through difficult situations.[26,27] It helps people deal with fear and uncertainty and enables them to envision positive outcomes.

Forgiveness

Ultimately a matter of self-healing, forgiveness is a deep need and hunger of the human experience. Religious beliefs, cultural traditions, family upbringing, and personal experience all help to shape an individual's attitudes about forgiveness, both given and received. Beliefs about the nature of God or the Sacred Source influence one's ability to offer and receive forgiveness. Difficulties with forgiving others, forgiving oneself, and accepting forgiveness from others often relate to a misunderstanding of the nature of forgiveness. Forgiveness is something one does for oneself, not for others. Forgiveness does not necessarily mean forgetting, condoning, absolving, or sacrificing; rather, it is a process of extending love and compassion to self and others.[28-30] An act of the heart, forgiveness is an internal process of releasing intense emotions attached to incidents from the past, releasing any need to carry grudges, resentments, hatred, self-pity, or desire to punish people who have done hurtful acts, and accepting that no punishment of others will promote internal healing. Forgiveness, a sign of positive self-esteem, allows a person to put the past in proper perspective, to free energy once consumed by grudges and resentments, to nurse unhealed wounds, and to use this energy for opening to healing and moving on with life.

Self-forgiveness—releasing the desire or need to berate or punish oneself for past actions—is an important part of forgiveness and is essential for spiritual growth and healing. Self-forgiveness is not about regret or guilt, but rather concerns acknowledgment of responsibility for one's choices and actions. Self-forgiveness is a gift to oneself that provides an opportunity to remove the energetic consequences from past actions and thoughts. Through acknowledgment of personal responsibility for past thoughts and actions, and the willingness to let go of any energetic attachment to these thoughts and actions, the cumulative energy of these actions is released so that they will not adversely affect the self. The notion of free will—that the actual or energetic result of one's actions and thoughts cannot be bypassed by God or the universe—is basic to self-forgiveness. The following analogy illustrates the self-forgiveness process: If you go for a walk and along the way get a sharp pebble in your shoe, every step from that point on is painful. The more you walk, the more it hurts. The pebble will cause pain and potential harm to the foot as long as it is in the shoe. Healing cannot take place as long as the pebble is irritating the foot; however, once the pebble is removed, the body can begin the healing process. Self-forgiveness, like taking the pebble out, enables the natural self-healing energy that is a part of the universe to begin and gives all of God's grace room to provide comfort.

Peace and Peacemaking

Peace, for many people, is inseparable from justice. Inner peace reflects a way of being, a space from which one is able to live and be in ways that nurture and heal. This peace does not depend on external circumstances; it flows from the connections that sustain us. Spiritual practices from many traditions sustain people and help them align with an inner peace in the midst of trials and hardships. Today as in the past many people throughout the world are experiencing brutal trials. Living as peacemakers in times and places of uncertainty, fear, injustice, and war is a spiritual challenge facing all citizens of the world, and it demands courageous and creative solutions. The work of peacemaking is grounded in the awareness that:

> There is an inherent power in rightness, in goodness in love, and in love of peace, and that if even a single individual chooses to act rightly and truthfully and peacefully in the midst of tempting and contrary choices, the power of that act and aspiration can change the world. By extension, if untold numbers of single individuals love peace enough, seek peace enough, stand for

peace enough, are themselves persons of peace, the ideal of peace will become the world's transforming reality.[31]

As persons appreciate and live in the reality of their connection with others and all creation across distance, time, and space, the possibility of peace with justice grows.

Grace

Experiences of grace contain elements of surprise, awe, mystery, and gratitude. Grace is often experienced as a support that is unplanned and unexpected. An experience of grace may touch one's spirit in deep and profound ways and may be life changing. Grace opens one's awareness to the experience of wholeness, healing, and connectedness. Grace is reflected in statements such as the following:

- He just showed up at the door right when I needed him.
- I didn't know how I was going to pay for everything; then, this check arrived.
- I don't know why my spirits lifted that morning; perhaps it was the rain after such a long drought.
- I didn't think I could stand another bout of chemotherapy, but my friend said she will go with me and we'll take one day at a time.
- My CT scan was clear for the third time, something that the doctors didn't expect and that I didn't dare hope for.

Although some see such happenings as coincidence or chance, others sense something deeper that connects persons within the web of life and enables us to find acceptance, courage, peace, and endurance beyond our own making or understanding. Grace is often spoken of as a gift from the Sacred Source, or from Life itself, that enables, assists, and empowers a person in the midst of difficult and sometimes seemingly overwhelming circumstances. The experience of grace as a blessing that comes into one's life unearned calls forth a response of gratitude.

Prayer

An expression of the spirit, prayer is a deep human instinct that flows from the core of one's being where the longing for and awareness of one's connectedness with the source of life are blended. Prayer represents a longing for communion or communication with God or the Sacred Source. The most fundamental, primordial, and important language that humans speak, prayer is an endeavor that starts and ends without words. In this understanding, prayer flows from yearnings of the soul that rise from a place too deep for words and move to a space beyond words.

Forms and expressions of prayer are as varied as the people who pray. Prayer, which is intrinsic to many religious traditions and rituals, may be public or private, individual or communal. It is not always a fully conscious activity. Speaking (sometimes silently), singing, chanting, listening, waiting, moaning, being attuned to what is going on in the present moment, and being silent can all be elements of prayer. Prayer includes petition, intercession, confession, lamentation, adoration, invocation, thanksgiving, being, and showing care and concern for others. Some people incorporate processes and techniques such as relaxation, quieting, breath awareness, focusing, imagery, and visualization into their prayer. Movement such as walking, dancing, or drumming may be expressions of prayer. A reminder of our nonlocal, unbounded nature, prayer is infinite in space and time. It is divine, the universe's affirmation that we are not alone.[32]

That prayer is an appropriate consideration for nursing is grounded in the writings of Florence Nightingale.[33,34] Research affirms the truth that people have known for ages: Prayer can affect healing.[35-37] Both directed prayer, which focuses on a specific outcome, and nondirected prayer, which focuses on the greatest good of the organism, can affect healing and other outcomes, although nondirected prayer may be more effective. Even at a distance, prayer alters processes in a variety of organisms, including plants and people. Furthermore, the observed effects of prayer do not depend on what the one prayed for thinks. In his book *Be Careful What You Pray For*, Dossey reminds us that prayer is a potent force that is best used thoughtfully, with care and discernment.[38]

Spiritual and Psychological Dimensions

The term *psyche* means soul or spirit, reflecting the relationship between the spiritual and the psychological that is evident even in the spoken language. Before the time of Freud, phenomena of the sentient realm that could not be explained physically often were considered matters of the spirit and viewed in religious terms. With the advent and ongoing development of psychology, matters of the soul often have been subsumed into psychological theory and frequently interpreted as pathology. Within a holistic paradigm, spiritual and psychological elements are interconnected because the bodymindspirit is an integrated whole. Failing to differentiate the spiritual and psychological dimensions, however, can lead nurses to miss cues regarding spiritual concerns and thus inappropriately label spiritual issues as psychopathology. Although spiritual awakenings and deepenings may be accompanied by elements of psychological distress, the "dark night of the soul" may be a very important part of the process of moving to greater awareness and enlightenment. Fortunately, many contemporary psychological models address the spiritual dimension.

Unlike Eastern and indigenous traditions around the world, Western traditions have only a limited familiarity and comfort with the spiritual nature of different levels of awareness. The misinterpretation of behaviors, emotions, and reactions associated with individual experiences and expressions of the spiritual is keenly evident in the life of Florence Nightingale and the many interpretations of her life.[34,39,40] Some have interpreted the behaviors and health concerns evident throughout her life after her return from the Crimea as psychological pathology, such as anxiety, neurosis, malingering, depression, and stress burnout. Approaching Nightingale's life from a spiritual as well as psychological perspective, however, allowed Dossey to recognize Nightingale for the mystic that she was.[34,39] In a similar vein, appreciating the difference between spiritual and psychological domains enables nurses to assess spiritual cues and spiritual crises more effectively, as well as to recognize opportunities to foster spiritual growth.

■ SPIRITUALITY IN HOLISTIC NURSING

Nurturing the Spirit

The way that nurses care for and nurture themselves influences their ability to function effectively in a healing role with another. The spiritual path is a life path. Attentiveness to one's own spirit is a key component of living in a healing way and is foundational to integrating spirituality into clinical practice. Care of their spirit or soul requires nurses to pause for reflecting and taking in what is happening within and around them; to take time for themselves, for relationships, and for other things that animate them; and to be mindful about nourishing their spirits. The many ways nurses nurture their spirits and respond to their spiritual concerns are the same as those that they suggest to their patients.

Care of the spirit is a professional nursing responsibility and an intrinsic part of holistic nursing. Within a holistic perspective, providing spiritual care is an ethical obligation, which, if ignored, deprives patients of their dignity as human beings. As an interpersonal, intuitive, altruistic, and integrative expression, spiritual caregiving draws on the nurse's awareness of the transcendent dimension and is grounded in the patient's reality.[41] Nurses must become competent and confident with spiritual caregiving, expanding their skills in assessing the spiritual domain and developing and implementing appropriate interventions. A persistent barrier to incorporating spirituality into clinical practice is the fear of imposing particular religious values and beliefs on others. Nurses who integrate spirituality into their care of others recognize that although each person acts out of and is informed by her or his own spiritual perspective, acting from this foundation is not the same as imposing these beliefs and values on another. In fact, many practitioners believe that the more they are grounded in an awareness of their own spiritual journey, the less likely they are to impose their values and beliefs on others.

Assessing and Investigating Spirituality in Practice and Research

The literature reflects attempts to make sense of spirituality within a scientific frame of reference, and clinicians and researchers continue to struggle with the inherent difficulties of assessing and measuring a phenomenon that defies definition. Many researchers approach the study of spirituality primarily through examining religious beliefs and practices. This approach can be problematic, however, in that many people do not express their spirituality within a religious tradition; conversely, religious practices do not necessarily indicate a person's true spirituality. Some assessment scales used in research on spirituality reflect a strong bias toward Judeo-Christian beliefs, suggesting that those who do not ascribe to these traditions may not be spiritual.

Developing credible quantitative instruments for spiritual inquiry may facilitate a more formal integration of spirituality assessment into health care by including such instruments in a patient's medical record. However, attempts to quantify spirituality, even with more broadly applicable scales, are at best a reflection of a particular perspective of spirituality as understood through the lens of the concepts included in the scale. Appreciating the allusive nature of spiritual phenomena, nurses recognize that an individual's spiritual journey may have many facets and meanings that are not captured within the limitations of a particular scale. Providing opportunities to explore personal meaning and understanding with patients is essential to effective spirituality assessment. A goal of holistic nursing is to know a person in the fullness and complexity of her or his wholeness. Knowledge obtained about a person through any process of assessment is not an end in itself; rather, it is useful inasmuch as it contributes to understanding and knowing more of the essence of the person. Listening and intentional presence are key in exploring individual meanings associated with a patient's spiritual journey.

Listening and Intentional Presence

Attentive listening and focused presence are at the heart of caring for the spirit, and they are essential in any approach to spirituality assessment. This concept is simple in many ways, but is not always easy. Good therapeutic communication skills facilitate the exploration of spiritual issues. Broad, open-ended questions are often useful. Questions and statements such as "Tell me more about . . . ," "Help me to understand what you need," "I don't understand what you are trying to say," and "What was that like for you?" are useful as nurses seek a deeper understanding of their patients. Creating a sacred space in which spirituality can be expressed and being clear about one's own spiritual perspective enhance a nurse's facility with spirituality assessments. Practicing spiritual disciplines such as prayer, centering, awareness, and meditation make it easier for nurses to be fully present, available to be with and listen to another. In the face of distractions from within and without, the nurse's ability to focus on the relationship with a particular person in a particular moment is an important aspect of being a healing presence, one that greatly enhances spiritual care.

One of the gifts of intentional, active listening is that the client, in sharing with an open-hearted and fully present listener, often hears herself or himself with greater clarity and understanding. Such a listener provides a safe space for expression of negative as well as positive feelings and experiences. The contradictions, pains, questions, and struggles can be heard without judgment or advice. The person is able to express and often to recognize and better understand the situation's richness and complexity and move toward the future with more awareness.

Holistic nurses assess their own abilities as listeners and consider barriers to intentional listening that are part of their personal journeys. There may be topics that make one uncomfortable. Although discomfort alone need not make one an unsuitable listener, being aware of one's discomfort, and its source and manifestations, is an important part of a self-evaluation. Nurses should consider how external distractions such as the environment or time pressures affect their ability to listen. In addition, they should be attentive to how body posture conveys presence and attention. A hospice patient illustrated an experience of intentional listening and presence in describing his relationship with one of the hospice workers on his team:

> It just makes me feel good to see him come in. One day he and I both fell asleep, kind of took a nap for a bit. He probably knows as much about me as anyone—because he's the kind of guy who's interested in everything I talk about, my family, my worries, my sickness. Sometimes he asks a question, but mostly he just listens—but I mean really listens, like he wants to know about whatever is on my mind.

Intentional listening and presence foster authenticity in the nursing process. Such listening and presence demand a recognition of both verbal and nonverbal cues in communication, and the validation by the patient of any of the nurse's interpretations. In reflecting on personal experiences of intentional listening, nurses might ask themselves the following questions: When have I been intentionally present for another, listening with my whole being and with an open heart? What factors, internal and external, help me to listen attentively or make that difficult for me? When have I been in the presence of one who was fully present for me? How did I recognize that full presence? How did that affect me?

The core of active listening and healing presence lies in the intention and attention of the nurse who recognizes all persons as spiritual beings. **Exhibit 32-1** lists important considerations for nurses as they strive to listen in healing ways to their clients. According to Bruchac, "It all begins with listening. There are stories all around us, but many people don't notice those stories because they don't take the time to listen."[42]

Using Story and Metaphor in Spiritual Care

Recognizing all persons, including themselves, as ongoing and unfolding stories offers nurses a valuable perspective from which to approach spiritual caregiving.[2,43-45] Story and metaphor often provide a language and form for conveying the richness of one's spirituality when factual statements of experience fail to do so. Stories bring people enjoyment, teach them to solve problems, help them form identities, and are wonderful teachers. Sharing stories helps people to understand themselves and their world. Through the vehicle of story, people learn to know each other and themselves from many perspectives. Stories reveal experiences of relationships, emotions, conflicts, struggles, and responses that are at once personal and universal. Nurses become part of the life stories of those for whom they care. Nurses' own life stories inform and form them, and understanding those stories deepens the awareness with which they hear another's story.

Listening and encouraging people to share their stories can be both assessment and intervention in spiritual care. Stories make it possible to move beyond physical symptoms, diagnoses, and theoretical constructs, which may be similar for any number of patients. Attentiveness to story allows nurses another glimpse into the wholeness and uniqueness of each person and the particular way in which he or she fits into the family and community. As an assessment approach, story and metaphor provide insight into spiritual concerns such as supportive and

EXHIBIT 32-1   Listening in Healing Ways

- Be intentionally present.
- Maintain focus on the patient/client as a whole person.
- Set aside the need to fix, answer, or correct.
- Learn to be with another in silence.
- Interrupt as little as possible, recognizing that even what is not said at a particular time has meaning and that the way and sequence in which a story is told are part of the story.
- View the other as embodied spirit, an ongoing and unfinished story.
- Hear the journey, the relationships, and the meanings in the story.
- Listen with all your senses.
- Do not prematurely diagnose.
- Let the conversation flow, being with silence as well as words.
- Breathe!

Source: M. G. Nagai-Jacobson and M. Burkhardt, © 1997.

disruptive relationships, questions of meaning, values and purpose, issues of forgiveness, hope and hopelessness, and experiences of grace. Listening is a reminder that life stories are ongoing and unfinished.

The sharing of story and metaphor can also be a nursing intervention. In sharing with a fully present listener, patients hear their own stories with new insights and appreciation for their own lives—affirmations and validations, conflicts and struggles, questions of meaning and dark times—life in its variety and fullness. In a safe space, patients can express fears and perceived failures, hopes and wonderings, disappointments and achievements, as they consider pages of their life stories. Through this process, patients come to see themselves more clearly and, in an atmosphere of acceptance, accept themselves in their full humanity. From such a stance, patients are able to participate more consciously in the present situation.

The case of Mr. M. is an example of the power of the story:

> Mr. M. has been diagnosed with probable cancer of the lungs and is scheduled for exploratory surgery in a few days. Several times he has asked the nurse, "How serious do you think this is?" After he asks once again, the nurse says, "Mr. M., you seem to be asking me more than how serious this is. Can you tell me more about what is concerning you?" He responds, "Well, to be honest, I've been thinking about telling the kids . . . especially my son in Chicago. You see, we haven't been on very good terms." And so begins an important story for Mr. M. to tell, and for the nurse to hear. The medical information about Mr. M.'s illness is but one piece of the greater fabric of his life as a family man and father. The nurse now hears Mr. M. talk about his concerns for his family and the relationships within the family as his upcoming surgery and uncertain future affect them. In telling his story, Mr. M. participates in both the assessment and intervention related to his spiritual care. The nurse learns about his relationships and his

concerns surrounding them, and Mr. M. begins to understand what the most important aspects of his situation are from his unique perspective. With that understanding, he can begin to plan what he will do and what help he will seek. The nurse becomes a partner in his plan, which will be revised and updated as his story continues to unfold.

Sharing a story brings the listener face to face with quandaries, insights, struggles, joy, suffering, pain, and healing moments. Stories may make the listener feel helpless in the face of perceived hopeless situations or help the listener recognize the hope that lies in such a situation. Stories challenge nurses to understand the wholeness of a person and to listen for the meaning of a life. One nurse commented,

> I used to think that people who told me stories about their lives were just wasting my time and theirs, but now I realize that they are telling me about what is really important. I've learned to listen and to use what they say to help them see who they really are, what they can really do. Even when they tell me things that are really hard to hear, or even to understand, it seems like they just want me to know that it is part of their life, too.

Stories help the nursing process fit the patient rather than requiring the patient to fit the process.

Some shared wonderings and questions that may help others share their stories include the following:

- If you were writing your life story, what would be the title?
- What is the title of the current chapter?
- Who are some of the heroines and heroes of your story?
- How would you like this chapter to turn out?
- Tell me more about how you handled your child's accident.
- I wonder where you get your spunk.
- I wonder what it's like to live with your physical limitations.
- You've mentioned several times that your sister is ill, and you seem worried.

Nurses can affirm the sharing of stories through statements such as "Your sharing has helped me see this in a different light." As nurses encourage clients to share their stories, it is helpful to encourage the significant people in the clients' lives to participate in the process. The exercises presented in **Exhibit 32-2** may increase attentiveness to story, both among nurses themselves and with clients.

Using Guides and Instruments to Facilitate Spirituality Assessment

Different approaches to assessing spirituality are available to facilitate the integration of spirituality into holistic care. When incorporated into a clinical setting, spirituality assessment guides are a means of gaining a deeper understanding of a person from a holistic perspective. Rather than considering the completion of an instrument to be an end point, nurses can use the questions of an assessment guide as openings or reference points for discussing spirituality with patients and thus come to know and understand them better as unique persons. Furthermore, nurses can adapt the various guides to the specific situation and person. Assessing a person's understanding of spirituality and ways of expressing spirituality includes exploring the role and influence of important connections in the present circumstances; issues related to meaning and purpose; important beliefs, values, and practices; prayer or meditation styles; and desire for connection with religious groups or rituals. The following are a few examples of different approaches to assessing spirituality.

The Spiritual Assessment Tool (**Exhibit 32-3**) is based on a conceptual analysis of spirituality derived from Burkhardt's critical review of the literature.[46] This instrument poses open-ended, reflective questions that assist nurses in developing awareness of spirituality for themselves and others. These questions are meant to be prompts to focus on pertinent spiritual concerns. Similar types of questions are equally appropriate. Some areas may be addressed more fully than others, depending on a particular client's needs. This instrument is meant to be a guide for nurses, to support and enhance their comfort and skills with spirituality assessment, and is not designed as a self-administered survey.

EXHIBIT 32-2 Exercises to Facilitate Awareness of Story

1. Take a few moments to become quiet, perhaps using some breath awareness. In this quiet space, allow yourself to remember, in as much detail as possible, something about yourself, some event or incident that comes to mind. How has this experience or event become a part of who you are? What meaning does it have for your life at this moment?

2. Keep a journal in which you record events, feelings, experiences, insights, and questions in your life. Periodically review your writings, noting themes flowing through your story. Reflect on your story as it keeps evolving.

3. Think about books, stories, songs, fairy tales, movies, plays, or works of art that have special meaning for you. Take time to consider why and how they hold that meaning for you. Think about the images, characters, colors, and sounds that are found in each of these and how they are reflective of your own story. What meanings do you find that provide insight into your own unfolding journey?

4. Write an autobiography for your eyes only. Take your time. Reread and reflect on it. Are there parts you want to share? With whom would you share? What new awareness and insights into yourself and your life journey have come to you?

5. Look at some old family photos or photos of friends. What story do they tell? What memories and feelings come with these pictures? Do you want to tell someone else about them? What do you want to say? Would you like to hear someone else's story about these same photos?

Source: M. Burkhardt and M. G. Nagai-Jacobson, © 1997.

EXHIBIT 32-3   Spiritual Assessment Tool

To facilitate the healing process in clients/patients, families, significant others, and yourself, the following reflective questions assist in assessing, evaluating, and increasing awareness of the spiritual process in yourself and others.

Meaning and Purpose: These questions assess a person's ability to seek meaning and fulfillment in life, manifest hope, and accept ambiguity and uncertainty.
- What gives your life meaning?
- Do you have a sense of purpose in life?
- Does your illness interfere with your life goals?
- Why do you want to get well?
- How hopeful are you about obtaining a better degree of health?
- Do you feel that you have a responsibility in maintaining your health?
- Will you be able to make changes in your life to maintain your health?
- Are you motivated to get well?
- What is the most important or powerful thing in your life?

Inner Strengths: These questions assess a person's ability to manifest joy and recognize strengths, choices, goals, and faith.
- What brings you joy and peace in your life?
- What can you do to feel alive and full of spirit?
- What traits do you like about yourself?
- What are your personal strengths?
- What choices are available to you to enhance your healing?
- What life goals have you set for yourself?
- Do you think that stress in any way caused your illness?
- How aware were you of your body before you became sick?
- What do you believe in?
- Is faith important in your life?
- How has your illness influenced your faith?
- Does faith play a role in regaining your health?

Interconnections: These questions assess a person's positive self-concept, self-esteem, and sense of self; sense of belonging in the world with others; capacity to pursue personal interests; and ability to demonstrate love of self and self-forgiveness.
- How do you feel about yourself right now?
- How do you feel when you have a true sense of yourself?
- Do you pursue things of personal interest?
- What do you do to show love for yourself?
- Can you forgive yourself?
- What do you do to heal your spirit?

These next questions assess a person's ability to connect in life-giving ways with family, friends, and social groups and to engage in the forgiveness of others.
- Who are the significant people in your life?
- Do you have friends or family in town who are available to help you?
- Who are the people to whom you are closest?
- Do you belong to any groups?
- Can you ask people for help when you need it?
- Can you share your feelings with others?
- What are some of the most loving things that others have done for you?
- What are the loving things that you do for other people?
- Are you able to forgive others?

(continues)

EXHIBIT 32-3 Spiritual Assessment Tool *(continued)*

These next questions assess a person's capacity for finding meaning in worship or religious activities and a connectedness with a divinity or universe.
- Is worship important to you?
- What do you consider the most significant act of worship in your life?
- Do you participate in any religious activities?
- Do you believe in God or a higher power?
- Do you think that prayer is powerful?
- Have you ever tried to empty your mind of all thoughts to see what the experience might be like?
- Do you use relaxation or imagery skills?
- Do you meditate?
- Do you pray?
- What is your prayer?
- How are your prayers answered?
- Do you have a sense of belonging in this world?

These next questions assess a person's ability to experience a sense of connection with all of life and Nature, an awareness of the effects of the environment on life and well-being, and a capacity or concern for the health of the environment.
- Do you ever feel at some level a connection with the world or universe?
- How does your environment have an impact on your state of well-being?
- What are your environmental stressors at work and at home?
- Do you incorporate strategies to reduce your environment stressors?
- Do you have any concerns for the state of your immediate environment?
- Are you involved with environmental issues such as recycling environmental resources at home, work, or in your community?
- Are you concerned about the survival of the planet?

Source: Based on M. Burkhardt, "Spirituality: An Analysis of the Concept," *Holistic Nursing Practice* 3, no. 3 (1989): 69. Reprinted from B. M. Dossey, *AHNA Core Curriculum for Holistic Nursing* (Aspen Publishers, 1997): 46–47.

Howden's Spirituality Assessment Scale (SAS; **Exhibit 32-4**) is a 28-item instrument based on a conceptualization of spirituality as a phenomenon represented by four critical attributes.[47] These attributes and the corresponding items on the scale are as follows:

1. *Purpose and meaning in life.* The process of searching for or discovering events or relationships that provide a sense of worth, hope, or reason for existence (Items 18, 20, 22, 28)
2. *Innerness or inner resources.* The process of striving for or discovering wholeness, identity, and a sense of empowerment, manifested in feelings of strength in times of crisis and calmness or serenity in dealing with uncertainty in life, a sense of being guided in living and being at peace with oneself and the world, and feelings of ability (Items 8, 10, 12, 14, 16, 17, 23, 24, 27)
3. *Unifying interconnectedness.* The feeling of relatedness or attachment to others, a sense of relationship to all of life, a feeling of harmony with self and others, and a feeling of oneness with the universe or Universal Being (Items 1, 2, 4, 6, 7, 9, 19, 25, 26)
4. *Transcendence.* The ability to reach or go beyond the limits of usual experience; the capacity, willingness, or experience of rising above or overcoming body or psychic conditions; or the capacity for achieving wellness or self-healing (Items 3, 5, 11, 13, 15, 21)

The SAS is a six-point response-rating scale that uses the following numerical rating: strongly disagree (SD) = 1; disagree (D) = 2; disagree more than agree (DM) = 3; agree more than disagree

EXHIBIT 32-4   Spirituality Assessment Scale

DIRECTIONS: Please indicate your response by circling the appropriate letters indicating how you respond to the statements.

MARK:

SA   if you STRONGLY AGREE

A   if you AGREE

AM   if you AGREE MORE than DISAGREE

DM   if you DISAGREE MORE than AGREE

D   if you DISAGREE

SD   if you STRONGLY DISAGREE

There is no right or wrong answer. Please respond to what you think or how you feel at this point in time.

1. I have a general sense of belonging.	SA	A	AM	DM	S	SD
2. I am able to forgive people who have done me wrong.	SA	A	AM	DM	S	SD
3. I have the ability to rise above or go beyond a physical or psychological condition.	SA	A	AM	DM	S	SD
4. I am concerned about destruction of the environment.	SA	A	AM	DM	S	SD
5. I have experienced moments of peace in a devastating event.	SA	A	AM	DM	S	SD
6. I feel a kinship to other people.	SA	A	AM	DM	S	SD
7. I feel a connection to all of life.	SA	A	AM	DM	S	SD
8. I rely on an inner strength in hard times.	SA	A	AM	DM	S	SD
9. I enjoy being of service to others.	SA	A	AM	DM	S	SD
10. I can go to a spiritual dimension within myself for guidance.	SA	A	AM	DM	S	SD
11. I have the ability to rise above or go beyond a body change or body loss.	SA	A	AM	DM	S	SD
12. I have a sense of harmony or inner peace.	SA	A	AM	DM	S	SD
13. I have the ability for self-healing.	SA	A	AM	DM	S	SD
14. I have an inner strength.	SA	A	AM	DM	S	SD
15. The boundaries of my universe extend beyond usual ideas of what space and time are thought to be.	SA	A	AM	DM	S	SD
16. I feel good about myself.	SA	A	AM	DM	S	SD
17. I have a sense of balance in my life.	SA	A	AM	DM	S	SD
18. There is fulfillment in my life.	SA	A	AM	DM	S	SD
19. I feel a responsibility to preserve the planet.	SA	A	AM	DM	S	SD
20. The meaning I have found for my life provides a sense of peace.	SA	A	AM	DM	S	SD
21. Even when I feel discouraged, I trust that life is good.	SA	A	AM	DM	S	SD
22. My life has meaning and purpose.	SA	A	AM	DM	S	SD
23. My innerness or an inner resource helps me deal with uncertainty in life.	SA	A	AM	DM	S	SD
24. I have discovered my own strength in times of struggle.	SA	A	AM	DM	S	SD
25. Reconciling relationships is important to me.	SA	A	AM	DM	S	SD
26. I feel a part of the community in which I live.	SA	A	AM	DM	S	SD
27. My inner strength is related to belief in a Higher Power or Supreme Being.	SA	A	AM	DM	S	SD
28. I have goals and aims for my life.	SA	A	AM	DM	S	SD

Source: Copyright © 1992, Judy W. Howden.

(AM) = 4; agree (A) = 5; strongly agree (SA) = 6. There is no neutral option. It is scored by summing the responses to all 28 items; subscale scores may be obtained by summing the responses to subscale items.

Another quantitative assessment, the Spirituality Scale (SS; **Exhibit 32-5**), was developed by Delaney as a way to holistically assess beliefs, practices, lifestyle choices, intuitions, and rituals that represent the human spiritual dimension.[48] The SS is a 23-item questionnaire designed to measure the essence of spirituality and guide spiritual interventions in diverse nursing settings. The SS focuses on three domains of spirituality: self-discovery—related to meaning and purpose in life (4 items); relationships—connections with others based on respect and reverence for life (6 items); and eco-awareness—connection with Nature based on belief that Earth is sacred (13 items). Delaney suggests that the scores of the SS (range 23–138) indicate the relative importance of spirituality to the person, with high scores suggesting that spirituality is more evident in the person's life.

The usefulness of numerical scores derived from quantitative spirituality assessment instruments may be more apparent within the context of a research study. In a clinical setting, however, scales such as the SAS or SS can enable a nurse to gain an overall sense of a person's spirituality, either when administering the instrument or when discussing it with a client who has already completed it. The pattern of responses to individual items, more than a numerical score, provides nurses with insights into areas of spiritual strengths and concerns, enabling them to support the strengths and address the concerns. For example, discovering that a person may be experiencing a lack of kinship with others and a lack of connection to life enables the nurse to explore these concerns further and plan appropriate interventions. In the clinical arena, nurses need to remember that a quantitative measure should be an adjunct to, but not a replacement for, listening presence.

Barker offers yet another approach to spirituality assessment in her Personal Spiritual Well-Being Assessment (PSWBA) and Spiritual Well-Being Assessment (SWBA), presented in **Exhibit 32-6**.[49,50] These instruments, which originate in her clinical experiences and research, were developed initially as a short process for assessing spiritual well-being among cancer patients. The SWBA is intended for use by clinicians as they elicit information about the patient's place in the spiritual walk. The PSWBA was originally intended for use by clinicians in determining and clarifying their own spiritual well-being prior to addressing the spiritual well-being of others, but may be useful with patients as well. The respondent is asked to verbalize thoughts regarding the key guide questions. Each instrument uses four broad facets of spiritual well-being: relationship to self, relationship to God/Creative Source, relationship to others, and relationship to Nature. Although this type of assessment format can be self-administered, a greater depth of information and insight can be gained from an interactive process that allows for an exploration of responses.

Barker cautioned nurses to be aware of certain barriers related to spiritual well-being assessment. These barriers include believing that there is not enough time to do the assessment, being embarrassed about asking the questions, thinking that doing the assessment means that the nurse has to solve all of the patient's problems (rescue fantasy), doubting that the nurse can make a difference in the patient's life, feeling responsible for the patient's place in the cosmos, and accepting responsibility for the patient's choices. When experiencing such reactions, nurses can utilize the PSWBA or other processes to explore their own understanding of spirituality, to develop the necessary skills, and to become comfortable with this area of holistic nursing care.

Burkhardt's Care and Nurture of the Spiritual Self—Personal Reflective Assessment (PRA) is derived from qualitative research and broad study of spirituality.[2] This assessment process is designed for personal and clinical use, offering healthcare professionals and patients an opportunity to reflect on the spiritual nature of their life journeys. The PRA encourages persons to take a deeper look at what gives meaning to their lives and important connections with the self, the Sacred Source, others, Nature, and the balance between rest and activity that shapes their spiritual journey. The questions are designed to assist persons in becoming more aware of and attentive to spiritual needs, concerns, supports, and direction at the present time, acknowledging

EXHIBIT 32-5   Spirituality Scale

Please indicate your level of agreement to the following statements by circling the appropriate number that corresponds with the answer key.

Key:
  1. Strongly disagree
  2. Disagree
  3. Mostly disagree
  4. Mostly agree
  5. Agree
  6. Strongly agree

1. I find meaning in my life experiences.	1	2	3	4	5	6
2. I have a sense of purpose.	1	2	3	4	5	6
3. I am happy about the person I have become.	1	2	3	4	5	6
4. I see the sacredness in everyday life.	1	2	3	4	5	6
5. I meditate to gain access to my inner spirit.	1	2	3	4	5	6
6. I live in harmony with nature.	1	2	3	4	5	6
7. I believe there is a connection between all things that I cannot see but can sense.	1	2	3	4	5	6
8. My life is a process of becoming.	1	2	3	4	5	6
9. I believe in a Higher Power or Universal Intelligence.	1	2	3	4	5	6
10. I believe that all living creatures deserve respect.	1	2	3	4	5	6
11. The earth is sacred.	1	2	3	4	5	6
12. I value maintaining and nurturing my relationships with others.	1	2	3	4	5	6
13. I use silence to get in touch with myself.	1	2	3	4	5	6
14. I believe that nature should be respected.	1	2	3	4	5	6
15. I have a relationship with a Higher Power or Universal Intelligence.	1	2	3	4	5	6
16. My spirituality gives me inner strength.	1	2	3	4	5	6
17. I am able to receive love from others.	1	2	3	4	5	6
18. My faith in a Higher Power or Universal Intelligence helps me cope during challenges in my life.	1	2	3	4	5	6
19. I strive to correct the excesses in my own lifestyle patterns/practices.	1	2	3	4	5	6
20. I respect the diversity of people.	1	2	3	4	5	6
21. Prayer is an integral part of my spiritual nature.	1	2	3	4	5	6
22. At times, I feel at one with the universe.	1	2	3	4	5	6
23. I often take time to assess my life choices as a way of living my spirituality.	1	2	3	4	5	6

Note: Those interested in using the Spirituality Scale for clinical or research purposes are asked to contact Dr. Colleen Delaney, RN, PhD, AHN-BC, Associate Professor, University of Connecticut, 231 Glenbrook Rd., Storrs, CT 06269-2026, Colleen.Delaney@uconn.edu.

Source: © Copyright 2003, C. Delaney.

EXHIBIT 32-6   Spiritual Well-Being Assessment Instruments

Personal Spiritual Well-Being Assessment

Relationship to Self

Overall, in the last month, I feel _____ about myself.

Overall, this feeling is _____.

Overall, my "well" feels _____.

Relationship to God/Creative Source

Overall, in the last month, my sense of connection to God/my Creative Source is _____
_____.

Overall, I feel a purpose to being where I am today _____.

Overall, I feel _____ about my place in the world.

Relationship to Others

I feel most connected to _____.

This connection feels _____.

Overall, my relationships are _____.

I have one intimate relationship _____.

This relationship brings me _____.

Relationship to Nature

My favorite part of creation is _____.

The last time I was able to experience this part of creation was _____.

When I experienced this part of creation, I felt _____.

Spiritual Well-Being Assessment

What is (the illness or other concern) _____ like for you?

What do you do to cope with (the illness or other concern)? _____

What makes you smile? _____.

If you could be anywhere, where would you be? _____

What relationships are most important to you? _____

How can I help? _____.

Source: Copyright © 1996, Elizabeth R. Barker.

---

that responses, needs, and insights to a particular question may vary with each visit. Because it is a reflective process, persons are encouraged to focus on those questions that speak to them at the present time. The following are examples of questions included in the PRA:

- *Purpose and meaning.* What principles, values, or beliefs guide your life? How are your life choices congruent with what you consider to be your spiritual path?

- *Connection with self.* What helps you become more aware of who you are, your purpose in being, your place in the cosmos? How do you express your spirit through your physical body? How has your intuitive knowing supported your spiritual journey?

- *Connection with the Sacred Source.* What is most sacred for you? How do you seek and experience relationship with the Divine? What is prayer for you?

- *Connection with others.* Where is forgiveness needed in your life and relationships? How do you nurture your spirit through service to others? Which relationships allow you to be who you are, and to receive as well as to give?

- *Balance of rest and recreation.* How do you incorporate Sabbath time—balance between activity and rest—into your life?

- *Connection with Nature.* How is your spirit nurtured through Nature? What kinds of connection with Nature enliven you?

- *Reflecting on the journey.* As you reflect on your Soul journey, what is the next thing you wish or need to do to support or attune to your wholeness, your self-becoming? How can you make this step real in your life?

The reflective nature of the PRA encourages persons to identify spiritual strengths and supports, as well as needs and concerns, in caring for the spiritual self, and to commit to processes or actions that will assist and support them on the spiritual journey. Nurses can use this process personally and with patients to explore where they are on the spiritual journey, where they feel their path is leading them, where they might like to be going, and what their next step might be in the process.

Each of the assessment guides that have been discussed provides a process for exploring the elements of spirituality. For example, spirituality involves relationships, and each instrument offers a different way in which a nurse may enhance the patient's awareness of significant relationships. The Spiritual Assessment Tool addresses the area of harmonious interconnectedness; Howden's work asks the patient to consider questions related to unifying interconnectedness; Delaney's scale asks about nurturing relationships with others; Barker asks what relationships are most important to the patient; and Burkhardt explores relationships that need mending as well as those that provide support. As nurses become more at home with the concept of spirituality and its language, they will form their own questions and make their own observations in understanding another person as a whole being whose essence is spirit.

■ HOLISTIC CARING PROCESS CONSIDERATIONS

Spiritual caregiving requires an understanding of the holistic caring process that is integrative, in which assessment and intervention may well be the same process, and where description is more useful than labeling. Identification of needs in the area of spirituality does not necessarily indicate pathology or impairment. Research on spirituality and health continues to highlight the importance of describing the human spirit in the language of each person's unique experience and expression and exploring individual meaning within the context of the person's life story. Holistic nurses recognize that spirituality is an important dimension of any health concern, and they use the evolving nursing diagnoses regarding spirituality appropriately. Nurses collaborate with clients and their families in determining appropriate outcomes, developing a plan, and organizing overall care to ensure the incorporation of each person's selfhood, values, and worldview. Nurses facilitate this process when they promote an atmosphere that is accepting and encouraging of spiritual expression in its many and varied forms.

Tending to the Spirit

Care of the spirit, a fundamental aspect of holistic nursing care, takes place in the context of the significant connections in a person's life. The nurse, for a time, enters the patient's world and, through intentional presence in this relationship, may facilitate healing. Assessment, diagnosis, planning, and intervening are all experienced within a unique and particular relationship. Recognizing that all persons are spiritual beings provides the basis for being alert to the many and varied ways in which persons express their spirituality. Often, simply hearing and validating questions and concerns of the spirit are not only part of the assessment, but a part of the intervention as well. Simply giving clients the opportunity to discuss and reflect on spiritual concerns enables them to become more aware of their spirituality and personal spiritual journeys.

Awareness of and care for self as a spiritual being is an important aspect of holistic nursing care. Spiritual co-counseling among colleagues who also deal with spiritual issues and consciously pursue a spiritual path can nurture a nurse's spirit. Forming spiritual companionship, mentoring, or support groups within the work environment, even with one or two colleagues, can help nurses maintain their spirits in the midst of the daily demands on their energies.

Regular practices of prayer, centering, mindfulness, meditation, or starting the day with intention assist nurses in both maintaining and drawing from their own wholeness, and grounds their practice of intentional presence with each patient encounter. With intentionality and consciousness, busy nurses can use common activities as processes or rituals for leaving past situations behind to be more fully present in a current client encounter. For example, when washing hands between patients, nurses can release the concerns of the previous patient and, thus, be more open to those of the next patient. Similarly, by consciously taking a breath before entering an examination room, nurses can clear themselves of other distractions so as to focus on the person to be seen. Pausing to center and focus; "stepping back" from a confusing, distressing situation to reenter from a point of calmness; and being silent as one listens deeply are skills that develop as nurses attend to spirit. With awareness and creativity, nurses can use almost any activity as a way to foster spiritual presence.

Touching

Physical contact through touch in its myriad forms may foster connection. Sensitivity to the meaning of touch for each person is essential in using touch therapeutically. When appropriate, a hand on the shoulder can provide support, a handclasp can convey understanding and presence, an arm around the waist can literally and figuratively give a lift! One patient described a nurse's support in saying, "When the doctor came in to give me the news, she was standing beside me and I could feel her hand on my arm the whole time he was talking. I was so glad that she was just there with me." At times when words cannot be found, or in circumstances where persons are more comfortable with physical expression than with words, touch is a powerful expression of spirit and instrument of healing.

Fostering Connectedness

Relationships are a major aspect of spirituality. Awareness and an appreciation of important relationships in the patient's life enable the nurse to help strengthen meaningful and supportive bonds. Some family members may need encouragement and guidance in visiting and calling. Patients may need assistance in sharing some aspects of their situation with others—even when they very much want to explain what is happening to them and express their feelings about it. Nurses can remind patients of their network of care and support by recognizing and affirming the support of significant others. Statements such as, "You seem especially close to Marta" may provide an opportunity for sharing about a special relationship. Photographs, artwork, and memorabilia of loved ones provide reminders of connections beyond the confines of illness or injury. Pictures or discussions of special places or pets are evidence of other special connections. Visits from pets may be as spiritually uplifting for some people as those from human companions! Using imagery, pictures, and stories can help persons connect with important places, people, and experiences.

Contact with persons from religious, social, business, neighborhood, school, hobby, or interest groups may provide reminders of connections with and participation in the larger community and world. In some healthcare settings, such as intensive care or long-term care facilities, bonds of mutual caring develop among various patients, families, and caregivers. These networks of support can become very significant in the lives of all those involved. Holistic care implies a recognition of the healing potential in such relationships and impels nurses to foster the development of such relationships.

The client's sense of connection with the environment may be an important source of comfort and strength. For persons to be able to feel the wind, see the stars, smell the flowers, touch the trees, and simply to experience the world may be a significant aspect of healing. Is there a window with a view of Nature? Can the patient spend some time outside? Is there a photograph of a scene from Nature on the wall or one of a special place that can be placed at the bedside? Would the patient enjoy a plant, a bouquet of flowers, or a single rose? Some people enjoy audiotapes of music or of nature sounds. Spiritual uplifting can occur when visitors share the progress of the vegetable garden, the news of a recent fishing trip, or reflect on the weather conditions.

Spirituality often calls to mind one's relationship with the sacred. People have unique and personal understandings and experiences of the sacred, and language may pose a problem when talking about this aspect of spirituality. Those who are comfortable with the Judeo-Christian tradition of God or Lord, or the Islamic Allah, may find themselves less comfortable with understandings expressed as Higher Power, Tao, Universal Light, or Absolute. The reverse may also be true. For some people, "new age" is a relevant term that connotes spiritual growth and expansion; for others, however, anything "new age" is suspect and can be spiritually distressing. Listening beyond specific words to hear what is most sacred for this person and how his or her relationship with the sacred may be nurtured is important in addressing spiritual concerns. Are particular words of importance to this person? What is the place of formal religion, and a person's own rabbi, priest, shaman, minister, imam, or spiritual leader in their spiritual journey? How do music, prayer, sacred texts, books, particular objects, foods, or rituals nurture the spirit of this person?

Sensitivity to and appreciation of persons who profess atheism (i.e., disbelief in the existence of a supreme being) or agnosticism (i.e., doubt surrounding the existence of God or ultimate knowledge) involve moving beyond what is not believed. Instead, the nurse listens for that which gives meaning and purpose to the patient's life, including that which brings joy and satisfaction, the nature of hopes and fears, and the recognition of important relationships. How does this particular health crisis fit into the patient's understanding of her or his life, and how is she or he dealing with it? For example, an astronomer who noted that she was not religious and did not believe in God described her understanding and awe in regard to the evolution of the universe as a cause of deep wonder to her that all that had gone before led to this particular time. This sense gave her a feeling "that I belong." The words voiced were not traditionally religious language, but her expressions of appreciation, awe, wonder, and meaning spoke of spirituality.

Nurses who attend to spiritual concerns are willing to be present with mystery, uncertainty, pain, or suffering, seeking not to fix or to answer, but to be in the mystery with another. Letting the client know that they are willing, with their whole being and intention, to stay the course through times of difficulty, pain, and mystery provides encouragement when nurses can only say, "I don't understand this either." This willingness on the part of the nurses may help family and friends to understand that, when they feel that there is nothing they can do, their presence and expressions of love and care are important and valuable components of their healing support.

As nurses learn to understand the relationships and connections that frame a client's life, they become more aware of recurring themes and concerns. When such themes are noted, the nurse reflects on and validates them with the client. Statements such as, "It seems I have often heard you speak of . . . with great concern" gives the client the opportunity to hear the nurse's perceptions and to validate or correct them. In general, it is reassuring to the client to know that the nurse is indeed listening and responding to deep concerns.

Using Rituals to Nurture the Spirit

Rituals serve as reminders to allow sacred time and space in our lives. Both the ritual behavior and the mindfulness that accompanies it are important aspects of ritual. Achterberg and colleagues describe three phases of ritual.[51] The first phase is the symbolic breaking away from everyday busyness. The second phase is the transition phase, which calls for the identification and focus on areas of life that need attention. The third and final phase, referred to as the return phase, is the reentry into everyday life. In essence, ritual gives a person time apart so that he or she may return to the world in a clearer, more centered way. Ritual then can enable nurses to be more intentionally present in healing ways with another. **Exhibit 32-7** provides an example of a ritual that can enhance the healing process.

Either shared with others or highly personalized, rituals are significant aspects of various

EXHIBIT 32-7   The First Ritual Guide to Getting Well

This ritual helps you decide what to do if you are diagnosed with the unknowable, the unthinkable, the awful, or the so-called incurable. By doing this, you can better determine how to survive treatment, yourself, your friends and family, and life in general.

1. Find a quiet place, a healing place, and go there. This might be a corner of your favorite room where you have placed gifts, pictures, a candle, or other symbols that signal peace and inner reflection to you. Or it might be in a park, under an old tree, or in a special place known for its spirit, such as high on a sacred mountain or on the cliffs overlooking a coastline or in the quiet magnificence of a forest.

2. Ask questions of your inner self about what your diagnosis or treatment means in your life. How will life change? What are your resources, your strengths, your reasons for staying alive? These deeply philosophical or spiritual issues often come to mind when problems are diagnosed. Listen with as quiet a mind as possible for any answers or messages that come from within, or from your higher source of guidance.

3. Take this time, knowing that very few problems advance so quickly that you must rush into making decisions about them immediately, without first gaining some perspective.

4. Find at least one friend or advocate who can be levelheaded when you think you are going crazy, who can be positive for you when you are absolutely certain you are doomed, and who can listen when your head is buzzing with uncertainty.

5. Love yourself. Ask yourself moment by moment whether what surrounds you is nurturing and life-giving. If the answer is no, back off from it. Kindly tell all negative-thinking people that you will not be seeing them while you are going through this. You may need never to see them again, and this is your right and obligation to yourself.

6. Assess your belief system. What do you believe? How did you get to believe it in the first place? What is really happening inside you and outside you? How serious is it? What will it take to get you well?

7. Gather information, keeping an open mind. Everyone who offers to treat you or give you advice has their life invested in what they tell you. Stand back and listen thoughtfully.

8. Now go and hire your healing team. Remember, you hired them—you can fire them. They are in the business of performing a service for you, and you are paying their salaries. Sometimes this relationship gets confused. Make sure they all talk to each other. You are in command. You are the captain of the healing team.

9. Don't let anyone talk you into treatment you don't believe in or don't understand. Keep asking questions. Replace anyone who acts too busy to answer your questions. Chances are, they're also too busy to do their best work for you.

10. Don't agree on any diagnostic or lab tests unless someone you trust can give you good reasons why they are being ordered. If the tests are not going to change your treatment, they are an expensive and dangerous waste of your time.

11. Sing your own song, write your own story, take your own spiritual journey through a journal or diary. A threat to health and well-being can be a trigger to becoming and doing all those things you've been putting off for the "right" time.

12. Consider these maxims in your journey:
    - Everything cures somebody, and nothing cures everybody.
    - There are no simple answers to complex issues, like why people get sick in the first place.
    - Sometimes disease is inexplicable to mortal minds.

EXHIBIT 32-7   The First Ritual Guide to Getting Well *(continued)*

13. You will not be intimidated by the overbearing world of medicine or alternative health know-it-alls but can thoughtfully take the best from several worlds.

14. You can teach gentleness and compassion to the most arrogant doctor and the crankiest nurse. Tell them that you need your mind and soul nurtured, as well as the best medical treatment possible in order to get well. If they are not up to it, you'll find someone someplace who is.

Source: From *Rituals of Healing: Using Imagery for Health and Wellness*, by J. Achterberg, B. Dossey, and L. Kolkmeier. Copyright © 1994 by Jeanne Achterberg, Barbara Dossey, and Leslie Kolkmeier. Used by permission of Bantam Books, a division of Bantam Doubleday Dell Publishing Group, Inc.

religious traditions and cultures. Rituals come in many shapes and forms. Routine morning walks, daily prayer time, sharing of the day's experiences with family over dinner, or a soothing bath can all be rituals. Anything done with awareness may serve as a ritual. Rituals provide a rich resource in caring for the spirit, and attending to rituals in one's life can be an important aspect of self-care.

Developing Centering, Mindfulness, and Awareness

Spiritual disciplines are those practices that cause people to pause in the midst of their activities and busyness to attend to matters of the spirit or soul. The practice of spiritual disciplines requires intention and attention. Eastern and many indigenous traditions around the world emphasize the importance of mindfulness and awareness as disciplines that permeate all of life. Similar to the practice of centering prayer in Judeo-Christian traditions, the mystical path of many traditions calls one to quietness. Making the intentional decision to pause and be mindful of the present moment and all that it holds nurtures the ability to be centered and aware. Taking the time to observe what is going on within oneself, without judgment or elaboration, and to note thoughts, feelings, physical sensations, and distractions, provides valuable experiences in the practice of awareness. Observing what is going on in the environment, attending to all senses, and experiencing all sensations enhance a person's full presence in the moment.

Processes of relaxation and imagery facilitate awareness and centering and assist patients in accessing their own Sacred Space. The practice of spiritual disciplines provides access to a centered space from which the nurse and client can work together, confronting significant life experiences in an environment that is often busy and complex. Questions such as, "Have you ever tried any particular methods of relaxing?" or "What kinds of activities help you find calm in the middle of a busy day?" may facilitate a person's practice of spiritual disciplines in a more intentional way.

Praying and Meditating

Prayer and meditation are spiritual disciplines practiced in many traditions, both cultural and religious. Appreciating the personal nature of these disciplines, the nurse, with respect and sensitivity, can help patients remember or explore ways in which they reach out to and listen for God or the Sacred Source. Recalling the place and meaning of prayer, and the ways in which they experience the presence of and communion with God or the Sacred Source, provides patients with a rich resource. In the clinical setting, both the nurse's and the patient's understanding of prayer will determine the role of prayer. Clarifying the patient's understanding of and need for prayer is a part of holistic care. Some patients want others to pray with or for them, while others do not believe in prayer. Supporting each patient's requests and needs for prayer may mean inviting others to take part in various forms of prayer with and for the patient or simply praying with the patients themselves. The nurse can encourage expression of the patient's desire for shared prayer, for participation in religious worship, or for quiet, uninterrupted periods of time for personal spiritual practices. Facilitating the appreciation and practice of prayer in a patient's life is an important aspect of caring for the spirit.

Exploring as many aspects of the prayer experience as possible enriches both the nurse's and the patient's understanding of the nature and place of prayer for a particular individual. Sacred or inspirational readings, music, drumming, movement, light or darkness, aromas, and time of day are among the many factors that may be important considerations in one's prayer life. The patient's prayer life, in all of its fullness and meaning, nurtures the spirit, and the nurse may be able to support the patient's prayer needs by facilitating changes in the environment or schedule. It is wise to remember that merely the process of listening to and appreciating the prayer life of another nurtures the spirit and acknowledges the spiritual dimension of that person.

Ensuring Opportunities for Rest and Leisure

Integral aspects of holistic living and care of the spirit, rest, leisure, and Sabbath time enhance growth, creativity, and renewal.[52-54] Leisure is an attitude of the heart that facilitates connection with the inner self and the Sacred Source and opens one to reflect on and envision a life of doing to allow for more Being. Authentic leisure implies an approach to living that allows one to relax into a level of being that deepens self-awareness, nourishes one's wholeness, and enriches connections with the Sacred Source and other people. Assisting persons to consider the place of rest and leisure in their lives is part of holistic nursing. Taking stock of how they integrate rest and leisure into their own lives is a necessary part of self-care for nurses as well. In an increasingly busy society—where filling each moment is viewed in terms of productivity, where even leisure time is scheduled—the notion of rest and leisure deserves thoughtful consideration.

Holistic nurses try to enhance patients' conscious awareness of how rest and leisure are, or are not, part of their lives. Such awareness makes those areas available for intentional evaluation and, if desired, change. Observations and questions that may be helpful in the exploration of this aspect of spirituality include the following:

- I notice that you read a lot. What does reading do for you?
- You say you just can't rest. When have you been able to rest? Are there things that usually help you to rest?
- What is a real vacation like for you?
- What time of the day (year, season, week) is most restful or peaceful for you?
- How do you relax?
- Some people just help us to relax; who does that for you?
- Is there something I can do to help you to relax?

Regular exercise, music, imagery, a specific time for rest and quiet, and the commitment to incorporating these experiences into daily life encourage rest and leisure. Validating the importance of rest and leisure and encouraging a commitment to making time for renewal an essential part of one's life are important aspects of holistic care.

■ ARTS AND SPIRITUALITY

The arts have a role in the life of the spirit. Many persons find that various forms of artistic endeavor are doors to and expressions of the spirit. The term *artist* can include anyone who creates—the homemaker who cooks and sews and the carpenter who designs and builds, as well as the more easily recognized persons whose works are heard in symphonies or seen in galleries. As an expression of her or his wholeness, an artist's work is also a reflection of spirituality. L'Engle expresses this well:

> As I listen in the silence, I learn that my feelings about art and my feelings about the Creator of the Universe are inseparable. To try to talk about art and about Christianity is for me one and the same thing, and it means attempting to share the meaning of my life, what gives it, for me, its tragedy and its glory. It is what makes me respond to the death of an apple tree, the birth of a puppy, northern lights shaking the sky, by writing stories.[55]

Literature contains life stories, both real and fictional, to which people relate and from which they learn, gain comfort, and garner encouragement. Poetry contains deep truths, often in a few well-chosen words, a rhythm, and spaces for silence. Music expresses feelings that are beyond words. Songs bring back memories or capture what people would like to say. Pottery awakens the senses of touch and sight as one forms a vessel or holds a favorite mug. Dance moves people, literally and figuratively, in space and time. Photography connects individuals and sometimes moves their hearts for those known only through the images seen all over the world. Drumming awakens deep, basic yearnings and calls some to worship. Gardens nourish not only the body, but also the senses of sight, touch, taste, and smell. Cave drawings are reminders of civilizations past and awaken a sense of wonder.

Providing an atmosphere that, as much as possible, is pleasing to the sensibilities of the patient may promote rest and relaxation. It may also facilitate the use of other interventions, such as imagery. Encouraging and facilitating opportunities for people to engage in or share stories of their creative endeavors is one of the ways that nurses include spirituality in care.

■ CONCLUSION

Because all persons, nurses as well as patients, are spiritual beings, care of the spirit is integral to holistic nursing care. Care of the spirit requires the evolution of language to express this dimension of ourselves better and an approach to the nursing process that is integrative rather than linear. Spirituality assessment and intervention, which are often the same process, require intentional listening, presence, and a willingness to hear another's story. Spiritual care is based on a recognition that people express and experience their spirituality in and through relationships with the Sacred Source, others, Nature, and self.

Spiritual care may incorporate "experts," such as representatives of particular religious traditions or other spiritual support people, but nurses need to do more than merely refer matters of the spirit to these persons. Although

spiritual matters are both deep and personal, they often come to the forefront of life when health crises cause a person to stop, to take stock, to experience anxieties and fear, and to seek that which is at the heart of his or her life. Nurses offer spiritual support as they are able to be present with mystery and the life questions of others. Tending to matters of the spirit may include incorporating ritual, prayer, meditation, rest, art, and any activity that enhances awareness of oneself and one's place in the world.

Directions for
FUTURE RESEARCH

1. Further explore the influence of spirituality in health and illness across cultures and in different age groups, using both qualitative and quantitative methodologies.
2. Explore the role of spirituality in reducing stress and promoting positive health outcomes.
3. Investigate ways to support nurses in integrating spirituality into clinical practice.

Nurse Healer
REFLECTIONS

After reading this chapter, the nurse healer will be able to answer or to begin a process of answering the following questions:

- In recognizing my wholeness, how would I describe my relationship with my physical being, my emotional being, and my spiritual being?
- What signals spiritual distress in my own life?
- How do I nurture my spirit?
- How do nurture and make time for the most important connections in my life?
- What areas of the spirit need intentional care in my own life, perhaps because of pain or distress, or because there are areas in which I want to focus and grow?
- How have my life experiences contributed to the growth and development of my spirit?
- How have I experienced intentional presence?

For a full suite of assignments and additional learning activities, use the access code located in the front of your book to visit this exclusive website: http://go.jblearning.com/dossey. If you do not have an access code, you can obtain one at the site.

NOTES

1. L. Tzu, *Tao Te Ching* (London, England: Penguin Books, 1988).
2. M. A. Burkhardt and M. G. Nagai-Jacobson, *Spirituality: Living Our Connectedness* (Albany, NY: Delmar Thompson Learning, 2002).
3. L. Chiu et al., "An Integrative Review of the Concept of Spirituality in the Health Sciences," *Western Journal of Nursing Research* 26 (2004): 405–428.
4. B. McBrien, "A Concept Analysis of Spirituality," *British Journal of Nursing* 15, no. 1 (2006): 42-45.
5. M. Lewis et al., "African American Spirituality: A Process of Honoring God, Others, and Self," *Journal of Holistic Nursing* 25, no. 1 (2007): 16–23.
6. L. Y. F. Chung et al., "Relationship of Nurses' Spirituality to Their Understanding and Practice of Spiritual Care," *Journal of Advanced Nursing* 58, no. 2 (2007): 158–170.
7. E. Mok et al., "The Meaning of Spirituality and Spiritual Care Among the Hong Kong Chinese Terminally Ill," *Journal of Advanced Nursing* 66, no. 2 (2010): 360–370.
8. J. C. Engebretson and J. H. Headley, "Cultural Diversity and Care," in *Holistic Nursing: A Handbook for Practice*, 6th ed., ed. B. M. Dossey and L. Keegan (Burlington, MA: Jones & Bartlett Learning, 2013).
9. M. A. Burkhardt, "Becoming and Connecting: Elements of Spirituality for Women," *Holistic Nursing Practice* 8 (1994): 12–21.
10. B. McBrien, "A Concept Analysis of Spirituality," *British Journal of Nursing* 15, no. 1 (2006): 42-45.
11. C. M. Lemmer, "Recognizing and Caring for Spiritual Needs of Clients," *Journal of Holistic Nursing* 2, no. 3 (2005): 310–322.
12. A. Noble and C. Jones, "Getting It Right: Oncology Nurses' Understanding of Spirituality," *International Journal of Palliative Nursing* 16, no. 11 (2010): 565–569.
13. C. Craig et al., "Spirituality, Chronic Illness, and Rural Life," *Journal of Holistic Nursing* 24, no. 1 (2006): 27–35.
14. I. Tuck, R. Alleyne, and W. Thinganjana, "Spirituality and Stress Management in Healthy Adults," *Journal of Holistic Nursing* 24, no. 4 (2006): 245–253.
15. L. M. Lewis et al., "African American Spirituality: A Process of Honoring God, Others, and Self," *Journal of Holistic Nursing* 25, no. 1 (2007): 16–23.
16. T. Berry and M. E. Tucker, *The Sacred Universe: Earth, Spirituality, and Religion in the Twenty-First Century* (New York, NY: Columbia University Press, 2009).
17. P. Woodruff, *Reverence—Renewing a Forgotten Virtue* (Oxford, England: Oxford University Press, 2001).
18. B. Plotkin, *Nature and the Human Soul* (Novato, CA: New World Library, 2008).
19. S. Jeffers, *Brother Eagle, Sister Sky* (New York, NY: Dial Books, 1991).
20. M. A. Burkhardt, "Healing Relationships with Nature," *Complementary Therapies in Nursing and Midwifery* 6 (2000): 35–40.
21. M. McKivergin, "The Nurse as an Instrument of Healing," in *Holistic Nursing: A Handbook for Practice*, 5th ed., pp. 721–737, ed. B. M. Dossey and L. Keegan (Sudbury, MA: Jones & Bartlett, 2009).
22. J. Watson, *Caring Science as Sacred Science* (Philadelphia, PA: F. A. Davis, 2005).
23. E. Tolle, *A New Earth: Awakening to Your Life's Purpose* (New York, NY: Dutton, 2005).
24. A. Hankey, "The Thermodynamics of Healing, Health, and Love," *Journal of Alternative and Complementary Medicine* 13, no. 1 (2007): 5–7.
25. B. R. Ferrell and N. Coyle, "The Nature of Suffering and the Goals of Nursing," *Oncology Nursing Forum* 35, no 2 (2008): 241–247.
26. S. Johnson, "Hope in Terminal Illness: An Evolutionary Concept Analysis," *International Journal of Palliative Nursing* 13, no. 9 (2007): 451–459.
27. T. R. Pipe et al., "A Prospective Descriptive Study Exploring Hope, Spiritual Well-Being, and Quality of Life in Hospitalized Patients," *MEDSURG Nursing* 17, no. 4 (2008): 247–257.
28. B. L. Seaward, *Quiet Mind, Fearless Heart: The Taoist Path Through Stress and Spirituality* (Hoboken, NJ: John Wiley, 2005).
29. W. Grossman, *To Be Healed by the Earth* (New York, NY: Seven Stories Press, 2007).
30. G. Recine, et al., "Concept Analysis of Forgiveness with a Multi-cultural Emphasis," *Journal of Advanced Nursing* 59, no. 3 (2007): 308–316.
31. M. Arnold, B. Ballif-Spanvill, and K. Tracy, eds., *A Chorus for Peace—A Global Anthology of Poetry by Women* (Iowa City, IA: University of Iowa Press, 2002): xv.
32. L. Dossey, *Prayer Is Good Medicine* (San Francisco, CA: Harper, 1996).
33. M. D. Calabria and J. A. Macrae, eds., *Suggestions for Thought by Florence Nightingale: Selections and Commentaries* (Philadelphia, PA: University of Pennsylvania Press, 1994).

34. B. M. Dossey, *Florence Nightingale: Mystic, Visionary, Healer* (Springhouse, PA: Springhouse Corporation, 2000).

35. A. Narayanasamy and M. Narayanasamy, "The Healing Power of Prayer and Its Implications for Nursing," *British Journal of Nursing* 17, no. 6 (2008): 394–398.

36. M. B. Helming, "Healing Through Prayer: A Qualitative Study," *Holistic Nursing Practice* 25, no. 1 (2011): 33–44.

37. M. J. Breslin and C. A. Lewis, "Theoretical Models of the Nature of Prayer and Health: A Review," *Mental Health, Religion & Culture* 11, no. 1 (2008): 9–21.

38. L. Dossey, *Be Careful What You Pray For* (San Francisco, CA: HarperCollins, 1997).

39. B. M. Dossey, "Florence Nightingale: A 19th-Century Mystic," *Journal of Holistic Nursing* 28, no. 1 (2010): 10–35.

40. B. M. Dossey, "Florence Nightingale: Her Crimean Fever Chronic Illness," *Journal of Holistic Nursing* 28, no. 1 (2010): 38–53.

41. R. Sawatzky and B. Pesut, "Attributes of Spiritual Care in Nursing Practice," *Journal of Holistic Nursing* 23, no. 1 (2005): 19–33.

42. J. Bruchac, *Tell Me a Tale* (New York, NY: Harcourt, Brace, 1997): 1.

43. M. P. R. Liehr and M. J. Smith, "Story Theory," in *Middle Range Theory for Nursing*, 2nd ed., ed. M. J. Smith and P. R. Liehr (New York, NY: Springer, 2008).

44. H. L. Gaydos, "Understanding Personal Narratives: An Approach to Practice," *Journal of Advanced Nursing* 49, no. 3 (2005): 254–259.

45. M. Stibich and L. Wissow, "Meaning Shift: Findings from Wellness Acupuncture," *Alternative Therapies in Health and Medicine* 12, no. 2 (2006): 42–48.

46. M. A. Burkhardt, "Spirituality: An Analysis of the Concept," *Holistic Nursing Practice* 3 (1989): 69–77.

47. J. W. Howden, *Development and Psychometric Characteristics of the Spirituality Assessment Scale* (unpublished doctoral dissertation, Texas Woman's University, Denton, 1992).

48. C. Delaney, "The Spirituality Scale: Development and Psychometric Testing of a Holistic Instrument to Assess the Human Spiritual Dimension," *Journal of Holistic Nursing* 23, no. 2 (2005): 145–167.

49. E. R. Barker, *Patient Spirituality Assessment: A Tool That Works* (paper presented at the Uniformed Nurse Practitioners Association Meeting, Seattle, WA, November 1996).

50. E. R. Barker, *How to Do Research, Get Finished, and Not Lose Your Balance* (presentation at the Nursing Research Symposium, San Diego, CA, 1998).

51. J. Achterberg et al., *Rituals of Healing: Using Imagery for Health and Wellness* (New York, NY: Bantam Books, 1994).

52. W. Mueller, *Sabbath: Restoring the Sacred Rhythms of Rest* (New York, NY: Bantam Books, 2000).

53. S. Grafanaki et al., "Sources of Renewal: A Qualitative Study on the Experience and Role of Leisure in the Life of Counselors and Psychologists," *Counseling Psychology Quarterly* 18, no. 1 (2005): 31–40.

54. P. Heintzman, "Leisure-Spiritual Coping: A Model for Therapeutic Recreation and Leisure Services," *Therapeutic Recreation Journal* 42, no. 1 (2008): 56–73.

55. M. L'Engle, *Walking on Water: Reflecting on Faith and Art* (Wheaton, IL: Harold Shaw Publishers, 1980): 16.

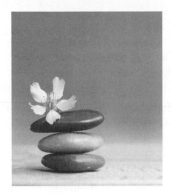

Chapter 33

Energy Healing

Victoria E. Slater

Nurse Healer
OBJECTIVES

Theoretical

- Name and describe three major energetic structures.
- Discuss one view of chakras.
- Describe electromagnetic induction and entrainment and how they might operate in energy healing.
- Discuss the role of intention in creating healing space.
- Discuss one problem in energy healing research.

Clinical

- Find an expert healer and determine what makes this person an expert healer. What made you decide this person was an expert? If this person is a nurse practicing energy healing, how does she integrate them?

Personal

- Use the intuitive exercises in the chapter to explore auras, chakras, and meridians.
- Experience a laying on of hands modality.
- Explore the effect of your presence.
- Experience an essential oil, flower essence, and/or homeopathic preparation that might be useful for you.

- Experience the effects of music you do not like. Stand a few feet away from it as you listen to it for a few minutes. Gradually, over several weeks, move closer.

DEFINITIONS

Aura: An atmosphere; a vague, luminous glow surrounding something. It may be an information-containing electromagnetic field and can be likened to the data contained within a computer.

Capacitor: A device that stores electric charge.

Centering: An altered state of consciousness that results in the centered person's hands emitting measurable extra-low-frequency magnetic pulses of 0.3–3.0 hertz (Hz), that is, cycles per second.

Chakra: An energy center in the subtle, or energetic, body that is described as a whirling vortex of light.

Electromagnetic induction: The causing or inducing of voltage, a change in an electrical current.

Energy healing: The deliberate process of using an external energy field to induce a change in one's own or another's field for the purpose of physical, mental, emotional, and spiritual healing. Energy healing may involve the presence of a caring person.

Entrainment: The phenomenon of rhythmic processes synchronizing with each other.

Synchronization is recognized in pendulum clocks, planets, music, an organism adjusting to the light/dark cycle, brain waves, social groups, and more.

Intention: Purpose, aim, or objective; the choice to act or think in a certain way.

Meridian: Microvolt electrical conduits organized in an electrical mesh that permeates the body and precedes development of vessels and organs. In Eastern philosophies, the meridians are said to conduct *chi*, or universal energy.

Resistor: Part of an electrical device that resists the flow of charge.

Subtle energies: Barely noticeable electrical and magnetic fields of living organisms that may be related to internal electrical and magnetic activity.

Voltage: A measurement related to the difference in potential energy between two adjacent areas.

■ THEORY AND RESEARCH

Energy healing is often described as "woo-woo" or wishful thinking. This chapter is an attempt to offer physics explanations for healing approaches that make no sense from a biological or physiological perspective. How can laying on of hands modalities such as Reiki, Healing Touch, and Therapeutic Touch, among others, work? How do aromatherapies, flower essences, homeopathy, and even music, sound, and light work as healing modalities? This chapter proposes that electromagnetic induction is involved in many of the results of laying of hands modalities and that entrainment contributes to the effects of aromatherapies, flower essences, homeopathies, some music, sound, and light.

Physicists teach that until there is experimental and mathematic proof of something, it is a theory, not a fact. That is the state in which we find ourselves with energy healing modalities—laying on of hands treatments *act* like they involve electromagnetic induction; other types of healing modalities *act* like they involve entrainment, but there is no experimental proof or mathematic support for these theories. However, a theory must be presented before it can be tested. This chapter attempts to do that—to

present the idea that well-known, basic physics principles are involved in energy therapies.

To accomplish this goal, the chapter presents the three-part energy anatomy of aura, chakras, and meridians from a traditional viewpoint and then compares those views to physical structures they resemble. Once the reader has the understanding that these seemingly esoteric structures might be just pieces of an electromagnetic structure, the physics principles of electromagnetic induction and of entrainment are discussed. An understanding of these principles opens the possibility that the *presence* of the nurse might even be an electromagnetic and entrainment event and that the mere presence of a caring person can be healing.

Researching the effects of applied electromagnetic induction techniques (laying on of hands modalities) and of entrainment (homeopathy) requires a new look at standard research methodology. If the presence of another person is healing, then the experimental/control research methodology to test laying on of hands modalities is questionable. How do you isolate the effect of the presence of the experimental and sham providers versus the treatment protocol? Perhaps you can't. Typical research questions then may become: "How do you teach nurses to maximize an electromagnetic event, such as laying on of hands? How do you teach a nurse how to maximize *presence*? When are energy therapy modalities appropriate and in what combination with standard treatment?" These are just a few of the research questions that come to mind when one begins to imagine how to research phenomena that may be based in principles of physics, rather than the sciences nurses have studied for decades.

We begin the study of energy healing by defining it and looking at two ways to categorize energy modalities.

■ DEFINITIONS AND CATEGORIZATION OF ENERGY HEALING

Energy healing describes healing that alters the subtle flow of energy within and around a person or organism. Many people believe that the state of this subtle flow of energy determines the biological and psychological health of the organism; if it is not flowing properly, you hurt. You hurt physically, you hurt emotionally, and you hurt spiritually. Many cultures have developed methods to heal that flow, including the Chinese *ChiKung* (qi gong), the Hawaiian *Huna*, Tibetan meditations, Hindu yoga, and Native American drumming, among others. The energy is called by many names, including *chi, ki, qi, mana, prana*, and *etheric*; modalities using these energies are classified as "laying on of hands," "biofield therapy," and "subtle energy healing." Other forms of subtle energy healing use light, sound, aromas, homeopathy, and flower essences.

As people have been exposed to different cultures and experiences, energy healing modalities have become more common and accepted in the United States. Therapeutic Touch was one of the first energy healing modalities brought to nursing. Krieger, an American nurse, developed this popular Western adaptation of the Indian laying on of hands practice of Pranic healing.[1] Other traditional forms of laying on of hands healing are Reiki and qi gong, which are from Japan and China. New versions of laying on of hands modalities have evolved, such as Polarity and Healing Touch, which blend traditional and scientific concepts. Many nurses have adopted these and other subtle energy modalities as part of their nursing practices.

Energy healing may or may not be the same thing as the widely used term *energy medicine*. *Energy healing* seems more appropriate for holistic nurses because so much of nursing is about the use of *presence*, and many forms of healing involve the active presence of a caring person. Energy medicine is one of five National Center for Complementary and Alternative Medicine (NCCAM) categories; the others are mind–body medicine, natural product–based therapies, manipulative and body-based practices, and whole medical systems.[2]

NCCAM places various modalities in each of these categories, but in this chapter the modalities are not approached from the five categories, but are viewed from the perspective of the physics that might underpin them. For example, laying on of hands modalities such as qi gong, Healing Touch, and Reiki are listed as energy therapies in the NCCAM categories; in this chapter they are considered electromagnetic induction techniques. NCCAM puts homeopathy under Alternative (Whole) Medical Systems; here it is considered an entrainment technique.

■ ENERGY ANATOMY

The Aura

The discussion of the aura begins with exploring some traditional explanations of the nature of the aura, moves to a discussion of the small amount of scientific research on the human aura, considers the possibility that the aura acts like an electromagnetic field, and concludes with some intuitive exercises the reader can use to explore his/her own aura.

Traditional Explanations of the Aura

The aura is traditionally described as an oval of golden light surrounding the body. It seems to be denser closer to the body, thus easier to sense, and less dense and more difficult to sense as you move farther away from the body. A person's aura is slightly larger than the person is when he or she stands with the arms extended.

There are a number of diverse understandings of the aura. Two well-known ones are Brennan's and Kunz's. Brennan's system includes seven layers divided into three planes: physical, astral, and spiritual. The astral body is "the state between energy and matter."[3] According to Brennan, each layer interpenetrates the others as well as the physical body, which is considered the densest layer. Her model also reflects chakra functions, with each auric level associated with a chakra.

Kunz defines the aura as dense light—a 12- to 18-inch-thick, multicolored, elastic oval light that interpenetrates and surrounds the body.[4] It is composed of an upper and a lower hemisphere linked by a green band that encircles the middle of the physical body. She taught that chakras are an integral part of the aura.

Although the two descriptions differ, they have several similarities. Both describe two planes linked by a narrower band and both authors believe that chakras are integral to the aura. It would appear that Kunz and Brennan describe the same phenomenon from different perspectives.

The differences between these two interpretations may be explained by Benor's discovery that multiple healers making simultaneous intuitive diagnoses of the same person sense different things. Each believes that he or she "perceived THE true picture of each patient's condition, rather than one out of many possible pictures of this reality."[5] He proposes that intuitive diagnosticians obtain their impressions through a "window of observation" and that individual healers may have "blind spots." Just as Benor's healers saw different information in the same aura, perhaps Brennan, Kunz, and others see different aspects of the aura.

The aura, it is believed, can be damaged, which leads to a host of physical, emotional, and social problems, including post-traumatic stress disorder syndrome (PTSD). Damage can be caused by accidents, surgery, radiation therapy, hateful stares, not speaking your own truth, combat, and innumerable other traumas. Such damage can lead to stress, fatigue, pain, depression, and other problems; energy healing can lead to relief of these problems along with increased energy, peace, and, eventually, a deeper relationship with loved ones and with the Divine.

Research into the Aura

Scientific research into the aura is difficult. How do we study something many people do not believe exists? Two types of cameras have been designed that show movement within the aura. Harry Oldfield invented Polycontrast Interference Photography (PIP), a computer imaging system that shows the energy moving around the body.[6] The colored bands of light reveal areas where the energy is diminished or not flowing and even where the body is leaking energy. Chakras and meridians are visible and the details in the photographs give information about the level of their functioning. The International Society for the Study of Subtle Energies and Energy Medicine (ISSSEEM) gave Oldfield the 2006 Alyce and Elmer Green Award for Innovation for his camera.[7] Enter the term "Harry Oldfield" in a search engine on the Web to see videos available on YouTube.

At the 2010 ISSSEEM conference, another camera was demonstrated, the Electrophotonic Camera (EPC). This one is based on Gas Discharge Visualization analysis. The theory is that exposure to electrical fields causes the body to emit gases that can be photographed and analyzed.[8] The result allows for viewing of real-time changes in the energy field of humans and other organisms.[9]

Scientific Explanations of the Aura: Comparing the Aura to an Electromagnetic Field

The human aura mimics an electromagnetic (EM) field (see **Table 33-1**), which has the following properties:

1. An electromagnetic field gives us power to do work we could not do by ourselves. It can lift cars in junk yards and is used to create the motors we use in many aspects of life.

2. One way to create an electromagnetic field is to place current carrying wires close together. When electricity is flowing, it creates an electromagnetic field surrounding the flow. When current-carrying wires are close to each other, their electromagnetic fields combine and the result is a stronger field. Engineers do this by tightly coiling an electrical wire around some kind of core, such as an iron rod, creating the effect of a series of adjacent wires even though it is one long electric wire.

3. The amount of power created is determined by the number of times the electric wire is wound around the core, meaning the more adjacent electric currents, the more work that can be done with the same amount of electricity.

4. Although it is not exactly the same, you can visualize an electromagnetic field by sprinkling iron filings randomly on a piece of paper. Place a bar magnet in the middle of the iron filings and notice how they instantly move to take a more or less oval shape around the magnet. (You may need to tap the piece of paper to help the iron filings move a bit.) This oval shape demonstrates the magnetic field emitted by the magnet. If you have the equipment, coil an electric wire around an iron core, sprinkle iron filings next to it, and turn on the electricity. You will see that the iron filings arrange themselves in a pattern around the wire/iron core device. More filings are closer to the core than farther

TABLE 33-1 Similarities Between an Electromagnetic Field and the Human Aura	
An Electromagnetic Field	**The Human Aura**
A magnetic field can be created by using a core, often iron or ceramic, that is surrounded by a current carried by coiled wires.	Hemoglobin contains iron and it constantly circulates in the arteries, veins, and capillaries. This iron mesh is intertwined by the electrical field of neurons, meridians, and the pulsing of each cell.
When electricity flows through the wiring around the core, a magnetic field is created that is somewhat oval shaped.	The human aura can be sensed as an oval-shaped area that surrounds the body. (See **Figure 33-1**.)
The EM field decreases in strength farther from the core.	The aura is more difficult to discern farther from the body.
EM fields can carry information, just as they do in computers and around telephone wires.	The aura stores our information: our personal history, thoughts, emotions, hopes, fears, and more.
Only a small amount of electrical power properly configured is needed to create a powerful magnetic field at a certain location.	The human being (a certain location) is surprisingly powerful for just a collection of bones, muscles, tissue, blood, neurons, and meridians.

EM = electromagnetic.

Source: Material on EM fields interpreted from P. G. Hewitt, *Conceptual Physics*, 10th ed. (San Francisco, CA: Pearson-Addison Wesley, 2006): 464–469; P. Xiong-Skiba, personal communication, March–April 2007; material on the human aura from V. Slater's personal observations (copyright © 2011, Victoria Slater).

away, suggesting that the field is stronger closer to the core than it is farther away.

The Human Aura

The human aura closely resembles an electromagnetic field in the following ways:

1. Human blood contains hemoglobin, which contains iron. The vascular system of heart, arteries, veins, and capillaries results in an intricate tubular iron core that is surrounded by or, more accurately, intertwined by three electrical fields: neurons, meridians, and the minute electrical pulses of each single cell. Because of the electrical flow around the body's iron core, the body must put out an electromagnetic field.

   Medical science uses the magnetic nature of the human body for diagnoses. The magnetocardiogram (MCG) measures the heart's magnetic field, and the magnetoencephalogram (MEG) assesses the head's magnetic field. The well-known

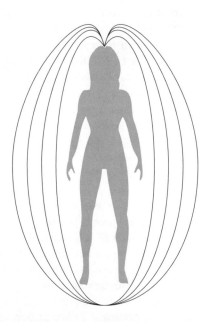

FIGURE 33-1   The Electromagnetic Human
Source: Copyright © 1999, Carol Eckert.

MRI (magnetic resonance imaging) produces pictures of the body at the cellular level.[10]

2. People who are anemic have too little iron in their bloodstreams and are weak. Perhaps this is because their iron core is diminished, and, even with an unchanged electrical field, they emit less electromagnetic power and have less power to do work.

3. If you choose to sense a person's electromagnetic field, notice that it is easier to sense closer to the person than farther away. You may be able to sense a layer-like pattern with different characteristics at different distances from the body. Some areas are thick, others moist, some bumpy; each is likely to be different from the next.

Intuitive Experiences of the Aura

The best way to understand the electromagnetic nature of the aura is to experience it. Take a moment to sense your own electromagnetic field.

Rub your hands vigorously until you feel heat. Separate them slightly and notice the amount of pressure, heat, or other sensations between them. Slowly, move your hands apart and then together. Do you feel changes in the density, heat, or other sensations between your hands?

Sense another person's electromagnetic field by moving your hands around their head and shoulders and down their bodies. Is everyone's field the same or do they differ? Compare an area that hurts to one that doesn't. Notice the differences in the fields of an athletic person versus a sedentary one, of a man and a woman, and of a child and an adult. Sense your pet's field. What did you discover about the aura of your family, friends, pets, and yourself?

Chakras

The word "chakra" is becoming more widespread in the Western world, but their functions have been recognized in a number of psychological theories well known to nurses, including Maslow's Hierarchy of Needs. In this section, we explore traditional understandings of chakras, including their location, function, and maturation. Chakra functioning is looked at from traditional and psychological viewpoints. Research on chakras and the possible physics that underpins them is followed by exercises the reader can do to explore chakras, perhaps to prove to themselves that they exist.

Traditional Explanations of Chakras

In Sanskrit, *chakra* means vortex, or wheel of light. Chakra lore is varied, but there are two commonalities: Chakras exist within the body, and they are ports for energy and information exchange with the environment. They receive the information that surrounds them and transform it so that it is meaningful to the person. The chakras, then, broadcast the person's unique interpretations of the initial data. People share their emotions and thoughts through their chakras and their aura; one never has to say what she or he is feeling for people around that person to know. This is likely the basis of the famous "nurse's intuition."

Beliefs vary about chakra locations in and around the body. Many traditions simply identify seven major chakras, five found along the spine and two in the brain, and all located near large collections of nerves or neuroendocrine glands. (See **Table 33-2**.) Leadbeater, who was the first person to bring chakra lore to the Western world, taught the Hindu model where one of the chakras is not along the spine, but at the spleen.[11] Joy added a chakra at the manubiosternal joint (just below the neck at the junction of the collar bones) that he called the "high heart."[12] At least one tradition teaches that there are 12 primary chakras, 7 within the physical body and 5 above and below the body. These five are believed to provide access to higher levels of spirituality.[13]

In addition, there are numerous minor chakras: the palm, the sole of the foot, the base of the skull, and all joints in the body, including the spinal joints, which Gimbel describes as five octaves of chakras.[14] Every joint has the same job as the seven major chakras—to gather and transform data. It helps if you can imagine an animal standing on all four paw chakras. These chakras bring in data from the pulses flowing through the Earth. The flow of information moves quickly from the sole of the paw, to the ankles, knees, and hip joints and into the central chakra chain. The animal uses the accumulated information to choose how to respond to its environment.

Human beings do this, too. We collect data with the soles of our feet and palms of our

TABLE 33-2   Traditional Chakra Locations, Associated Organs and Nervous Structures, and Attributes

Chakra Location	Structure	Nervous System Function	Gland	Color	Tone
7 Crown of head	Pineal gland	Spiritual	Pineal or pituitary	Violet/white	B
6 Brow	Pituitary gland Carotid plexus	Intuition, insight	Pituitary or pineal	Indigo (red-blue)	A
5 Throat and shoulders	Pharyngeal plexus	Expression Speak own truth	Thyroid	Blue	G
4 Heart and knees	Carotid plexus	Heart, love	Thymus	Green	F
3 Stomach	Solar plexus	Emotions	Adrenals	Yellow	E
2 Lower abdomen Wrists and ankles	Pelvic plexus	Reproduction, creativity, passion	Lymphatic tissue	Orange	D
1 Groin Palms and soles	Coccygeal plexus	Survival, security	Gonads	Red	C

Source: Data from B. A. Brennan, *Hands of Light: A Guide to Healing Through the Human Energy Field* (Bantam Books, 1987): 48; R. L. Bruyere, *Wheels of Light: A Study of the Chakras*, vol. 1 (Sierra Madre, CA: Bon Productions, 1989): 42; R. Gerber, *Vibrational Medicine: New Choices for Healing Ourselves* (Rochester, VT: Bear & Company, 1988): 130; A. Judith, *Wheels of Life: A User's Guide to the Chakra System* (Woodbury, MN: Llewellyn Publications, 1990): 23; Z. F. Lansdowne, *The Chakras and Esoteric Healing* (Samuel Weiser, 1978): 56; A. E. Powell, *The Etheric Double* (Theosophical Publishing House, 1978): 56; C. W. Leadbeater, *The Chakras* (Theosophical Publishing House, 1927): 40–41.

hands, move it up through the joints in the arms and legs, to the hips and shoulders, and to the central chakra chain. In the major–minor chakra scheme, there are more than 360 chakras in the human body, which enables a person to gather and process the minute details of every experience.[15] Very little crucial data are likely to escape detection by such a finely crafted system.

People who see and hear chakras describe them as emitting various colors and tones. One well-known model assigns to them the colors of the rainbow (red, orange, yellow, green, blue, indigo, and violet) and tones of an octave (middle C, D, E, F, G, A, B) (see Table 33-2).[16] In this model, the root chakra is seen as red and is heard as the note middle C. Leadbeater describes a Hindu chakra model of colors and hues that are not related to the rainbow of colors produced by the refraction of light.[11] Likewise, the Hindu model attributes different tones to the chakras, ones that reflect

a 12-tone musical tradition. Probably both are partially true because, as Benor points out, we sense through a window of observation. If you are familiar with the 12-tone scale, you are likely to hear more tones than someone who is more comfortable with the smaller 8-tone scale of Western music. Chakras are probably more tonally complex than either scale.

The orderly increase in frequencies of the colors and tones ascribed to the chakras suggests that each chakra processes information that is on a higher frequency than the one below it. Each higher chakra adds information, creating a type of information tree. For example, you first must survive (lowest chakra), which enables you, eventually, to speak your own truth (a throat chakra function), a more complex task than surviving. Your relationship with your Spirit and with the Holy (a crown chakra function) is even more complex.

Everyone who writes about chakras gives them somewhat different functions, but all organize them from the concrete to the complex and abstract (Table 33-2). There is widespread agreement on the functions of five of the seven chakras: the first chakra (at the base of the spine) relates to survival, the fourth (at the heart) to love, the fifth (at the throat) to expression; the sixth (at the brow) to insight, and the seventh (at the crown) to spirituality. Interpretations of the second and third chakras vary widely.

Four popular chakra perspectives are displayed in **Table 33-3**: Bruyere's and Brennan's energy models, Maslow's[17] well-known hierarchy of needs, and Covey's[18] Seven Habits Paradigm. Maslow's psychological and Covey's organizational success models are not generally recognized as such, but when compared to chakra functioning, it is clear that they are chakra models.

Chakras mature; they exist and work even while you are in utero. However, just as the arms, legs, and intelligence of the child must mature, so must chakras. A person cannot do the tasks of a chakra well until it matures. For example, you can emote and communicate even as an infant (throat chakra functioning), but you cannot "speak your own truth" until the throat chakra matures. Communicating and speaking your own truth are not the same. It is as if Nature kindly gave us enough time to master each chakra task before we are faced with mastering the task of the next highest chakra.

Once again, there are different models of chakra development. Bruyere gives one model of chakra maturity.[19] She teaches that the first chakra matures between birth and ages 3 or 4 years, the second between ages 4 and 7 years, the third between 8 and 12 years old, the heart chakra during the teenage years of 13 to 19, and

TABLE 33-3   Four Perspectives of Chakra Functions

	Bruyere	Brennan	Maslow	Covey
7th Chakra	Release, surrender	Integration of total personality, spiritual aspects	Aesthetics needs, wonder, beauty, harmony	
6th Chakra	Inspiration, insight	Visualization, carry out ideas	Need to know and understand	Interdependence
5th Chakra	Expression	Sense of self, taking in and assimilating	Self-actualization, realize one's potential growth, autonomy	
4th Chakra	Secondary feeling (usually contrary to first feeling)	Love, openness to life, ego will	Self-esteem, self-worth, feeling dignity, self-reliance, self-respect, independence	Independence
3rd Chakra	Opinion	Healing who you are in the universe	Love and belonging, intimacy	
2nd Chakra	Feeling	Pleasure, sexual energy	Safety	Dependence
1st Chakra	Concept, original idea	Physical energy, will to live	Survival	

Source: Data from R. L. Bruyere, *Wheels of Light: A Study of the Chakras,* vol. 1 (Sierra Madre, CA: Bon Productions, 1989): 43; B. A. Brennan, *Hands of Light: A Guide to Healing Through the Human Energy Field* (New York, NY: Bantam Books, 1987): 47–54; A. H. Maslow, *Motivation and Personality* (New York, NY: Harper & Bros., 1954): 35–51; A. H. Maslow, *Psychological Review,* no. 50 (1943): 370–396; S. R. Covey, *The 7 Habits of Highly Effective People: Restoring the Character Ethic* (New York, NY: Free Press, 2004): 53.

the fifth chakra from 19 to 25 years. Insight, the abstract and complex function of the sixth chakra, matures between 25 and 35 years of age. The crown chakra, which includes the ability to have a mature relationship with the Divine, matures after age 35 (see **Table 33-4**).

A second developmental pattern is suggested by the Fibonacci number sequence. The pattern of 0-1-1-2-3-5-8-13-21-34-55-89-144 and so on is consistent throughout nature. Each number after the first is the sum of the two preceding numbers. This sequence is seen in the emergence of biological structures, such as DNA, RNA, the branching of trees, and the branching of dendrites throughout the nervous system.[20] For example, in the spring, a tree has no leaves. One will emerge, then a second, then two emerge at the same time, then three, then five, and so on. To make this more visible, go to http://britton.disted.camosun.bc.ca/fibslide/jbfibslide.htm. If the Fibonacci number sequence is a pattern that Nature finds useful, perhaps chakras develop along the same pattern.

Research into Chakras

When Valerie Hunt, a retired professor of physical therapy at the University of California, Los Angeles (UCLA), placed electromyographic-like (EMG) electrodes on the skin of chakra areas,

she found regular, high-frequency, wave-like signals from 500 to 20,000 cycles per second (Hz), which is higher than any previously recorded human body frequency.[21] Other known human frequencies are brain waves between 1 and 100 Hz, muscle frequencies up to 225 Hz, and heart frequencies as high as 250 Hz.

Gerber reports that Motoyama also recorded the electrical state and changes over chakra areas. He measured control subjects, advanced meditators, and people with histories of psychic experiences. Chakras that the meditators believed were "awakened" showed electrical readings of increased frequency and amplitude when compared to control subjects' chakras. Subjects who could consciously project energy through their chakras displayed significant electrical field disturbances over the activated chakras. Gerber says that "ability to activate and transmit energy through one's chakras is a reflection of a rather advanced level of consciousness development and concentration by the individual."[15pp128-130] He suggests that Motoyama's finding that advanced meditators could consciously project energy through their chakras indicates that people can deliberately control their own energy.

Curtis, Zeh, Miller, and Rich measured chakra functioning and found that people with more

TABLE 33-4   Theoretical Ages of Chakra Development

Chakra	Chakra Function	Age Based on Fibonacci Number	Age Based on Bruyere Oral Teaching
1st, Root, Sacrum	Survival	1 year (conception/birth)	Birth to 3 or 4 years
2nd, Pelvic plexus	Reproduction, creativity	1 to 2 years (first cell division) and age 2 to 3 years ("terrible twos")	4 to 7 years
3rd, Solar plexus	Emotion	3 to 5 to 8 years	8 to 12 years
4th, Heart	Love	13 to 21 years	13 to 19 years
5th, Throat	Expression	21 to 35 years	19 to 25 years
6th, Brow	Insight	35 to 55 years	25 to 35 years
7th, Crown	Spiritual	55 to 89 years	35+ years

Fibonacci numbers are calculated by adding the previous two numbers together. The Fibonacci number sequence begins with 1, 1, 2, 3, 5, 8, 13, 21, 34, 55, 89, 144 . . . .

psychological symptoms had more poorly functioning chakras.[22] As they point out, although this is consistent with chakra theory, it is impossible to determine whether impaired chakras contribute to depression, anxiety, hostility, and other symptoms or the symptoms themselves contribute to chakra dysfunction.

Scientific Explanations of Chakras: Comparing Chakras to Electrical Components

The chakra models in Table 33-3 identify stages of the growth of a human ability. They begin with the simplest stage, move through increasingly more complex ones, and end with a highly sophisticated ability that few people attain. This progression suggests that the human being is designed to develop in stages of some kind, as if we must master a simpler behavior to master the next, a more difficult one. This mastery is cumulative, and each stage builds on the next. This is what chakras help us do.

Chakras act as if they are designed to process specific information; some chakras can process only fairly simple information and some process such complex information that it takes a long lifetime to even appreciate it. Each chakra receives only the information with which it can work, process that information according to Nature's protocol and add in the person's specific choices, and then forward the bundle of information to the next chakra. The repetitive process of receiving information, adding new information, processing and forwarding the result creates a complex body of data available to the person. Even if everyone experienced the same thing, this chakra process gives individuals the ability to interpret their experiences differently and respond in their own unique ways.

Chakras resemble types of electrical equipment found in radios, televisions, and computers. (See **Table 33-5**.)

1. Radios contain circuits, equipment that allows the radio to receive a variety of frequencies but gives listeners the ability to listen to only one of the many stations (frequencies) at a time. Because of these LCR circuits, people don't have to listen to overlapping stations but only to the ones they choose. LCR stands for inductance (L), capacitance (C), and resistance (R). (It would have been an ICR circuit, but the "I" was already taken.)

   a. Induction (i.e., inductance) is the ability of an electromagnetic field to cause or induce an electric current in a nearby electric wire without them touching but because there is a change in the first device. Remember the coiled electric wire around an iron core? When the current is flowing through the wire, each coil *induces* an electric current in adjacent coils. Invisible signals received by your radio or TV induce information-laden electric currents in your set that results in a program you can enjoy.

   b. Capacitors have the capacity to store electrical charge (i.e., electrons). A capacitor holds on to electrons until it reaches its capacity, and then releases the charge. This allows a flow of electricity.

   c. Resistors do exactly what their name suggests—they resist the flow of something. In electrical devices, good resistors (i.e., poor conductors), such as rubber, restrict the amount of charge that can flow. A poor resistor (i.e., a good conductor), such as copper, allows more charge to cross it.

   Capacitors and resistors work together. The capacitor holds on to the electrons until they begin to flow, but the resistor can prevent them from flowing in the wrong direction. In this way, you get electricity where you want it, such as in your home, car, TV, radio, computer, or cell phone, rather than scattered around randomly accomplishing little or nothing.

2. Radio, TV, and cell phone towers transmit information across long distances.

3. Computers and cell phones are limited by the condition (the health) of their hardware and software and by the information you put in them. When you write or text/tweet, your computer or cell phone reproduces exactly what you have written. You can share your ideas with your friends by e-mail, Facebook, texting, or talking. All of this sharing occurs across distances by invisible means.

TABLE 33-5   Similarities Between Electrical Components and Chakras

Chakras resemble electrical components and systems:
LCR circuits, receivers and transmitters, capacitors, and computers

Electrical Devices	Chakras
LCR circuits are components in radios and TVs that can be tuned to receive a specific frequency.	Each chakra receives the information on only a limited range of sound and electromagnetic frequencies.
Radio and television signals are transmitted by one instrument and received by another.	Chakras receive information from the environment and transmit your unique information to those around you.
Capacitors store electrical charge up to their capacity, and then release it. They can be recharged.	Chakras store electrical charge, and then release it to the adjacent chakras and to the world.
An electrical resistor is part of an electrical device that resists the flow of charge through the device. It prevents damage and helps direct the flow of electricity to where you want it.	Chakras protect you by resisting the flow of unfamiliar information.
Modern computers are able to store large amounts of data and do complex logical operations. They can do only what they are programmed to do. They can be linked to process more information than any one of them alone. They also break down.	Each chakra processes different information from that of the other chakras and your history partially determines the result. The chakra chain is like a series of linked computers. Chakras are delicate but strong systems that can be damaged by strong, hostile emotions and by traumas such as combat, tornados, and abuse of all types.

Source: Material on electrical components and systems interpreted from P. G. Hewitt, *Conceptual Physics,* 10th ed. (San Francisco, CA: Pearson-Addison Wesley, 2006); P. Xiong-Skiba, personal communication, March–April 2007; material on the chakras from V. Slater's personal observations (copyright © 2011, Victoria Slater).

Chakras resemble these electrical components and systems in the following ways:

1. Each chakra receives, processes, and transmits only a limited range of frequencies from the vast range that bombards it. As in your computer, these frequencies are arranged in such a way that they are "energy in formation," or information, not just a range of frequencies. Chakras receive such information (induction) from the surrounding environment and nearby chakras, hold on to new and old information (capacitor), and resist (resistor) letting go of old information and receiving new information.

2. Chakras release information. It may be one way that nurses know when a patient is not saying what he or she really needs to say or when a patient looks unchanged but is in trouble.

3. Chakras make it relatively easy to respond in habitual ways. Your automatic responses are ones you have stored in the software-like programs in your chakras, which are part of their resistor function. You have learned some of these responses from family, friends, and culture and you have created others. Some of those programs include what is safe, familiar, and what you like, making most decisions relatively

easy. Some of these are useful, but some interfere with healthy growth and maturation. For example, if you grew up in an alcoholic family, your chakra programming will include how to live with or be an alcoholic. You learned those skills at your "mother's (or father's) knee." They are so basic to you that you don't even know they are there. These laws will interfere with your ability to reach the more complex possibilities of the higher chakras because you will be stuck in a feedback loop of how to be an adult child of some problem. As you mature, you may choose to override your earlier programs, create new ones, and respond differently.

Chakras can be damaged. They are tough, but also delicate sound and electromagnetic management systems that abuse, hostile emotions, extremely loud noises, combat, and other traumas can damage. These are the same events that can damage the aura. Such damage is physical; it is as if the chakras' components break from overload or violence. Damaged chakras prevent you from responding in new ways because your information flow cannot reach the higher chakras. Chakras can be repaired with energy healing and your habitual information changed with counseling, meditation, and other life experiences.

Intuitive Experiences of Chakras

The following exercise can help you become aware of your own chakra energy.

EXERCISE

Place one hand lightly over your perineum (i.e., first or root chakra) and the other hand below your umbilicus. Your second hand will be resting near your second chakra (i.e., sacral plexus). Ask the chakra under one hand to close. What do you notice? Ask that chakra to open. What changes? Open and close your chakra several times.

Leave your hand at the sacral plexus chakra and place your other hand on your solar plexus over your stomach (the solar plexus chakra). Tune in to the subtle responses under your hand, in your body, and in your emotions as you ask

the chakra beneath your lower hand to close and open. As it opens, notice how the energy flows from the lower chakra to the upper one. Are you more comfortable when your chakras are open or closed?

The heart chakra (i.e., fourth chakra) is located in the center of your chest about where you would do closed-chest cardiac massage. As you place your hand over it, ask it to open and close several times. What happens to your breathing? Are there changes in the tension in your back?

Your throat or fifth chakra is in the area of the Adam's apple and suprasternal notch. It is the smallest of the seven major chakras, and about the size of a 50-cent piece. Put your hands over it and ask it to close and open. What happens?

By this time, you may have noticed that each time you ask a chakra to open and close, you feel a slight sensation or a change of pressure or temperature under your hands. You may feel a movement like a flower opening. When your chakras are closed, you may feel tense or have pain and you may be more relaxed when they are open.

Your sixth chakra, also called the third eye, is in the center of your forehead. Place a hand lightly over it, and ask the chakra to close and open. What happens? Your seventh chakra is at the crown of your head where your soft spot was. Sense your body and emotions as you ask it to close and open. What do you experience?

You may find it interesting to close all of your chakras at the same time, from your tailbone to the crown of your head. Is this a familiar sensation? Open them all. One way to help them to open is to imagine seeing the colors of the rainbow in turn—red, orange, yellow, green, blue, indigo, and violet/white. What is different when your chakras are closed or open?

Give yourself a chakra treatment.[12] Place one hand over your first chakra, at your groin area, and the other hand over the second chakra. For 60 seconds, visualize universal love flowing through your hands into your chakras. Fill your second and third chakras, above and below the umbilicus, with love. Do the same for the third and fourth, fourth and fifth, fifth and sixth, and sixth and seventh chakras. How do you feel?

Meridians

There is more research on meridians than on the aura or chakras. The data suggests that the meridian structure may be fundamental, perhaps preceding the vascular and nervous systems.

Traditional and Not So Traditional Explanations of Meridians

Meridians are described as 12 pairs of pathways that carry subtle energy throughout the body. The Chinese call this energy *chi*, and the Japanese, *qi*. Although the meridians have names like the organs, they feed all of the organs along their path, not just the one they are named for. For example, the liver meridian refers to the sphere of influence of that meridian, not the organ. When the energy flow is compromised, illness is believed to result in the parts of the body fed by that meridian.[23p47] The meridians have acupoints along them; these pressure- and light-sensitive areas are used in acupuncture and acupressure to change the flow of chi.

Unlike the chakras, which rapidly carry and process the details of complex information, the meridians appear to slowly carry the complete picture throughout the body. To tune into the meridian data, we must patiently wait as the gestalt reveals itself. The chakras give us instant information; the meridians complete information. Complex organisms need both.

Meridians act like a very slow, but complete, messenger system that may be an expansion of the information processing of single cells. A microvolt pulse of less than 1-billionth of an ampere[24] might be just the right power and speed for a single-celled organism to get all the information it needs to respond reflexively to its environment. If meridians are an expansion of the electrical and information processing ability of single cells, then they may play a fundamental role in the health of complex, multicellular organisms.

Research into Meridians

Gerber, in *Vibrational Medicine*, summarizes the data on the location, function, and hormonal content of meridians.[15pp122–127] He reports that the meridian system is a continuous mesh that precedes the development of even the most rudimentary organs. The electrical flow and the elec-

tromagnetic field that results exist before the organs, vessels, nerves, and layers of skin. Like a river that continually diverges into smaller channels to water the land, meridians divert electrical flow into ever-smaller channels, terminating with meridian fibrils flowing energy into each cell's nucleus. It is almost as if the cells are the flower of the meridian tree; when the tree is damaged, the cells do not work optimally.

Gerber reports that meridians are 0.5 to 1.5 microns in diameter, which is smaller than a single human hair. Becker states that the current flow in a meridian is between 1-billionth and 1-trillionth of an ampere (the rate at which electricity flows per second) into the central nervous system and that acupoints have the electrical characteristics needed for boosters of such a weak current.[24] He discovered that the Schwann cell sheath (perineural cells) surrounding every neuron appears to conduct the current and that broken bones will heal only after the perineural sleeve mends.

The emerging evidence indicates that meridians act like "biological fiberoptic light cables"[23p225] and conduct microvolt electromagnetic frequencies throughout the body. Because they appear to be electromagnetic, they should be capable of inducing current in and having it induced by other nearby electromagnetic forces.[25p238] They also appear to conduct sound waves, which may mean that every cell is bathed in sound.[26]

Motoyama has been researching meridians for years and has designed the Apparatus for Meridian Identification (AMI) that measures the electrical charge in the meridians. It is being used more frequently for research in subtle energies and healing, such as in Tsuchiya and Motoyama's study of the effect of Pranic healing in a breast cancer patient.[27] The authors conclude that the AMI measurements supported the healer's sense of the changes that occurred during the Pranic healing session. Motoyama believes there is a relationship between the chakras and meridians.[28]

Acupuncture is the most researched of all meridian modalities; in the 2 years between 2006 and 2008, 985 articles were published about its results, safety, proper needle placement, ethics, and neurochemical basis.[29] Acupuncture has been found to be useful in a wide range of conditions, including stroke rehabilitation, infectious disease, angina pectoris, and immunomodulation in cancer patients.[30] It is reputed to bring a body into balance, or equilibrium. For example, the same acupuncture technique given to both a hyperthyroid patient and a hypothyroid patient brings each closer to normal thyroid functioning.

Scientific Explanations of Meridians: Comparing Meridians to Electric Currents

Meridians carry a complex flow of electric current. Their intricate structure involves a series of up, down, and diagonal flows of very weak electrical current that flows close to the iron containing blood vessels, creating an electromagnetic effect. As in any electromagnet, the result is more power available to a person than the weak electrical flow would provide on its own. Because they carry an electrical current, meridians can be influenced by nearby electromagnetic fields, possibly including people. The electromagnetic field produced by the interaction of meridians and hemoglobin may contribute to the aura.

Meridians also carry information, but not in the same way that chakras do. Because meridian tendrils reach into the nucleus of every cell, meridians may bring information from the external environment to every cell allowing the entire body to interpret events. (See **Table 33-6.**)

Intuitive Experiences of Meridians

The meridian system appears to act like part of the body's defense system. The ability to gather information in a gestalt and send it to each cell may be primitive, but it could be effective, even for humans. Meridians can be healthy, hyperalert, or sluggish.

Imagine your skin receiving information from the room, different information from what you gather by your five senses. What nuances are you aware of that you did not notice before? Notice how your skin information changes when you are around different people.

To discover the meridians' slow, information processing capability, shake hands with someone. Set a timer for 15–30 minutes. When it goes off, become quiet and ask to be aware of what you learned about that person. Be patient. Do not expect the information to be crystal clear; it will be more like an impression.

TABLE 33-6   Similarities Between Electric Currents and Simple Computers and Meridians

Meridians resemble electric currents and simple computers.	
Electrical Devices	**Meridians**
Electric currents exist when electrons flow from areas with lots of electrons to areas with few. Some electric currents flow in one direction only.	Meridians carry a unidirectional current within a complex mesh that is embedded throughout our body and that reaches into every cell.
Resistance to an electrical current can occur when the wire is long and narrow. Such an electric current requires periodic boosting to maintain the signal.	Meridians are very long and very narrow, 0.5 to 1.5 micron in diameter. Without boosting at regular intervals, the signal dies out.
A current is induced in one electric wire when a current changes in a nearby one.	Meridians are a series of adjacent electrical currents. Each is constantly changing and being changed by the nearby meridians.
The original computers of the 1940s were not able to conduct complex information or carry it as quickly as modern computers can. They could not be used to do the complex calculations that computers now can.	Meridians act like our early computers; they carry simple information slowly and don't perform complex logical functions. Chakras act like our high-speed modern computers.

Source: Material on electrical components and systems interpreted from P. G. Hewitt, *Conceptual Physics,* 10th ed. (San Francisco, CA: Pearson-Addison Wesley, 2006); P. Xiong-Skiba, personal communication, March–April 2007. (Copyright © 2011, Victoria Slater.)

Summary of Energy Anatomy

The three-part aura, chakra, and meridian system is a sophisticated data gathering, processing, storage, and transmission system. The system resembles computers in a number of ways. Computers contain software programs, memory, and tiny wires that carry very weak electrical signals throughout the machine. Similarly, your chakras process the data based on your software, your aura stores your entire history, and meridians carry very weak electrical signals through your body. Chakras give you information rapidly with both simple and complex data that may be too much to handle in a second; meridians provide the gestalt, the big picture; and the aura stores it all so that you can review it later. From the perspective of the survival of the individual and the human species, this might be a good system, one that may be so fundamental that its importance has largely been overlooked.

■ LAYING ON OF HANDS MODALITIES, THE HEALER, ELECTROMAGNETIC INDUCTION, AND PRESENCE

One of the questions practitioners of laying on of hands modalities are often asked is, "How does this work?" Usually we say, "We don't know, but it does. Try it for yourself." This section is an attempt to propose an answer to that question.

The answer may be electromagnetic induction, a physics phenomenon that is so common it is involved in many of the tools we use to make our lives simpler. As will be discussed in this section, laying on of hands modalities may be applied electromagnetic induction, which may lead to healing. One human may induce healing in another just be being present. Every human to human interaction, every nurse-patient interaction may have the potential to be healing because of electromagnetic induction.

Laying on of Hands and the Healer

People who do laying on of hands modalities learn a method to enter into a healing state. That method is often a ritual or a meditative state; the meditative state results in slower breathing, heart rate, and, often, slower brain waves. As healers become relaxed, their electromagnetic field may change. Zimmerman found that when Therapeutic Touch (TT) practitioners entered a relaxed state called centering, which is a type of an altered state of consciousness, their hands began to emit an electromagnetic signal that pulsed from 0.3 to 30 Hz, and mostly in the 7- to 8-Hz range.[31] These are the brain wave frequencies present during meditative and other contemplative states. The signals were not found before the TT practitioners entered the altered state of consciousness or in nonhealers. Waechter and Sergio found the same results with qi masters.[25pp233,246]

More recently, Moga and Bengston tested laying on of hands with caged mice who had been injected with cancer.[32] Bengston did a few laying on of hands sessions near the cages without touching the mice. When he went home, he continued to give long-distance healing sessions from a different part of the country. (The mice did well; 75% were tumor free at 12 weeks.) When the investigators tried to measure the magnetic field around Bengston as he did the healing, there were no changes. However, they found changes adjacent to the mice cages and then within the cages where Bengston has directed his attention. The magnetic field showed waves that dropped to 8–9 Hz, to less than 1 Hz, and then reversed direction, which is similar to the signals reported by Zimmerman. Overall, the waves lasted 60–120 seconds. The pattern existed during both hands-on treatments and long-distance ones.

Unlike the Therapeutic Touch practitioners, Bengston did not enter a meditative state; rather, his method speeds up brain functioning. If he felt an emotion, he just observed it rather than being caught up in it. Second, he imagined positive images such as a healthy body, healing being complete, and visions of success such as the lab personnel toasting the results of an experiment. These images were things that Bengston wanted to happen in his life. Other healers report holding equally positive images of what they want.

Bengston adds another twist to the role of the healer.[33] In the 1970s, when he had his first experience giving laying on of hands healing, he discovered that healers do not have to be trained to center. The healer in an experiment had to leave before giving any treatments. The mice had already been injected with the cancer, so Bengston was persuaded to try what he had learned from the healer. He made a list of 20 specific outcomes he wanted in his life, created and memorized an image for each, then, during the healing just scrolled through his images as if they were on a film loop. He paid little attention to the hands-on work, but to the images in his mind. He would even carry on a conversation or read while treating the mice. The six mice were fully cured.

When he tried the same experiment again, he recruited four individuals to give the treatments; none of them believed that healing of this type was possible. Again, all of the mice were cured. When the mice were again injected with the cancer, it did not take; they remained immune to cancer during their entire natural life span of 2 years. When cells were taken from these immune mice and injected into cancerous mice, the sick mice got well. Bengston wonders if this means we can design healing vaccines.

A surprising result of the study was that the mice in the control group were healed if they were kept in the same room as the treated mice or if healers came in contact with them. Without treatment, both groups had a 100% death rate. It appeared that the experimental and control groups were not independent of each other, even though separated.

Bengston concludes that neither belief nor a positive attitude is necessary to do healing. Rather, he thinks that healers who believe that a healing will work can interfere because they tend to try to help and get in the way. Ritual may even get in the way.

What does all of this say about energy healers and about expert healers? Recipients report having long-lasting and occasionally permanent pain relief from an expert energy practitioner, but only transient changes after receiving a single laying on of hands treatment from novices.[34] This suggests that those who have worked to perfect their skills do bring something different to energy healing.

Expert energy practitioners have studied and practiced their skills and are examples of Benner's expert nurses who transcend technique; they are the artisans of healing.[35] Even Bengston and his four skeptics practiced their approach by planning, memorizing, and perfecting it. Bengston may be correct when he claims that

someone who believes that energy healing will work might interfere with the results. Expecting a modality to work in a particular way may limit the possible outcomes. It might be more effective to use the protocol of your modality, which might include centering or scrolling 20 positive scenes through your mind, but truly having no expectations about how the energy will work for the recipient or what the outcome will be.

Electromagnetic Induction

The continuing question about energy healing is "How does it work?" Part of what may be getting in the way of finding an answer is the use of the word *energy*. Xiong, a physics professor in Tennessee, says that the use of the word *energy* in the phrase "energy healing" is incorrect because *energy* is not being used as physics defines it.[36] If you shouldn't use the word *energy*, what physics concept would describe laying on of hands work? *Electromagnetic induction*. (In this chapter, we continue to talk about energy healing rather than electromagnetic induction healing. It is simpler.)

As described earlier, electromagnetic induction is the ability of one device to induce or cause an electric current or a surge of current in another device without direct contact between the two. The key is the *change* in the primary one; the changing field transforms the electrical flow in the secondary one.[37]

These changes sound like the electric surges that were found in healers. In the 1990s, several studies showed that healers develop a buildup of charge in their bodies and discharge it periodically; this charge–discharge sequence was seen in long-distance healing as well as person–person healing. Tai chi students have also been found to release accumulated charge. Moga and Bengston propose that this electrical phenomenon may not be limited to healers, but may be a basic part of health and healing, bioenergy therapies, and mind–body practices.[32pp405,407-408]

Imagine two people sitting side by side. As discussed earlier, each is an electromagnet because they have iron cores (hemoglobin) surrounded by electrical fields (neurons and meridians). Each person creates an electromagnetic field that interacts or interferes with the other, causing a change in the state of the other's electrical current. If one is more active electromagnetically, perhaps creating more charge–discharge than the other, this person may create more change in the other person than he receives.

What makes one person more electromagnetically active than another? Bengston's and Zimmerman's work suggests that part of the answer is "what one is thinking." A healer is imagining results she wants, such as celebrating a success or being still within and/or communing with the Holy. The more vivid the images, the more charge–discharge the healer may create, which may enable the person (or mouse) nearby to change (electromagnetic induction) in a way that ultimately may be healing.

Because everything electrical is susceptible to changing electromagnetic fields, our meridians and chakras will respond to changes in a nearby electromagnet, which might be a person. An electrical surge in the meridians may help reduce obstructions in the meridian flow to organs and tissues allowing them to function more normally. Chakras may be able to reduce their resistance to change when in the presence of an electromagnetic field of the right strength. Muscles, fascia, and connective tissue also have electrical characteristics and may be influenced by changes in nearby electromagnets and by the charge–discharge occurring in nearby people. This may lead to the relaxation that people consistently report after receiving a laying on of hands treatment.

Presence

If electromagnetic induction is a factor between people, it may contribute to the effect of *presence*. Nurses are taught that their presence makes a difference. Many of us have learned that sometimes the best thing to do is sit with a person and be quiet. Just be there. Just be present. Perhaps our caring and wishing good things for this person create a change in us that can induce a change in their electromagnetic field. That change may not be recognized as healing, it may just be called "comfort."

If presence is an electromagnetic event, then the presence of a sham healer can be healing. This may explain the confusing results of many of the Healing Touch and Therapeutic Touch studies; the experimental and sham groups both show healing.[34,38]

OTHER FORMS OF ENERGY HEALING

Holistic nurses use a variety of other forms of energy healing than the laying on of hands. Homeopathy, flower essences, aromatherapy, and sound, music, and light therapies are potent energy healing modalities.

Homeopaths prepare many of Nature's plants, animals, and gases in a specific way so that they support the body's healing efforts. The theory is that the human body knows how to treat problems. The symptoms of a problem, such as fever or rash, reflect how the body is trying to heal itself, so a homeopath selects a remedy that creates the same symptoms as the problem the body is fighting. The army might call it "force multiplying." Homeopathic preparations contain no molecules of the original plant. The remedy is created by repeatedly diluting and vigorously shaking (called succussion) until the correct number of dilutions and succussions has occurred. Most homeopathic remedies are oral, either in small tablet form or liquid, but some are injected.

Lenger measured the magnetic fields of various homeopathic preparations using spectrum analysis and discovered that the dilution and succussion process changes the substance into magnetic photons with high energy.[39] The megahertz (MHz) resonance frequency of each remedy she tested increased with higher numbers of succussions from, for example, a low of 9.3 MHz after relatively few succussions of Argentum metallic to 501.19 MHz with thousands of succussions.

Flower essences are another energetic preparation of plants, animals, and minerals. The original substance, such as a rose, is placed in water in the sun. The theory is that the sun's electromagnetic frequency causes the "essence" of the plant to be transferred to the water, which is then diluted, mixed with a stabilizing substance such as alcohol or vinegar, and ingested when appropriate.[23p186] It may be that the changing electromagnetic vibration of the sun's rays causes an induction of a very, very weak current between the rose and the water. By drinking the final preparation, a person takes in the original substance's magnetic frequency, which interacts with and changes the individual's energetic state.

Aromatherapy, which is described in an earlier chapter, is also an energy healing modality. Although essential oils are most often used for their biological properties, some holistic nurses also use them for their energy patterns. For example, cedar and cypress act as if they help a person access deeply hidden memories that can then be released, much like unzipping and deleting a computer file. Any means of delivery, including inhalation, topical application, or infusion in the air provides a person with the healing properties of essential oils.

Homeopathy, flower essences, and aromatherapy utilize many of the same substances, but prepare them differently, which creates three different methods of healing. None of these are understood scientifically, but a number of people are convinced they are effective and that an individual has invisible work going on for as long as the frequency of that flower essence, essential oil, or shaken water remains in the person, which can be for hours or months. These modalities may give the person the experience of gently and gradually healing with little conscious effort.

Sound is an ancient form of healing exemplified by the American Indian use of drums and flutes, as well as in Tibetan bowls, which are often tuned to stimulate chakras. Jenny found that various sound wave frequencies create highly complex patterns in liquids.[40] Some look like the skeletons of simple animals, and some look almost exactly like Leadbeater's descriptions of traditional Hindu chakras.[11] A frequency of 6,250 cycles per second (cps) creates a pattern that resembles pictures of the heart chakra, 8,200 cps forms a pattern resembling the brow chakra, and 16,000 cps produces a pattern resembling the crown chakra. Such data suggest that sound creates the chakras and/or that chakras respond to sound.

Two popular sound therapy programs are InnerSound[41p272] and Acutonics.[42] Both use tuning forks to create external sound that may transform the client's internal state. The InnerSound's tuning forks deliver a series of musical fifths and are held by the ears, close to the cranial bones, which are in direct contact with the cerebral spinal fluid. The cranial bones provide a gateway for sound waves to enter the cerebral spinal fluid and change its vibration, possibly creating a change deep within the body. The Acutonics program applies their unique tuning forks directly to acupuncture points, trigger points, and points of pain, creating a vibration that is believed to assist tissues to relax and help relieve pain.

Music has long been used to comfort the dying, to inspire, to create unity within a group, and to relax. According to Wilken, music can also be used to heal energy blockages.[41pp274-275] She teaches that when a person does not like particular music, the music is stimulating an energy blockage within the body. As a person exposes him- or herself to that music, the sound waves cause the blockage to release. Physical and emotional pain often disappears, and the person learns to like the music.

The music we listen to might leave us relaxed, with a sense of well-being, or it may leave us energized or on edge. Well-crafted symphonies and other music that moves sound waves through the entire chakra chain leaves the listener with that sense of well-being. Music at some rock concerts can do just the opposite; they stimulate fans' root chakras, but don't assist the energy to move through the chakra chain and out the crown chakra. It appears that the unrelenting percussive sound waves build up pressure in the lower chakras, which must be released somehow. This may be one reason for violence after some events.

The therapeutic value of drumming is being more widely recognized.[43] A 1-hour drumming session has been shown to cause a statistically significant increase in an individual's natural killer cell activity and reduce the level of stress. First-year nursing students who participated in multiple drumming sessions had a 28.1% improvement in total mood scores. Long-term care workers also showed improvement (46%), followed by a lower turnover than expected. The residents of a long-term care facility reported that after drumming they were more able to deal with their grief and that the effects were preferable to antidepressants. At-risk adolescents who participated in REMO's HealthRHYTHMS adolescent protocol showed improvement in behavior. Genetic changes have been demonstrated following drumming.

Light also has a long history in healing. In the past, tuberculosis patients were treated with sunlight, as were patients with certain skin disorders. Gerber reviews new forms of healing that utilize light and colors and reports that "innovative light therapies have proven effective in treating depression, mental and emotional problems, seizure disorders, and memory problems, as well as difficulties with concentration and attention span."[23p223] He suggests that light deprivation may cause some anxiety, as seen in seasonal affective disorder (SAD).

The eyes may not be the only portals for light to enter the body; the pineal gland appears to be light sensitive and may be a true "third eye." Acupoints appear to allow light to enter and stimulate meridians. Having light sensitive eyes, pineal gland, and multiple acupoints suggest that our system is designed to receive sunlight. Sitting in the sun for a short time each day may be a useful self-care technique.

Color therapies, which use the different frequencies of light, are increasing in use. A useful color therapy for holistic nurses is to imagine a particular color and let the body be filled with that color. Simply thinking about the different colors of the rainbow—red, orange, yellow, green, blue, indigo, and violet—seems to offer a person a simple self-healing treatment.

Intuitive Experiences of Aromas, Flower Essences, Sound, Light, and Color

Explore aromatherapy, homeopathy, and flower essences. Select a problem you would like addressed and use an essential oil (i.e., aromatherapy), a flower essence, and a homeopathic preparation that are specific for that issue. Use them at different times and notice their effects on your body, mind, emotions, and spirit. You might find it interesting to use the same flower or herb in its homeopathic, flower essence, and aromatherapy form.

Give yourself an aromatherapy experience. Some essential oils are caustic, so for this experience you may choose to just smell your aroma of choice. Frankincense has been used in churches for centuries because it opens the sixth chakra, the third eye, and opens the person to insight and spiritual experiences. Basil helps relax the tension in the chest and lungs and is useful for asthmatics and people having difficulty breathing. Smell these or any other essential oil and discover how your body, mind, and emotions respond to the aroma.

Experiment with flower essences. Discover what they are used for then try one for a week or more. Notice any changes in your body, mind, emotions, attitude, and spirit. Do your experiences match the descriptions?

Experience music you do not like. Stand at a distance and keep the music at a low volume. Each time you listen, move a little closer. When you are ready, gradually increase the volume. As you do this a number of times over several days or weeks, notice how your response to the music changes? What else changes? For example, is your back more relaxed or are you more patient? Has your attitude toward something changed?

Go outside and let your eyes be bathed in the light of the day and the dark light of the night. Don't wear glasses even on a sunny day; instead, find a shady place to be while still receiving the light. All 12 meridian pairs are present in your eyeballs; when you let light into your eyes, the meridians get an electric surge. Notice how you feel after you spend 10 minutes bathing your meridians in light.

Play with color. Collect seven pieces of colored cloth or paper so that you have red, orange, yellow, green, blue, indigo, and violet pieces. Put each hand on a different color at the same time. Notice how the vibrations under your hands differ. Your body responds to these subtle differences in a consistent manner. How do your chakras and your entire body respond to those colors?[44]

Give yourself a color therapy treatment. Become quiet and for 1 minute see the color red. Notice how you respond as the color fills your body. Follow red with orange, and then yellow, green, sky blue, indigo, and violet. Give each at least 1 minute to fill you before you move on to the next color. Finish by filling yourself with peach, apricot, and pink. How do you feel physically and emotionally after an entire chakra treatment?

■ ENTRAINMENT

Many people know about entrainment; it is witnessed when clocks swing their pendulums in unison, even when they started out at different rates, or when heart cells beat in unison when brought close to each other. Holistic nurses may be more interested in the human aspects of entrainment, including social entrainment and/or interactional synchrony. Social entrainment proposes that much of human behavior is regulated by endogenous, cyclical processes and that people synchronize those processes, such as women who live together all having their menses at the same time. Interactional synchrony describes how skilled and empathic listeners naturally adjust their posture and natural speech rhythms to match the person with whom they are speaking. An excellent review of entrainment is "In Time with the Music: The Concept of Entrainment and Its Significance for Ethnomusicology" by Martin Clayton, Rebecca Sager, and Udo Will (you can find this article at http://ethnomusicology.osu.edu/EMW/Will /InTimeWithTheMusic.pdf).[45]

To help you get a picture of entrainment, imagine two things beating or pulsating at different rates. For them to entrain, the faster one must slow down, the slower one must speed up, or each must move toward the other's rate. Somehow, they will match frequencies. If one of them cannot change its frequency, the other must do all the work.

This phenomenon may be part of the reason for the effectiveness of aromatherapy, flower essences, homeopathy, and even light, sound, and music. Aromatherapy, flower essences, and homeopathy are preparations of natural products; their frequencies will not change. If you make a preparation of a rose, it will have the frequency of the rose and it will not change; you must. The same thing happens when you use any homeopathy, flower essence, or aromatherapy; you must do the work to entrain. Because you change, you may have the opportunity to release some old patterns easily and painlessly.

Music has a rhythm that is fairly steady, or it would be noise. You know how you react to sound such as drumming or construction noise; skillful drumming can excite you, but equally loud construction noise can be irritating. Entrainment may have something to do with Wilken's conclusion that you do not like particular music because it is activating emotional blockages. As you entrain to the music, you flow in the same rhythm and the blockage can lose its tension.

Summary of the Holistic Nurse, Entrainment, Electromagnetic Induction, and Presence

The holistic nurse who is talking with a patient is very likely involved in interactional synchrony, entrainment, electromagnetic induction, and healing, all at the same moment. The nurse who is being present to the patient may well be leaning forward or somehow letting her body broadcast her interest in the patient, listening intently, and adjusting her speech patterns to the patient's (entrainment). She also may be focused intently on the patient while wishing good things for him (electromagnetic induction). We would just call this good nursing and good listening skills. It may be more; it may also be healing.

■ INTENTION

The nature of the space in which healing happens is not often discussed; the room in which something is done is just a given. But McTaggart helps us understand that how space is used is important. When a space is used regularly for the same activity that activity becomes easier to do.[46] Perhaps this explains why Bengston's mice, both experimental and control, were healed. The space, itself, became healing.

The sad events at Abu Ghraib are an example of intent changing a space. The American soldiers who mistreated the Iraqi prisoners were merely "going with the flow" of the actions of generations of prison guards. Although this dramatic example of the energy signature of a space is an unfortunate one, it points out how powerfully a space can be prepared for an activity.

Because clients seem to experience changes at a much faster rate in a space that is used exclusively for healing than in one that is used for many things, healing space should be dedicated to healing. Ideally, holistic nurses whose healing rooms are in their homes use that room only for healing. Rooms that are not used exclusively for healing can be cleaned. Because so much pain, grief, and death are common in hospitals, clinics, and nursing homes, they should be frequently cleaned of prevailing energy. You might consider cleaning the energy in your home regularly. This might be the reason so many people do "spring cleaning"; not only do the corners of the rooms get dusted, the energy in the house is cleared.

There are many ways to clean a room of its history, but the easiest is to be in it and invite the Holy to clean it and fill it with Love, Light, Joy, Comfort, or whatever seems appropriate for who will use the room next. Try this with a room in your home.

■ RESEARCH AND RESEARCH IMPLICATIONS

Researching energy healing is not an easy task. Forty years of researching laying on of hands modalities may have taught us more about how not to research them than about their results. We have learned that the experimental-control research design is inappropriate and that sham providers do healing.[47] It seems that the presence of the sham provider is healing in itself. This means that we need to test energy modalities against other modalities, test against no additional treatment, use the participants as their own controls, or find a methodology that does not require a person to be in the room with a control participant.

We have learned that the effects attained by an expert healer can be quite different from those of a novice and that space can be "prepared" for a particular result, thus both the nature of the treatment provider and of the space in which the research is conducted can influence study results.

We know that the effects of all energy modalities are cumulative, so the immediate result may be quite different from the effect of many treatments; we could also expect that acute problems would respond differently from chronic ones. The initial effects of energy healing are often attitudinal and then emotional; physical changes may emerge later.[48] For example, even if the back pain didn't go away, did the participant change an attitude? Most studies have looked for short-term effects, and often physical ones. We need to take into account the tier effect of laying on of hands treatments.

Electromagnetic induction may be responsible for all of these findings. When you use the experimental-control research design to study laying on of hands modalities, a person must be close to the people receiving the experimental and the sham treatments. If presence, indeed, is healing, then one should expect that a caring person giving attention to a patient would be healing. To truly measure the effects of a treatment modality that includes the effect of presence, you need to test it against a treatment that does not require the presence of another person.

Expert healers have been shown to generate and release a charge and to emit a pulsating current; the research on non-energy healing practitioners is limited but suggests that they do not have the same powerful electromagnetic effect as the expert energy healer. Therefore, the effect of expert healers, novices, and untrained individuals needs to be identified and research studies need to take into account the possible different effects of the three groups.

If laying on of hands modalities are, in fact, electromagnetic events, the electromagnetic changes might create small but permanent changes in the electrical flow of the meridians, within chakras, and across the muscles, fascia, and connective tissue. Each change is built on the last, creating a gentle, cumulative effect. This suggests people who receive regular energy healing treatments may be healthier than others of the same age.

Homeopathy, flower essences, and aromatherapy appear to be entrainment modalities and they, too, have been difficult to research. The individual preparations within all of these modalities have been shown to have specific effects and many people just look up their problem in books and take what is recommended. The popularity of the modalities suggests that people find them useful.

However, the expert practitioner takes a history that will help identify the correct essence, homeopathy or essential oil. Some of the questions a homeopath might ask, for example, seem odd, such as "Which side of your body do you sleep on, your right or your left side?" The goal is to discover enough about the person to fit the right remedy to that person. If entrainment is involved, then the expert practitioner is seeking the remedy that the patient can entrain to that will move her toward healing. Entrainment modalities may be more difficult to research in depth than electromagnetic ones as we do not have a clear understanding of how to measure such subtle entrainment.

Directions for
FUTURE RESEARCH

Directions for future research in energy healing therapies require assistance from physicists. We need to discover if there is an electromagnetic induction effect between humans, or is this just a tantalizing theory? The scientists who study this will be challenged by Becker's[24] finding that meridians carry a current that is in the nano-ampere and microvolt range. If this minute current is standard within meridians, then the degree of induction is likely to be in this range. Once they have learned how to measure such a miniscule current, they will be able to discover if there is an electromagnetic change between nearby individuals and how that change influences the electrical flow within meridians and across tissues of each individual.

If such an effect were proven, we will be able to discover the electromagnetic effect of the presence of one person on another, such as an energy healing practitioner on the client or any nurse with any patient. Other relationships that could then be studied might be the role the sham provider plays in a research study. What about a person just sitting with someone, or holding the hand of a loved one or a patient. What is the electromagnetic effect of a loved pet? Is presence more than a theoretical concept or a real physical phenomenon?

As discussed previously, comparing the electromagnetic presence of expert healers, novices, and the untrained might be an enlightening study. Entrainment studies may be difficult unless there are tools to measure frequencies of solutions, such as homeopathy and flower essences. These preparations may have impacts other than through their frequencies, and those will need to be identified.

In addition to the studies that will require the expertise of physicists, the immediate and long-term effects of energy healing modalities need to be identified. Is there a difference in effects in acute and chronic problems? Is there a relatively consistent pattern to changes seen during a series of treatments, such as attitudinal changes occurring before physical ones? Is there a difference in effects between different modalities, i.e., does Reiki have a different effect on a problem than Therapeutic Touch?

One might also compare energy therapies with other modalities, not to discover if one is better than the other but to discover how their effects differ. Does the order in which treatments are given make a difference? For example, is it more beneficial to a joint replacement patient to have occupational therapy before or after an energy therapy? How much more mobility does an arthritic have if hot wax treatments are preceded or are followed by an energy therapy? Do stroke patients have a different recovery picture when receiving energy therapies in addition to standard treatment?

A study that might capture the imagination of many people would be to look at the health of expert energy healers compared to people who do not give and receive energy therapies. Are the energy therapy practitioners healthier than the average? If expert healers get sick, do they get as sick as other people with the same problem and do they get well faster? What is the health of the clients of these healers?

Perhaps the most immediate research need is to discover the ideal methodology to use for studying modalities that may be electromagnetic in nature, rather than biological or psychological. We know that studies cannot use sham providers to give treatments; they are effective, which may say more about the provider than the modality. So, how do you adequately study a phenomenon that may be founded in physics, rather than in the sciences that nurses usually study and one in which the provider applying the modality may be more important than the modality itself?

Nurse Healer
REFLECTIONS

After reading this chapter, the nurse healer will be able to answer or to begin a process of answering the following questions:

- I am a holistic nurse. What change does my presence create in those around me?
- What type of people am I drawn to; does their presence make me happy or sad and grumpy (entrainment)?
- How does just being at the American Holistic Nurses Association's annual conference change me?

- Which energy modality interests me, if any? Do I just want to play with it, which is okay, or do I want to put in the time to become an expert? Do I want to add one to my self-care routine?

 For a full suite of assignments and additional learning activities, use the access code located in the front of your book to visit this exclusive website: http://go.jblearning.com/dossey. If you do not have an access code, you can obtain one at the site.

NOTES

1. D. Krieger, *The Therapeutic Touch* (New York, NY: Prentice Hall, 1979).
2. National Center for Complementary and Alternative Medicine, "What Is Complementary and Alternative Medicine?" http://nccam.nih.gov/health/whatiscam/.
3. B. A. Brennan, *Hands of Light: A Guide to Healing Through the Human Energy Field* (New York, NY: Bantam Books, 1987): 49.
4. D. v. G. Kunz, *The Personal Aura* (Wheaton, IL: Quest Books, 1991): 39.
5. D. J. Benor, "Intuitive Diagnosis," *Subtle Energies* 3, no. 2 (1992): 41–64.
6. F. Brock, "Taoism to Harry Oldfield: Subtle Energies in China" *Bridges Magazine* 3 (2010): 20.
7. International Society for the Study of Subtle Energies and Energy Medicine, "Alyce and Elmer Green Award." http://www.issseem.org/greenaward.cfm.
8. B. O. Williams, "Imaging the Human Energy Field," *EdgeScience Magazine* 4 (July–September 2010): 17–19.
9. K. G. Korotkov, P. Matravers, D. V. Orlov, and B. O. Williams, "Application of Electrophoton Capture (EPC) Analysis Based on Gas Discharge Visualization (GDV) Technique in Medicine: A Systemic Review," *Journal of Alternative and Complementary Medicine* 16, no. 1 (2010): 13–25.
10. K. Hobbie and B. J. Roth, *Intermediate Physics for Medicine and Biology* (New York, NY: Springer Sciences + Business Media, 2007): xvi.
11. C. W. Leadbeater, *The Chakras* (Wheaton, IL: Quest Books, 1927).
12. W. B. Joy, *Joy's Way: A Map for the Transformational Journey. An Introduction to the Potentials for Healing with Body Energies* (Los Angeles, CA: J. P. Tarcher, 1987).
13. Concept: Synergy, "The Power of Our Chakras: Removing Blockages to Our Success," Cassette Recording No. 567. (Orlando, FL: NPN Publishing, 1996).
14. T. Gimbel, *Form, Sound, Colour and Healing* (Essex, England: Daniel Company Limited, 1987): 65.
15. R. Gerber, *Vibrational Medicine: The #1 Handbook of Subtle-Energy Therapies* (Rochester, VT: Bear & Company, 2001).
16. R. L. Bruyere, *Wheels of Light: A Study of the Chakras*, Vol. 1 (New York, NY: Fireside, 1994): 42.
17. A. H. Maslow, *Motivation and Personality* (New York, NY: Harper, 1954).
18. S. R. Covey, *The 7 Habits of Highly Effective People: Powerful Lessons in Personal Change* (New York, NY: Free Press, 2004).
19. R. L. Bruyere, oral teachings.
20. Platonic Realms, "The Fibonacci Sequence." http://www.mathacademy.com/pr/prime/articles/fibonac/index.asp.
21. V. V. Hunt, *Infinite Mind: The Science of Human Vibrations* (Malibu, CA: Malibu Publishing, 1995): 19–21.
22. R. Curtis et al., "Examining the Validity of a Computerized Chakra Measuring Instrument: A Pilot Study," *Subtle Energies and Energy Medicine* 15, no. 3 (2004): 209–223.
23. R. Gerber, *Vibrational Medicine for the 21st Century: The Complete Guide to Energy Healing and Spiritual Transformation* (New York, NY: HarperCollins, 2000).
24. R. Becker and G. Selden, *The Body Electric: Electromagnetism and the Foundation of Life* (New York, NY: William Morrow/Quill, 1985): 142, 234–239.
25. R. L. Waechter and L. Sergio, "Manipulation of the Electromagnetic Spectrum Via Fields Projected from Human Hands: A Qi Energy Connection?" *Subtle Energies and Energy Medicine* 13, no. 3 (2002).
26. C. L. Zhang, "Skin Resistance vs. Body Conductivity: On the Background of Electronic Measurement on Skin," *Subtle Energies and Energy Medicine* 14, no. 2 (2003): 161–162.
27. K. Tsuchiya and H. Motoyama, "Study of Body's Energy Changes in Non-Touch Energy Healing 1. Pranic Healing Protocol Applied for a Breast Cancer Subject," *Subtle Energies and Energy Medicine* 20, no. 3 (2010): 15–29.
28. H. Motoyama, *Karma and Reincarnation, the Key to Spiritual Evolution and Enlightenment* (Encinitas, CA: CIHS Press, 2009): 125–134.
29. H.-Y. Li, L. Cui, M. Cui, and Y-Y Tong, "Active Research Fields of Acupuncture Research: A Document Co-citation Clustering Analysis of Acupuncture Literature," *Alternative Therapies* 16, no. 6 (2010): 38–45.

30. S. S. Knox, "Physics, Biology, and Acupuncture: Exploring the Interface," *Frontier Perspectives* 9, no. 1 (2000): 12–17.

31. J. Zimmerman, "Laying-on-of-Hands Healing and Therapeutic Touch: A Testable Theory," *BEMI Currents: Journal of the Bio-Electro-Magnetics Institute* 2 (1990): 8–17.

32. M. M. Moga and W. F. Bengston, "Anomalous Magnetic Field Activity During a Bioenergy Healing Experiment," *Journal of Scientific Exploration* 24, no. 3 (2010): 397–410.

33. W. F. Bengston, "Breakthrough: Clues to Healing with Intention," *EdgeScience Magazine* 2 (January–March 2010): 5–9.

34. V. E. Slater, *Safety, Elements, and Effects of Healing Touch on Chronic Non-Malignant Abdominal Pain* (doctoral dissertation, University of Tennessee, Knoxville, 1996).

35. P. Benner, *From Novice to Expert* (Menlo Park, CA: Addison-Wesley, 1984).

36. P. Xiong, personal conversation, May 2008.

37. P. G. Hewitt, *Conceptual Physics*, 10th ed. (San Francisco, CA: Pearson-Addison Wesley, 2006): 483–484.

38. J. F. Quinn, "Building a Body of Knowledge: Research on Therapeutic Touch 1974–1986," *Journal of Holistic Nursing* 6, no. 1 (1988): 37–45.

39. K. Lenger, "Homeopathic Potencies Identified by a New Magnetic Resonance Method: Homeopathy—An Energetic Medicine," *Subtle Energies and Energy Medicine* 15, no. 3 (2004): 225–243.

40. H. Jenny, *Cymatics: A Study of Wave Phenomena and Vibration* (Newmarket, NH: MACROmedia, 2001).

41. A. Wilken and J. Wilken, "Our Sonic Pathways," *Subtle Energies and Energy Medicine* 16, no. 3 (2005).

42. E. Franklin and D. Carey, "From Galaxies to Cells: Bridging Science Sound Vibration and Consciousness Through the Music of the Spheres," *Subtle Energies and Energy Medicine* 16, no. 3 (2005): 287.

43. REMO, "HealthRhythms." http://remo.com/portal/pages/hr/research/index.html

44. S. Lutz, oral teachings, March 2007.

45. M. Clayton, R. Sager, and U. Will, "In Time with the Music: The Concept of Entrainment and Its Significance for Ethnomusicology," *ESEM CounterPoint* 1 (2004): 1–82. http://ethnomusicology.osu.edu/EMW/Will/InTimeWithTheMusic.pdf.

46. L. McTaggart, *The Intention Experiment: Using Your Thoughts to Change Your Life and the World* (New York, NY: Free Press, 2007): 113–123.

47. D. Wardell, personal conversation, June 2010.

48. V. Slater, personal observations.

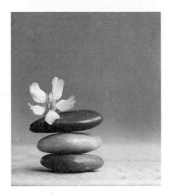

Chapter 34

Holistic Nursing Research: Challenges and Opportunities

Rothlyn P. Zahourek

Nurse Healer
OBJECTIVES

Theoretical

- Discuss ways holistic philosophy and theoretical frameworks are reflected in holistic nursing research (HNR) priorities.
- Discuss the recent NCCAM strategic plan and its impact on holistic nursing research.
- Discuss the complexity of determining adequate evidence for holistic nursing research.
- Explore the challenges for holistic nursing research.
- Compare and contrast a variety of research methods.

Clinical

- Explore how holistic nursing research questions can be developed in your clinical setting.
- Read a research article related to a modality you use in your holistic nursing practice.
- Collect data from various clients who are participating in some form of holistic therapy to determine their subjective evaluations of the experience and outcome.
- Discuss ways to enhance practice through holistic research with colleagues and nurse researchers.
- Devise a holistic nursing research question and propose a method of research that would best explore that question.

Personal

- Contemplate how a conceptual framework of holism is the foundation for holistic nursing research and practice.
- Clarify your own personal definition of holism and holistic nursing.
- Consider that you do research every day in clinical practice as you assess patients and their situations, make diagnoses, plan and follow through on actions, and evaluate those actions.
- Plan time to learn how to form a research question.
- Attend a research conference or a section on research at the American Holistic Nursing Association (AHNA) annual conference or at a local networking meeting.

DEFINITIONS

Bias: Having preconceived ideas and expectations about a research study's outcome. May be overt or more subtle as a hope or expectation.

Bracketing: Characteristic of qualitative research. The researcher outlines in writing his or her philosophies, biases, or concerns and expectations about the research project process and/or outcome.

Credibility: A term used in qualitative research that accounts for the researcher's trustworthiness in demonstrating the process of data collection and interpretation of results.

Hawthorne effect: When people know they are being observed in a study, their behavior is affected simply by being observed.

Healing: Both a process and result; defined by the individual as perception of shift or meaningful change. The central concept in holistic nursing research.

Healing relationship: The quality and characteristics of interactions between healer and the one being healed (healee) that facilitate healing, including empathy, care, love, warmth, trust, confidence, honesty, courtesy, respect, and communication, as well as compassion, presence, intent, and intentionality.

Heisenberg's Uncertainty Principle: The principle that observation of phenomena or objects changes the nature of what is studied.

Integral: The appreciation for the interactions and interrelationships of the many parts within the whole of a system.

Meta-analysis: A statistical technique that combines the results of many studies related to one topic to establish an overall estimate of the therapeutic effectiveness of an intervention.

Mixed methods research: A type of research that combines paradigms, philosophies, and methods on a specific topic to grasp a more complete representation of reality and/or confirm the credibility of the research findings; also may be referred to as triangulation.

Placebo: A medically inert medication, preparation, treatment, technique, or ritual that has no intended effects on the person and no actual therapeutic value. The fact that the placebo is inert is now in question based on the impact of suggestion and intention.

Praxis: The bringing together of practice and research. It is a synthesizing and reflective process in which theory is dynamic and practice reflects research and theory in a unified whole.

Qualitative research: A systematic, subjective research approach that describes life experiences and searches for how participants find meaning in their experiences;

based on philosophical, psychological, and sociological theory; focuses on understanding the whole, which is consistent with the philosophy of holistic nursing.

Quantitative research: A systematic, formal, reductionistic, objective approach in which numerical data are used to obtain and interpret information about the world. It embodies the principles of the scientific method and describes variables, examines relationships among variables, determines cause-and-effect interactions between variables, and predicts future responses.

Reductionism: The approach of breaking down phenomena to their smallest possible parts; also called positivism and equated with the linear, logical nature of the scientific method.

Reliability: Generally associated with quantitative research and the ability of a scale or a tool to consistently measure a phenomenon when used repeatedly.

Research: A diligent, systematic inquiry or investigation to validate and refine existing knowledge and generate new knowledge.

Systematic review: A specific form of review of research studies that yields more convincing evidence. Several methods exist; these are invaluable in discovering what has already been discovered about a particular phenomenon.

Translational research: Taking basic bench highly reductionist (molecular or cellular) research and translating that into clinical application. It generates new research questions that are fed back to the bench. More broadly, translating any research into practice.

Unitary: The recognition that parts cannot be separated from the whole because the whole is greater than, and different from, the parts; contention that separating phenomenon into parts undermines the understanding of the whole.

Validity: Generally associated with quantitative research; internal and external; relates to the interpretation of data; meaningful, appropriate, and useful results are required for validity. Internal validity is related to the controls placed on the research design and process and ensures that the effects of the independent variable are causing the results in the dependent variable. External validity ensures that the results are generalizable to other populations, settings, and times and depends on internal validity.

■ HOLISTIC NURSING RESEARCH

As human beings, we are driven to explore. We strive to understand ourselves and our world and thereby construct belief systems that we want others to accept and act on. Historically, mystics and shamanic healers believed in the healing power of ecstatic experiences of a unified cosmic whole. Pagans believed that all matter, living and nonliving, had spirit and a life force that could communicate. Now philosophers, theoretical physicists, and behavioral scientists study "subtle energy" and theorize about the nature of and actions by consciousness.[1]

In the 1600s, Descartes' notion of reductionism separated soul from body by breaking down every research subject into its smallest parts. This liberated medicine from religion and advanced the use of the scientific method in medical research. Since then, *science* developed and humans become smug about being rational creatures. Depending on the logic of the scientific method, A plus B has to equal C; such logical relationships have to behave predictably to be considered credible and valid. Impassioned controversy wages between a belief in only that which is visible and proven, and faith in what is unseen, experienced, but poorly understood. Is the world flat as it appears to the naked eye, round as the globe in the classroom, or egg shaped as seen from space? Does energy exist as quantifiable sound waves, electrons colliding, or as something nonlocal that we cannot see, touch, or, at present, measure? Surprisingly, invisible cyberspace e-mail messages become visible when they are transduced into images on a computer screen.

Holistic nursing research (HNR), as well as the fields of complementary and integral medicine and complementary and integral nursing, are on the cusp of such a conundrum. Much of what nurses value in interventions and holistic nursing process can't be seen or measured. Often, effects take time to be realized and are unpredictable. Many concepts that nurses want

to study remain ill defined, and some holistic practices appear to others as based in mysticism, magic, or paranormal phenomena. Others use nursing theories to explain holistic nursing practice as well as abstract theories from quantum physics and evolving theories on the nature of consciousness and reality. Although holistic nurses may continue to believe in the power of spirit and unexplained forces, we have a duty to understand the nature of such phenomena and to ethically demonstrate their safety and efficacy in clinical practice. The nurse's primary mission is to foster healing and, therefore, we must develop a body of credible, reliable, and valid research and sound scholarship.

In 2003, a stellar multidisciplinary group of scholars met to determine the definitions and standards for healing research. Their work continues to influence holistic nursing research. The authors insisted that the healing relationship be the focus for healing research. Healing is both a process and result. "Those physical, mental, social, and spiritual processes of recovery, repair, renewal, and transformation that increase wholeness, and often (though not invariably), order and coherence. Healing is the emergent process of the whole system."[2] Healing is perceived by the individual as a shift, meaningful change, or transformation and is experienced as restored balance or sense of wholeness.[3] Quinn and nurse colleagues provide a definition of healing relationship for nursing research: "the quality and characteristics of interactions between healer and healee that facilitate healing. Characteristics of this interaction involve empathy, caring, love, warmth, trust, confidence, honesty expectation, courtesy, respect, and communication."[4] Holistic nurses also consider compassion, presence, and intent and intentionality as components of the relationship and process of healing.

The purpose of this chapter is to provide a matrix framework for HNR that is based on definitions of wholeness and healing, and nursing theories that are based on ways of knowing and viewing the world. We consider the third National Center for Complementary and Alternative Medicine (NCCAM) strategic plan for 2011–2015 and its influence on HNR, review the status of HNR and approaches to HNR, and consider the challenges and opportunities for the future. In addition to the standard approaches of qualitative, quantitative, and mixed methods designs, other approaches are discussed.

■ WHAT IS HOLISTIC NURSING RESEARCH?

How do we understand and connect science and spirit? How do we explore the healing relationship and healing itself? What is different about holistic nursing research? Enzman-Hagedorn and Zahourek emphasize that although holistic nurses use a variety of integrative and complementary modalities, HNR must occur within a framework of theory and practice that accepts holism as its base.[5,6] The American Holistic Nurses Association (AHNA) white paper on holistic nursing research adopts this caveat: "Solid evidence for the effectiveness of these approaches is often dependent on the interplay of relationships, the passage of time, and interaction of many variables some of which are not easily controlled using standard methods or a conventional scientific frame work."[7]

Simply evaluating a modality or providing evidence of safe, effective practice is not necessarily true HNR. The AHNA recognizes two definitions of holism: The whole is viewed as a relational integration of parts (i.e., *integral*), or the whole is separate from and greater than the parts (i.e., *unitary*).[8] A researcher using the *integral* framework values interactions, influences, and outcomes and most often utilizes quantitative, mixed methods, evidence-based practice research, meta-analyses, and surveys. The *unitary* researcher recognizes that separating phenomena into parts undermines total understanding. Research in this framework is most often qualitative, including hermeneutic, phenomenologic, ethnographic, and grounded theory methods, as well as mixed methods and aesthetic, historical, and other approaches. For nursing research to be holistic, it must clearly incorporate one of these frameworks into the question, design, method, analysis, and interpretation of findings. Integrating one framework or developing a unique definition of holism should be evident in the research question and interpretation of results.

The research gold standard, the randomized controlled trial (RCT), is reductionistic as opposed to holistic in nature. However, such a study could be considered holistic if the researcher acknowledges that there is a whole context, or experience, that is greater than, and possibly different from, the smaller interactions of specific variables. The researcher might skillfully qualitatively study a phenomenon by describing the individuals' experiences and interpreting results in a holistic framework. For example, several patients react positively to Healing Touch treatments. Their reactions remain for that selected population. From such data, however, a beginning theory or hypothesis might emerge. When we use observations and descriptors, devise measurement tools, and quantitatively measure outcomes, we have increasingly reliable, valid, and generalizable results. However, we may have missed understanding the nature of a person's total experience and the subsequent implications for practice.

■ BASICS OF HOLISTIC NURSING RESEARCH: WAYS OF KNOWING AND NURSING THEORIES

Holistic nursing research is based in a holistic paradigm. Nurse theorists such as Rogers, Newman, Parse, Watson, and Leininger developed a wealth of unitary and integral theories as they struggled to understand caring, healing, and the nature of the whole. (See Chapter 5.) In addition, they and their protégés created methodologies and tools to conduct research. For example, Margaret Newman developed the theory of Health as Expanding Consciousness (HEC). Newman conceptualizes a unitary time framework that illuminates "the meaning of a person's present situation within the context of the past and anticipating future action."[9] She proposes a qualitative "hermeneutic, dialectic method," which is used to "allow the pattern of the person and environment to reveal itself without disrupting the unity of the pattern. The process culminates in intuitive apprehension and expression."[10] For Newman, research is *praxis* and, therefore, based in practice. Research emanates from the nurse's engagement with participants during important events and within significant relationships; it "enables pattern recognition and expanding consciousness to occur."[9] Pattern recognition acknowledges the whole. In a classic text on research based on Newman's work, Jones and Picard present numerous research examples using Newman's framework including the pattern of letting the past go in order to move on for parents of persons with bipolar illness[11] and recognizing life patterns in women with multiple sclerosis.[12] Measurement tools are beginning to appear to document behaviors that illustrate caritas in Jean Watson's evolving Theory of Caring.[13,14]

Richard Cowling has developed a research framework, Unitary Appreciative Inquiry, based on Martha Rogers's Science of Unitary Man. This framework considers the pattern of the unitary whole as the orientation and process for "uncovering human wholeness and discovering life patterning in individuals and groups"[15] His unitary pattern recognition with women experiencing despair utilizes data synopses rather than data analysis.

Worldviews and Ways of Knowing

All research is based on a philosophy or worldview. Although differing in language, these systems all tend to view a bifurcated, or particulate, reality in which humans and their world are portrayed through such descriptors as *subjective* and *objective*; *individual–intrapersonal*; *interpersonal* and *cultural*; and *aesthetic* and *ethical*. Few paradigms try to address the whole other than by describing parts and their relationships. *Pattern* may be one concept that captures a unitary whole. However, when posing a research question, choosing one of the following ways of knowing can help researchers frame their studies. (See Chapter 1 for more discussion on ways of knowing.)

The AHNA recognizes various patterns of knowing including rational or scientific, intuitive, and aesthetic. Intuitive and aesthetic are emphasized because these approaches are needed to understand the "multidimensional nature of our work, which encompasses the art of care; the wholeness of the client's experiences and meaning of patterns that emerge; the beauty of authentic interaction; and the knowledge of that which is perceived through nonverbal, nonobjective expression."[16]

Historically, nursing research and theory generation have been based on Carper's classical work. She proposed a system of *four ways of knowing*:[17]

1. *Empirical:* Objective, logical, and positivistic science
2. *Ethical*: Obligations, what should be done in a given situation; what is acceptable

practice; requires openness to differences in philosophical positions[18p12 13]
3. *Personal:* Self-knowledge; determined by ability to self-actualize; comfort with ambiguity; commitment to patience and self-care
4. *Aesthetic*: Artful knowledge; abstract; defies formal description and measurement; understanding of subjective experiences; creative pattern

Porter recently argued that these patterns are linear and hierarchical rather than holistic.[18pp3-14] He critiques both evidence-based practice and Carper's framework as reductionist, linear, and too weighted in the empirics and simplistic in logic. He believes that too little weight has been given to the personal, aesthetic, and ethical, all of which fall into the ineffable. He advocates for "practice based evidence"[18p12] in which "nonempirical patterns of knowing animate practice" and become documented and thereby empirical. The role of empirics, then, is demonstrative rather than deterministic.[18p13]

Fawcett developed a classic paradigmatic system that describes three frameworks of increasing degrees of abstractness:[19]

1. *Particulate–deterministic.* Reductionist, concrete
2. *Interactive–integrative.* Reality is multidimensional and contextual; reciprocal relationships
3. *Unitary–transformative.* Human beings are unitary, evolving, self-organizing fields, and defined by pattern; highly abstract[19]

Nurse theorists Watson, Newman, Parse, and Rogers are associated with the unitary–transformative paradigm. Enzman-Hagedorn and Zahourek developed an integrated model that combines Carper's and Fawcett's paradigms with specific research approaches for holistic nursing research.[20]

Mariano provides a slightly different framework described as four "attributes of scholarship": wide awake, reflective, caring, and humorous.[21] By keeping ourselves wide awake, we become aware of our place in humanity, are open to possibility, are attentive to others, and are conscious of our evolving experiences. In research, we are sensitized to ask unexplored questions with which we discover the unique and novel. Reflection is an introspective thoughtful process in which one's philosophical stance, values, assumptions, biases, and decision-making process become more evident. The third attribute for scholarship is caring. Drawing from Jean Watson,[22] Mariano explains that our research should be ethical, moral, and based on pressing human needs. We must be intellectually empathic, just, and fair minded. Finally, she states that true scholars have a sense of humor. We should expect and embrace the unexpected, keep our goals and accomplishments in perspective, and be willing to admit when we are wrong.[21]

Munhall describes one additional worldview useful to HNR: the *pattern of unknowing*. Unknowing captures intuitive experiences.[23] Knowledge is shaped, but not completely defined, by the process or context in which it occurs. Larry Dossey continues to discuss the local and nonlocal aspects of healing, arguing that we must grapple with these areas of mystery to understand such fundamental concepts as compassion and intentionality.[24] Schwartz and Dossey discuss the unexpected confounds of the *observer effect* and intention on prayer, "distant healing," and intention research outcomes.[25] Braud and Anderson developed transpersonal research methods based on such alternative ways of knowing as altered levels of consciousness, intuition, setting intention, knowing through art, feminine spirituality, and knowing through movement and through listening.[26] Jonas and Crawford analyzed more than 220 reports on nonlocal healing effects (122 controlled laboratory studies and 80 randomized controlled trials).[27] Their results support that these unexplainable phenomena do exist, but inconsistently. Any energy-based research must struggle with the inability to see and measure process and effects accurately and consistently. Finally, Ken Wilber developed yet another integral model of how people experience their world that is useful for holistic nurses.[28] (See Dossey's Theory of Integral Nursing in Chapter 1 for a full discussion of this model.)

These frameworks provide a malleable matrix on which to ground HNR. Each framework acknowledges holism and reductionism. All include experiential qualitative approaches that enrich our understanding of complex phenomena as well as the quantitative comparative approaches, program evaluation, and other forms of evidence from practice. We need better

and more diversified approaches and more sensitive instruments to assess and document the interactive nature of holistic nurses with each client's bio-psycho-social-spiritual patterns in wellness and in illness. **Table 34-1** summarizes these paradigms and provides a reference for holistic nurse researchers' planning, executing, and interpreting their research. In addition, research frameworks from the behavioral and social sciences and psychoneuroimmunology provide useful methods, theories, and models for HNR.

■ IMPACT OF THE NCCAM 2011 STRATEGIC PLAN

The National Center for Complementary and Alternative Medicine (NCCAM) is the agency dedicated to scientific research on complementary and alternative medicine (CAM). CAM is defined by NCCAM as a group of diverse medical and healthcare interventions, practices, products, and disciplines that are not generally considered part of conventional medicine.[29p1] Early in 2011, NCCAM released its new strategic plan. Because many of the interventions classified as CAM are also holistic nursing interventions, this plan has implications for holistic nurse researchers. The plan will shape not only what NCCAM and other government agencies fund but also the national direction and focus of research for the next few years. In her introduction, NCCAM Director Josephine Briggs states that the previous plans emphasized that CAM research focus on basic evidence to discover biological properties of interventions and conduct RCTs to ensure effectiveness and safety. In this current plan, translational research, effectiveness and outcomes research, and real-world results are emphasized. Training new researchers and multidisciplinary teams is encouraged.

NCCAM Strategic Plan: Goals and Objectives

Within the strategic plan are three goals and five strategic objectives. The three overarching goals are the following:

1. Advance the science and practice of symptom management.
2. Develop effective, practical, personalized strategies for promoting health and wellbeing.

TABLE 34-1 Summary: Ways of Knowing Theoretical Frameworks

Research Approach	Carper's Ways of Knowing:	Fawcett's Paradigms	Wilber's Integral Model	AHNA's Way of Knowing	Mariano's Attributes of Scholarship
Quantitative: RCT, EBP, experimental, quasi-experimental, descriptive	**Empirical:** Objective, logical, positivistic; provides measurement and generalizability	**Particular-Deterministic:** Reductionist, concrete	Objective "it," material body, biochemistry, behaviors, scientific observations on time and space	Rational/Scientific	
Quantitative: Descriptive, correlational Mixed methods		**Interactive and Integrative:** Multidimensional reality, contextual, reciprocal relationships	Objective "its," collective exterior, social systems, regulatory structures	Rational/Scientific	**Being Wide Awake:** Thinking about our place in humanity, open to possibility, attentive to others and conscious of our evolving experiences, posing questions from descriptive data
TRANSITION **Qualitative:** Postmodern feminist mixed method approaches	**TRANSITION** **Ethical:** Obligation about what should be done, open to different philosophies	**TRANSITION** **Interactive and Integrative or Unitary Transformative:** Human beings are unitary, evolving self-organizing fields defined by patterns	**TRANSITION** Subjective "I" and subjective "we," imagination, internal experience	**TRANSITION** Intuition	**TRANSITION** **Caring:** Ethics, fair mindedness, human and society needs, intellectually empathic
Qualitative: Reflective, transpersonal Mixed methods	**Personal:** Self-knowledge, ability to self-actualize, comfort with ambiguity, commitment to patience and self-care	**Unitary Transformative:** Human beings are unitary, evolving self-organizing fields defined by patterns	Subjective "I" and subjective "we," shared values and meaning		**Reflective:** Introspection, displays one's thought process, values, biases, ethics, etc., to others; critical thinking
Qualitative: Transpersonal, aesthetic creative approaches	**Aesthetic:** Artful knowledge, abstract, defies formal description, creative	**Unitary Transformative:** Human beings are unitary, evolving self-organizing fields defined by patterns	Subjective "I" and subjective "we," changing states of consciousness and emphasis	Aesthetic	**Humor:** Expect and embrace the unexpected, willingness to admit when we are wrong or failed

3. Enable better evidence-based decision making regarding CAM use and its integration into health care and health promotion.

These goals resonate with holistic nursing philosophy, research, and practice. The plan stresses research to understand more clearly how, and if, interventions augment other treatments. For example, does yoga practice augment standard approaches for treating back pain? According to the NCCAM plan, recent epidemiologic data indicate that people who use CAM engage in other health-seeking behaviors.[29p5] At present, this remains a good hypothesis that needs further testing. Health promotion is a standard nursing (especially holistic) practice, goal, and activity on which we also are compiling research evidence. Currently, the term *evidence based* is being expanded to include multidisciplinary research teams conducting research "across the continuum of basic, translational and efficacy and effectiveness research."[29p11] The definitions of those terms according to the new strategic plan are useful in that they are now used with increasing frequency:[29p11]

1. *Basic science:* Investigates biological effects and mechanisms of action; it clarifies hypotheses and answers the question: "How does it work?"
2. *Translational research:* May identify markers of biological effect; develops and validates measures of outcome; develops algorithms and preliminary clinical efficacy; estimates sample size for future studies. Answers the question: "Can it be studied in people?"
3. *Efficacy studies:* Highly controlled studies to determine specific effects of an intervention. Answers the question, "What are the specific effects?"
4. *Effectiveness and outcome studies:* What is the usefulness and safety of the intervention in general populations and healthcare settings? Answers the question: "Does it work in the real world?"

The five strategic objectives of the 2011–2015 NCCAM plan are as follows:

1. Advance research on mind and body interventions, practices, and disciplines.
2. Advance research on CAM natural products.

3. Increase understanding of real-world patterns and outcomes of CAM use and its integration into health care and health promotion.
4. Improve the capacity of the field to carry out rigorous research.
5. Develop and disseminate objective, evidence-based information on CAM interventions.

Holistic nurse researchers already are addressing many of these strategies. The following discussion gives specific examples of selected strategies. Researchers, educators, and clinicians are all encouraged to become aware of this plan as it relates to a portion of what holistic nurses do and how they might consider crafting their research. Recognizing national trends helps frame potential problems to be studied and provides additional research methods to use. The following discusses the strategic objectives and provides examples of related holistic nursing research.

Strategic Objective 1: Advance the Research on Mind–Body Interactions

This objective includes elucidating biological effects and mechanisms of action. Developing a greater understanding of the placebo response, the influence of expectancy and the relationship, and discovering creative and innovative research designs that account for issues of treatment burden and the ethics of random assignment are included in this category. Coakley and Duffy report a pilot study to investigate the effect of a single Therapeutic Touch treatment on pain perception and biological markers of stress such as cortisol and natural killer cells (NKCs) in patients recovering from vascular surgery.[30] The design incorporated both physiologic measures as well as subjective reports of pain. Their sample included 21 patients, 12 in the experimental group and 9 in the control usual treatment group. After adjusting their statistics using standard approaches, the results indicated that preoperative pain and cortisol levels dropped significantly and NKC levels increased significantly. The authors recommend that further study be done in a more controlled fashion.

Comparative effectiveness research (CER) is a priority established by both the Institute of Medicine (IOM) and NCCAM. According to the

IOM, "CER is the generation and synthesis of evidence that compares the benefits and harms of alternative methods to prevent, diagnose, treat and monitor a clinical condition, or to improve delivery of care."[31] This research focuses on effectiveness, which evaluates results in real-world situations. According to Coulter, CER offers an approach to studying phenomena that are not easily studied in the blinded controlled situation of the RCT.[32] It allows for individual variability and as a result yields more clinically relevant data. It describes what works, not how it works. Researchers using this framework recognize that the double-blind placebo controlled study does not reflect the real world of integrative or holistic research where many factors including intention, relationship, context, and culture influence and confound results. CER has numerous implications for real-world nursing and particularly holistic nursing research.

Many holistic nursing studies are based on real clinical situations. Often these are pilot or small studies that need to be expanded into a larger venue and/or replicated.

Strategic Objective 2: Advance Research on CAM Natural Products

Some nurses are studying the effects of herbs and supplements as well as aromatherapy. The emphasis in the current NCCAM strategic plan is basic molecular research, the effects of probiotics, and the anti-inflammatory action of omega-3 fatty acids. Nurses have traditionally been involved in largely using research results as they advise their patients regarding supplements and herbs. Libster provides us with a historical review of Shaker nurse–herbalists from 1830–1860.[33] Nurses have actively researched aromatherapy. In an aromatherapy therapy study, McCaffrey et al. investigated the use of lavender and rosemary with students to manage test anxiety and found that both reduced test anxiety measures, pulse rate, and personal statements.[34] Muzzarelli, Force, and Sebold also studied aromatherapy with 118 patients waiting for endoscopy procedures.[35] They measured pre and post anxiety using the standard State Trait Anxiety Inventory (STAI; a frequently used measure in many holistic nursing studies). They also used lavender and inert oil as placebo. They found no statistical differences on pre and post

measures of anxiety in either group. (See Chapter 25 for more references on aromatherapy.) Research results from large national studies and systematic reviews on herbs and supplements can be found on the NCCAM and Cochrane review websites: nccam.nih.gov and www.cochrane.org/cochrane-reviews.

Strategic Objective 3: Increase Understanding of Real-World Patterns and Outcomes of CAM Use and Its Integration into Health Care and Health Promotion

Such studies address how and why individuals use CAM, the benefits and risks as well as the cost-effectiveness of CAM and how CAM approaches influence healthy lifestyles. Guarneri, Horrigan, and Pechura provide an extensive review of medical research conducted at universities, studies done in corporate-sponsored wellness centers, and pilot health promotional studies done by insurance companies on the relationship between integrative health programs and costs.[36] These studies focused on lifestyle changes, nutritional interventions, resiliency, moderate exercise, and programs that fostered greater love and intimacy, and emotional well-being. The authors' contention was that these programs mitigated and sometimes reversed the progression of chronic conditions. If such practices were initiated more broadly, millions of healthcare dollars could be saved. The study focused on the impact of such interventions as mindfulness-based stress reduction, Transcendental Meditation, cognitive therapies, and other mind–body interventions on overall healthcare cost savings. The emphasis is treating the whole person, often with multifaceted interventions. Based on the review, the authors advocate for the integration of life-change programs for people with chronic illness, integrative interventions for those with depression, and preventive strategies for all populations.

Many studies continue to appear in the literature regarding the use of CAM by specific populations. Eschiti used a cross-sectional, retrospective, explanatory secondary analysis of the 2002 National Health Interview Survey data set to describe the personal factors of 725 women with female-specific cancers and the types and prevalence of their use of CAM modalities.[37]

The presence of pain and anxiety and depression or having more than two types of cancer was associated with high use of CAM. The most common modality for this group was prayer followed by herbs and deep breathing. Because herbal use may be contraindicated because of interactions with mainstream treatments, nurses need to assess for this. This and other such studies help predict who might be most likely to use CAM modalities, which modalities are most common, and as a result what nurses caring for such patients need to be knowledgeable about.

Strategic Objective 4: Improve the Capacity of the Field to Carry Out Rigorous Research

As nurses receive advanced education, "research" is taught. Increasingly, nurses are learning the various types of research and how to read a research report. Some learn how to formulate a problem statement as well as how to plan and initiate a study. AHNA provides support for developing researchers in the form of small research grant funding, consultation, mentorship, and a regular Internet-based newsletter that addresses specific research issues for holistic nursing. Although the Doctor of Nursing Practice (DNP) is not a research degree, many programs teach interpretation and application of research. DNP programs often require program evaluation projects by students. These foster looking at and evaluating real-world clinical effectiveness and outcomes.

Strategic Objective 5: Develop and Disseminate Objective, Evidence-Based Information on CAM Interventions

The research section on the AHNA website is a growing resource for holistic nursing. This site includes guidelines for developing qualitative, quantitative, and mixed method studies; glossary of research terms; and articles that have been solicited on such topics as systematic reviews, what evidence is, protection of human subjects, and complexity theory. A library of research articles is available as well as lists of references on topics specific to holistic nursing. Links to resources are also available. The research committee produces a regular e-mail newsletter. Each issue has a theme and features a noted holistic nurse researcher. The website is available to nonmembers as well as members and is a growing resource for holistic nurse researchers (www.ahna.org).

Two primary holistic nursing journals (*Journal of Holistic Nursing* and *Holistic Nursing Practice*) regularly publish holistic nursing research. Nursing journals and publications devoted to complementary and integrative medicine also publish relevant research by and for nurses as do other scholarly nursing journals.

■ THE CURRENT STATUS OF HOLISTIC NURSING RESEARCH

Since the last edition of this text, holistic nursing research has flourished. Although we continue to have unpublished master's theses and doctoral dissertations, many of these become the basis for more elaborate pilot and follow-up studies that later appear in the established literature. Pilot studies may be feasibility studies to prepare for a larger project or to refine and revise a research methodology.[38] Often, pilot studies are published but not expanded into full research projects even though evidence exists that a more extensive study would yield more convincing results. As more holistic nurses obtain advanced degrees including the Doctor of Nursing Practice (DNP), the wealth and breadth of research will grow to include action-oriented and program evaluation projects.

AHNA enthusiastically supports the development of HNR. The 2007 revision of the position statement on research states,

> AHNA endorses and supports nursing scholarship relevant to learning, documenting, and comprehending that which is the science and art of holistic nursing with the goal of producing dependable and relevant information to practitioners and the public. . . . Holistic Nursing Research includes descriptive, explanatory, and exploratory designs that expand our understanding of holistic practice and enhance the evidence base for practice. . . . [It] may be conducted using qualitative, quantitative, mixed methods, or other approaches that further our understanding of such

phenomena as the complexity of the human condition, healing, and/or nursing process and intervention.[16]

In 2009, the White Paper Research in AHNA expanded that statement and is available on the website.[7]

Holistic nursing research has become increasingly diverse and includes standard RCTs and other quantitative approaches as well as qualitative and mixed method studies. Some researchers investigate the elusive aspects of our practice including the effect of Reiki on work-related stress,[39] healing through prayer,[40] effect of therapeutic touch on postoperative patients,[41] and healing through the lens of intentionality.[42]

Studies have ranged in method and approach. For example (see **Table 34-2**):

1. Research using randomized controlled trials to evaluate mindfulness-based stress reduction for solid organ transplant patients[43]
2. A quasi-experimental pre–post intervention design evaluating the effect of live music on patients' experience of pain, anxiety, and muscle tension[44]
3. Mixed method study on garden walking for depressed elders[45]
4. A qualitative historical study on the nature of the caring relationships in Florence Nightingale's writing[46]
5. A descriptive hermeneutic phenomenologic investigation of the transformational and extraordinary experiences of nurse healers[47]
6. A phenomenologic study of eco-spirituality exploring the experience of environmental meditation in patients with cardiovascular disease[48]

Researchers propose new models such as a unitary praxis model and the method of appreciative inquiry in the study of women and despair.[49] Additional methods and tools continue to be developed to investigate holistic nursing issues. For example, a tool to measure caring and caritas based on Jean Watson's Theory of Caring has recently been modified.[50] New research addresses the difficulty in studying such elusive phenomenon as therapeutic touch. Monzillo and Gronowicz in their study of therapeutic touch effects on normal human cells and osteosarcoma developed a method to more readily control for practitioner

variability by quantifying the basic level of skill and maturity of the practitioner.[51] They enlisted several other controls: Practitioners kept a journal that helped them stay centered and able to replicate their treatments over several months, several types of blinding and controlling for cell type and cell behavior, and standard protocols for performing therapeutic touch. More research evaluating practice and programs that integrate holistic nursing principles into hospitals and other healthcare facilities is being funded and conducted.[52]

■ HOLISTIC RESEARCH METHODS

Research is diligent, systematic inquiry to validate and refine existing knowledge and to generate new knowledge.[53] No longer limited to qualitative and quantitative approaches, methods now include triangulation and mixed methods, aesthetic, postmodern, feminist, reflective, participatory action, transpersonal, meta-analyses, and methods based on specific nurse theorists such as Parse, Watson, and Newman (see earlier section), as well as others. First, this section briefly reviews the two most conventional research paradigms (i.e., qualitative and quantitative) and then discusses additional approaches as they are relevant in HNR. Readers are encouraged to explore various methods and philosophical bases with experienced nurse researchers and social scientists, keeping in mind the need for a unitary or integral perspective.

Quantitative Research

Quantitative research is a systematic, formal, objective process based on the scientific method in which numerical data are used to obtain information about the world. Quantitative research involves the following: (1) descriptive research, which describes phenomena; (2) correlational research, which examines relationships between and among variables; (3) quasi-experimental research, which explains relationships, examines causal relationships, and clarifies the reasons for events; and (4) experimental research, the randomized controlled trial (RCT), which examines cause-and-effect relationships between variables.[53pp167–203]

Because nurses are engaged in healthcare systems we must recognize both the value of and

TABLE 34-2   Some Examples of Holistic Nursing Research

Example	Author and Reference	Summary
Theoretical: Rogerian	H. Butcher, "Unitary Pattern-Based Praxis: A Nexus of Rogerian Cosmology, Philosophy, and Science," *Visions: Journal of Rogerian Science* 14, no. 2 (2006): 8–33.	A detailed description of Rogerian theory implications for research; synthesis of Barrett's and Cowling's practice methodology into one model.
Mixed Theories	J. Engebretson, "A Heterodox Model of Healing," *Alternative Therapies* 4, no. 2 (1998): 37–42.	The heterodox model of healing that emerged from a prior ethnographic study of healers using forms of Healing Touch is described and implications for practice and research are discussed—a classic.
Theoretical: Watson	M. Hemsley, N. Glass, and J. Watson, "Taking the Eagle's View: Using Watson's Conceptual Model to Investigate the Extraordinary and Transformative Experiences of Nurse Healers," *Holistic Nursing Practice* 20, no. 2 (2006): 85–94. Also as M. Hemsley and N. Glass, "Sacred Journeys of Nurse Healers," *Journal of Holistic Nursing* 24, no. 4 (2006): 256–268.	Watson's conceptual model of caring, healing, and transpersonal understanding was used to underpin a hermeneutic–phenomenologic study of extraordinary and transformational experiences of nurse healers. The five essential themes were belonging and connecting, opening to spirit, summoning, the wounding and healing journey, and living as a healer. The unity of meaning was "Walking Two Worlds."
Theoretical: Newman	L. P. Finch et al., "Research-As-Praxis: A Model of Inquiry into Caring in Nursing," *International Journal of Human Caring* 10, no. 2 (2006): 28–31.	Useful comprehensive article integrating research-as-praxis methodology and Caring Theory; uses a study of interactive dialogue between nurse practitioner (NP) and clients' experiences of caring; phenomenologic.
Mixed Theories	J. Engebretson, "A Heterodox Model of Healing," *Alternative Therapies* 4, no. 2 (1998): 37–42.	The heterodox model of healing that emerged from a prior ethnographic study of healers using forms of Healing Touch is described and implications for practice and research are discussed—a classic.
Mixed Theories	M. Enzman-Hagedorn and R. Zahourek, "Research Paradigms and Methods for Investigating Holistic Nursing Concerns," *Nursing Clinics of North America* (42, no. 2 (June 2007): 335–353.	Reviews the status of HNR and the paradigms underlying that course of study.
Methods Quantitative Studies: Quasi-experimental	M. J. Walker, "The Effects of Nurses' Practicing of HeartTouch Technique on Perceived Stress, Spiritual Well-Being, and Hardiness," *Journal of Holistic Nursing* 24, no. 2 (2006): 164–175.	Although there were not statistically significant results between groups, within-group results indicated the technique resulted in changed perceptions and feeling states.

TABLE 34-2   Some Examples of Holistic Nursing Research *(continued)*

Example	Author and Reference	Summary
Survey	J. Shreffler-Grant, W. Hill, C. Weinert, E. Nichols, and B. Ide, "Complementary Therapy and Older Rural Women: Who Uses It and Who Does Not?," *Nursing Research* 56, no. 1 (2007): 28–33.	Telephone interviews. A direct logic regression analysis; 26.6% of women used complementary and alternative medicine (CAM). The specific characteristics of these women are described.
Pilot experimental	A. T. Vitale and P. C. O'Connor, "The Effect of Reiki on Pain and Anxiety in Women with Abdominal Hysterectomies: A Quasi-Experimental Pilot Study," *Holistic Nursing Practice* 20, no. 6 (2006): 263–272.	A small pilot; experimental group had less pain, less anxiety, and reported few needs for analgesia in post op.
Quantitative	J. Mahoney, "Do You Feel Like You Belong? An Online Versus Face-to-Face Pilot Study," *Visions* 14, no. 1 (2006): 16–25.	Using a Rogerian framework, this study challenges the notion of space and presents data and interpretations of the data that online courses may produce the same sense of belonging and connectedness as face-to-face classes. Interesting unitary implications for HNR.
Qualitative Method: Qualitative phenomenology	B. Raingruber and J. Milstein, "Searching for Circles of Meaning and Using Spiritual Experiences to Help Parents of Infants with Life Threatening Illness Cope," *Journal of Holistic Nursing* 25, no. 1 (2007): 39–49.	A phenomenologic study to identify the interactions with healthcare workers that were helpful and not. Parents were helped by identifying "circles of meaning."
Qualitative phenomenologic descriptive	M. Gunther and S. P. Thomas, "Nurses' Narratives of Unforgettable Patient Care Events," *Journal of Nursing Scholarship* 38, no. 4 (2006): 370–376.	Unstructured interviews; caregiver experiences resulted in residue of moral and existential distress from their life-altering experiences. Implications for how the holistic nurse integrates experience.
Qualitative grounded theory	L. Lewis et al., "African American Spirituality: A Process of Honoring God, Others, and Self," *Journal of Holistic Nursing* 25, no. 1 (2007): 16–23.	Need to address definitions of spirituality from participants, take into account cultural differences. Three categories of spirituality identified love in action, relationships and connections, and unconditional love.
Qualitative aesthetic approaches	G. J. Mitchell and N. D. Halifax, "Feeling Respected–Not Respected: The Embedded Artist in Parse Method Research," *Nursing Science Quarterly* 18, no. 2 (2006): 105–112.	Research project involving researchers, artists, and participants to explore the use of artwork to enhance understanding the phenomenon of feeling respected or not.

(continues)

TABLE 34-2 Some Examples of Holistic Nursing Research *(continued)*		
Example	**Author and Reference**	**Summary**
Qualitative aesthetic approaches	G. J. Mitchell, C. Jonas-Simpson, and V. Ivonofski, "Research-Based Theater: The Making of 'I'm Still Here,'" *Nursing Science Quarterly* 19, no. 3 (2006): 198–206.	Researcher and directors and playwrights partnered to craft a script about dementia and living with dementia. The article is an evaluation of the project.
Qualitative aesthetic approaches	R. McCaffrey, "The Effect of Healing Gardens and Art Therapy on Older Adults with Mild to Moderate Depression," *Holistic Nursing Practice* 21, no. 2 (2007): 79–84.	Using focus group interviews, study evaluated effects of garden walks alone, with guided imagery, and art therapy on depression in older adults.
Qualitative critical incident and focus groups	L. Sharoff, "A Qualitative Study of How Experienced Certified Holistic Nurses Learn to Become Competent Practitioners," *Journal of Holistic Nursing* 24, no. 2 (2006): 116–124.	A naturalistic study of how nurses learn to become expert. Characteristics of and challenges for these practitioners identified.
Qualitative historical	B. M. Dossey, *Florence Nightingale: Mystic, Visionary, Healer* (Springhouse, PA: Springhouse, 2000).	Historical life of Nightingale and implications for holistic nursing practice.
Triangulated	A. Brathovde, "A Pilot Study of Reiki for Self-Care of Nurses and Healthcare Providers," *Holistic Nursing Practice* 20, no. 2 (2006): 95–101.	A methodological triangulated pilot study; based on Watson's theoretical caritas framework, uses a caring efficacy scale. Interviews and self-report caring scale to assess effectiveness of Reiki as a self-care approach for nurses and healthcare providers.

Note: Many examples of holistic nursing research (HNR) currently are being published. This is a small sample of what is currently available in the literature.

the controversies surrounding RCT and, recently, evidence-based practice (EBP) research. The RCT employs randomized sampling, an experimental intervention, a control or placebo group, and *blinding* (neither the client nor the investigator knows whether the experimental treatment is real or placebo). When well designed and controlled, the RCT fosters inference about cause-and-effect relationships and ensures that results could be generalized to similar client populations and replicated in similar studies. Positive results in such studies may reassure us that we know what is effective and safe most of the time.

Many criticize the positivist, reductionist nature of quantitative research and advocate for combined or triangulated studies that include the individual's experience of healing and wholeness as well as standard measures of change such as blood pressure or number of inpatient hospital days.[54] NCCAM's 2011 strategic plan acknowledges what many have been emphasizing for years:

1. Distinctive features of unique individuals may be lost in aggregate means, standard deviations, and various statistical analyses.[55]
2. Many complementary therapies are not testable under blinded and sham conditions, and the choice of an appropriate control condition is not always clear.[56]
3. In highly controlled research, it is difficult to include the individualistic whole human being response to variables.

Zahourek recently reviewed two articles that questioned hallowed statistical significance.[57] Both articles focus on the work of a Greek physician–mathematician, Dr. Ioannidis, who has done work at Tufts, Johns Hopkins, and the National Institutes of Health (NIH). When statistically reviewing well-accepted studies, he found many variables that were in fact influencing the results of those studies. He notes such factors as decay over time and the impact of subtle variables such as the fashionability of the topic, funding resources, and difficulty in publishing negative results.[58]

Presently, healthy debate rages regarding the applicability of evidence-based practice research to study the complexity of healing.[59] (See Chapter 35 for full discussion of EBP.) According to some, because EBP relies heavily on RCT and systematic reviews[60] the approach provides "limited guidance to critically consider evidence from the diversity of researcher methods found within nursing literature and other related disciplines relevant for nursing practice."[61] Eriksson suggests a new and more holistic concept of evidence as "truth, reality and being in the world; it involves seeing, realizing, making visible and clothing thoughts into words" and includes "envisioning, seeing, knowing, attesting, and revising."[62] While the theoretical conflict continues, we in holistic nursing need all kinds of research approaches to learn more about the process of healing as well as the effectiveness and safety of our practice.

Qualitative Research

Holistic nurses embrace several philosophies of science and research methods that are compatible with investigating humanistic, unitary, and integral phenomena. Qualitative methods are appropriate when little information is known about a phenomenon or when phenomena are difficult to measure.[63] Qualitative research systematically describes and promotes understanding of human experiences such as health, healing, energy, intention, caring, comfort, and meaning. The context of this approach is meaning of observed patterns. This produces rich, articulate, in-depth, and coherent understanding of phenomena.

Qualitative research includes: (1) phenomenology: focuses on experience as the whole person

lives it; (2) hermeneutics: seeks to understand meaning and the individual's sociocultural experiences; (3) ethnography: describes a culture and the people within the culture; (4) grounded theory: uncovers psychosocial problems and how people manage; and (5) historical research: describes or analyzes past events to better understand the present.[53pp206-226] Qualitative approaches also include narrative and aesthetic forms of inquiry.

■ ENHANCING HOLISTIC RESEARCH

Additional Methods: Mixed Methods and Triangulation

Triangulation and mixed methods research involves multidimensional approaches to collect and evaluate data. These approaches attempt to capture a more complete representation of reality and strengthen the credibility of the research results. Mixed methods may include multiple data sources, methodologies, investigators, theories, and triangulated analyses.

According to Flemming,[64pp41-51] adopting the third paradigm—mixed methods—promotes a "ceasefire to the 'paradigm wars' that have raged since the 20th century" and that have "hindered the development of holistic nursing knowledge."[64p44] Such "binary opposition" does not address the nature of most nursing questions that are multifaceted and involve quantitative evidence of change or influence and qualitative holistic experience of the healing process.[64p43]

Giddings and Grant caution that mixed methods research may be a Trojan horse for positivism.[65p83] They contend that too often qualitative research is done poorly, tacked on with little acknowledgment of paradigmatic perspective, and relegated to the position of "handmaiden to the quantitative findings."[65p58] We need "radical theoretical flexibility" and "layering complexity" to expand our ways of knowing to make them more useful.[65p58] Although combining methods provides a broader focus and richer descriptions, "messiness" may occur when researchers do not acknowledge their "paradigmatic positions."[65pp58-59]

Sometimes mixed methods research yields conflicting results as in Ironside's sequential mixed methods study of implementing and evaluating narrative pedagogy with students.[66] When statistical data did not correspond with the qualitative narrative data, Ironside evaluated the conflicting results and posed new research questions. Finding conflicting results and discovering additional influencing factors are common in holistic nursing and CAM research. The research on prayer is another example. Some studies yield positive results, others no results, and some negative results; investigator intention seems to also play a major part in results.[25] What does this mean for understanding the phenomenon, the intervention, and the methods of research, data collection, analysis, and interpretation? Contradictions shift how we understand conventional research constructs and practices and keep us aware that we want to understand a complex world in which we want to promote healing.

Additional Methods: Synthesis, Systematic Reviews, and Meta-Analysis

Increasingly, meta-analyses, systematic reviews, and syntheses of research studies are published. At the top of the hierarchy of evidence are the systematic reviews and meta- analyses. According to Rew:

> A systematic review of literature is done not only to provide the evidence to guide current practice, but it is also an essential step in conducting research on new and innovative ideas for practice. In particular, conducting a systematic review of literature can be helpful in identifying tools to measure specific constructs in a planned study.[67]

In 1996, NCCAM formed a section of the Cochrane Collaboration to prepare, maintain, and disseminate systematic reviews on CAM and, when possible, meta-analyses. There are currently more than 400 Cochrane reviews on CAM including therapeutic touch and other touch therapies that are frequent modalities practiced by holistic nurses. See www.cochrane.org/cochrane-reviews for a complete list. Similar information can be found directly in the NCCAM site: Projects: Awarded Grants and Projects at http://nccam.nih.gov/research/extramural/awards/.

These reviews are resources for researchers and clinicians. However, Fonnebo critiques these reviews, stating that many were performed by people unfamiliar with CAM teaming up with CAM clinicians who know little about research methods.[60] Three weaknesses exist related to clinical relevance:

1. Primary trials that do not reflect clinical or best practices are included.
2. Primary trials that represent mutually exclusive treatment traditions are combined.
3. Primary trials that address different research questions are combined.[60p53]

Findlay and colleagues conducted a systematic review on the "return investment to hospitals that implement programs aimed at enhancing healing relationships."[68] Of the 80 studies reviewed, they found only 10 to be strong methodologically. Problematic issues that they encountered related to language and the differing definitions of *healing* and the lack of standards for rigorous program evaluation in hospitals. Qualitative studies, however, produced themes of what might constitute a healing relationship.

Rew completed an extensive review of studies on intuition in nursing.[69] Her presentation of results is exemplary for other researchers who want to do a synthesis on a particular topic of concern. Baldwin, Vitale, and associates have assembled three teams to collect and systematically review the research on Reiki.[70] This is the Touchstone Process. To date, 26 Reiki articles have been reviewed for strengths and weaknesses. Their results have been presented on an accessible website: www.centerforreikiresearch.org. Only 12 articles were based on robust experimental design and utilized adequate outcome measures.

Meta-analysis is a statistical technique that establishes an overall estimate of the therapeutic effectiveness of an intervention by combining and synthesizing the results of many small, but meaningful, experiments. The final conclusions are stronger than those provided in systematic reviews because meta-analysis considers sample size, strength of the experimental methods, and threats to internal and external validity, using both qualitative and quantitative approaches.[71] Meta-analyses allow inferences to be made about the current known effectiveness of a treatment, providing valuable information to clinicians and researchers planning future clinical studies.

In 1999, Winstead-Fry and Kijek completed a meta-analysis of therapeutic touch (TT).[72] The analysis compared 29 outcome studies; of those, 19 supported all or some of the hypotheses and 10 did not. Of the studies that reported means and standard deviations for control and treatment groups, 13 of 16 studies revealed an average effect size, weighted for sample size, of 0.39; this is considered a moderate effect. Meta-analyses may be inconclusive but still identify problems to be addressed in future studies. The authors identified the following difficulties: inadequate description of the study sample and intervention, not reporting statistical values for insignificant results, use of healthy subjects, overuse of a standard anxiety measure (State Trait Anxiety Inventory [STAI]), and an unusually brief TT treatment. These difficulties are useful caveats for future researchers investigating therapeutic touch.

Several nursing reviews address such topics as relaxation interventions for pain,[73] Healing Touch,[74] research based on the Rogerian Science of Unitary Human Beings,[75] energy healing and pain,[76] and an integrative review of self-concept in older adults.[77] Freysteinson completed an intriguing creative integrative review in therapeutic mirror interventions.[78] Qualitative and quantitative strategies were used in addition to a narrative synthesis approach.

A recent review has significance for HNR.[79] The researchers used a best evidence synthesis approach to evaluate 66 research studies on biofield therapies including therapeutic touch, qi gong, Reiki, Healing Touch, Johire, and others using a specific critical review checklist. Most of the studies were of average to minimum quality for randomization, use of controls, and statistical methods. The outcome measures were pain-related disorders. Strong evidence was found that pain intensity was reduced and general functioning increased as a result of these biofield therapies. Related disorders of anxiety and depression and long-term benefits were equivocal. Readers are encouraged to read this study for excellence in methodology and results.

Additional Methods: Aesthetic, Transpersonal

Numerous approaches to research exist and should be considered by holistic nurse researchers. The caveat remains: The method evolves from the question being asked and what the researcher hopes to find as an outcome.

Aesthetic and transpersonal methods are qualitative methodologies that value the researcher's reactions and interpretation. Margo Ely and colleagues[80] and Lee Gaydos[81] developed classic aesthetic methods that many have incorporated into data collection and interpretation. Aesthetic expressions can be used as data as well as can aid in the process of explaining ineffable phenomena such as healing and caring. Kongsuwan and Locsin use drawing to illuminate the experience of Thai ICU nurses caring for people experiencing a peaceful death.[82] Through the drawings, the unique meaning for these nurses of "caring for" could be articulated. Such expressions serve as sources of lived experience that is expressed in ways that may be communicated more readily by participants. Butcher developed the "field pattern portrait" as an aesthetic way of knowing.[83]

The transpersonal approach is based in a worldview that recognizes, values, and seeks to understand our fundamental oneness with each other and with all life. Implicit in this approach is a sense of "wonderment about the commonplace, an acceptance of life as precious, and recognition of the miraculous strata of all experiences."[84] Transpersonal research methods include intuition, storytelling, imagery, meditation, direct knowing, creative means of expressions, dreams, trance states, and describing uncommon experiences that are used as possible "strategies and procedures at all phases of the research inquiry."[84pxxx] If we reflect on our unusual experiences, we are led to "transcendent realities beyond the limits of our egos and personalities. Reflected in these realities, we can become more integral and whole, finding our more authentic and creative selves."[84pxvii] An example of this method can be found in a poem Zahourek wrote following a dream. The poem illuminates concepts that later became part of her theory of intentionality in healing.[42] Because these approaches are currently out of the norm for research methodology, it is less likely that currently traditional funding agencies would consider such methodology valid.

■ CONFOUNDS FOR HOLISTIC NURSING RESEARCH

Numerous challenges confront HN researchers.[85] First is language. What do we mean by such terms as *caring, healing, holism, presence,* and especially *spirit(uality)* and *energy*? How do we communicate those meanings to the established healthcare community and the public? When these terms are used casually, outsiders may view our research as superficial and vague, and therefore not credible or valid.

Many confounding variables need to be considered for holistic nursing research. Coakley and Duffy in their study of therapeutic touch on post vascular surgery pain discuss the difficulties of doing such a real-world study on a busy surgical unit.[41] Patients were often at rehabilitation or a test or were too tired when the researcher wanted to meet and do a treatment. The researcher provided the treatment, which can be a confound in causing the expectancy effect. In addition, the study required the use of an angiocatheter to draw blood pre and post therapeutic touch treatment; some potential participants refused because they wanted to avoid this procedure. Would they have reacted differently to the therapeutic touch treatment alone? Many question, "What is the adequate most effective 'dose' for a therapeutic touch treatment?" How often should the treatment be given and for how long? Additional confounds include but are not limited to the following:

1. The passage of time; the impact of many interventions is not observable or measurable immediately and may develop over time
2. The qualitative interpretation and meaning of an experience that may not be measured physiologically
3. Other intervening life experiences
4. Environmental impacts (e.g., natural and human-made disasters)
5. Cultural influences (e.g., an Hispanic as opposed to Chinese interpretation of an experience)
6. Personality temperament influences
7. Standardization of method (e.g., can therapeutic touch be standardized?), variation in method, approach, and skill used by individual practitioners
8. Sensitivity and reliability of tools and instruments to measure change
9. Placebo and expectation effect (valuable in one's personal experience of being healed, but a problem in conducting controlled research)

10. The Heisenberg principle and the Hawthorne effect
11. The impact of the interpersonal relationship and the intentions of healer and healee

The Placebo Response

Although the placebo response can be a nuisance and an unreliable factor that distorts research results, it is probably present in all clinical situations. The placebo response demonstrates the holistic communication between expectation (i.e., mind) and physiologic response (i.e., body). Placebo elements in the healing relationship that enhance therapeutic response and confound RCTs include expectation, degree of suffering, healing rituals (taking a temperature, writing a prescription) and symbols (e.g., the stethoscope, the white coat), the impact of being an expert, and providing an explanation for a malady.[86]

Questions of Objectivity in Scientific Investigation

Objectivity must govern scientific inquiry. Heisenberg, while studying the properties of an electron, discovered that it is impossible to look at a physical object without changing it.[87] Holistic researchers accept his uncertainty principle, realizing as participants in a research process that their presence affects the results. A word, a facial expression, a touch, or simply their presence influences observational data. Discovered in industrial research, the Hawthorne effect is described as the fact that the awareness of being observed changes the relationship, what is being measured, and the subsequent results of a research project.[88] Blinding is one method to control for this confound as well as for placebo response.

■ HOW IS HOLISTIC NURSING RESEARCH DIFFERENT?

The shift in emphasis to understanding the healing relationship through a holistic (unitary or integral) model has motivated holistic nurses to reexamine research priorities, methodologies, and findings. The current mandate to use the best evidence to direct our clinical decisions and actions is sculpted by the goal of achieving safe, effective, and holistic outcomes. Because most holistic therapies are in need of investigation, more and varied research needs to be conducted so that we can establish a comprehensive evidence base to support integrative healing practices.

Certain phenomena related to holistic research may not be accessible to reductionist scientific investigation because they cannot be objectively measured. The individual who experiences certain effects in a holistic nursing relationship may be unable to conceptualize, express, translate, or communicate these effects to another. Likewise, the researcher may be unable to interpret the effects because he or she lacks experience with these effects or because our language is inadequate for describing and communicating these phenomena. However, as we accumulate a database that includes various approaches and methodologies our body of supportive evidence grows.

The holistic care of clients must be based on research that clarifies and develops the holistic conceptual framework from which we practice. Some of our practice continues to be based on tradition, ritual belief systems and the way we were taught, with little supportive research evidence. For research to be holistic, we must articulate and explicate our view of holism as we plan, initiate, and interpret research. Holistic nursing research not only evaluates the effects of alternative and complementary modalities but also puts that evaluation into the context of a whole. What do we consider the "whole"? What worldview do we use to understand holism? Holistic nursing research is different because it simply is based in a holistic paradigm.

■ CONCLUSION

What will the future bring? More research in multidisciplinary teams? Investigators working on a similar problem or concept at multiple sites? It will bring a marriage between highly technical and skilled research that maps our molecular-chemical selves and our energetic make-up with a more profound appreciation for, and understanding of, the range of human experience in which we participate and hope to enhance and repair to promote growth and healing.

In summary and conclusion, Margaret A. Chesney, deputy director of NCCAM and director of its Division of Extramural Research and Training, in her 2006 keynote address said:

We have a long way to go, but there is much to discover, and we have an agenda rich in research challenges. . . . Be bold in what you try, cautious in what you claim, and thoughtful about what you do. Express your purpose in a way that inspires commitment, innovation, and courage. We need you to contribute your part to the whole, as we work together to add to the fabric of CAM [and holistic nursing] and create a new, comprehensive health care.[89]

Our challenges are great and the opportunities to explore new frontiers of investigation and understanding of what we do are thrilling.

Directions for
FUTURE RESEARCH

1. Evaluate a holistic nursing therapy that may promote wellness and healing in a specific client population.
2. Ask both healers and the one being healed how they experience and understand healing and the healing relationship.
3. Determine whether holistic therapies can be combined to augment their effectiveness in achieving desired client outcomes (e.g., combine Reiki with imagery or music therapy with therapeutic touch).
4. Determine the most effective way to integrate holistic therapies with traditional modes of therapy to achieve optimal outcomes.
5. Identify which standard health-related outcomes (e.g., in cardiology, rehabilitation, or during pregnancy) are most influenced by a healing relationship.

Nurse Healer
REFLECTIONS

After reading this chapter, the nurse healer will be able to answer or to begin a process of answering the following questions:

- How do I view healing and holism?
- How do I feel about the importance of research in advancing holistic nursing practice?
- What is my role in nursing research?
- How can I become more involved in holistic clinical research?

For a full suite of assignments and additional learning activities, use the access code located in the front of your book to visit this exclusive website: http://go.jblearning.com/dossey. If you do not have an access code, you can obtain one at the site.

NOTES

1. G. I. Viamontes & B. D. Beitman,"Neurobiology of the Unconscious: Relating Psychodynamic Principles to Scientific Studies of the Brain," *Psychiatric Annals* 37, no. 4 (2007).
2. L. Dossey, "Samueli Conference on Definitions and Standards in Healing Research: Working Definitions and Terms," *Alternative Therapies in Health and Medicine* 9, no. 3, suppl. (2003): A11.
3. R. P. Zahourek, "Healing Through the Lens of Intentionality," *International Journal of Healing and Caring* 9, no 2 (May 2009).
4. J. F. Quinn et al., "Research Guidelines for Assessing the Impact of the Healing Relationship in Clinical Nursing," *Alternative Therapies in Health and Medicine* 9, no. 3, suppl. (2003): A75.
5. R. P. Zahourek, "What Is Holistic Nursing Research? Is It Different?" *Beginnings* 26, no. 5 (2006): 4–6.
6. M. Enzman-Hagedorn and R. P. Zahourek, "Research Paradigms and Methods for Investigating Holistic Nursing Concerns," *Nursing Clinics of North America* 42, no. 2 (June 2007): 335–353.
7. White Paper Research in AHNA. http://www.ahna.org/Portals/4/docs/Research/WHITE%20PAPER%20RESEARCH%20IN%20AHNA.pdf
8. American Holistic Nurses Association, "What Is Holistic Nursing?" AHNA Position Statements, Flagstaff, Az., *AHNA Leadership Council Handbook* (2003, 2006): 61.
9. D. A. Jones, "The Impact of HEC: Concluding Thoughts and Future Directions," in *Giving Voice to What We Know; Margaret Newman's Theory of Health as Expanding Consciousness in Nursing Practice, Research and Education Studies*, ed. C. Picard and D. Jones (Sudbury, MA: Jones and Bartlett, 2005): 222.
10. M. A. Newman, Health as Expanding Consciousness. http://www.healthasexpandingconsciousness.org.
11. C. Picard, "Parents of Persons with Bipolar Disorder and Pattern Recognition," in *Giving Voice to What We Know; Margaret Newman's Theory of Health as Expanding Consciousness in Nursing Practice, Research and Education Studies*, ed. C. Picard

12. J. Neill, "Recognizing Patterns in the Lives of Women with Multiple Sclerosis," in *Giving Voice to What We Know; Margaret Newman's Theory of Health as Expanding Consciousness in Nursing Practice, Research and Education Studies*, ed. C. Picard and D. Jones (Sudbury, MA: Jones and Bartlett, 2005): 153–165.
13. J. Watson, *Assessing and Measuring Caring in Nursing and Health Science*, 2nd ed. (New York, NY: Springer, 2008).
14. P. P. DiNapoli and J. Nelson, "Measuring the Caritas Processes: Caring Factor Survey," *International Journal of Human Caring* 14, no. 4 (2010): 15–20.
15. R. Cowling and E. Repede, "Unitary Appreciative Inquiry: Evolution and Refinement," *Advances in Nursing Science* 33, no. 1 (2010): 64.
16. American Holistic Nurses Association, "Position Statement on Holistic Nursing Research and Scholarship." http://www.ahna.org/Resources/Publications/PositionStatements/tabid/1926/Default.aspx#P3.
17. B. Carper, "Fundamental Patterns of Knowing in Nursing," *Advances in Nursing Science* 1, no. 13 (1978): 13–23.
18. S. Porter, "Fundamental Patterns of Knowing in Nursing; The Challenge of Evidence-Based Practice," *Advances in Nursing Science* 33, no. 1 (2010).
19. J. Fawcett, *Analysis and Evaluation of Nursing Theories* (Philadelphia, PA: F. A. Davis, 1993): 10–12.
20. M. Enzman-Hagedorn and R. P. Zahourek, "Research Paradigms and Methods for Investigating Holistic Nursing Concerns Nursing," in *Nursing Clinics of North America* 42, no. 2 (2007): 335–353.
21. C. Mariano, "The Many Faces of Scholarship," *Beginnings* 26, no. 5 (2006): 3.
22. J. Watson, "Caring Knowledge and Informed Moral Passion," *Advances in Nursing Science* 12, no. 1 (1990): 15–24.
23. P. Munhall, "Unknowing: Toward Another Pattern of Knowing in Nursing," *Nursing Outlook* 41 (1993): 125–128.
24. L. Dossey, "Compassion," *Explore: Journal of Science and Healing* 3, no. 1 (2007): 1–5.
25. S. A. Schwartz and L. Dossey, "Nonlocality, Intention and Observer Effects in Healing Studies: Laying a Foundation for the Future," *Explore* 6, no. 5 (2010): 295–307.
26. W. Braud and R. Anderson, *Transpersonal Research Methods for the Social Science: Honoring Human Experience* (Thousand Oaks, CA: Sage, 1998).
27. W. B. Jonas and C. C. Crawford, *Healing Intention and Energy Medicine: Science, Research Methods and Clinical Implications* (Edinburgh, Scotland: Churchill Livingstone, 2003).
28. K. Wilber, *Integral Psychology: Consciousness, Spirit, Psychology, Therapy* (Boston, MA: Shambhala, 2000).

29. National Center for Complementary and Alternative Medicine, "National Center for Complementary and Alternative Medicine Exploring the Science of Complementary and Alternative Medicine: Third Strategic Plan: 2011–2015." http://nccam.nih.gov/about/plans/2011/index.htm/.

30. A. B. Coakley and M. E. Duffy, "The Effect of Therapeutic Touch on Post Operative Patients," *Journal of Holistic Nursing* 28, no. 3 (2010): 193–200.

31. H. C. Sox and S. Greenfield, "Comparative Effectiveness Research: A Report of the Institute of Medicine," *Annals of Internal Medicine* 15, no. 3 (2009): 203–205.

32. I. D. Coulter, "Comparative Effectiveness Research: Does the Emperor Have Clothes?" *Alternative Therapies* 17, no. 2 (2011): 8–15.

33. M. M. Libster, "A History of Shaker Nurse-Herbalists, Health Reform, and the American Botanical Medical Movement (1830–1860)," *Journal of Holistic Nursing* 27, no. 4 (2009): 222–231.

34. R. McCaffrey, D. Thomas, and A. Orth Kinzelman, "The Effects of Lavender and Rosemary Essential Oils on Test-Taking Anxiety Among Graduate Nursing Students," *Holistic Nursing Practice* 23, no. 2 (2009): 88–93.

35. L. Muzzarelli, M. Force, and M. Sebold, "Aromatherapy and Reducing Preprocedural Anxiety: A Controlled Prospective Study," *Gastroenterology Nursing* 29, no. 6 (2006): 466–471.

36. E. Guarneri, B. J. Horrigan, and C. M. Pechura, "The Efficacy and Cost Effectiveness of Integrative Medicine: A Review of the Medical and Corporate Literature," *Explore* 6, no. 5 (2010): 308–312.

37. V. Eschiti, "Complementary and Alternative Modalities Used by Women with Female-Specific Cancers," *Holistic Nursing Practice* 22, no. 3 (2008): 127–138.

38. J. Kilanowski, "Pilot Studies: Helmsman on the Ship of Research Design," *American Nurse Today* 6, no. 4 (2011).

39. C. L. Cuneo, M. R. Cooper, C. S. Drew, et al., "The Effect of Reiki on Work-Related Stress of Registered Nurses," *Journal of Holistic Nursing* 29, no. 1 (2011): 33–43.

40. M. B. Helming, "Health Through Prayer: A Qualitative Study," *Holistic Nursing Practice* 25, no. 1 (2011): 33–44.

41. A. B. Coakley and M. E. Duffy, "The Effect of Therapeutic Touch on Postoperative Patients," *Journal of Holistic Nursing* 28, no. 3 (2010): 193–200.

42. R. P. Zahourek, *Intentionality: The Matrix of Healing: A Qualitative Theory for Research, Education and Practice* (Saarbrucken, Germany: VDM Verlag, 2009).

43. C. R. Gross et al., "Mindfulness-Based Stress Reduction for Solid Organ Transplant Recipients: A Randomized Controlled Trial," *Alternative Therapies in Health and Medicine* 12, no. 4 (2010): 30–38.

44. K. Sand-Jecklin and H. Emerson, "The Impact of a Live Therapeutic Music Intervention on Patients' Experience of Pain, Anxiety and Muscle Tension," *Holistic Nursing Practice* 24, no. 1 (2010): 7–15.

45. R. McCaffrey, C. Hansen, and W. McCaffrey, "Garden Walking for Depression: A Research Report," *Holistic Nursing Practice* 24, no. 5 (2010): 252–259.

46. D. Wagner and B. Whaite, "An Exploration of the Nature of Caring Relationships in the Writings of Florence Nightingale," *Journal of Holistic Nursing* 28, no. 4 (2010): 225–234.

47. M. Hemsley, N. Glass, and J. Watson, "Taking the Eagle's View: Using Watson's Conceptual Model to Investigate the Extraordinary and Transformative Experiences of Nurse Healers," *Holistic Nursing Practice* 20, no. 2 (2006): 85–94.

48. C. Delaney and C. Barrere, "Ecospirituality: The Experience of Environmental Meditation in Patients with Cardiovascular Disease," *Holistic Nursing Practice* 23, no. 6 (2009): 361–369.

49. W. R. Cowling, "A Unitary Healing Praxis Model for Women in Despair," *Nursing Science Quarterly* 19, no. 2 (2006): 123–132.

50. P. P. DiNapoli et al., "The Effect of Reiki on Work-Related Stress of Registered Nurses," *Journal of Holistic Nursing* 29, no. 1 (2011): 33–43.

51. E. Monzillo and G. Gronowicz, "New Insights on Therapeutic Touch: A Discussion of Experimental Methodology and Design That Resulted in Significant Effects on Normal Human Cells and Osteosarcoma," *Explore* 7, no. 1 (2011): 44–51.

52. V. Andrus, M. Shannahan, and M. J. Assi, "A Research Study to Enrich the Professional Practice Environment for RNs," *Beginnings* 26, no. 5 (2006): 10–11.

53. D. F. Polit, C. T. Beck, and B. P. Hungler, *Essentials of Nursing Research: Methods, Appraisal, and Utilization*, 5th ed. (Philadelphia, PA: Lippincott, 2001).

54. O. Caspi and K. O. Burleson, "Methodological Challenges in Meditation Research," *Advanced Mind Body Medicine* 2, no. 1 (2005): 4–11.

55. D. Lukoff et al., "The Case Study as a Scientific Method for Researching Alternative Therapies," *Alternative Therapies in Health and Medicine* 4, no. 2 (1998): 44–52.

56. A. Margolin et al., "Investigating Alternative Medicine Therapies in Randomized Controlled Trials," *Journal of the American Medical Association* 280, no. 18 (1998): 1626–1628.

57. R. P. Zahourek, "Does the Empress Wear Clothes?" *Connections in Holistic Nursing* 3, no. 2 (February 2011). http://www.ahna.org/portals/4/docs/Research/Enews/Connections_R-eNews_2-11.htm.

58. D. H. Freedman, "Lies, Damned Lies, and Medical Science," *Atlantic Monthly* (November

2010). http://www.theatlantic.com/magazine/archive/2010/11/lies-damned-lies-and-medical-science/8269/.

59. D. Holmes et al., "Deconstructing the Evidence-Based Discourse in Health Sciences: Truth, Power and Fascism," *International Journal of Evidence-Based Health Care* 4 (2006): 180–186.

60. V. Fonnebo, "Cochrane CAM Reviews Commentary: Is There More to Quality Than the Research Method Itself?" *Explore* 7, no. 1 (2011): 53–54.

61. S. R. Kirckbaum et al., "Knowledge Development and Evidence-Based Practice: Insight and Opportunity from a Postcolonial Feminist Perspective for Transformative Nursing," *Advances in Nursing Science* 30, no. 1 (2007): 28.

62. K. Eriksson, "Evidence: To See or Not to See," *Nursing Science Quarterly* 23, no. 4 (2011): 275.

63. M. Sandelowski, "Rigor or Rigor Mortis: The Problem of Rigor in Qualitative Research Revisited," *Advances in Nursing Science* 16, no. 2 (1993): 1–8.

64. K. Flemming, "The Knowledge Base for Evidence-Based Practice: A Role for Mixed Methods Research," *Advances in Nursing Science* 30, no. 1 (2007): 41–51.

65. L. S. Giddings and B. M. Grant, "A Trojan Horse for Positivism?: A Critique of Mixed Methods Research," *Advances in Nursing Science* 30, no. 1 (2007).

66. P. Ironside, "Trying Something New: Implementing and Evaluating Narrative Pedagogy Using a Multimethod Approach," *Nursing Education Perspective* 24, no. 30 (2003): 122–128.

67. L. Rew, "How to Conduct a Systematic Review of Literature," *AHNA Research Enews* (April 2010). http://www.ahna.org/Portals/4/docs/Research/Library/Conduct-systematic-review.pdf.

68. B. Findlay et al., "Methodological Complexities Associated with Systematic Review of Healing Relationships," *Alternative Therapies* 16, no. 5 (2010): 40–46.

69. L. Rew, "State of the Science: Intuition in Nursing: A Generation of Studying the Phenomenon," *Advances in Nursing Science* 30, no. 1 (2007): E15–E25.

70. A. L. Baldwin et al., "The Touchstone Process: An Ongoing Critical Evaluation of Reiki in the Scientific Literature," *Holistic Nursing Practice* 24, no. 5 (2010): 260–276.

71. R. J. Gatchell and A. M. Maddrey, "Clinical Outcomes Research in Complementary and Alternative Medicine: An Overview of Experimental Design and Analysis," *Alternative Therapies in Health and Medicine* 4, no. 5 (1998): 41.

72. P. Winstead-Fry and J. Kijek, "An Integrative Review and Meta-analysis of Therapeutic Touch Research," *Alternative Therapies in Health and Medicine* 5, no. 6 (1999): 58–67.

73. K. L. Kwekkeboom and E. Gretarsdottir, "Systematic Review of Relaxation Interventions for Pain," *Journal of Nursing Scholarship* 38, no. 3 (2006): 269–277.

74. D. W. Wardell and K. F. Weymouth, "Review of Studies of Healing Touch," *Journal of Nursing Scholarship* 36, no. 2 (2004): 147–154.

75. T. S. Kim, "Science of Unitary Human Beings: An Update on Research," *Nursing Science Quarterly* 21, no. 4 (2008): 294–299.

76. D. L. Fazzino, M. T. Quinn Griffin, Sr., R. McNulty, and J. J. Fitzpatric, "Energy Healing and Pain: A Review of the Literature," *Holistic Nursing Practice* 24, no. 2 (2010): 79–88.

77. V. T. Cotter and E. W. Gonzales, "Self-Concept in Older Adults: An Integrative Review of Empirical Literature," *Holistic Nursing Practice* 32, no. 6 (2009): 335–348.

78. W. M. Freysteinson, "Therapeutic Mirror Interventions: An Integrated Review of the Literature," *Journal of Holistic Nursing* 27, no. 4 (2009): 241–252.

79. S. S. Janin and P. Mills, "Biofield Therapies: Helpful or Hype? A Best Evidence Synthesis," *International Journal of Behavioral Medicine* 17 (2010): 1–16.

80. M. Ely et al., *On Writing Qualitative Research: Living by Words* (London, England: Falmer Press, 1997).

81. H. L. Gaydos, "Making Special: A Framework for Understanding the Art of Holistic Nursing," *Journal of Holistic Nursing* 22, no. 2 (2004): 152–163.

82. W. Kongsuwan and R. C. Locsin, "Aesthetic Expressions Illuminating the Lived Experience of Tai ICU Nurses Caring for Persons Who Had a Peaceful Death," *Holistic Nursing Practice* 24, no. 3 (2010): 131–141.

83. H. K. Butcher, "The Unitary Field Pattern Portrait Research Method: Facets, Processes, and Findings," *Nursing Science Quarterly* 1, no. 4 (2005): 293–297.

84. W. Braud and R. Andersen, *Transpersonal Research Methods for the Social Sciences: Honoring Human Experience* (Thousand Oaks, CA: Sage, 1998): xxii.

85. R. P. Zahourek, "What Is Holistic Nursing Research?" *Beginnings* 26, no. 5 (2006).

86. W. A. Brown, "Understanding and Using Placebo Effect," *Psychiatric Times* 23, no. 11 (2006): 15–17.

87. W. Heisenberg, *Physics and Philosophy* (New York, NY: Harper & Row, 1978): 42.

88. D. Polit and C. T. Beck, *Nursing Research: Generating and Assessing Evidence for Nursing Practice*, 9th ed. (Philadelphia, PA: Lippincott Williams & Wilkins, 2012).

89. M. A. Chesney, *International Research Conference Highlights Progress, New Directions* (keynote address, North American Research Conference on Complementary and Integrative Medicine, Edmonton, Alberta, Canada, May 24–27, 2006). *NCCAM Newsletter* 13, no. 3 (2006).

Chapter 35

Evidence-Based Practice

Carol M. Baldwin, Alyce A. Schultz,
Bernadette Mazurek Melnyk,
and Jo Rycroft-Malone

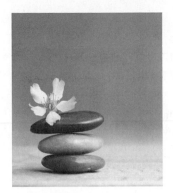

Nurse Healer
OBJECTIVES

Theoretical

- Explore the concept of evidence-based practice (EBP).
- Review the historical underpinnings of EBP.
- Compare and discriminate between individual and system-wide models of EBP.
- Discuss ways in which EBP has redirected priorities for evaluating best practices in nursing research.
- Compare and contrast the barriers to and strengths of evidence-based care.
- Examine international approaches to EBP in holistic nursing practice

Clinical

- Describe the five steps to searching for the best evidence.
- Apply the EBP process to a peer-reviewed journal article and assess the evidence for making a decision or practice change.
- Identify resources that can be used to incorporate EBP in your clinical setting.
- Discuss ways in which EBP can be adapted at your clinical setting to enhance best practices in the holistic caring process.
- Practice framing a clinical issue of interest into a standardized clinical question, such as the PICOT format in your clinical setting.
- Define and describe ways in which EBP informs comparative effectiveness research.

Personal

- Set aside time to learn more about how EBP can enhance the holistic caring process.
- Attend an EBP conference or workshop.
- Develop expertise in EBP through an online course or program of study.
- Search online resources to appreciate the application of EBP in clinical practice nationally and internationally.

DEFINITIONS

Comparative effectiveness research (CER): The conduct and synthesis of research that compares the benefits and harms of various interventions and strategies for preventing, diagnosing, treating, and monitoring health conditions in real-world settings. The purpose of this research is to improve health outcomes by developing and disseminating evidence-based information to patients, clinicians, and other decision makers about which interventions are most effective for which patients under specific circumstances.

Evidence-based practice (EBP): The conscientious use of the best available evidence combined with the clinician's expertise and judgment and the patient's preferences and values to arrive at the best decision that leads to high-quality outcomes.

PICOT: A standardized format for asking the searchable, answerable question: population of interest (P); the intervention or issue of interest (I); the comparison intervention, if relevant (C); the outcome (O); and time frame (T), if relevant.

■ HOLISTIC NURSING AND EVIDENCE-BASED PRACTICE

The science and art of holistic nursing honor an individual's subjective experience about health, health beliefs, and values and develop therapeutic partnerships with individuals, families, and communities that are grounded in nursing knowledge, theories, research expertise, intuition, and creativity.[1] Evidence-based practice (EBP) is the conscientious use of the best available evidence combined with the clinician's expertise and judgment and the patient's preferences and values to arrive at the best decision that leads to high-quality outcomes.[2,3] Research has shown that when these conceptual components of EBP are integrated within a context of caring (**Figure 35-1**), components that are consonant with the science and art of holistic nursing, they lead to the best clinical decision making, as well as best outcomes for patients, families, communities, and populations.[4]

■ HISTORICAL UNDERPINNINGS OF CURRENT EVIDENCE-BASED PRACTICE

Knowledge translation or the use of research evidence to improve clinical outcomes is not a 21st-century phenomenon. Neither is the difficulty with or resistance to the application of new scientific knowledge to practice. For example, the usefulness of citrus juice for the treatment of scurvy was noted in the 16th century, although it would be another 100 years for these findings to be put into practice by the British Admiralty.[5] Another example is that of the work of Ignatz Semmelweis, who recognized that obstetricians were carrying the contagion for puerperal fever from the morgue to the delivery room.[5] His recommendation to reduce maternal mortality by hand-washing was rejected by the Viennese medical society in the mid-18th century with a mantra used today that contradicts evidence to practice, "Because we've always done it that way."

As the disease transmission theory was being rejected by practicing physicians, Florence Nightingale, as a nurse in the Crimean War

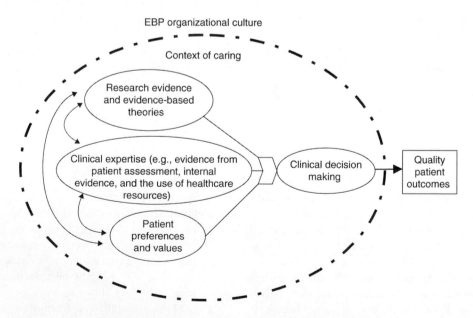

FIGURE 35-1   Evidence-based practice conceptual framework.
Source: Adapted from B. Melnyk and E. Fineout-Overholt, *Evidence-Based Practice in Nursing and Healthcare: A Guide to Best Practice*, 2nd edition (Philadelphia, PA: Wolters/Kluwer Lippincott Williams & Wilkins, 2005)

(1853–1856), found that washing hands between patients along with other public health measures reduced morbidity and mortality among the soldiers.[6] Recognized as the first nurse to conduct and use research, Nightingale showed that the quality of care can be improved through sanitary conditions, careful data collection, and critical thinking.[7] More than 150 years later, Nightingale's insight into the need for research laid the groundwork for evidence-based practice in holistic nursing when she wrote:

> In dwelling upon the vital importance of *sound* observation, it must never be lost sight of what observation is for. It is not for the sake of piling up miscellaneous information or curious facts, but for the sake of saving life and increasing health and comfort.[8]

■ NURSING RESEARCH INTO EVIDENCE-BASED PRACTICE

For 75 years, research has been recognized as important for improving nursing education and practice. Sigma Theta Tau International (STTI), the only nursing honor society, offered the first nursing research grant in 1936. Thirty-five years later, research became a required course in baccalaureate nursing programs. As research skills and knowledge became a requirement for the professional nurse, concern for use of research findings in practice and strategies to increase research utilization became a top priority. In the mid-1970s, federal grants supported the Western Interstate Commission on Higher Education (WICHE) Regional Program for Nursing Research Development, the Conduct and Utilization of Research in Nursing (CURN), and Nursing Child Assessment Satellite Training (NCAST).[9] The Regional Program for Nursing Research Development was conducted in the 13 western states to teach practicing nurses how to identify researchable practice issues, critique the current research literature, initiate and lead practice changes, and evaluate their outcomes.[10] The CURN project was designed to develop practice protocols based on the synthesis of the best available science. Ten research-based protocols were completed and evaluated for their applicability.[11] NCAST, based on the early findings of

Dr. Kathryn Barnard, focused on teaching cues to maternal-child interaction to nurses in Washington using the new satellite system. Stetler and Marram, as young doctoral students, published the original version of their research utilization model for use by advanced practice nurses as leaders and mentors for changing clinical nursing practice.[12] An early meta-analysis showed that patients who received research-based interventions experienced outcomes that were 28% better than patients receiving routine care.[13] These findings strongly supported the efforts to increase the use of research by direct care providers.

Despite this foundation of nursing knowledge built on practice based on evidence, Ketefian concluded that nurses who conducted research and nurses who practiced at the bedsides lived in separate "subcultures" and that to narrow this gap, researchers must publish research findings in a format that practicing nurses could read and use.[14] It was apparent that even though individual nurses learned and supported the concepts of research utilization, there were many barriers to actually implementing and maintaining research-based practice changes.[15-17]

Further studies exploring barriers to and facilitators of research use were conducted in the 1980s, the 1990s, and continue today.[9,18] Funk and colleagues, using the concepts within Rogers' Diffusion of Innovation model, explored the individual and the organizational challenges to the use of research in the early 1990s. They reported barriers associated with the characteristics of the adopter, the organization, the innovation itself, and the communication and dissemination of the findings. These findings encouraged the development of models and programs addressing organizational and dissemination barriers. Using the Dissemination Model, Funk et al. held a series of national conferences on use of research in practice.[19] Cronenwett implemented research utilization conferences at Dartmouth-Hitchcock Hospitals that focused on integrative reviews for promoting research use by direct care nurses.[20] An early model for addressing organizational challenges was implemented in a rural Iowa hospital that was later adapted at the University of Iowa Hospitals and Clinics.[21] Four educational videos on research utilization for direct care nurses were developed to support the Organizational Process Research

Utilization Model.[22-25] Titler and colleagues expanded on this organizational model in their development of the Iowa Model for Research in Practice.[26] Rutledge and Donaldson received federal funding to develop and implement the Orange County Research Utilization in Nursing (OCRUN) project, focusing on building organizational capacity as a tool for increasing research utilization.[27]

As it became evident that much of nursing care was based on best practice and the methodology for and emphasis on quality improvement was increasing, more forms of evidence began to be used as the basis for practice. In the early 1990s, Sackett and colleagues coined the term *evidence-based medicine* to add credibility to internal quality improvement data and common practices that were providing good patient outcomes.[28] *Evidence-based practice* soon became the term used to describe practices by all healthcare professionals. One of the early interdisciplinary models for evidence-based practice was developed at the University of Colorado to provide the framework for quality improvement activities.[29] From the mid-1990s to the present, a number of new quality improvement and evidence-based practice models and frameworks have been developed.

■ CONCEPTUAL MODELS FOR EVIDENCE-BASED PRACTICE

From these early underpinnings, a variety of conceptual models has emerged for EBP, including models that focus on the EBP process for individual clinicians, such as the model of DiCenso and colleagues,[30] the Stetler Model,[31] and the Clinical Scholar Model.[32] Several models focus on system-wide implementation of EBP, including the Iowa Model,[33] the Promoting Action on Research Implementation in Health Services (PARIHS) Model,[34] and the Advancing Research and Clinical Practice Through Close Collaboration (ARCC) Model.[4] Although these models are useful in conceptually guiding the implementation of EBP for individuals and within systems, there is a pressing need for further testing to support them empirically. Exemplars for the individual system-wide models are described in this chapter.

Exemplar: The DiCenso Model

The DiCenso Model of EBP,[30] adapted from Haynes,[35] promotes the use of research findings within the context of an evidence-based decision-making framework.[4] The individual clinician integrates the best research evidence with the patient's clinical status, preferences, action, and circumstances; available healthcare resources; and clinical expertise to decide on the interventions or type of care to be delivered. Aspects of this approach are described using a clinical scenario and an exemplar analysis when the principles of the EBP process are used to critically appraise an article from the *Journal of Holistic Nursing* later in this chapter.

Exemplar: The Clinical Scholar Model and Program

Clinical scholars are agents of change whether through promoting the spirit of inquiry in the areas where they work, translating new knowledge into practice using internal and external evidence, or generating new knowledge through the conduct of research. The Clinical Scholar Model and Program provides a framework and process for these agents of change.

Seeds for the Clinical Scholar Model were sown in 1980 when Dr. Janelle Krueger in her keynote address at one of the first national nursing research conferences, Promoting Nursing Research as a Staff Nursing Function, emphasized that staff nurses could "use" and "do" research.[10] She argued that research utilization and conduct should be an expectation of bedside nurses because they are the link between research and practice and can identify problems that need to be researched. During the 1990s, staff nurses at Maine Medical Center in Portland with the mentorship of a doctorally prepared nurse researcher learned how to apply research findings to practice and answer their own burning clinical questions by conducting their own studies. The Clinical Scholar Program was developed to facilitate larger cohorts of professional nurses who were interested in improving quality of care through the use of internal and external evidence.

The Clinical Scholar Model is inductive, decentralized, and predicated on "building a community" of clinical scholars to serve as mentors anywhere patient care is provided.[32] The clinical scholar is always questioning whether a procedure needs to be performed at all and, if so, whether there is a more efficient and effective way of providing the same care. Clinical scholarship, as described in a Sigma Theta Tau International position paper,[36] is an intellectual process, steeped in curiosity that challenges traditional nursing practice through observation, analysis, synthesis, application, and dissemination, concepts that form the structure of the Clinical Scholar Model.[32,37] Qualitative and quantitative studies are reviewed for applicability to practice and knowledge generation research designs are based on the clinical inquiry.

The Clinical Scholar Program, based on the Clinical Scholar Model, is a series of six interdisciplinary all-day workshops, generally presented one month apart. The goals of the program are to: (1) promote a culture of EBP and clinical scholarship through a program of interdisciplinary clinical research and EBP at the bedside, extending work that has already been initiated in a clinical setting; and (2) prepare a cadre of direct care providers as clinical scholars to implement change and evaluate practice based on evidence. The clinical scholars serve as mentors/champions to other staff.

The Clinical Scholar Model serves as the framework for several academic and community healthcare facilities across the country including Scottsdale Healthcare System; John C. Lincoln North Mountain Hospital; St. Joseph's Hospital in Marshfield, Wisconsin; Maine Medical Center; St. Joseph Medical Center in Kansas City, Missouri; the James Comprehensive Cancer Center at The Ohio State University; Banner Del E. Webb Medical Center; and Phoenix Children's Hospital.[38-40] Concepts of the Clinical Scholar Model have been adapted into models within nursing departments at Baylor Health Care System and Mayo Clinic and also serve as the underlying framework for the Maine Nursing Practice Consortium in northern Maine and the Texas Christian University Evidence-Based Practice and Research (EBPR) Collaborative among urban hospitals in the Dallas-Fort Worth area.[41-42]

Exemplar: Promoting Action on Research Implementation in Health Services (PARIHS) Model

If implementation was straightforward, the production and dissemination of evidence in the form of guidelines, followed by an education or teaching package, would lead to an expectation that practitioners would automatically integrate them into their everyday practice. Politically and educationally, there has been a focus on developing the skills and knowledge of individual practitioners to appraise research and make rational decisions. As such, the emphasis has been placed on developing the skills of individual nurses to be able to find and critically appraise research evidence in the hope that this will influence its use in practice.

Despite these efforts and considerable investment, for the most part, research evidence is still not used routinely in practice. Over recent years, there has been a shift to recognize that, in fact, the process of implementing evidence into practice is more complex than some rational or linear models and approaches to implementation imply. The individual nurse cannot be isolated from all the bureaucratic, political, organizational, and social factors that affect change.[43-47] The implementation of research-based practice depends on an ability to achieve significant and planned behavior change involving individuals, teams, and organizations.[48]

Stetler and colleagues conducted a study in which the importance of organizational context in the routine use of EBP was highlighted.[47,49] Their research shows that some key contextual features enable the institutionalization of EBP. These features include leadership in EBP at all levels of the organization from chief nursing officer to staff nurse, a supportive organizational culture, effective multidisciplinary team work, and coherent policies and procedures. This research supports the idea that although it is critical to have reflective and inquiring nurses, their ability to practice in an evidence-based way may be more or less facilitated by the context in which they work.

The PARIHS framework was developed to represent the complexities involved in implementing evidence into practice.[19,34] The successful implementation (SI) of evidence into practice is a function (f) of the nature and type of evidence (E), the qualities of the context (C) in which the evidence is to be implemented, and the way the process is facilitated (F); therefore, SI = $f(E,C,F)$. It provides a practical and conceptual heuristic to guide implementation and practice improvement activity, which takes multiple factors into account and acknowledges the dynamism in implementation processes. This conceptual and theoretical framework has been used for research and evaluation, the basis for tool development, modeling research utilization, and evaluating the facilitation of interventions.[34]

Exemplar: Advancing Research and Clinical Practice Through Close Collaboration (ARCC) Model for System-wide Implementation and Sustainability of EBP

In 1999, Bernadette Melnyk conceptualized the ARCC Model as part of a research strategic planning initiative involving faculty from a school of nursing and school of medicine. The purpose was to launch an initiative that would closely integrate clinical practice and research to advance EBP within an academic medical center and healthcare community.[50-51] The ARCC Model has expanded to include multiple strategies for advancing EBP within healthcare organizations. The key element for implementing and sustaining system-wide EBP in the model is a cadre of EBP mentors who facilitate clinician and organizational culture change to EBP.[4] The ARCC Model has been implemented in several healthcare systems and agencies, including the Visiting Nurse Service of New York, Pace University, SUNY Upstate Medical Center, the University of Rochester, the National Institutes of Health Clinical Center, and Washington Hospital Healthcare System.[4] These liaisons have fostered empirical testing of the model, and findings from studies support multiple aspects of the ARCC Model at the preceding institutions.[50-51]

Within the conceptual framework of the ARCC Model (see Figure 35-1), the first step to system-wide implementation is the assessment of an organization's strengths and limitations in advancing EBP. Once strengths and limitations are identified, a key implementation strat-

egy in the ARCC Model, the development of a cadre of EBP mentors, is initiated. The EBP mentor is typically an advanced practice nurse with in-depth EBP knowledge and skills. The mentor possesses individual behavior and organizational change skills, provides mentorship, and facilitates improvement in clinical care and patient outcomes through EBP implementation, quality improvement, and outcomes management projects. Goals of the ARCC Model include (1) promoting EBP among both advanced practice and staff nurses as well as transdisciplinary clinicians, (2) establishing a cadre of EBP mentors to facilitate system-wide implementation of EBP in healthcare organizations, (3) disseminating and facilitating use of the best evidence from well-designed studies to advance an evidence-based approach to clinical care, (4) designing and conducting studies to evaluate the effectiveness of the ARCC Model on the process and outcomes of clinical care, and (5) conducting studies to evaluate the effectiveness of the EBP implementation strategies.[3,50]

Empirical evidence supports the various relationships within the ARCC Model. Nurses and clinicians who report having greater knowledge of EBP and who hold positive beliefs about their ability to implement EBP are more likely to implement it and teach it to others. Nurses who have an EBP mentor are more likely to implement evidence-based care.[52] In addition, supportive EBP cultures are related to more positive beliefs about EBP and greater EBP implementation. Having more positive cognitive beliefs about EBP is related to increased group cohesion and job satisfaction.[53] Construct validity of three instruments that measure important aspects of the ARCC Model (the EBP Beliefs Scale, the EBP Implementation Scale, and the Organizational Culture and Readiness for System-wide Integration of Evidence-Based Practice Survey) has been supported, and internal consistency reliabilities for each of the three scales has consistently been above .80 with multiple samples. These measures can be applied to successful understanding of and orientation to the EBP process at the individual and system-wide levels.[52-56]

Several intervention studies have been conducted to test the efficacy of the ARCC Model on the process and outcomes of care. A pilot study was completed that tested the efficacy of the ARCC Model within a visiting nurse service.[56] Findings indicated that nurses who received the ARCC intervention program, in comparison to nurses who received a placebo control program, not only reported stronger beliefs about the value of EBP and their ability to implement it, but also reported higher EBP implementation and stronger group cohesion. These findings suggest that knowledge of EBP leads to a higher quality of care and may contribute to reduced nurse turnover rates at a time when the United States is facing its most severe shortage in the history of nursing. Another study indicated that participating in a structured mentorship program based on the ARCC model led to more positive beliefs among nurses about organizational culture and EBP, which were related to greater EBP implementation.[57] Furthermore, implementation of the ARCC Model at a community hospital system resulted in more positive beliefs and increased EBP implementation by clinicians and substantially improved patient outcomes that included reductions in length of intensive care unit stay, decreased infection rates, and fewer rehospitalizations.

■ CHALLENGES TO AND STRENGTHS OF EVIDENCE-BASED CARE

There are several barriers to providing care based on the latest evidence, including lack of searching skills, inability to critically appraise studies, insufficient institutional support, as well as negative attitudes toward research.[54,58] Based on a nationwide sample of 1,097 randomly selected registered nurses in the United States, the Nursing Informatics Expert Panel of the American Academy of Nursing found that almost half of the respondents were not familiar with the terms *evidence-based practice* and *EBP*, more than half of the respondents reported that they did not believe their colleagues used research findings in practice, only 27% of the respondents had been taught how to use electronic databases, most of the respondents did not search information databases (e.g., Medline and CINAHL) to gather practice information, and respondents who did search these resources did not believe they had adequate searching skills.[58]

Similar survey data have been collected at several Pan American Health Organization (PAHO)-sponsored conferences in Argentina, Ecuador, Panama, and Spain. The leading individual barriers reported by U.S. nurses include lack of value for research in practice, lack of knowledge of electronic database organization and structure, and difficulty accessing research materials. Pan American nurses rated lack of research knowledge, synthesis skills, and library access as their leading individual barriers. Both U.S. and Pan American nurses rated presence of goals with higher priority and organization budget for acquisition of information resources as their first and third leading institutional barriers, whereas U.S. nurses rated difficulty in recruiting and retaining nursing staff as second compared to Pan American nurses rating the organization's perception of lack of nurse preparation for EBP as second among institutional barriers.[59]

For several years, however, empirical evidence has shown that patient outcomes are at least 28% better when clinical care is based on rigorously designed research studies rather than care that is steeped in tradition.[13] Studies also suggest that clinicians who use research evidence in their practice are more satisfied with their roles.[53,60-61] Anecdotal reports indicate that evidence-based care renews the professional spirit of the nurse, a key variable in professional satisfaction. Nurses who incorporate EBP into their care report that it gives them a voice, allows them to reclaim their authentic selves as real nurses, and supports them in becoming patient advocates to improve the quality of care given to patients and families.[62] As holistic nurses embrace EBP, it will be important for them to have a sound understanding of strategies to reduce barriers when implementing EBP to nurture the holistic caring process based on evidence that can empirically support the science and art of holistic nursing.[63]

■ MAGNET RECOGNITION AND EVIDENCE-BASED PRACTICE

The Magnet Recognition Program, developed in the early 1990s by the American Nurses Credentialing Center (ANCC), added impetus to the EBP movement, particularly in nursing.[64] Originally, the Magnet Program was based on

14 "Forces of Magnetism" derived from research findings characterizing hospital nursing departments that were able to attract and retain excellent nurses during a time of nursing shortage.[65] From its beginning, the Magnet Program expectations were based on the American Nurses Association (ANA) *Nursing Administration: Scope and Standards of Practice.*[65] These standards of practice have always expected that nurses will be involved in the conduct and utilization of research. The expectation for nurses in Magnet facilities to be actively generating new knowledge through the conduct of research has increased in the past decade.[64] Likewise, there is the expectation that nurses at all levels of practice will apply research-based evidence (the science) and utilize practice-based evidence as appropriate. Practice-based evidence is defined in the Magnet Program as interventions that have been shown effective in improving outcomes but have not been scientifically validated.[66] The number of Magnet recognized facilities around the globe is approaching 400, including designated facilities in Lebanon, Singapore, and Australia.[67] The expectation that Magnet facilities will demonstrate excellence through the use of internal and external data is continuously increasing.

■ APPLYING EBP TO THE HOLISTIC CARING PROCESS STEP BY STEP

Holistic nurses may believe that barriers, such as time, search skills, knowledge of research, or minimal support in their working environment, may preclude them from incorporating EBP into their professional practice. The seven-step EBP process (**Table 35-1**), however, can become as natural a part of holistic nursing care as it is to utilize a 5-minute relaxation technique. The EBP process requires that the holistic nurse: (0) cultivate a spirit of inquiry; (1) determine a clinical issue of interest and formulate a searchable, answerable question; (2) perform an efficient, focused search to find an answer to the clinical question (akin to an abbreviated literature search); (3) assess the article using rapid critical appraisal techniques; (4) apply the valid and reliable evidence; (5) evaluate the outcomes of the implementation of evidence; and (6) disseminate the outcomes of the EBP decision or change.[4,68-71] This is not unlike the holistic caring process. To understand better the EBP process, this chapter includes a peer-reviewed publication drawn from the *Journal of Holistic Nursing* to provide a scenario[72] and an exemplar journal article appraisal[73] for applying the seven steps according to the ARCC Model.

Clinical Scenario: Music for Reducing Dyspnea and Anxiety in Patients with COPD[72]

Imagine a clinical scenario in which the holistic nurse is caring for a client who has chronic obstructive pulmonary disease (COPD).

Step 0: Cultivating a Spirit of Inquiry

Clinical judgment leads the holistic nurse to think that perhaps some of the dyspnea may be associated with anxiety or stress related to difficulty breathing and wants to know if there are nonpharmacologic holistic approaches, such as music therapy, that can be used in conjunction

---

TABLE 35-1   The EBP Process[4]
0.   Cultivate a spirit of inquiry.
1.   Ask the clinical question (PICOT).
2.   Collect the most relevant and best evidence.
3.   Critically appraise and synthesize the evidence.
4.   Integrate all evidence based on the holistic nurse's clinical expertise and the patient's preferences and values in making a practice decision or change.
5.   Evaluate the practice decision or change.
6.   Disseminate the outcomes of the EBP decision or practice change.

with oxygen and/or medication. The holistic nurse knows that the organization in which she works is a Magnet recognized facility that supports inquiry, that EBP is part of her practice repertoire, and that the EBP process can assist in finding answers for best practices in providing holistic care.

Step 1: Asking the Clinical Question

In step 1 of the EBP process—asking the searchable, answerable question—the holistic nurse is encouraged to use a standardized format when determining the clinical issue of interest.[70] PICOT is one such recommended format that consists of the population of interest (P); the intervention or issue of interest (I); the comparison intervention, if relevant (C); the outcome (O); and time frame (T), if relevant (**Table 35-2**). For this clinical scenario, the clinical question using the PICOT format is, "In patients with COPD, how does music therapy compared to anxiolytics reduce anxiety and subsequent dyspnea?"

Step 2: Searching for the Best Evidence to Answer the Question

To find the best evidence to answer the sample question, the nurse implements a thorough efficient search.[70] In this clinical scenario, two interventions are being compared, music therapy and anxiolytics. When looking at which intervention leads to the most desired outcome, a systematic review or meta-analysis of all relevant randomized controlled trials (RCTs) or practice guidelines based on RCTs, Level 1 evidence, would provide the strongest evidence to

guide practice. Levels of evidence are ranked by the type of design or methodology that answers the question with the least amount of error and provides the most reliable findings.[4] Level 2 evidence derives from at least one well-designed RCT; Level 3 from controlled trials without randomization; Level 4 from case-control or cohort studies; Level 5 from descriptive and qualitative systematic reviews; Level 6 from a single descriptive or qualitative study; and Level 7 from expert opinion or committee reports.[4] For example, epidemiological studies are best suited to questions about disease risk (Level 4 or 5), while qualitative or descriptive studies might best answer questions of personal meaning or experience (Level 5, 6, or 7).

Frequently, RCTs are not available to answer intervention questions in holistic nursing literature, and other evidence may be helpful in guiding holistic practice. The initial search begins with the key words from the PICOT question. In this scenario, the search words are *COPD*, *music therapy*, *anxiolytics*, *anxiety*, and *dyspnea*. It is important for the holistic nurse to choose databases carefully to gather all relevant evidence. In this case, the nurse searches the Cochrane Database of Systematic Reviews, Medline, CINAHL, and PsychINFO databases using keywords and controlled vocabulary headings, which provide a mechanism to gather more relevant evidence.[4,70] In the search, the nurse uses a combination of keywords and headings that are based on the questions to reduce the number of studies gathered to answer the given question.[70] While reviewing the results of the search, the holistic

TABLE 35-2	Applying the Standardized Format (PICO) for Formulating a Searchable, Answerable Question	
PICO Format	**Clinical Scenario:[72]** (McBride et al., 1999)	**Exemplar:** (Bormann et al., 2005)
Population of interest:	Patients with COPD	Ambulatory veterans
Intervention of interest:	Music therapy	Frequent mantra repetition
Comparison of interest:	Anxiolytics	None
Outcome of interest:	Reduce anxiety and subsequently reduce dyspnea	Reduce stress and anxiety and improve spiritual well-being
Time frame:	5 weeks	21 months

nurse identifies a study that examined the use of music to reduce dyspnea and anxiety in 24 home-dwelling patients with COPD.[72]

Step 3: Critical Appraisal of Evidence

The article is an intervention study, which could provide an answer to the clinical question.[72] Because it is a level 4 quasi/experimental (cohort) study, it is important for the nurse to determine the best available evidence and related implications for holistic practice; therefore, she performs a rapid critical appraisal of this study using standardized criteria.[69] The rapid critical appraisal checklist for quasi-experimental studies (**Table 35-3**) contains pointed questions that

address the validity of this design, the size and precision of the treatment effect, and how to assess the applicability of the study findings.

The holistic nurse finds that the study used a mixed-method repeated measures quasi-experimental design in which 24 participants with COPD provided information for 5 weeks about how music of their preference affected their anxiety and dyspnea.[72] The abstract indicates that two research questions were addressed: (1) "What is the effect of music therapy on dyspnea and anxiety in COPD patients?" and (2) "What is the effect of music therapy compared to anxiolytics on the perception of anxiety and dyspnea of COPD patients?" Pre- and posttest

---

TABLE 35-3   Rapid Critical Appraisal Checklist for Quasi-Experimental Studies

	Yes	No	N/A	Unknown
1. Are the study findings valid?				
Were the subjects randomly assigned to the experimental and control groups?	❑	❑	❑	❑
Were the follow-up assessments conducted long enough to fully study the effects of the intervention?	❑	❑	❑	❑
Did at least 80% of the subjects complete the study?	❑	❑	❑	❑
Was random assignment concealed from the persons who were first enrolling subjects to the study?	❑	❑	❑	❑
Were the subjects analyzed in the group to which they were randomly assigned?	❑	❑	❑	❑
Was the control group appropriate?	❑	❑	❑	❑
Were the subjects and providers kept blind to the study group(s)?	❑	❑	❑	❑
Were the instruments used to measure the outcomes valid and reliable?	❑	❑	❑	❑
Were the subjects in each of the groups similar on demographic and baseline clinical variables?	❑	❑	❑	❑
2. What are the results of the study and are they important?				
How large is the intervention or treatment effect, effect size, and level of significance?	❑	❑	❑	❑
How precise is the intervention or treatment (CI)?	❑	❑	❑	❑
3. Will the results help in caring for patients?				
Are the results applicable to my clients?	❑	❑	❑	❑
Were all clinically important outcomes measured?	❑	❑	❑	❑
Is the treatment feasible in my clinical setting?	❑	❑	❑	❑
▪ What are the risks and benefits of the treatment?				
▪ What are my client's/family's values and expectations for the outcome that is trying to be prevented and the treatment itself?	❑	❑	❑	❑

repeated outcome measures included the Spielberger State Trait Inventory (STAI) and a Visual Analogue Dyspnea Scale (VADS). Patients also kept a music diary in which they documented their level of dyspnea just before and immediately after listening to the music, and a qualitative questionnaire listing the effects of listening to the music. Each patient was allowed to select the music that he or she played while experiencing dyspnea.

The validity of the study is reflected in the reported information on the sample, sample selection, number of dropouts, the validity and reliability of the outcome measures, the intervention, the collection of qualitative data, the use of qualitative and quantitative data, and the followup. It is important to note that the researchers incorporated patient preference (i.e., patients selected the music that they played while experiencing dyspnea) as a variant of the intervention to make a difference in outcomes. After reading the study and further assessing markers of validity (Table 35-3), which can serve as a rapid critical appraisal in holistic nursing practice, the holistic nurse determines that this study is valid and may apply to holistic practice.

It is noted that the anxiety and dyspnea findings are statistically significant, and that both measures showed moderate effect sizes (**Table 35-4**), indicators of the amount of treatment effect. Because this study was a repeated measures design, pre- and posttest correlations were not available to calculate confidence intervals.

Hence, assumptions can be made only about the effect size parameters in this particular study, but the precision of the effect cannot be interpreted. This is not the usual case with other studies that use two or more groups, and it is important for holistic nurse researchers to include this information in study reports so that readers can determine both statistical and clinical significance. The reported analysis of participants' perceptions of levels of dyspnea before and after listening to the music was also insufficient to determine clinical meaningfulness of the results because no pre- and posttest mean anxiety scores and standard deviations were reported. This further underscores the importance for researchers to include sufficient data to determine both statistical and clinical significance.

Based on the evaluation of the qualitative data, it is apparent that clients benefited from music therapy (**Table 35-5**). Participant comments suggest that the music assisted them in pacing their breathing, thereby reducing their demand for oxygen, which allowed them to accomplish their goals. It is noted that their comments do not indicate that they felt anxious, or that music decreased their anxiety, if it existed. From these data, the expected relationship between anxiety and dyspnea is not apparent. Based on the participant information, it is not known whether music therapy reduced anxiety and, subsequently, dyspnea. Participants reported a perceived reduction in oxygen

TABLE 35-4   Effect Sizes for Anxiety and Dyspnea

Indicator(s)	Mean ± SD	Effect Size
Spielberger State Trait Inventory (STAI)		
Pretest	7.75 ± 3.03	0.511
Posttest	6.38 ± 2.32*	
Visual Analogue Dyspnea Scale (VADS)		
Pretest	2.83 ± 2.01	0.501
Posttest	1.88 ± 1.87**	

*$P < .05$.
**$P < .01$.
Source: Adapted from S. McBride et al., "The Therapeutic Use of Music for Dyspnea and Anxiety in Patients with COPD Who Live at Home," *Journal of Holistic Nursing* 17 (1999): 229–250.

TABLE 35-5 Qualitative Statements and Music Diary Documentation	
Music Effectiveness Questionnaire Comments	**Music Diary**
"Decreased my concentration on breathing"	Music helped to make daily household chores achievable.
"Dulled the sound of oxygen"	Music helped to accomplish outdoor activities, making the work less strenuous.
"Gave me time to gain control"	Music helped to adapt to a slower pace and more efficient use of oxygen during outdoor activities.

Source: Adapted from S. McBride et al., "The Therapeutic Use of Music for Dyspnea and Anxiety in Patients with COPD Who Live at Home," *Journal of Holistic Nursing* 17 (1999): 229–250.

demand after listening to their chosen music therapy that allowed them a better quality of life. This leaves the second research question unanswered ("What is the effect of music therapy compared to anxiolytics on the perception of anxiety and dyspnea of COPD patients?"), which brings into question the applicability of this study's findings to practice.

Step 4: Implementing the Evidence into Holistic Nursing Care

Step 4 of the EBP process highlights the integration of all the evidence obtained from the critical appraisal combined with the holistic nurse's clinical expertise and patient preferences and values to make a practice decision or change. The holistic nurse knows that some of the dyspnea may be associated with anxiety or stress related to difficulty breathing and wants to determine whether there are nonpharmacologic holistic approaches, such as music therapy, that can be used in conjunction with oxygen and/or medication. A reduction in anxiety is desirable, whether or not it leads to a reduction in dyspnea. The holistic nurse recognizes that there are numerous approaches to reduce anxiety, such as massage, relaxation training, and Healing Touch. Regardless of the modality, each approach would require empirical support to determine effectiveness in reducing anxiety-associated dyspnea, as well as the client's perception of the intervention. The holistic nurse is aware that several of these holistic interventions require advanced education and/or certification, and the holistic

nurse may or may not have the required training. However, the music therapy used in the study was driven by patient preference,[2] is readily available, and does not require certification; therefore, it has great potential as an intervention to reduce dyspnea in patients with COPD.

The qualitative information provided by the participants also lends insight into their lived experiences with dyspnea and reinforces the idea that holistic nurses need to be considerate regarding clients' music preferences and the potential effects on dyspnea, such as assisting patients to achieve their goals. The quantitative findings were both statistically and clinically significant. Hence, moving from critical appraisal of the evidence to action, the holistic nurse decides to incorporate music therapy into care of patients with COPD, emphasizing the music is to be selected by the clients.

Step 5: Evaluating the Decision or Practice Change

The holistic nurse is cognizant of the fact that incorporating interventions, such as music therapy, into clinical practice leads to step 5 of the EBP process, to evaluate the practice change or decision.[50] Evaluation requires valid and reliable measurement of outcomes—the same outcomes that were designated in the PICOT question. After incorporating patient-preferred music therapy into the clinical plan for patients with COPD, the holistic nurse continues to collect information on anxiety, perceived dyspnea, oxygen demand, and perceived quality of life.

These outcome indicators will assist in evaluating the success of, or need for changes in, the patient-preferred music therapy program. The holistic nurse also recognizes that music therapy may have actions other than decreasing anxiety and subsequently reducing oxygen demand. Perhaps client-preferred musical selections influence respiratory muscle relaxation separate from anxiety, allowing clients to pace their goal setting, thereby enhancing their quality of life. As these practice-based data provide information about how well music therapy influences dyspnea and anxiety in patients with COPD, the holistic nurse is continually looking for empirical evidence to further establish the relationships among music therapy, oxygen demand, quality of life, and other clinical outcome indicators.

Step 6: Disseminating the Outcomes of the EBP Change

The holistic nurse knows that implementing a practice change or decision is not the sum total of the EBP process. A critical component of the EBP process for the nurse both professionally and personally is that of disseminating the change to colleagues, the organization, and peers nationally and, if culturally relevant, internationally. Venues that the holistic nurse can utilize for disseminating the outcomes of the practice change, whether positive or negative, include organizational in-services, paper and poster presentations at the American Holistic Nurses Association annual conference, publishing an article on the change in the *Journal of Holistic Nursing*, and presenting the practice change at the annual Honor Society of Nursing, Sigma Theta Tau International Nursing Research Conference.

■ EBP AND HOLISTIC NURSING PRACTICE, EDUCATION, AND SCHOLARSHIP

On average, it takes 17 years to translate research findings into clinical practice.[74] Based on this report, leading professional and healthcare organizations and policymakers have placed a major emphasis on accelerating EBP in the educational, practice, and research settings. In the landmark document *Crossing the Quality Chasm*, the Institute of Medicine (IOM) emphasizes that one of the

10 "rules for health care" is evidence-based decision making.[75] Additionally, the five core competencies for educational programs for healthcare professionals deemed essential by the IOM's Health Professions Educational Summit include employing EBP.[76] EBP must be the foundation of practice, education, and research. Holistic nursing requires valid evidence-based practice that is conducted to assist clinicians at the point of care to have the latest and best information upon which to base their care.[10,50]

■ GLOBAL HEALTH, HOLISTIC CULTURE CARE, AND EBP

The teaching, implementation, and application of EBP are shared concerns globally, according to the Sigma Theta Tau International (STTI) *Resource Paper on Global Health and Nursing Research Priorities*.[77] In addition to EBP, the global development initiative outlines common priorities among regions, such as health promotion, health policy, advocacy, patient-centered care, palliative care, genetic testing, and professional issues, that are relevant to transcultural and international care from a holistic nursing perspective. Each of these priorities would benefit from an understanding and application of EBP principles and practices. To guide all nurses toward understanding the implications and applications of EBP internationally, the peer-reviewed journal *Worldviews on Evidence-Based Nursing: Linking Evidence to Action* is an information resource for nurses worldwide that is published on a quarterly basis under the auspices of STTI. The Joanna Briggs Institute (JBI) is an international not-for-profit research and development organization based within the Faculty of Health Sciences at the University of Adelaide, South Australia.[78] The institute collaborates internationally with more than 60 entities around the world, including in Singapore, Canada, China, and the United States. The institute and its collaborating entities promote and support the synthesis, transfer, and utilization of evidence through identifying feasible, appropriate, meaningful, and effective healthcare practices to assist in the improvement of healthcare outcomes globally. The EBP process has been disseminated throughout the

Americas via a technical agreement between the Pan American Health Organization (PAHO) and the Arizona State University College of Nursing and Health Innovation. Pre-colloquiums and paper and poster presentations held in such PAHO-determined venues as Mexico, Central and South America, and Spain highlight the emphasis placed on the role of EBP in the global arena and support best practices for holistically based culture care.[59,73] Three series of Clinical Scholar Program workshops were conducted through Boromarajonani College of Nursing Nakhon Lampang (BCNLP), Thailand, under the auspices of a Fulbright grant. The grant resulted in 40 ongoing evidence-based clinical practice projects in hospitals in northern Thailand. Components of the model form the basis for evidence-based applications in Bogota, Colombia, and Santiago, Chile. As the ARCC, Clinical Scholar, PARIHS, and other models are adapted as frameworks for EBP and clinical research around the globe, more empirical research regarding clinician and patient outcomes as well as organizational changes are needed.

■ EBP AND COMPARATIVE EFFECTIVENESS RESEARCH

It is important for holistic nurses to know the advances in moving evidence forward to inform national and global health policy and to support informed consumer choices.[79-80] In these matters, EBP and comparative effectiveness research (CER) are not mutually exclusive. Initiated as a focal activity by the National Institutes of Health and the Institute of Medicine in 2009,[81-82] the purpose of CER is to improve health outcomes by developing and disseminating evidence-based information to patients, clinicians, and other decision makers about which interventions are most effective for which patients under specific circumstances at individual and population levels.[80]

Characteristics of CER studies include, but are not limited to: (1) directly informing clinical or health policy decisions, (2) comparing at least two alternatives, each with the potential to be best practices, (3) results are generated at population and subgroup levels, (4) outcome measures are important to patients, (5) meth-

ods and data sources (qualitative and/or quantitative) are appropriate for the decision of interest, and (6) are conducted in real-world settings. Interventions may include medications, procedures, medical and assistive devices and technologies, diagnostic testing, holistic practices, behavioral change, and delivery system strategies. The implementation of CER necessitates the development, expansion, and use of a variety of data sources and methods to assess comparative effectiveness and disseminate the results. Sample topics relevant to holistic nursing might include a comparison of the effectiveness of primary prevention methods, such as tai chi exercise and balance training versus clinical treatments in preventing falls in older adults with varying degrees of risk. At the organizational level, a sample topic might compare the effectiveness of comprehensive care coordination programs, such as the medical home, and usual care in managing children and adults with severe chronic disease, especially in populations with known health disparities. A focus of CER is to implement practice- and cost-effective interventions to improve health outcomes in large patient populations.

■ CONCLUSION

Holistic nursing scholarship grounded in empiricism is necessary to determine the "(1) basic mechanisms of nursing actions and integrative therapies; (2) clinical safety, efficacy, and treatment outcomes of holistic modalities; and (3) the interactive nature of body-mind-spirit."[1] EBP supports a culture of best practices across multiple settings within a holistic nursing framework to improve health care, client outcomes, and systems. It is essential for holistic nursing to adopt EBP as a culture in education, practice, and research for the ultimate purposes of improving the quality of health care and patient outcomes, as well as empowering holistic nurses to implement best practices, which result in a higher level of professional care and personal satisfaction. Future directions for EBP in holistic nursing practice include the understanding and application of EBP into CER for health policy changes at the national and global levels.

Directions for
FUTURE RESEARCH

1. Using the EBP process, evaluate holistic, complementary, alternative, integrative, and folk therapies that may promote healthy lifestyles based on client preferences in specific client populations.

2. Using the EBP process, synthesize evidence from literature searches on such topics as body-mind-spirit healing modalities to determine statistically significant and clinically meaningful best practices.

3. Implement quantitative and/or qualitative studies of nurse retention, satisfaction, creativity, and well-being in clinical settings that have and have not implemented system-wide EBP.

4. Implement quantitative and/or qualitative studies of patient and family satisfaction, well-being, and outcomes in clinical settings that have and have not implemented system-wide EBP.

5. Examine the quality of health care, healthcare delivery, and health outcomes from a global perspective as EBP becomes utilized by nurses around the globe as the gold standard for best practices.

6. Develop a working knowledge of the ways in which EBP and CER work in concert to make policy changes at the national and global levels taking into consideration needs and preferences of diverse populations.

Nurse Healer
REFLECTIONS

After reading this chapter, the nurse healer will be able to answer or to begin a process of answering the following questions:

- What is my role in establishing an evidence-based holistic nursing practice?
- How do I feel about the importance of EBP in advancing holistic nursing practice?
- What are my personal and clinical barriers to adopting EBP, and what can I do to reduce these barriers?

- What are my personal and clinical strengths that would support EBP, and what can I do to enhance these strengths?
- What models are suited to my private or clinical practice and how can I facilitate the interweaving of a model to improve holistic clinical care?
- How can I become more involved in EBP?
- How can I become more involved in CER to effect policy change?

■ ACKNOWLEDGMENT

We wish to gratefully acknowledge Kimberly Sidora-Arcoleo, PhD, MPH, Associate Professor, Director, Graduate Programs for Clinical Research Management and Translational Science and Associate Director, Masters in Public Health Program, Arizona State University College of Nursing and Health Innovation for her comments on CER and EBP.

> *For a full suite of assignments and additional learning activities, use the access code located in the front of your book to visit this exclusive website: http://go.jblearning.com/dossey. If you do not have an access code, you can obtain one at the site.*

NOTES

1. American Holistic Nurses Association (AHNA), "What Is Holistic Nursing?" http://www.ahna.org/AboutUs/WhatisHolisticNursing/tabid/1165/Default.aspx.

2. B. Melnyk and E. Fineout-Overholt, "Consumer Preferences and Values as an Integral Key to Evidence-Based Practice," *Nursing Administration Quarterly* 30 (2006): 123–127.

3. E. Fineout-Overholt et al., "Transforming Healthcare from the Inside Out: Advancing Evidence-Based Practice in the 21st Century," *Journal of Professional Nursing* 21 (2005): 335–344.

4. B. Melnyk and E. Fineout-Overholt, *Evidence-Based Practice in Nursing and Healthcare: A Guide to Best Practice* (Philadelphia, PA: Lippincott Williams & Wilkins, 2011).

5. S. Doherty, "History of Evidence-Based Medicine. Oranges, Chloride of Lime and Leeches: Barriers to Teaching Old Dogs New Tricks," *Emergency Medicine Australasia* 17 (2005): 314–321.

6. B. M. Dossey, *Florence Nightingale: Mystic, Visionary, Healer*, Commemorative ed. (Philadelphia, PA: V. A. Davis Company, 2010).

7. H. Stringer, "The Evolution of Evidence-Based Practice," *Nursing Spectrum & NurseWeek, Commemorating Nightingale's Legacy*, 2010, 70–72.

8. F. Nightingale, *Notes on Nursing: What It Is, and What It Is Not* (Mineola, NY: Dover Publications, 1860/1969): 125.

9. S. G. Funk et al., "Barriers and Facilitators of Research Utilization," *Nursing Clinics of North America* 30 (1995): 395–407.

10. J. C. Krueger, "Utilization of Nursing Research. The Planning Process," *Journal of Nursing Administration* 8 (1978): 6–9.

11. J. A. Horsley et al., *Using Research to Improve Nursing Practice: A Guide* (Orlando, FL: Green & Stratton, 1983).

12. C. B. Stetler and G. Marram, "Evaluating Research Findings for Applicability to Practice," *Nursing Outlook* 24 (1976): 559–563.

13. B. S. Heater et al., "Nursing Intervention and Patient Outcomes: A Meta-analysis of Studies," *Nursing Research* 37 (1988): 303–307.

14. S. Ketefian, "Application of Selected Nursing Research Findings into Nursing Practice: A Pilot Study," *Nursing Research* 24 (1975): 89–92.

15. K. T. Kirchhoff, "Using Research in Clinical Practice: Should Staff Nurses Be Expected to Use Research?" *Western Journal of Nursing Research* 5 (1983): 245–247.

16. C. A. Lindeman, "Priorities in Clinical Nursing Research," *Nursing Outlook* 23 (1975): 693–698.

17. J. R. Miller and S. R. Messenger, "Obstacles to Applying Nursing Research Findings," *American Journal of Nursing* 78 (1978): 632–634.

18. S. G. Funk et al., "Application and Evaluation of the Dissemination Model," *Western Journal of Nursing Research* 11 (1989): 486–491.

19. J. Rycroft-Malone et al., "An Exploration of the Factors That Influence the Implementation of Evidence into Practice," *Journal of Clinical Nursing* 13 (2004): 913–924.

20. L. R. Cronenwett, "Research Reflections: Research Utilization in a Practice Setting," *Journal of Nursing Administration* 17 (1987): 9–10.

21. C. J. Goode and G. M. Bulechek, "Research Utilization: An Organizational Process That Enhances Quality of Care," *Journal of Nursing Care Quality* (1992): 27–35.

22. C. J. Goode, Using Research in Clinical Nursing Practice (videotape, Ida Grove, IA: Horn Video Productions, 1987).

23. C. J. Goode and J. Cipperley, *Research Utilization: A Process of Organizational Change* (videotape, Ida Grove, IA: Horn Video Productions, 1989).

24. C. J. Goode, *Research Utilization: A Study Guide* (videotape, Ida Grove, IA: Horn Video Productions, 1991).

25. C. J. Goode and J. Cipperley, *Reading and Critiquing a Research Report* (videotape, Ida Grove, IA: Horn Video Productions, 1991).

26. M. G. Titler et al., "Infusing Research into Practice to Promote Quality Care," *Nursing Research* 43 (1994): 307–313.

27. D. N. Rutledge and N. E. Donaldson, "Building Organizational Capacity to Engage in Research Utilization," *Journal of Nursing Administration* 25 (1995): 12–16.

28. D. L. Sackett et al., *Evidence-Based Medicine: How to Practice and Teach EBM* (New York, NY: Churchill Livingstone, 2000).

29. C. J. Goode and F. Piedalue, "Evidence-Based Clinical Practice," *Journal of Nursing Administration* 29 (1999): 5–21.

30. A. DiCenso et al., *Evidence-Based Nursing. A Guide to Clinical Practice* (St. Louis, MO: Mosby, 2005).

31. C. B. Stetler, "Updating the Stetler Model of Research Utilization to Facilitate Evidence-Based Practice," *Nursing Outlook* 49 (2001): 272–278.

32. A. A. Schultz et al., "Advancing Evidence into Practice: Clinical Scholars at the Bedside [Electronic version]," *Excellence in Nursing Knowledge* (February 2005).

33. M. G. Titler, "Use of Research in Practice," in *Nursing Research: Methods, Critical Appraisal and Utilization*, ed. G. LoBiondo and J. Haber (St. Louis, MO: Mosby, 2002).

34. J. Rycroft-Malone, "Promoting Action on Research Implementation in Health Services (PARIHS)," in *Models and Frameworks for Implementing Evidence-Based Practice: Linking Evidence to Action*, ed. J. Rycroft-Malone and T. Bucknall (Oxford, England: Wiley Blackwell/STTI, 2010).

35. R. B. Haynes et al., "Clinical Expertise in the Era of Evidence-Based Medicine and Patient Choice," *ACP Journal Club* 136 (2002): A11–A14.

36. Clinical Scholarship Task Force, *Sigma Theta Tau International Clinical Scholarship White Paper* (1999). http://www.nursingsociety.org/aboutus/Position Papers/Documents/clinical_scholarship_paper.pdf

37. T. D. Strout et al., "Development and Implementation of an Inductive Model for Evidence-Based Practice: A Grassroots Approach for Building Evidence-Based Practice Capacity in Staff Nurses," *Nursing Clinics of North America* 44 (2009): 93–102.

38. B. B. Brewer et al., "A Collaborative Approach to Building the Capacity for Research and Evidence-Based Practice in Community Hospitals," *Nursing Clinics of North America* 44 (2009): 11–25.

39. C. Honess et al., "The Clinical Scholar Model: Evidence Based Practice at the Bedside," *Nursing Clinics of North America* 44 (2009): 117–130.

40. C. Mulvenon and M. K. Brewer, "From the Bedside to the Boardroom: Resuscitating Nursing Research," *Nursing Clinics of North America* 44 (2009): 145–152.

41. A. E. Sossong et al., "Renewing the Spirit of Nursing by Embracing Evidence-Based Practice," *Nursing Clinics of North America* 44 (2009): 33–42.

42. S. M. Weeks et al., "Development of an Evidence-Based Practice and Research Collaborative Among Urban Hospitals," *Nursing Clinics of North America* 44 (2009): 7–31.

43. S. Dopson and L. Fitzgerald, *Knowledge into Action* (Oxford, England: Oxford University Press, 2005).

44. J. Gabbay et al., "A Case Study of Knowledge Management in Multi-agency Consumer-Informed 'Communities of Practice': Implications for Evidence-Based Policy Development in Health and Social Services," *Health* 7 (2003): 283–310.

45. T. Greenhalgh et al., "Diffusion of Innovations in Service Organizations: Systematic Review and Recommendations," *Milbank Quarterly* 82 (2004): 584–629.

46. J. Rycroft-Malone, "Evidence-Informed Practice: From Individual to Context," *Journal of Nursing Management* 16 (2008): 404–408.

47. C. B. Stetler et al., "Institutionalizing Evidence-Based Practice: An Organization Case Study Using a Model of Strategic Change," *Implementation Science* 4 (2009): 78.

48. J. Rycroft-Malone, "The Politics of Evidence-Based Practice: Legacies and Current Challenges," *Journal of Research in Nursing* 11 (2006): 95–108.

49. C. Stetler et al., "Improving Quality of Care Through Routine, Successful Implementation of Evidence-Based Practice at the Bedside: An Organization Case Study Using the Pettigrew and Whipp Model of Strategic Change," *Implementation Science* 2 (2007): 3. doi:10.1186/1748-5908-2-3

50. B. Melnyk and E. Fineout-Overholt, "Putting Research into Practice," *Reflections on Nursing Leadership* 28 (2002): 22–25.

51. B. Melnyk et al., "Outcomes and Implementation Strategies from the First U.S. Evidence-Based Leadership Summit," *Worldviews on Evidence-Based Nursing* 2 (2005): 113–121.

52. B. Melnyk et al., "Nurses' Perceived Knowledge, Beliefs, Skills, and Needs Regarding Evidence-Based Practice: Implications for Accelerating the Paradigm Shift," *Worldviews on Evidence-Based Nursing* 1 (2004): 185–193.

53. B. M. Melnyk et al., "Correlates Among Cognitive Beliefs, EBP Implementation, Organizational Culture, Cohesion and Job Satisfaction in Evidence-Based Practice Mentors from a Community Hospital System," *Nursing Outlook* 58 (2010): 301–308.

54. B. Melnyk, "Strategies for Overcoming Barriers in Implementing Evidence-Based Practice," *Pediatric Nursing* 28 (2002): 159–161.

55. B. Melnyk et al., "Sparking a Change to Evidence-Based Practice in Health Care Organizations," *Worldviews on Evidence-Based Nursing* 1 (2004): 83–84.

56. B. Melnyk, "The Latest Evidence on Factors Impacting Nurse Retention and Job Satisfaction," *Worldviews on Evidence-Based Nursing* 3 (2006): 201–204.

57. G. R. Wallen, et al., "Implementing Evidence-Based Practice: Effectiveness of a Structured Multifaceted Mentorship Programme," *Journal of Advanced Nursing* 66 (2010): 2761–2771.

58. D. S. Pravikoff et al., "American Academy of Nursing Publication Advisory Committee Evidence-Based Practice Readiness Study Supported by Academy Nursing Informatics Expert Panel," *Nursing Outlook* 53 (2005): 49–50.

59. C. M. Baldwin et al., *Individual and Institutional Barriers to Implementing EBP in Clinical Practice: A Comparison of Pan American and U.S. Nurses* (paper presented at the 10th Annual National/International EBP Conference, Phoenix, AZ, February 20, 2009).

60. R. Maljanian et al., "Evidence-Based Nursing Practice, Part 2: Building Skills Through Research Roundtables," *Journal of Nursing Administration* 32 (2002): 85–90.

61. A. Retsas, "Barriers to Using Research Evidence in Nursing Practice," *Journal of Advanced Nursing* 31 (2000): 599–606.

62. T. Strout, "Curiosity and Reflective Thinking: Renewal of the Spirit," *Online Journal of Excellence in Nursing Knowledge* 2 (2005): 39. http://www.nursingknowledge.org.

63. B. Melnyk, "Calling All Educators to Teach and Model Evidence-Based Practice in Academic Settings," *Worldviews on Evidence-Based Nursing* 3 (2006): 93–94.

64. B. S. Reigle et al., "Evidence-Based Practice and the Road to Magnet Status," *Journal of Nursing Administration* 38 (2008): 97–102.

65. M. L. McClure et al., *Magnet Hospitals: Attraction and Retention of Professional Nurses* (Washington, DC: American Nurses Association, 1983).

66. American Nurses Credentialing Center, *Magnet Recognition Program, Application Manual* (Silver Springs, MD: ANCC, 2008).

67. American Nurses Credentialing Center, Magnet Program. http://www.nursecredentialing.org/Magnet.aspx.

68. C. M. Baldwin and E. Fineout-Overholt, "Evidence-Based Practice as Holistic Nursing Research," *Beginnings* 25 (2005): 16.

69. B. Melnyk, "Finding and Appraising Systematic Reviews of Clinical Interventions: Critical Skills for Evidence-Based Practice," *Pediatric Nursing* 29 (2003): 147–149.

70. B. Melnyk and E. Fineout-Overholt, "Key Steps in Implementing Evidence-Based Practice: Asking Compelling, Searchable Questions and Searching for the Best Evidence," *Pediatric Nursing* 28 (2002): 161–162, 266.

71. B. Melnyk and E. Fineout-Overholt, "Rapid Critical Appraisal of Randomized Controlled Trials (RCTs): An Essential Skill for Evidence-Based Practice (EBP)," *Pediatric Nursing* 31 (2005): 50–52.

72. S. McBride et al., "The Therapeutic Use of Music for Dyspnea and Anxiety in Patients with COPD Who Live at Home," *Journal of Holistic Nursing* 17 (1999): 229–250.

73. C. M. Baldwin et al., "Práctica Basada en la Evidencia (PBE): Una Introducción a la Revisión de la Evidencia para Mejorar el Resultado en los Pacientes (Evidence-Based Practice (EBP): An Introduction to Reviewing the Evidence to Improve Patient Outcomes) [Abstract]," in *Proceedings of the 10th Coloquio Panamericano de Investigacion en Enfermeria* (Buenos Aires, Argentina: Office of Pan American Health Organization, 2006): 41.

74. E. A. Balas and S. A. Boren, "Managing Clinical Knowledge for Healthcare Improvements," in *IMIA Yearbook of Medical Informatics*, ed. V. Schattauer (Chicago, IL: American Health Information, 2000): 65–70.

75. Committee on Quality of Health Care in America, Institute of Medicine, *Crossing the Quality Chasm: A New Health System for the 21st Century* (Washington, DC: National Academy Press, 2001).

76. A. Greiner and E. Knebel, eds., *Health Professions Education: A Bridge to Quality* (Washington, DC: National Academic Press, 2003).

77. Sigma Theta Tau International (STTI) Honor Society in Nursing. *Global Development*. http://www.nursingsociety.org/aboutus/PositionPapers/Documents/policy_development.doc

78. Joanna Briggs Institute. http://www.joannabriggs.edu.au/.

79. J. G. Bauer and F. Chiappelli, "Transforming Scientific Evidence into Better Consumer Choices," *Bioinformation* 7 (2011): 297–299.

80. K. Chalkidou et al., "Comparative Effectiveness Research and Evidence-Based Health Policy: Experience from Four Countries," *Milbank Quarterly* 87 (2009): 339–367.

81. J. K. Iglehart, "Prioritizing Comparative Effectiveness Research. IOM Recommendations," *New England Journal of Medicine* 361 (2009): 325–238.

82. E. Nabel, *Role of the NIH in Comparative Effectiveness Research* (presentation at the National CER Summit, Washington, DC, 2009). http://www.ehcca.com/presentations/compeffective1/nabel_1.pdf.

■ EBP RESOURCES

Annual national and international EBP conferences and workshops offer intensive sessions on EBP. Some of these venues include STTI's yearly international EBP/research congress, annual EBP conferences held by the Academic Center for Evidence-Based Practice (ACE) at the University of Texas Health Sciences Center's San Antonio School of Nursing, and the University of Iowa Hospitals and Clinics. Following is a selection of national and international EBP, clinical scholar, and Magnet online resources:

- Academic Center for Evidence-Based Practice, University of Texas: http://www.acestar.uthscsa.edu/.
- Agency for Healthcare Research and Quality Evidence-based Practice Centers: http://www.ahrq.gov/clinic/epc/.
- The Cochrane Collaboration: http://www.cochrane.org/.
- Joanna Briggs Institute: http://www.joannabriggs.edu.au/.
- Magnet Program: http://www.nursecredentialing.org/Magnet.aspx.
- Maine Medical Center: http://www.mmc.org/nursing_body.cfm?id=4658.
- NIH Library Evidence Based Practice Resources: http://nihlibrary.ors.nih.gov/jw/ebp.html.
- PARIHS Centre Website: http://www.parihs.org/.
- Sigma Theta Tau International Evidence-based Nursing Position Statement: http://www.nursingsociety.org/aboutus/PositionPapers/Pages/EBN_positionpaper.aspx
- Student Nurse Connections Evidence-Based Practice: http://studentnurseconnections.com/Links29.html.

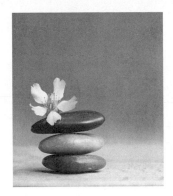

Chapter 36

Teaching Future Holistic Nurses: Integration of Holistic and Quality Safety Education for Nurses (QSEN) Concepts

Cynthia C. Barrere

Nurse Healer

OBJECTIVES

Theoretical

- Describe how holistic concepts and quality safety education for nurses (QSEN) competencies complement each other.
- Design effective pedagogical teaching/learning methodologies that emphasize holistic concepts and QSEN competencies throughout an undergraduate nursing curriculum.

Clinical

- Explore ways to initiate successful teaching strategies that integrate the teaching of holistic concepts and quality safety requirements into the class, skills laboratory, simulation laboratory, and clinical learning environments as well as integrate holism and quality safety into nonclinical courses.

Personal

- Determine how holistic and quality safety clinical practice support an instructor's ability to teach these important concepts to nursing students.
- Explore ways in which an instructor is a role model in the practice and teaching of caring, healing, and quality safety.
- Strengthen commitment to teaching holistic concepts and quality safety to nursing students.

DEFINITIONS

Holistic nursing learning activities: Learning activities in which students are encouraged to reflect on ways to interface nontraditional healing therapies with traditional medical therapies to help patients heal in mind, body, and spirit.

Quality safety education for nurses (QSEN): A project in which the overall goal is to meet the challenge of preparing future nurses who will have the knowledge, skills, and attitudes (KSAs) necessary to continuously improve the quality and safety of the healthcare systems within which they work.[1]

▪ INTRODUCTION

A plethora of studies and evidence-based practice initiatives supports the consideration of various holistic approaches in nursing practice.[2-11] Patient satisfaction surveys conducted to evaluate the quality of care received indicate caring interventions, such as active listening and compassion by healthcare providers, make a positive difference in the healing process of patients[12,13] whereas noninclusion of the patient and family in the care process can lead to devastating outcomes.[14] In addition, the provision of complementary and alternative modalities (CAM) in many healthcare institutions, and the expanding consumer demand for such alternative modalities, continues to proliferate.[15] The realization of the importance of holistic nursing as essential to effective nursing practice is increasing as demonstrated by the recognition of holistic nursing as a specialty by the American Nurses Association (ANA)[16] and the merging of the American Holistic Nurses Association and ANA scope and standards of practice (see Chapter 2). Despite this evidence supporting the need for nurses to provide high-quality, whole-person caring, room for improvement exists.[17]

Rather than waiting until after graduation to teach holistic and quality concepts, schools of nursing are encouraged to integrate this content in undergraduate curricula. The revised 2008 *Essentials of Baccalaureate Education for Professional Nursing Practice* advocates the preparation of the baccalaureate graduate to practice from a holistic caring framework.[18] It recognizes the importance of baccalaureate nursing curricula content including reflective practice, self-care engagement, CAM, patient teaching and health promotion, spirituality, and caring, healing interventions. Similarly, a National Nursing Advisory Board and the American Association of Colleges of Nursing, funded by the Robert Wood Johnson Foundation, developed six quality and safety education for nurses competencies: patient-focused care, teamwork–collaboration, informatics, safety, quality improvement, and evidence-based practice.[19,20] These competencies provide a framework to enhance the amount of quality and safety content addressed in undergraduate nursing programs. The Institute of Medicine (IOM) in its most recent 2010 report echoes the sentiments regarding new graduate nurse preparation.[17]

Holistic caring and QSEN competencies are closely aligned and complement one another in emphasizing compassionate and respectful care in a safe, healing environment. Students need to learn holistic nursing and quality safety as fundamental to practice. The incorporation of holistic and QSEN concepts in an undergraduate curriculum is not adding new content but refers to teaching content in different ways so as to enable students to enhance their clinical reasoning skills creatively to facilitate patient healing and quality safety. This chapter provides nursing faculty with selected teaching/learning strategies that can be used to integrate holistic healing and QSEN concepts into an undergraduate nursing curriculum. Section headings of the chapter reflect the six QSEN competencies. Section content offers nursing faculty examples of effective approaches to teaching/learning holistic and quality safety activities currently incorporated into a class, simulation lab, or clinical component of selected undergraduate nursing courses at Quinnipiac University (QU).

■ PATIENT-FOCUSED CARE

Literature documents a growing interest in patient-focused care.[21-26] QSEN highlights patient-focused care as one of the essential competencies for nursing and defines it as the "recognition of the patient or designee as the source of control and full partner in providing compassionate and coordinated care based on respect for a patient's preferences, values, and needs."[27] Holistic nursing subscribes to a similar definition: "Patient-focused and family focused care actively involves patients and family members or significant others, as the patient desires, in the care process. This type of care provides services based on patient's needs."[28] These definitions complement one another by demonstrating the blending of Eastern and Western schools of thought and emphasizing the importance of patient empowerment to facilitate healing.

Nursing students at QU begin their initial junior clinical rotation at a long-term care or rehabilitation facility. The first year these sites were used for clinicals, the course coordinator and clinical faculty noted student boredom after 3 weeks as evidenced by negative comments regarding their experiences. Upon asking the students to describe their experiences, a number of them replied working with "old people" was not fun or rewarding. The course coordinator was dismayed by their negativity and decided to design a reflective teaching/learning strategy that would assist students in realizing the individualism, fascination, and wisdom of older adults. Before reviewing the assignment, she entered the classroom and read the following poem to the students:

Sunshine Acres Living Center
The first thing you see up ahead is Mr.
Polanski, wedged in the
Arched doorway, like he means absolutely
To stay there, he who shouldn't
Be here in the first place, put in here
by mistake, courtesy of that grandson
who thinks himself a hotshot, and too busy
raking in the dough to find time for an old
man. If Polanski had anyplace
to go, he'd be out
instantly, if he had any
money. Which he doesn't, but he does have
a sharp eye, and intends to stay in that
doorway, not missing
a thing, and waiting
for trouble. Which of course
will come. And could be
you—you're handy, you look
likely, you have
the authority. And
you're new here, another young
whippersnapper, doesn't know
ass from elbow, but has been given
the keys. Well he's
ready, Polanski. Mr. Polanski, good
morning—*you say it in Polish,*
which you learned a little of
when you were little, and your grandmother
taught you a little song about lambs, frisking
in a pen, and you danced a silly little dance
with your grandmother, while the two of you
sang. So you sing it
for him, here in the dim, institutional
light of the hallway, light which even you
find insupportable, because even those who just
work here, and can leave when their
shift ends, deserve light to
see by, and because it reminds you
of the light in the hallway
outside the room
where, when your grandmother
died, you were three thousand miles
away. So that you're singing the little song
and remembering the silly little dance
to console yourself, and to pay your grandmother
tribute, and to try to charm Polanski,
which you do: you sing, and Mr. Polanski,

he who had set himself against the doorjamb
to resist you, he who had made of himself
a fist, Mr. Polanski,
contentious, often
combative and always
and finally
inconsolable
hears that you know
the song. And he steps out
from the battlement
of the doorway, and begins to
shuffle
and sing along.[29]

As the poem was read, not a sound could be heard. A few of the students began to cry as the concepts of authentic presence, patient-focused care, and the nurse as an instrument of healing were brought to life by the interventions used by the nurse in the poem. After reading the poem, the course coordinator assigned the students a writing activity titled "Healing Others" in which each student needed to describe one example of how he or she was an instrument of healing with a patient at the clinical site during the next few weeks. This reflective assignment taught the students the power of caring as they learned how small acts of kindness led to patient smiles and nurse–patient connections that were equally as important and, at times, more healing than medications or treatments. One student beautifully illustrated her reflections in the following poem she wrote:

Healing Others
Ginny was missing home you could see it on
   her face,
She missed all of her friends and wanted out of
   this place.

A horrible hip fracture landed her in this
   rehab center,
The injury needed to take time to heal and
   get stronger.

Disappointment she felt because she was not able
   to leave,
For there is no right way for a person to grieve.

There were so many rules she had to learn to obey,
It seemed to put Ginny in dismay.

*No crossing your legs, you must always wear
   your brace,
Were just a few of the rules in her case.*

*All of these factors seemed to make her frustrated
   and miserable,
Just adding on to her existing feeling of dismal.*

*I knew there had to be a way to relieve her stress,
And it was not going to be through a game of chess.*

*Ginny needed some relaxation and amour,
So I kindly offer her a manicure.*

*Her face lit up, I could see the stress fading away,
With such a simple gesture I was able to make
   her day.*

*I cut her nails, painted them purple too,
But it was the hand massage that made her renew.*

*Ginny's spirit was lifted—her mind was at ease
She asked to take me home, she said
   "pretty please."*

*Then she laughed at her comment and along
   came a smile,
Something many have not seen in a while.*

*All it took was some loving tender care,
To bring Ginny out of her state of despair.*[30]

In this course, students learn the meaning of holistic patient-centered care and have many opportunities to practice the art of nursing as an instrument of healing. A student nurse who has learned how to use the whole self as an instrument of healing will likely be more sensitive to cues from others and make a profound healing difference in someone's life in a very short time using his or her expanded repertoire of healing interventions.

■ INFORMATICS

Nursing informatics is a more recently recognized competency for nursing that supports safe, patient-centered care.[31,32] It is a competency in which students lack knowledge—including how to evaluate the quality of health-related websites and search electronic scientific databases.[33] Therefore, inclusion of informatics in an undergraduate nursing curriculum is necessary. The QSEN definition of informatics is: "use information and technology to communicate, manage knowledge, mitigate error, and support decision making."[27] Although technology tends to be considered a Western approach to practice, holistic nurses use technology for example: when documenting their individualized care plans on computers, when calling patients, or when searching the web for health information

CAM therapies are often available in healthcare facilities. Selected CAM approaches specific to the older adult population serve as examples here of incorporating informatics into an undergraduate nursing curriculum. Nurses need to be knowledgeable of the more common CAM interventions and be able to locate information on modalities less often used. Also, nurses need to support or refute the use of a selected modality based on the evidence. To accomplish this, nurses must be able to conduct literature reviews. As nursing students at QU enter the professional component of the nursing curriculum, they are exposed to selected healthcare library resources they will use throughout junior and senior years. A learning activity was designed to introduce them to selected aspects of the library technological resources. One library resource is RefWorks, an online bibliographic management program that allows users to create individual database reference lists in a variety of formats such as the American Psychological Association (APA) and the American Medical Association (AMA) styles. Another library resource is the CINAHL database, the comprehensive Cumulative Index to Nursing and Allied Health Literature.

The teaching/learning activity Complementary and Alternative Modalities and Older Individuals is assigned as part of the clinical experience in the nursing fundamentals course. This teaching/learning activity offers nursing students an opportunity to work in pairs in their clinical groups to locate information about one of the following CAM topics often used in the long-term care and/or rehabilitation settings:

- Pet Therapy and Older Adults
- Music Therapy and Older Adults
- Games and Older Adults
- Dancing and Older Adults
- Art and Older Adults

Once the student pairs have their topics they proceed to discover how their CAM intervention is/can be used in clinical practice with older adults by conducting a search using the CINAHL database. In some cases, their assigned CAM is also available on their clinical units, enabling them to observe the modality directly in use. After they locate two or three articles of interest about their CAM topic, they develop an annotated bibliography and save their information using RefWorks. To complete the assignment, student pairs share their reflections and learning about their CAM topics with their clinical instructors and classmates at a post conference. Clinical instructors are amazed at the transition in thinking students demonstrate as they describe interest and enthusiasm in the CAM intervention they pursued for the project.

■ TEAMWORK–COLLABORATION

Teamwork and collaboration among interprofessionals are necessary for high-quality patient care, yet are challenging to achieve.[34,35] The QSEN definition of teamwork–collaboration is "function effectively within nursing and inter-professional teams, fostering open communication, mutual respect, and shared decision-making to achieve quality patient care."[27] From a holistic perspective, relationship-centered philosophies such as practitioner-to-practitioner relationships are a priority to enhance the creation of healing environments.[36] (See also Chapters 4 and 20.)

Interprofessional education during preprofessional licensure education programs has been identified as one way to improve communication, collaboration, and trust after graduation (see Chapter 3). Nursing students find clinical simulation, a teaching/learning strategy in which students interact with a high-fidelity mannequin, an effective way to practice "performing in the moment" as they demonstrate psychomotor skills, therapeutic nurse–patient interaction, clinical reasoning, and caring.[37] Clinical simulation offers a wonderful opportunity for the practical application of teamwork and collaboration as well. Van Soeren et al. are currently designing a research study to examine the effectiveness of clinical simulation as an interprofessional teaching strategy for preprofessionals.[38] A number of schools of nursing use this teaching pedagogy in collaboration with students from other disciplines. For example, real-life clinical simulation scenarios provide nursing students and physician assistant (PA) students with actual opportunities to communicate and collaborate in much the same way they will work together in the future. Running a code is one common example where students have a chance to use teamwork as expected to occur in practice.

A particularly instructive teaching moment often occurs spontaneously. At QU, Cynthia Booth Lord, clinical associate professor of Physician Assistant Studies and PA program director in the School of Health Sciences, and Mary Ann Cordeau, assistant professor in the School of Nursing and coordinating faculty of the Simulation Laboratory at QU, built in a unique simulation planned-spontaneity strategy to teach nursing and PA students to work together on behalf of a patient. The spontaneity occurs during a simulation scenario when a clinical emergency arises and the student nurse determines a call to the student PA is necessary. **Exhibit 36-1** provides an example of an interprofessional teamwork/collaboration clinical simulation scenario.

During the debriefing session that follows all clinical simulation experiences, the nursing and PA students reflect on their communication and critique themselves and one another. The instructor facilitates the discussion and can play back video snippets of the interaction as needed. Outcomes from this type of on-the-spot interprofessional interaction reinforces in students the need for teamwork and collaboration. Student nurses learn to have their patient phone reports complete and organized as well as have solid rationales for the nursing interventions carried out prior to calling the PA. The PA student learns to appropriately address emergent issues by phone when interrupted—much like will occur upon graduation.

■ QUALITY IMPROVEMENT

Engaging nurses in quality improvement processes is critical to delivering excellent patient care.[39] In QSEN, the definition of quality improvement is "use data to monitor the outcomes of care processes and use improvement methods to design and test changes to continuously improve the quality and safety of health care systems."[27] A comparable definition from a holistic perspective is the use of reflective practice

EXHIBIT 36-1   Sample of Interprofessional Teamwork/Collaboration Clinical Simulation

It is 8:15 a.m. The student nurse walks into the simulation room of Michelle Duncan (sim mannequin) prepared to check that her breakfast tray arrived. Michelle is a 72-year-old female with diagnoses of hypertension, chronic obstructive pulmonary disease (COPD), type 2 diabetes and is one day post-op partial sigmoid resection for acute diverticulitis. As the student nurse approaches Michelle's bed, she realizes Michelle is not responding to her greetings. The student asks Michelle if she is okay. Michelle says she feels dizzy and faint and her head is spinning. Her vital signs are: T = 98.4, P = 110 weak, R = 14, BP = 92/58 mm Hg (was 138/90 mm Hg 45 minutes earlier), oxygen saturation = 90% on room air, and eyes are half shut. The student nurse recalls Michelle received Lopressor (metoprolol tartrate) at 7:30 a.m. The nurse lowers the head of the bed and calls the on-call PA student on her cell phone. The PA student may be in the middle of class; however, when the cell phone goes off, she immediately and quietly leaves the classroom to take the call and address the student nurse's concern. The nursing and PA students converse about Michelle's condition and determine the appropriate way to proceed. If the PA student feels the patient warrants a visit by her, she comes to the simulation lab to interact face to face with the student nurse and patient.

in the holistic caring process.[40,41] (See also Chapter 7.) After the nurse reflects on the information, the nurse can make practice changes as necessary. An individual nurse can apply reflective techniques by thinking back to a specific patient situation to contemplate whether interventions were effective or ineffective and to consider how she or he might do things differently in the future. A group of nurses can also use reflective techniques by considering ways to improve care for a group of patients on an inpatient unit or in the community. Quality improvement (QI) and reflective practice dovetail with evidence-based practice when nurses examine ways to "do things better" by evaluating data and current research that leads to more effective nursing interventions.

Many nursing schools are enhancing QI content in undergraduate nursing curricula to better prepare new nurses in practice for active participation in QI activities.[42] At QU, CoryAnn Boyd, associate professor and accelerated track coordinator, designed a holistic quality safety activity to teach students about QI and reflective practice. This activity is completed as part of the medical-surgical hospital clinical rotation during the spring of the junior year. Alternatively, this activity could be carried out in any healthcare facility or community agency clinical site. Students work in small clinical groups for this project to examine the influence of research and actual observed data on guiding practice in the clinical

setting. First, a student group determines the clinical question its members would like to answer. Once the group decides on the question, students collect the most relevant and best evidence (systematic reviews, meta-analyses, and evidence-based clinical practice guidelines). Second, using RefWorks, they prepare an annotated bibliography for distribution to the other students at their clinical site and a copy for their clinical instructor. At this point in the curriculum, they are familiar with a number of healthcare databases and know how to use RefWorks. Third, students compare their findings from the evidence with the clinical agency's existing practice policy and/or observed practice. Fourth, students reflect on their findings from the comparisons they made, and if a change in practice is warranted for improvement, they share one way a nurse or group of nurses might go about making the change occur. Fifth, the students in the group present a critique of their findings based on their study of the current research, the written agency procedure or policy, and their observations of data, sharing their reflections about whether or not a change in clinical practice is indicated.

One clinical group worked with the infection control nurse on a staff hand hygiene project. Students assisted in recording the hand washing practices of physicians, nurses, and other healthcare staff as they entered and exited patient rooms. They quickly observed that the hand hygiene policy was not followed consistently. For those caregivers/providers who did not follow the hand hygiene policy, they documented the reasons the caregivers/providers gave for not following the practice. The most frequently cited reasons for not following the essential hand hygiene practice protocol were: "I forgot" and "My hands were full." Students were previously aware of the ongoing hand hygiene issue and the risk of infection when caregivers/providers did not wash their hands upon entering and exiting a patient's room. Upon reflecting on this practice issue information and the data they directly observed, they developed a keen awareness of the importance of individual adherence to essential practice protocols and guidelines. They observed first-hand one reason infection rates remained high. The outcome of their project led to the development of a positive reinforcement strategy they shared with the unit manager for consideration. They also designed a poster presentation of their work to share at the Interprofessional Student Poster Session sponsored by the School of Health Sciences, School of Nursing, and School of Medicine at QU.

■ EVIDENCE-BASED PRACTICE

Nurses must embrace evidence-based practice (EBP) as the underpinning for nursing interventions to provide optimal patient care.[43] The QSEN definition for EBP is "integrate best current evidence with clinical expertise and patient/family preferences and values for delivery of optimal health care."[27] Holistic standards concur with this interpretation: "The conscientious use of the best available evidence combined with the clinician's expertise and judgment and the patient's preferences and values to arrive at the best decision that leads to quality outcomes."[44]

Creative teaching and learning activities for nursing students about EBP are intended to foster attitudes of understanding and appreciation of the importance of examining the literature and other appropriate information when making clinical decisions.[45] Elizabeth McGann, professor of nursing at the School of Nursing at QU, designed a unique student assignment that focuses on the promotion of understanding and appreciation of EBP for senior-level students

in the nursing research course. Drawing on students' prior knowledge and skills of reviewing the literature in their junior year, an evidence-based project is assigned to teams of five or six students. For this project, intensive librarian support for database searching and the use of bibliographic software is provided. Multiple group drafts are reviewed and students receive feedback that enables them to modify their work and learn that writing is an iterative process. No team leader is identified. Working in a common document makes everyone responsible and accountable for his or her own work and the overall product, which is an annotated bibliography.

Each student group works with a community Magnet hospital collaboratively to devise clinical questions on a single topic such as Assessment and Management of Cognitively Impaired Elders in the Acute Care Setting, then present their work in a symposium format. Unlike earlier assignments at the junior level in which students were introduced to the process of doing a literature review, this search is carried out at a higher level appropriate for seniors: students need to critique each research study, addressing its strengths as well as its limitations. This approach assists them to determine whether there is support for a current practice or whether a practice change is needed.

Upon project completion, findings are shared via a live net-meeting. Students in each group present their findings to nurses at the community hospital they worked with, while nurses at the community hospital listen. Each presentation is followed by a lively interactive question and answer period. The net-meeting component is another way in which this assignment raises the bar for senior-level students and exposes them to an innovative way to communicate across settings. Rather than simply sharing in small clinical groups, students present to a professional audience. The grading aspect of the project is also part of the net-meeting. Each student group has faculty and student raters who listen to the presentations and score them using a predetermined set of guidelines and grading rubric. The ratings contribute to the group's overall presentation grade. At the conclusion of the net-meeting, students have one more opportunity to make final corrections. Their individual annotated bibliographies with embedded icons of the primary source articles are disseminated to the Magnet hospital's director of education. The intent is to provide the director of education with a useful product outcome for evidence-based protocol creation or revision.

Success of this distinctive teaching/learning strategy is not only measured by the student grading process and students' evaluations of their learning, but also by clinical practice changes that can take place based on a project. One student group annotated bibliography project on measurement of orthostatic vital signs led to staff education at the facility and protocol review and standardization throughout the institution. The teaching/learning strategy used for this EBP research project wonderfully blends the Eastern (creative and experiential) and Western (use of technology) schools of thought.

■ SAFETY

Management commitment to a patient safety culture is crucial in keeping patients safe while healing takes place.[46] QSEN defines the safety competency as that which "minimizes risk of harm to patients and providers through both system effectiveness and individual performance."[27] Holistic healing occurs in many ways. The concept of safety is included in discussion of healing environments: "With both attention and intention, the environment can become one in which the client can feel safe and explore the dimensions of self in the healing moment."[47]

The literature documents that there are opportunities for improvement in patient safety curricula in schools of nursing.[48,49] One of the holistic patient safety learning activities assigned in the QU undergraduate nursing curriculum is titled "No Prescription Needed: Take Ma Huang and Call Me in the Morning." This assignment is part of the nursing pharmacology course. Many individuals ingest herbal preparations on a sporadic or regular basis. Herbal preparations are easily available over the counter at pharmacies and vitamin stores. The purpose of this group activity is to examine the holistic safety implications of taking an herbal preparation. Activity instructions include learning about the assigned herb, visiting a pharmacy to find out the approximate cost of

the herb, and writing about the research, experience, and learning that occurs using the following knowledge and reflective questions as a guide:

1. Briefly describe the history of your assigned herb. From where does it originate? What is its intended purpose? Why do people take it?
2. How does this herb work in the body? What body system(s) does it affect and how does it affect it/them?
3. Explain the benefits of taking this herb. What literature supports these benefits?
4. What is the recommended dose of this herb? What literature supports the dosing schedule?
5. Explain the risks of and precautions about taking this herb. What literature documents these risks?
6. Visit a pharmacy or health food store and find out the approximate cost of this herb and whether or not the cost is covered by insurance. What instructions are provided to customers about this herb (either on the container label or in a pamphlet). How is this information similar to or different from what you discovered about this herb in the literature?
7. How is this herb marketed/advertised? Are there any ethical issues?
8. What implications does the evidence you collected have for you in your role as a nurse?

Students enjoy this learning activity because it is partially experiential. They are often surprised at the information they learn about the herb they investigate. Also, especially for those students who take herbal preparations themselves, this activity solidifies the importance of patient education and empowerment.

■ CONCLUSION

Holistic quality and safety initiatives are a vital part of clinical nursing practice. Nursing students who graduate from schools in which holistic quality and safety learning activities are integrated throughout the curriculum are better prepared to join in improvement projects or suggest topics for improvement to enhance patient caring and healing.

Directions for
FUTURE RESEARCH

1. Evaluate the effectiveness of the integration of holism and quality safety into the curriculum of nursing schools as a mechanism to enhance the transformation of nurses as healers and safe practitioners.
2. Determine the impact of the role of graduate nurses in the healthcare environment after graduation from schools of nursing in which holism and quality safety are integral parts of their program.

Nurse Healer
REFLECTIONS

After reading this chapter, the nurse healer will be able to answer or to begin a process of answering the following question:

- How can I incorporate these suggestions of teaching healing concepts into my own curriculum design?

 For a full suite of assignments and additional learning activities, use the access code located in the front of your book to visit this exclusive website: http://go.jblearning.com/dossey. If you do not have an access code, you can obtain one at the site.

NOTES

1. Quality and Safety Education for Nurses, "About QSEN." http://www.qsen.org.
2. J. Casida and S. A. Lemanski, "An Evidenced-Based Review on Guided Imagery Utilization in Adult Cardiac Surgery," *Clinical Scholars Review* 3 (2010): 22–30.
3. L. Chiang, W. Ma, J. Huang, and K. Hsueh, "Effect of Relaxation-Breathing Training on Anxiety and Asthma Signs/Symptoms of Children with Moderate-to-Severe Asthma: A Randomized Controlled Trial," *International Journal of Nursing Studies* 46 (2009): 1061–1070.
4. L. Clukey, "'Just Be There,' Hospice Caregivers' Anticipatory Mourning Experience," *Journal of Hospice and Palliative Nursing* 9 (2007): 150–158.
5. J. Costello, "Spirituality and Nursing Care: A Holistic Approach to the Dying Patient," *Healing Ministry* 17 (2011): 36–40.
6. S. Cutshall, D. Derscheid, A. G. Miers, S. Ruegg, B. J. Schroeder, S. Tucker, and L. Wentworth, "Knowledge, Attitudes, and Use of Complementary and Alternative Therapies Among Clinical Nurse Specialists in an Academic Medical Center," *Clinical Nurse Specialist: The Journal of Advanced Nursing Practice* 24 (2010): 125–131.
7. D. Doherty et al., "Therapeutic Touch and Dementia Care: An Ongoing Journey," *Nursing Older People* 18 (2006): 27–30.
8. H. Gregory and M. C. Watson, "The Effectiveness of Tai Chi as a Fall Prevention Intervention for Older Adults: A Systematic Review," *International Journal of Health Promotion and Education* 47 (2009): 94–100.
9. K. Kwekkeboom, M. Bumpus, and B. Wanta, "Factors Influencing Oncology Staff Nurses' Use of Non-Drug Pain Interventions in Practice," *Oncology Nursing Forum* 34 (2007): 202.
10. D. Selimen and I. I. Andsoy, "The Importance of a Holistic Approach During the Perioperative Period," *AORN Journal* 93 (2011): 482–490.
11. C. Valdez, C. Locke, and N. Sloan, "Healing Touch (HT) as an Innovative Method of Care for Patients: 2011 Annual Conference of the National Association of Clinical Nurse Specialists," *Clinical Nurse Specialist: The Journal for Advanced Nursing Practice* 25 (2011): 45.
12. U. Eriksson and M. Svedlund, "Struggling for Confirmation—Patients' Experiences of Dissatisfaction with Hospital Care," *Journal of Clinical Nursing* 16 (2007): 438–446.
13. M. R. London and J. Lundstedt, "Families Speak About Inpatient End-of-Life Care," *Journal of Nursing Care Quality* 22 (2007): 152–158.
14. C. Jackson, "Magnet Status—Does It Promote Holistic Health Care?" *Holistic Nursing Practice* (July/August 2011): 175–183.
15. J. P. Clement et al., "Are Consumers Reshaping Hospitals? Complementary and Alternative Medicine in U.S. Hospitals, 1999–2003," *Health Care Management Review* 31 (2006): 109–118.
16. C. Mariano, "Holistic Nursing Achieves ANA Specialty Status" (AHNA press release, December 14, 2006).
17. Institute of Medicine, *The Future of Nursing: Leading Change, Advancing Health* (Washington, DC: National Academies Press, 2010). http://www.iom.edu/nursing.
18. American Association of Colleges of Nursing, *The Essentials of Baccalaureate Education for Professional Nursing Practice* (Washington, DC: AACN, 2008).
19. D. S. Brady, "Using Quality Safety Education for Nurses (QSEN) as a Pedagogical Structure for

Course Redesign and Content," *International Journal of Nursing Education Scholarship* 8 (2011): 1–18.

20. T. M. Chenot and L. G. Daniel, "Frameworks for Patient Safety in the Nursing Curriculum," *Journal of Nursing Education* 49 (2010): 559–568.

21. A. Kjornsberg, L. Karlsson, A. Babra, and B. Wadensten, "Registered Nurses' Opinions About Patient Focused Care," *Australian Journal of Advanced Nursing* 28 (2010): 35–44.

22. H. Laitinen, M. Kaunonen, and P. Astedt-Kurki, "Patient-Focused Nursing Documentation Expressed by Nurses," *Journal of Clinical Nursing* 19 (2010): 489–497.

23. R. E. O'Hara, J. G. Hull, K. D. Lyons, M. Bakitas, M. T. Hegel, Z. Li, and T. A. Ahles, "Impact on Caregiver Burden of a Patient-Focused Palliative Care Intervention for Patients with Advanced Cancer," *Palliative and Supportive Care* 8 (2010): 395–404.

24. K. McCauley and R. S. Irwin, "Changing the Work Environment in Intensive Care Units to Achieve Patient-Focused Care: The Time Has Come," *American Journal of Critical Care* 16 (2006): 541–548.

25. J. Scullion, "Patient Focused Outcomes in Chronic Obstructive Pulmonary Disease," *Nursing Standard* 22 (2008): 50–56, 58, 60.

26. V. M. Boscart, "A Communication Intervention for Nursing Staff in Chronic Care," *Journal of Advanced Nursing* 65 (2009): 1823–1832.

27. Quality and Safety Education for Nurses, "Quality/Safety Competencies." http://www.qsen.org/competencies.php.

28. N. Moore and J. Hanson, "Relationship-Centered Care and Healing Initiative in a Community Hospital," in *Holistic Nursing: A Handbook for Practice*, 5th ed., ed. B. M. Dossey and L. Keegan (Sudbury, MA: Jones and Bartlett, 2009): 503.

29. M. Krysl, *Midwife and Other Poems on Caring* (New York, NY: NLN Press, 1989): 35–36.

30. D. Tarello, *Healing Others* (unpublished reflective class assignment, 2010).

31. M. Kleib, A. E. Sales, I. Liama, M. Andrea-Baylon, and A. Beaith, "Continuing Education in Informatics Among Registered Nurses in the United States in 2000," *Journal of Nursing Continuing Education* 41 (2010): 329–336.

32. J. Murphy, "Nursing Informatics: The Intersection of Nursing, Computer, and Information Services," *Nursing Economics* 28 (2010): 204–207.

33. S. Jette, D. S. Tribble, J. Gagnon, and L. Mathieu, "Nursing Students' Perceptions of Their Resources Toward the Development of Competencies in Nursing Informatics," *Nurse Education Today* 30 (2010): 742–746.

34. L. Rose, "Interprofessional Collaboration in the ICU: How to Define?" *Nursing in Critical Care* 16 (2011): 5–10.

35. K.-L. Miller, S. Reeves, M. Zwarenstein, J. D. Beales, C. Kenaszchuk, and L. G. Conn, "Nursing Emotion Work and Interprofessional Collaboration in General Internal Medicine Wards: A Qualitative Study," *Journal of Advanced Nursing* 64 (2008): 332–343.

36. I. Gaboury, M. Lapierre, H. Boon, and D. Moher, "Interprofessional Collaboration Within Integrated Healthcare Clinics Through the Lens of the Relationship-Centered Care Model," *Journal of Interprofessional Care* 25 (2011): 124–130.

37. M. A. Cordeau, "The Lived Experience of Clinical Simulation of Novice Nursing Students," *International Journal for Human Caring* 14 (2010): 8–14.

38. M. Van Soeren, K. MacMillan, S. Cop, C. Kenaszchuk, and S. Reeves, "Development and Evaluation of Interprofessional Care Practices Through Clinical Simulation," *Journal of Interprofessional Care* 23 (2009): 304–306.

39. M. P. Albanese, D. A. Evans, C. A. Schantz, M. Bowen, M. Disbot, J. S. Moffa, P. Piesieski, and R. C. Polomano, "Engaging Clinical Nurses in Quality and Performance Improvement Activities," *Nursing Administration Quarterly* 34 (2010): 226–245.

40. R. J. Beam, R. A. O'Brien, and M. Neal, "Reflective Practice Enhances Public Health Nurse Implementation of Nurse–Family Partnership," *Public Health Nursing* 27 (2010): 131–139.

41. F. Lange, "Nursing Management of Subarachnoid Haemorrhage: A Reflective Case Study," *British Journal of Neuroscience Nursing* 5 (2009): 463–470.

42. D. T. Sullivan, D. Hirst, and L. Cronenwett, "Assessing Quality and Safety Competencies of Graduating Pre-licensure Nursing Students," *Nursing Outlook* 57 (2009): 323–332.

43. M. B. F. Makic, K. T. VonRueden, C. A. Rauen, and J. Chadwick, "Evidence-Based Practice Habits: Putting More Sacred Cows Out to Pasture," *Critical Care Nurse* 31 (2011): 38–61.

44. B. M. Melnyk and C. M. Baldwin, "Evidence-Based Practice," in *Holistic Nursing: A Handbook for Practice*, 5th ed., ed. B. M. Dossey and L. Keegan (Sudbury, MA: Jones and Bartlett, 2009): 34.

45. H. Smith-Strom and M. W. Nortvedt, "Evaluation of Evidence-Based Methods Used to Teach Nursing Students to Critically Appraise Evidence," *Journal of Nursing Education* 47 (2008): 372–375.

46. X. Q. Feng, L. Acord, Y. J. Cheng, J. H. Zeng, and J. P. Song, "The Relationship Between Management Safety Commitment and Patient Safety Culture," *International Nursing Review* 58 (2011): 249–254.

47. M. McKivergin, "The Nurse as an Instrument of Healing," in *Holistic Nursing: A Handbook for Practice*, 5th ed., ed. B. M. Dossey and L. Keegan (Sudbury, MA: Jones and Bartlett, 2009): 730.

48. E. L. Smith, L. Cronenwett, and G. Sherwood, "Current Assessments of Quality and Safety Education in Nursing," *Nursing Outlook* 55 (2007): 132–137.

49. T. M. Chenot and L. G. Daniel, "Frameworks for Patient Safety in the Nursing Curriculum," *Journal of Nursing Education* 49 (2010): 559–568.

CORE VALUE 5

Holistic Nurse Self-Care

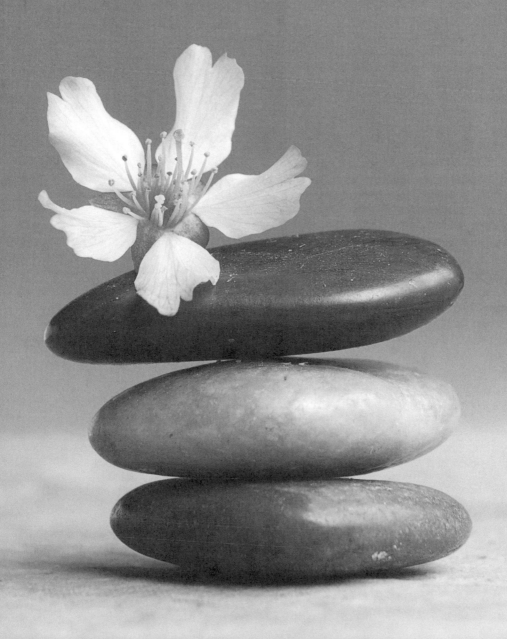

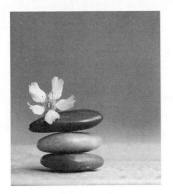

Chapter 37

The Nurse as an Instrument of Healing

Deborah McElligott

Nurse Healer
OBJECTIVES

Theoretical

- Discuss the importance of self-care related to health promotion efforts on a national and international level.
- Review the integration of nursing theory into self-care fostering the nurse as an instrument of healing.
- Define the concepts of self-care, health promotion, health/wellness, and healing.
- Review the qualities of self-care as the core of healing relationships and health promotion.
- Describe the dynamics between self-care, healing, and health promotion.

Clinical

- Identify components of a holistic self-assessment.
- Describe benefits of a holistic self-care plan.
- Describe the qualities and the nurse's role in a healing intervention.
- Discuss the role of the nurse coaching others in self-care.

Personal

- Complete a holistic self-assessment tool.
- Develop weekly, monthly, and long-term self-care goals.
- Develop self-care practices to expand self-awareness and enhance presence, intuition, and healing abilities.

- Identify and mobilize a self-care support team.
- Routinely reassess and set priorities and time for healing of self to align with the qualities of being an instrument of healing.

DEFINITIONS

Healing: Healing is a positive, subjective, unpredictable process involving transformation to a new sense of wholeness, spiritual transcendence, and reinterpretation of life.[1] Healing involves the process of the right relationships forming on any or all levels of the human experience—a goal of holistic nursing.[2p93]

Health: The actualization of inherent and acquired human potential through goal-directed behavior, competent self-care, and satisfying relationships with others, while adjustments are made as needed to maintain structural integrity and harmony with relevant environments.[3p23]

Health promotion: "Behavior motivated by the desire to increase well-being and actualize human health potential."

Inner wisdom: The innate inner knowledge or knowing that one can access through meditation, mindfulness, and other methods that connect to the subconscious.

Intuition: Sudden insight or knowing without the perceived use of logic or analysis. Often called a right brain activity, intuition may be enhanced through the senses and is often used to guide integrative treatments including energy work.[2p34]

Self-care: The practice of engaging in health-related activities, using health-promoting, desired behaviors to adopt a healthier lifestyle and enhance wellness.[4]

Self-care plan: A plan developed with a goal of actualizing behaviors and actions to promote one's health, wellness, and healing.

Transpersonal caring: A caring presence where the nurse acknowledges and appreciates the total body, mind, and spirit connection between each interaction with self and others. The relationships occur on sacred ground, and both the nurse and client become part of something larger than themselves. This is the embodiment of the nurse as an instrument of healing.[5]

■ THEORY AND RESEARCH

It is fitting that the chapter on self-care is the last chapter in this text because for nurses to practice this core value, they need to incorporate the other core values as well—truly a holistic approach. Previous discussions of nursing theory, holistic self-assessment, coaching, self-reflection, nutrition, exercise, integrative therapies, healing environment, therapeutic communication, diversity, spirituality, evidence-based practice, and education could easily be repeated in the context of self-care and enhancing the role of the nurse as an instrument of healing.

The *Scope and Standards of Practice* of the American Holistic Nurses Association and American Nurses Association (see Chapter 2) reiterates the necessity of nurses being on their own healing journeys if they are to be instruments of healing as they partner with others. This lifelong process requires education, practice, and self-work, translating into the very knowledge, skills, presence, and attitude of holistic nurses. Along with the focus on self-care is the focus on health versus illness on a continuum where the individual, a microcosm of the universe, and society are constantly fluctuating in various stages of health and illness. There is no stasis in the universe, in Nature, or in humans: no static state of health that may be achieved and never lost. Hence, the concept of self-care is continuous, with the goal of a healthy lifestyle being a life-

long practice. The self-care work of the holistic nurse involves continual holistic self-assessment and the redefining of self-care plans to facilitate balance in one's life. The nurse's ability to focus on and provide attention to self-care is affected by health, personal thoughts, practices, behaviors and actions, others, and the environment. Each nurse's life, in constant interaction with the universe, evolves as the nurse participates in transpersonal caring throughout life's journey. Thus, the practice of self-care involves the development of lifelong health-promoting behaviors.

The holistic nurse uses more than laboratory results and physical parameters in assessment of self and others and freely incorporates modern medicine, functional medicine, and evidence-based practices with other traditional forms of healing. Evidence-based practices such as energy work, acupuncture, imagery, and body work may be used in assessment, treatment, and promotion of self-care and wellness. Additional healing paradigms include whole medical systems, both ancient such as Traditional Chinese Medicine (TCM) and ayurvedic medicine, and modern systems such as homeopathy and naturopathy.[6] From a holistic standpoint, the focus is balancing, healing, partnering with, and coaching to reach the person's potential. The other end of the spectrum may involve support as the person transitions from this life. The standards of holistic nursing practice guide self-care, recommending that nurses identify at-risk patterns; develop practices that enhance whole-person healing; recognize the individual capacity to heal; create a conscious awareness and understanding of their purpose, meaning, and connection with a greater being/force; and develop an understanding that crisis creates opportunity as they continually evolve.[7p88]

■ INTERNATIONAL AND NATIONAL TRENDS

A focus on self-care, involving health promotion and healthy behaviors, reflects both international and national trends. On an international level, the United Nations (UN), formed in 1945, created the World Health Organization (WHO) 3 years later to meet global health goals. The UN and the WHO continue to partner and recently formed the Eight Millennium Development

Goals. These goals focus on global health problems and aim to improve well-being by 2015 in eight different areas.[8]

In the United States, *Healthy People 2020* builds on 3 decades of prevention and wellness activities with a vision of a society where everyone lives long, healthy lives. The Institute of Medicine (IOM) Committee on Leading Health Indicators for *Healthy People 2020* developed recommendations that integrate the life course model with a model of health determinants and health outcomes.[9] These indicators and objectives guide the national agenda. Many of these topics include areas of self-care: healthy behaviors, healthy physical environment, healthy social environment, positive mental health, responsible sexual behavior, and avoidance of tobacco use. One of four goals of *Healthy People 2020* is a life course perspective to "promote quality of life, healthy development and healthy behaviors across all life stages."[9p8] Additional indicators and objectives in *Healthy People 2020* include a focus on quality of life (QOL). Overall, QOL is conceptualized as well-being, which may be described as thriving and flourishing; it is assessed through happiness and life satisfaction tools.[10]

Thus, through both international and national agendas the need to focus on health, healthy behaviors, and responsibility for self-care is highlighted. Nurses, as instruments of healing, must follow the recommendations for consumers and assume responsibility for self-care and health promotion.[7] Nurses—in the most trusted profession—now have the opportunity to model self-care for others and assist in coaching the nation and the world in self-care.

■ NURSING THEORY

In the development and evaluation of self-care for wellness activities and programs, it is important to be guided by nursing theories and use valid evaluation tools to support evidence-based practice. Earlier discussions address grand nursing theories such as the Science of Unitary Human Beings, Caring Science, and Integral Nursing, which individually and collectively support the concept of self-care and the caring process. These theories direct nursing assessment, reflection, presence, coaching, therapeutic relationships, holistic communication, healing environments, and nursing education and research. They support the nurse as an instrument of healing, honoring therapeutic presence, intuition, caring science, and the integral role of the nurse in relationship with others, society, and the world. Grand nursing theories define many methods of assessment on both physical and energetic levels and support the concept of "being" with the client as opposed to the frequent focus on "doing." In holistic nursing, it is paramount to honor and support the individual's goals based on that person's situation, culture, beliefs, and capabilities. The "being" is further enhanced because the theories support the concept of coaching, or working with an individual to hold the space to allow the person's inner wisdom to unfold and guide the development of a personal wellness plan. Advances in science support the wisdom of the energetic effect a therapeutic presence can have on self and others, identifying basic cellular changes resulting from "heart-based living" (feelings of love and appreciation vs. anger and stress).[11] The plan for self-care can be as varied as the grand nursing theories that support each of the many strategies used to heal body, mind, and spirit.

Programs focusing on self-care are also supported by midrange theories such as the Health Promotion Model.[3] The Health Promotion Model offers a holistic approach to self-care as perspectives from nursing and behavioral sciences are integrated into factors that may influence health behaviors. Nurses can practice and direct these practices, identifying interpersonal influences, interventions for health behavior change, and individual needs in tailoring the path to reach the necessary and desired changes. This model is congruent with holistic nursing because it guides data collection, processing, nursing activities, and possible client outcomes.[12]

In the Health Promotion Model, the motivation for behavior is neither fear nor threat and is not disease or injury specific. The approach seeks to expand the potential for health, not prevent the occurrence of imbalances or disease. Health is influenced by multidimensional factors and is viewed as greater than the absence of disease. The person's desire for an active role in promoting health is honored because the individual can express his or her own unique health potential, assess his or her own competencies, value growth in positive directions, achieve balance, and desire to regulate his or her own behaviors.[3p7] This description of health promotion may be applied to an individual or family, community, or society. Health may be improved as risks are assessed and interventions are suggested to change perceptions, decrease barriers, gather support, and improve health-promoting behaviors. The Health-Promoting Lifestyle Profile Tool (HPLPII), often used in this model, identifies six behaviors or subscales to measure interpersonal relations, nutrition, health responsibility, physical activity, stress management, and spiritual growth.[13] Evaluating, addressing, and incorporating health-promoting behaviors into daily activities creates a lifestyle representing self-care or self-management of health promotion.

■ CONCEPTS RELATED TO SELF-CARE

Concept of Health

Health may be defined from various perspectives; for example, the absence of illness; the capacity to adapt; the ability to fulfill a role; the ability to incorporate the importance of wholeness, peacefulness, and meaningfulness;[14] and "the actualization of inherent and acquired human potential through goal directed behavior, competent self-care, and satisfying relationships with others, while making adjustments to maintain structural integrity and harmony with relevant environments."[3p23] Optimal health is viewed as a dynamic balance of all aspects of the whole person—physical, emotional, social, and spiritual. Health is therefore enhanced through goal-directed behavior, self-care, satisfying relationships, spiritual wellness, and harmony/balance within the self and with the environment. Health is often viewed as one end of a continuum where illness is on the other end (**Figure 37-1**). From a holistic perspective, health is recognized as a fluid balance of the body, mind, and spirit within and with the environment. Most people fluctuate between the two states. Health is often taken for granted and is not noticed when an individual functions as a whole in daily activities without pain or discomfort; at this point, the person may focus little on self-care because he or she feels fine.

When an individual notices a "part" separate from the whole and feels an imbalance, the person begins to move away from the health end of the spectrum. Slight symptoms may occur, presenting the person the opportunity to address the issue and seek a new wholeness. If these symptoms are ignored, they usually progress to an actual disease and the focus shifts from finding the source of the disease or imbalance to alleviation of symptoms or cure of disease. Today, many chronic conditions are the result of slight symptoms that were ignored or only slightly alleviated. In contrast, a focus on health involves treating minor symptoms, adjusting lifestyle as needed, discovering the cause, and preventing further imbalances.

Concept of Health Promotion

Health promotion, the effort or activity adopted to achieve health, is centered on self-care. Definitions of health promotion include "behavior motivated by the desire to increase well-being

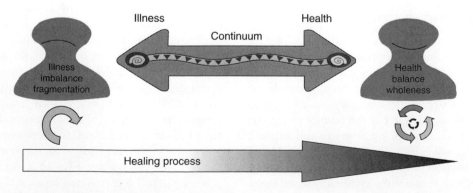

FIGURE 37-1   Illness/health continuum.
Source: D. McElligott, © 2011.

and actualize human health potential"[3p7] and "the science and art of helping people change their lifestyle to move towards a state of optimal health."[15] Operationally, this term can be defined as the practice of health-promoting behaviors.

Concept of Self-Care

Self-care has been discussed from many perspectives and directly relates to health promotion. Orem describes self-care as the "practice of activities that individuals initiate and perform on their own behalf in maintaining life, health and well-being."[16] *Self-care* implies deliberate action and may occur as one maintains health and recognizes and treats symptoms. Learned behavior is inherent in self-care, making it naturally culturally specific and necessitating individualization of recommendations for activities. Self-care may be operationalized through the examination of health-promoting or healthy, desired behaviors and activities as listed on various wellness worksheets, web-based programs, and standardized validated tools such as the HPLPII.[17]

From a holistic perspective, the path to health was traditionally a focus on body, mind, and spirit, seeking to rebalance the system when imbalances occurred. As theories progress, we have begun to recognize that there is no one state of balance that is recovered, but a new dynamic state of balance is achieved because each person continually evolves. The recommended path to self-care is as complicated as the many tools, programs, books, and audios sold commercially that promise to enhance health. To support health on a physical level, an individual must experience health on the emotional and spiritual levels as well. Numerous tools categorize the body, mind, and spirit into additional areas in attempts to pinpoint the imbalance and focus activities on areas needed to achieve wellness and health.

With a renewed international focus on health, the need for self-care, closely tied to self-responsibility, is a priority. Statistics show that societies face increased numbers of chronic diseases, many of which can be prevented, modified, or eradicated by healthier lifestyles. Beginning in 1979 and continuing until today, the U.S. Surgeon General's office has set goals of developing a healthy and fit nation.[18] The current focus is on nutrition, physical activity, and stress management across the life span of the population, from childhood to senior years.

Many past efforts were aimed at education, but failed to sustain long-term results in helping people improve their health. Newer efforts use continuing education programs to engage people in overall health assessment, goal setting, skill building, experiential activity, demonstration, and opportunities for feedback. The area of coaching (see Chapter 9) is expanding as one method of enhancing self-care. The coaching process, using more "evocative than didactic approaches," supports the individual as a partner in achieving higher levels of wellness.[19] The technique frequently includes the development of a self-care plan that lists specific, measurable, achievable goals for both the short and long terms. These goals, realistic in day-to-day living, are based on the individual's inner knowledge, current assessment, and priorities. Opportunities for peer, family, and community support are identified.

Concept of Healing

Aspects of healing, the goal of nursing care, have been discussed throughout this text. Here, healing is described as a process of self-care in the quest for health and wellness. For this purpose, healing may be defined as a positive, subjective, unpredictable process involving a transformation to a new sense of wholeness, spiritual transcendence, and reinterpretation of life.[1] As one experiences healing, suffering is transcended, and feelings of serenity, interconnectedness, gratitude, and a new sense of meaning emerge. Quinn sums it up as the development of a right relationship.[20]

Suffering may occur on many levels including physical, emotional, spiritual, and social.[21] Because it is a subjective experience, an individual's perception of suffering warrants attention no matter how it appears to others—if it is perceived, we honor it as real. Whereas theories on health promotion arise from a desire to actualize wellness and health, the motivation for self-care may also come from suffering, discord, or imbalances in the person's system, such as a newly diagnosed disease or disorder.

Mediators in healing may be internal or external, involving traits of the patient or traits of the environment and the nurse. Both internal and external traits influence the degree to which the individual accepts and participates in the transpersonal caring process. The nurse, through transpersonal caring, becomes the healing environment as a caring moment is created, and both the soul of the nurse and the soul of the patient are changed.[5] The healing relationship occurring as the internal and external environments rebalance to a new level is characterized by various qualities, as described in **Table 37-1**.[20]

In summary, the concept of healing may be defined by describing the antecedents, mediators, attributes, and consequences of healing, as described in **Figure 37-2**.

Client and Self-Healing

The goal in this era of self-responsibility and self-care is for the nurse to partner in the healing process, to motivate and enable each person to develop skills and behaviors on the healing journey toward health.[22] Modeling, memory, and perspective are three ways to support clients in the healing process. Modeling brings intention, education, and reassurance to the relationship. Memory identifies internal resources. Perspective models acceptance and supports change.

Often, the nurse identifies the patient's need for healing separate from the medical diagnosis. At these times, the nurse can introduce additional methods of self-assessment and through transpersonal caring elicit the patient's story and support the expression of the patient's inner wisdom. The nurse realizes that healing is a subjective, unpredictable process and the client has his or her individual path. Although

transpersonal caring and the nurse as an instrument of healing support the process, the outcome cannot be predicted. By creating a sacred, safe space for the client to harness inner wisdom, the path to self-care and healing may be identified for the first time.

Because healing is a mutual process, the internal and external environments of both the nurse and client change and interact. The role and influence of the nurse vary during the process, moving from one of support to becoming a bystander as the person gains a new relational system. It is important for the nurse to recognize the partnership in this experience; although nurses are often referred to as healers, the patient is not passive and control of the healing is not in the nurse's hands. The goal is to support the patient's beliefs and innate healing ability, thereby enhancing the opportunity for healing. For example, if a patient's pain is diminished after a nurse provides guided imagery, it may seem that the nurse healed the person. In actuality, the nurse, using "energetic patterns of consciousness, intentionality and authentic presence," guided the patient in imagery and allowed the person's own inner wisdom and self-healing patterns to emerge with solutions to assist in pain management.[5]

■ SELF-CARE IN NURSES

Although self-care is important for everyone, its importance is underscored for those who are caregivers, including nurses. How can nurses care and support others if they do not have the energy, presence, or ability to support themselves? There are many reports of nurses who are wounded healers as a result of personal and professional experiences, with documented needs for self-healing. For decades, nurses have been giving their last bit of strength, ignoring their individual needs, and burying feelings of grief, moral distress, and anxiety—feeling it was the noble thing to do. How did we arrive at this place? When did this shift occur?

More than a hundred years ago, Florence Nightingale emphasized the need for nurses to focus on self-care as well as the care and support of other nurses (the *esprit de corps*) and the environment.[23] She discussed the need for environments to support healing. She highlighted

| TABLE 37-1 | Qualities of the Nurse in Transpersonal Caring/ Partnering with the Client in Self-Care/Healing |

love	gratitude	intentionality
acceptance	presence	mindfulness
compassion	awareness	trust
empathy	self-care	respect

Source: © D. McElligott, 2011 (adapted from Quinn, 2000; Schmidt, 2004; Watson, 2005).

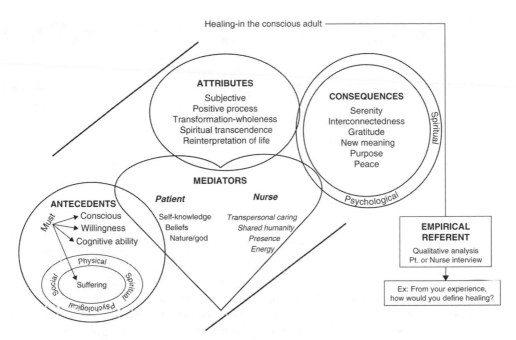

FIGURE 37-2   Healing in the conscious adult.
Source: D. McElligott, © 2011.

spiritual self-care in letters directing nurses to develop a sacred space for reflection, to gain support from a Being greater than themselves, and to see that reflection in each and every person.

How strong is your focus on self-care after working a 60-hour week or a 16-hour day or leaving work only to face the challenges of family life or caring for an aging parent? These are real challenges facing the nursing population and are no longer unique to women as a greater number of men enter the profession. For many nurses, 12-hour shifts provide the opportunity—or the issue—of working two jobs or balancing school and work. As the life expectancy increases in the United States, many nurses, similar to the general public, are caring for aging parents in addition to family and work responsibilities.

Holistic nursing focuses on health promotion, viewing the individual as a whole, body, mind, and spirit. Whereas nurses may use holistic approaches to counsel patients about health promotion, they often neglect their own care. Poor health-promoting behaviors are linked to stress, illness, increased healthcare costs, obesity, job turnover, errors, and poor-quality care.[24-26]

The importance of self-care in nurses is further highlighted when one realizes there are more than 15 million nurses globally. Nurses form the largest group of employees in hospitals, yet the profession is projected to have a shortage of more than a million by 2020.[27] Studies on nurses' actual health status and health-promoting behaviors range from good general overall health ratings[28] to overall poor health-promoting behaviors on standardized tools,[29] including poor diet, lack of physical activity, obesity,[25] stress, and compassion fatigue.[30] From a business perspective, promoting health in nurses and their work environment can decrease the cost of turnover, disability, and employer health care[26] and improve quality of care.[24,30,31] Many practices and strategies can be incorporated into a self-care plan, as shown in **Table 37-2**.

Process of Self-Care

Self-care begins with assessment and the identification of patterns that put one at risk for disease and imbalances. This includes identifying unhealthy lifestyle behaviors, including risky behaviors such as living or working in toxic environments, using tobacco and alcohol, working long hours, experiencing stress, and lack of sleep. The individual must recognize and believe in his

TABLE 37-2   Self-Care Practices That Enhance Whole Person Healing

Holistic Self-Assessment	Nurse Coaching	Appreciative Inquiry	Self-Reflection
Healthy nutrition	Daily exercise	Yoga/Tai Chi/QiGong	Meditation
Humor, Laughter, Play	Relaxation	Affirmations	Mindfulness
Music, Art therapy	Massage/bodywork	Reflexology	Imagery
Acupuncture	Aromatherapy	Therapeutic communication	Spirituality
Energy healing	Song & Dance	Journaling	Storytelling
Creative practice	Volunteering		

Source: © D. McElligott, 2011

or her own innate healing ability, realizing the power of emotions, thoughts, and practices to influence the body-mind-spirit. Practices that enhance self-care are developed and incorporated into a daily lifestyle with a goal of reaching the greatest potential of one's health.

To provide care to others in a meaningful way, nurses must be able to focus, be present, and resonate positive feelings such as love and appreciation. Consciousness toward one's purpose, which adds meaning to one's life, is a powerful component of self-care, guiding one from daily to lifelong living. The development of meaning in one's life is directly related to a sense of meaning and connection to a force greater than oneself. This force can range from God or a Supreme Being to Nature or Mother Earth. Within this framework, change is viewed as part of the joy of living, where opportunity may arise from crisis. As one embodies self-care, purpose, and meaning, the environment, and all those around are affected; patient care is enhanced through one's presence.

As nurses partner with patients in the healing journey, nursing knowledge, skills, and caring are required. The skills of reflection, presence, therapeutic relationship, and communication are not available in a nurse who is avoiding self-care, who is stressed and constantly multitasking. A lifestyle building resilience through meditative practices, healthy nutrition, exercise, supportive relationships, and ongoing assessment is crucial to the ability to participate as an instrument of healing. As the nurse pursues self-

care, it is often a challenge to assess oneself with the same loving compassion used for clients. It is vital for nurses as caregivers to balance compassion ("opening the heart to suffering") with equanimity ("the state of being non-partial"). (p. 44). In other words nurses need a "soft front, but strong back") (p. 14, Halifax). Because nursing is a calling and healing is the essence of nursing, healing and self-care must be a central core of every nurse's life.

Themes of self-care goals from a study on nursing health promotion behaviors included the following: increasing physical activity, stress management, healthy diet, health responsibility, and time management related to self-care and relaxation.[32] Respondents listed personal strengths including the traits of caring, calmness, patience, and humor. Spirituality, interpersonal skills, organizational skills, and teamwork were also listed as strengths. Challenges to wellness included time management, stress management, lack of physical activity, diet and weight management, working the night shift, responsibilities for dependants, and interpersonal relations. Support identified by participants included family, friends, peers, significant others, and God. Action plans identified by participants included increasing activity, managing time more effectively, learning relaxation techniques, being educated regarding wellness, planning healthy meals, and teamwork. **Table 37-3** lists excerpts from the top three scores that were reported in each category.

TABLE 37-3   Self-Care Plan Themes Table (Excerpts)

Self-Care Goal N=51/52	n	Strength n=26/52	n	Challenge n=46/52	n	Support n=44/52	n	Action n=45/52	N
Physical activity	23	Personal traits: patience, calm caring, humor	12	Time mgmt	15	Family	26	Increase activity	12
Stress mgmt	13	Spiritual values	5	Stress mgmt	9	Friends	16	Time mgmt	9
Diet	9	Interpersonal skills	3	Physical activity	6	Peers	13	Relax	7

Source: © D. McElligott, 2009, unpublished.

■ SELF-CARE IN THE WORKPLACE

Whereas the value of self-care has been recognized in terms of health benefits, increased quality of life, and decreased health expenditures, the effect of self-care on work teams, productivity, and quality care is now being acknowledged. This recognition occurred with the IOM reports highlighting poor communication and lack of teamwork as major contributors to errors in the workplace.[24] The ability of a team to work together is directly related to the wellness of the team. Stress has been known to affect the body, mind, and spirit, influencing judgment, caring, and communication—key elements of the person's wellness and job performance. Because the 2011 national patient safety goals highlight the importance of communication among healthcare team members, stress management and communication skills are now the focus of many workplace programs.[33] To encourage participation in employee wellness programs and self-care activities, workplaces, including hospitals, are harnessing both peer and leadership support.

Holistic nursing recognizes the complexity of wellness and the challenges of nursing—each area of nursing has unique requirements that demand unique solutions. For example, when comparing three different groups of hospital nurses, Hooper et al. found that emergency room nurses scored lowest in compassion satisfaction, ICU nurses were at risk for burnout, and oncology nurses were at risk for compassion fatigue.[30] While the obstacles may be unique to each area, generic solutions may

include individual and team assessment, identification of stressors, perceived barriers to and benefits of health promotion activities, and situational influences on health behaviors. Assessment could include individual wellness tools and the development of individual wellness plans; unit/group discussions regarding issues affecting health (stressful situations, employee illness or sudden death, difficult patient situations, unit relationships and staffing patterns, personal family issues, etc.); and the development of group wellness plans and opportunities. Themes that cross units and services may require institutional changes or programs. This can be as substantial as establishment of an on-site gym, meditation/healing room, massage program, acupuncture program, and on-site employee wellness clinics or can include small-scale projects based on institutional resources, as discussed in the following case study.

Barriers to health promotion in the nursing population are identified as excessive work demands, injustices, and unsafe work environments.[34] Anecdotal data identify additional barriers to health promotion in the nursing population as environmental, lack of time, lack of education regarding strategies, and lack of social support.[35]

Synthesis of the literature provides strategies to address the variables, specific barriers, and the direction for programs to assist in worksite health promotion for nurses. Participants in holistic programs who developed a self-care plan report significantly increased overall health-promoting lifestyle behavior scores as measured by the HPLPII over time.[29,36] These programs, ranging from one day in the acute care setting to one semester in academia, offer ongoing support, structured time for self-care, and time for change. Participants' individual self-care plans focused on the areas of physical activity, stress management, and health responsibility, with diet and time management as additional needs.

Recommendations for successful worksite programs include decreasing perceived barriers to health promotion, providing convenient time and location for interventions, encouraging holistic self-assessment, considering employee preferences, strengthening social support, and encouraging involvement and use of a holistic approach.[7,29] Holistic approaches at the worksite present the opportunity to decrease identified barriers to health promotion, enabling nurses to increase health-promoting behaviors, thus preventing the costly results of poor behaviors.[37] Nurses can align their institutional values with the core values of the American Holistic Nurses Association and use nursing theory to guide and evaluate holistic programs focusing on self-care and health promotion. The goal is to increase well-being and actualize human health potential for staff, and then for patients. As holistic programs provide interventions to address the many aspects of health promotion, results may appear as improved health, productivity, and satisfaction and reduced healthcare costs.[26]

Case Study 1

Setting: Acute care institution

Clients: Individual RN; nursing unit; institution

Pattern/Challenges/Needs: Self-care deficits

The individual nurse completes the wellness tool and identifies a need to improve stress management, diet, and exercise. She develops a self-care plan related to improving stress management, diet, and exercise.

The nursing unit staff members identify similar needs for the unit in a group meeting. They plan a weekly meeting with a healthy lunch and a nursing unit retreat on two separate days.

The acute care facility identifies themes consistent across the institution and discusses them at an organizational meeting. Staff from various areas are interested in healthy eating, stress man-

agement, and improving exercise. They plan institutional development of the following items:

- A walking path and discounted gym membership
- A "healthy corner" in the cafeteria with healthy meal options and calories posted
- Scheduled on-site retreats conducted by holistic nurses (see the description in the list that follows)[37]

As described, desired individual self-care practices in the workplace often have similar themes. Although staff may complete individual wellness assessments, especially if supported by an organization, discussions in groups assist in identifying themes and supporting workplace programs. Lunch and learns, staff meetings, 4-hour workshops, or full-day retreats can be facilitated by holistic nurses to gather group themes, develop self-care plans, and then harness peer support.

Possible Agenda for a 1-Day Holistic Program

- Opening ritual to create sacred space
- Overview of day, guidelines to therapeutic communication in sharing circle
- Alignment of institutional values with values of AHNA and holistic nursing theory
- Mindful breathing and imagery exercise (followed by individual reflection through art/journaling)
- Group discussion (based on common need)
- Experience self-care modalities (reflexology, aromatherapy, energy work, massage)
- Healthy lunch
- Meditative walk on hospital grounds—experience healing environment (trees, waterfall, meditation room)
- Yoga/tai chi/Qigong
- Appreciative inquiry as a method of change
- Development of care plan
- Sharing circle—one thing to take back to work[38]

(McElligott © 2011)

■ SELF-CARE USING THE HOLISTIC CARING PROCESS

Holistic Assessment and Identification of Patterns/Challenges/Needs

The development of self-care plans naturally follows the holistic caring process (as described in Chapter 7). Assessment for the purpose of developing a self-care plan incorporates both Western and traditional assessment tools and patterns and may occur in collaboration with a healthcare practitioner or be conducted by individuals themselves. Common practices and tools include the standard physical, history, and review of systems based on guidelines used in most healthcare institutions and outpatient settings. Although the purpose of these practices is to develop a medical diagnosis, they can be useful for care plan development even though they may provide only a part of the person's story. Assessments may also occur through dialogue, imagery, art, various physical and biofield exams, and manipulative practices, common in many integrative practices.

As discussed elsewhere, numerous tools and methods are available for self-assessment. The choice of which to use must fit with the individual. Individuals may use written tools such as questionnaires that examine health-promoting behaviors, quality of life and satisfaction, physical wellness, recent lab and radiology exams, medications, and compliance with and effectiveness of medical regimen. With these assessment tools, integrative health practitioners seek the occurrence and correlations of responses to situations, behaviors, foods, and activities as they evaluate the person as a whole being. Information obtained in the written form helps to initiate the relationship and complements other methods of assessment. The development of the relationship and comprehensive assessment has been identified as one of the reasons for the increase in people seeking health care from integrative health providers.

Case Study 2

Setting: Employee wellness clinic where staff pay for a massage

Client: JL, a 32-year-old nurse practitioner

Pattern/Challenges/ Needs:

1. Fatigue
2. Frequent upper respiratory infections
3. Negative medical workup

JL recently started working as a nurse practitioner in an oncology unit working 12-hour shifts. As JL received a massage, the health practitioner noted tenderness on JL's lateral aspect of both fore-arms, with increased tenderness on lung points in the antecubital area. The practitioner asked JL whether there are any physical reasons for this tenderness, and there are none. The practitioner asked further regarding the emotions of grief and sadness, and JL began to cry, explaining the loss of her grandparent 3 years ago and the difficult "stories of her patients" she hears when they describe them during imagery sessions. JL replays these images in her mind at night. Both her dreams and sleep are being affected, leaving her exhausted.

The practitioner explains to JL the correlation in Chinese medicine of emotions to the energy channels (meridians) in the body. When energy is blocked, imbalances occur and may be noted during massage as a difference in the channel or pulses and tenderness in the channel and various points. For more than 3,000 years, energy channels in Traditional Chinese Medicine have been recognized as part of an organ system pair and are assigned a particular emotion that is believed to be active in specific channels. The emotion attached to the lung (and colon) channel is grief and sadness.[39] From a TCM perspective, this manifestation of grief in the lung channel with associated weakness in the lung energy affects the whole person. In JL, it manifested as fatigue, frequent upper respiratory infections, and difficulty sleeping.

During the treatment, the practitioner held open the sacred space for JL to cry and express her grief. Following the massage, JL continued to talk and highlight the wonderful relationship she enjoyed with her grandmother, the influence her grandmother had on her career, and how she never had the time to grieve the loss or discuss it with her family. JL felt like she strongly connected to the many losses experienced by her patients and their families. She identified that although patients were greatly comforted by her presence and imagery work, she would replay their troubling stories in her head at night and she was unable to sleep.

JL recognized that she needed to process her own grief and identified journaling and joining the hospital bereavement group for peer support as first steps. She also identified the need to practice centering skills prior to working with clients and the need for additional education in self-care strategies. She would continue massage weekly for 2 more weeks.

Her initial self-care plan included the following activities: journal daily for 2 weeks, massage weekly for 2 weeks, daily practice of centering skills through meditation, and join a bereavement group.[38]

Integrative Assessment

The preceding case study is just one example of the power of integrative assessment. The self-care plan that develops from this assessment is completely different from one that would be developed from a strict medical model. Integrative assessment provides the opportunity for the client to adopt health-promoting behaviors, initiate a healing journey, and reach for a new level of health, with a greater awareness of the body-mind-spirit connection. Practitioners using integrative models, instruments, and techniques may also assess energetic levels (for example, acupuncture channels, chakras, biofields).

In this age of technology, a number of online tools are available for assessment and generation of a self-care plan. Some even include built-in daily reminders. Many insurance companies provide discounts on premiums for participants who complete online health assessment programs. These tools may be used for individual assessment or by a practitioner. For example, the goal may be stress management, and the practitioner may use a type of computer program or biofeedback to assess heart coherence. With biofeedback, the client can instantly visualize the changes that occur with a change in feelings from stress to love and appreciation. A practitioner may use a computer probe to assess a client's energy channels related to nutritional needs so as to make a recommendation for supplements.

The development of self-awareness is paramount. It is important for individuals to know when self-assessment is sufficient and when further assessment from a credentialed healthcare provider is needed. Daily assessment may take the form of self-inventory through the use of practices such as mindfulness, meditation, journaling, self-reflection, movement therapies, energy work, or any other practice of going inward to access inner wisdom, identify imbalances, and rebalance. Finally, self-awareness may be enhanced through dialogue with a coach who asks the powerful questions and listens while holding and safeguarding the space for the client to unfold inner wisdom.

Therapeutic Care Plan and Interventions

The next step in the caring process in self-care is the actual development of a self-care plan: personalizing a plan of care to fit individual needs. The self-care plan outlines the steps to achieving individual health goals while considering recommendations from a healthcare provider. Developing the self-care plan is often challenging, especially if one completes a lengthy complicated tool and identifies numerous activities that are important for health. The self-care plan is an ongoing process, as fluid as the relationship with self and the healthcare provider.

The care plan developed in the case study about the nurse practitioner JL is just a start; the practitioner can develop numerous strategies for JL and devise a longer plan of care that includes nursing rationales. The care plan described was JL's self-care plan based on the immediate needs she identified. In future weekly visits, evaluation (the final part of the holistic caring process) would occur. The practitioner and JL would discuss the self-care plan and modify it based on accomplishments and identified needs.

Developing a self-care plan in this way resonates with the field of coaching, as described earlier and in the next section. Techniques used in coaching involve the caring process, intuition to ask powerful questions, active listening, presence, and caring. Coaching can be incorporated into many integrative techniques as long as the practitioner follows the coaching principles. The area of coaching has made great strides in assisting clients to create realistic, attainable self-care plans that continually build on weekly successes so that the client feels successful and remains motivated.

■ COACHING THE CORE VALUE OF SELF-CARE FOR PATIENTS/ CLIENTS AND THE COMMUNITY

Using the information acquired from assessment to design self-care plans positions nursing to model health promotion for other disciplines, patients, and the community. The information used for nursing and client self-care can easily be adapted to use by communities, caregiver groups, and other support groups (cardiac, diabetes, oncology). No matter the culture, language, or diagnosis, *general* wellness and self-care guidelines are universal. It is important to note that although education is necessary to promote self-care, the task of nursing is larger than education. Many populations are knowledgeable regarding healthy behaviors, yet their knowledge does not translate into action. A fitting example is nursing: nurses often coach patients on self-care practices but do not incorporate these health-promoting behaviors into their own routines.

Holistic nurses are well positioned to devise creative opportunities for communities to meet the mandate to improve self-care across the life span. Whereas programs designed for teens will most likely be different from programs for older adults, creativity may allow combining groups to enrich experiences. From a coaching perspective, nurses need to provide the space, ask the right questions, consider health literacy and cultural diversity, and partner with communities to develop self-care programs. Often, opportunities to experience massage, movement, reflexology, and energy work attract curious participants. Working with community leaders, from politicians to religious leaders, from Girl Scouts troops to senior centers, nurses can identify groups seeking information and ways to enhance their well-being. Presenting information in a simple format or as a short overview is often all that is needed to start conversations that lead to care plan development.

Possible Talking Points for Community Presentations and Dialogue

Although it is recognized that the body-mind-spirit is a continuum, it may be helpful to separate these entities for initial self-care and wellness discussions. Nurses can highlight the fact that improving one "part of the whole" enhances other "parts," just as caring for one family member in some way affects the whole family. Simple questions to ask are as follows:

- *For body/physical wellness:* How is/are your . . . sleep, nutrition, exercise (aerobic, strength, flexibility), habits, physical exams/screenings, home and work environments?
- *For mind/emotional wellness:* Have you ever tried . . . affirmations, appreciative inquiry,

breath work, meditation, being creative, use of imagination, learning something new, cognitive therapy, self-reflection, journaling, humor, relaxation, open communication, or stress management?
- *For spirit/social wellness:* How are your relationships with family and friends? Do you give and feel love and appreciation? What gives your life meaning? Do you feel connected to something greater as well as to others? Can you forgive? Do you use your intuition, laughter, play? Do you have a sense of community?

■ SUPPORTING THE CORE VALUE OF SELF-CARE FOR THE ENVIRONMENT

As holistic nurses practice self-care, attention to the environment is a natural progression as we realize that we are in constant interaction with our environment. Recent research highlights the impact of toxic environments. Environmental issues that must be addressed include chemical pollutants, radiation, noise, pollution, technology (for example, cell phone usage), and their relationships to health and illness. The need to conserve and protect our planet and natural resources, including water and energy, are all issues that affect self-care.

Healing environments with soothing sounds, nature scenes, and aromas are beneficial in the healing process. The creation of a sacred space in one's home, a place for quiet meditation/reflection, is often a part of nurses' self-care plan. The effect of the work environment on staff has been the focus of many institutions as they "go green" and recognize the value of a healing environment. Self-care environmental action for the nurse may include recycling, buying organic when possible, avoiding foods with added chemicals and artificial coloring, prudent energy use, and partnering with community activists to increase safeguarding of the environment.

■ CONCLUSION

Although Florence Nightingale emphasized the importance of supporting self-care and health promotion, the actual practices are underutilized in the nursing workforce, patient population, and community. Nursing requires a broad spectrum of knowledge and skills, from presence and the fostering of caring relationships to the ability to multitask. Caring begins with self-care of the nurse through assessment and health-promoting behaviors. Holistic nursing recognizes the complexity of wellness and the challenges facing nursing. The core values of holistic nursing provide a structure to support self-care and the mandate to practice. Practicing self-care allows nurses to model health promotion for other disciplines, patients, and community. Studies that support holistic models of care and report significant outcomes will ensure that healing and health promotion remain integral components of nursing.

As nurses focus on self-care and model caring behaviors in the workplace, communication, relationships, and patient care may be improved. When quality measures and national patient care standards are met and exceeded, institutional support closely follows. Through assessment, education, and a focus on self-care and health promotion, institutions may assist employees in identifying self-care needs and support health promotion behaviors. Outcomes from studies on self-care and health promotion provide knowledge for local, national, and international programs. Understanding and practicing the core value of self-care strengthens holistic nursing practice. Holistic nursing, grounded in holistic nursing theory, resonating transpersonal caring, focusing on whole-person healing and health promotion, supports not only the future health of the nursing profession, but that of our clients, communities, and the world.

Directions for
FUTURE RESEARCH

1. Evaluate the health-promoting behaviors of nurses in your institution, analyze themes, and develop holistic programs to address identified needs.
2. Develop an ongoing holistic worksite wellness plan and evaluate the long-term effects on finances, retention, quality indicators, and patient experiences
3. Complete a qualitative analysis on a healing intervention.
4. Evaluate the impact of self-care classes incorporated into nursing school curricula.

5. Evaluate the outcomes of 1-day nursing retreats on teamwork, caring, and productivity.
6. Evaluate the long-term effects of holistic programs on patient populations in the community.
7. Examine the effects of coaching on the development and adherence to self-care plans for different age groups and culturally diverse communities.
8. Examine the implications of peer/family support on self-care practices.

Nurse Healer
REFLECTIONS

After reading this chapter, the holistic nurse will be able to answer or to begin a process of answering the following questions:

- What is the interaction between self-care, health, healing, and health promotion?
- What activities can I incorporate into my self-care plan to strengthen my ability to care for patients?
- How can I balance the need for multitasking with the desire to be present for my patients?
- What is the difference between coaching a patient on self-care and prescribing a self-care regimen?
- How can I sustain my focus on the need and benefits of therapeutic presence when I am addressing the complex medical needs of patients?

 For a full suite of assignments and additional learning activities, use the access code located in the front of your book to visit this exclusive website: http://go.jblearning.com/dossey. If you do not have an access code, you can obtain one at the site.

NOTES

1. D. McElligott, "Healing: From Concept to Nursing Practice," *Journal of Holistic Nursing* 28 no. 4 (2010): 251–259.
2. B. M. Dossey, L. Keegan, and C. Guzzetta, *Holistic Nursing: A Handbook for Practice*, 5th ed. (Sudbury, MA: Jones and Bartlett, 2009).

3. N. Pender, C. Murdaugh, and M. Parsons, *Health Promotion in Nursing Practice,* 5th ed. (Upper Saddle River, NJ: Prentice Hall, 2006).

4. G. Acton and P. Malathum, "Basic Need Status and Health Promoting Self-Care Behavior in Adults," *Western Journal of Nursing Research* 22, no. 7 (2000): 796–811.

5. J. Watson, *Caring Science as Sacred Science* (Philadelphia, PA: F. A. Davis, 2005).

6. National Institute of Health, National Center for Complementary and Alternative Medicine, "What Is Complementary and Alternative Medicine?" http://nccam.nih.gov/health/whatiscam/.

7. American Holistic Nurses Association and American Nurses Association, *Holistic Nursing: Scope and Standards of Practice* (Silver Spring, MD: NurseBooks.org, 2007).

8. World Health Organization, "Millennium Developmental Goals (MDGs)." http://www.who.int/topics/millennium_development_goals/about/en/index.html.

9. Institute of Medicine, *Leading Health Indicators for Healthy People 2020: Letter Report* (Washington, DC: National Academies Press, 2011).

10. J. F. Helliwell, 2005. *Well-Being, Social Capital and Public Policy: What's New?* (paper presented at the special session on well-being at the Annual Meetings of the Royal Economic Society, Nottingham, March 21, 2005). http://www.gpiatlantic.org/conference/papers/helliwell.pdf.

11. D. Childre, *Heart-Based Living* (2005). http://www.heartmathbenelux.com/doc/Heartbasedliving.pdf.

12. S. Peterson and T. Bredow, *Middle Range Theories: Application to Nursing Research* (Philadelphia, PA: Lippincott Williams & Wilkin, 2004).

13. S. N. Walker and D. Hill-Polrecky, "Psychometric Evaluation of the Health Promoting Lifestyle Profile II," in *Proceedings of the 1996 Scientific Session of the American Nurse Association's Council of Nurse Researchers* (Washington, DC: American Nurses Foundation, 1996).

14. J. Smith, "The Idea of Health: A Philosophical Inquiry," *Advanced Nursing Science* 3 (1981): 43–50.

15. M. P. O'Donnell, "Definition of Health Promotion 2.0: Embracing Passion, Enhancing Motivation, Recognizing Dynamic Balance, and Creating Opportunities," *American Journal of Health Promotion* 24, no. 1 (September–October 2009): iv.

16. D. Orem, *Nursing: Concepts of Practice*, 6th ed. (St. Louis, MO: Mosby, 2001).

17. S. N. Walker, K. Sechrist, and N. Pender, *Health Promoting Lifestyle Profile II*. Omaha: University of Nebraska Medical Center, College of Nursing 1995.

18. U.S. Department of Health and Human Services, *The Surgeon General's Vision for a Healthy and Fit Nation* (Rockville, MD: U.S. Department of

Health and Human Services, Office of the Surgeon General, January 2010).

19. M. Moore and B. Tschannen-Moran, *Coaching Psychology Manual* (New York, NY: Wolters Kluwer/Lippincott Williams & Wilkins, 2010).

20. J. F. Quinn, "The Self as Healer: Reflections from a Nurse's Journey," *AACN Clinical Issues* 11, no. 1 (2000): 17–26.

21. T. Egnew, "Suffering, Meaning and Healing: Challenges of Contemporary Medicine," *Annals of Family Medicine* 7, no. 2 (2009): 170–175.

22. S. Bolles and M. Maley, "Designing Relational Models of Collaborative Integrative Medicine That Support Healing Processes," *Journal of Alternative and Complementary Medicine* 10 (2004): S61–S69.

23. B. M. Dossey, L. Selanders, D. M. Beck, and A. Attewell, *Florence Nightingale Today: Healing Leadership Global Action* (Silver Spring, MD: American Nurses Association, 2005).

24. Institute of Medicine, *Keeping Patients Safe: Transforming the Work Environment of Nurses* (2003). http://www.iom.edu/CMS/3809/4671/16173.aspx.

25. J. M. Zapka, S. C. Lemon, R. P. Manger, and J. Hale, "Lifestyle Behaviors and Weight Among Hospital-Based Nurses," *Journal of Nursing Management* 17, no. 7 (2009): 853–860.

26. R. Z. Goetzel et al., "Promising Practices in Employer Health and Productivity Management Efforts: Findings from a Benchmarking Study," *Journal of Occupational Environmental Medicine* 49, no. 2 (2007): 111–130.

27. Health Resources and Services Administration, *What Is Behind HRSA's Projected Supply, Demand and Shortage of Registered Nurses?* (2004). http://dwd.wisconsin.gov/healthcare/pdf/behind_the_shortage.pdf.

28. S. J. Tucker, M. R. Harris, T. B. Pipe, and S. R. Stevens, "Nurses' Ratings of Their Health and Professional Work Environments," *Journal of the American Association of Occupational Health Nursing* 58, no. 6 (2010): 253–267.

29. D. McElligott, K. Capitulo, D. Morris, and E. Click, "The Effect of a Holistic Intervention on the Health Promoting Behaviors of Registered Nurses (CNE Activity)," *Journal of Holistic Nursing* 28, no. 3 (2010): 174–186.

30. C. Hooper, J. Craig, D. R. Janvrin, M. A. Wetsel, and E. Reimeis, "Compassion Satisfaction, Burnout, and Compassion Fatigue Among Emergency Nurses Compared with Nurses in Other Selected Inpatient Specialties," *Journal of Emergency Nursing* 36, no. 5 (2010): 420.

31. American Nurses Association, *ANA's Health System Reform Agenda* 2008: 1–21. Silver Spring, Maryland.

32. D. McElligott, An Intervention to Increase Health Promotion in Hospital Nurses. Frances Payne Bolton School of Nursing, Case Western Reserve

University (unpublished data from dissertation, 2009).

33. Joint Commission, *2011 National Patient Safety Goals.* http://www.jointcommission.org/assets/1/6/2011_NPSG_Hospital_3_17_11.pdf.

34. C. P. Buerhaus, K. Donelan, B. Ulrich, and C. Desroches, "Trends in the Experiences of Hospital-Employed Registered Nurses: Results from Three National Surveys," *Nursing Economics* 25, no. 2 (2007): 69-79.

35. D. McElligott, S. Siemers, and L. Thomas, "Nursing Wellness: Is There a Healthy Nurse in the House?" *Applied Nursing Research* 22, no. 3 (2009): 211-215.

36. M. Stark, J. Manning-Walsh, and S. Vliem, "Caring for Self While Learning to Care for Others: A Challenge for Nursing Students," *Journal of Nursing Education* 44, no. 6 (2005): 266-270.

37. T. Richards, D. Oman, J. Hedberg, C. Thorensen, and J. Bowden, "A Qualitative Examination of a Spirituality Based Intervention and Self-Management in the Workplace," *Nursing Science Quarterly* 19, no. 3 (2006): 231-239.

38. McElligott, 2011.

39. G. Maciocia, *The Foundations of Chinese Medicine* (London, England: Churchill Livingston, 1989).

40. J. Halifax, *Being with Dying* (Boston: Shambala, 2009).

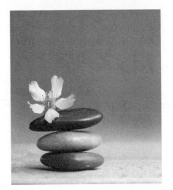

Index

Exhibits, figures, and tables are indicated by e, f, and t following the page number.